Gross and Microscopic Pathology of the Skin

Second Edition

GROSS and MICROSCOPIC PATHOLOGY of the SKIN

SECOND EDITION

MILTON R. OKUN, M.D.

Clinical Professor of Dermatology and Pathology, Boston University School of Medicine; Lecturer in Dermatology, Tufts University School of Medicine; Chairman, Board of Trustees, Dermatopathology Foundation; Director, Boston Dermatopathology Laboratory; Diplomate, American Board of Dermatology; Certified for Special Qualification in Dermatopathology.

LEON M. EDELSTEIN, M.D.

Clinical Professor of Dermatology and Pathology, University of California (Davis) Medical School; Clinical Associate Professor of Dermatology, Stanford Medical School; Diplomate, American Boards of Anatomic and Clinical Pathology; Diplomate, American Board of Dermatology.

BENJAMIN K. FISHER, M.D., F.R.C.P.(C)

Chief, Division of Dermatology, The Wellesley Hospital, Toronto, Ontario, Canada; Associate Professor of Medicine (Dermatology), University of Toronto Medical School, Toronto, Ontario, Canada; Diplomate, American Board of Dermatology; Certified for Special Qualification in Dermatopathology.

In Two Volumes
Volume One: Non-Tumors

Dermatopathology Foundation Press, Inc.
P.O. Box 377
Canton, MA 02021 U.S.A.
(Telephone: (617) 821-0648)

Second Edition

Library of Congress Catalog Card Number: 87-71751
ISBN 0-9618536-0-3

PRINTED IN THE UNITED STATES OF AMERICA

General Editor

WENDY CHRISTISON

Office Manager, Dermatopathology Foundation and Press

Medical Copy Editor

INTA A. GROTS, M.D.

Associate, Boston Dermatopathology Laboratory; Formerly Associate Clinical Professor of Dermatology, Boston University School of Medicine; Diplomate, American Board of Dermatology.

Acknowledgments

The authors acknowledge with gratitude:

1. The extraordinary persistence of Wendy Christison, the General Editor, in tying this whole project together.
2. The careful copy editing of Dr. Inta Grots.
3. The generosity of Dr. Walter F. Lever for the use of numerous clinical photographs from his personal collection.
4. The diligence of Marian Munroe, Vickie Kohler, and Nino LaBadessa for their assistance in preparing the bibliography.
5. The contributions of Barbara Donnellan, S. Henry Pearson, Mary Ann Piotrowicz, Patricia Ayoub,and Marie Galvin in preparing microscopic slides used in this book.
6. The important contribution of Dr. Ken Hashimoto to Chapter 1.
7. The important contributions of Dr. John Walter and Dr. Denis Bailey to Chapter 27.
8. The suggestions of Dr. Robert Collins for Chapter 27.
9. The assistance of Janice Geary, Carol Fritz, Marion Levine, and Dr. Robert Bain for their contribution in helping prepare the First Edition.

Preface

We have attempted to produce a reference work in pathology of the skin in which illustrations and text are given equal weight, and gross and microscopic material are carefully integrated.

The clinical photographs and microscopic slides were selected, from our own files and those of many others, from the standpoints of accuracy and technical quality.

The books were designed to facilitate retrieval of information, with illustrations and related text on facing pages.

We have tried to present essential morphologic features in concise language, without omitting subtleties of morphologic detail.

We have also tried to include enough current information on pathogenesis and enough selected references to enhance the morphologic material and put it in perspective. Reference categories follow the order of material in the text, with articles of greatest morphologic interest taking precedence.

In the second edition, the original format and approach have been retained, but there has been a major revision, with updating of concepts, inclusion of additional entities, improvement of existing illustrations, and inclusion of numerous new illustrations, especially new color illustrations.

Histopathologic analysis of skin lesions: Sampling and limitations

Histologic examination is an important diagnostic technique in dermatology. In some instances a diagnosis is unequivocally established on the basis of biopsy alone; in other instances a combination of histologic, clinical, and other laboratory data can establish a diagnosis. Even negative and nonspecific information from biopsies can be helpful.

While it is important for the clinician to be aware of the potential of a skin biopsy, it is also important to be aware of its limitations.

Ideally, the skin specimen should be of sufficient size and integrity to reveal optimally pathologic patterns. Ideally, the specimen or specimens should be taken from representative areas. In the case of widespread lesions, multiple biopsies may be required to show characteristic microscopic features. In the case of tumors, complete removal of the lesion with sections through the block may be required to show the key features.

It is important to keep in mind that the pattern in one portion of a lesion does not necessarily reflect the pattern in the remainder. This is especially true in melanocytic neoplasms; malignant melanoma may be a focus within a benign nevus.

Generally, mature or well-developed lesions are most likely to show characteristic features, but this is not true of bullous lesions, which tend to show diagnostic features in their early stages.

Lesions with spreading active borders, such as ringworm, are most likely to show diagnostic features if the edge is biopsied.

Specimens can be removed by scalpel excision, punch biopsy, shave biopsy, or curettage.

Scalpel excision, including subcutaneous fat is ideal; the other methods are compromises that can be adequate for certain situations. In shave biopsy, the upper portion of the lesion is shaved with a scalpel and submitted for examination. This is often done in the case of benign-looking nevi since malignant change usually (but not always) begins at the epidermal-dermal junction. Curettage is the least advantageous method, since architecture is not preserved and cellular appearance can be distorted. In some lesions, such as keratoacanthoma, architectural preservation is essential.

If panniculitis or other deep process is suspected, it is essential to include subcutaneous fat in the specimen.

Specimens should be handled with care and put in fixative immediately after removal. Use of electrosurgery should be after the specimen has been removed. Electrosurgical current can produce severe tissue damage.

Even if tissue is ideally visualized, there are limitations to microscopic analysis. Some microscopic patterns are specific; some are not. Some are suggestive. The clinician understandably wants a definite answer from the pathologist. When this is not possible, the pathologist is under pressure to give a definite answer when this is not warranted. Succumbing to this pressure is bad for all concerned.

The greatest pressure of this type and the most widespread abuse is in the area of melanocytic neoplasms. Definite diagnoses are sometimes dispensed when neither the tissue sample nor the microscopic pattern warrant this. Unfortunately, there is a "gray zone" in microscopic patterns of melanocytic neoplasms in which biologic behavior cannot be predicted with certainty.

Accuracy in dermatologic diagnosis is increased by correlation of clinical and laboratory information. The clinician has an obligation to provide the pathologist with an adequate skin specimen and adequate clinical information.

Contents

Contents

VOLUME ONE

Contents

VOLUME TWO

Gross and Microscopic Pathology of the Skin

Second Edition

Chapter 1
Staining Procedures Used in Dermatopathology

Fixation

For most purposes, 10% neutral phosphate-buffered formalin is the recommended fixative. Specimens 4 mm thick should be fixed for at least 8 hours before routine processing for paraffin sections. Thicker specimens require longer fixation.

Although some authors have recommended fixation in either basic lead acetate or absolute alcohol for preservation of mast cell granules, formalin fixation is usually adequate.

Fixation in absolute alcohol helps preserve the structure of urate crystals in routinely processed tissue.

Winter mailing may cause freeze-thaw damage to tissue. We have found that addition of 50% alcohol to the formalin (resulting in a 10% solution of 50% alcohol by volume) has satisfactory antifreeze properties and preserves morphology well. Phosphate for buffering is not used in such solutions since the phosphate precipitates.

Tissue fixed in Karnovsky's fixative (a solution of formaldehyde and glutaraldehyde) can be used for light microscopic or electron microscopic processing. For subsequent electron microscopic processing, it is best to keep the fixative at 4°C.

"Routine" Stains

HEMATOXYLIN AND EOSIN

A mixture of these dyes is the most commonly used routine stain. Hematoxylin is a natural dye which requires the presence of metal ions (e.g., aluminum) and an oxidizing agent (e.g., hydrogen peroxide; potassium permanganate) to stain tissue. The blue color is produced by the oxidation product of the dye (which is basic). Hematoxylin stains nuclei. Eosin is used as a counterstain for cytoplasm.

GIEMSA STAIN (pp. 45, 265)

Giemsa stain is a mixture of polychrome methylene blue and eosin. Polychrome methylene blue is a basic dye (it stains acidic substrates) which has the property of metachromasia. With Giemsa stain, nuclei stain blue. Cytoplasm may also stain various shades of blue, depending on the amount of RNA or other acidic substances. Acid mucopolysaccharides (see pp. 45, 265) are stained metachromatically with Giemsa stain. Metachromasia is the shift in color of a blue dye towards red, when combined with substrate. Eosin stains cytoplasm.

Giemsa stain is believed to produce good cytologic detail and is useful in evaluating sections for lymphoma. It is also useful in examining sections for Leishman bodies and *Histoplasma capsulatum*.

Connective Tissue Stains: Collagen

MASSON TRICHROME STAIN (p. 1073)

Mature collagen stains blue. Immature collagen, muscle fibers, nerve fibers, and keratin stain red. Nuclei stain black.

VAN GIESON STAIN

Mature collagen stains red. Immature collagen, muscle fibers, nerve fibers, and keratin stain yellow. Nuclei stain bluish-black.

Connective Tissue Stains: Elastic Fibers

VERHOEFF STAIN (pp. 621, 623)

Elastic fibers stain bluish-black.

WEIGERT'S RESORCIN-FUCHSIN STAIN

Elastic fibers stain bluish-black.

ACID ORCEIN GIEMSA STAIN (pp. 247, 685)

Elastic fibers stain brown to black.

GOMORI'S ALDEHYDE FUCHSIN STAIN

Elastic fibers stain deep purple.

Connective Tissue Stains: Reticulum (p. 33)

Methods for reticulum depend on silver impregnation. Silver nitrate is used together with a reducing agent (e.g., sodium metabisulfite). Two widely used methods are *Foot's stain* and *Snook's stain*. Structures stained by silver impregnation are called *argyrophil*. Reticulum appears black.

Stains for Mucopolysaccharides and Polysaccharides

NEUTRAL MUCOPOLYSACCHARIDES AND POLYSACCHARIDES: PAS STAIN (pp. 33, 341, 753)

The periodic acid-Schiff stain has two main components—periodic acid and Schiff reagent. Periodic acid oxidizes adjacent hydroxyl groups in 1,2 glycols, and the Schiff reagent (fuchsin-sulfuric acid) reacts with the resultant aldehyde groups, producing a red color.

The PAS stain is useful for staining glycogen, neutral mucopolysaccharides of the basement zone, and neutral mucopolysaccharides in the wall of fungi. Glycogen can be differentiated from other PAS-positive material by prior digestion of sections with diastase. (Human saliva can serve as the source of diastase.) Glycogen is diastase-labile.

STAINS FOR ACID MUCOPOLYSACCHARIDES

Stains for these substances combine with acidic groupings in the polymer.

Hyaluronic acid can be distinguished from sulfated acid mucopolysaccharides (e.g., heparin, chondroitin sulfate B) by prior digestion with hyaluronidase.

Specificity of the staining methods cited can be controlled by pH. Acid mucopolysaccharides maintain their stainability at acid pH. Sulfated acid mucopolysaccharides are most resistant to extinction in acid media.

Metachromatic stains (pp. 45, 265)

Metachromatic dyes shift in color from blue to violet after combining with substrate. Examples: polychrome methylene blue (incorporated in Giemsa stain); toluidine blue.

Nonmetachromatic stains

Copper phthalocyanin dyes

Examples: alcian blue; astrablau. These stain acid mucopolysaccharides blue; there is no metachromasia.

Hale's colloidal iron stain (p. 665)

Sections are exposed to colloidal iron, which is then stained by the ferrocyanide-HCl method. A blue color indicates a positive reaction for acid mucopolysaccharides.

Mucicarmine stain

Mucicarmine stain is another nonmetachromatic stain for acid mucopolysaccharides. It can be used to stain epithelial mucin or the mucinous capsule of Cryptococcus neoformans. Mucin stains pink to red.

Stains for Pigment

The chemical structure of melanin and other pigments found in the skin is not fully understood, and histochemical methods of identification are not entirely specific.

MELANIN: FONTANA-MASSON AMMONIATED SILVER NITRATE STAIN (p. 1247)

This method stains melanin and premelanin black due to the reduction of silver nitrate to free silver. Substances reducing silver salts to free silver are called *argentaffin*. (Melanin is also *argyrophil*—it can be stained with silver impregnation methods.)

The Fontana-Masson technique is erroneously considered specific for melanin. Hemosiderin can also show a positive (but less intense) reaction. It is possible that some hemosiderin may represent melanin-containing stainable iron (possibly derived from peroxidase).

HEMOSIDERIN: PERLS STAIN (PRUSSIAN BLUE REACTION) (p. 981)

A deep blue color is produced by iron that becomes available for reaction with ferrocyanide in an acid medium. Hemosiderin is intensely positive; however, melanin may sometimes also be moderately positive.

FORMALIN PIGMENT AND LIPOFUSCIN (LIPOMELANIN)

Formalin pigment forms from hemoglobin in sections fixed in formalin with a pH below 6. It does not show a positive reaction with the Fontana-Masson stain or with Perls stain. Formalin pigment consists of dark brown microcrystalline particles, mainly among red blood cells and also within phagocytes. It may be removed by several methods, such as Verocay's method.

Lipofuscin is not generally observed in the skin. There is now extensive evidence that it represents a combination of melanin and lipid. Therefore, it will show histochemical reactions for melanin, as well as for lipid (e.g., with acid fast stains).

Stains for Lipids (p. 1271)

Examination for lipids is generally performed on formalin-fixed frozen sections, since the alcohol and xylene used in routine processing remove most lipids.

The demonstration of lipids with lipid-soluble dyes is a physicochemical process, in contrast to other staining procedures, which generally involve chemical reactions. "Staining" is due to the presence of dye between the solvent and the lipid substrate. Boundary surface absorption plays an important role in this process. Stains in this category include *scarlet red, oil red O,* and *Sudan black B.*

On the other hand, *osmium tetroxide* stains lipids by a chemical mechanism whereby it is reduced (blackened) by unsaturated carbon linkages. Osmium tetroxide is useful in differentiating animal and vegetable fats (which contain these linkages) from mineral oil (which does not).

Stains for Nerve Fibers

Nerve fibers are *argyrophil.* They are stained by silver impregnation techniques. One example is *Bodian stain,* which contains protargol and uses hydroquinone as a reducing agent.

Stains for Nucleic Acids

DNA

The *Feulgen reaction* stains DNA a magenta color by a process involving mild acid hydrolysis followed by reaction with Schiff's reagent.

RNA

The *methyl green-pyronin* method is generally used. Pyronin stains RNA-containing structures (e.g., nucleoli) pink, and methyl green stains DNA green. The mechanism of differential staining by this method is not understood.

Stains for Amyloid

Amyloid is a complex carbohydrate-containing protein. Some methods for demonstrating amyloid are listed below.

CONGO RED STAIN (p. 685)

This can be performed on routine sections, but a better reaction is obtained with frozen sections. Amyloid stains brick red. The stained amyloid may show orange or green birefringence with polarized light (dichroism), depending on the rotation angle. Although dichroism is considered an important feature for identifying amyloid, it may not be demonstrable, possibly due to the variability of amyloid or thinness of the sections.

Colloid has histochemical reactions similar to amyloid.

METHYL VIOLET STAIN

This stain is best performed on frozen sections. Amyloid stains red to violet. The color is not permanent.

FLUORESCENCE MICROSCOPY WITH THIOFLAVIN T

This can be performed on routine sections, but frozen sections are preferable. Sections are stained with thioflavin T and examined with ultraviolet illumination. Amyloid fluoresces shades of blue or green.

ACID ORCEIN GIEMSA STAIN (p. 685)

With this stain, amyloid stains sky blue. It can be performed on routine sections. Solar elastotic material can be distinguished from amyloid with this stain, since it stains brown to black.

Stains for Calcium (p. 713)

In the *Von Kossa* method, silver replaces calcium in the calcium salt, and then the silver salt is reduced to free silver (black granules).

Stains for Bacteria

Various modifications of the Gram stain are used (e.g., *MacCallum-Goodpasture stain*). Cocci and bacilli also usually can be well-visualized with acid orcein Giemsa stain. Mycobacteria are stained with acid-fast stains. Staining is based on the ability to retain carbol fuchsin in an acid alcohol medium. The *Fite stain* is superior to the *Ziehl-Neelsen stain* for demonstrating lepra bacilli and certain strains of Nocardia (p. 319).

Enzyme-Histochemical Stains

Enzyme histochemical stains are not frequently used in diagnostic dermatopathology. The dopa and peroxidase reactions are commonly used.

Most enzyme-histochemical reactions require fresh frozen sections. Some can be performed on frozen sections from formalin-fixed tissue, and others can be performed on formalin-fixed routine sections.

DOPA REACTION (pp. 27, 1247)

The dopa reaction is used to help identify amelanotic melanomas. Fresh frozen sections or frozen sections fixed briefly in formalin are incubated in DL-dopa. A positive reaction is indicated by deposits of grayish-black dopa melanin. Cells containing aerobic *L-dopa oxidase* ("tyrosinase") and/or peroxidase give a positive reaction. Melanocytes contain either or both enzymes. The reaction is not specific for melanocytes, since other peroxidase-containing cells will also give a positive reaction (e.g., granulocytes, mast cells).

Preincubation with thiol compounds can differentiate a positive dopa reaction due to peroxidase from that due to aerobic dopa oxidase. Copper-dependent aerobic dopa oxidase is inhibited by such treatment, while peroxidase is unaffected. The presence of aerobic dopa oxidase indicates that the cell is a melanocyte.

TYROSINE-DOPA REACTION; TYROSINE-DHF REACTION

These reactions can be used to demonstrate conversion of tyrosine to melanin by peroxidase in fresh frozen sections or briefly fixed frozen sections. In the tyrosine-dopa reaction, a saturated solution of tyrosine, containing a much smaller concentration of dopa as a cofactor, is used along with a control solution containing dopa alone. Differential melanin formation in the presence of tyrosine indicates conversion of tyrosine to melanin.

In the tyrosine-DHF reaction, dihydroxyfumaric acid (a nonmelanogenic compound) is used as cofactor. Formation of melanin indicates oxidation of tyrosine by peroxidase.

Nonautoradiographic methods using tyrosine alone as substrate are of no value in demonstrating melanogenic enzymes.

Enzyme-Histochemical Stains of Value in Diagnosing Granulocytic Leukemia

PEROXIDASE

Methods using benzidine and its variants (e.g., DAB) as chromogenic substrates have been used. Since these substances are carcinogenic, other chromogenic substrates, such as 3-amino and 9-ethyl carbazole have been substituted. The dopa reaction, controlled with inhibitors (see above) can be used.

CHLOROACETATE ESTERASE

This stain is positive in myelocytes but negative in myeloblasts and eosinophilic myeloid cells. The antilysozyme immunoperoxidase reaction is positive in myeloblasts and eosinophilic myeloid cells, as well as in myelocytes.

Comment

1. *Polariscopic examination* is not a staining procedure, but it is useful in dermatopathologic diagnosis. With this procedure, two polarizing discs are used; one is placed in the eyepiece, and the other is placed below the condenser. The element in the eyepiece is rotated until the field is dark. Doubly refractile substances such as silica, talcum powder, wood, suture material, sodium urate crystals, and certain lipids have a brilliant whitish appearance (see p. 429).
2. *Cytologic methods.* The main cytologic method used in dermatopathology is the Tzanck smear (see p. 391), employed in the diagnosis of vesicular viral diseases and acan tholytic dermatoses. The base of a vesicle or bulla is scraped with a surgical blade and smeared onto a glass slide. After air-drying and fixation with 95% alcohol, the preparation is stained with Giemsa stain, Wright's stain, or Papanicolaou stain.

Immunological Methods Used in Dermatopathology

Ken Hashimoto, M.D., Milton R. Okun, M.D.

Immunological testing has become increasingly important in dermatopathologic diagnosis. However, routine light microscopic examination remains the mainstay of dermatopathologic analysis. Immunologic tests can be important adjuncts in making a diagnosis.

IMMUNOFLUORESCENCE TESTING

Immunofluorescence testing is of greatest value in certain vesiculobullous diseases and in connective tissue diseases. With direct immunofluorescence testing, fluorescein-labeled antibodies react with sections from human tissue; then the sections are exposed to fluorescein-labeled antibodies to human immunoglobulin. Direct immunofluorescence testing detects tissue-bound antibody. With indirect immunofluorescence testing, sections of animal tissue are exposed to human serum. Then the sections of animal tissue are exposed to fluorescein-labeled antibodies to human immunoglobulin. Indirect immunofluorescence testing is usually used to detect circulating antibody. Tissue for direct immunofluorescence testing can be transported in special holding solution (Michel's solution).

IMMUNOPEROXIDASE TESTING

Immunoperoxidase testing is similar to immunofluorescence testing except that antibodies are conjugated to peroxidase rather than fluorescein. Enzyme histochemical reactions for peroxidase, such as the diaminobenzidine method (DAB), are then used to visualize the presence of immunoglobulins fixed to tissue. Carbazole or naphthol compounds can be used instead of DAB. An advantage of the immunoperoxidase technique is that it can be performed on some of the formalin-fixed tissues with trypsin digestion or with amplifying methods such as PAP; the slides can be stored permanently. Another advantage of immunoperoxidase testing is that it does not require the special fluorescence microscope.

Important applications of immunoperoxidase testing:

1. Antibodies against S100 protein can assist in the diagnosis of malignant melanoma or neural tumors.
2. Antibodies against carcinoembryonic antigen (CEA) can identify Paget's cells and distinguish them from pagetoid malignant melanoma cells.
3. The lectin UEA-1, used in peroxidase-conjugated form, is a useful endothelial cell marker.
4. Antibodies against B and T cells can assist in distinguishing B and T cell lymphomas.
5. The use of antibodies to alpha and beta subunits of S100 protein can help distinguish between histiocytosis X and juvenile xanthogranuloma. The beta subunit is present in histiocytosis X; the alpha subunit is present in juvenile xanthogranuloma.
6. Antibodies to human papillomavirus antigen can help distinguish between bowenoid papulosis and Bowen's disease.
7. The lectin PNA, in peroxidase-conjugated form, can help distinguish malignant from benign keratinocytes. The reaction is positive in benign keratinocytes, and in malignant keratinocytes the reaction is mostly negative.
8. Immunoperoxidase testing, like immunofluorescence testing, can be used to identify *in vivo* bound immunoglobulins or complement. Immunoperoxidase testing has the advantage of being applicable to electron microscopy.

9. Immunoperoxidase testing can help identify cell types by identifying characteristic intermediate filaments that make up the cytoskeleton of cells. The most important intermediate filament in dermatopathology is cytokeratin, characteristic of true epithelia. Antibodies to this filament can help identify spindle cell squamous cell carcinoma. Vimentin is found in mesenchymal cells. Neurofilaments are present in most neuronal cells. Desmin is present in most muscle cells.

The following is a suggested scheme for using immunoperoxidase techniques to identify undifferentiated skin tumors:

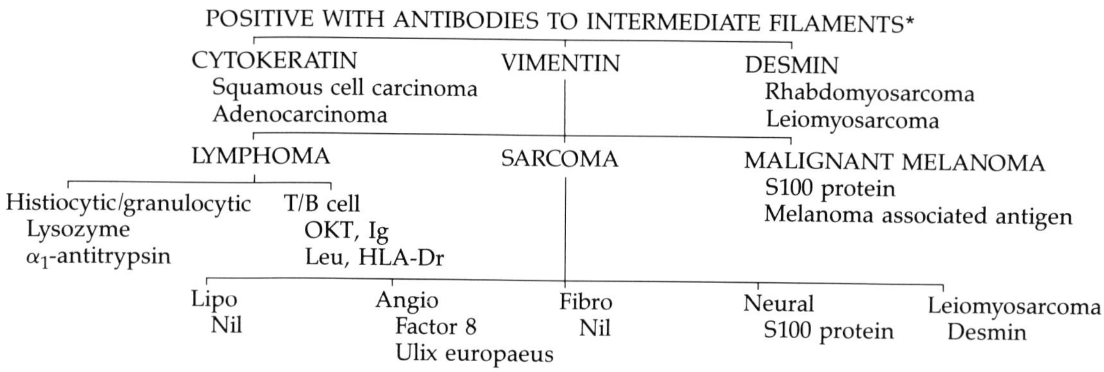

Scheme for evaluation by immunoperoxidase staining of undifferentiated tumors involving the skin, showing results of immunostaining of skin tumors. In other tissues, additional cytokeratin-, vimentin-, and desmin-positive tumors would have to be considered as possible diagnoses.

*from Kahn, H., Baumal, R., From, L. Role of immunohistochemistry in the diagnosis of undifferentiated tumors involving the skin. *J. Am. Acad. Dermatol.* 14:1063, 1986.

Cytopathologic Analysis

The criteria developed using smear or imprint technology can be applied to tissue sections and are important in assessing possible malignant changes:

1. Departure from normal in size, shape, and density of: a) nuclei, b) nucleoli, c) nuclear envelope, d) chromatin clumps or bodies.
2. Variation of number of nuclei or nucleoli.
3. Variation in cell size.
4. Intranuclear cross-bridging between nucleoli, chromatin, and nuclear envelope.

DNA Probe

Modern DNA probe methods can identify viral nucleic acid components in tumors, such as HPV 16 and 18 in bowenoid papulosis, condyloma acuminatum, and carcinoma of the cervix. These methods can also identify evidence of acquired genetic mutations in certain tumors.

Suggested Reading

Staining Procedures Used in Dermatopathology

Ackerman, A. and Penneys, N. Formalin pigment in the skin. *Arch. Dermatol.*, 102:318, 1970.

Baker, J. *Principles of Biologic Microtechnique.* New York, John Wiley and Sons, 1958.

Beutner, E., Chorzelski, T. and Bean, S. *Immunopathology of the Skin.* 2nd Ed., New York, John Wiley and Sons, 1979.

Kahn, H., Baumal, R. and From, L. Role of immunohistochemistry in the diagnosis of undifferentiated tumors involving the skin. *J. Am. Acad. Dermatol.*, 14:1063, 1986.

Kardasewitsch, B. Eine Methode zur Beseitigung der Formalin-Sedimenta aus mikroskopischen Präparaten. *Z. Wiss. Mikr.*, 42:322, 1925.

Lillie, R. *Histopathologic Technic and Practical Histochemistry.* 4th Ed., New York, McGraw-Hill Book Co., 1976.

Luna, L. *Manual of Histologic Staining Methods of the Armed Forces Institute of Pathology.* 3rd Ed., New York, McGraw-Hill Book Co., 1968.

McClung-Jones, R. *Microscopical Technique.* 3rd Ed., New York, P. B. Hoeber, Inc., 1950.

Neiman, R. et al. Granulocytic sarcoma. *Cancer*, 48:1426, 1981.

Okun, M. et al. Dopa compared with dihydroxyfumarate as co-factor in peroxidase-mediated oxidation of tyrosine to melanin: Histochemical studies with neutrophils, eosinophils, mast cells, melanoma cells, and neurons. *Histochemie*, 27:331, 1971.

Okun, M. et al. The histochemical tyrosine-dopa reaction for tyrosinase and its use in localizing tyrosinase activity in mast cells. *J. Invest. Dermatol.*, 53:39, 1969.

Pearse, A. *Histochemistry, Theoretical and Applied.* Vol. I, 4th Ed., New York, Churchill Livingstone, 1980.

——. *Histochemistry, Theoretical and Applied.* Vol. II, 4th Ed., New York, Churchill Livingstone, 1985.

Preece, A. *A Manual for Histologic Technicians.* 3rd Ed., Boston, Little, Brown and Co., 1972.

Schaumburg-Lever, G. Immunoenzyme technique in dermatopathology. *Internat. J. Dermatol.*, 25:217, 1986.

Takahashi, S. et al. Immunohistochemical localization and distribution of S-100 proteins in the human lymphoreticular system. *Am. J. Pathol.*, 116:497, 1984.

Valenzuela, R., Bergfeld, W. and Deodhar, S. *Interpretation of Immunofluorescent Patterns in Skin Diseases.* Chicago, Amer. Soc. of Clin. Path. Press, 1984.

Verocay, J. Beseitigung der "Formolniederschläge" aus mikroskopischen Schnitten. *Zentralbl. Allg. Pathol.*, 19:769, 1908.

Chapter 2
Normal Histology of the Skin

Normal histology of the skin

There are two major architectural components of the skin: the epidermis and the dermis (cutis). When viewing the cross-sectional architecture, however, it is advantageous to include the adjoining subcutaneous fat.

The diagram illustrates the cross-sectional architecture of the skin. The epidermis (E) covers the dermis, which is divided into an upper part (pars papillaris-P) and lower part (pars reticularis-R). The subpapillary capillary plexus (CP) is at the interface between the pars papillaris (papillary dermis) and pars reticularis (reticular dermis). Fibrous trabeculae extend downward from the pars reticularis and divide the subcutaneous fat (F) into lobules.

Cutaneous appendages (A) lie within the dermis and are surrounded by loose connective tissue, similar to that of the papillary dermis. In some instances, parts of appendages may extend into the subcutaneous fat (e.g. hair follicles and eccrine glands).

Striated muscle in the regions of the face and neck extends through the subcutaneous fat into the dermis and can sometimes be observed in sections of skin from these regions. Smooth muscle is present as arrectores pilorum and as dermal fibers in skin of the areolae and external genitals.

There is considerable variation in the skin with anatomic region, age, sex, and race, and it is important to be familiar with these variations in order to separate the normal from the abnormal in pathologic interpretation.

Examples of Variations in the Normal Histology of the Skin

I. With region
   a. The dermis of the back extends deeply and shows particularly coarse collagen bundles in the pars reticularis. A misdiagnosis of borderline scleroderma can be made in sections from this region if this normal variation is not considered. (By contrast, the dermis of the eyelids is relatively thin.)
   b. The horny layer of the epidermis is thicker and more compact in the palms and soles than elsewhere, and shows a prominent stratum lucidum.
   c. Large terminal hairs are most abundant on the scalp and, in post-adolescent males, in the beard area; vellus hairs are abundant on the helix of the ear.
   d. Eccrine glands are most abundant on the palms and soles.
   e. Sebaceous glands are large and abundant in the center of the face after adolescence.
   f. Apocrine glands are found principally in the axillae and anogenital areas.
   g. Specialized nerve endings are found on the volar aspects of the palms and soles: Meissner corpuscles in the papillae and Vater-Pacini corpuscles in the subcutaneous fat.

II. With age
   a. The dermis decreases in thickness with age.
   b. Solar elastosis is primarily a function of cumulative ultraviolet exposure, but the latter increases with age.

III. With sex
   a. Terminal hairs are not present in significant numbers on the beard area of post-adolescent females.

IV. With race
   a. Epidermal melanization is more intense in Negroid and Mongoloid races than in Caucasians.

NORMAL HISTOLOGY OF THE SKIN

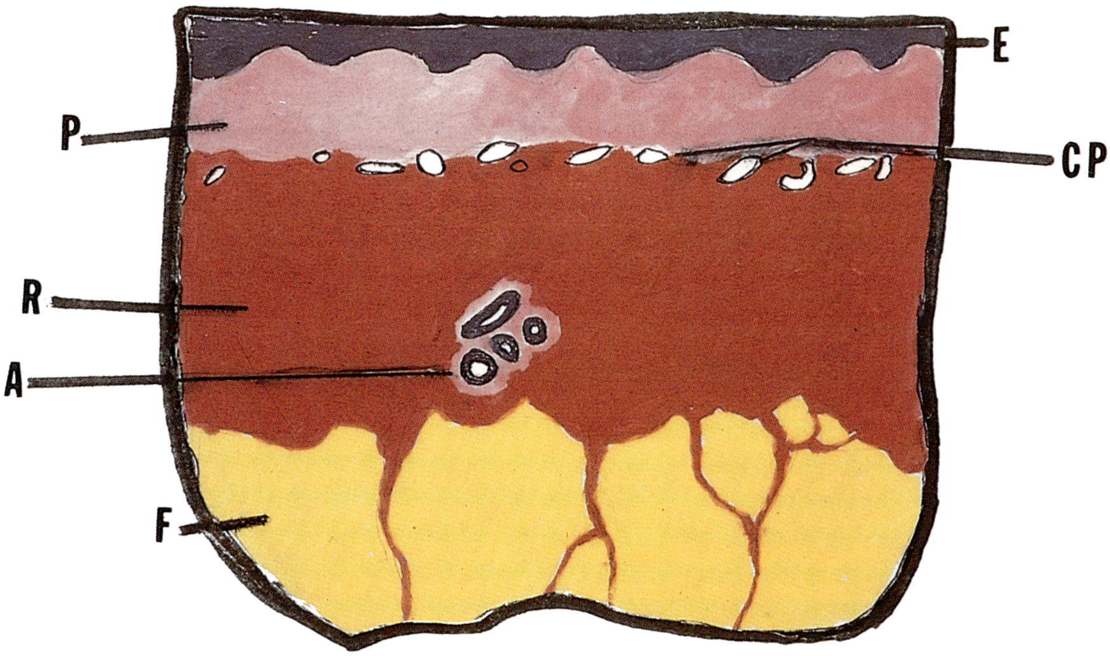

A

Epidermis

The epidermis has an undulating lower border with downward projections (rete ridges [R–Figs. A,C]) alternating with the dermal papillae (P–Figs. A,C).

Epithelial cells of the epidermis (keratinocytes) become increasingly keratinized as they approach the surface. There are four layers (from bottom to top): basal layer (B–Fig. B) (stratum germinativum); prickle cell layer (P–Fig. B) (stratum Malpighii); granular layer (G–Fig. B) (stratum granulosum); horny layer (H–Fig. B) (stratum corneum).

Basal cells (B–Fig. B) are cuboidal or columnar cells with relatively scant cytoplasm. Prickle cells (P–Fig. B) are polyhedral and have abundant cytoplasm. Granular cells (G–Fig. B) are fusiform and contain deeply basophilic cytoplasmic granules. These granules are called *keratohyaline granules*. They form the matrix that cements keratin fibrils as well as the marginal band of cornified cells. Fully cornified cells of the horny layer (Fig. B) lack a nucleus and are arranged in a loose meshwork (Figs. A,B) over most of the cutaneous surface. The horny layer is much more compact on the palms, soles, and lateral surfaces of the fingers and toes. (Figs. C,E). In these areas the stratum lucidum, a homogeneous eosinophilic zone, (Fig. C, Fig. E [arrow]) is easily visible at the lower border of the stratum corneum. The stratum lucidum is a transition zone between stratum corneum and stratum granulosum. It is seen with light microscopy only in thick epidermis. The stratum lucidum is rich in protein-bound phospholipids contained in Odland bodies (membrane-coating granules). The Odland bodies establish a barrier to water loss and mediate cohesion of cornified cells.

Keratinocytes are connected to each other by desmosomes. The prickles, (most evident when there is slight intercellular edema [Fig. D]), represent tonofibrils sweeping from the interior of the cell to the desmosomes. Slight thickening in the centers of the prickles (Bizzozero's nodules) represent desmosomes. Half-desmosomes also connect basal cells with the basement zone. Cohesion between keratinocytes also is mediated by intercellular cement substance, a gel-like material containing glycoproteins.

As the name indicates, keratinocytes produce the fibrous protein, keratin in increasing amounts as they migrate to the surface and differentiate. Ultrastructurally keratin is represented as tonofilaments. These connect with desmosomes, and in the granular layer, become cemented together by keratohyaline granules. Mitotic activity in normal keratinocytes is largely confined to the basal layer. It has been estimated that once a keratinocyte has been formed it will take 26 to 42 days for it to reach the surface.

The epidermis also contains three types of dendritic cells. The most important is the melanocyte (M–Fig. B) which is distributed at regular intervals along the basal layer. The other dendritic cells are the high-level clear cell (Langerhans cell) and the indeterminate dendritic cell. In the past the Langerhans cell has been regarded as an effete melanocyte. The histogenesis of Langerhans cells is uncertain. Embryologic evidence for and against a neural crest origin has been presented. It is now widely believed that they are involved in the processing of antigen and its conveyance to lymphocytes. Langerhans cells show a characteristic cytoplasmic granule, visible with electron microscopy. Langerhans cells are present in a variety of tissues. Cells with Langerhans type granules are present in histiocytosis X. T-zone histiocytes are cells with the morphology of Langerhans cells, which are present in T-cell areas of lymphatic tissue and in histiocytosis X. The indeterminate dendritic

EPIDERMIS

A X160

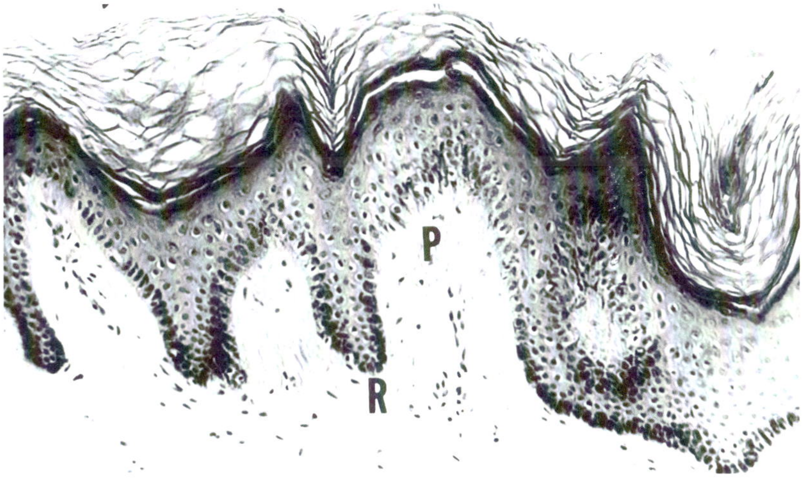

B X680

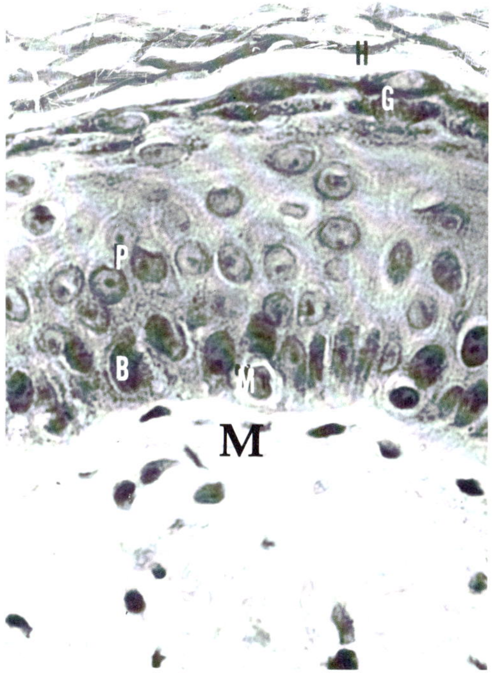

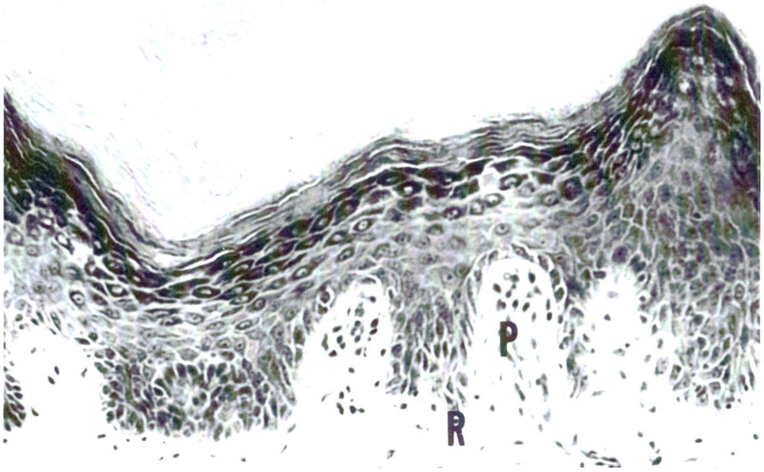

C
X220

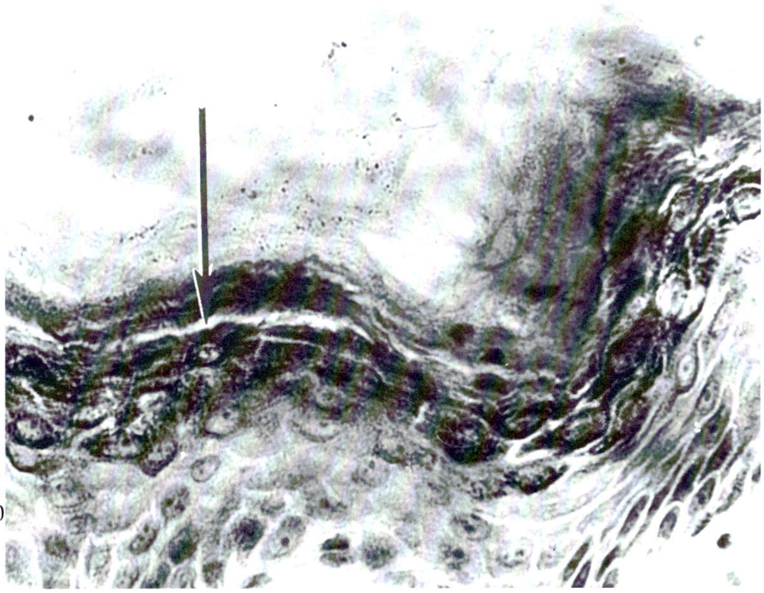

D X700

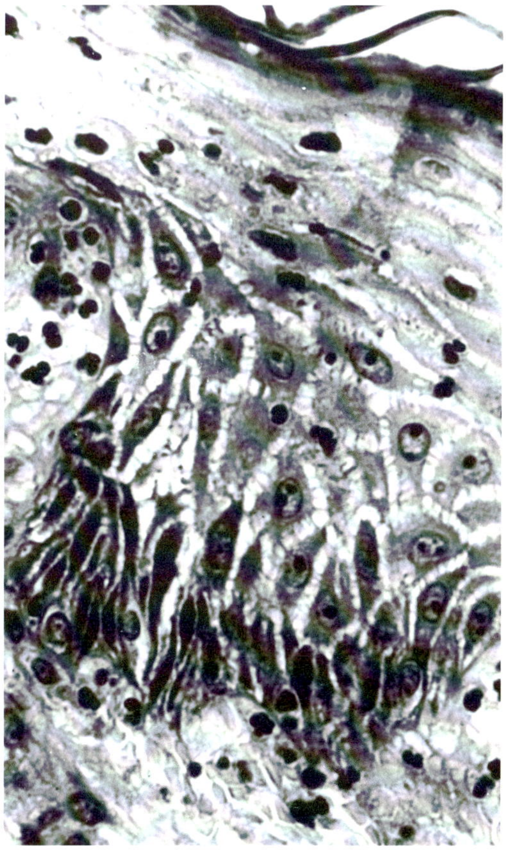

E
X610

EPIDERMIS continued

cell has no specific cytoplasmic organelles and may be a precursor of the other dendritic cells. It is usually found in the lower epidermis. Both Langerhans cells and indeterminate dendritic cells can be identified only by electron microscopy. Some believe the indeterminate dendritic cell is related to the Langerhans cell since it reacts with monoclonal antibody OKT6.

Comment

An additional cell type, seen occasionally with electron microscopy, is the Merkel cell, which is characterized by cytoplasmic organelles identical to norepinephrine granules of the adrenal medulla. It is believed to represent a specialized nerve ending.

Electron microscopic views of the epidermis

Fig. A shows a low power electron microscopic field of keratinocytes. Tonofilaments, prickles, and nodules of Bizzozero are visible.

Fig. B is a low magnification view of the epidermal-dermal junction. An indeterminate dendritic cell (I) is present. The cytoplasm contains neither melanosomes nor Langerhans granules.

ELECTRON MICROSCOPIC VIEWS OF THE EPIDERMIS

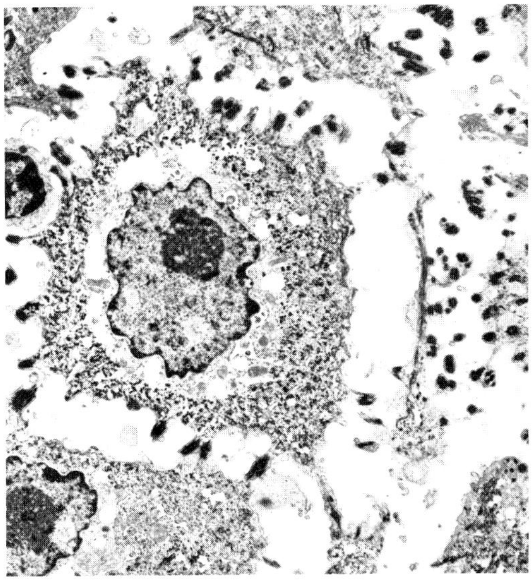

A
X3500

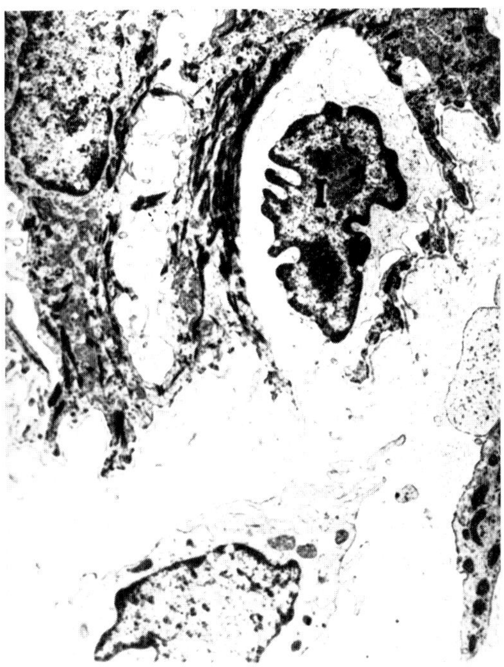

B
X3000

ELECTRON MICROSCOPIC VIEWS OF THE EPIDERMIS continued ⇨

Epidermis

Electron microscopic views

Fig. A shows a high magnification of desmosomes connecting keratinocytes. This complex structure consists of attachment plaques, intercellular contact layer, cell surface coat, trilaminar plasma membrane, and intercellular cement.

Fig. B. shows a high magnification view of the epidermal-dermal junction. A = anchoring fibrils; P = pinocytotic vesicle; LD = lamina densa or basal lamina; LL = lamina lucida; M = microfibrils; * = anchoring filaments spanning LL; arrowheads = subbasal dense plaque or dense plate; C = collagen fiber.

Determining cleavage site of subepidermal bullous dermatoses

Cleavage site of subepidermal bullous dermatoses can be determined by electron microscopy or by modified indirect immunofluorescence techniques delineating 3 components of the basement zone:

1. Bullous pemphigoid antibodies delineating the lamina lucida.
2. Anti type IV collagen antibodies, delineating a component of the basal lamina.
3. Antilaminin antibodies delineating a noncollagenous protein found throughout the basal lamina.

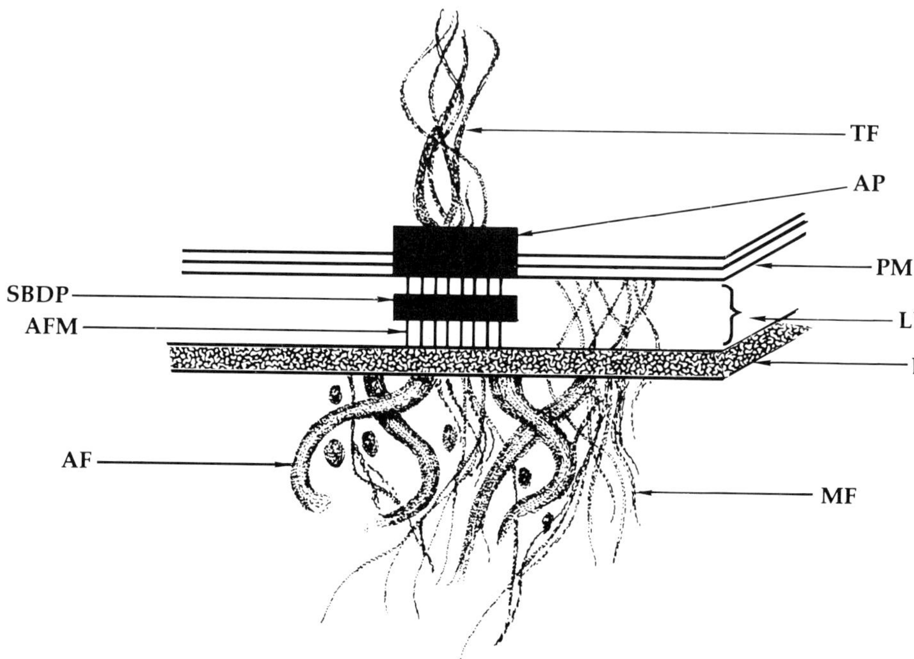

Schematic View of Epidermal-Dermal Junction

TF = Tonofilaments
AP = Attachment plaque of half-desmosome
PM = Trilaminar plasma membrane of basal cell
LL = Lamina lucida
BL = Basal lamina
MF = Microfilament
AF = Anchoring fibril
AFM = Anchoring filament
SBDP = Sub-basal cell dense plaque

ELECTRON MICROSCOPIC VIEWS OF THE EPIDERMIS

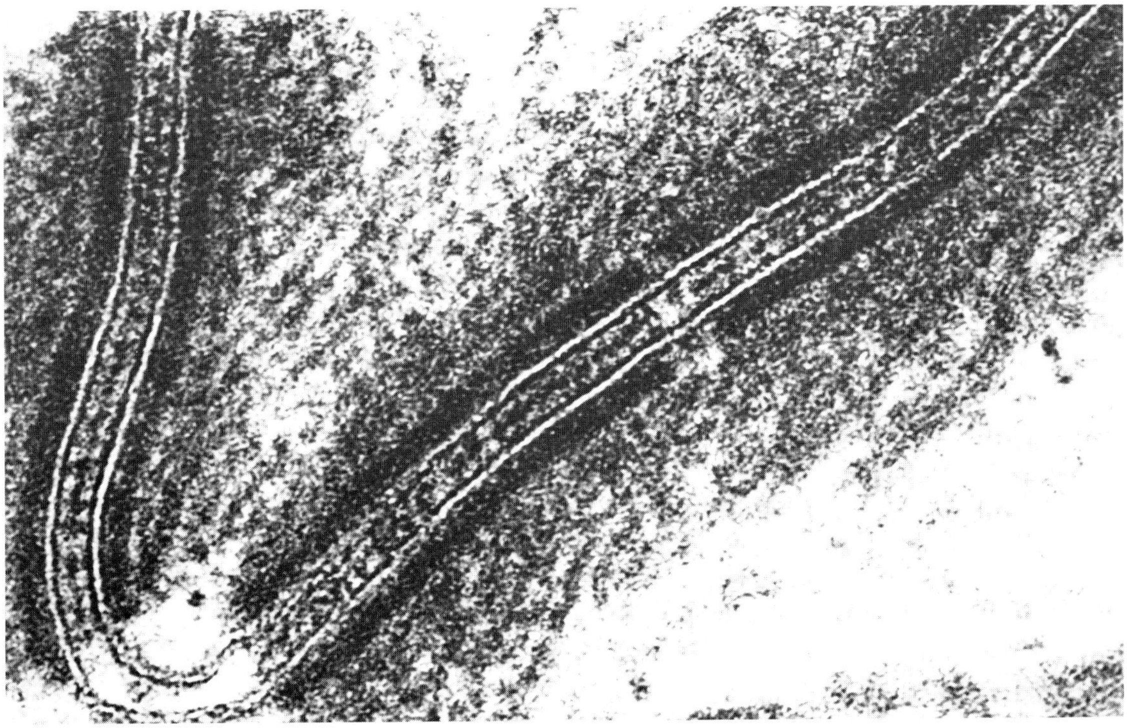

A
X120,000

Figs. A,B courtesy Dr. Ken Hashimoto

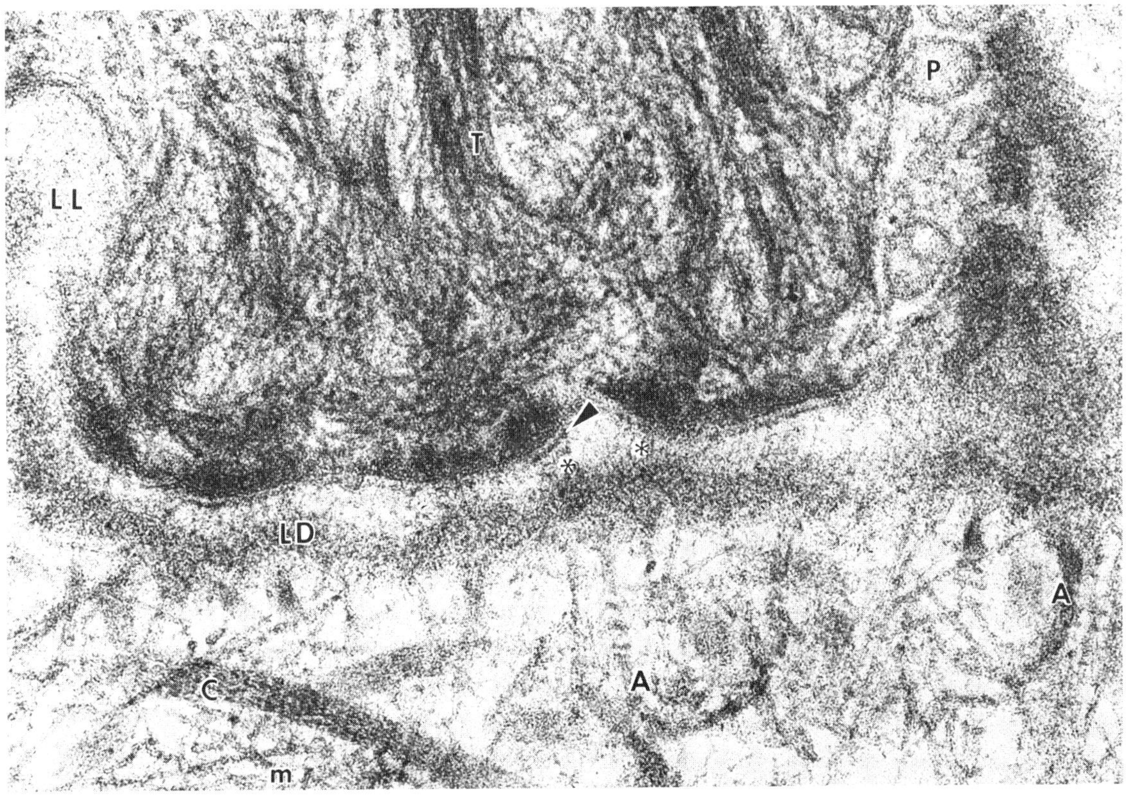

B
X80,000

ELECTRON MICROSCOPIC VIEWS OF THE EPIDERMIS continued

Epidermis

Electron microscopic views

Fig. A shows a high magnification of characteristic cytoplasmic organelles of Langerhans cells. They resemble tennis rackets. When not complete, the organelles resemble zippers.

ELECTRON MICROSCOPIC VIEWS OF THE EPIDERMIS

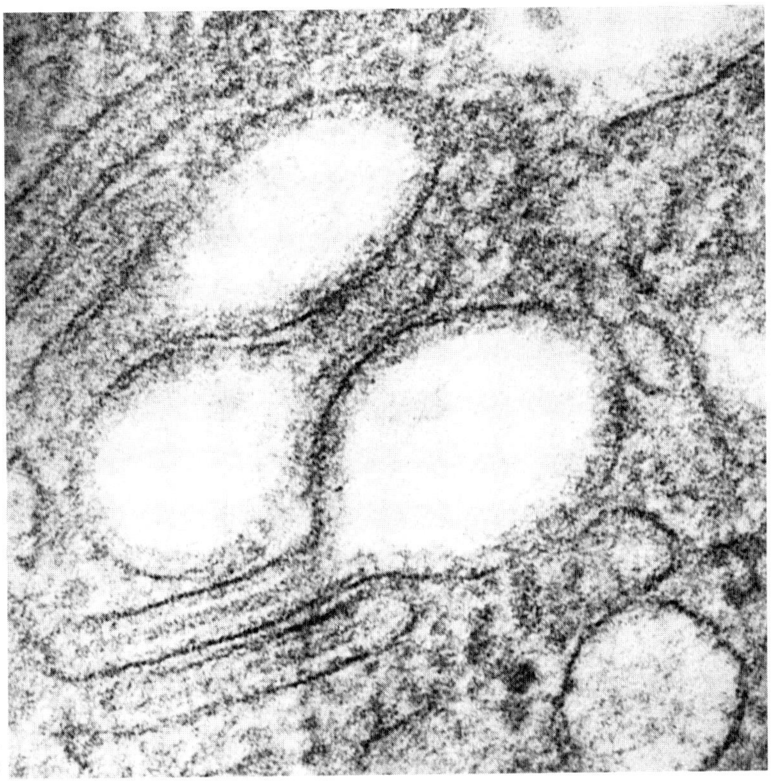

A
X120,000

Courtesy Dr. Ken Hashimoto

Mucous Membrane

Stratified squamous epithelium of mucous membrane, as seen in the oral mucosa (Fig. A), has a structure similar to that of epidermis. However, the keratinocytes show progressive vacuolization and shrinkage, with a parakeratotic surface layer. The granular layer is absent. The vacuolated appearance of the keratinocytes is largely due to their glycogen content.

MUCOUS MEMBRANE

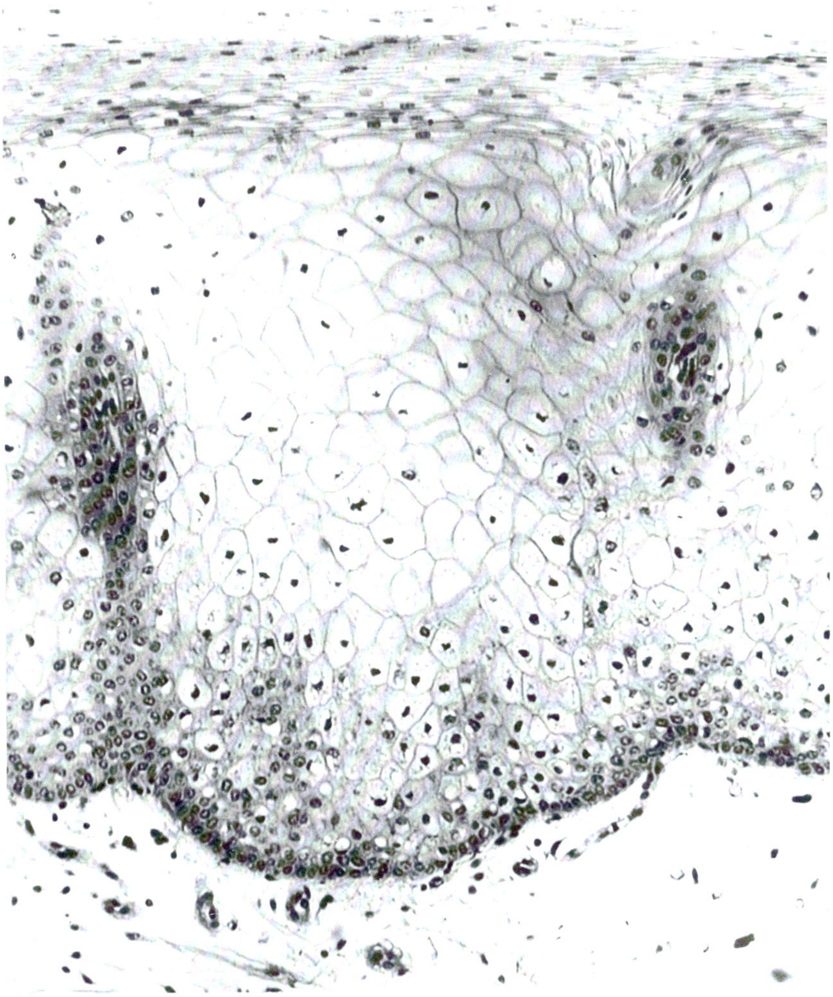

A
X750

Epidermis

MELANOCYTES

Melanocytes are distributed at regular intervals along the basal layer of the epidermis. In paraffin sections they appear to be surrounded by a clear zone (Fig. A [center]) and sometimes protrude downward into the dermis (Fig. A [left]). They are dendritic cells (Figs. A,B), and in heavily melanized normal skin (Fig. A) or certain pathologic conditions, such as melanoacanthoma (Fig. B), melanin granules are visible in the dendrites. Naturally formed melanin has a golden-brown color. Also, in certain pathologic conditions (Fig. B), the dendrites can form a dense, interlacing network.

Melanin granules are believed to be transferred from the melanocyte to the keratinocyte, which has no ability to synthesize melanin. The melanin granules accumulate in the supranuclear area of basal cells and are distributed throughout the rest of the epidermis as the basal cells divide to generate the upper layers. In heavily melanized epidermis, melanin granules can be observed even in the horny layer.

Melanogenic oxidase activity can be demonstrated in frozen sections of normal skin with the dopa reaction. Positive melanocytes show deposition of homogeneous grayish-black dopa melanin (Fig. C). The dopa reaction in melanocytes is the result of enzymatic activity of peroxidase and/or aerobic dopa oxidase ("tyrosinase"). Normal melanocytes in non-sun-exposed areas may show a negative dopa reaction due to very low enzymatic activity.

In normal (Fig. A) and pathologic skin, melanin-containing cells can also be observed in the dermis. Although it is widely believed that in humans these cells are phagocytes ("melanophages") which engulf melanin granules synthesized by epidermal melanocytes, there is evidence that at least some of these cells are dermal melanocytes which accumulate their own product by autophagy.

MELANOCYTES

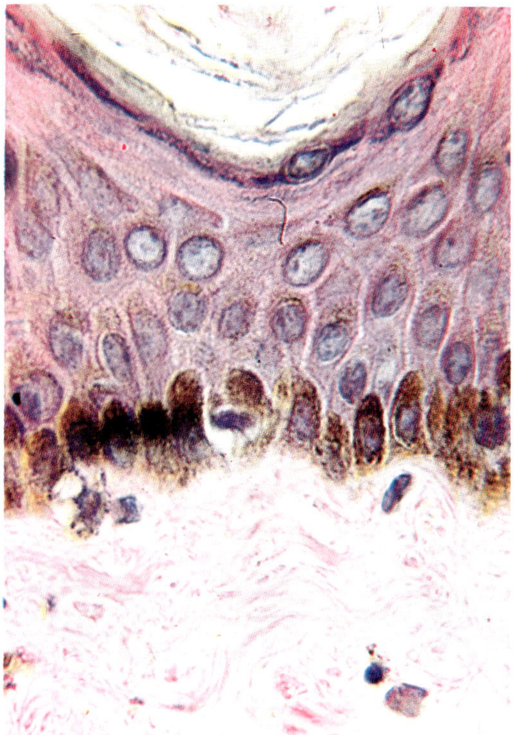

A
X1000

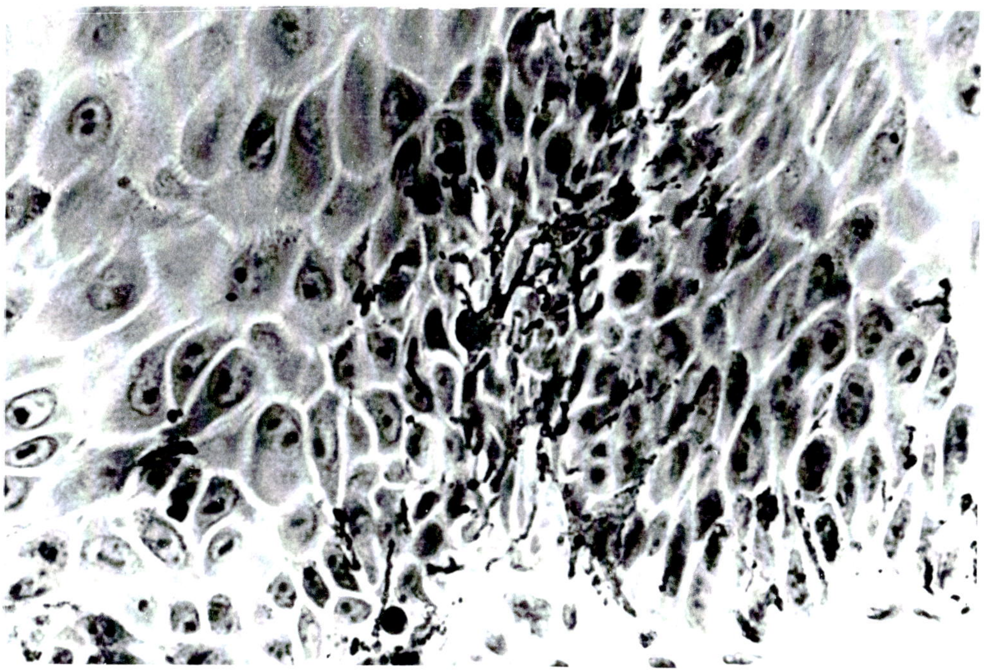

B
X730

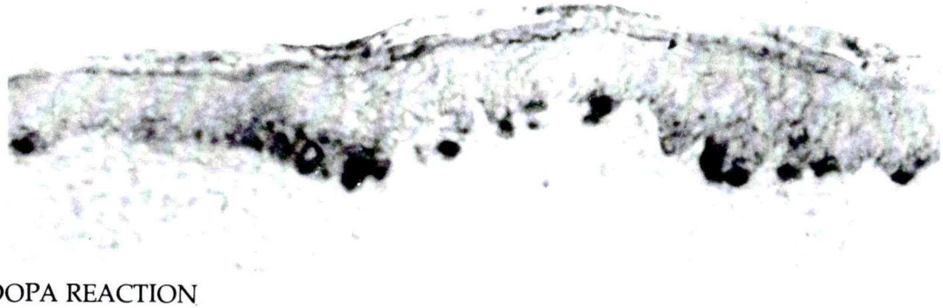

C
X130

DOPA REACTION

MELANOCYTES continued ⇨

Epidermis

Electron microscopic views of melanocytes

Fig. A shows a basal melanocyte (M) with cytoplasmic melanosomes. Fully melanized melanosomes are called melanin granules. Adjacent to it is a keratinocyte, whose cytoplasm shows tonofilaments and melanin granules. Melanin granules in Blacks tend to be dispersed singly in the cytoplasm of keratinocytes; in Caucasoids, melanin granules are largely within membrane-bound melanosome complexes in keratinocytes. Fig. B is a high magnification electron micrograph of a melanosome. Within it are cross-linked helical fibers. Increasing melanization is represented by accumulation of electron-dense material on the fibers. Fig. C shows a dermal "melanophage." In addition to melanin in membrane-bound melanosome complexes (secondary lysosomes), melanosomes in varying stages of melanization are present singly in the cytoplasm. Contrary to widespread belief, at least some "melanophages" may be dermal melanocytes which are accumulating and degrading melanin they have synthesized (autophagy).

Histogenesis of melanocytes and pigment cell tumors

The origin of melanocytes from embryonic neural crest is supported by extensive evidence. However, there is no scientific justification for the assumption that melanocytes are self-perpetuating and are histogenetically unrelated to surrounding tissue. It is well-established that much of the mesenchyme derives from neural crest rather than mesoderm; studies have shown that the connective tissue of the dermis is mainly of neural crest origin. We have proposed that melanocytes are not self-perpetuating, but continuously differentiate from pluripotential connective tissue cells of neural crest origin (mesectodermal cells). According to our hypothesis, therefore, pigment cell tumors represent tumors of mesectodermal origin, with principal differentiation in the direction of melanocytes. This hypothesis is supported by the presence of transitional forms between mast cells, nevus cells, and melanocytes, as well as histologic parallels between melanoma and canine mastocytoma.

Although it is generally acknowledged that dermal melanocytes are present in mammals (including primates), the anomalous belief persists that dermal melanocytes are not normally present in man. With the exception of neoplasms, it is assumed that all dermal melanin-containing cells are macrophages ("melanophages"). Enzymatic studies have indicated that at least some, and possibly most, "melanophages" are dermal melanocytes. It appears that melanosome complexes (observed with electron microscopy) in some "melanophages" are the result of autophagy rather than heterophagy.

ELECTRON MICROSCOPIC VIEWS OF MELANOCYTES

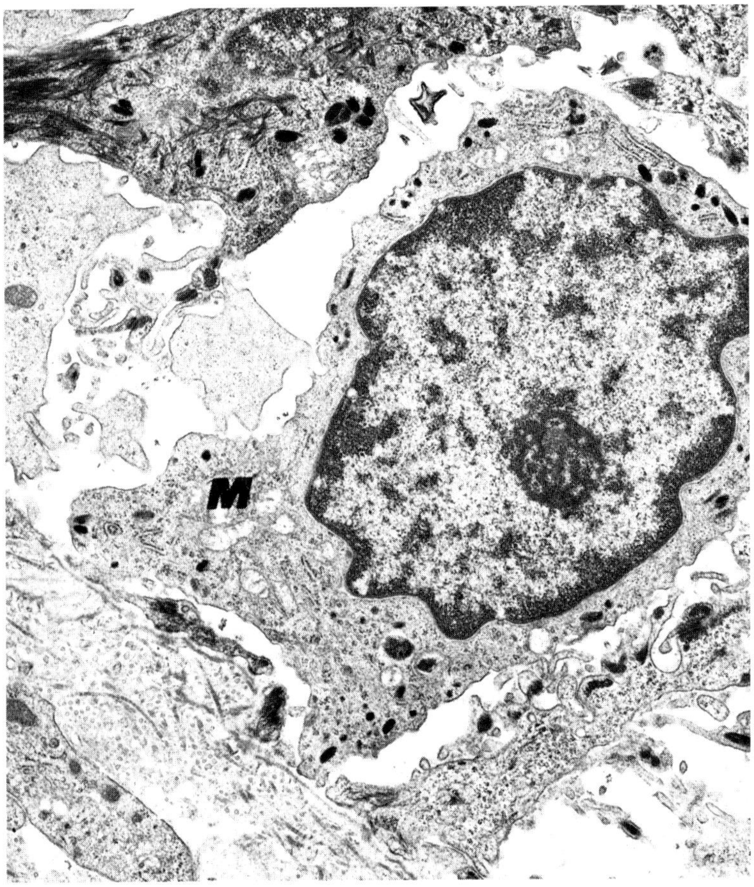

A X14,500

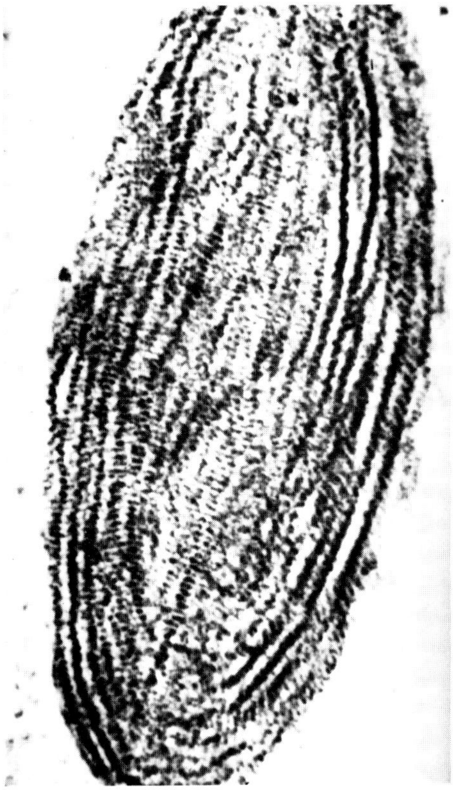

B
X300,000

Courtesy Dr. A. Breathnach

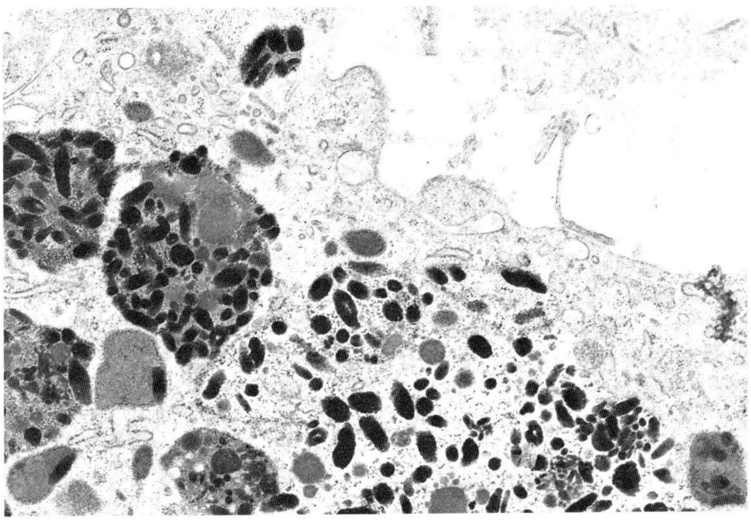

C
X14,500

Dermis

Fibroblast (Fibrocyte)

The fibroblast is the master cell of the dermis. It produces ground substance, collagen fibers, reticulum fibers, and elastic fibers. Fibroblasts (Fig. A) resemble histiocytes, but are more elongated and often have bipolar processes. Their nuclei are vesicular, with easily observed nucleoli.

There are multiple types of collagen, not all produced by fibroblasts.

The six collagens

Collagen type	Molecular formula	Main tissue location
I	$[a1\ (I)]_2\ a2$	Skin, tendon, bone
II	$[a1\ (II)]_3$	Cartilage
III	$[a1\ (III)]_3$	Fetal tissue, blood vessels, intestine
IV	$[a1\ (IV)]_3$	Basement membrane
V	$aA\ [aB]_2$	Placental membranes, epidermis
VI	$[a1\ (I)]_3$	Adult dermis

FIBROBLAST

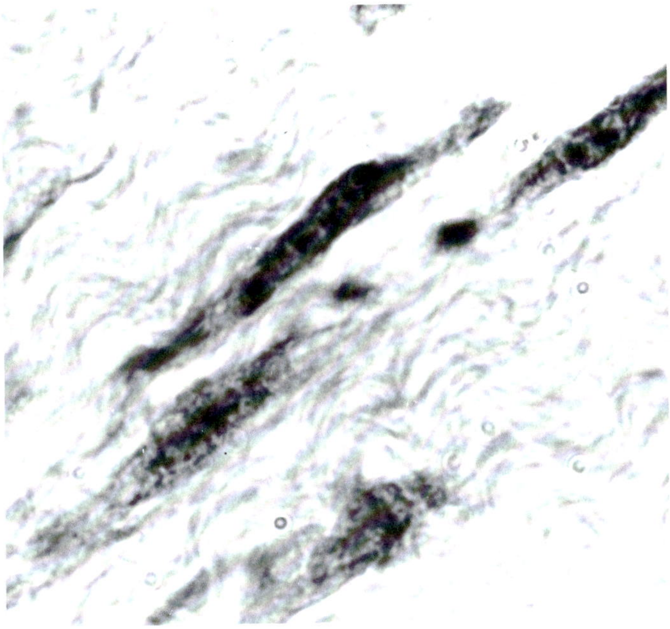

A
X1800

DERMIS continued ⇨

Dermis

The dermis extends from the epidermis to the subcutaneous fat and is composed of many parts. These include collagen fibers, elastic fibers, ground substance, blood vessels, nerves, fibroblasts, histiocytes, mast cells, and lymphocytes. Within the dermis are the cutaneous appendages.

With H&E stain, the most obvious component is the connective tissue, composed principally of collagen fibers. In the *papillary dermis* (P–Fig. A) (which includes the papillae and subpapillary layer), the collagen fibers constitute a fine meshwork. In the *reticular dermis* (R–Fig. A), the collagen fibers are much coarser and run in various directions in a plane parallel to the surface. The pars papillaris is more richly vascularized than the pars reticularis and contains superficial arterial and venous plexuses and their capillary loops. Fig. A, inset shows the papillary and reticular dermis with a lighter H&E stain. A fine meshwork of fibers also surrounds the cutaneous appendages and blood vessels. The component of the dermis with fine fibers is called *adventitial dermis*.

The ground substance of the dermis cannot be seen with H&E stain, but small foci can be seen with stains for acid mucopolysaccharides, which stain hyaluronic acid (the principal component of the ground substance) and sulfated acid mucopolysaccharides. The *interstitium* represents spaces between collagen and elastic fibers.

Similarly, the elastic fibers require special stains to be observed. Elastic fibers return distended skin to its original shape. Elastic fibers of the pars papillaris of the dermis (Fig. C,E) are much finer than those of the pars reticularis (Fig. E), and have a fragmented angular appearance.

Reticulum fibers represent immature collagen and can be demonstrated by silver impregnation stains (Fig. D). Reticulum fibers are present throughout the dermis. They are numerous around appendages.

With PAS stain (Fig. B), the basement membrane zone bordering the dermis can be seen. The PAS-positive material represents a condensation of neutral mucopolysaccharides beneath the basal lamina. The detailed structure of the epidermal-dermal junction can be seen only with electron microscopy. Adjacent components include the cell membrane of the basal cells, basal lamina, and anchoring fibrils. Cytoplasmic processes of basal cells alternate with corresponding dermal processes. The cell membrane of the basal cells is separated from the basal lamina by a narrow space, except where half-desmosomes connect them. A fine network of reticulum fibers extends downward from the basement zone (Fig. D). With elastic tissue stains, a fine brushwork of elastic fibers can be seen just beneath the basement zone (Fig. C); the fibers run perpendicular to the epidermis.

In normal skin, oval nuclei of fibroblasts and histiocytes are sparse. Lymphocytes and mast cells are present in small numbers, mainly in the loose connective tissue around blood vessels.

DERMIS

A X160

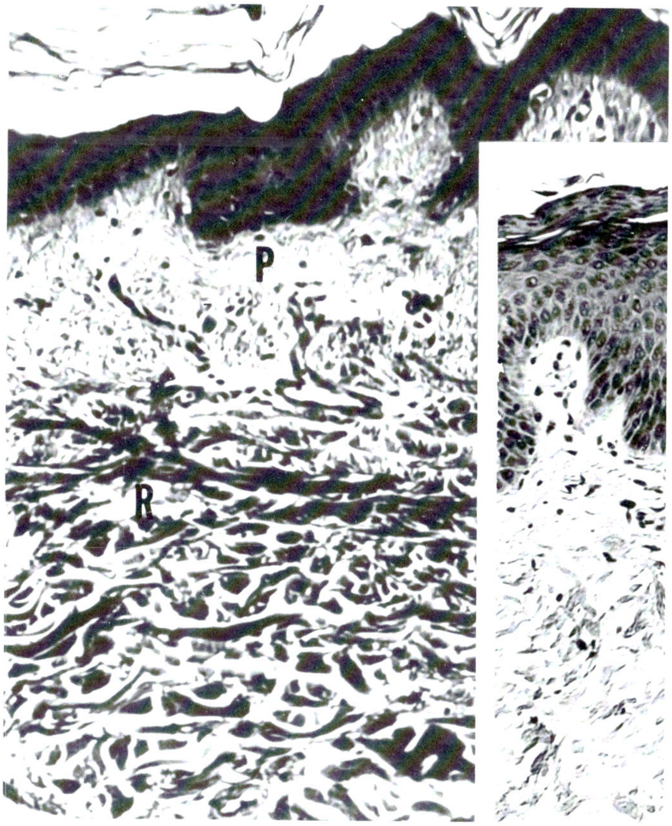

B X620 PAS STAIN

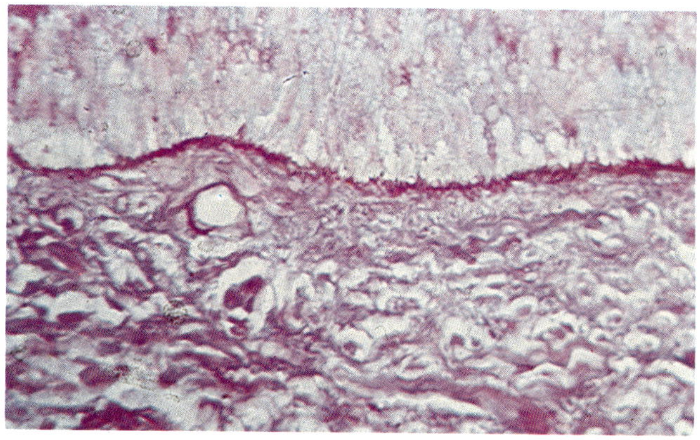

C X620 ACID ORCEIN GIEMSA STAIN

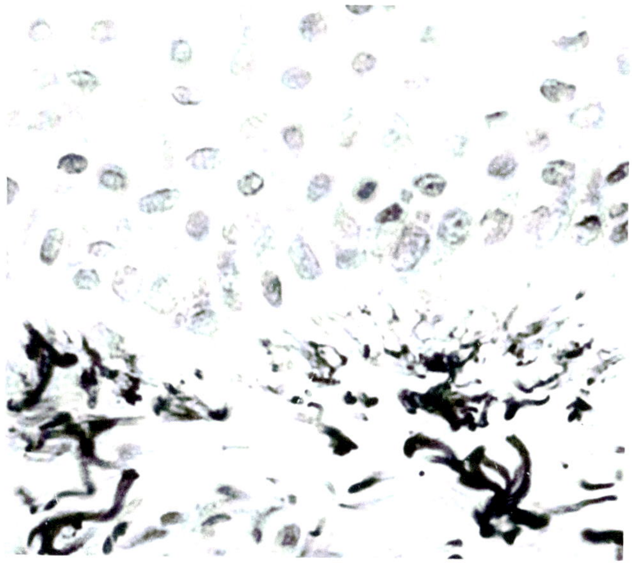

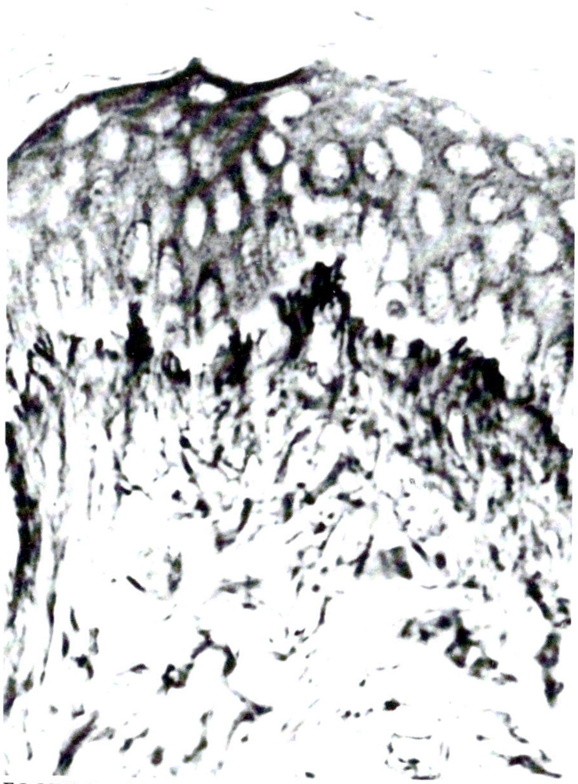

D
X810

FOOT'S RETICULUM STAIN

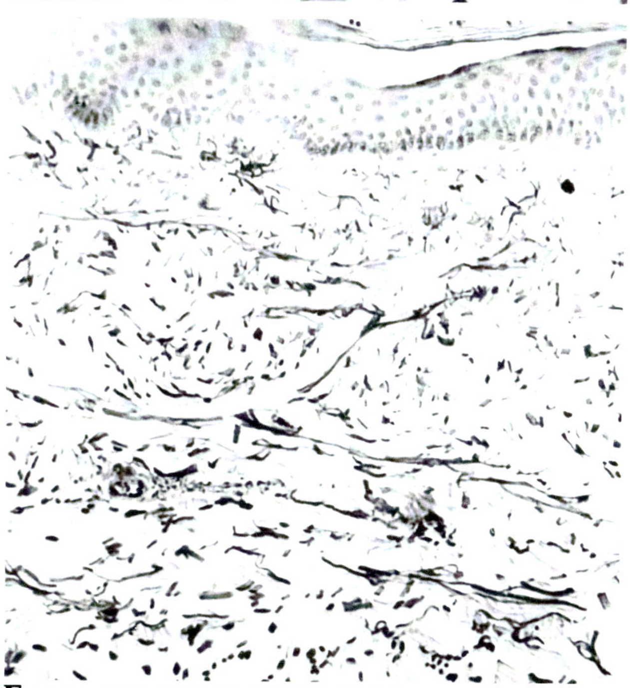

E X180 ACID ORCEIN GIEMSA STAIN

Striated Muscle

In some areas (e.g., face, scalp, neck) striated muscle fibers are located just beneath the subcutaneous tissue (Fig. A) and may extend into the dermis (Fig. B), particularly in the perioral area. Nuclei of striated muscle are at the periphery of the fibers.

Smooth Muscle

Smooth muscle is present in the skin as arrectores pilorum (see p. 55), as tunica dartos (Fig. C) of the external genitalia, and in the areola and nipples (Fig. D). Smooth muscle fibers do not have striations and have nuclei in the centers of the muscle cells.

STRIATED MUSCLE

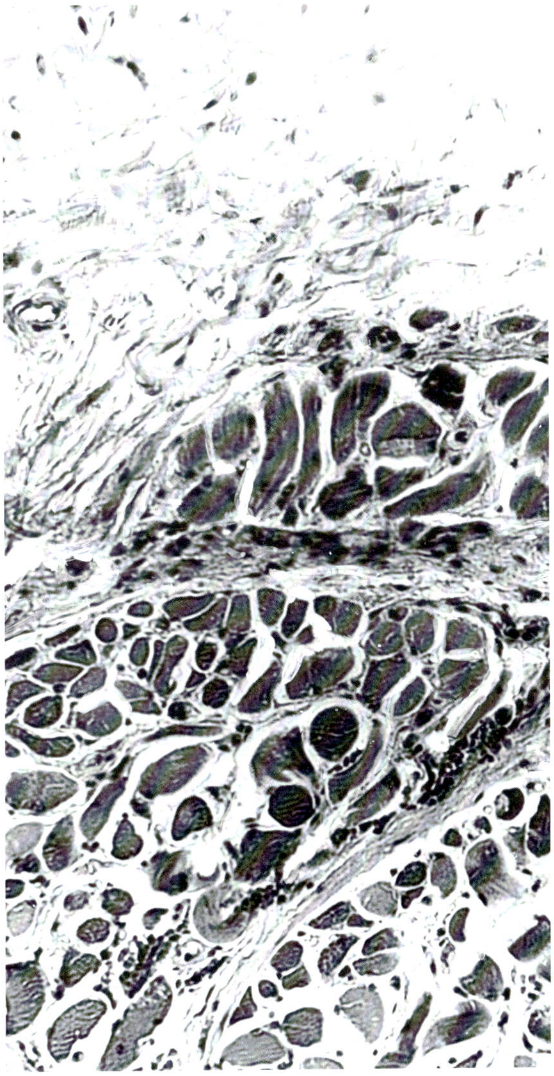

A
X260

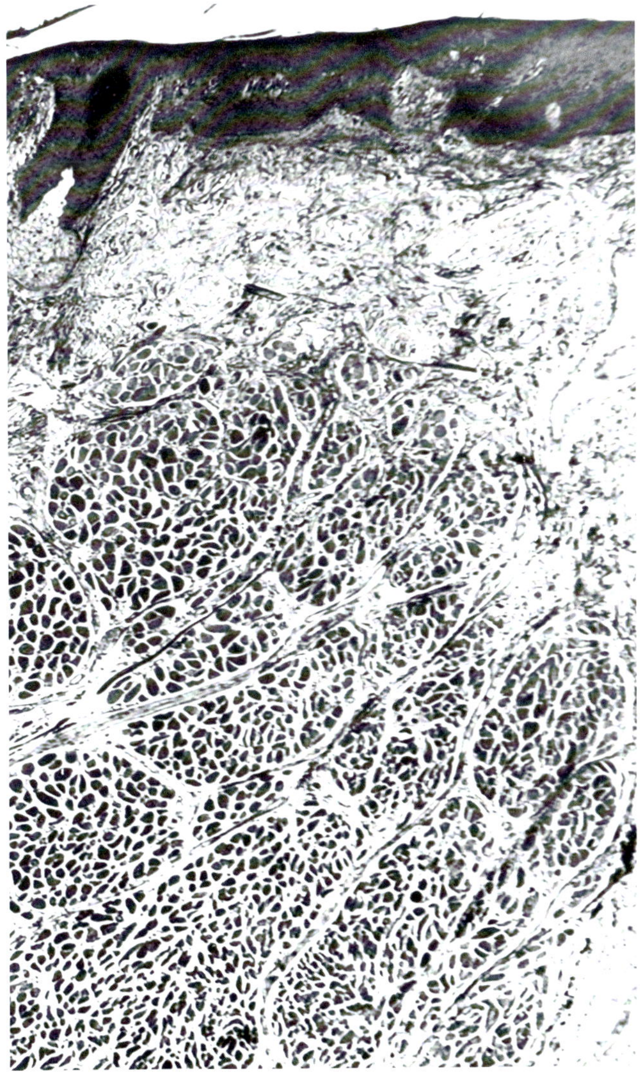

B
X70

SMOOTH MUSCLE

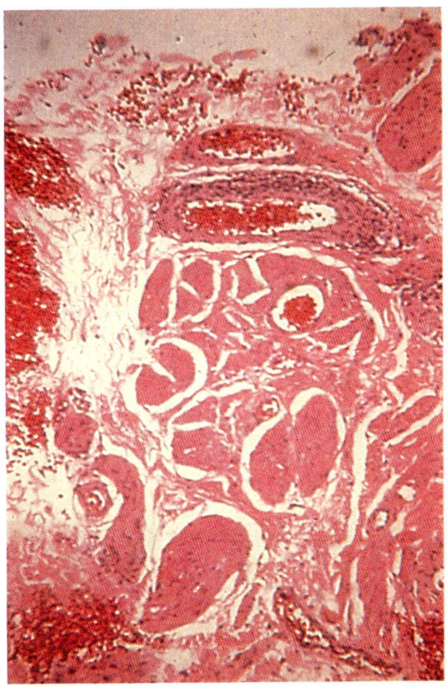

C
X125

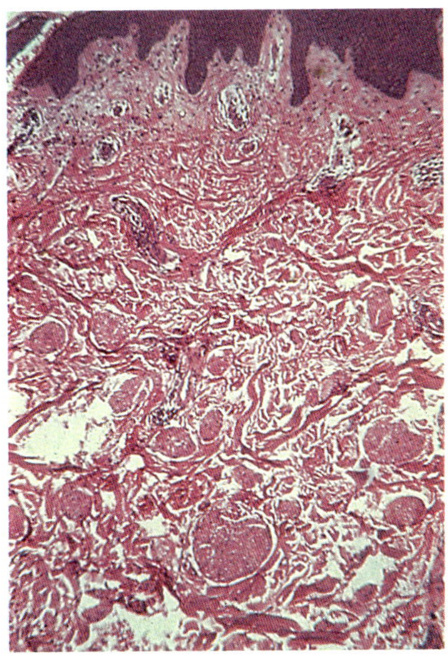

D
X60

Vasculature of the skin

The dermis contains capillaries, arterioles, venules, lymph capillaries, and post-capillary lymph vessels.

There are subcutaneous (Fig. C) and subpapillary (Fig. A) plexuses. Capillary loops (Fig. B) extend into the dermal papillae from the subpapillary plexuses. There are also plexuses around hair follicles and eccrine glands.

The capillaries are lined by a layer of endothelial cells surrounded by an incomplete layer of pericytes. The pericytes are enmeshed in reticulum fibers. The reticulum fibers make up the basement membrane.

VASCULATURE OF THE SKIN

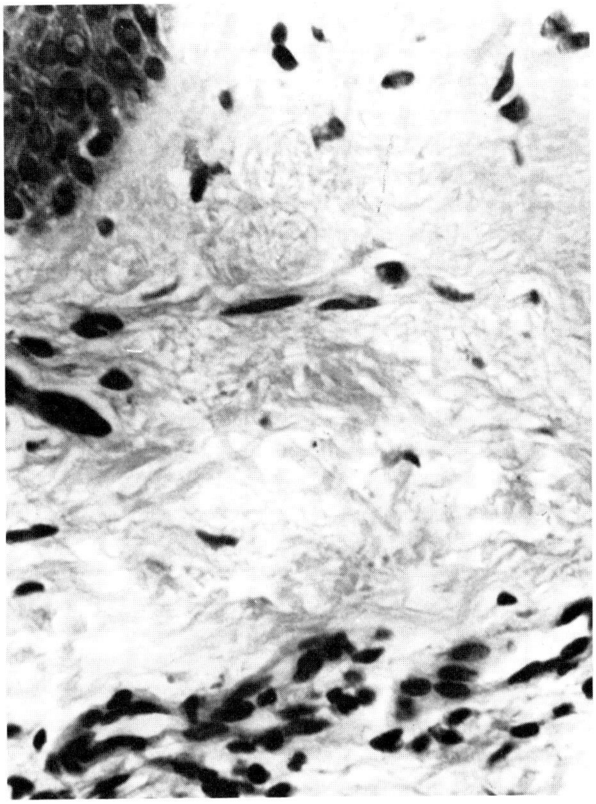

A
X520

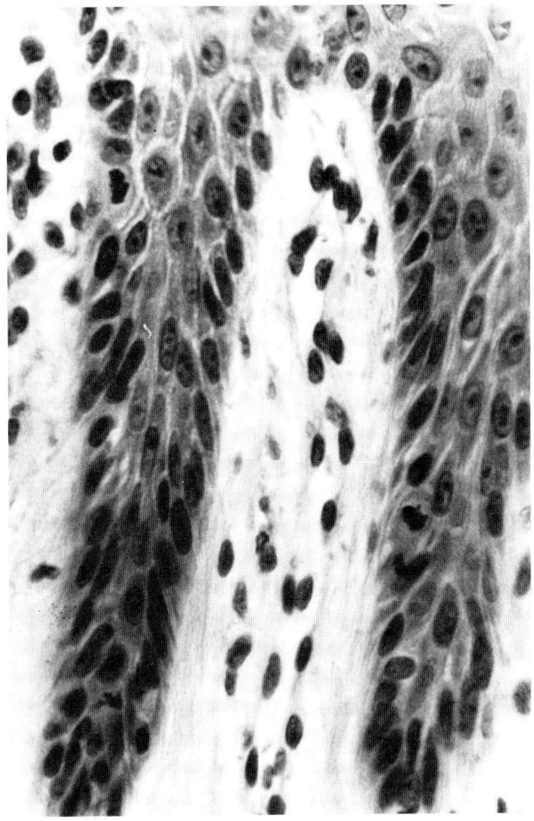

B
X520

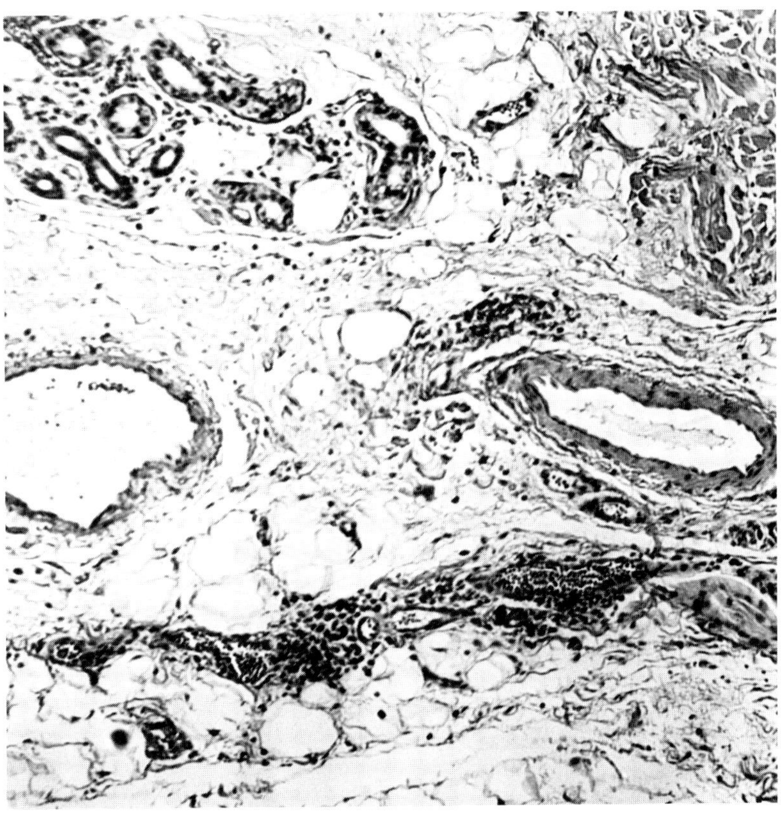

C
X96

VASCULATURE OF THE SKIN continued

Vasculature of the skin

The arterioles (Fig. A) are composed of three layers: a) the intima, which contains endothelial cells and an internal elastic lamina (Fig. B); b) the media, which contains smooth muscle cells; c) the adventitia, which contains connective tissue. A basement membrane composed of reticulum fibers is at the periphery. The reticulum fibers surround pericytes.

The venules (Fig. C) have a structure similar to that of arterioles, but have thinner walls, with less distinct layers.

Lymph capillaries differ from blood capillaries by an absence of pericytes and a basement membrane. They are surrounded by a loosely arranged zone of collagen and elastic fibers. Postcapillary lymph vessels have a similar structure, but have larger lumina and thicker walls. Lymph capillaries are not visible in sections of normal skin.

The glomus (Fig. D) is a specialized vascular structure which is present in certain areas: nailbeds, pads of the fingers and toes (and elsewhere on the volar aspects of the hands and feet), ears, and center of the face. It is a shunt connecting arterioles and venules, concerned with temperature regulation. The arterial segment of the shunt (Fig. D) is called the Suquet-Hoyer canal; its endothelial layer is surrounded by reticulum fibers, and its media is composed of multiple layers of contractile glomus cells, resembling epithelioid cells.

VASCULATURE OF THE SKIN

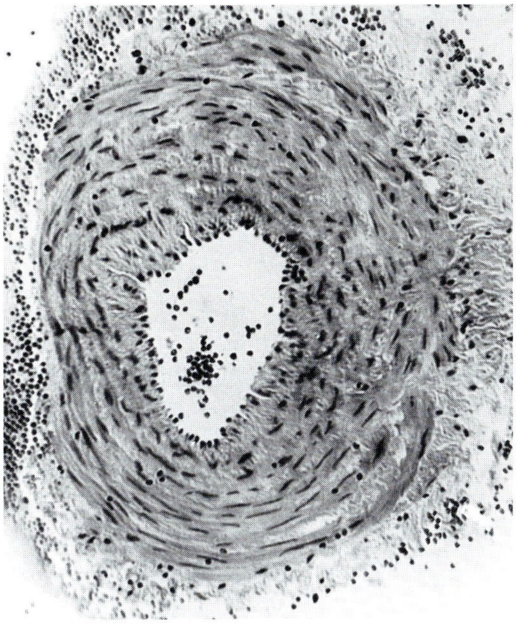

A
X130

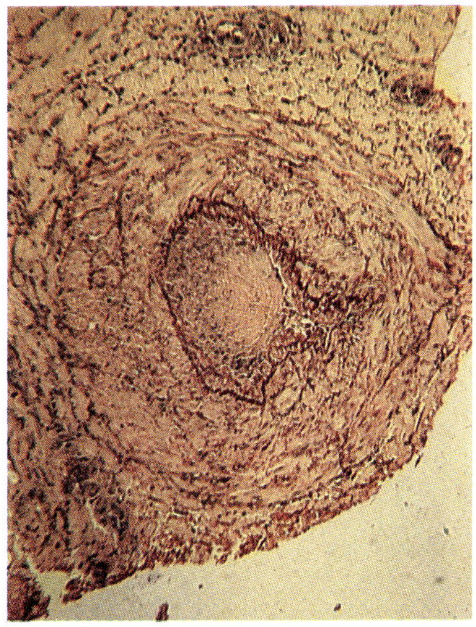

B
X80

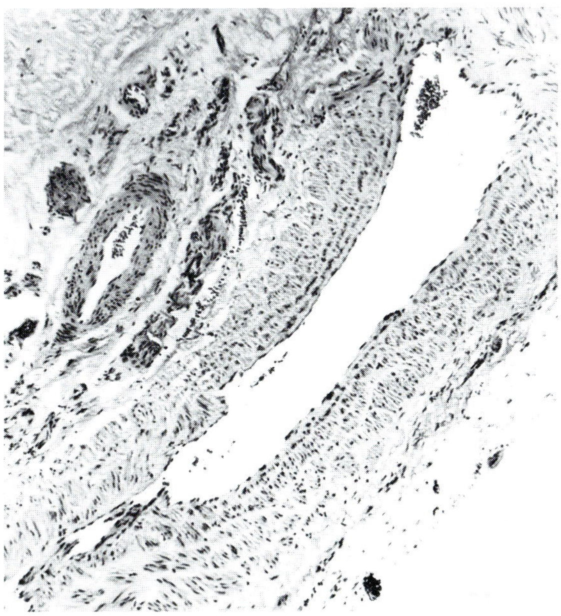

C
X180

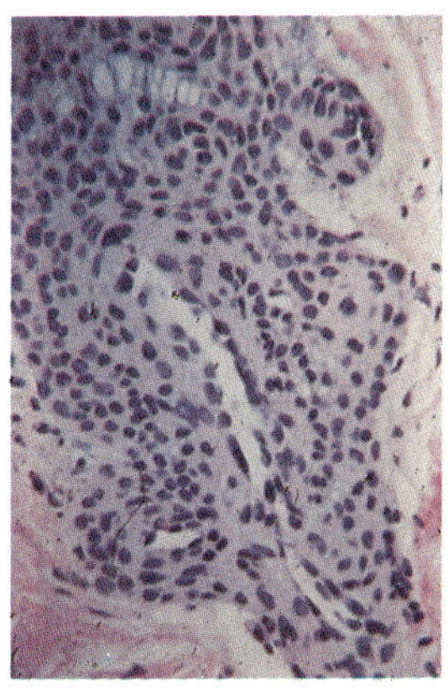

D
X200

Tissue Cytology of Inflammatory Cells

Lymphocyte

With light microscopy, B lymphocytes and T lymphocytes look alike. The average diameter is 8 to 10 microns, and a dense, basophilic nucleus occupies virtually all of the cross-sectional area (L–Fig. A). Larger lymphocytes may be indistinguishable from tissue monocytes with routine stains.

Monocyte and Histiocyte (Macrophage)

Monocytes circulate in the blood and enter tissue. They can be transformed into histiocytes on proper stimulation.

Histiocytes have amphophilic or eosinophilic cytoplasm and a large, vesicular nucleus with a visible nucleolus. They are 15 to 25 microns in diameter (H–Fig. A).

Epithelioid cell

Epithelioid cells are transformed histiocytes, with abundant, ill-defined cytoplasm which is usually eosinophilic. They occur in compact groups, and their indistinct cell walls suggest cell fusion (Fig. B).

Comment

1. Immunologically stimulated lymphocytes enlarge and develop a darker nucleus, resulting in a resemblance to an atypical cell.
2. Epithelioid cells become giant cells by fusion.

Tissue Inflammatory Cells

Cell type	*Important Functions*
I. LYMPHOID CELLS	
A. Lymphocytes	
1. B lymphocytes	humoral immunity often via transformation into plasma cells
2. T lymphocytes	cell-mediated immunity
B. Monocytes	phagocytosis, when transformed into histiocytes; antigen processing
II. GRANULOCYTIC CELLS	
A. Neutrophils	phagocytosis
B. Eosinophils	phagocytosis, including immune complexes
C. Mast cells	synthesis of heparin and histamine and other mediators of inflammation; receptor for immune complex

TISSUE CYTOLOGY OF INFLAMMATORY CELLS

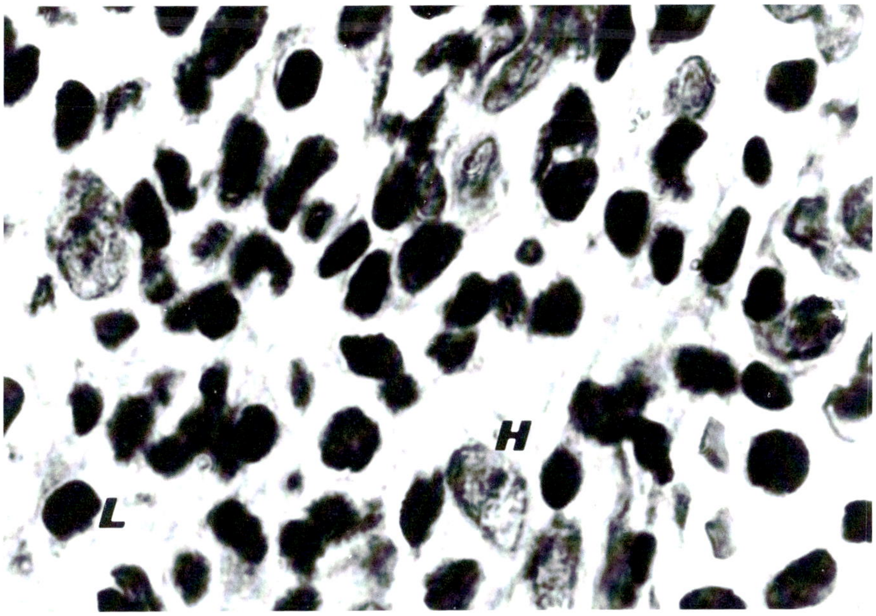

A
X1800

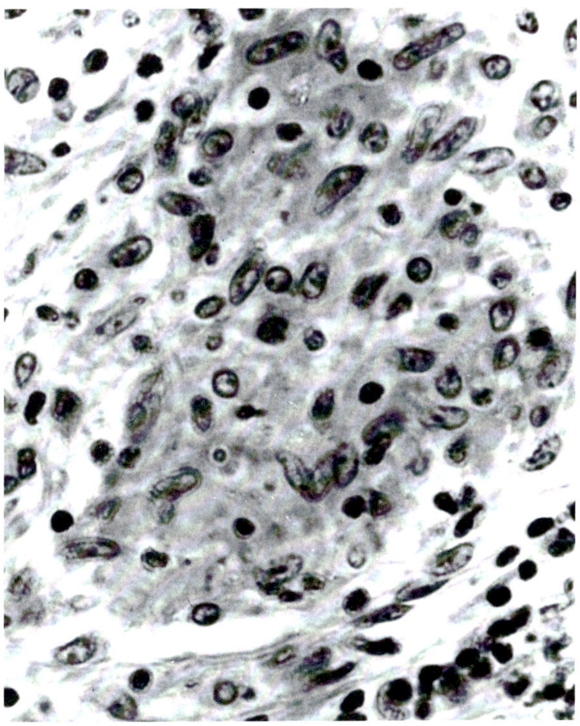

B
X900

TISSUE CYTOLOGY OF INFLAMMATORY CELLS continued ⇨

Tissue Cytology of Inflammatory Cells

Foreign Body Giant Cell

These are multinucleated giant histiocytes. The diameter can reach 100 microns. Nuclei are relatively small and randomly arranged (Fig. A).

Langhans Giant Cell

These differ from the foreign body giant cells by the arcuate arrangement of their nuclei (Fig. B).

Plasma Cells

Plasma cells range from 10 to 20 microns in diameter and have an eccentric nucleus, a perinuclear halo (Golgi complex), and abundant amphophilic or basophilic cytoplasm. The nuclear heterochromatin is attached to the nuclear membrane, giving it a "cartwheel" appearance (Fig. C). Plasma cells develop from antigenically stimulated B lymphocytes.

TISSUE CYTOLOGY OF INFLAMMATORY CELLS

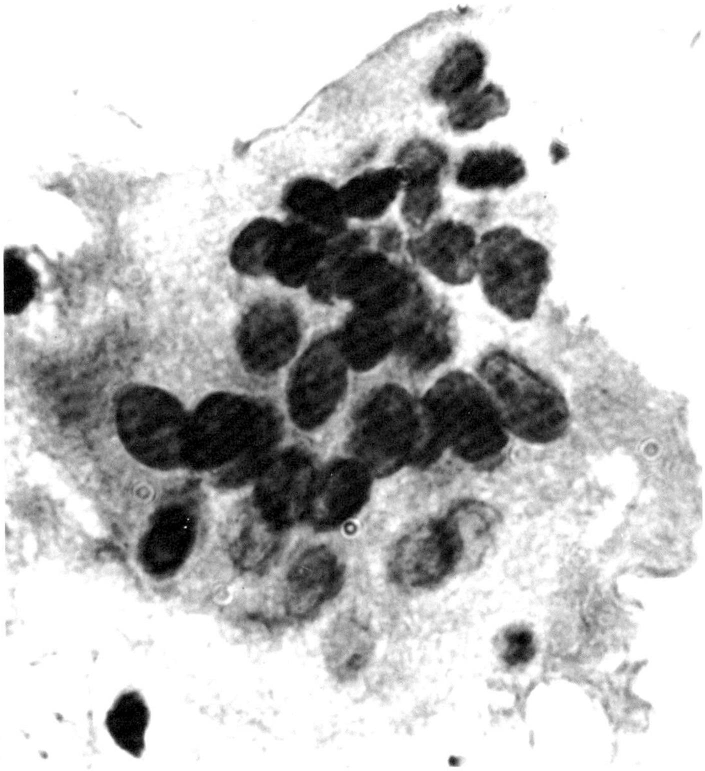

A
X1800

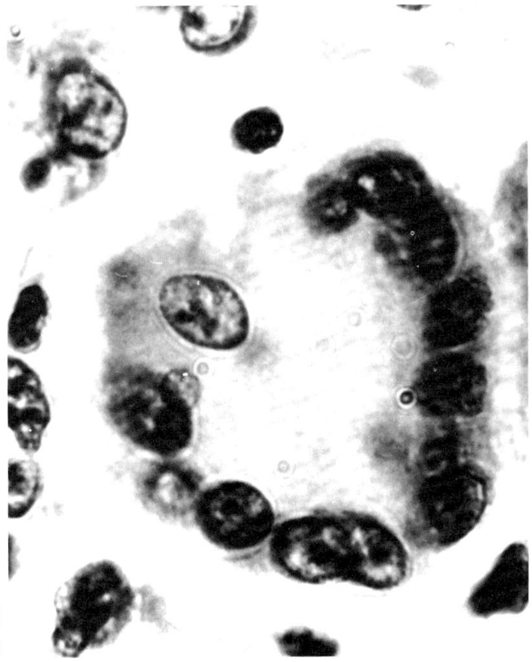

B
X1800

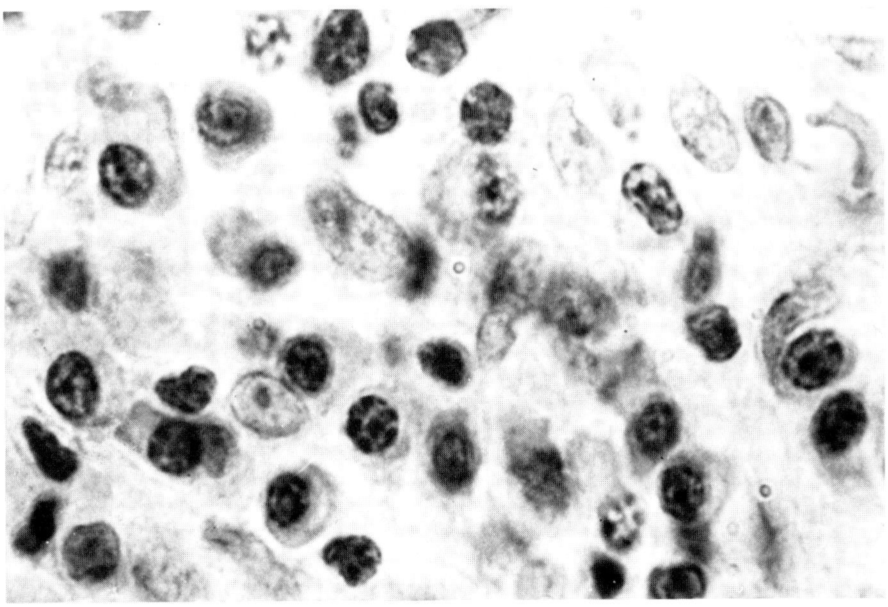

C
X1800

TISSUE CYTOLOGY OF INFLAMMATORY CELLS continued

Tissue Cytology of Inflammatory Cells

Mast Cell

With H&E stain, mast cells cannot always be identified. Their shape can resemble that of histiocytes, fibroblasts, or melanocytes. Mast cells with a polyhedral shape can resemble type A epithelioid nevus cells (Fig. A). The compact, central nucleus is often indented and is surrounded by an amphophilic cytoplasm. Definitive identification of mast cells is accomplished with stains for acid mucopolysaccharides (Fig. B), which have an affinity for the mast cell granules. Figs. A,B show cuboidal mast cells in nodular mastocytosis. The cytoplasm is filled with purple metachromatic granules. Basophils have similarities to mast cells. They can be distinguished from mast cells in one micron sections of tissue prepared for electron microscopy, but not in routine sections.

Eosinophil

It is slightly larger than the neutrophil, and the granules are coarser than neutrophil granules; they are brilliantly eosinophilic. Nuclei of eosinophils are bilobed (Fig. C). The crystalloid core of eosinophil granules contains some melanin. Therefore, eosinophils show a positive Fontana-Masson silver stain (Fig. C, inset).

Neutrophil

The average diameter ranges from 7 to 10 microns. The nucleus has 3 to 5 lobes. Cytoplasmic granules are amphophilic (Fig. D).

TISSUE CYTOLOGY OF INFLAMMATORY CELLS

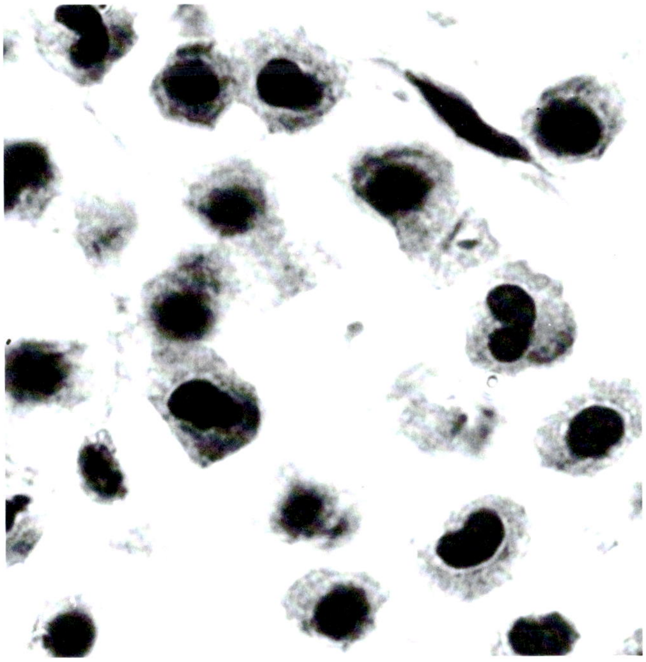

A
X1800

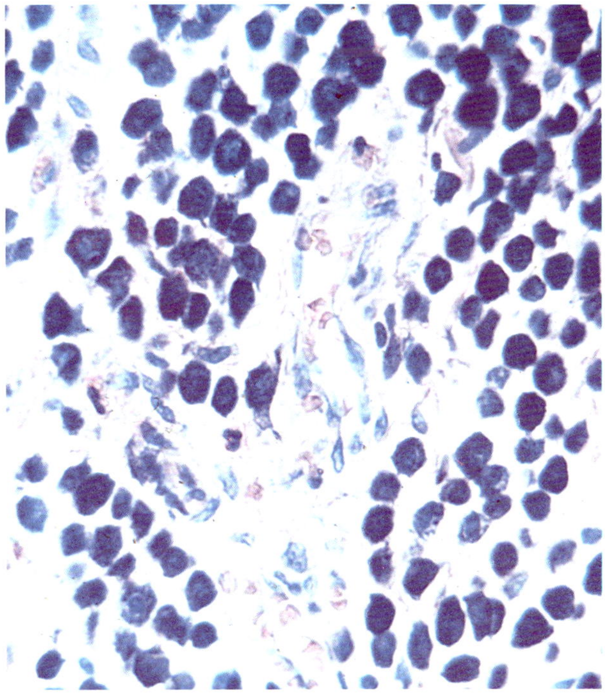

B
X760

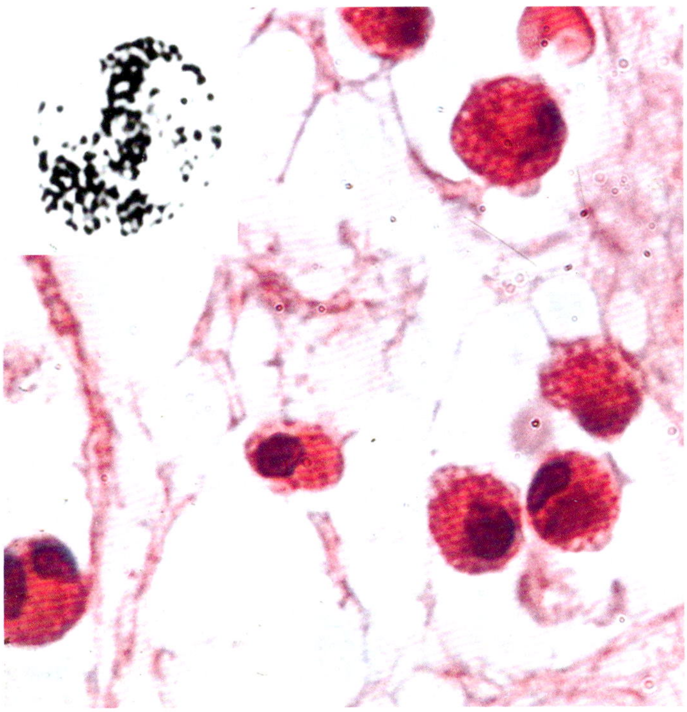

C X1800
INSET: FONTANA-MASSON STAIN
(NO COUNTERSTAIN)
INSET: X3600

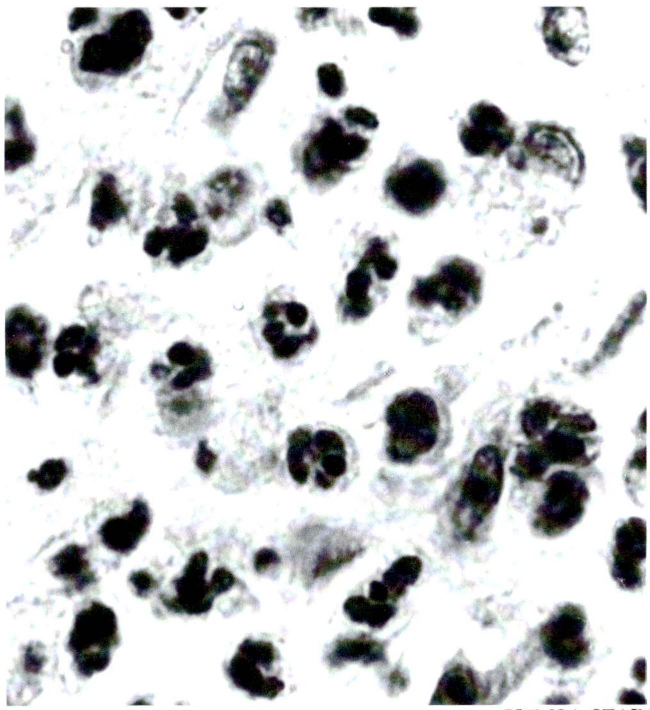

D X1800
GIEMSA STAIN

Hair

The Pilary Complex

Hairs are part of the pilary complex, which also includes the sebaceous glands and apocrine glands. The pilary complex develops from the embryonic primary epithelial germ. There are two principal types of hair: terminal hair and vellus hair. Terminal hairs are larger, coarser, and more heavily pigmented than vellus hairs. Terminal hairs of the scalp extend into the subcutaneous fat. Terminal hairs of the body of the adult male extend into the lower dermis. Vellus hairs extend to the upper dermis. A special type of vellus hair is the sebaceous follicle. At puberty the sebaceous glands of sebaceous follicles become large and well-developed. They are numerous on the face; they are the target organs of acne vulgaris.

Hairs have a cyclic pattern of growth and regression. Actively growing hairs are called anagen hairs; the stage of regression is called catagen; the resting stage is called telogen.

The diagram (Fig. A) illustrates a pilary complex containing a hair in anagen. Emptying into the hair follicle are the duct of the sebaceous glands (S) and apocrine duct (AD). The apocrine duct leads to the apocrine coil (C). The hair follicle is divided into segments as follows: the infundibulum is above the sebaceous duct; the isthmus is between the insertion of the arrectores pilorum (AP) and the sebaceous duct; the inferior segment is below the insertion of the arrector pili muscle.

Extending the length of the follicle is the outer root sheath (O). The upper portion of the outer root sheath can be regarded as an extension of the epidermis, and is histologically identical to it, unlike the cells of the lower portion of the outer root sheath (L), which do not keratinize and appear clear due to the presence of large amounts of glycogen.

The germinative cells that give rise to the hair shaft (H) make up the hair matrix (M), which also gives rise to the inner root sheath (I). Within the matrix are dendritic melanocytes. The expansion of the lower part of the hair follicle is termed the hair bulb. An invagination of connective tissue at the lower pole of the hair bulb is the hair papilla (P), analogous to the dermal papilla adjacent to epidermal rete ridges. The epithelial structures of the hair follicle are enclosed by a glassy membrane (G), beyond which is a connective tissue sheath.

HAIR

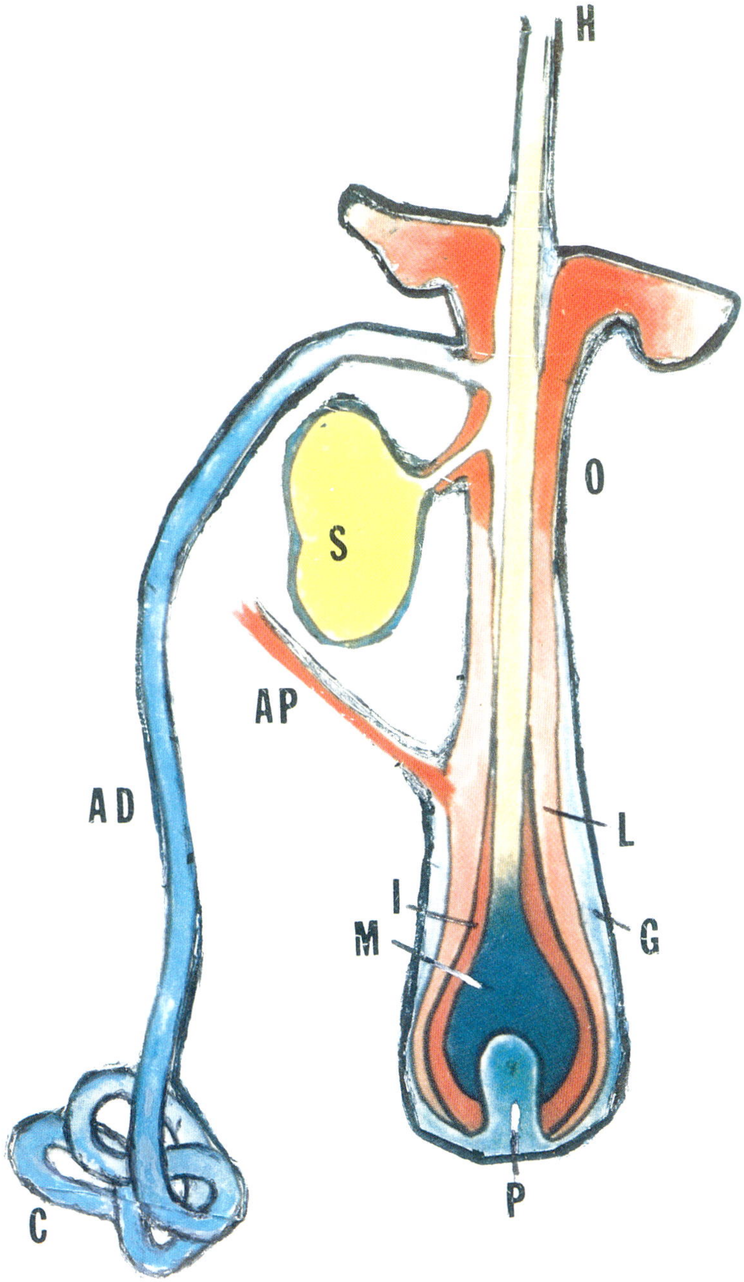

A

HAIR continued ⇨

Hair Cycle

Fig. A illustrates the hair cycle. Since anagen persists far longer than catagen or telogen at any given time, most hairs are in anagen.

During the phase of regression (catagen), the inferior segment of the hair (broken line in diagram on the left) disappears, producing the club hair of telogen, with a fully cornified outer root sheath, and which contains a focus of undifferentiated epithelial cells (U) on its undersurface.

When a new anagen phase begins (diagram on the right), the papilla (P) makes contact with the undifferentiated cells, and a new hair matrix (M), inner root sheath, and hair shaft are generated, descending along the fibrous sheath remaining from the old anagen hair. The new hair shaft dislodges the old hair shaft, in its upward ascent.

HAIR CYCLE

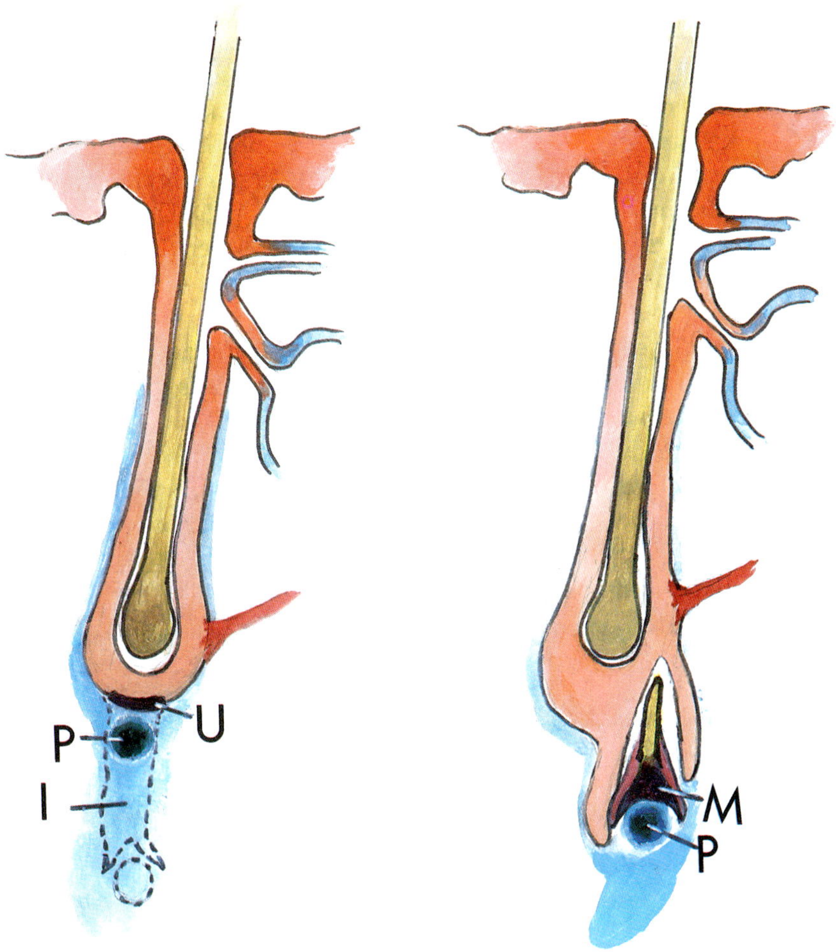

A

HAIR continued

Hair

Illustrated are areas of a terminal hair in anagen (Figs. A,B,D,E). The scanning view (Fig. A) shows the infundibulum (If) and isthmus (Is) of the hair follicle. The infundibulum (upper portion of the outer root sheath) has a structure similar to that of the epidermis, with active basal melanocytes. Also shown are sebaceous gland lobules (S), cortex of the hair shaft (C), lower portion of the outer root sheath (in isthmus area [Is]), inner root sheath (I), and hair bulb (B). The outer root sheath is lined by a vitreous layer beyond which is the fibrous root sheath.

Fig. B shows the lower part of the hair with higher magnification. Symbols correspond to those of Fig. A. Cells of the outer root sheath below the entrance of the sebaceous duct (O – Fig. B) have a clear cytoplasm because of their glycogen content. Inactive melanocytes, demonstrable with methylene blue are present in this part of the outer root sheath. The upper part of this segment of the outer root sheath forms homogeneous keratinized cells without the production of keratohyaline granules (*trichilemmal* keratinization). (Trichilemma = outer root sheath.)

Area of the inset with higher magnification (Fig. D) illustrates layers of the follicle. From outside in, arrows indicate (1) vitreous layer, (2) outer root sheath, (3) Henle layer of the inner root sheath, (4) Huxley layer of the inner root sheath, (5) inner root sheath cuticle, and (6) hair cuticle.

In all three layers of the inner root sheath, keratinization is associated with eosinophilic trichohyalin* granules. The hair cortex cells (C) however, keratinize without the production of trichohyalin granules.

Higher magnification of the hair bulb (Fig. E) shows the hair matrix cells (M), which resemble basal cells of the epidermis, and connective tissue papilla (P). Numerous dendritic melanocytes are interspersed among the hair matrix cells.

Fig C shows a telogen hair, with fully cornified outer root sheath and a focus of undifferentiated epithelial cells on its lower surface.

*The eosinophilic trichohyalin granules contrast with the basophilic keratohyalin granules of the epidermis.

HAIR

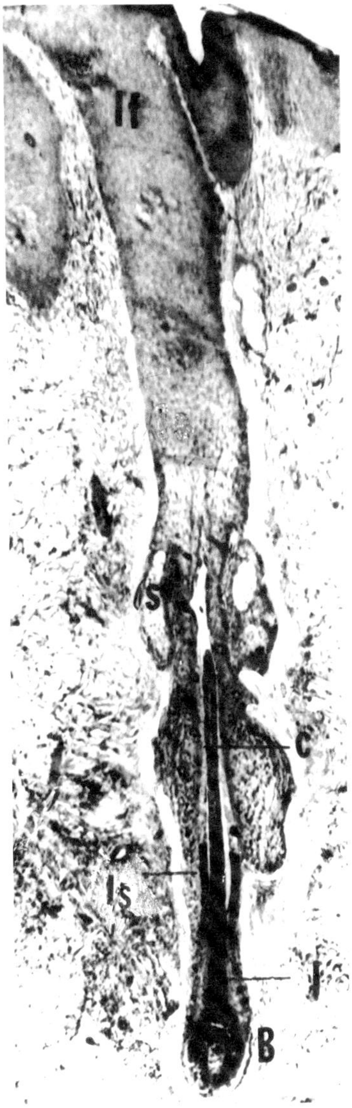

A
X55

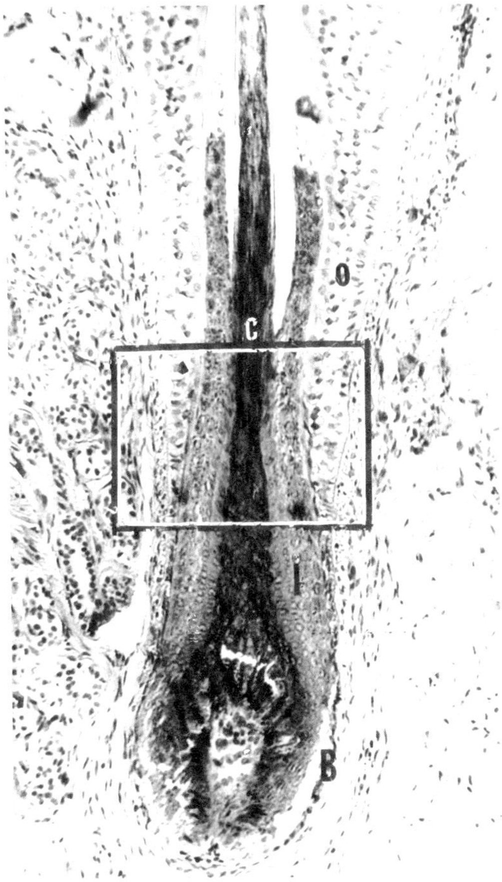

B
X190

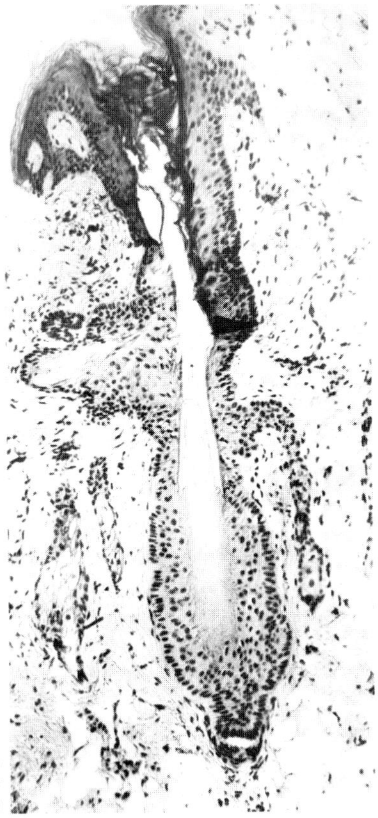

C
X120

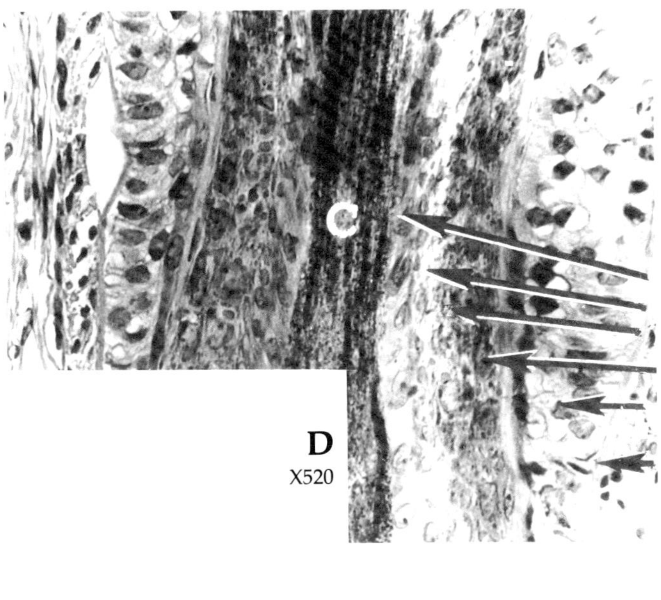

D
X520

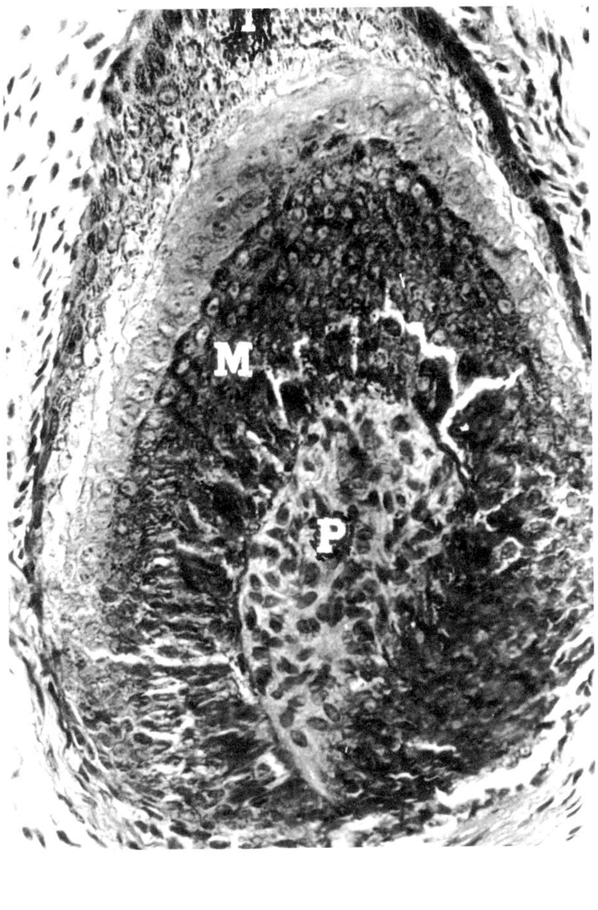

E
X420

HAIR continued ⇨

VELLUS HAIRS

Vellus hairs are small (Fig. A). They extend to the upper dermis. The illustration shows vellus hairs from the ear in cross-section.

SEBACEOUS FOLLICLES

Sebaceous follicles are variants of vellus hairs. At puberty the sebaceous glands emptying into these follicles become large and well-developed (Fig. B). Sebaceous follicles are most numerous on the face. They are the target organs of acne vulgaris.

VELLUS HAIRS

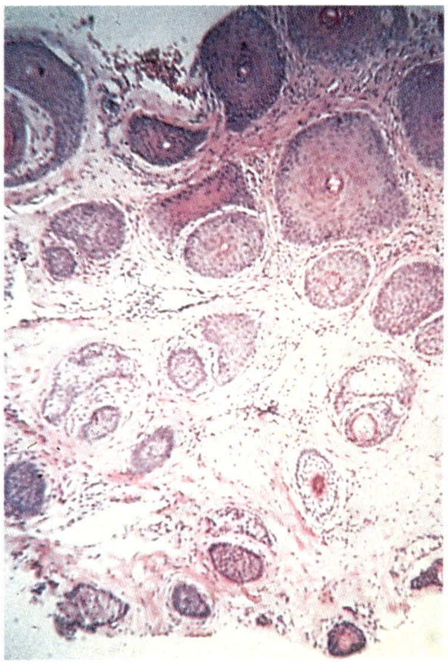

A
X60

SEBACEOUS FOLLICLES

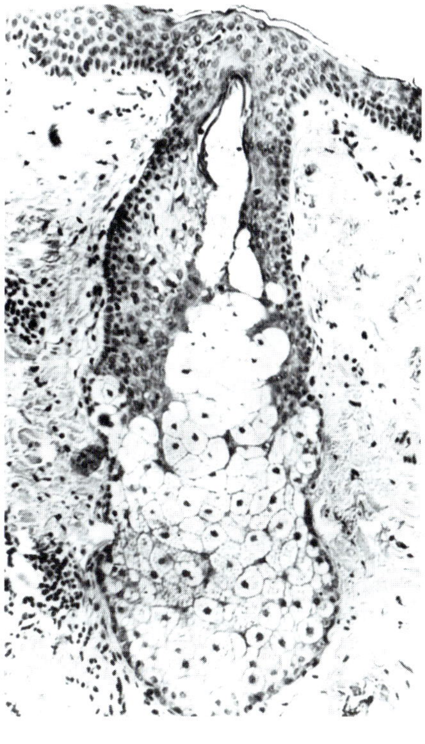

B
X150

Arrectores Pilorum

The smooth muscle fibers have a centrally placed nucleus and no cross striations. Nuclei typically have blunt ends; the cytoplasm is often vacuolated. Arrectores pilorum originate in the upper dermis (Fig. A) and attach to the outer hair sheath at a point below the sebaceous duct (Figs. A,B). The zone between the entrance of the sebaceous duct and the attachment of the arrectores pilorum is called the isthmus of the hair follicle.

ARRECTORES PILORUM

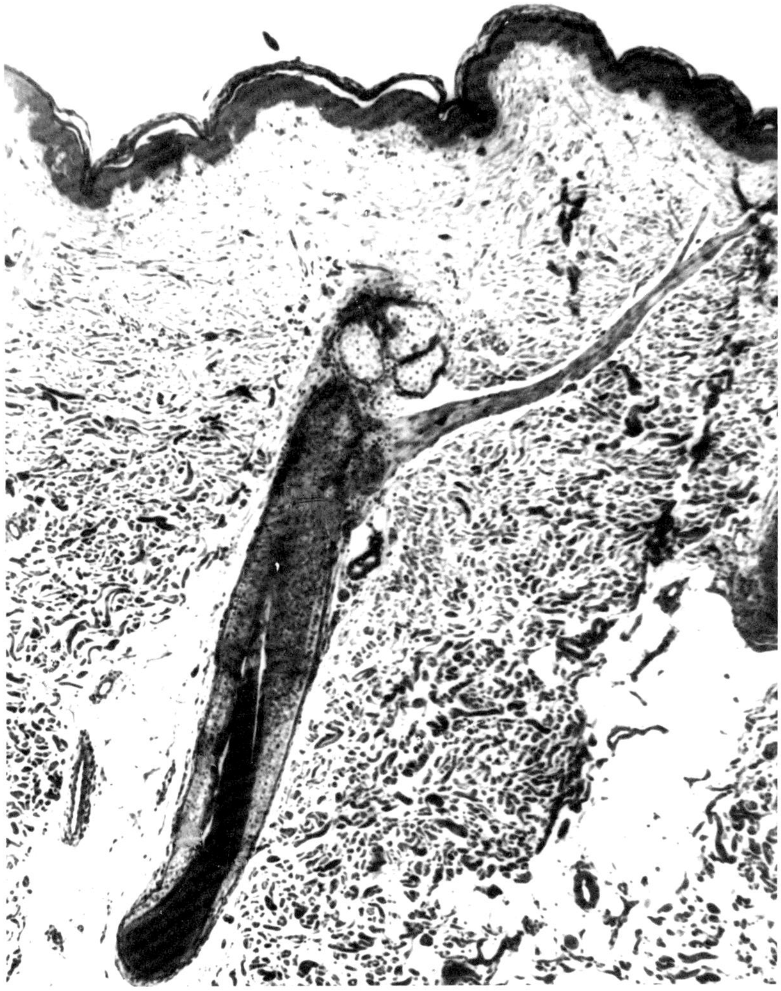

A
X50

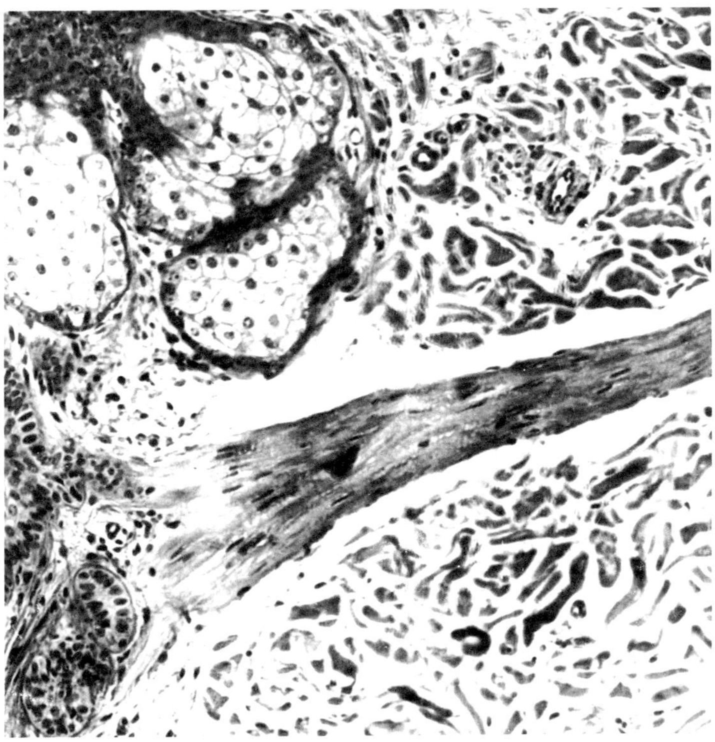

B
X230

Sebaceous Glands

Sebaceous glands are part of the pilary complex. They are holocrine glands in which the secretory product is formed by cellular disintegration.

Before puberty, sebaceous glands are very small. Sebaceous glands are absent on the palms and soles. They are rare on the glans penis. The skin of the central face has the largest sebaceous glands, and in this area hairs may be very small or absent. The meibomian glands of the eyelids are modified sebaceous glands. Ectopic sebaceous glands may occur on the vermilion border of the lips and oral mucosa. (Fordyce condition.)

Sebaceous glands are composed of one or more lobules which empty into a duct lined by stratified squamous epithelium (Fig. A), which in turn, empties into the pilosebaceous follicle (Fig. A).

Lobules are composed of large lipidized cells with a central nucleus and a peripheral layer of flattened, basophilic cells (Figs. A,C). In routine sections, the lipidized cytoplasm has a foamy appearance (Fig. C).

Brownish pigment can be occasionally observed in the cytoplasm and nucleus of lipidized sebaceous cells. This pigment is strongly positive with Perls stain (Fig. B), indicating the possible presence of hemosiderin.

SEBACEOUS GLANDS

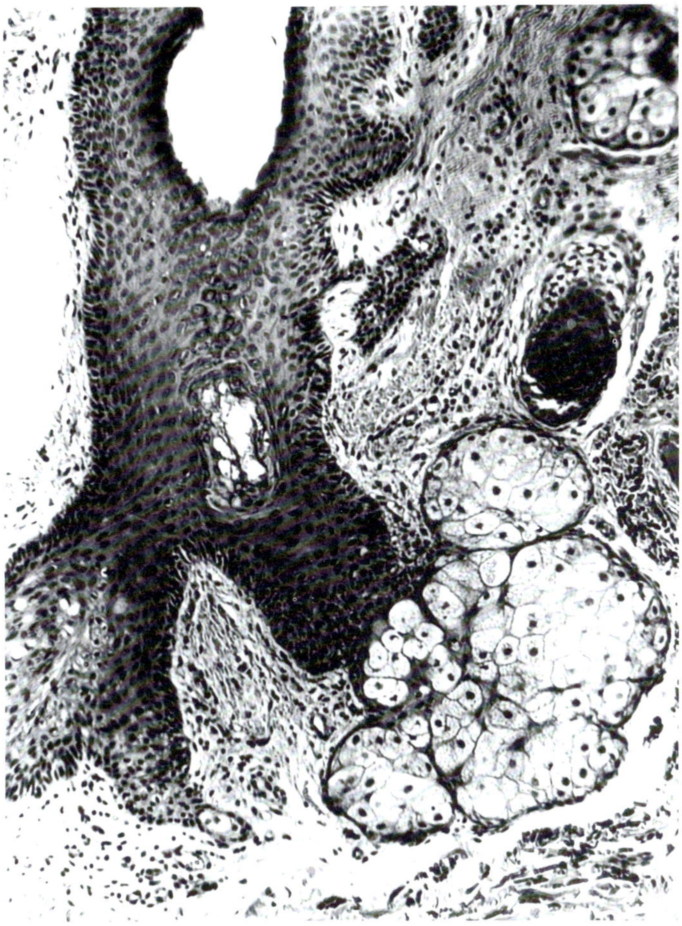

A
X165

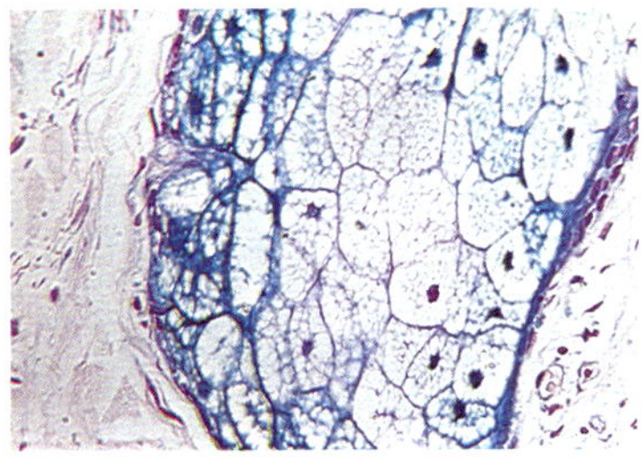

B
X230

PERLS STAIN

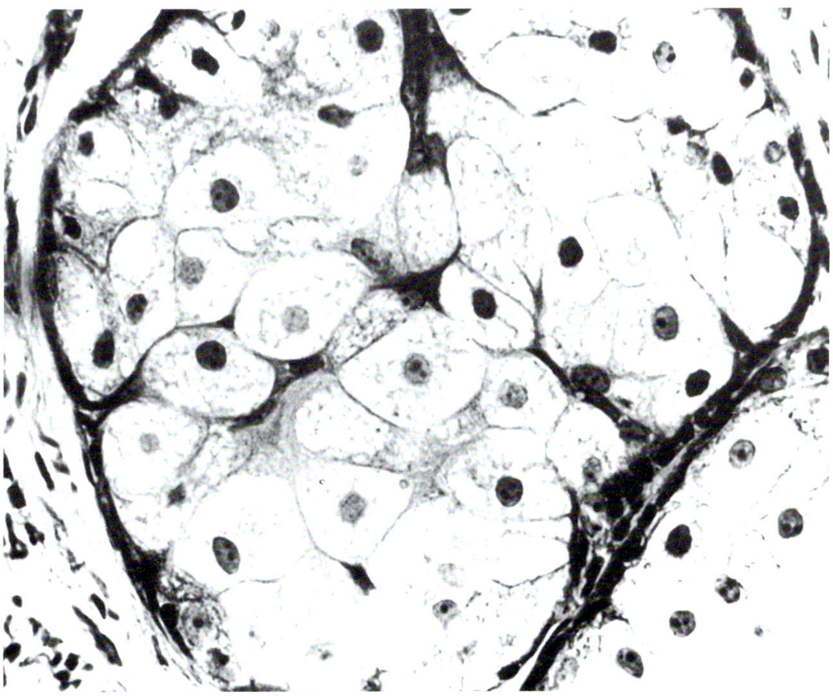

C
X520

Apocrine Glands

Apocrine glands constitute the third component of the pilary complex. The term *apocrine* refers to decapitation secretion—a process in which the apical portions of the secretory cells become detached. Whether this actually occurs or whether this is a morphologic illusion has been controversial. Recent studies have suggested that apocrine, holocrine, and merocrine secretion all take place in apocrine glands. Apocrine glands are believed to represent scent glands.

The ceruminous glands of the external ear canal, Moll's glands of the eyelids, and the mammary glands are modified apocrine glands.

Before puberty, apocrine glands are difficult to find. After puberty, fully developed apocrine glands are most numerous in the axillae, female breasts, and anogenital areas. They are also scattered over other parts of the body and occur in moderate numbers on the face and scalp.

The ducts of the apocrine glands empty into the pilosebaceous follicle at a level above the sebaceous duct. Occasional ducts have independent openings on the cutaneous surface near the pilosebaceous follicles. Apocrine ducts have a structure similar to that of eccrine ducts. The wall is composed of two layers of cuboidal epithelial cells, and there is a periluminal eosinophilic cuticle (Fig. A).

The secretory portion of the apocrine gland is lined by one layer of cells (Figs. A,B) whose height varies with the stage of secretion. Actively secreting cells are high columnar cells with apical projections (Fig. B). Secretory cells contain PAS-positive, diastase-resistant granules and often also contain granules which stain positively for iron.

A layer of flattened, elongated myoepithelial cells (Fig. B [arrow]) is present peripheral to the secretory cells, and peripheral to the myoepithelial cells is a hyaline basement membrane.

APOCRINE GLANDS

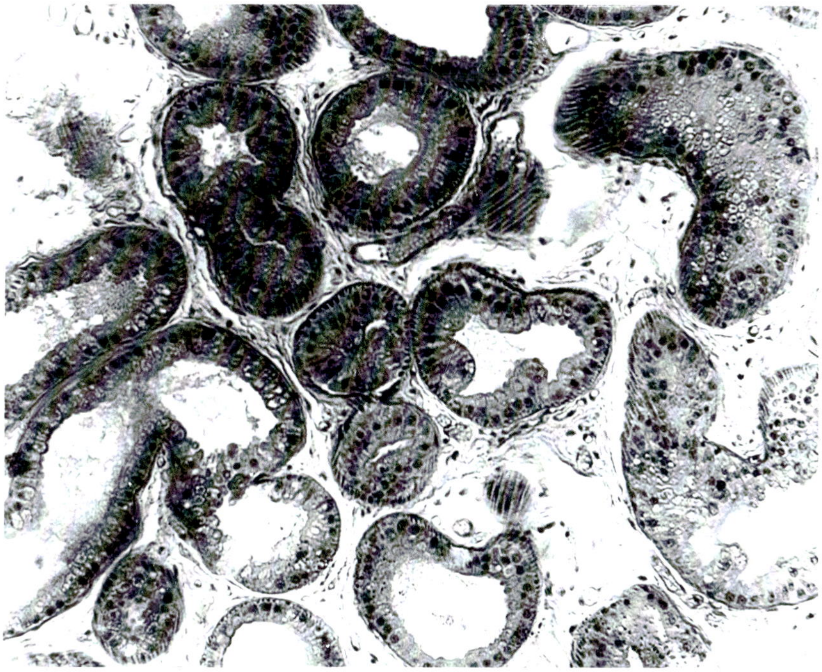

A
X150

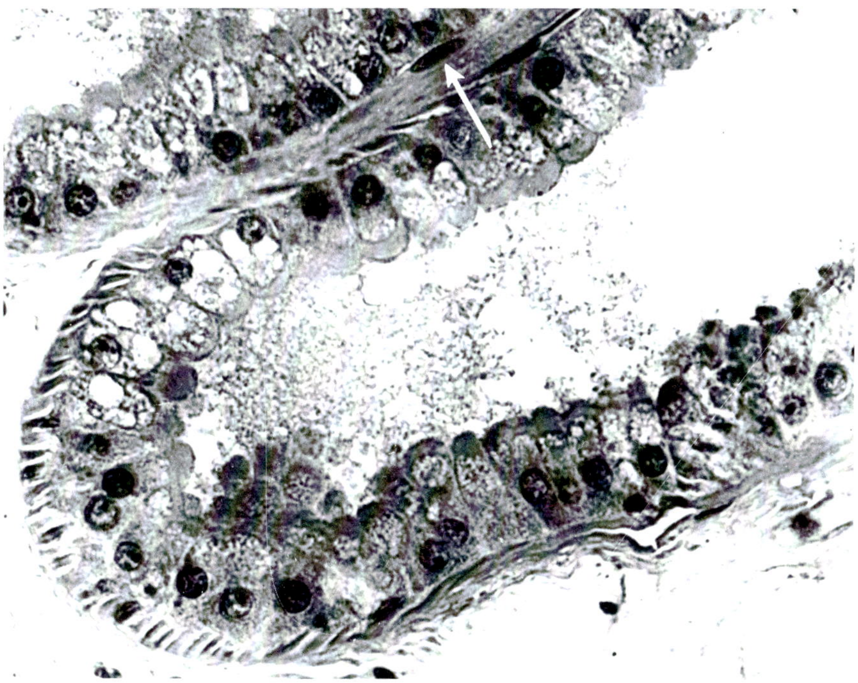

B
X520

Eccrine Glands (Sweat Glands)

Eccrine glands are characterized by merocrine secretion, which leaves the secretory cell intact. Secretion is not visible with H&E stain. Eccrine glands are widely distributed and are most numerous on the palms and soles and in the axillae. They are not present on the vermilion border of the lips, the external ear canal, the glans penis, the inner surface of the prepuce, the labia minora, and the nail bed.

Eccrine glands are composed of two principal parts: a duct and a secretory portion. The duct opens directly onto the skin surface, and the lowermost part of the secretory portion is located either at the border of the dermis and subcutaneous fat or in the lower dermis.

Temperature regulation is the principal function of eccrine glands.

Intraepidermal Part of the Duct (Acrosyringium)

The epidermal portion of the duct maintains a spiral configuration (Figs. A,B) throughout all levels, including the stratum corneum (Fig. A). From inside out it is lined by (1) an eosinophilic cuticle, (2) an inner layer of squamous epithelial cells, and (3) several outer layers of squamous epithelial cells (Figs. B,C). The cuticle is PAS-positive and diastase-resistant. The lining cells keratinize with the production of keratohyaline granules (Fig. C). Melanin is usually not present in these cells.

INTRAEPIDERMAL PORTION OF ECCRINE DUCT

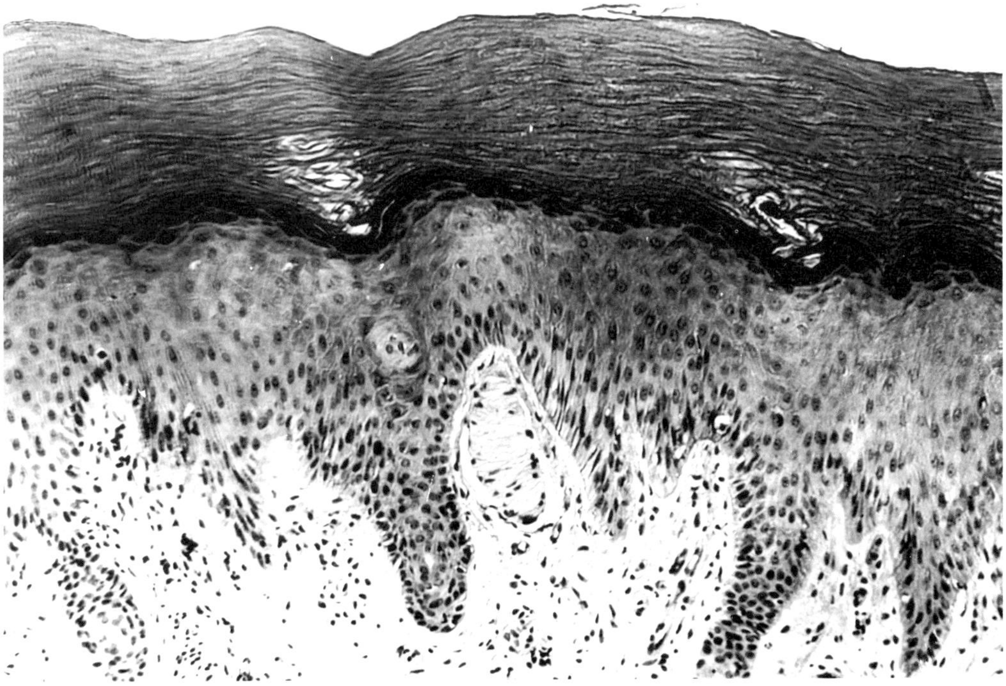

A
X190

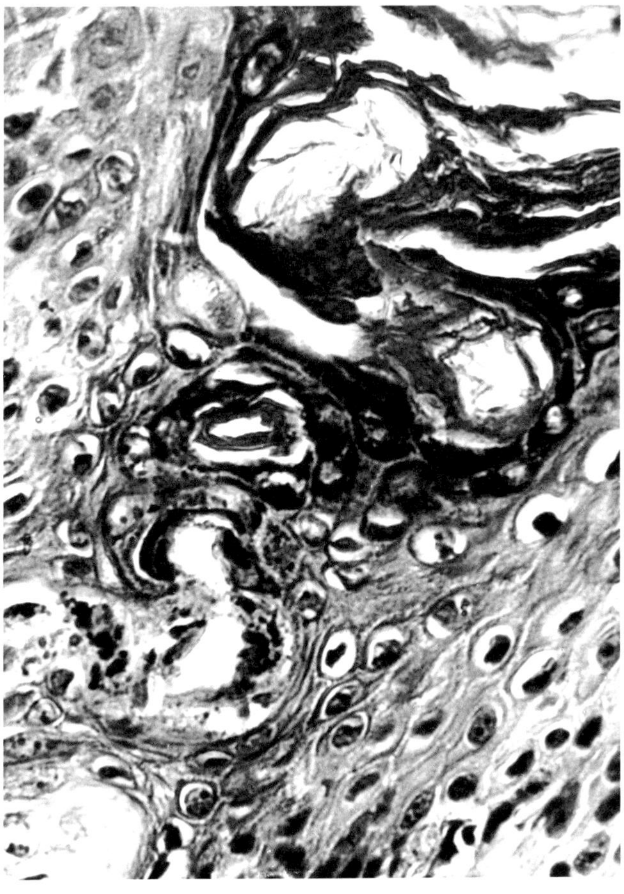

B
X900

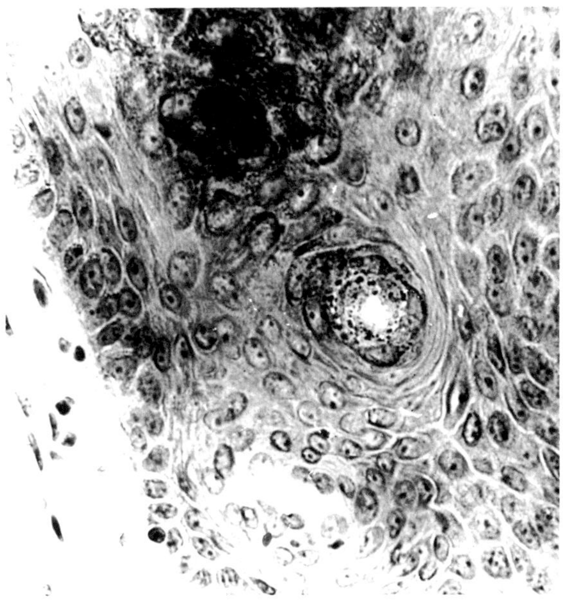

C
X520

ECCRINE GLANDS continued ⇨

Eccrine Glands

Intradermal Part of the Duct

The upper portion of the intradermal part of the eccrine duct is rather straight (Figs. A,B), but its terminal lower portion forms about one half of the terminal coil of the eccrine gland. A dilated ampulla is present at its distal end.

The intradermal part of the eccrine duct has a periluminal cuticle similar to that observed in the intraepidermal part and is lined by two rows of cuboidal epithelial cells (Figs. A,B).

INTRADERMAL PORTION OF ECCRINE DUCT

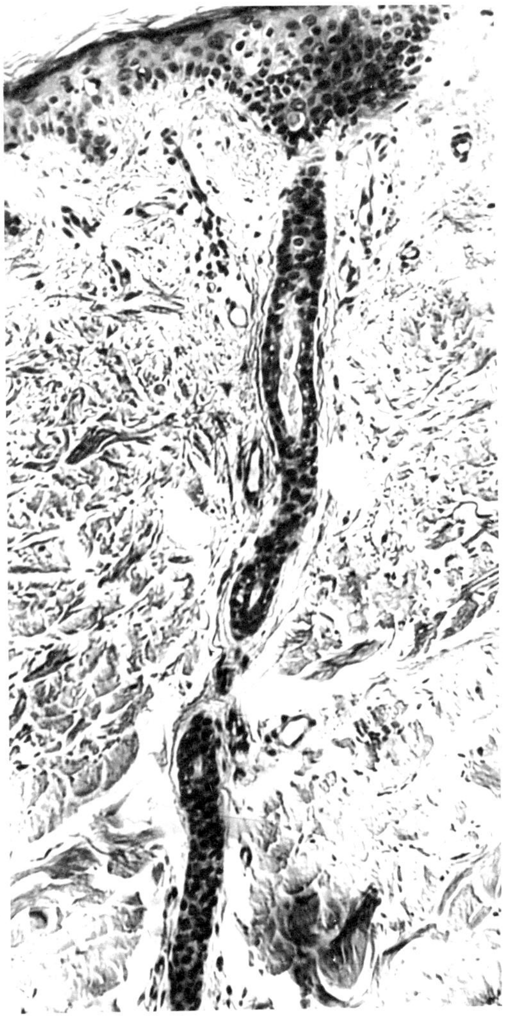

A
X190

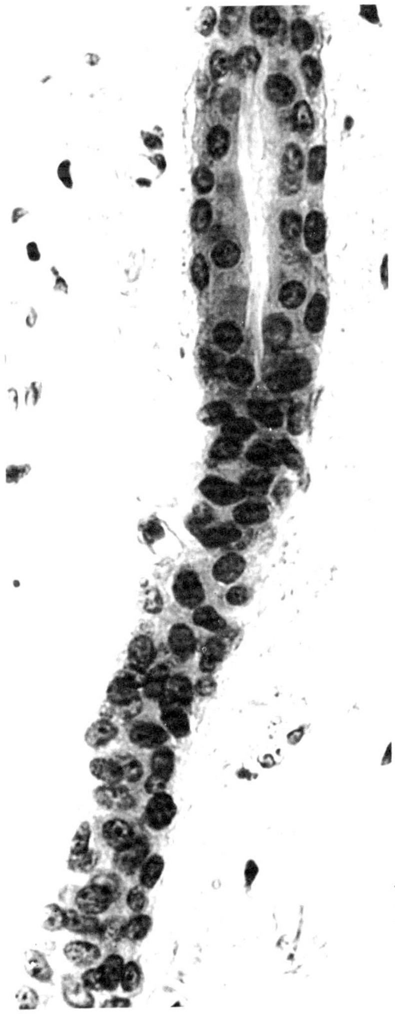

B
X670

ECCRINE GLANDS continued

Eccrine Glands

Terminal coil

The terminal coil is located at the junction of the dermis and subcutaneous fat (Figs. A,B) or in the lower dermis. The proximal half of the coil is formed by the duct and the distal half by the secretory portion. Therefore, in cross section, ducts (D–Fig. C) and secretory coils (S–Fig. C) can be seen.

Secretory coils (S–Fig. C) have no inner cuticle and are lined by a single layer of columnar epithelial cells. These are of two types: (1) clear cells with their apices at the lumen and (2) dark cells with their bases at the lumen. The clear cells are larger than the dark cells and contain eosinophilic granules. They show a diastase-labile PAS reaction, indicating the presence of glycogen. The dark cells contain basophilic granules and PAS-positive, diastase-resistant neutral mucopolysaccharides.

A layer of myoepithelial cells (arrow–Fig. C) is peripheral to the secretory cells and a PAS-positive, diastase-resistant basement zone containing fibroblasts is peripheral to the myoepithelial cells.

TERMINAL COIL OF ECCRINE GLAND

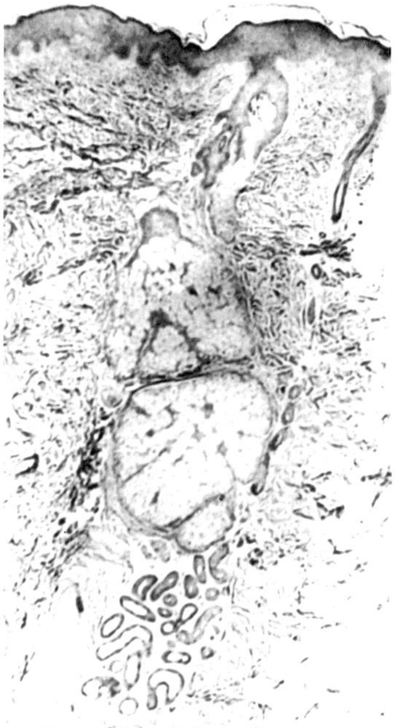

A
X30

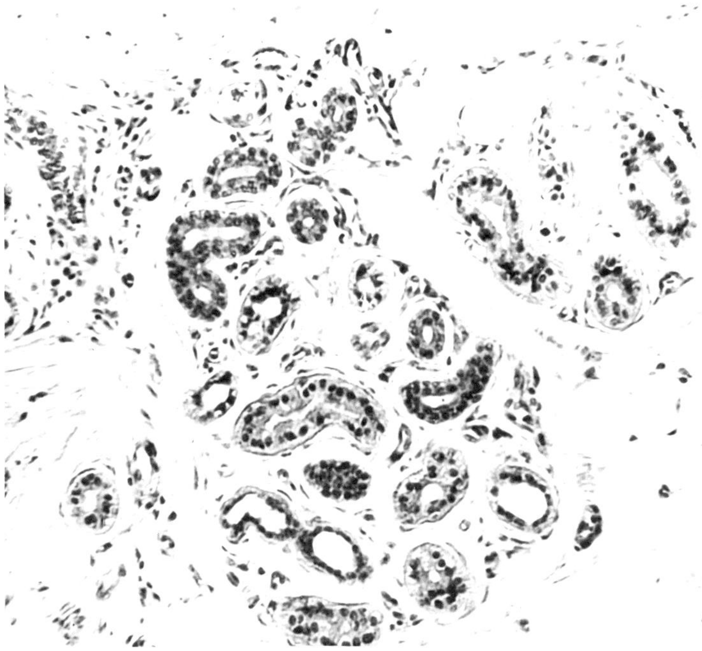

B
X190

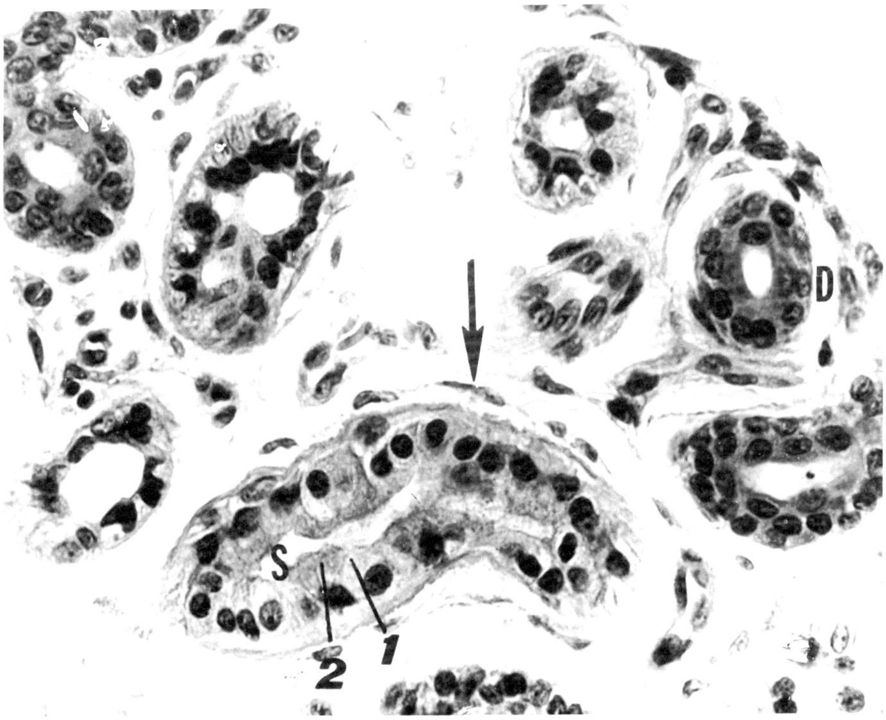

C
X670

Nails

The structure of the nail is illustrated by this schematic sagittal section (Fig. A). The nail plate (NP) is a fully cornified structure produced by cells of the nail matrix (M) via orthokeratosis, without a transitional granular zone. It is inserted into the lateral (la) and posterior (p) nail folds, and its free edge is adjacent to the hyponychium (h). The hyponychium is a narrow zone of skin, structurally similar to the adjacent volar skin (from which it is separated by a groove).

The nail plate lies on the nail bed (dotted line just below NP), extending from the nail matrix to the hyponychium. The epidermis of the nail bed keratinizes via parakeratosis.

The ventral surface of the proximal nail fold produces the nail cuticle via orthokeratosis (with the presence of an intermediate granular layer). The anterior end of the posterior nail fold is called the eponychium.

The lunula (L), a whitish zone which represents the distal portion of the nail matrix, is normally present in the thumbnail, absent in the fifth fingernail, and variably present in the other fingernails.

This sagittal section (Fig. B) of the nail shows the posterior nail fold, nail matrix, nail plate, and nail bed. The dermis of the nail bed is very vascular and contains glomus formations.

NAILS

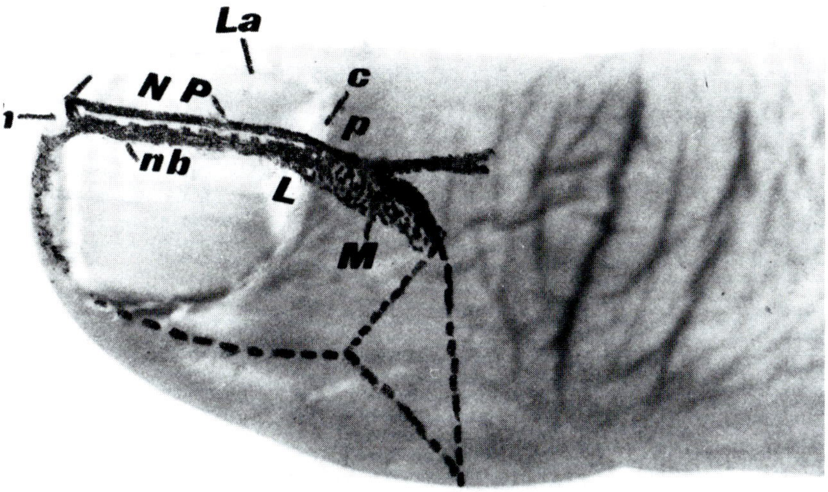

A

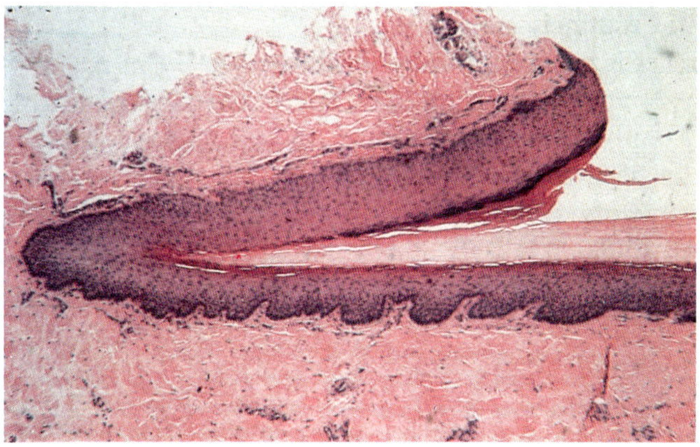

B
X120

Nerves

The dermis contains both sensory and autonomic nerves. Autonomic nerves are principally sympathetic and innervate blood vessels, smooth muscle, apocrine glands, and eccrine glands.

With H&E stain only the Schwann cells, perineurium, and endoneurium of the nerve bundles can be seen. Axons require special staining techniques, such as impregnation with silver salts or vital staining with methylene blue.

With H&E stain, nerves resemble smooth muscle-bundles in longitudinal (Fig. A) and cross section (Fig. B).

Nerve End-Organs

Meissner corpuscles are specialized end-organs that mediate the sense of touch. They are located in the dermal papillae (Fig. C) on the volar surfaces of the hands and feet and are most numerous in the fingertips. Meissner corpuscles are encapsulated and contain Schwann cells arranged parallel to the short axis (Fig. C).

Vater-Pacini corpuscles are specialized end-organs that mediate the sense of pressure. They are very large structures up to 900 microns in diameter (Fig. D) located in the subcutaneous tissue, most commonly the subcutaneous tissue of the palms and soles. The central bulb is surrounded by up to 50 concentric lamellae (Fig. D). Adjacent to the body proper of the Vater-Pacini corpuscle is the nerve stalk (arrow – Fig. D).

Mucocutaneous end-organs are present in the subpapillary dermis at mucocutaneous junctions; they are composed of irregular coils of nerve fibers. They cannot be seen in routinely stained sections.

Merkel cells are present above the basement membrane in the epidermis and oral mucosa. A meniscoid neural terminal that covers the basal portion is demonstrable in silver-impregnated sections as the Merkel disc. A sensory nerve terminates at the disc. It is believed that the Merkel cell is a touch receptor. Merkel cells contain cytoplasmic organelles identical to the norepinephrin-containing granules of the adrenal medulla. It is likely that the Merkel cells belong to the APUD system (APUD = amino precursor uptake and decarboxylation).

NERVES AND NERVE END-ORGANS

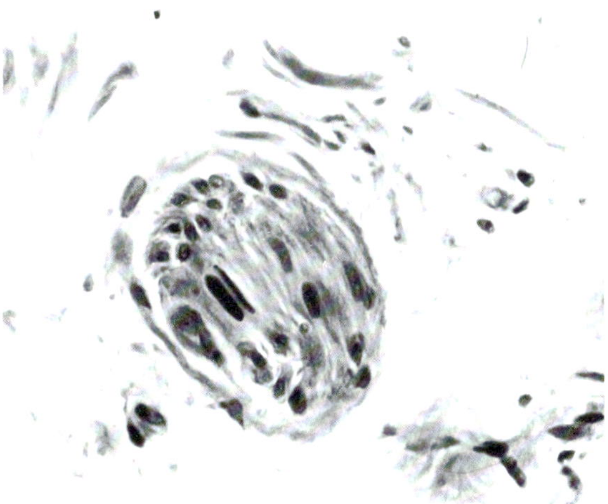

A
X680

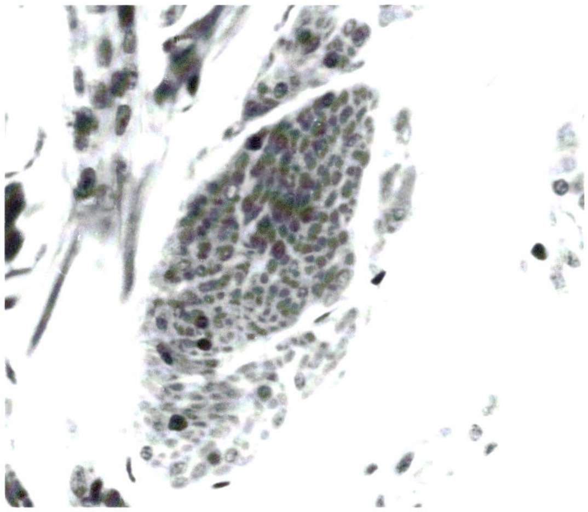

B
X680

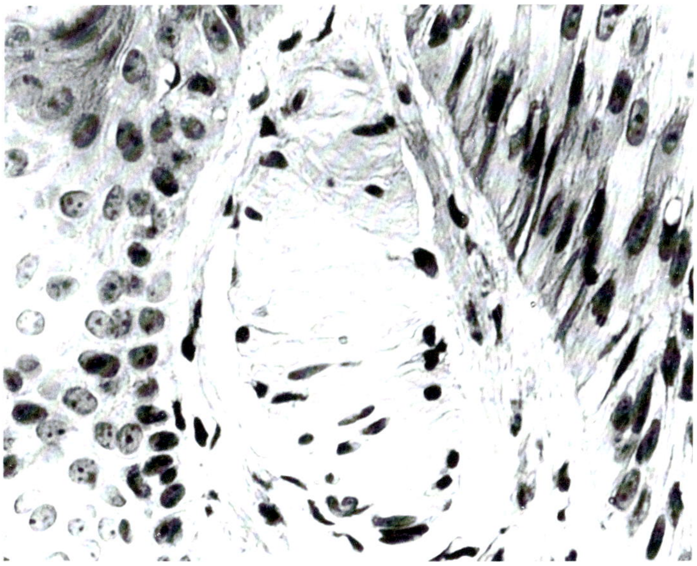

C
X700

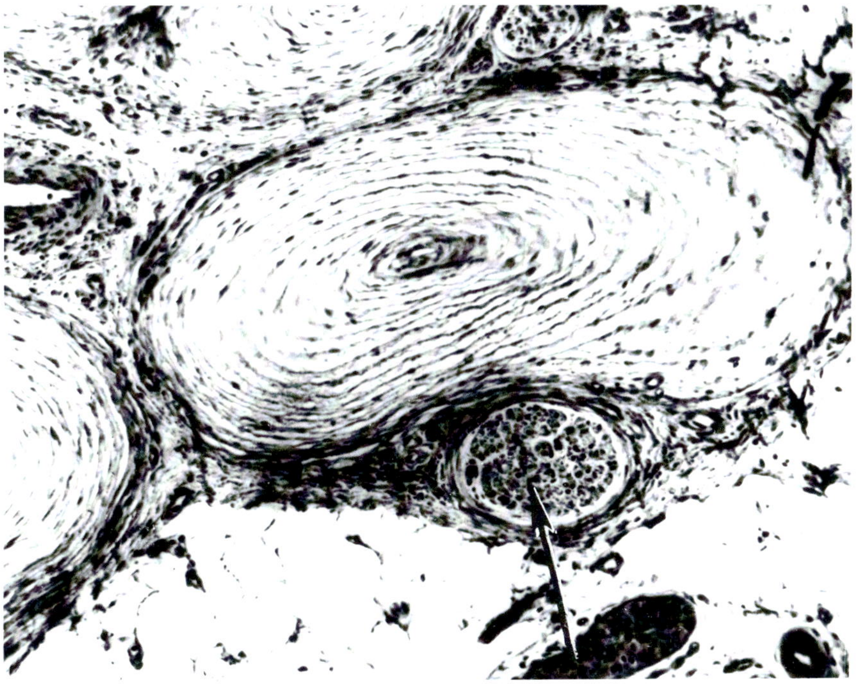

D
X150

Some Common Artifacts

Freeze-Thaw Damage

Specimens exposed to very low temperatures in mail transit may freeze, with resultant vacuolization due to ice crystal formation (Figs. A,B). Fixation before exposure to freezing temperatures will not prevent this type of artifact unless it is prolonged. We have found that addition of 50% alcohol (10% by volume) to the formalin has satisfactory antifreeze properties and preserves morphology well.

Compression

Compression due to forceps (Fig. C) is commonly observed, with the most pronounced effects on tissue components close to the surface.

COMMON ARTIFACTS

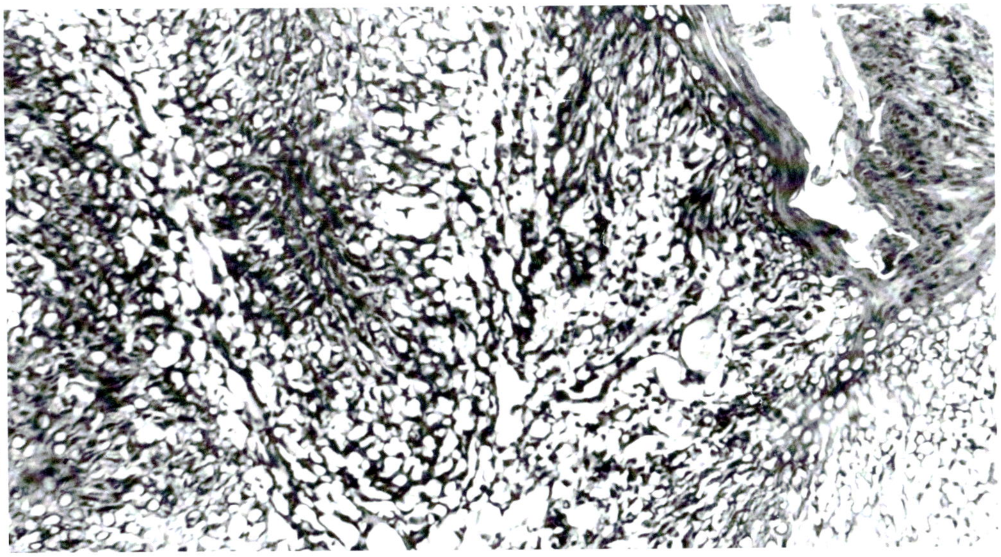

A
X160

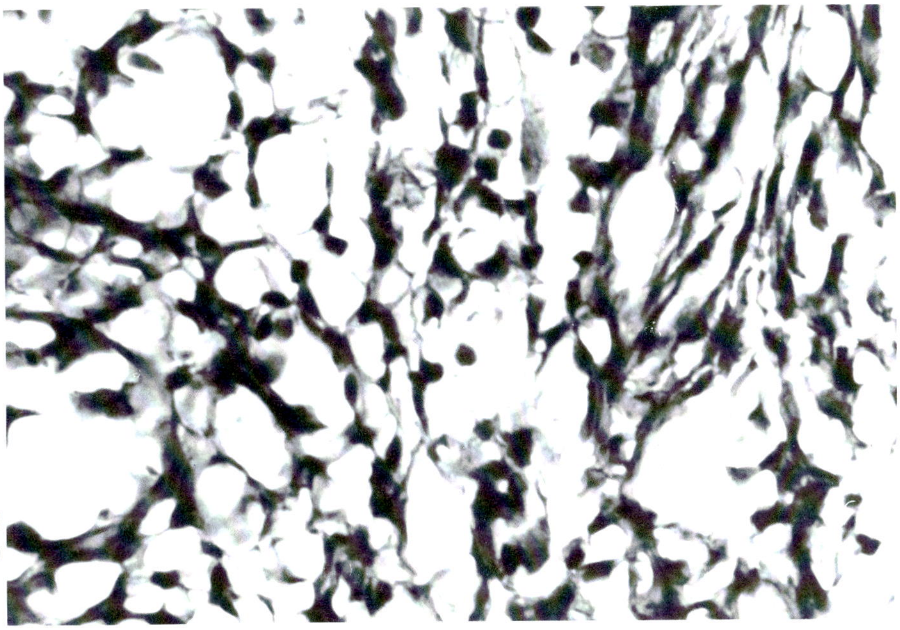

B
X620

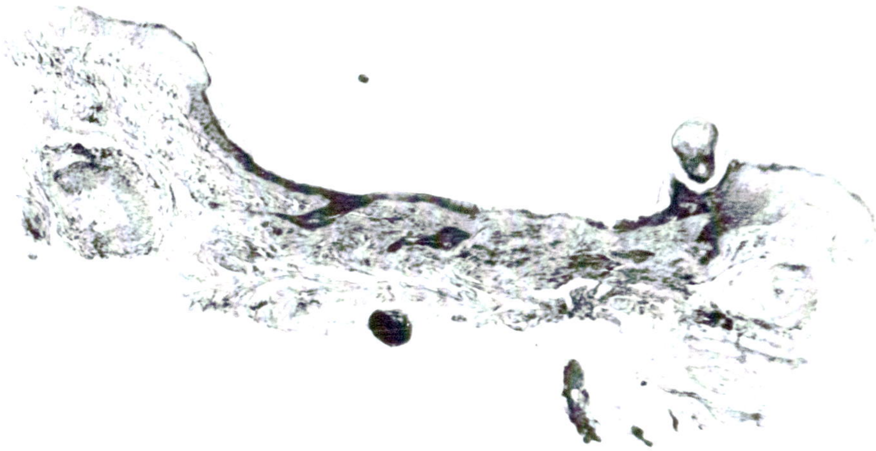

C
X45

COMMON ARTIFACTS continued ⇨

Some Common Artifacts

Inadequate Dehydration

Inadequate exposure to dehydrating agents (e.g., alcohol) in processing, results in difficulty in sectioning. Sections are thick and fragmented (Figs. A,B).

Tangential Cut

When blocks of skin are cut tangentially (Fig. C) an illusory acanthosis is the result. However, the artifact can usually be recognized, since the "acanthotic" epidermis contains many completely enclosed dermal papillae.

Burn Artifact

Contact with the electrosurgical needle produces an electrothermal burn with coagulation necrosis and elongation of epidermal cells (Fig. D).

Water Droplets in Mounting Medium

When there is high humidity, water droplets may be present in the mounting medium of paraffin sections (Fig. E).

Chatter

A dull microtome knife can produce multiple parallel fissures in sections. This phenomenon is called *chatter*.

COMMON ARTIFACTS

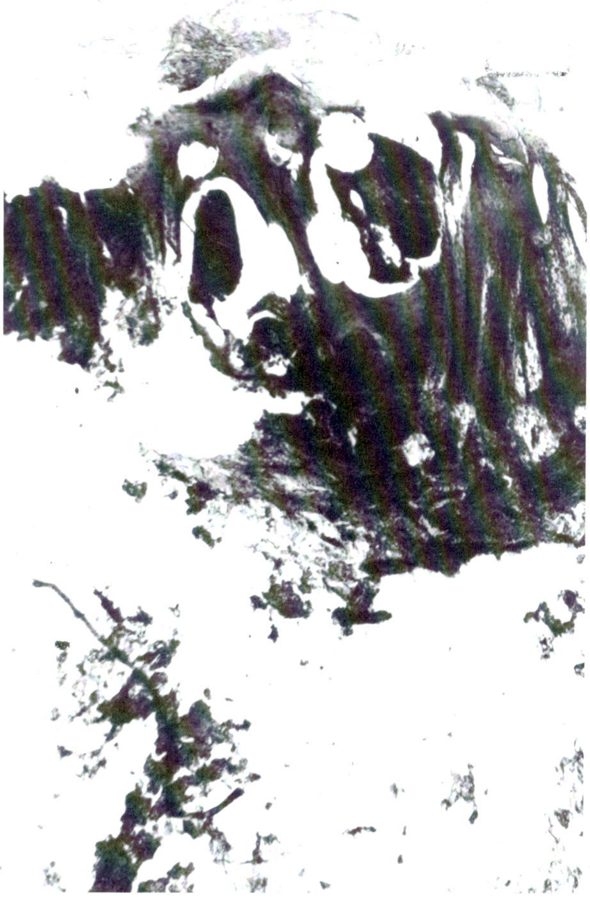

A
X50

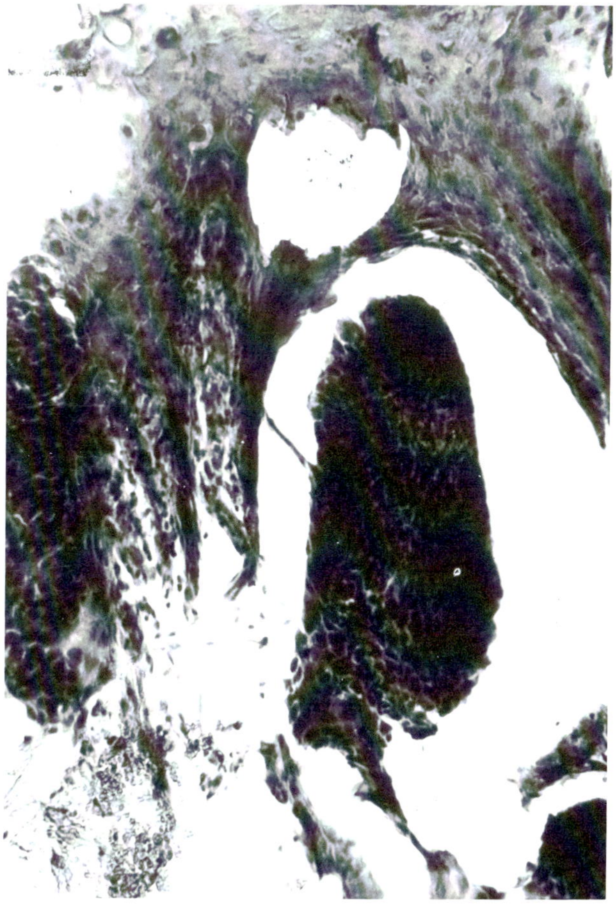

B
X180

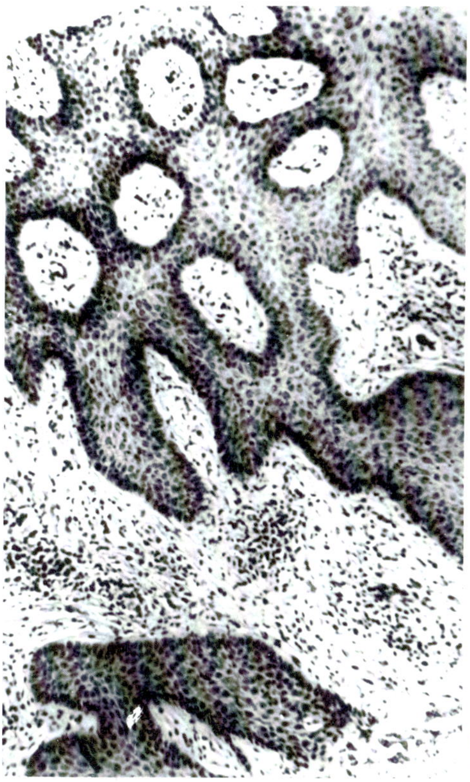

C
X100

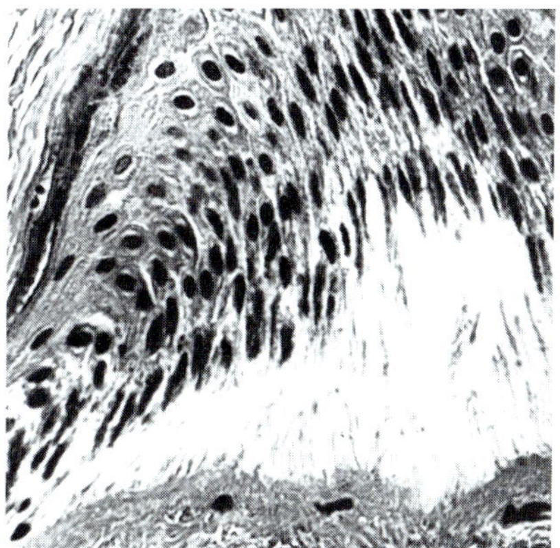

D
X350

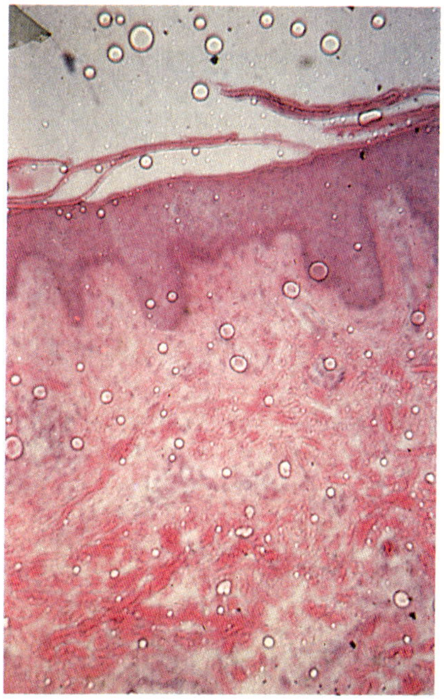

E
X130

Suggested Reading

Normal Histology of the Skin

General References

Bloom, W. and Fawcett, D. *A Textbook of Histology.* 11th Ed., Philadelphia, W. B. Saunders Co., 1986.
Breathnach, A. *An Atlas of the Ultrastructure of Human Skin.* London, Churchill, 1971.
Copenhaver, W., Bunge, R. and Bunge, M. *Bailey's Textbook of Histology.* 17th Ed., Baltimore, Williams and Wilkins, 1978.
Fenske, N. and Lober, C. Structural and functional changes of normal aging skin. *J. Am. Acad. Dermatol.*, 15:571, 1986.
Lyne, A. and Short, B. *Biology of the Skin and Hair Growth.* Sydney, Australia, Angus and Robertson, (Publishers), 1965.
Mishima, Y., Van Scott, E. and Tanioku, K. Pathobiology of the skin. *Acta Derm. Venereol.*, 53 (73, suppl.), 1973.
Montagna, W. and Parakkal, P. *Structure and Function of the Skin.* 3rd Ed., New York, Academic Press, 1974.
Rothman, S. *Physiology and Biochemistry of the Skin.* Chicago, Univ. of Chicago Press, 1954.
Rushmer, R. et al. The skin. *Science,* 154:343, 1966.
Zelickson, A. *Ultrastructure of Normal and Abnormal Skin.* Philadelphia, Lea and Febiger, 1967.

Epidermis

Bell, R. and Kellum, R. Early formation of keratohyalin granules in rat epidermis. *Acta Derm. Venereol.*, 47:350, 1967.
Billingham, R. and Silvers, W. Studies on the conservation of epidermal specificities of skin and certain mucosas in adult mammals. *J. Exp. Med.*, 125:429, 1967.
Briggaman, R., Biochemical composition of the epidermal-dermal junction and other basement membranes. *J. Invest. Dermatol.*, 78:1, 1982.
Briggaman, R., Dalldorf, F. and Wheeler, C. Formation and origin of basal lamina and anchoring fibrils in adult human skin. *J. Cell Biol.*, 51:384, 1971.
Briggaman, R. and Kelly, T. Continuous thymidine labeling studies of normal human skin growth on nude mice: Measurement of cycling basal cells (abstr.). *J. Invest. Dermatol.*, 78:359, 1982.
Briggaman, R. and Wheeler, C., Jr. The epidermal–dermal junction. *J. Invest. Dermatol.*, 65:71, 1975.
——. The epidermal-dermal junction. *J. Invest. Dermatol*, 65:71, 1975.
Brody, I. The modified plasma membranes of the transition and horny cells in normal human epidermis as revealed by electron microscopy. *Acta Derm. Venereol.*, 49:128, 1969.
Caputo, R. and Perluchetti, D. The junctions of normal human epidermis: A freeze-fracture study. *J. Ultrastruct. Res.*, 61:44, 1977.
Cerimele, E., Del Forno, C. and Serri, F. Histochemistry of the intercellular substance of the normal and psoriatic human epidermis. *Arch. Dermatol. Res.*, 262:27, 1978.
Clark, W., Jr., Watson, M. and Watson, B. Two kinds of "clear" cells in the human epidermis. *Am. J. Pathol.*, 39:333, 1961.
Cochran, A. The incidence of melanocytes in normal skin. *J. Invest. Dermatol.*, 55:65, 1970.
Dale, B. et al. Assembly of stratum corneum basic protein and keratin filaments in macrofibrils. *Nature,* 276:729, 1978.
Elias, P. Epidermal lipids, barrier function, and desquamation. *J. Invest. Dermatol.*, 80 (suppl.):44s, 1983.
Elias, P., Goerke, J. and Friend, D. Mammalian epidermal barrier layer lipids: Composition and influence on structure. *J. Invest. Dermatol.*, 69:535, 1977.
Freinkel, R. and Traczyk, T. Acid hydrolases of the epidermis: Subcellular localization and relationship to cornification. *J. Invest. Dermatol.*, 80:441, 1983.
Gelfant, S. Psoriasis versus cancer: Adaptive versus iatrogenic human cell proliferative diseases. *Internat. Rev. Cytol.*, 81:145, 1983.

Green, H. The keratinocyte as a differentiated cell type. *Harvey Lect.*, 74:101, 1979.

Grove, G. Epidermal cell kinetics in psoriasis. *Internat. J. Dermatol.*, 18:111, 1979.

Hartschuh, W. and Weihe, E. Fine structural analysis of the synaptic junction of Merkel cell-axon-complexes. *J. Invest. Dermatol.*, 75:159, 1980.

Hashimoto, K. Fine structure of the Merkel cell in human oral mucosa. *J. Invest. Dermatol.*, 58:381, 1972.

——. Langerhan's cell granule: An endocytic organelle. *Arch. Dermatol.*, 104:148, 1971.

Hashimoto, K. and Tarnowski, W. Some new aspects of the Langerhans cells. *Arch. Dermatol.*, 97:450, 1968.

Hodge, S. and Freeman, R. The basal lamina in skin disease. *Internat. J. Dermatol.*, 17:261, 1978.

Jimbow, K., Chiba, M. and Horikoshi, T. Electron microscopic identification of Langerhans cells in the dermal infiltrates of mycosis fungoides. *J. Invest. Dermatol.*, 78:102, 1982.

Juhlin, L., ed. The Langerhans cell and contact dermatitis. *Acta Derm. Venereol.* (Stockh.), (79, suppl.):1, 1978.

Juhlin, L. and Shelley, W. New staining techniques for the Langerhans cell. *Acta Derm. Venereol.*, 57:289, 1977.

Katz, S. The role of Langerhans cells in immunity. *Arch. Dermatol.*, 116:1361, 1980.

Katz, S. et al. Epidermal Langerhans cells are derived from cells orginating in the bone marrow. *Nature*, 282:324, 1979.

Kefalides, N. Basement membranes: Structural and biosynthetic considerations. *J. Invest. Dermatol.*, 65:85, 1975.

Kidd, R., Krawczyk, W. and Wilgram, G. The Merkel cell in human epidermis: Its differentiation from other dendritic cells. *Arch. Derm. Forsch.*, 241:374, 1971.

Kiistala, U. and Mustakallio, K. The presence of Langerhans cells in human dermis with special reference to their potential mesenchymal origin. *Acta Derm. Venereol.* (Stockh.), 48:115, 1968.

Klein-Szanto, A. Clear and dark basal keratinocytes in human epidermis. *J. Cutan. Pathol.*, 4:275, 1977.

Kobayasi, T. Anchoring of basal lamina to elastic fibers by elastic fibrils. *J. Invest. Dermatol.*, 68:389, 1977.

——. Dermoepidermal junction of normal skin. *J. Dermatol.* (Tokyo), 5:157, 1978.

Lavker, R. and Sun, T. Epidermal stem cells. *J. Invest. Dermatol.*, 81:121, 1983.

——. Heterogeneity in basal keratinocytes: Morphological and functional correlations. *Science*, 15:1239, 1982.

Lonsdale-Eccles, J. et al. A phosphorylated keratohyalin-derived precursor of epidermal stratum corneum basic protein. *J. Biol. Chem.*, 255:2235, 1980.

Mackie, R. and Turbitt, M. The use of a double-label immunoperoxidase monoclonal antibody technique in the investigation of patients with mycosis fungoides. *Br. J. Dermatol.*, 106:379, 1982.

Matoltsy, A. Desmosomes, filaments, and keratohyaline granules: Their role in stabilization and keratinization of the epidermis. *J. Invest. Dermatol.*, 65:127, 1975.

Montagna, W. Histology and cytochemistry of human skin. XXXIV. The eyebrows. *Arch. Dermatol.*, 101:257, 1970.

Montagna, W. and Lobitz, W. *The Epidermis.* New York, Academic Press, 1964.

Penneys, N. et al. Location of proliferating cells in human epidermis. *Arch. Dermatol.*, 101:323, 1970.

Sauder, D. et al. Langerhans cell production of interleukin-1. *Clin. Res.*, 32:258A, 1984.

Saurat, J. et al. A human monoclonal antibody reacting with Merkel cells: Immunofluorescence, immunoperoxidase, and immunoelectron microscopy. *J. Invest. Dermatol.*, 81:249, 1983.

Serri, F. and Montagna, W. The structure and function of the epidermis. *Pediatr. Clin. N. Am.*, 8:917, 1961.

Silberberg, I., Baer, R. and Rosenthal, S. The role of Langerhans cells in allergic contact hypersensitivity: A review of findings in man and guinea pig. *J. Invest. Dermatol.*, 66:210, 1976.

Silberberg-Sinakin, I., Baer, R. and Thorbekke, G. Langerhans cells. A review of their nature with emphasis on their immunologic functions. *Prog. Allergy*, 24:268, 1978.

Sjöberg, S. et al. A new method for the visualization of the epidermal Langerhans cell and its application on normal and allergic skin. *Acta Derm. Venereol.* (Stockh.), (79, suppl.):23, 1978.

Squier, C. and Hopps, R. A study of the permeability barrier in epidermis and oral epithelium using horseradish peroxidase as a tracer *in vitro*. *Br. J. Dermatol.*, 95:123, 1976.

Tamaki, K., Stingi, G. and Katz, S. The origin of Langerhans cells. *J. Invest. Dermatol.*, 74:309, 1980.
Toker, C. Trabecular carcinoma of the skin. *Arch. Dermatol.*, 105:107, 1972.
Ugel, A. Bovine keratohyalin: Anatomical, histochemical, ultrastructural, immunologic and biochemical studies. *J. Invest. Dermatol.*, 65:118, 1975.
Wessells, N. Differentiation of epidermis and epidermal derivatives. *New Eng. J. Med.*, 277:21, 1967.
Winkelmann, R. The Merkel cell system and a comparison between it and the neurosecretory or APUD cell system. *J. Invest. Dermatol.*, 69:41, 1977.
Winkelmann, R. and Breathnach, A. The Merkel cell. *J. Invest. Dermatol.*, 60:2, 1973.
Wolff, K. Epidermal lysosomes. Electron microscopic cytochemical studies. *Arch. Dermatol.*, 101:276, 1970.
Wolff, K. and Wolff-Schreiner, E. Trends in electron microscopy of skin. *J. Invest. Dermatol.*, 67:39, 1976.
Wolff-Schreiner, E. Ultrastructual cytochemistry of the epidermis. *Internat. J. Dermatol.*, 16:77, 1977.
Yaoita, H., Foidart, J. and Katz, S. Localization of the collagenous component in the skin basement membrane. *J. Invest. Dermatol.*, 70:191, 1978.
Zelickson, A. and Mottaz, J. Epidermal dendritic cells. *Arch. Dermatol.*, 98:652, 1968.

Epidermis

MELANOCYTES

Duchon, J., Fitzpatrick, T. and Seiji, M. Melanin 1968: Some definitions and problems. In: *1967–1968 Year Book of Dermatology.* Chicago, Year Book Medical Publishers, 1968.
Edelstein, L. et al. Inability of murine melanosomal "tyrosinase" (L-dopa oxidase) to oxidize tyrosine to melanin in polyacrylamide gel systems. *J. Invest. Dermatol.*, 64:364, 1975.
Fitzpatrick, T. and Szabó, G. The melanocyte: Cytology and cytochemistry. *J. Invest. Dermatol.*, 32:197, 1959.
Montagna, W. and Hu, F. *Advances in Biology of the Skin,* Vol. 8: *The Pigmentary System,* Oxford, Pergamon Press, 1967.
Mottaz, J. and Zelickson, A. Melanin transfer: A possible phagocytic process. *J. Invest. Dermatol.*, 49:605, 1967.
Okun, M. Dermal dopa-positive cells in lichen planus. *Arch. Dermatol.*, 106:422, 1972.
——. Histogenesis of melanocytes. *J. Invest. Dermatol.*, 44:285, 1965.
Okun, M. and Zook, B. Histologic parallels between mastocytoma and melanoma. *Arch. Dermatol.*, 95:275, 1967.
Okun, M. et al. Dopa compared with dihydroxyfumarate as co-factor in peroxidase-mediated oxidation of tyrosine to melanin: Histochemical studies with neutrophils, eosinophils, mast cells, melanoma cells and neurons. *Histochemie,* 27:331, 1971.
Okun, M. et al. Histochemical differentiation of peroxidase-mediated from tyrosinase-mediated melanin formation in mammalian tissues: The biologic significance of peroxidase-mediated oxidation of tyrosine to melanin. *Histochemie,* 23:295, 1970.
Okun, M. et al. Histochemical studies of conversion of tyrosine and dopa to melanin mediated by mammalian peroxidase. *Life Sci.*, (II) 9:491, 1970.
Okun, M. et al. Oxidation of tyrosine and dopa to melanin by mammalian peroxidase: The possible role of peroxidase in melanin and catecholamine synthesis *in vivo.* In: *Pigmentation: Its Genesis and Biologic Control.* Riley, V., ed., New York, Appleton-Century-Crofts, 1972, p. 571.
Okun, M. et al. A revised concept of mammalian melanogenesis: The possible synergistic functions of aerobic dopa oxidase and peroxidase: A review. *Yale J. Biol. Med.*, 46:535, 1973.
Okun, M. et al. The role of peroxidase vs. the role of tyrosinase in enzymatic conversion of tyrosin to melanin in melanocytes, mast cells and eosinophils: An autoradiographic-histochemical study. *J. Invest. Dermatol.*, 55:1, 1970.
Okun, M. et al. Subcellular demonstration of peroxidatic oxidation of tyrosine to melanin using dihydroxyfumarate as a co-factor in mouse melanoma cells. *J. Invest. Dermatol.*, 61:60, 1973.
Okun, M. et al. Subcellular localization of peroxidase-mediated oxidation of tyrosine to melanin. In: *Pigment Cell: Mechanisms in Pigmentation.* Vol. 1, McGovern, V., ed., Basel, Karger, 1973, p. 98.

Patel, R. et al. Biochemical studies of the peroxidase-mediated oxidation of tyrosine to melanin: Demonstration of the hydroxylation of tyrosine by plant and human peroxidases. *Biochem. J.*, 124:439, 1971.
Patel, R. et al. Inability of murine melanoma "tyrosinase" (dopa oxidase) to oxidize tyrosine in the presence or absence of dopa or dihydroxyfumarate co-factors. *J. Invest. Dermatol.*, 61:55, 1973.
Porta, G. and Muhlbock, O. *Structure and Control of the Melanocyte.* Berlin, Springer-Verlag, 1966.
Seiji, M., Fitzpatrick, T. and Birbeck, M. The melanosome: A distinctive subcellular particle of mammalian melanocytes and the site of melanogenesis. *J. Invest. Dermatol.*, 36:243, 1961.
Szabó, G. et al. Racial differences in the fate of melanosomes in human epidermis. *Nature,* 222:1081, 1969.
Toda, K. et al. Alteration of racial differences in melanosome distribution in human epidermis after exposure to ultraviolet light. *Nature (New Biol.),* 236:143, 1972.

Dermis

Bentz, H. et al. Isolation and partial characterization of a new human collagen with an extended triple-helical structural domain. *Proc. Natl. Acad. Sci. USA,* 80:3168, 1983.
Breathnach, A. *An Atlas of the Ultrastructure of Human Skin.* London, Churchill, 1971, p. 174.
Breathnach, S. et al. A unique epithelial basement membrane antigen defined by a monoclonal antibody (KF-I). *J. Invest. Dermatol.*, 80:392, 1983.
Burgeson, R. Genetic heterogeneity of collagens. *J. Invest. Dermatol.*, 79 (suppl.):25s, 1982.
Fisher, B. The Ehlers-Danlos Syndrome. *Weekly Update: Dermatology,* 1:1, 1980.
Foidart, J. and Yaar, M. Type IV collagen, laminin and fibronectin at the dermoepidermal junction. *Front Matrix Biol.*, 8:175, 1981.
Grant, M. and Prockop, D. The biosynthesis of collagen. *N. Eng. J. Med.*, 286:194, 1972.
Hashimoto, K. Normal and abnormal connective tissue of the human skin . I. Fibroblast and collagen. *Internat. J. Dermatol.*, 17:457, 1978.
Holbrook, K. et al. The structure and function of dermal connective tissue in normal individuals and patients with inherited connective tissue disorders. *Scan Electron Microsc.*, (part IV): 1731, 1982.
Jacques, J. and Cameron, H. Changes in the ground-substance of healing wounds. *J. Pathol.*, 99:337, 1969.
Johnson, W. and Helwig, E. Histochemistry of the acid mucopolysaccharides of the skin in normal and in certain pathologic conditions. *Am. J. Clin. Pathol.*, 40:123, 1963.
Kleinman, H. et al. Role of collagenous matrices in the adhesion and growth of cells. *J. Cell Biol.*, 88:473, 1981.
Kobayasi, T. Electron microscopy of the elastic fibres and the dermal membrane in normal human skin. *Acta Derm. Venereol.*, 48:303, 1968.
Lapière, C. The molecular basis of connective tissue pathology. *Br. J. Dermatol.*, 89:87, 1973.
Lapière, C. and Pierard, G. Skin procollagen peptidase in normal and pathologic conditions. *J. Invest. Dermatol.*, 62:582, 1974.
Lazarus, G. Collagen, collagenase and clinicians. *Br. J. Dermatol.*, 86:193, 1972.
Liotta, L. et al. Metastatic potential correlates with enzymatic degradation of basement membrane collagen. *Nature,* 284:67, 1980.
Meigel, W., Gay, S. and Weber, L. Dermal architecture and collagen type distribution. *Arch. Dermatol. Res.*, 259:1 , 1977.
Montagna, W., Bently, J. and Dobson, R. *The Dermis.* In: *Advances in Biology of Skin.* Vol. 10, New York, Appleton-Century-Crofts, 1970.
Sandberg, L. et al. Structure of the elastic fiber: An overview. *J. Invest. Dermatol.*, 79 (suppl.):128s, 1982.
Smith, J. The dermal elastoses. *Arch. Derm. Venereol.*, 88:382, 1963.
Stanley, J. et al. Laminin and bullous pemphigoid antigen are distinct basement membrane proteins synthesized by epidermal cells. *J. Invest. Dermatol.*, 78:456, 1982.
Stenn, K. Collagen heterogeneity of skin. *Am. J. Dermatopathol.*, 1:87, 1979.
Swanson, J. and Helwig, E. Special fibrils of human dermis. *J. Invest. Dermatol.*, 50:195, 1968.
Timpl, R. and Martin, G. Components of basement membranes. In: *Immunochemistry of the Extracellular Matrix,* Vol. II, edited by H. Furthmayr. Boca Raton, FL, CRC Press, 1982, p. 119.
Woodley, D. et al. Localization of basement membrane components after dermal-epidermal junction separation. *J. Invest. Dermatol.*, 81: 149, 1983.

Muscles of the Skin

Adams, R., Denny-Brown, D. and Pearson, C. *Diseases of Muscle.* 2nd Ed., New York, Harper and Row, 1967.

Breathnach, A. *An Atlas of the Ultrastructure of Human Skin.* London, Churchill, 1971, p. 330.

Vasculature of the Skin

Braverman, I. and Yen, A. Ultrastructure of the human dermal microcirculation. II. *J. Invest. Dermatol.*, 68:44, 1977.

Cormia, F. Vasculature of the normal scalp. *Arch. Dermatol.*, 88:692, 1963.

Davis, M. and Lawler, J. The capillary circulation of the skin. *Arch. Dermatol.*, 77:690, 1958.

Higgins, J. and Eady, R. Human dermal microvasculature: Its segmental differentiation. Light and electron microscopic study. *Br. J. Dermatol.*, 104:117, 1981.

Mescon H., Hurely, H. and Moretti, G. The anatomy and histochemistry of the arteriovenous anastomosis in human digital skin. *J. Invest. Dermatol.*, 27:133, 1966.

Montagna, W. and Ellis, R. *Blood Vessels and Circulation.* In: *Advances in Biology of Skin.* Vol. 2, New York, Pergamon Press, 1961.

Mortimer et al. The importance of elastic fibers in skin lymphatics. *Br. J. Dermatol.*, 108:561, 1983.

Ryan, T. The lymphatics of the skin. In: *The Physiology and Pathophysiology of the Skin,* Vol. V, edited by A. Jarrett. New York, Academic Press, 1978, p 1755.

Weber, K. and Braun-Falco, O. Ultrastructure of blood vessels in human granulation tissue. *Arch. Derm. Forsch.*, 248:29, 1973.

Tissue Cytology of Inflammatory Cells

GENERAL REFERENCES

Caro, W. and Helwig, E. Cutaneous lymphoid hyperplasia. *Cancer,* 24:487, 1969.

Carr, I. The cellular basis of reticulo-endothelial stimulation. *J. Pathol.*, 94:323, 1967.

Dienes, L. and Mallory, T. Histological studies of hypersensitive reactions. *Am. J. Pathol.*, 8:689, 1932.

Glynn, L. and Holborow, E. *Autoimmunity and Disease.* Philadelphia, F. A. Davis, 1965.

Lawrence, H. *Cellular and Humoral Aspects of the Hypersensitive States.* New York, P.B. Hoeber, 1959.

Montagna, W. and Billingham, R. *Immunology and the Skin.* In: *Advances in Biology of Skin.* Vol. 11, New York, Appleton-Century-Crofts, 1971.

Nowell, P. and Wilson, D. Lymphocytes and hemic stem cells. *Am. J. Pathol.*, 65:641, 1971.

Robb-Smith, A. The reticular tissue and the skin. *Br. J. Dermatol.*, 56:151, 1944.

LYMPHOCYTES AND PLASMA CELLS

Gell, P. and Benacerraf, B. Studies on hypersensitivity. IV. The relationship between contact and delayed sensitivity: A study on the specificity of cellular immune reactions. *J. Exp. Med.*, 113:571, 1961.

Gowans, J. Life-span, recirculation and transformation of lymphocytes. *Internat. Rev. Exp. Pathol.*, 5:1, 1966.

Montagna, W. and Billingham, R. *Immunology and the Skin.* In: *Advances in Biology of Skin.* Vol. 11, New York, Appleton-Century-Crofts, 1971.

Nowell, P. and Wilson, D. Lymphocytes and hemic stem cells. *Am. J. Pathol.*, 65:641, 1971.

Rebuck, J. *The Lymphocyte and Lymphocytic Tissue.* New York, P. B. Hoeber Co., 1960.

Seligmann, M. B-cell and T-cell markers in lymphoid proliferations. *New Eng. J. Med.*, 290: 1483, 1974.

Yoffey, J. The mammalian lymphocyte. *Biol. Rev.*, 25:314, 1950.

HISTIOCYTES, MACROPHAGES, EPITHELIOID CELLS, FOREIGN-BODY AND LANGHANS GIANT CELLS AND FIBROBLASTS

Allgöwer, M. *The Cellular Basis of Wound Repair.* Springfield, IL, Thomas, 1956.

Black, M. and Epstein, W. Formation of multinucleate giant cells in organized epithelioid cell granulomas. *Am. J. Pathol.*, 74:263, 1974.

Carr, I. The cellular basis of reticulo-endothelial stimulation. *J. Pathol.*, 94:323, 1967.
Downey, H. The development of histiocytes and macrophages from lymphocytes. *J. Lab. and Clin. Med.*, 45:499, 1955.
Hartwell, S. *The Mechanism of Healing in Human Wounds.* Springfield, IL, Thomas, 1955.
Maximow, A. The morphology of the mesenchymal reactions. *Arch. Pathol. Lab. Med.*, 4:557, 1927.
Montagna, W. and Billingham, R. *Wound Healing.* In: *Advances in Biology of Skin.* Vol. 5. New York, Pergamon Press, 1964.
Papadimitriou, J., Sforsina, D., and Papaelias, L. Kinetics of multinucleate giant cell formation and their modifications by various agents in foreign body reactions. *Am. J. Pathol.*, 73:349, 1973.
Papadimitriou, J. and Spector, W. The origin, properties and fate of epithelioid cells. *J. Pathol.*, 105:187, 1971.
Slome, D. *Wound Healing.* New York, Pergamon Press, 1961.
Spector, W. and Heesom, N. The production of granulomata by antigen-antibody complexes. *J. Pathol.*, 98:31, 1969.
Stossel, T. Phagocytosis: The department of defense. *N. Eng. J. Med.*, 286:776, 1972.

MAST CELLS

Asboe-Hason, G. The mast cell in health and disease. *Acta Derm. Venereol.*, 53 (73, suppl.):139, 1973.
Benditt, E. and Lagunoff, D. The mast cell: Its structure and function. *Progr. Allerg.*, 8:195, 1964.
Mikhail, G. and Miller-Milinska, A. Mast cell population in human skin. *J. Invest. Dermatol.*, 43:249, 1964.
Okun, M. Histogenesis of melanocytes. *J. Invest. Dermatol.*, 44:285, 1965.
Okun, M. and Chorzelski, T. Metachromatic granules in dendritic cells within epithelial structures in alopecia mucinosa. *J. Invest. Dermatol.*, 45:129, 1965.
Okun, M. and Donnellan, B. Ultrastructural relationship of melanocytes to mast cells and "melanophages" in a lesion of alopecia mucinosa. *J. Invest. Dermatol.* 59:211, 1972.
Okun, M. et al. Latency of the dopa reaction in mast cells. *Histochemie,* 25:1, 1971.
Sagher, F. and Even-Paz, Z. *Mastocytosis and the Mast Cell.* Chicago, Yearbook Medical Publishers, 1967.
Schwartz, L. and Austen, K. Enzymes of the mast cell granule. *J. Invest. Dermatol.*, 74:349, 1980.
Schwartz, L. et al. Cell association of complexes of chymase, heparin, proteoglycan and protein after degranulation by rat mast cells. *J. Immunol.*, 126:2071, 1981.
Selye, H. *The Mast Cells.* London, Butterworths, 1965.
Soter, N. Mast cells in cutaneous inflammatory disorders. *J. Invest. Dermatol.*, 80:225, 1983.
Uvnäs, B. Chemistry and storage function of mast cell granules. *J. Invest. Dermatol.*, 71:76, 1978.

NEUTROPHILS AND EOSINOPHILS

Archer, R. The eosinophil and its functions. *Trans. St. John's Hosp. Dermatol. Soc.*, 50:112, 1964.
——. *The Eosinophil Leukocytes.* Philadelphia, F. A. Davis Co., 1963.
——. On the functions of eosinophils in the antigen-antibody reaction. *Br. J. Haematol.* 11:123, 1965.
Boggs, D. The kinetics of neutrophilic leukocytes in health and disease. *Seminars in Hematol.*, 4:359, 1967.
Elek, S. *Staphylococcus Pyogenes.* Edinburgh, E. S. Livingstone, 1959.
Henson, P. Pathologic mechanisms in neutrophil-mediated injury. *Am. J. Pathol.*, 68:593, 1972.
Litt, M. Studies in experimental eosinophilia. VI. Uptake of immune complexes by eosinophils. *J. Cell Biol.*, 23:355, 1964.
Mann, P. An electron-microscope study of the relations between mast cells and eosinophilic leukocytes. *J. Pathol.*, 98:183, 1969.
Okun, M. et al. Melanin: A normal component of human eosinophils. *Lab. Invest.*, 30:681, 1974.
Parish, W. Effects of neutrophils on tissues. *Br. J. Dermatol.*, 81:28, 1969.
Poole, J. Electron microscopy of polymorphonuclear leukocytes. *Br. J. Dermatol.*, 81:11, 1969.

Hair

Garn, S. The examination of the hair under the polarizing microscope. *Ann. N. Y. Acad. Sci.*, 53:649, 1951.

Holbrook, K. and Odland, G. Structure of the human fetal hair canal and initial hair eruption. *J. Invest. Dermatol.*, 71:385, 1978.

Kligman, A. The human hair cycle. *J. Invest. Dermatol.* 33:307, 1959.

Montagna, W. and Dobson, R. *Hair Growth.* In: *Advances in Biology of Skin.* Vol. 9, New York, Pergamon Press, 1969.

Montagna, W. and Ellis, R. *Biology of Hair Growth.* New York, Academic Press, 1958.

Parakkal, P. and Matoltsy, A. A study of the differentiation products of the hair follicle cells with the electron microscope. *J. Invest. Dermatol.*, 43:23, 1964.

Staricco, R. The melanocytes and the hair follicle. *J. Invest. Dermatol.*, 35:185, 1960.

Weedon, D. and Strutton, G. Apoptosis as the mechanism of the involution of hair follicles in catagen formation. *Acta Derm. Venereol.* (Stockh.), 61:335, 1981.

Arrectores Pilorum

Dolnick, E. Comparative study of skin of fur bearers: Functional role of some connective tissue elements. In: *Biology of the Skin and Hair Growth.* Lyne, A. and Short, B., eds., New York, American Elsevier Publishing Co., Inc., 1965, p. 155.

Domonkos, A. *Andrews' Diseases of the Skin.* 7th Ed., Philadelphia, Saunders, 1982.

Fisher, W. and Helwig, E. Leiomyomas of skin. *Arch. Dermatol.*, 88:510, 1963.

Sebaceous Glands

Botelho, S., Brooks, F. and Shelley, W. *Exocrine Glands,* Philadelphia, Univ. of Pennsylvania Press, 1969.

Cashion, P., Skobe, Z. and Nalbandian, J. Ultrastructural observations on sebaceous glands of the human oral mucosa (Fordyce's disease). *J. Invest. Dermatol.*, 53:208, 1969.

Epstein, E. and Epstein W. New cell formation in human sebaceous glands. *J. Invest. Dermatol.*, 46:453, 1966.

Kellum, R. Isolation of human sebaceous glands. *Arch. Dermatol.*, 93:610, 1966.

Montagna, W., Ellis, R. and Silver, A. *The Sebaceous Glands.* In: *Advances in Biology of Skin.* Vol. 4, New York, Pergamon Press, 1963.

Niizuma, K. Lipid droplets of the sebaceous glands: Some observations from tannic acid fixation. *Acta Derm. Venereol.* (Stockh.), 59:401, 1979.

Strauss, J. and Pochi, P. Histology, histochemistry and electron microscopy of sebaceous glands in man, *Normale und Pathologische Anatomie der Haut I.* In: *Jadassohn Handb. Haut-Geschlechtskr. Bd. I/1.* Gans, O. and Steigleder, G. eds., Berlin. Springer-Verlag, 1968.

Suskind, R. The chemistry of the human sebaceous gland. I. Histochemical observations. *J. Invest. Dermatol.*, 17:37, 1951.

Sweeny, T. et al. Effect of estrogen and androgen on sebaceous gland turnover time. *J. Invest. Dermatol.*, 53:8, 1969.

Apocrine Glands

Biempica, L. and Montes, L. Secretory epithelium of the large axillary sweat glands. *Am. J. Anat.*, 117:47, 1965.

Hashimoto, K., Gross, B. and Lever, W. Electron microscopic study of apocrine secretion. *J. Invest. Dermatol.*, 46:378, 1966.

Hurley, J. and Shelley, W., *The Human Apocrine Sweat Gland in Health and Disease.* Springfield, IL, Thomas, 1960.

Schaumburg-Lever, G. and Lever, W. Secretion from human apocrine glands. *J. Invest. Dermatol.*, 64:38, 1975.

Smith, D. Jr., Peter, T. and Donegan, W. Montgomery's areolar tubercle. *Arch. Pathol. Lab. Med.*, 106:60, 1982.

Eccrine Glands

Botelho, S., Brooks, F. and Shelley, W. *Exocrine Glands.* Philadelphia, Univ. of Pennsylvania Press, 1969.

Dobson, R. and Sato, K. The secretion of salt and water by the eccrine sweat gland. *Arch. Dermatol.*, 105:366, 1972.

Dobson, R. et al. Some histochemical observations on the human eccrine sweat gland. III. The effect of profuse sweating. *J. Invest. Dermatol.*, 31:147, 1958.

Hashimoto, K., Gross, B. and Lever, W. Electron microscopic study of the human adult eccrine gland. I. The Duct. *J. Invest. Dermatol.*, 46:172, 1966.

Holyoke, J. and Lobitz, W., Jr. Histologic variations in the structure of human eccrine sweat glands. *J. Invest. Dermatol.*, 18:147, 1952.

Kunyo, Y. *Human Perspiration.* Springfield, IL, Thomas, 1956.

Montagna, W., Chase, H. and Lobitz, W., Jr. Histology and cytochemistry of human skin. IV. The eccrine sweat glands. *J. Invest. Dermatol.*, 20:415, 1953.

Montagna, W., Ellis, R. and Silver, A. *Eccrine Sweat Glands and Eccrine Sweating.* In: *Advances in Biology of Skin.* Vol. 3, New York, Pergamon Press, 1962.

Nails

Hashimoto, K. The marginal band: A demonstration of the thickened cellular envelope of the human nail cell with the aid of lanthanum staining. *Arch. Dermatol.*, 103:387, 1971.

Lewin, K. The normal finger nail. *Br. J. Dermatol.*, 77:421, 1965.

Lewis, B. Microscopic studies of fetal and mature nail and surrounding soft tissue. *Arch. Dermatol.*, 70:732, 1954.

Norton, L. Incorporation of thymidinemethyl-H^3 and glycine-$2H^3$ in the nail matrix and bed of humans. *J. Invest. Dermatol.*, 56:61, 1971.

Pardo-Castello, V. and Pardo, O. *Diseases of the Nails.* 3rd Ed., Springfield, IL, Thomas, 1960.

White, C. and Laipply, T. Histopathology of nail diseases. *J. Invest. Dermatol.*, 1952.

Zaias, N. Embryology of the human nail. *Arch. Dermatol.*, 87:37, 1963.

——. The movement of the nail bed. *J. Invest. Dermatol.*, 48:402, 1967.

Zaias, N. and Alvarez, J. The formation of the primate nail plate: An autoradiographic study in squirrel monkey. *J. Invest. Dermatol.*, 51:120, 1968.

Nerves and Nerve End-Organs of the Skin

Arthur, R. and Shelley, W. The innervation of human epidermis. *J. Invest. Dermatol.*, 32:397, 1959.

Cauna, N. Fine morphological characteristics and microtopography of the free nerve endings in human digital skin. *Anat. Rec.*, 198:643, 1980.

Hashimoto, K. Fine structure of the Meissner corpuscle of human palmar skin. *J. Invest. Dermatol.*, 60:20, 1973.

Montagna, W. *Cutaneous Innervation.* In: *Advances in Biology of Skin.* Vol. 1, Oxford, Pergamon Press, 1960.

Orfanos, C. and Mahle, G. Ultrastructure and cytochemistry of human cutaneous nerves. *J. Invest. Dermatol.*, 61:108, 1973.

Pease, D. and Quilliam, T. Electron microscopy of the Pacinian corpuscle. *J. Biophys. Biochem. Cytol.*, 3:331, 1957.

Weddell, G., Pallie, W. and Palmer, E. The morphology of peripheral nerve terminations in the skin. *Quart. J. Micr. Sci.*, 95:483, 1954.

Winkelmann, R. *Nerve Endings in Normal and Pathologic Skin.* Springfield, IL, Thomas, 1960.

Winkelmann, R. and Osmet, L. The Vater-Pacinian corpuscle in the skin of the human finger tip. *Arch. Dermatol.*, 73:116, 1956.

Histologic Artifacts

Caro, M. Diagnostic pitfalls of dermal pathology. *Arch. Dermatol.*, 67:18, 1953.

Carpenter, C., Jr., Jolly, W., Jr. and Reed, R. Dermojet histopathological artifacts. *Arch. Dermatol.*, 92:304, 1965.

Mehregan, A. and Pinkus, H. Artifacts in dermal histopathology. *Arch. Dermatol.*, 94:218, 1966.

Okun, M., Ellerin, P. and Piotrowicz, M. Prevention of ice crystal damage to biopsy specimens in transport. *Arch. Dermatol.*, 105:458, 1972.

Smith, A. Tissue shrinkage caused by attachment of paraffin section to slides: Its effects on staining. *Stain Technol.*, 37:339, 1962.

Lichen striatus. This is an uncommon eruption consisting of lichenoid papules in linear arrangement. Lichen striatus generally occurs in children. Although lichen striatus generally shows only a nonspecific picture of dermatitis, dyskeratotic cells can sometimes be observed in the epidermis (see p. 96).

Seborrheic dermatitis. This is an idiopathic, scaling eruption with predilection for the scalp, face, and intertriginous areas (see p. 108).

Comment

1. Certain conditions which, in their most distinctive form or stage, have a characteristic histologic pattern, may at times show nonspecific dermatitis. These include psoriasis, seborrheic dermatitis, lichen planus, erythema multiforme, and the premycotic stage of mycosis fungoides.
2. *Exfoliative dermatitis* (exfoliative erythroderma) refers to widespread erythema and scaling. Various types of dermatitis as well as psoriasis may evolve into exfoliative dermatitis. Drugs can be implicated. In addition, exfoliative dermatitis may be a manifestation of lymphoma, pemphigus foliaceus, or lamellar ichthyosis. Mycosis fungoides, especially Sézary syndrome, is the usual form of lymphoma associated with exfoliative dermatitis (see p. 1342). The microscopic pattern in exfoliative dermatitis may be that of nonspecific dermatitis. In exfoliative dermatitis due to psoriasis, lymphoma, or pemphigus foliaceus, there may be microscopic evidence of psoriasis, lymphoma, or pemphigus foliaceus.
3. Any extensive dermatitis, particularly generalized exfoliative dermatitis, may produce a regional lymphadenopathy, most commonly of the cervical, axillary, or inguinal lymph nodes. This is called *dermatopathic lymphadenopathy* (lipomelanotic reticulosis). Dermatopathic lymphadenopathy may also be associated with exfoliative dermatitis caused by lymphoma. In such cases, the involved lymph nodes may show evidence of lymphoma (see pp. 112, 113).

Stages of Dermatitis

Dermatitis: A nonspecific inflammatory response with changes in epidermis and dermis.

Stages:

Acute
Gross: tense vesicles
Micro: spongiotic vesicles

Subacute
Gross: erythema, scale, crust, exudation
Micro: acanthosis, parakeratosis, spongiosis with small spongiotic vesicles, exocytosis

Chronic
Gross: papules, lichenification, exocytosis
Micro: acanthosis, hyperkeratosis, absence of spongiosis.

All stages show varying degrees of nonspecific dermal inflammation, mainly perivascular. Inflammatory cells are mainly lymphoid cells; in acute dermatitis there may be a fair number of neutrophils.

ACUTE DERMATITIS

Acute dermatitis is characterized by vesicles, bullae, and exudation, as in the illustrations of allergic contact dermatitis due to poison ivy (Figs. A,C), and vesicular stage of nummular dermatitis of the hands (Fig. D). In allergic contact dermatitis due to plants, vesicles often have a linear distribution.

Microscopic features

1. Intraepidermal vesicles, formed by spongiosis and intracellular edema are present. These may progress to form multilocular bullae, as a result of severe hydropic degeneration (reticular degeneration) of epithelial cells (Figs. B,E).
2. Spongiosis and intracellular edema are often present in the epidermis adjacent to the vesicles.
3. There is exocytosis of lymphoid cells and neutrophils (Fig. B,E).
4. The upper dermis (Fig. B) shows edema and a mixed perivascular infiltrate composed of mononuclear cells with some neutrophils and eosinophils. Capillaries are dilated.

ACUTE DERMATITIS

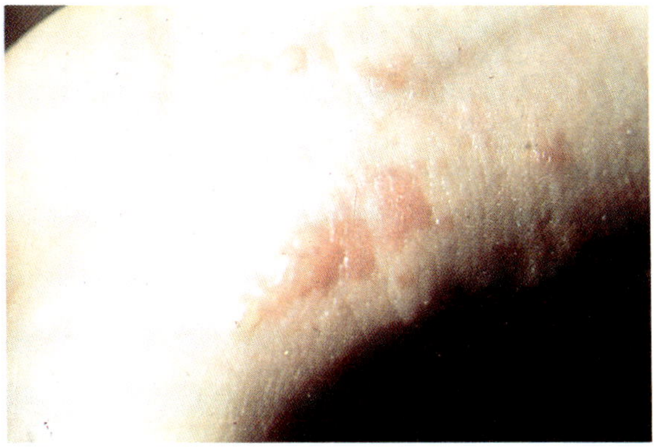

A

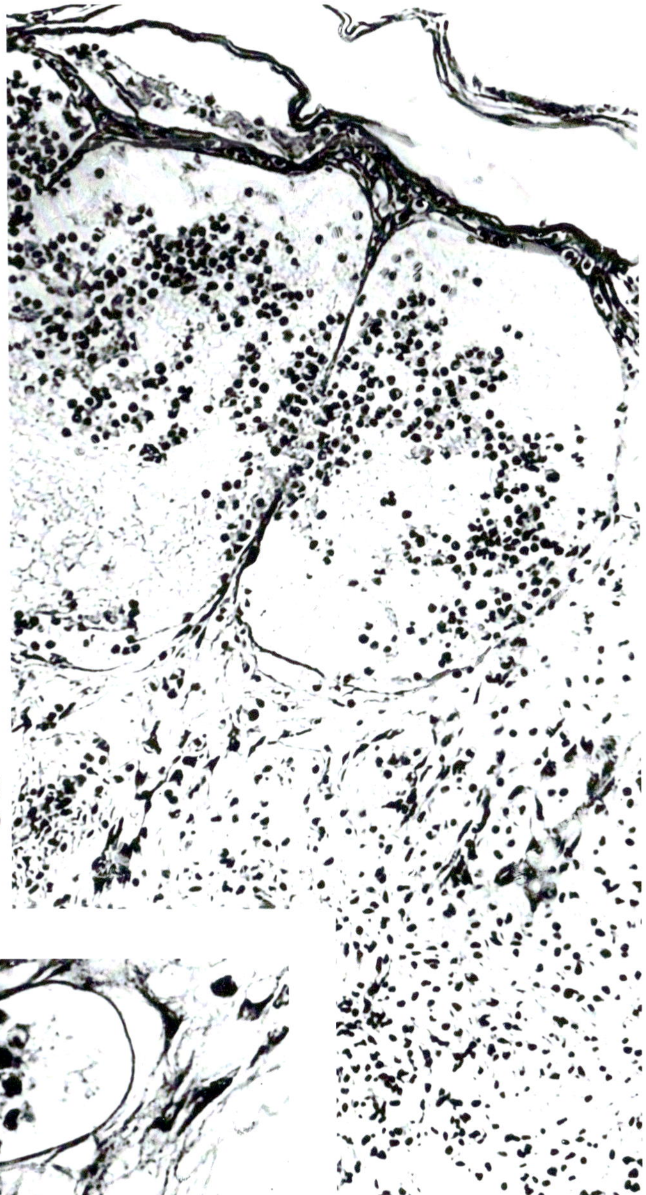

B

X160

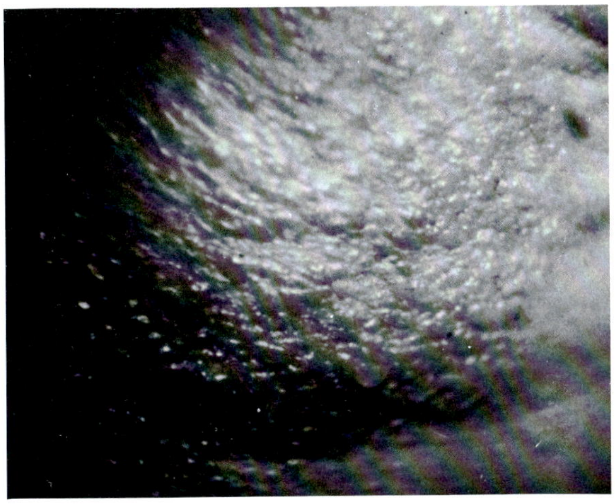

C

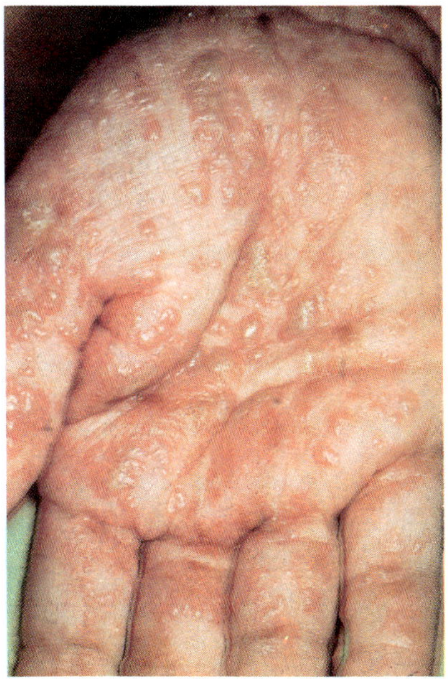

D

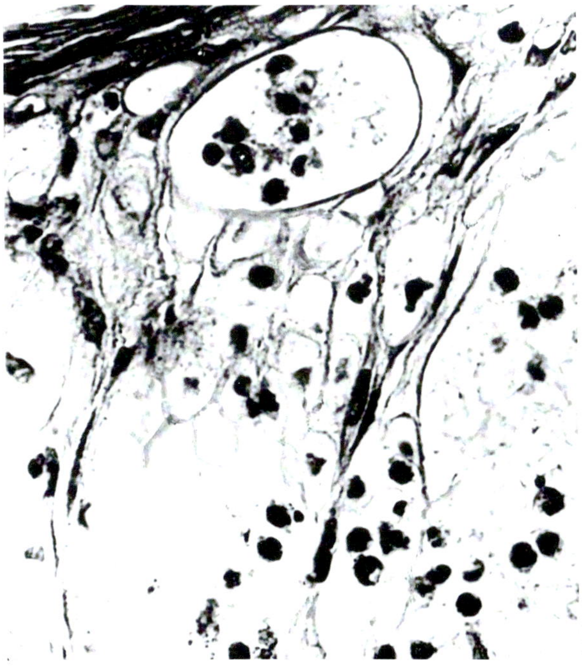

E

X520

DERMATITIS continued

SUBACUTE DERMATITIS

Subacute dermatitis is characterized by a spectrum of clinical features that may include erythema, moderate vesiculation, crusting, and scaling. Illustrated are examples of nummular dermatitis of the hands and leg (Figs. A,B) and allergic contact dermatitis of the face (Fig. C) and foot (Fig. D), due to nail polish and shoe components, respectively. As mentioned, nummular dermatitis is an idiopathic, patchy dermatitis. It may show pinpoint vesicles and erosions, as illustrated in the photograph of the leg.

Comment

Contact dermatitis may have allergic or nonallergic mechanisms. Nonallergic contact dermatitis is termed *primary irritant contact dermatitis*. Primary irritant contact dermatitis results from contact with substances that directly injure the skin, such as acid, alkali, soaps, detergents, and solvents. Reliable distinction between allergic and primary irritant contact dermatitis cannot be made on a histologic basis.

SUBACUTE DERMATITIS

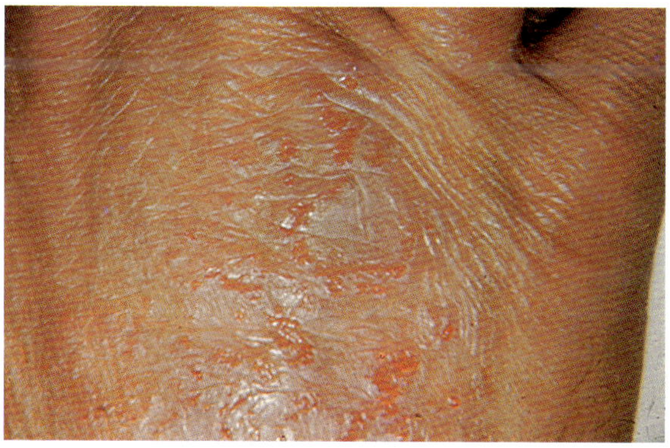
A

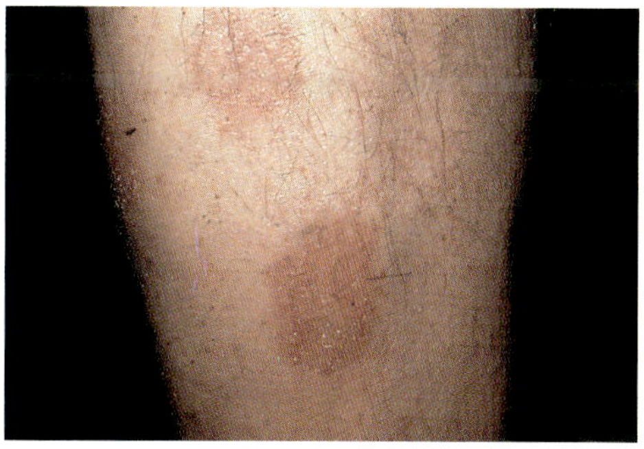
B

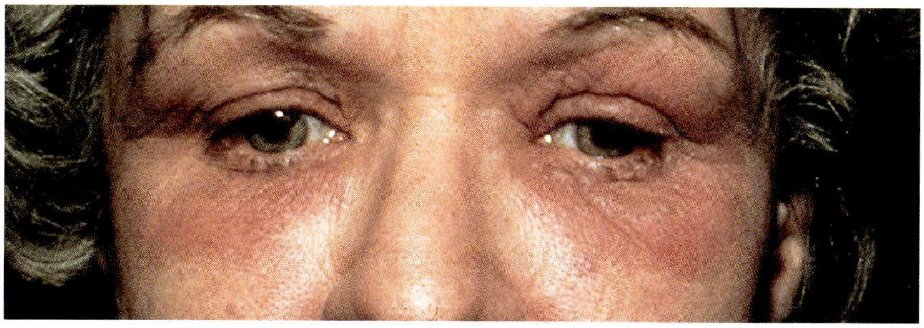
C

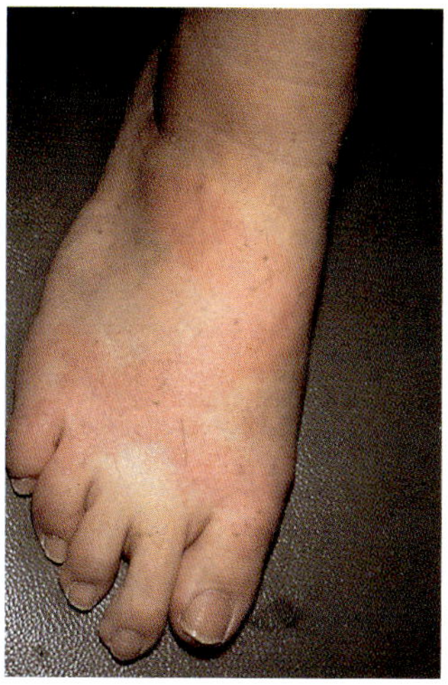
D

DERMATITIS continued

SUBACUTE DERMATITIS

Pityriasis rosea is an idiopathic condition characterized by an initial lesion—a large scaling patch (herald patch) with an active border and clearing center (Fig. B) resembling tinea corporis, and small scaling secondary lesions (Figs. A,B) which usually appear about one week after the herald patch. The secondary lesions are typically oval, with their long axes parallel to lines of cleavage (Fig. A). The scale is often peripheral in secondary lesions, but it may be central (Fig. B). In pityriasis rosea, involvement is mainly limited to the trunk. In most instances, the lesions disappear spontaneously in 6 weeks. Lesions of pityriasis rosea have a resemblance to lesions observed in secondary syphilis and to the early exanthem of AIDS (Fig. C), which precedes conversion to a positive test for antibodies. (A measles-like exanthem may occur at any stage of AIDS or ARC). A serologic test for syphilis should be carried out to aid in the distinction. A serologic test for AIDS should be performed when there is reason to suspect it.

SUBACUTE DERMATITIS

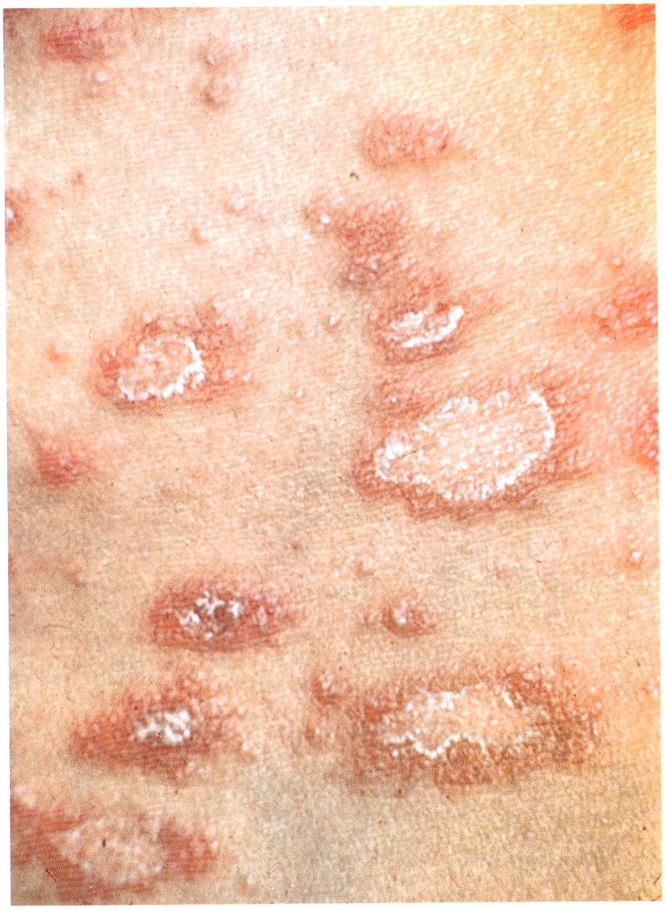

A

Courtesy Dr. K. Inaba

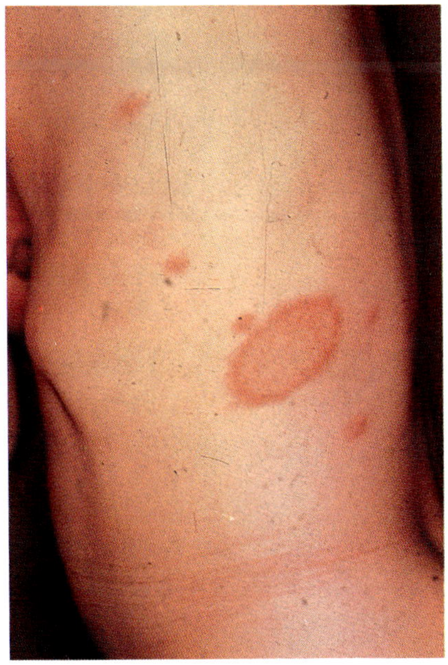

B

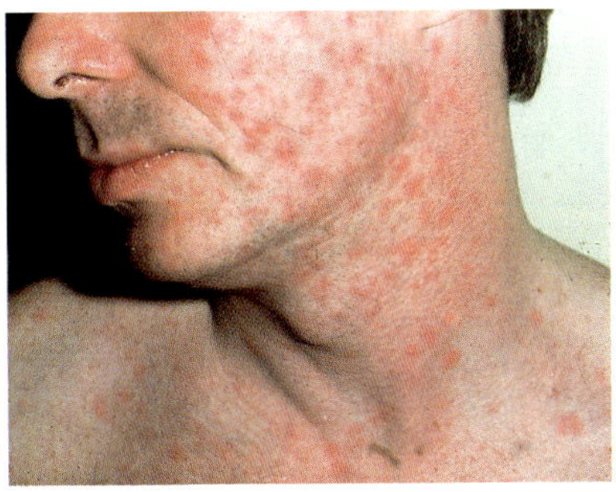

C

DERMATITIS continued ⇨

SUBACUTE DERMATITIS

Parapsoriasis. This is a term which has been the source of considerable confusion. Currently, parapsoriasis is divided into three types:

1. Small plaque type (digitate dermatosis)
2. Large plaque type
3. Parapsoriasis variegata

Small plaque parapsoriasis consists of elongated or oval patches of dermatitis (pink or yellowish) symmetrically distributed over the trunk (Fig. A) and proximal parts of the extremities (Fig. A). In large plaque parapsoriasis (Fig. B), the lesions are larger and more irregular in shape, and often have a brownish color. Parapsoriasis variegata (Fig. D) is an extensive eruption of reddish-brown, scaling lesions in net-like arrangement. Both large plaque parapsoriasis and parapsoriasis variegata may become poikilodermatous and may represent premycotic mycosis fungoides. Lesions of large plaque parapsoriasis may become infiltrated (Fig. C); this change may also be an indicator of evolving mycosis fungoides. Small plaque parapsoriasis as well as large plaque parapsoriasis in their early stages show a histologic picture of nonspecific dermatitis. When lesions of large plaque parapsoriasis or parapsoriasis variegata become poikilodermatous, they develop the histologic picture of poikiloderma atrophicans vasculare. Evolving mycosis fungoides in large plaque parapsoriasis or parapsoriasis variegata may be represented by the presence of mycosis cells (atypical T lymphocytes), with hyperchromatic, convoluted nuclei.

The relationship of parapsoriasis to mycosis fungoides is further discussed on p. 1330.

Comment:

Some authors include pityriasis lichenoides (see p. 146) in the category of parapsoriasis; this is a source of confusion.

SUBACUTE DERMATITIS: PARAPSORIASIS

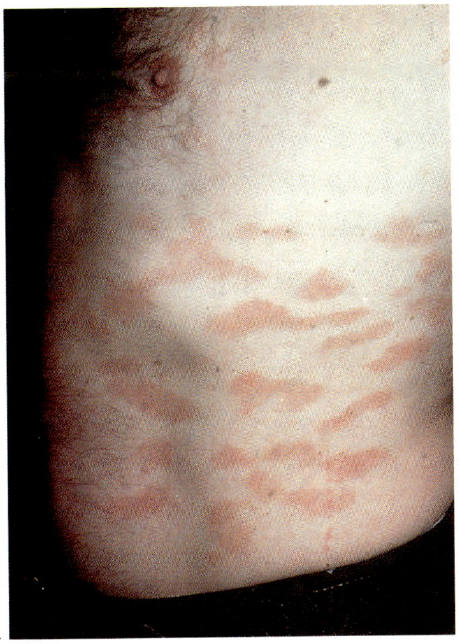

A

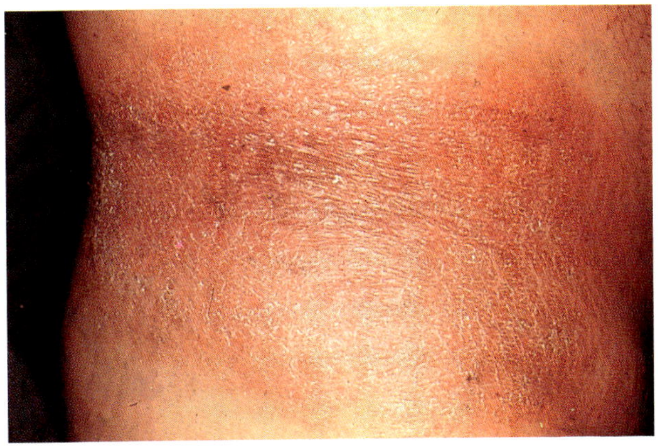

B

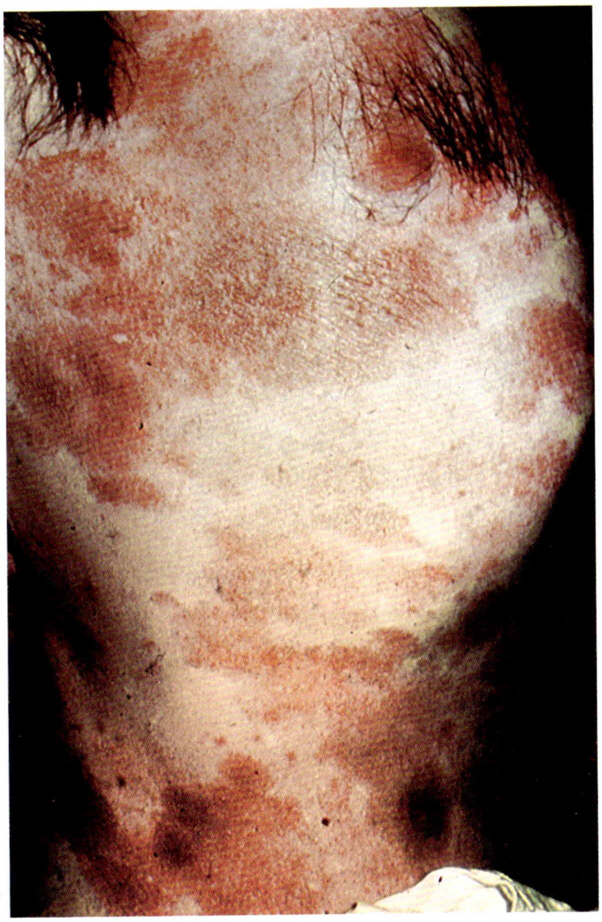

C

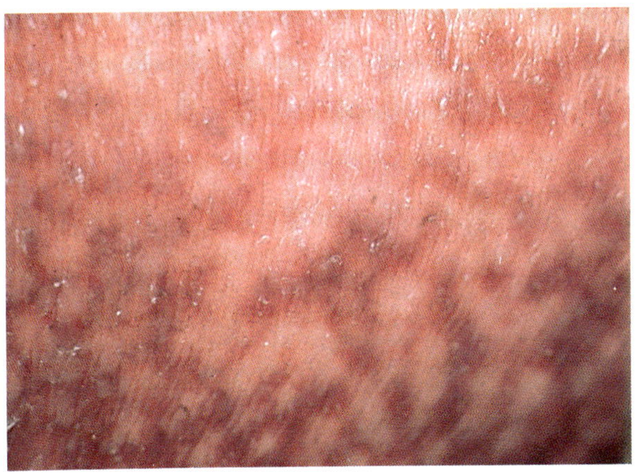

D

Courtesy Dr. Ramon Fusaro, Dr. J. Koh

DERMATITIS continued

SUBACUTE DERMATITIS

Lichen striatus. This is an uncommon (usually unilateral) eruption consisting of lichenoid, scaling papules in linear arrangement (Fig. A). Lichen striatus usually occurs in children; it is typically not pruritic. Disappearance in one year is the rule. Although the histologic picture is that of nonspecific dermatitis, occasionally a few dyskeratotic cells can be observed in the epidermis.

Comment:

Inflammatory linear verrucous epidermal nevus (see p. 748) (ILVEN) has clinical and histologic features virtually identical to lichen striatus, prompting some observers to believe these conditions represent the same disease. Others have cited the longer duration of ILVEN and its pruritic nature as justification for separating them.

SUBACUTE DERMATITIS: LICHEN STRIATUS

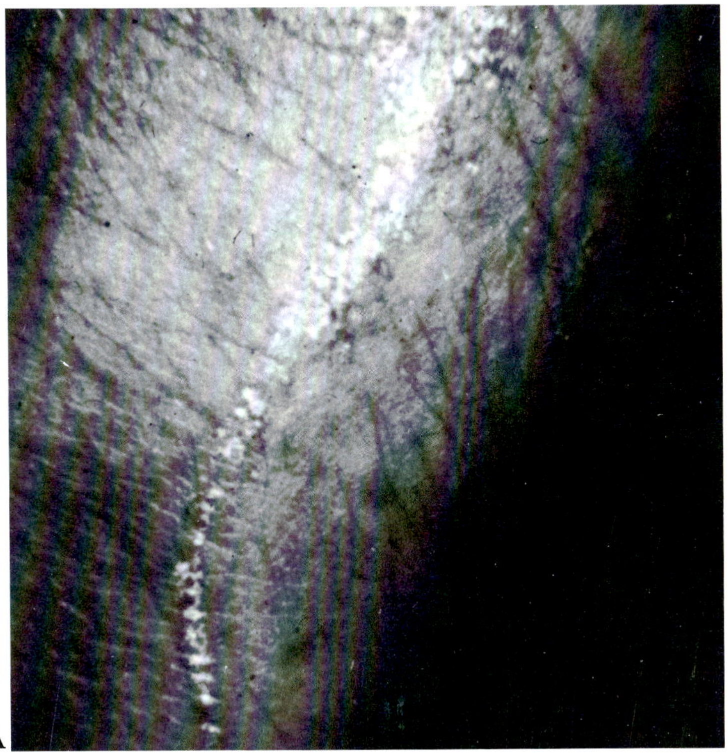

A

DERMATITIS continued

SUBACUTE DERMATITIS

Microscopic features

1. Vesicles may be present which are smaller than those of acute dermatitis (Fig. C).
2. Spongiosis and crusting are usually visible (Figs. A,C).
3. There is usually moderate acanthosis (Fig. A) and parakeratosis (Figs. C).
4. A dermal infiltrate is present similar to that of acute dermatitis (Fig. A). Exocytosis is often evident (Figs. A,B). Capillaries may be dilated.

SUBACUTE DERMATITIS

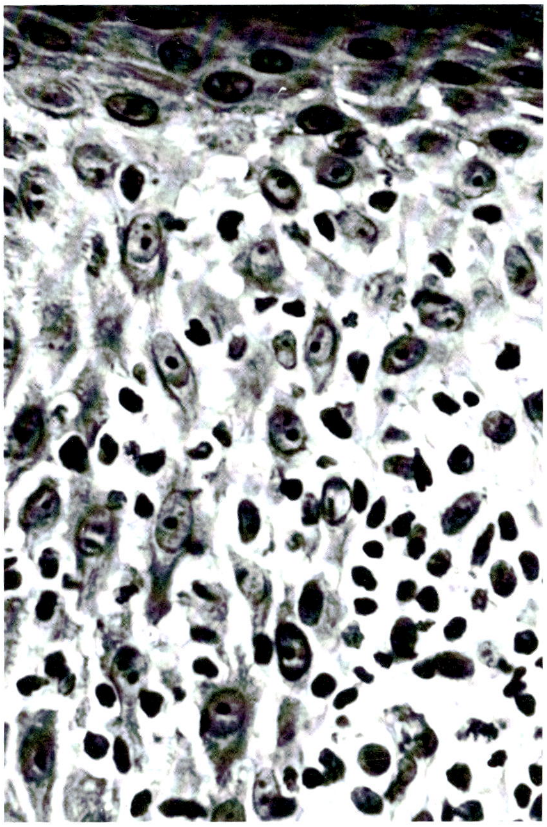

B
X780

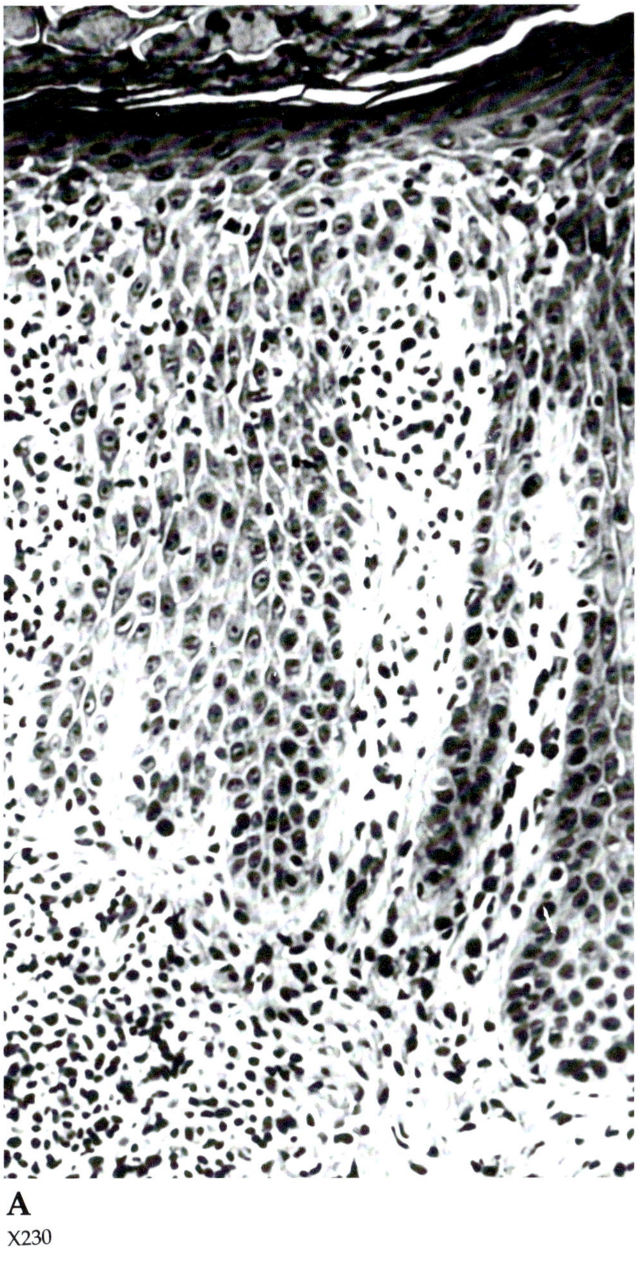

A
X230

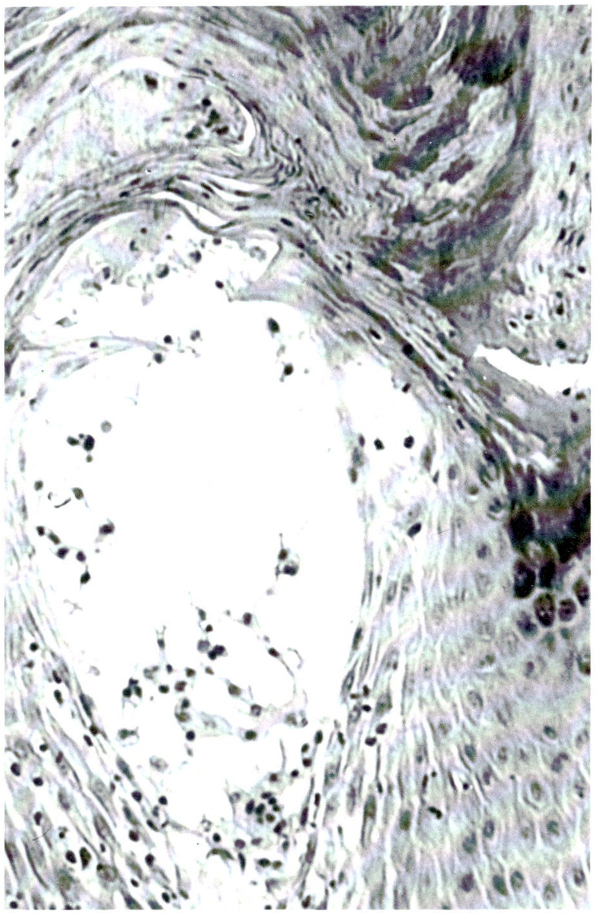

C
X310

DERMATITIS continued ⇨

CHRONIC DERMATITIS

Chronic dermatitis is characterized by scaling, fissuring, and lichenification, as in lichen simplex chronicus (Fig. A). Atopic dermatitis has a similar clinical appearance, but is often flexural in distribution (Fig. B). In infants, subacute to chronic atopic dermatitis is often present on the face (Fig. C).

Atopic dermatitis is a complex, genetically determined, relapsing disorder. The dermatitis is often linked to a personal and/or familial history of asthma or allergic rhinitis. Frequently there are elevated IgE levels.

Whether or not lichen simplex chronicus has a relationship to atopic dermatitis is uncertain. Common sites are ankles, wrists, anogenital area, and neck area.

Comment

1. *Prurigo nodularis* is regarded by some as a nodular variant of lichen simplex chronicus. The nodules are hyperkeratotic.
2. *Asteatotic eczema* (winter itch) is a common, dry dermatitis that occurs in middle-aged or elderly individuals. The legs are often affected. The clinical and histologic pictures grade into nummular eczema.

CHRONIC DERMATITIS

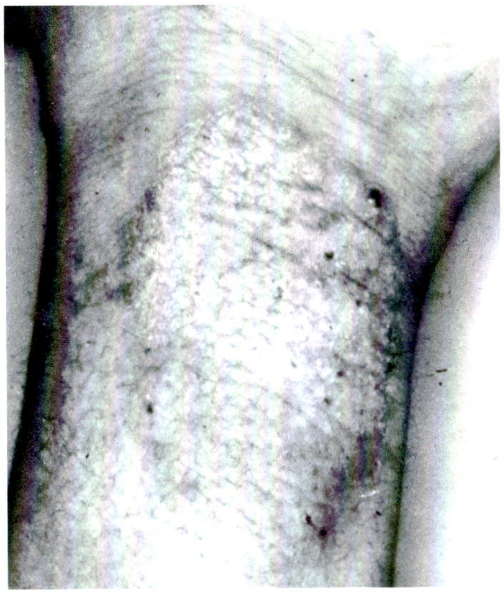

A

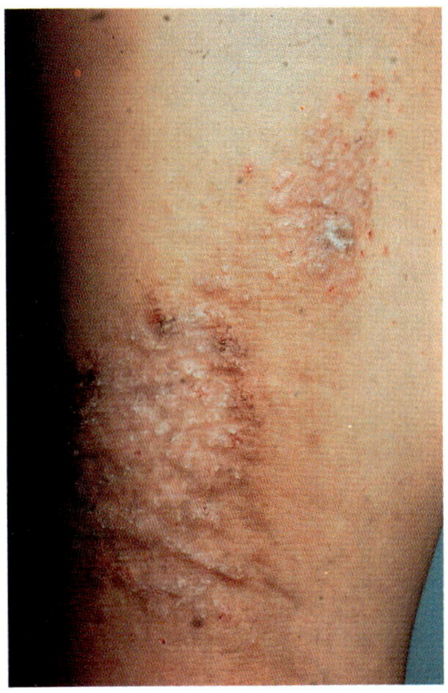

B

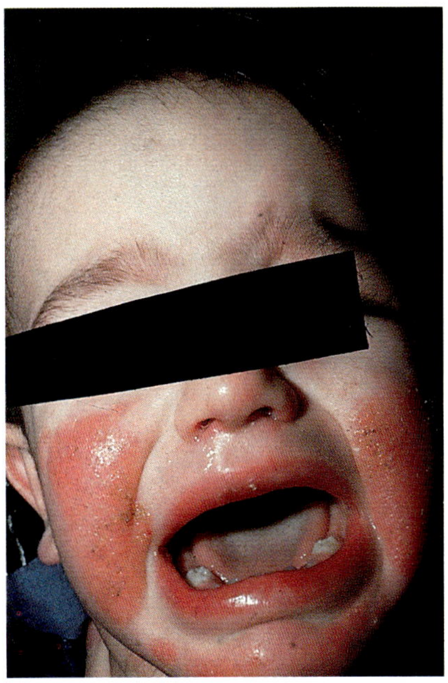

C

DERMATITIS continued ⇨

CHRONIC DERMATITIS

Microscopic features

1. Epidermal edema is minimal or absent (Fig. A).
2. Acanthosis is moderate (Fig. A) or pronounced.
3. A dermal infiltrate, similar to that observed in subacute dermatitis, is present (Figs. A,B).
4. An increased number of capillaries may be present.

CHRONIC DERMATITIS

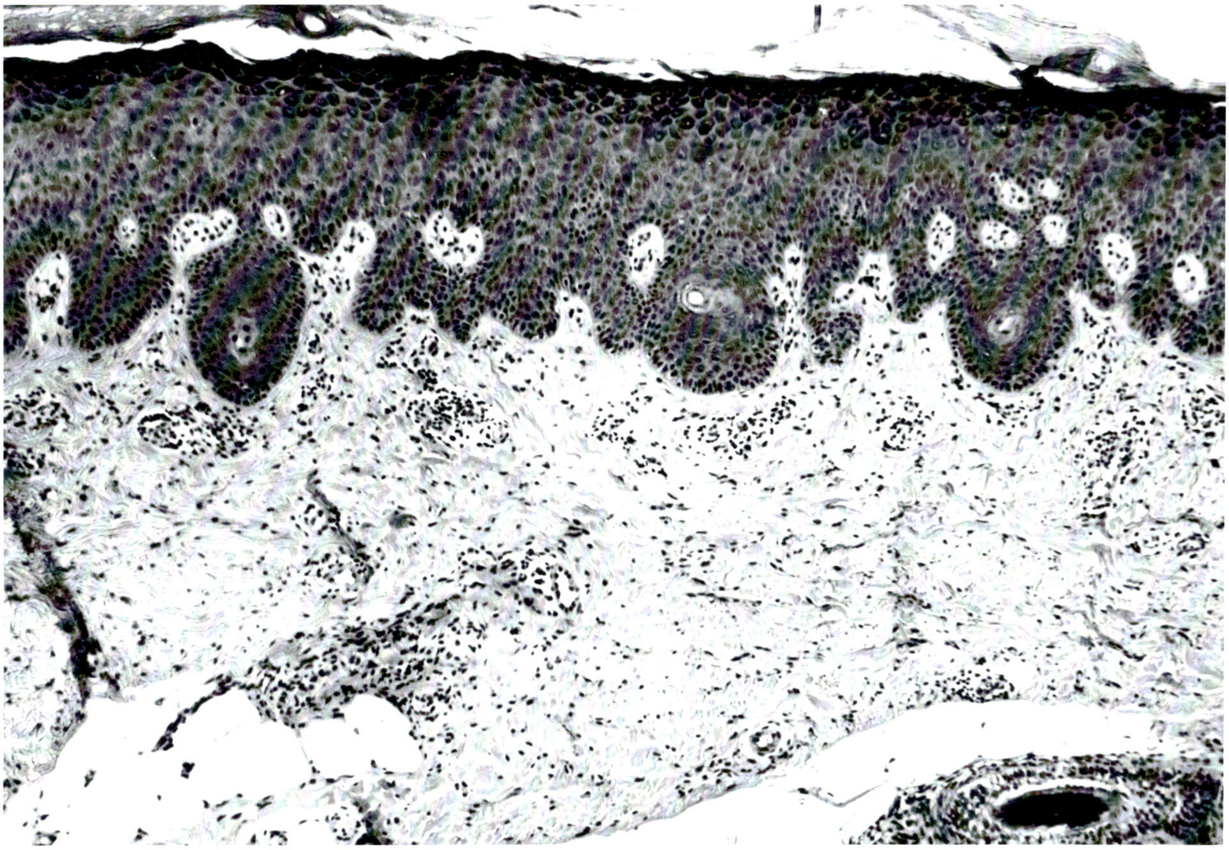

A
X110

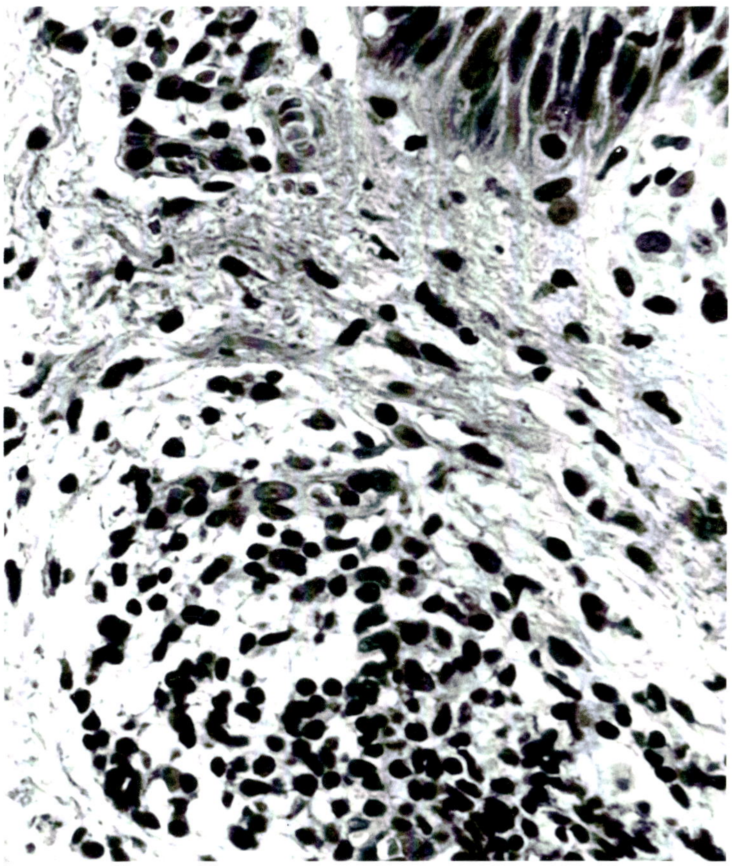

B
X500

DERMATITIS continued

CHRONIC DERMATITIS

Microscopic features

5. In some cases, such as lichen simplex chronicus (Fig. A), pronounced irregular acanthosis is present.
6. Hyperkeratosis (Fig. B) and/or parakeratosis (Fig. A) may be extensive.
7. Papillomatosis may be present.

CHRONIC DERMATITIS: POST-INFLAMMATORY HYPERPIGMENTATION AND HYPOPIGMENTATION.

Post-inflammatory hyperpigmentation may be a late sequel of chronic dermatitis or other cutaneous inflammation. It is characterized by mottled areas of increased melanization (Fig. C). Post-inflammatory hypopigmentation may also occur.

Microscopic features

1. In post-inflammatory hyperpigmentation, increased melanization may be present in the epidermis and/or dermis. Dermal melanization is characterized by accumulations of "melanophages" (Figs. D,E).
2. Post-inflammatory hypopigmentation is the result of partial loss of epidermal melanin.

CHRONIC DERMATITIS

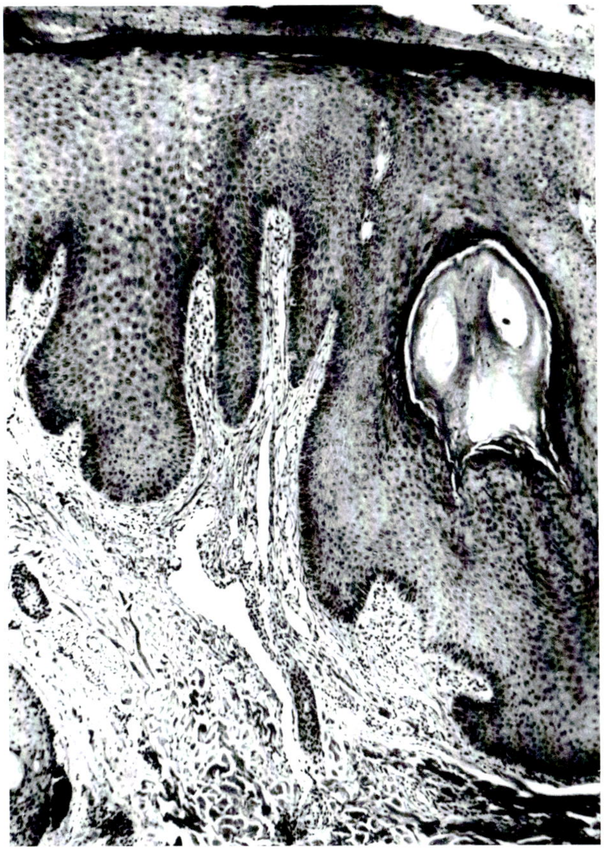

A
X65

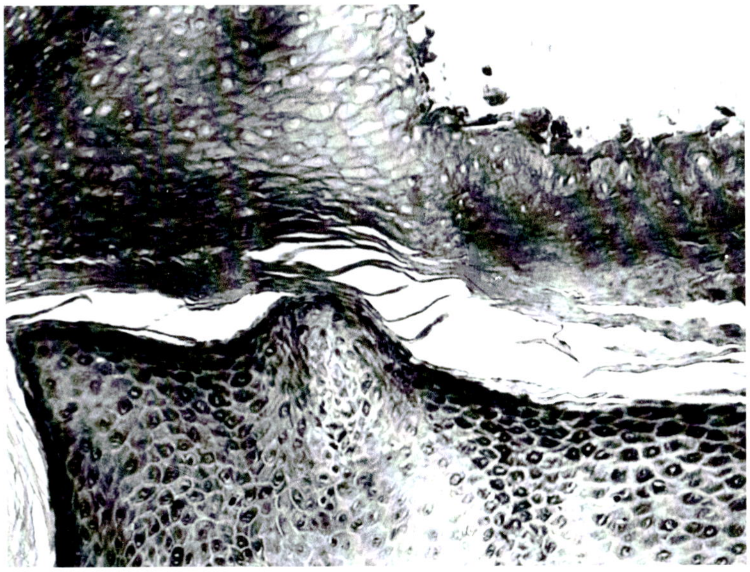

B X200

CHRONIC DERMATITIS: POST-INFLAMMATORY HYPERPIGMENTATION

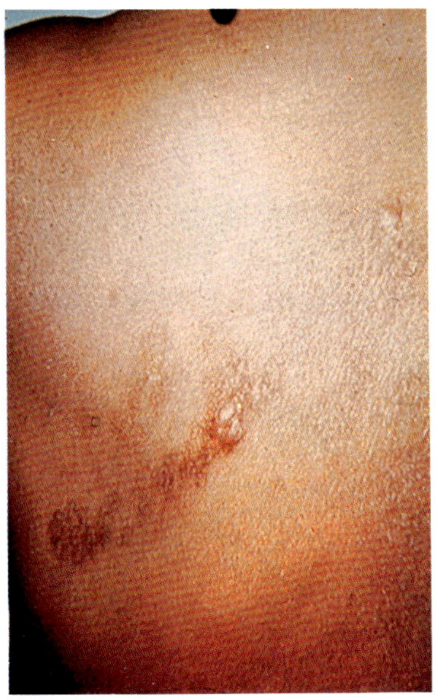

C

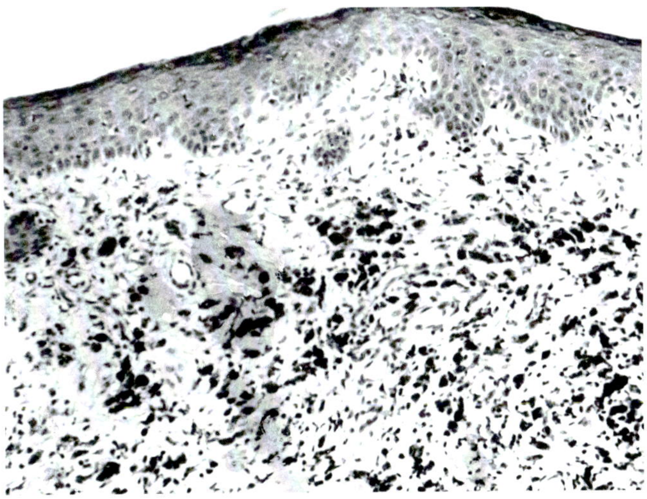

D X100

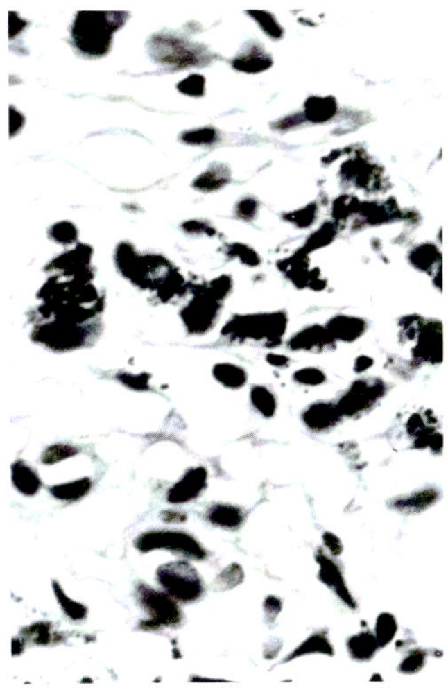

E X700

PITYRIASIS ALBA

Pityriasis alba is a common form of dermatitis (Fig. A). Dark-skinned races may be more frequently affected than others. There are focal, scaling, hypopigmented lesions. Pityriasis alba is an example of post-inflammatory hypopigmentation. The cause is unknown. It has been proposed that it is a variant of atopic dermatitis. The incidence is highest in children; the face and upper arms are common sites. The lesions resemble hypopigmented lesions of tinea versicolor. Distinction can be made by direct microscopic examination of scales in a KOH preparation. Early lesions of pityriasis alba may be pink in color.

PITYRIASIS ALBA

A
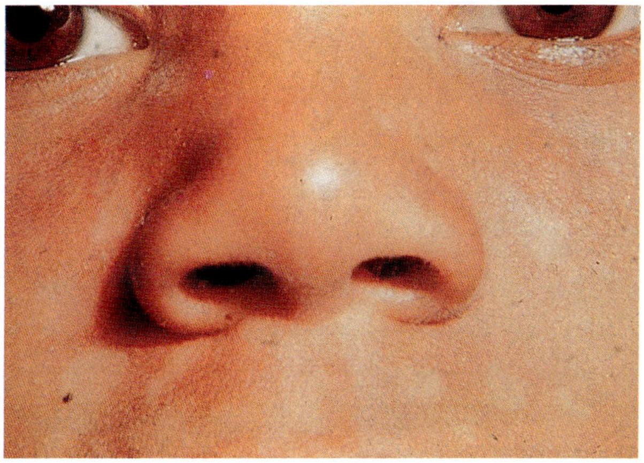

Microscopically Distinctive Forms of Dermatitis

SEBORRHEIC DERMATITIS

Seborrheic dermatitis is an erythematous, scaling eruption which is prevalent on the scalp, face (Fig. A), and intertriginous areas. It is of unknown cause. The distribution of seborrheic dermatitis appears to correspond to areas rich in sebaceous follicles, and there appears to be a correlation with high sebaceous gland activity. *Pityrosporum orbiculare* is present in large numbers in areas of seborrheic dermatitis, leading some to suggest an etiologic role for this organism. Severe variants in infants are cradle cap (Fig. C) and generalized exfoliative dermatitis (Leiner's disease) (Fig. B). There is a potentially fatal familial form of Leiner's disease associated with a dysfunction of C5. Clinical transitional forms between seborrheic dermatitis and psoriasis may occur. It is not uncommon for seborrheic dermatitis to show gradations approaching psoriasis ("seborrhiasis"). There is an association with Parkinsonism and AIDS.

Microscopic features

1. Although seborrheic dermatitis often shows microscopic features of nonspecific dermatitis, in some cases there are features resembling psoriasis.
2. In such instances, the epidermis shows a psoriasiform, regular acanthosis with clubbing of rete ridges (Fig. D), but differs from psoriasis by the presence of considerable intracellular edema and spongiosis (Fig. E). Parakeratosis is usually present (Figs. D,F), and there may be crusting (Fig. E).
3. The dermis shows a moderate chronic inflammatory infiltrate (Figs. E,F).

SEBORRHEIC DERMATITIS

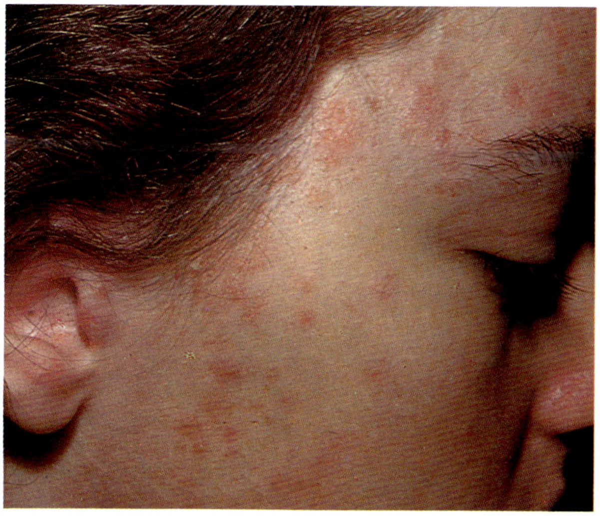

A

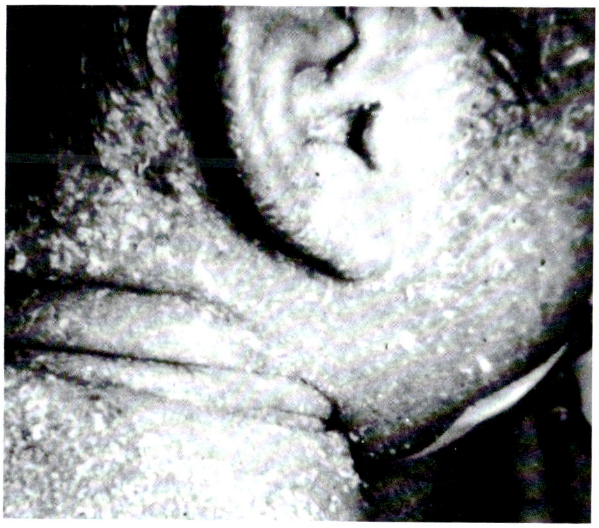

B

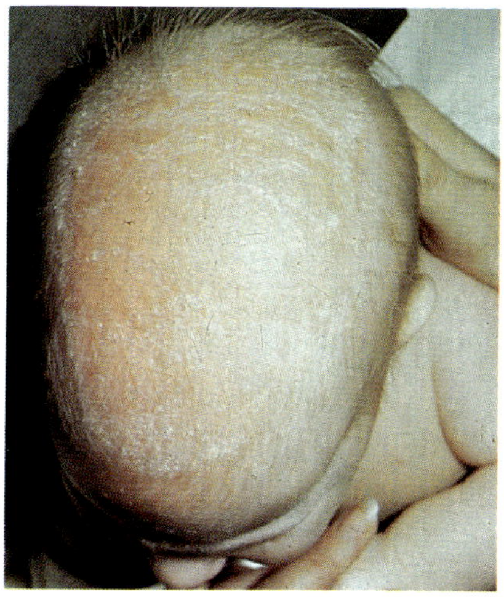

C

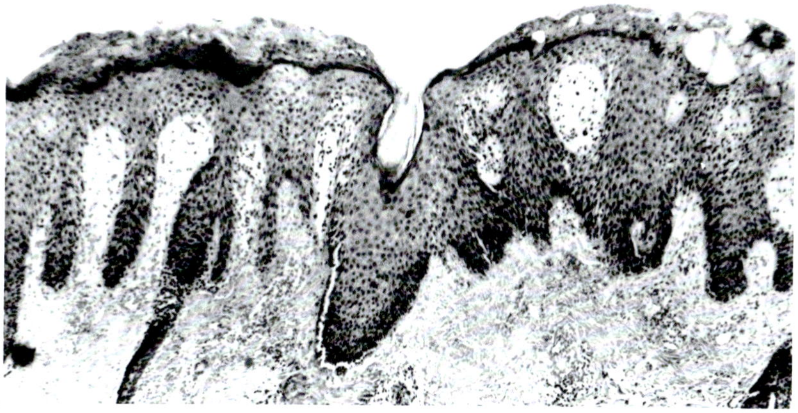

D
X64

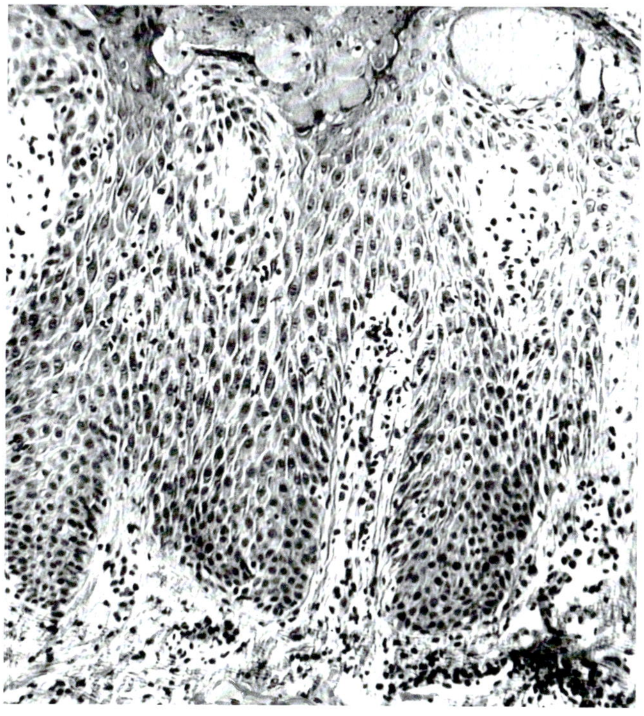

E
X230

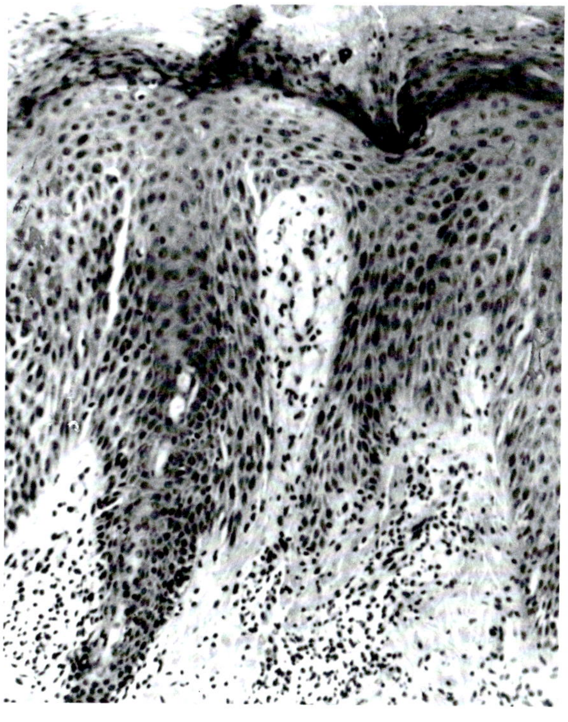

F
X230

Microscopically Distinctive Forms of Dermatitis

STASIS DERMATITIS

Stasis dermatitis involves the lower legs, particularly the malleolar areas (Fig. A). It is the result of venous stasis. The medial malleolar area is usually first involved. Hyperpigmentation (Fig. A) and ulceration (Fig. B) frequently occur. There may be edema or scarring.

Microscopic features

1. Subacute to chronic dermatitis is present, particularly in the early stages.
2. The inflammatory process usually involves the entire dermis, and sometimes the subcutaneous fat.
3. Deposits of hemosiderin are present in the dermis; these may be extensive (Figs. C,E). Hemosiderin deposits show a strong Perls reaction (Fig. D).
4. In late stages there is fibrosis (Fig. C), capillary proliferation (Fig. E), and thickening of the walls of capillaries and venules (Fig. E). Even in normal skin there is some thickening of vessel walls in the lower extremities.

Microscopic differential diagnosis

Stasis dermatitis has some resemblance to Schamberg's disease (see p. 148). However, the inflammatory process extends more deeply in stasis dermatitis, and there is usually more hemosiderin and fibrosis. Stasis dermatitis also has a resemblance to early Kaposi's sarcoma, and the frequency of Kaposi's sarcoma in the ankle area make differential diagnosis even more difficult. The presence of vascular slits and some atypia of endothelial cells can help identify Kaposi's sarcoma (see pp. 1050, 1052).

STASIS DERMATITIS

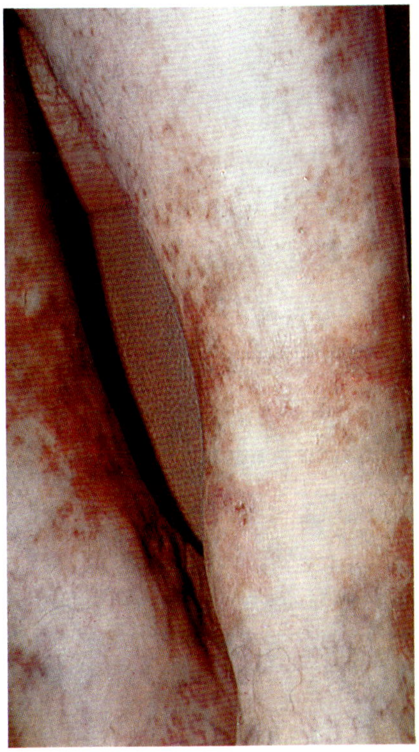

A

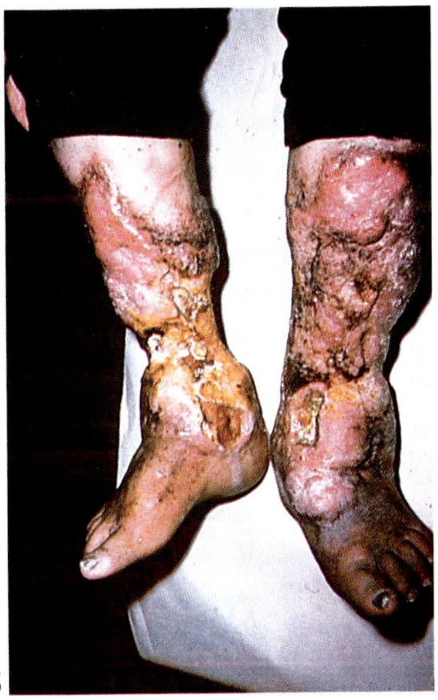

B

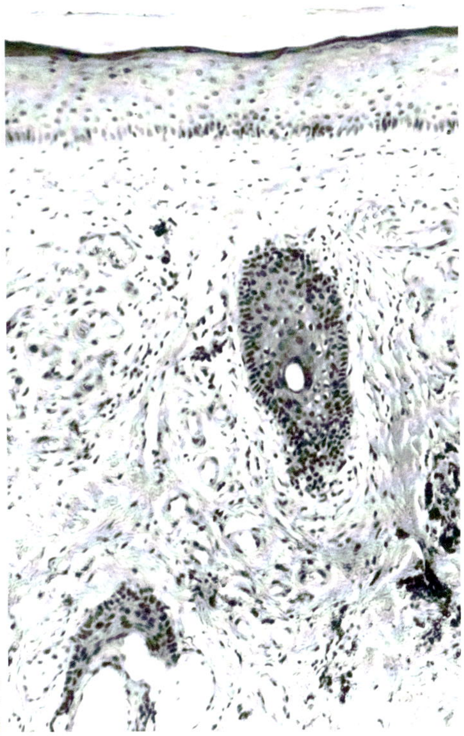

C
X170

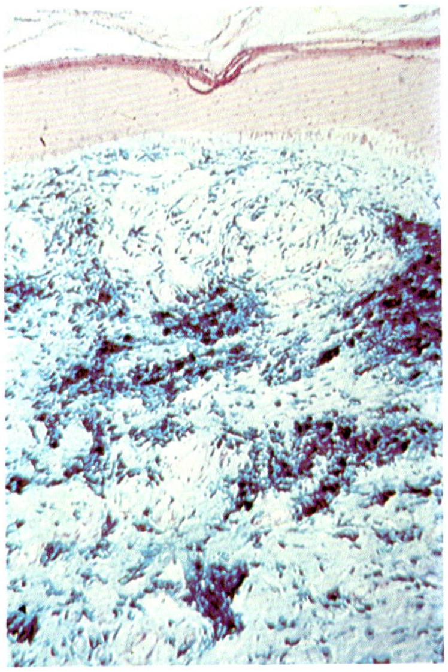

D
X100
PERLS STAIN

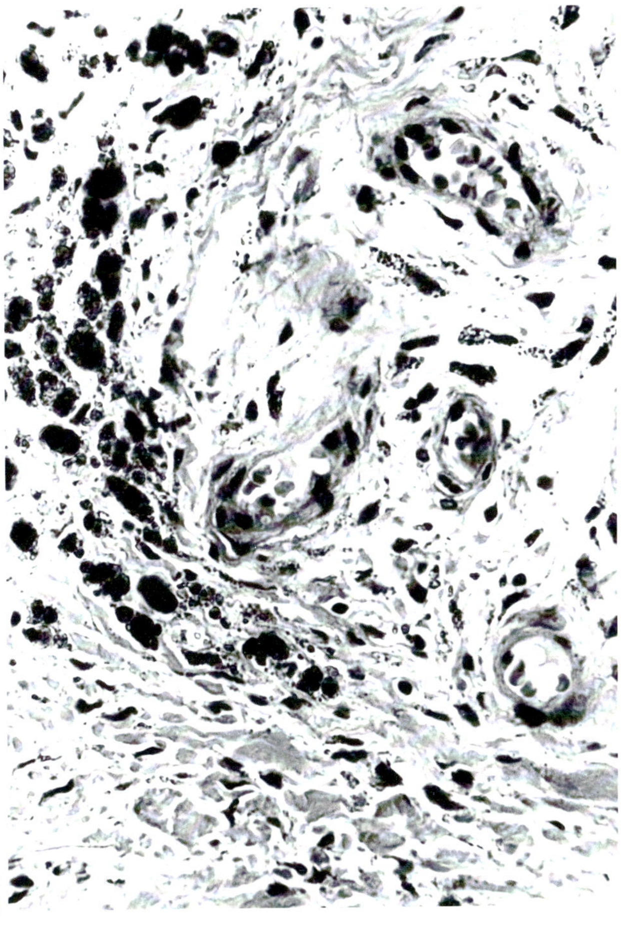

E
X700

DERMATOPATHIC LYMPHADENOPATHY (see p. 87)

Microscopic features

1. The cortical lymphoid follicles may appear normal (Fig. A) or hyperplastic.
2. There is a proliferation of paracortical cells replacing a substantial portion of the lymph node (Fig. A). These cells consist of immature lymphocytes and histiocytes, many of which contain melanin or hemosiderin (Fig. B). The lymphocytes may have cerebriform nuclei.

Distinction of dermatopathic lymphadenopathy from Hodgkin's and non-Hodgkin's lymphoma can usually be made on the basis of the absence of invasion of the lymph node capsule, preservation of lymph node architecture, and evidence of phagocytosis.

Distinction of dermatopathic lymphadenopathy from early mycosis fungoides of Sézary syndrome may be difficult. The picture of dermatopathic lymphadenopathy may undergo gradual transition into the picture of mycosis fungoides, with loss of lymph node architecture and accumulation of cells with atypical nuclei.

Comment

As mentioned, any widespread dermatitis, especially exfoliative dermatitis, may be associated with dermatopathic lymphadenopathy.

DERMATOPATHIC LYMPHADENOPATHY

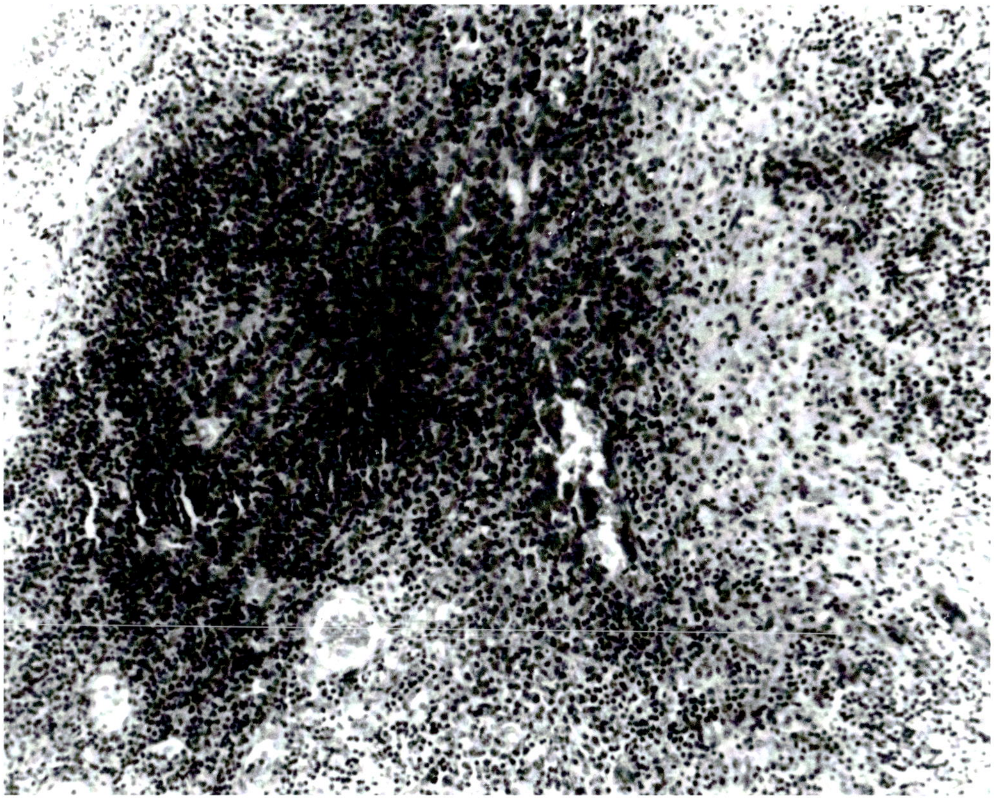

A
X240

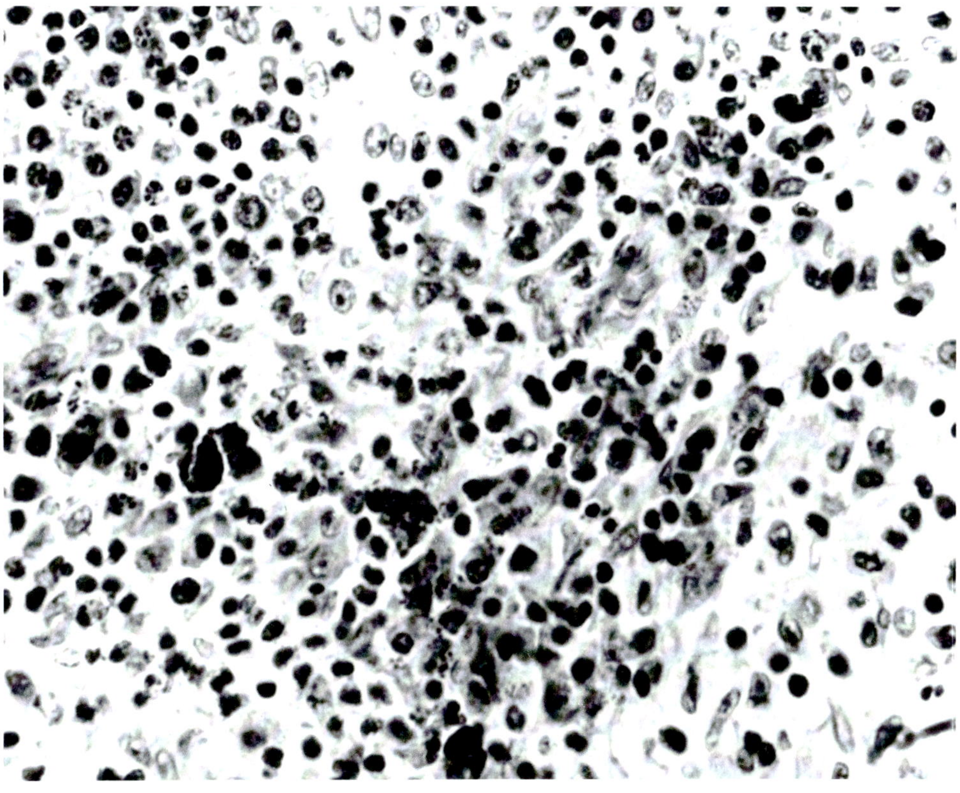

B
X750

Perivasculitis (Erythemas)

Perivasculitis consists of a group of disorders characterized by congestion of small vessels in the upper dermis, edema, a perivascular chronic inflammatory infiltrate, and lack of significant epidermal pathology. In contrast to vasculitis, the vessel walls are not significantly damaged. There may be endothelial edema. Gradation between perivasculitis and dermatitis may occur. Clinically, the lesions in this category are characterized by various degrees of erythema, with or without edema. When edema predominates, the lesions appear as wheals (urticaria). There are many disorders which have an element of perivasculitis, but, as defined, this category will be limited to those disorders in which perivasculitis is the sole or principal change.

Some disorders characterized by perivasculitis:

1. Allergic disorders
   a. Drug reactions (including fixed drug eruption)
   b. Food allergy
   c. Papular urticaria
2. Disorders caused by physical agents
   a. First degree burn
   b. Polymorphous light eruption
3. Disorders related to infectious agents
   a. Erysipelas
   b. Bacterial and viral exanthems
   c. Erythema marginatum
4. Hereditary disorders
   a. Familial angioneurotic edema
5. Idiopathic disorders
   a. Idiopathic urticaria
   Papular urticaria (lichen urticatus) is an eruption of papules and papulovesicles, commonly occuring in children. It is due to hypersensitivity to certain insect bites. In addition to perivasculitis, there may be some spongiosis.
   b. Erythema annulare centrifugum
   c. Erythema dyschromicum perstans
   d. Other figurate erythemas
   e. Nonspecific inflammatory reactions of pregnancy

Perivasculitis

Perivasculitis encompasses a wide range of entities, with clinical manifestations expressed as varying degrees of erythema and edema. Fig. A illustrates a drug reaction, with widespread, symmetrically arranged, bright red maculopapular lesions. Fig. B illustrates erysipelas (see pp. 288, 289), a superficial cellulitis, due to pathogenic streptococci. There is a well-demarcated lesion showing brawny edema and erythema. Fig. C illustrates urticaria, characterized by edematous plaques (wheals). Fig. D illustrates an infectious exanthem, scarlet fever (associated with pathogenic staphylococci or streptococci). There is diffuse erythema and punctate papular elevations.

Comment

Urticaria has a wide range of causes (see table below). Many cases have no known cause.

Classification of urticaria/angioedema

I. Immunologic urticaria/angioedema
  A. IgE-dependent
    1. Atopic diathesis
    2. Specific antigen sensitivity (foods, drugs, therapeutic agents, pollens, animal danders, *Hymenoptera* venom, helminths)
    3. Physical
      a. Dermographism
      b. Vibratory
      c. Cold
      d. Light
      e. Cholinergic
    4. Contact
  B. Complement-mediated
    1. Hereditary angioedema
    2. Acquired angioedema with malignant disorders
    3. Necrotizing vasculitis
    4. Serum sickness
    5. Reactions to blood products
II. Nonimmunologic urticaria/angioedema
  A. Direct mast cell-releasing agents
    1. Opiates
    2. Antibiotics
    3. Curare, d-tubocurarine
    4. Radiocontrast media
  B. Agents which presumably alter arachidonic acid metabolism
    1. Aspirin and nonsteroidal anti-inflammatory agents
    2. Azo dyes and benzoates
III. Idiopathic urticaria/angioedema

From Fitzpatrick, T. et al. *Dermatology in General Medicine*, McGraw-Hill, New York, p. 1284, 1987.

PERIVASCULITIS

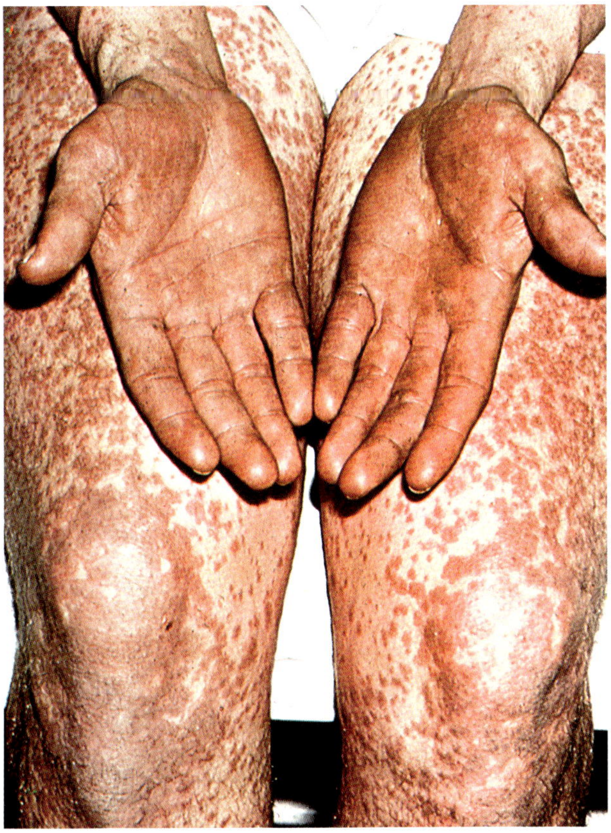

A

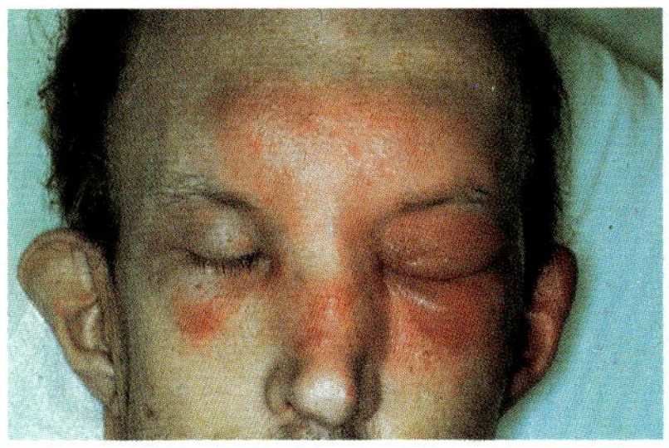

B

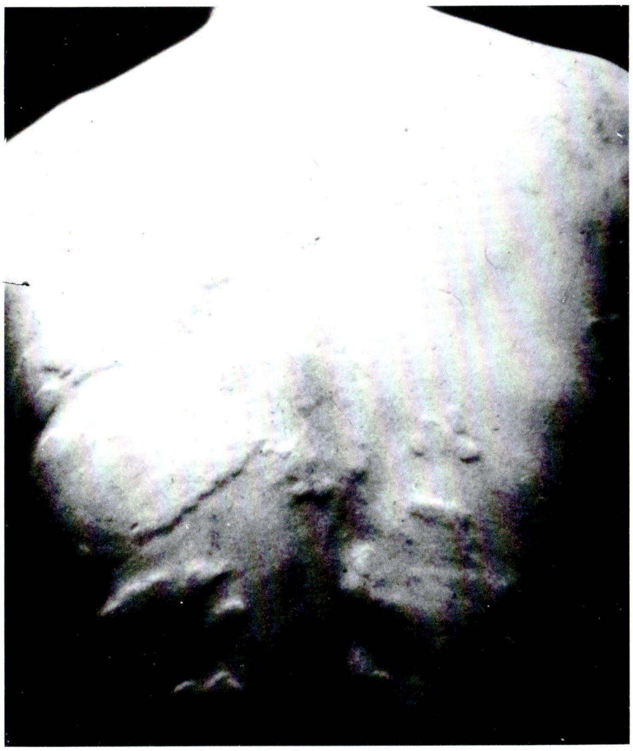

C

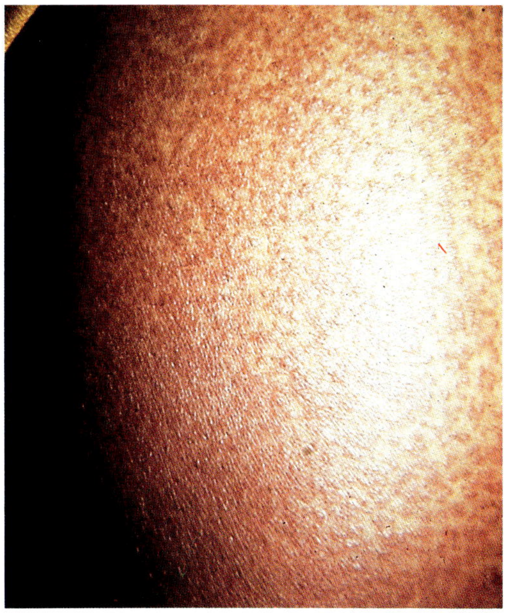

D

PERIVASCULITIS continued ⇨

PERIVASCULITIS

Comment

1. *Drug Reactions*

Drug reactions may have immunologic or nonimmunologic mechanisms. The clinical manifestations vary; they include urticaria, erythema, morbilliform eruptions, erythema multiforme, vasculitis, and erythema nodosum. Urticarial, erythematous, and morbilliform drug eruptions have the nonspecific histologic picture of perivasculitis. Erythema multiforme, vasculitis, and erythema nodosum are discussed elsewhere. Certain drug eruptions have special histologic and/or clinical patterns. These include fixed drug eruption, halide reactions, and argyria, which are discussed on pp. 472 to 480.

Drugs can produce reactions simulating lichen planus, lupus erythematosus, pemphigus vulgaris, or elastosis perforans serpiginosa. Dilantin can produce a pseudolymphoma syndrome, among other reactions. Inorganic trivalent arsenicals can produce premalignant cutaneous lesions having the histologic picture of Bowen's disease.

Birth control drugs can cause changes identical to porphyria cutanea tarda. The changes are reversible if drugs are withdrawn promptly.

2. *Inflammatory reactions of pregnancy*

A variety of inflammatory reactions have been described in association with pregnancy. These include prurigo gestationis, papular dermatitis of pregnancy, pruritic folliculitis of pregnancy, autoimmune progesterone dermatitis of pregnancy, pruritic urticarial papules and plaques of pregnancy (PUPPP), impetigo herpetiformis, and herpes gestationis. In addition, there is prurigo associated with benign recurrent intrahepatic cholestasis of late pregnancy. Perivasculitis is present in some of these disorders.

Papular dermatitis of pregnancy and prurigo gestationis are poorly defined, pruritic, papular eruptions. Papular dermatitis of pregnancy has been described as having elevated urinary gonadotropins. Pruritic folliculitis occurs during the last half of pregnancy. Autoimmune progesterone dermatitis of pregnancy is an extremely rare dermatosis with papules and pustules on extensor surfaces.

PUPPP is a common pruritic symmetrical eruption occurring late in the third trimester of pregnancy. Initially, there are numerous papules on the abdomen (Figs. A,B). These coalesce to form large erythematous plaques centered about the umbilicus. Urticarial and target-like lesions occur. Further extension results in involvement of buttocks and thighs. Other parts of the extremities may be involved. Often initial lesions are located in striae distensae. The histologic picture is that of a nonspecific perivasculitis. Eosinophils may be present.

Impetigo herpetiformis is a variant of pustular psoriasis (see p. 454) which occurs in pregnancy. It can be life-threatening to mother and fetus.Herpes gestationis is a vesiculobullous dermatosis which may be immunologically mediated. It is discussed on p. 568.

PRURITIC URTICARIAL PAPULES AND PLAQUES OF PREGNANCY (PUPPP)

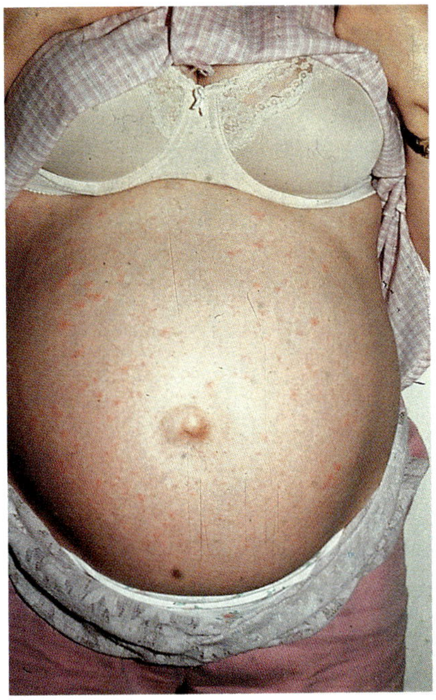

A

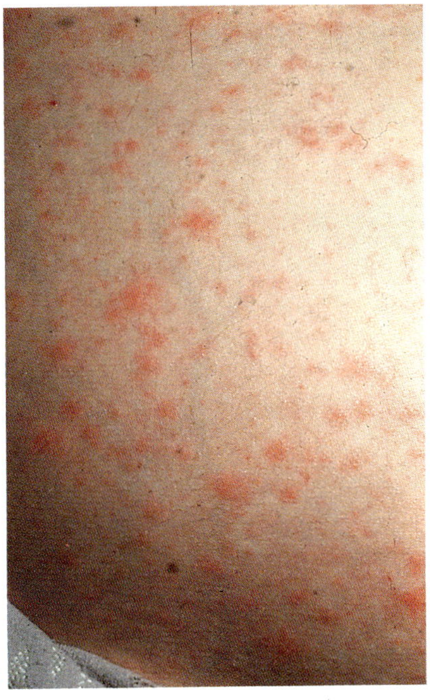

B

PERIVASCULITIS continued

PERIVASCULITIS

Microscopic features

1. Vascular dilation is present (Fig. B).
2. There is a perivascular inflammatory infiltrate of varying intensity composed principally of lymphoid cells (Figs. A,B).
3. There is a varying degree of edema, principally in the upper dermis (Fig. A), and around the small dermal vessels (Fig. B). In urticaria the edema is severe; in angioedema the edema extends into the subcutaneous tissue. Eosinophils and neutrophils may be present in urticaria.
4. Epidermal changes are generally absent (Fig. A).

Comment

1. Measles, in addition to general features of perivasculitis, may show multinucleated keratinocytes with overlying parakeratosis. Some of these multinucleated cells may show viral inclusions in the nucleus and/or cytoplasm.
2. Erysipelas has a large number of neutrophils in the infiltrate.
3. The morbilliform exanthem associated with AIDS shows atypical cells in the infiltrate.
4. *Eosinophilic cellulitis* (Wells' syndrome) is a rare entity characterized by sudden outbreaks of erythematous swellings that may be painful or pruritic. Blisters may be present. The early histopathologic picture shows an infiltrate composed mainly of eosinophils, with extensive degranulation. The infiltrate may extend deeply. After a few weeks, fibrinoid necrosis of collagen with surrounding eosinophils and histiocytes is observed. Such foci are called *flame figures*. As the lesions regress, granulomas form at sites of flame figures. Flame figures are not specific. They can be seen in insect bites and pseudolymphomas.

PERIVASCULITIS

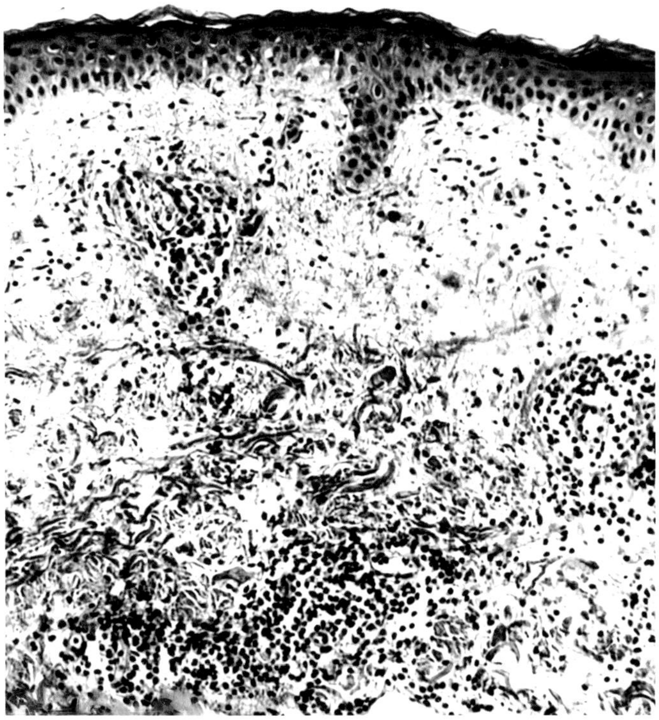

A
X200

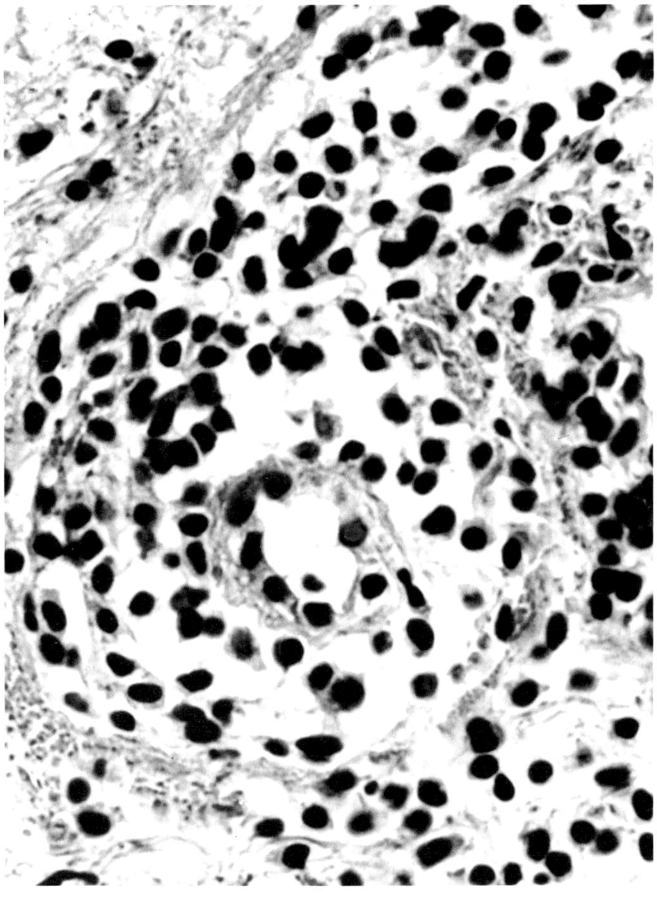

B
X1000

PERIVASCULITIS continued ⇨

Perivasculitis: Special Variants

FIGURATE ERYTHEMAS: ERYTHEMA ANNULARE CENTRIFUGUM

The figurate erythemas include a group of eruptions characterized by annular or polycyclic lesions, which may be fixed or migratory. Entities in this group include erythema annulare centrifugum, erythema gyratum repens, erythema chronicum migrans, necrolytic migratory erythema, and erythema dyschromicum perstans.

Erythema annulare centrifugum (Fig. A) is characterized by migrating annular, edematous, erythematous lesions. These disappear over a period of time and are replaced by new lesions. It is believed that erythema annulare centrifugum may represent an immunologic response to a variety of infectious and neoplastic antigens, but many cases remain totally unexplained. Superficial and deep variants have been described. The deep variant has no epidermal change; the superficial variant has scaling. *Erythema gyratum repens* has a very complex polycyclic pattern, resembling the grain of wood. Lesions tend to be scaling, to move very rapidly, and to involve large areas of the body. Most cases have been associated with internal malignancy. *Erythema chronicum migrans* is the cutaneous manifestation of Lyme disease, now known to be caused by a tick-borne spirochaete. Lesions are entirely dermal except for the bite site. *Necrolytic migratory erythema* is associated with glucagonoma, but can be seen in various combinations of essential fatty acid, zinc, and amino acid deficiencies. There are polycyclic areas of scaling, blistering, and erosive erythema, coupled with intertrigo and stomatitis.

Microscopic features

1. Erythema annulare centrifugum has the most distinctive histologic features of the figurate erythema group.
2. There is a dense perivascular infiltrate with a "coatsleeve" distribution (Figs. B,C).
3. The infiltrate is composed principally of lymphoid cells (Fig. C). Occasional histiocytes and eosinophils may be present.
4. In the superficial type of erythema annulare centrifugum there is spongiosis and parakeratosis; acanthosis may also be present. In the deep type, the epidermis is normal.
5. The other types of figurate erythema tend to have less compact perivascular inflammation. In erythema chronicum migrans, the causative spirochaete may be demonstrated in tissue sections. In necrolytic migratory erythema, there is much epidermal necrosis.

ERYTHEMA ANNULARE CENTRIFUGUM

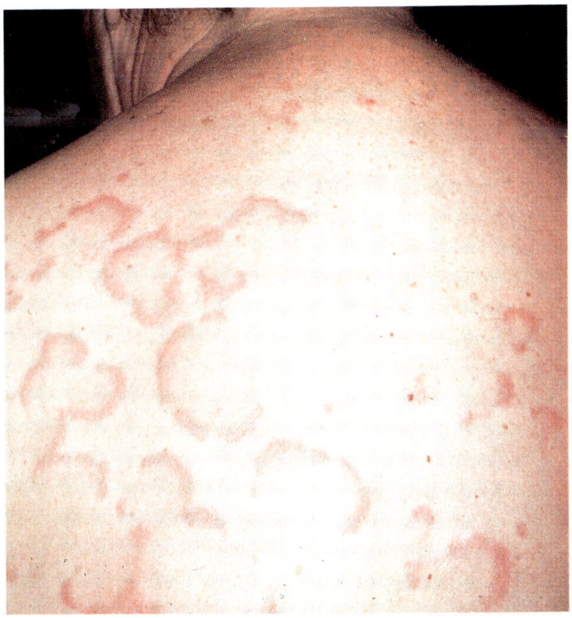

A

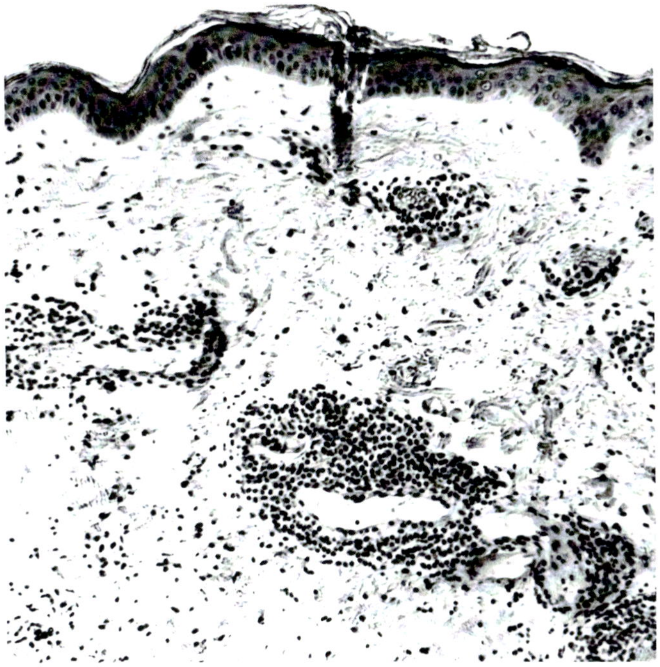

B
X220

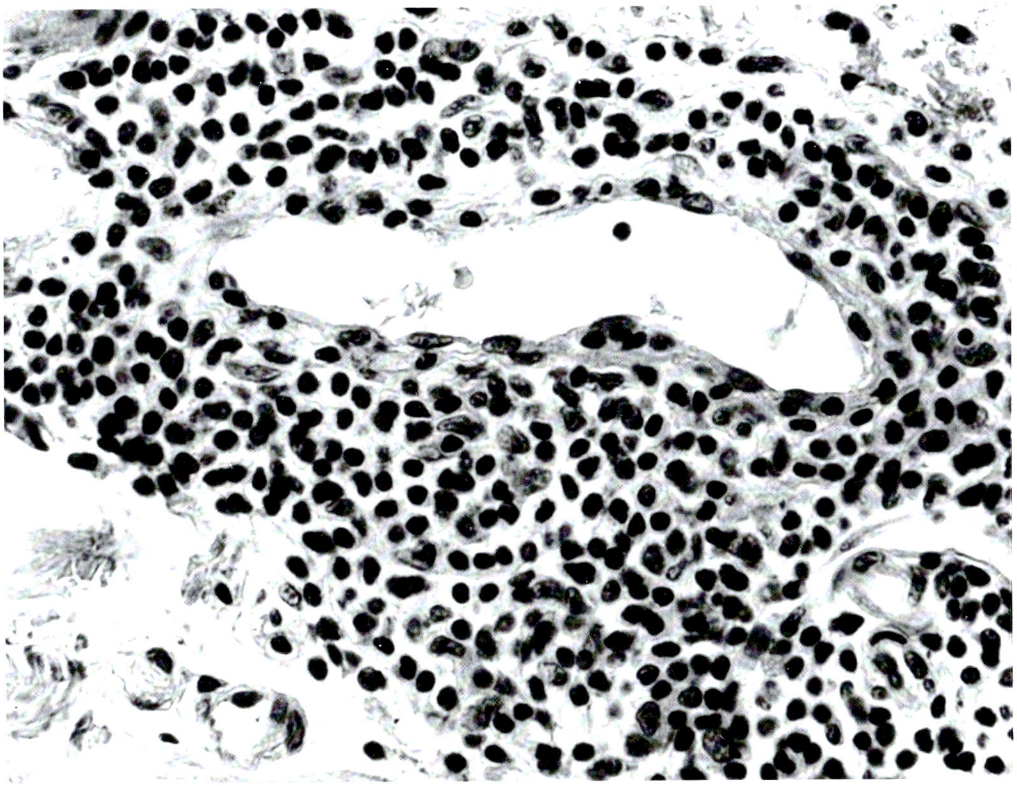

C
X720

PERIVASCULITIS continued ⇨

Perivasculitis: Special Variants

ERYTHEMA DYSCHROMICUM PERSTANS (ASHY DERMATOSIS)

Erythema dyschromicum perstans is a disorder of unknown origin characterized by slate-gray macules (Figs. A,B). Early lesions are erythematous; these eventually develop the typical slate-gray color. There is a resemblance to fixed drug eruption. Lesions tend to be located on the trunk, arms, and face. Most patients with this disorder have been from Latin America, but recent reports have described erythema dyschromicum perstans in northern Europeans and North Americans. Erythema dyschromicum perstans does not fit easily into standard categories. It has been suggested that it is a type of perivasculitis.

Microscopic features

1. The epidermis shows hydropic damage of the basal layer (Figs. C,D) and acanthosis (Figs. C,D).
2. A moderate nonspecific lymphocytic inflammatory infiltrate is present in the dermis (Figs. C,D); "melanophages" are usually numerous.
3. The late stage shows only "melanophages."

Microscopic differential diagnosis

1. The hydropic damage to the basal layer results in a resemblance to lupus erythematosus. However, hyperkeratotic plugging, atrophy of the epidermis, and a periappendageal dermal infiltrate are lacking. There is also some resemblance to lichen planus. Some believe that erythema dyschromicum perstans is a variant of lichen planus.
2. In lesions with minimal or absent hydropic damage of the basal layer, differentiation from other conditions showing dermal "melanophages" (e.g., fixed drug eruption, late stage of incontinentia pigmenti) cannot be made microscopically.

ERYTHEMA DYSCHROMICUM PERSTANS

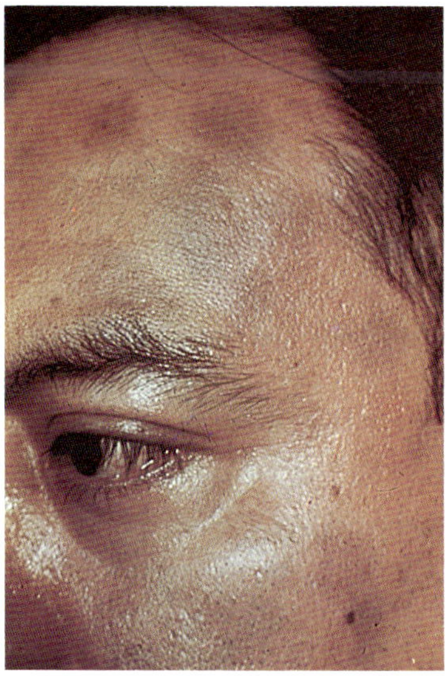

A

B

Figs. A,B courtesy Dr. John Knox

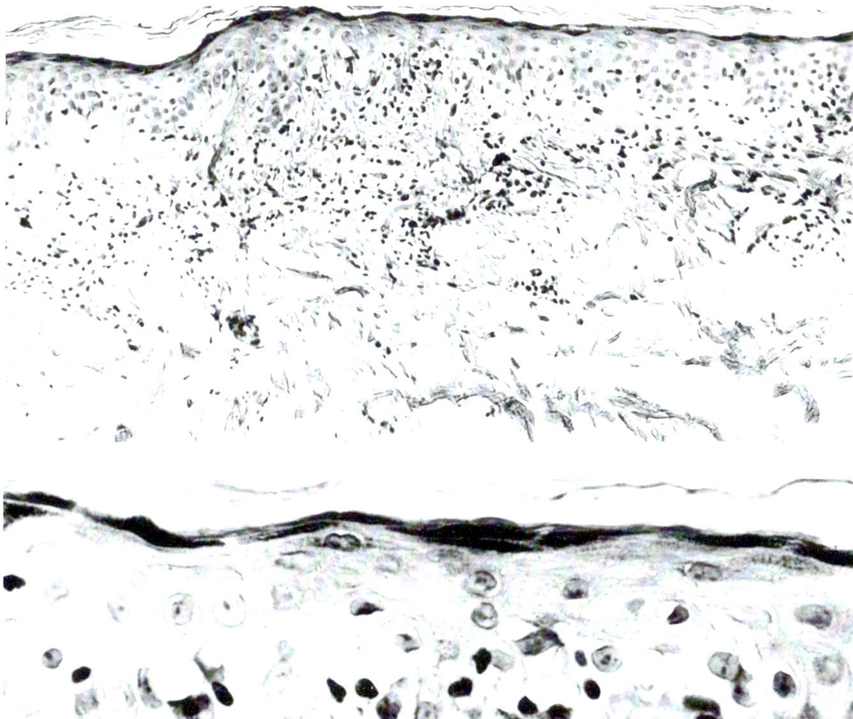

C
X150

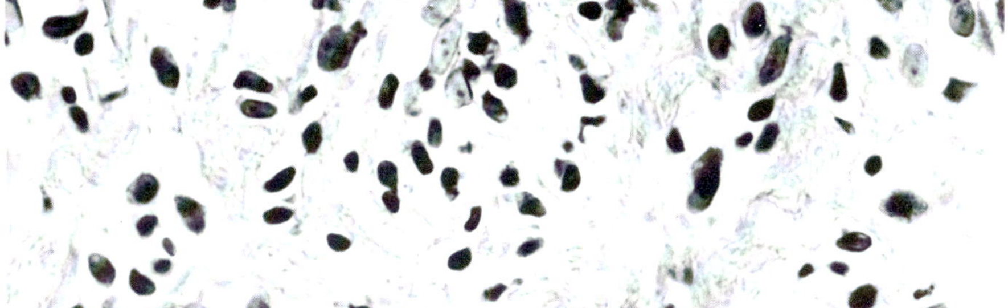

D
X650

Suggested Reading

Dermatitis and Perivasculitis

Dermatitis

GENERAL REFERENCES

Achten, G. and Delesoluse, J. Pathogenesis of allergic contact dermatitis. *Arch. Belg. Dermatol. Syph.*, 28:47, 1973.

Ackerman, A., Breza, T. and Capland, L. Spongiotic simulants of mycosis fungoides. *Arch. Dermatol.*, 109:218, 1974.

Aiba, S. and Tagami, H. Immunohistologic studies in pityriasis rosea: Evidence for cellular immune reaction in the lesional epidermis. *Arch. Dermatol.*, 121:761, 1985.

Altman, J. Parapsoriasis: A histopathologic review and classification. *Semin. Dermatol.*, 3:14, 1984.

Aoshima, T., Komura, J. and Ofuji, S. Virus-like particles in the herald patch of pityriasis rosea. *Dermatologica*, 162:64, 1981.

Baer, R. and Harris, H. Types of cutaneous reactions to drugs. *JAMA*, 202:710, 1967.

Bandmann, H. Histopathology of allergic cutaneous test reactions. *Acta Derm. Venereol.*, 45:3, 1965.

Bardach, H. and Raff, M. Poikilodermatische Parapsoriasis. *Hautarzt*, 28:542, 1977.

Barnes, P. and Moynahan, E. Zinc deficiency in acrodermatitis enteropathica: Multiple dietary intolerance treated with synthetic diet. *Proc. R. Soc. Med.*, 66:327, 1973.

Bassaly, M. et al. Studies on pityriasis alba. *Arch. Dermatol.*, 88:272, 1963.

Binazzi, M. Some research on parapsoriasis and lymphoma. *Arch. Dermatol. Res.* , 258:17, 1977.

Bonvalet, D. et al. Les différentes formes du parapsoriasis en plaques. *Ann. Dermatol. Venereol.* , 104:18, 1977.

Braun-Falco, O. and Burg, G. Celluläres Infiltrat und Capillaren bei Neurodermatitis diffusa. *Arch. Dermatol. Forsch.*, 249:113, 1974.

Braun-Falco, O. and Petry, G. Zur Feinstruktur der Epidermis bei chronischem nummulärem Ekzem. I. *Arch. Klin. Exp. Derm.*, 222:219, 1965. II. *Arch. Klin. Exp. Derm.*, 224:63, 1966.

Brocq, L. Les parapsoriasis. *Ann. Dermatol. Syphiligr.* (Paris), 3:433, 1902.

Bunch, L. and Tilley, J. Pityriasis rosea: A histologic and serologic study. *Arch. Dermatol.*, 84:79, 1961.

Carr, R., Scarpelli, D. and Greider, M. Allergic contact dermatitis: Light and electron microscopic study. *Dermatologica*, 137:358, 1968.

Charles, C., Johnson, B. and Robinson, T. Lichen striatus. *J. Cutan. Pathol.*, 1:265, 1974.

Chuang, T. et al. Pityriasis rosea in Rochester, Minnesota, 1969 to 1978: A 10-year epidemiologic study. *J. Am. Acad. Dermatol.*, 7:80, 1982.

Davies, J. Seborrheic eczema: An attempt to define the scope of the term. *Br. J. Dermatol.*, 64:213, 1952.

Dvorak, H., Mihm, M., Jr. and Dvorak, A. Morphology of delayed-type hypersensitivity in man. *J. Invest. Dermatol.*, 67:391, 1976.

Everett, M. and Handington, J. Parapsoriasis. *J. Cont. Educ. Dermatol.*, 17:12, 1978.

Fisher, A. *Contact Dermatitis.* 3rd Ed. Philadelphia, Lea & Febiger, 1986.

Fisher, J. and Cooke, R. Experimental toxic and allergic contact dermatitis. II. A histopathologic study. *J. Allergy*, 29:411, 1958.

Fleischmajer, R., Pascher, F. and Sims, C. Parapsoriasis en plaques and mycosis fungoides. *Dermatologica*, 131:149, 1965.

Fox, H. Partial depigmentation: Chiefly on the face in Negro children. *Arch. Dermatol. Syphilol.*, 7:268. 1923.

Frichot, B., III and Zelickson, A. Steroids, lysosomes and dermatitis. *Acta Derm. Venereol.*, 52:311, 1972.

Goldberg, L. Xantho-erythrodermia (Crocker). *Arch. Dermatol.*, 88:901, 1963.

Griffiths, W. Lichen striatus. *Proc. R. Soc. Med.*, 66:895, 1973.

Hagedorn, M. Electron microscopic findings in parapsoriasis en plaque (abstr.). *J. Cutan. Pathol.*, 5:295, 1978.

Hanifin, J. and Lobitz, W. Newer concepts of atopic dermatitis. *Arch. Dermatol.*, 113:663, 1977.

Heid, E. et al. Der Verlauf der Parapsoriasis en plaques (Brocq'sche Krankheit). *Z. Haut.*, 52:658, 1977.

Hendricks, A. and Lohr, J. Pityriasis rosea in infancy. *Arch. Dermatol.*, 115:896, 1979.

Hu, C. and Winkelmann, R. Digitate dermatosis. A new look at symmetrical small plaque parapsoriasis. *Arch. Dermatol.*, 107:65, 1973.

Jones, R. The histogenesis of eczema. *Clin. Exp. Dermatol.*, 8:213, 1983.

Karl, H., Burg, G. and Braun-Falco, O. Quantitative and qualitative dynamics of the epidermal and cellular inflammatory reaction in primary toxic and allergic dinitrochlorobenzene contact dermatitis in guinea pigs. *Arch. Derm. Forsch.*, 249:207, 1974.

Kirshbaum, B., Beerman, H. and Stahl, E. Drug eruption: A review of some of the recent literature. *Am. J. Med. Sci.*, 240:512, 1960.

Kligman, A. Poison ivy (Rhus) dermatitis: An experimental study. *Arch. Dermatol.*, 77:149, 1958.

Krestin, D. The seborrheic facies as a manifestation of postencephalitic parkinsonism and allied disorders. *Q. J. Med.*, 21:177, 1927.

Lambert, W. and Everett, M. The nosology of parapsoriasis. (Review) *J. Am. Acad. Dermatol.*, 5:373, 1981.

Laugier, P. et al. Parapsoriasis en plaques, de type poikilodermique avec infiltrat lymphohistiocytaire evolutif (étude ultrastructurale). *Ann. Dermatol. Venereol.* 106:507, 1979.

Lipman-Cohen, E. Pityriasis rosea. *Br. J. Dermatol.*, 79:533, 1967.

McCarthy, L. Differential diagnosis of parapsoriasis. *Arch. Dermatol. Syph.*, 45:81, 1942.

McMillan, E. et al. Identification of T-cells in parapsoriasis infiltrates: Use of an anti-human T-cell serum and the immunoperoxidase technique. *Arch. Dermatol.*, 118:238, 1982.

McMillan, E. et al. *In situ* demonstration of "T" cell subsets in atrophic parapsoriasis. *J. Am. Acad. Dermatol.*, 6:32, 1982.

McMillan, E. et al. *In situ* immunological phenotyping of mycosis fungoides. *J. Am. Acad. Dermatol.*, 6:888, 1982.

McMillan, E. et al. OKT 9 reactivity in mycosis fungoides and large plaque (atrophic) parapsoriasis. *Cancer*, 51:1403, 1983.

McPherson, A. et al. Is pityriasis rosea an infectious disease? *Lancet*, 2:1077, 1980.

Medenica, M. and Rostenberg, A., Jr. A comparative light and electron microscopic study of primary irritant contact dermatitis and allergic contact dermatitis. *J. Invest. Dermatol.*, 56:259, 1971.

Messenger, A. et al. Case clustering in pityriasis rosea: Support for role of an infective agent. *Br. Med. J.*, 284:371, 1982.

Michaelsson, G. Zinc therapy in acrodermatitis enteropathica. *Acta Derm. Venereol.*, 54:377, 1974.

Mihm, M., Jr. et al. The structure of normal skin and the morphology of atopic eczema. *J. Invest. Dermatol.*, 67:305, 1976.

Miller, C. Contact eczematous dermatitis and patch tests: A histologic study. *Arch. Dermatol. Syph.*, 56:678, 1947.

Moynahan, E. Acrodermatitis enteropathica: A lethal inherited human zinc disorder. *Lancet*, 2:399, 1974.

Musger, A. Zur Frage der nosologischen Stellung der Parapsoriasis lichenoides Brocq. *Hautarzt*, 17:280, 1966.

Nagarju, M., Adamson, D. and Rogers, J. Skin manifestations of folic acid deficiency. *Br. J. Dermatol.*, 84:32, 1971.

Nicolis, G. and Helwig, E. Exfoliative dermatitis. *Arch. Dermatol.*, 108:788, 1973.

O'Farrell, M. Pityriasis alba. *Arch. Dermatol.*, 73:376, 1956.

Ogawa, M. et al. IgE in atopic dermatitis. *Arch. Dermatol.*, 103:575, 1971.

Osmundsen, P. Parapsoriasis en plaques. *Acta Derm. Venereol.* (Stockh.), 48:345, 1968.

Panizzon, R. and Bloch, P. Histopathology of pityriasis rosea Gibert: Qualitative and quantitative light-microscopic study of 62 biopsies of 40 patients. *Dermatologica*, 165:551, 1982.

Perlman, H. and Lubowe, I. Pityriasis in children. *J. Pediatr.*, 40:109, 1952.

Pinkus, H. Lichen striatus and lichen planus. *J. Invest. Dermatol.*, 11:9, 1948.

Prose, P. Pathologic changes in eczema. *J. Pediatr.*, 66:178, 1965.

Prose, P. and Sedlis, E. Morphologic and histochemical studies of atopic eczema in infants and children. *J. Invest. Dermatol.*, 34:149, 1960.

Rachelefsky, G. et al. Defective T-cell function in atopic dermatitis. *J. Allergy Clin. Immunol.*, 57:569, 1976.

Reed, R., Meek, T. and Ichinose, H. Lichen striatus: A model for the histologic spectrum of lichenoid reactions. *J. Cutan. Pathol.*, 2:1, 1975.

Rees, R. *Dermatoses Due to Physical and Environmental Factors.* Springfield, IL, Thomas, 1962.

Sachs, W., Miller, C. and Gray, M. Neurodermatitic reaction. *Arch. Dermatol. Syph.*, 54:397, 1946.

Salley, G. et al. The late phase of the immediate wheal-and-flare skin reaction: Its dependence on IgE antibodies. *J. Clin. Invest.*, 58:408, 1976.

Samman, P. The natural history of parapsoriasis en plaques (chronic superficial dermatitis) and prereticulotic poikiloderma. *Br. J. Dermatol.*. 87:405, 1972.

——. Survey of reticuloses and premycotic eruptions: A preliminary report. *Br. J. Dermatol.*, 76:1, 1964.

Sanchez, J. and Ackerman, A. The patch stage of mycosis fungoides. *Am. J. Dermatopathol.*, 1:5, 1979.

Scheffer, E., Meijer, C. and Van Vloten, W. Dermatopathic lymphadenopathy and lymph node involvement in mycosis fungoides. *Cancer,* 45:137, 1980.

Shaffer, B. and Beerman, H. Lichen simplex chronicus and variants. *Arch. Dermatol. Syph.*, 64:340, 1951.

Silberberg-Sinakin, I. et al. Antigen-bearing Langerhans cells in skin, dermal lymphatics, and in lymph nodes. *Cell Immunol.*, 25:137, 1976.

Soeprono, F. et al. Seborrheic-like dermatitis of acquired immunodeficiency syndrome. *J. Am. Acad. Dermatol.*, 14:242, 1986.

Spangler, A. and Emerson, K. Estrogen levels and estrogen treatment in papular dermatitis of pregnancy. *Am. J. Obstet. Gynecol.*, 110:534, 1971.

Staricco, R. Lichen Striatus. *Arch. Dermatol.*, 79:311, 1959.

Stewart, M. et al. Lichen striatus. Critères histologiques. *Ann. Dermatol. Venereol.*, 104:132, 1977.

Thomsen, K. Seborrheic dermatitis and napkin dermatitis. *Acta Derm. Venereol.* (Stockh.), 61 (95, suppl.):40, 1981.

Uno, H. and Hanifin, J. Langerhans cells in acute and chronic epidermal lesions of atopic dermatitis, observed by L-dopa histofluorescence, glycol methacrylate thin section, and electron microscopy. *J. Invest. Dermatol.*, 75:52, 1980.

Vella Briffa, D., Warin, A. and Calnan, C. Parakeratosis variegata: A report of two cases and their treatment with PUVA. *Clin. Exp. Dermatol.*, 4:537, 1979.

Verbov, J. Purpuric pityriasis rosea. *Dermatologica,* 160:142, 1980.

Wantzen, G. et al. Acute HTLV-III infection associated with erythema, diagnosed by seroconversion. *Br. J. Dermatol.*, 115: 601, 1986.

Welbourn, E., Champion, R. and Parish, W. Nummular eczema with staphylococcal sensitivity. *Br. J. Dermatol.*, 93 (11, suppl.):40, 1975.

Wells, B. et al. Pityriasis alba: A ten year survey. *Arch. Dermatol.*, 82:183, 1960.

Wilkin, J. and Kirkendall, W. Pityriasis rosea-like rash from Captopril. *Arch. Dermatol.*, 118:186, 1982.

Winer, L. and Lipschultz, C. Comparative study of histology and cytology in vesiculating eruptions. *Arch. Dermatol. Syph.*, 65:270, 1952.

Wise, F. Discussion of Fox H: Partial depigmentation chiefly on the face in Negro children. *Arch. Dermatol. Syphilol.*, 7:268, 1923.

——. Parapsoriasis. *N. Y. State J. Med.*, 28:901, 1928.

Yates, V. et al. Early diagnosis of infantile seborrheic dermatitis and atopic dermatitis—clinical features. *Br. J. Dermatol.*, 108:633, 1983.

Young, E. Dyshidrotic (endogen) eczema. *Dermatologica,* 129:306, 1964.

Zaynoun, S. et al. Extensive pityriasis alba: A histological, histochemical, and ultrastructural study. *Br. J. Dermatol.*, 108:83, 1983.

SEBORRHEIC DERMATITIS

Pinkus, H. and Mehregan, A. The primary histologic lesion of seborrheic dermatitis and psoriasis. *J. Invest. Dermatol.*, 46:109, 1966.

Prieto, J. and Gonzalez, G. Histopathology of seborrheic dermatitis. *Med. Cutanea*, 2:223, 1968.

STASIS DERMATITIS

Arnoldi, C. and Linderholm, H. On the pathogenesis of the venous leg ulcer. *Acta Chir. Scand.*, 134:427, 1968.

Kulwin, M. and Hines, E., Jr. Blood vessels of the skin in chronic venous insufficiency: Clinical and pathologic study. *Arch. Dermatol. Syph.* 62:293, 1950.

DERMATOPATHIC LYMPHADENOPATHY

Adam, J. Exfoliative dermatitis. *Can. Med. Assoc. J.*, 99:661, 1968.

Hurwill, E. Dermatopathic lymphadenitis. *J. Invest. Dermatol.*, 5:197, 1942.

Laipply, T. Lipomelanotic reticular hyperplasia of lymph nodes: Report of six cases. *Arch. Int. Med.*, 81:19, 1948.

Nicolis, G. and Helwig, E. Exfoliative dermatitis. *Arch. Dermatol.*, 108:788, 1973.

Dermatitis and Perivasculitis

Perivasculitis

GENERAL REFERENCES

Ahmed, A. and Kaplan, R. Pruritic urticarial papules and plaques of pregnancy. *J. Am. Acad. Dermatol.*, 4:679, 1981.

Arndt, K. and Jick, H. Rates of cutaneous reactions to drugs. *JAMA*, 235:918, 1976.

Atkins, P. and Zweiman, B. Mediator release in local heat urticaria. *J. Allergy Clin. Immunol.*, 68:286, 1981.

Baer, R. and Harris, H. Types of cutaneous reactions to drugs. *JAMA*, 202:710, 1967.

Baughman, R. and Jillson, O. Seven specific types of urticaria. *Ann. Allerg.*, 21:248, 1963.

Beall, G. Urticaria: A review of laboratory and clinical observations. *Medicine*, 43:131, 1964.

Cahn, M. et al. Lupus erythematosus and polymorphous light eruption: An experimental study on their possible relationship. *J. Invest. Dermatol.*, 21:375, 1953.

Callen, J. and Hanno, R. Pruritic urticarial papules and plaques of pregnancy (PUPPP): A clinicopathologic study. *J. Am. Acad. Dermatol.*, 5:401, 1981.

Chafee, F. and Settipane, G. Aspirin intolerance. I. Frequency in an allergic population. *J. Allergy Clin. Immunol.*, 53:193, 1974.

Champion, R. et al. Urticaria and angio-oedema: A review of 554 patients. *Br. J. Dermatol.*, 81:588, 1969.

Charlesworth, E. Phenytoin induced pseudolymphoma syndrome. *Arch. Dermatol.*, 113:477, 1977.

Davidson, B. et al. Cimetidine: Associated exacerbation of cutaneous lupus erythematosus. *Arch. Int. Med.*, 142:101, 1982.

Derbes, V. The fixed eruption. *JAMA*, 190:765, 1964.

Doeglas, H. Reactions to aspirin and food additives in patients with chronic urticaria, including the physical urticarias. *Br. J. Dermatol.*, 93:135, 1975.

Donaldson, V. and Rosen, F. Hereditary angioneurotic edema: A clinical survey. *Pediatrics*, 37:1017, 1966.

Emmett, E. Phototoxicity from exogenous agents. *Photochem. Photobiol.*, 30:429, 1979.

Epstein, S. Chlorpromazine photosensitivity. *Arch. Dermatol.*, 98:354, 1968.

Girard, J. et al. Immunological mechanisms and diagnostic tests in allergic drug reactions. *Ann. Clin. Res.*, 3:74, 1976.

Grant, J. et al. Local heat urticaria/angioedema: Evidence for histamine release without complement activation. *J. Allergy Clin. Immunol.*, 67:75, 1981.

Jansen, C. Beta-carotene treatment of polymorphous light eruption. *Dermatologica*, 149:363, 1974.

Juhlin, L. Recurrent urticaria: Clinical investigation of 330 patients. *Br. J. Dermatol.*, 104:369, 1981.

Juhlin, L. and Michaelson, G. Blood vessel response in urticaria. *Br. J. Dermatol.*, 88:66, 1970.

Kirshbaum, B., Beerman, H. and Stahl, E. Drug eruption: A review of some of the recent literature. *Am. J. Med. Sci.*, 240:512, 1960.

Lawley, T. et al. Pruritic urticarial papules and plaques of pregnancy. *JAMA*, 241:1696, 1979.

Lawrence, C. et al. Cholinergic urticaria with associated angio-oedema. *Br. J. Dermatol.*, 105:543, 1981.

Leigh, I. Mepacrine (quinacrine) pigmentation in systemic lupus erythematosus, new data from an ultrastructural, biochemical and analytical electron microscopy investigation. *Br. J. Dermatol.*, 101:147, 1979.

Litwack, K., Hoke, A. and Borchardt, K. Rose spots in typhoid fever. *Arch. Dermatol.*, 105:252, 1972.

Maibach, H. and Johnson, H. Contact urticaria syndrome. *Arch. Dermatol.*, 111:726, 1975.

Miller, D., Freeman, G. and Akers, W. Chronic urticaria: A clinical study of 50 patients. *Am. J. Med.*, 44:68, 1968.

Moritz, A. Studies of thermal injury, III. The pathology and pathogenesis of cutaneous burns: An experimental study. *Am. J. Pathol.*, 23:915, 1947.

Neumann, H. and van Joost, T. Adverse reactions of the skin to metroprolol and beta-adrenergic-blocking agents. *Dermatologica*, 162:330, 1981.

Reinhardt, L. et al. Lichenoid eruption produced by captopril. *Cutis*, 31:98, 1983.

Rosen, F. and Austen, K. The "neurotic edema" (hereditary angioedema). *N. Eng. J. Med.*, 280:1356, 1969.

Sheffer, A. and Austen, K. Vascular responses: Urticaria and angioneurotic edema. In: *Dermatology in General Medicine.* Fitzpatrick, T. et al., eds. New York, McGraw-Hill Book Co. 1971, p.1261.

Sheffer, A. et al. Exercise-induced anaphylaxis: A distinct form of physical allergy. *J. Allergy Clin. Immunol.*, 71:311, 1983.

Soter, N. and Wasserman, S. Urticaria, angioedema. (Review) *Internat. J. Dermatol.*, 18:517, 1979.

Soter, N. et al. Cold urticaria: Release into the circulation of histamine and eosinophil chemotactic factor of anaphylaxis during cold challenge. *N. Eng. J. Med.*, 294:687, 1976.

Soter, N. et al. Mast cell mediator release and alterations in lung function in individuals with cholinergic urticaria. *N. Engl. J. Med.*, 302:604, 1980.

Soter, N. et al. Solar urticaria: Release of mast cell mediators into the circulation after experimental challenge. *J. Invest. Dermatol.*, 72:282, 1979.

Tappeiner, G. et al. Hereditary angioedema: Treatment with danazol. *Br. J. Dermatol.*, 100:207, 1979.

Tappeiner, J. and Pfleger, L. Zur Histopathologie cutaner Lymphgefässe beim chronisch-rezidivierenden Erysipel der unteren Extremitäten. *Hautarzt*, 15:218, 1964.

Tas, J. Chronic urticaria: Survey of 100 hospitalized cases. *Dermatologica,* 135:90, 1967.

Ulhin, S. Pruritic urticarial papules and plaques of pregnancy. *Arch. Dermatol.*, 117:238, 1981.

Warner, L. and Fisher, B. Cutaneous manifestations of the acquired immunodeficiency syndrome. *Internat. J. Dermatol.*, 25:337, 1986.

Warrington, R. et al. Drug hypersensitivities with special reference to penicillin. In: *Immediate Hypersensitivity, Modern Concepts and Developments,* edited by M. K. Bach, New York/Basel, Dekker, p.749, 1978.

Yancey, K. et al. Pruritic urticarial papules and plaques of pregnancy (PUPPP): Clinical experience in 25 patients. *J. Am. Acad. Dermatol.*, 10:473, 1984.

EOSINOPHILIC CELLULITIS (WELLS' SYNDROME)

Dijkstra, J. et al. Eosinophilic cellulitis associated with urticaria. *J. Am. Acad. Dermatol.*, 14:32, 1986.

Marks, R. Eosinophilic cellulitis. *Aust. J. Dermatol.*, 21:10, 1980.

Nielsen, T., Schmidt, H. and Søgaard, H. Eosinophilic cellulitis (Wells' syndrome) in a child. *Arch. Dermatol.*, 117:427, 1981.

Spigel, G. and Winkelmann, R. Wells' syndrome. *Arch. Dermatol.*, 115:611, 1979.

Wells, G. Recurrent granulomatous dermatitis with eosinophilia. *Trans. St. John's Hosp. Dermatol. Soc.*, 57:46, 1971.

Wells, G. and Smith, N. Eosinophilic cellulitis. *Br. J. Dermatol.*, 100:101, 1979.

Wood, C. et al. Eosinophilic infiltration with flame figures. *Am. J. Dermatopathol.*, 8:186, 1986.

Ashurst, P. Erythema annulare centrifugum. *Arch. Dermatol.*, 95:37, 1967.
Barber, P. et al. Erythema gyratum repens with pulmonary tuberculosis. *Br. J. Dermatol.*, 98:465, 1978.
Braunstein, B. Erythema annulare centrifugum and Graves' disease. *Arch. Dermatol.*, 118:623, 1982.
Bressler, G. and Jones, R., Jr. Erythema annulare centrifugum. *J. Am. Acad. Dermatol.*, 4:597, 1981.
Burgdorfer, W. et al. Lyme disease: A tick-borne spirochetosis? *Science,* 216:1317, 1982.
Copeman, P. Erythema something or other. *Br. Med. J.*, 1:111, 1980.
Darier, J. De l'erythème annulaire centrifuge. *Ann. Dermatol. Syphiligr.*, 6:57, 1916.
Ellis, F. and Friedman, A. Erythema annulare centrifugum (Darier). Clinical and histologic study. *Arch. Dermatol. Syph.*, 70:496, 1954.
Gammel, J. Erythema gyratum repens: Skin manifestations in a patient with carcinoma of the breast. *Arch. Dermatol.*, 66:494, 1952.
Gross, G. et al. Erythema chronicum migrans with purpura and polymorphonuclear infiltrates. *Arch. Dermatol.*, 115:873, 1979.
Hammar, H. Erythema annulare centrifugum coincident with Epstein-Barr virus infection in an infant. *Acta Paediatr. Scand.*, 63:788, 1974.
Harrison, P. The annular erythemas. *Internat. J. Dermatol.*, 18:282, 1979.
Hendricks, A. et al. Erythema annulare centrifugum associated with ascariasis. *Arch Dermatol.*, 117:582, 1981.
Holt, P. and Davies, M. Erythema gyratum repens: An immunologically mediated dermatosis? *Br. J. Dermatol.*, 96:343, 1977.
Krook, G. and Waldenström, J. Relapsing annular erythema and myeloma successfully treated with cyclophosphamide. *Acta Med. Scand.*, 203:289, 1978.
Lazar, P. Cancer, erythema annulare centrifugum, autoimmunity. *Arch. Dermatol.*, 87:246, 1963.
Leavell, U., Jr., Winternitz, W. and Black J. Erythema gyratum repens and undifferentiated carcinoma. *Arch. Dermatol.*, 95:69, 1967.
——. Erythema gyratum repens and undifferentiated carcinoma. *Arch. Dermatol.*, 95:343, 1977.
Mallinson, C. et al. A glucagonoma syndrome. *Lancet,* 2:1, 1974.
Mast, W. and Burrows, W. Erythema chronicum migrans in the United States. *JAMA,* 236:859, 1976.
Naversen, D. and Gardner, L. Erythema chronicum migrans in America. *Arch. Dermatol.*, 114:253, 1978.
Scrimenti, R. Erythema chronicum migrans. *Arch. Dermatol.*, 102:104, 1970.
Shelley, W. Erythema annulare centrifugum. *Arch. Dermatol.*, 90:54, 1964.
——. Erythema annulare centrifugum due to *Candida albicans. Br. J. Dermatol.*, 77:383, 1965.
Skolnick, M. and Mainman, E. Erythema gyratum repens with metastatic adenocarcinoma. *Arch. Dermatol.*, 111:227, 1975.
Smith, L. et al. Erythema chronicum migrans. *Cutis,* 17:962, 1976.
Sonck, C. Erythema chronicum migrans with multiple lesions. *Acta Derm. Venereol.* (Stockh.), 45:34, 1965.
Stankler, L. Erythema gyratum repens: Spontaneous resolution in a healthy man. *Br. J. Dermatol.*, 99:461, 1978.
Steere, A. and Malawista, S. Cases of Lyme disease in the United States: Locations correlated with distribution of *Ixodes dammini. Ann. Int. Med.*, 91:730, 1979.
Steere, A. et al. The spirochetal etiology of Lyme disease. *N. Eng. J. Med.*, 308:733, 1983.
Summerly, R. The figurate erythemas and neoplasia. *Br. J. Dermatol.*, 76:370, 1964.
Thomson, J. and Stankler, L. Erythema gyratum repens: Reports of two further cases associated with carcinoma. *Br. J. Dermatol.*, 82:406, 1970.
White, J. and Perry, H. Erythema perstans. *Br. J. Dermatol.*, 81:641, 1969.
Willis, W. The gyrate erythemas. *Internat. J. Dermatol.*, 17:698, 1978.

Byrne, D. and Berger, R. Erythema dyschromicum perstans: A report of two cases in fair-skinned patients. *Acta Derm. Venereol.*, 54:65, 1974.

Convit, J. et al. Erythema dyschromicum perstans: A hitherto undescribed skin disease. *J. Invest. Dermatol.*, 36:457, 1961.

Knox, J., Dodge, B. and Freeman, R. Erythema dyschromicum perstans. *Arch. Dermatol.*, 97:262, 1968.

Pinkus, H. Lichenoid tissue reactions: A speculative review of the clinical spectrum of epidermal basal cell damage with special reference to erythema dyschromicum perstans. *Arch. Dermatol.*, 107:840, 1973.

Soter, N., Wand, C. and Freeman, R. Ultrastructural pathology of erythema dyschromicum perstans. *J. Invest. Dermatol.*, 52:155, 1969.

Stevenson, J. and Meura, M. Erythema dyschromicum perstans (ashy dermatosis). *Arch. Dermatol.*, 94:196, 1966.

Tschen, J. et al. Erythema dyschromicum perstans. *J. Am. Acad. Dermatol.*, 2:295, 1980.

Verbov, J. and Borrie, P. Ashy dermatosis (erythema dyschromicum perstans). *Br. J. Dermatol.*, 84:185, 1971.

Vasculitis

Classification of Vasculitis

I. Leukocytoclastic vasculitis (allergic vasculitis)
  A. Small vessel
    1. Acute type (frequently associated with systemic manifestations).
      a. Schönlein's purpura—associated with arthralgia.
      b. Henoch's purpura—associated with crises of abdominal pain and melena.
      c. Hypersensitivity angiitis (Zeek)—associated with marked pulmonary and renal involvement.
    2. Chronic type (Gougerot-Ruiter)—not associated with systemic manifestations.
    3. Urticarial vasculitis—painful, purpuric, persistent urticarial lesions with a spectrum of systemic manifestations and hypocomplimentemia. Urticarial vasculitis may vary from mild disease to a severe form resembling systemic lupus erythematosus. Urticarial vasculitis may be associated with systemic lupus erythematosus.
    4. Systemic rheumatoid vasculitis—may develop in patients with long-standing rheumatoid arthritis. There are digital infarcts and cutaneous ulcers.
    5. Hypergammaglobulinemic purpura of Waldenström—petechiae are present (usually on the lower legs) in association with a polyclonal hypergammaglobulinemia.
    6. Bacterial vasculitides (e.g., meningococcemia; gonococcemia).
    7. Arthus phenomenon.
    8. Morphologically distinctive forms of small vessel leukocytoclastic vasculitis.
      a. Granuloma faciale
      b. Erythema elevatum diutinum
      c. Sweet's syndrome
  B. Large vessel
    1. Periarteritis nodosa
  C. Granulomatous vasculitis (see opposite page)
    1. Wegener's granulomatosis
    2. Allergic granulomatosis
    3. Lymphomatoid granulomatosis
    4. Midline granuloma of the face
    5. Temporal arteritis

II. Lymphocytic vasculitis
  A. Pityriasis lichenoides
    a. PLEVA
    b. Pityriasis lichenoides chronica
  B. Purpura pigmentosa chronica

GRANULOMATOUS VASCULITIS

Allergic granulomatosis (Churg-Strauss syndrome)

This has parallels to periarteritis nodosa, but differs by an initial period of respiratory symptoms, usually asthma, pronounced eosinophilia in blood and in lesions, pulmonary infiltrations, involvement of small arteries and veins, and by the presence of palisading granulomas with central necrosis. IgE levels may be elevated. Skin lesions showing necrotizing vasculitis and nodules are often present.

Microscopically, cutaneous lesions may show leukocytoclastic vasculitis, as well as palisading granulomas with central necrosis; giant cells may be present. Subcutaneous lesions may show similar palisading granulomas embedded in an inflammatory infiltrate rich in eosinophils.

Wegener's granulomatosis

This is characterized by three main features:

a. Necrotizing granulomas of the upper and lower respiratory tract.
b. Necrotizing vasculitis involving small arteries and veins, usually involving the lungs, but with involvement of other sites.
c. Renal disease, with necrotizing glomerulitis, necrotizing vasculitis, and extraglomerular granulomas.

Papulonecrotic, hemorrhagic skin lesions may be present, as well as ulcers of the oral mucosa.

Microscopically necrotizing vasculitis and necrotizing granulomas are observed. Necrotizing granulomas show central necrosis, surrounded by a mixed inflammatory infiltrate containing giant cells; eosinophils are few or absent.

Lymphomatoid granulomatosis

This has parallels to Wegener's granulomatosis, but differs by absence of glomerulitis and absence of lesions in the upper respiratory tract. It differs histologically by the presence of a dense, polymorphous inflammatory infiltrate containing lymphoid cells with atypical-appearing nuclei. Central nervous system involvement occurs in a significant percentage of cases. There is a histologic similarity to midline granuloma of the face, but the conditions differ clinically. Cutaneous lesions when present, are papules, plaques, and nodules with tendency to ulcerate.

Midline granuloma of the face

Midline granuloma of the face is a rapidly destructive and fatal process with similarities to lymphomatoid granulomatosis.

Temporal arteritis

Temporal arteritis involves large or medium-sized elastic arteries of the temporal region; it may also involve cerebral or retinal arteries. Elderly persons are affected. The primary event is degeneration of the internal elastic lamina. This is followed by digestion and phagocytosis of the degenerated material. Typically there is an inflammatory infiltrate with giant cells; however, giant cells may be absent. Temporal arteritis may be a variant of periarteritis nodosa.

Comment:

1. Erythema multiforme (see under *bullous dermatoses*) shows a spectrum of histologic features. Lymphocytic vasculitis is commonly observed in erythema multiforme. Although in the past it was believed that leukocytoclastic vasculitis could be a component of erythema multiforme, current concepts of classification exclude leukocytoclastic vasculitis from the spectrum of erythema multiforme.
2. Kawasaki's disease, a multisystem febrile disorder usually occurring in children, may have cutaneous lesions with histologic features of periarteritis nodosa.

Leukocytoclastic Vasculitis

SMALL VESSEL

The process involves capillaries, arterioles, and venules and is characterized by fragmentation of nuclei of neutrophils (karyorrhexis). A wide range of clinical syndromes has this histologic pattern (see outline). It is currently believed that all forms of leukocytoclastic vasculitis have a pathogenesis based on localization of immune complexes in or around the blood vessel walls. Interaction of these complexes with complement attracts neutrophils (leukotaxis) with resultant destruction of the vessel walls.

Leukocytoclastic vasculitis may be cutaneous or systemic. The dominant cutaneous lesions are purpuric papules (palpable purpura). Figs. A and C show purpuric papules, vesicles, and necrotic ulcers.

Microscopic features

1. There is swelling and degeneration of the endothelial cells and infiltration of the blood vessel walls by inflammatory cells (Figs. B,D).
2. The infiltrate is principally composed of neutrophils and their fragmented nuclei ("nuclear dust"). Varying numbers of eosinophils, as well as small numbers of lymphocytes and histiocytes are also present (Figs. B,D).
3. Hemorrhage is present, often accompanied by hemosiderin.
4. Deposition of "fibrinoid" material may be present in and about the vessel walls.
5. When vesicles and bullae occur, they are usually subepidermal.
6. Histologic changes are similar in the acute and chronic types of leukocytoclastic vasculitis, except that hemorrhage is less pronounced in the chronic type.
7. Direct immunofluorescence (Fig. E) shows IgG in vessel walls.

Comment

1. Changes of leukocytoclastic vasculitis may be present in dermatitis herpetiformis and bullous pemphigoid.
2. The "fibrinoid" material seen histologically consists of fibrin and/or immune complex and complement, as delineated by immunofluorescence examination.

LEUKOCYTOCLASTIC VASCULITIS

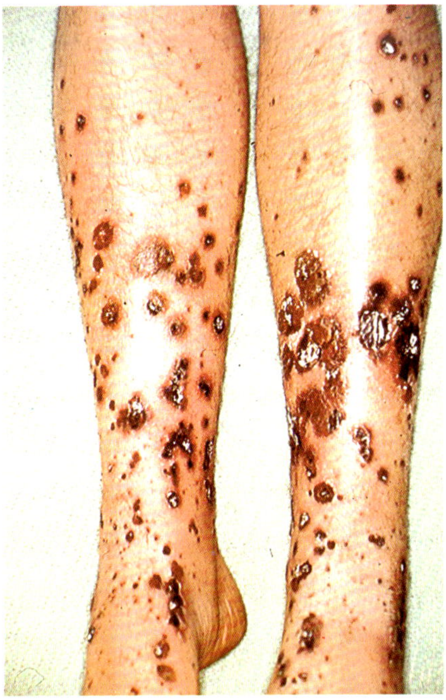

A

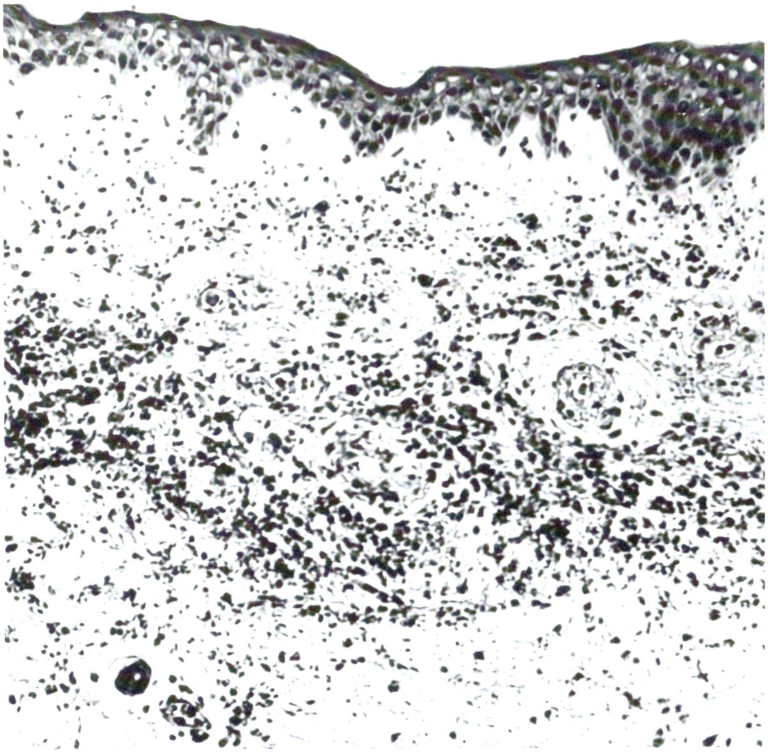

B
X200

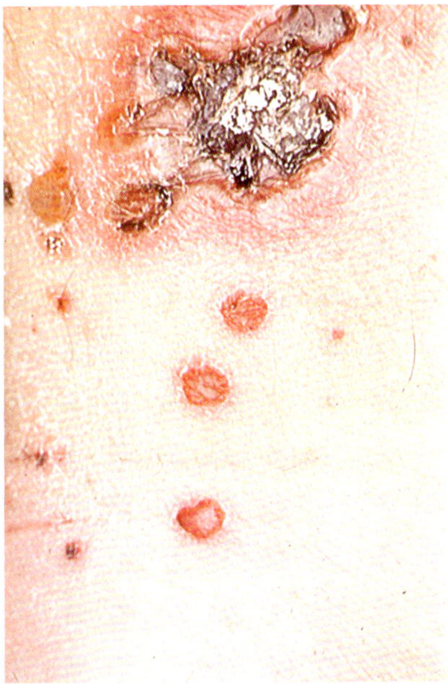

C

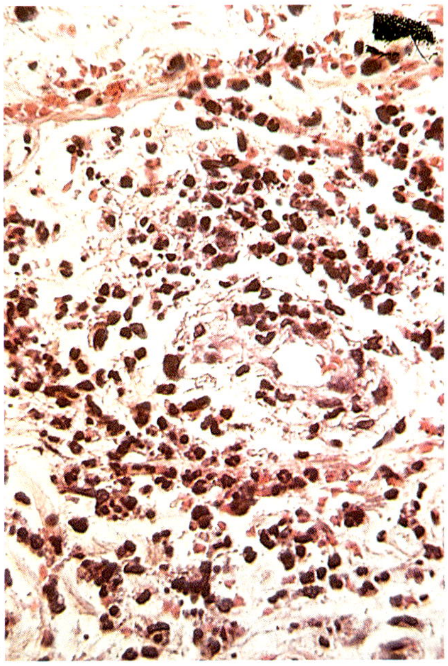

D
X890

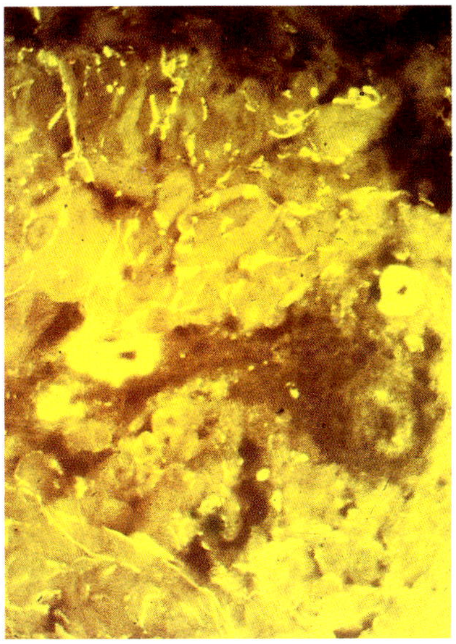

E
X510

IMMUNOFLUORESCENCE

LEUKOCYTOCLASTIC VASCULITIS continued

Morphologically Distinctive Forms of Small Vessel Leukocytoclastic Vasculitis

GRANULOMA FACIALE

Granuloma faciale is a disorder of unknown origin. It is characterized by the presence of brownish or violaceous nodules and plaques, principally on the face (Fig. B). Lesions have a smooth surface, but follicular orifices may be dilated. Onset is usually during middle age. Annular lesions may occur. Lesions do not have a tendency to regress spontaneously.

Microscopic features

1. A dense, confluent infiltrate is present in the dermis and is separated from the epidermis and cutaneous appendages by a distinct zone of normal collagen (grenz zone) (Fig. A).
2. Eosinophils predominate (Fig. C), but the infiltrate also includes neutrophils and histiocytes, as well as scattered lymphocytes, plasma cells, and mast cells.
3. Small vessel leukocytoclastic vasculitis is present (Fig. D), with resultant deposits of hemosiderin.
4. Fibrosis may develop (Fig. E).

Microscopic differential diagnosis

1. Granuloma faciale resembles polymorphous lymphomas (see pp. 1323, 1329), histiocytosis X (see p. 1272), and erythema elevatum diutinum (see pp. 140, 141).
2. Differentiation from lymphomas can be made by absence of atypical cells and by the presence of leukocytoclastic vasculitis. Differentiation from histiocytosis X (see pp. 1272–1281) can be made by absence of immature and lipidized histiocytes and presence of leukocytoclastic vasculitis. Differentiation from erythema elevatum diutinum can usually be made by the density and confluence of the infiltrate and by the predominance of eosinophils rather than neutrophils.
3. Even when fibrosis is present, granuloma faciale can usually be differentiated from other fibrosing conditions by the large number of remaining eosinophils.

GRANULOMA FACIALE

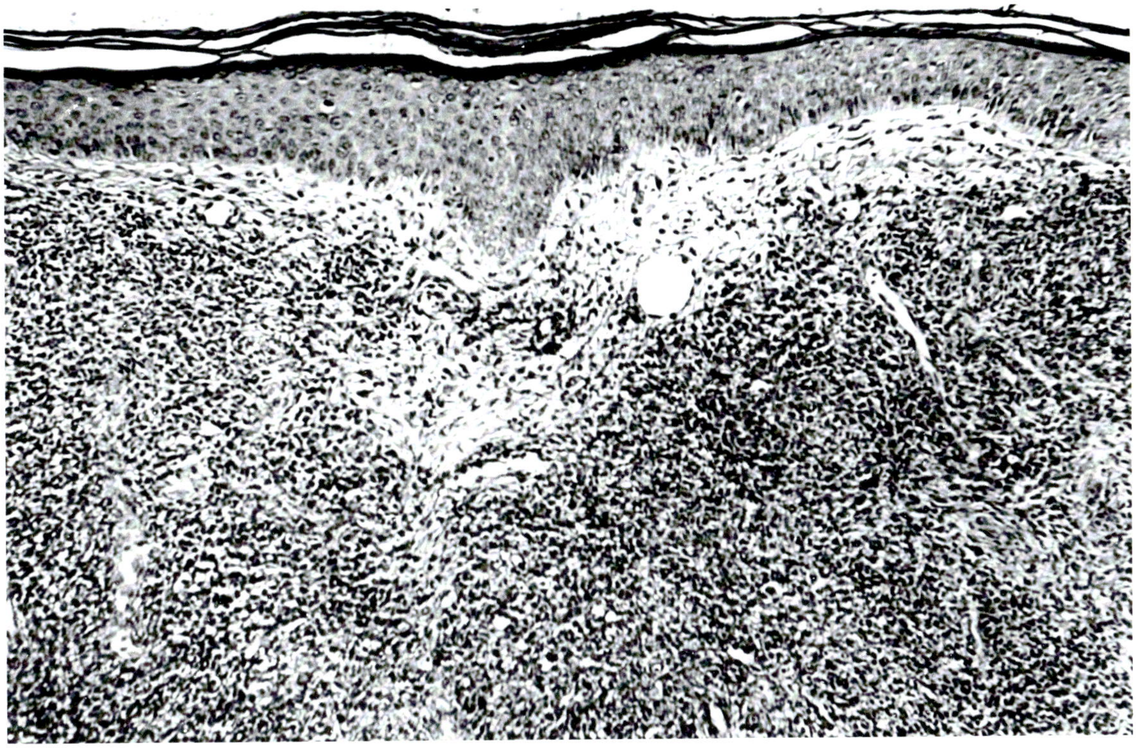

A
X270

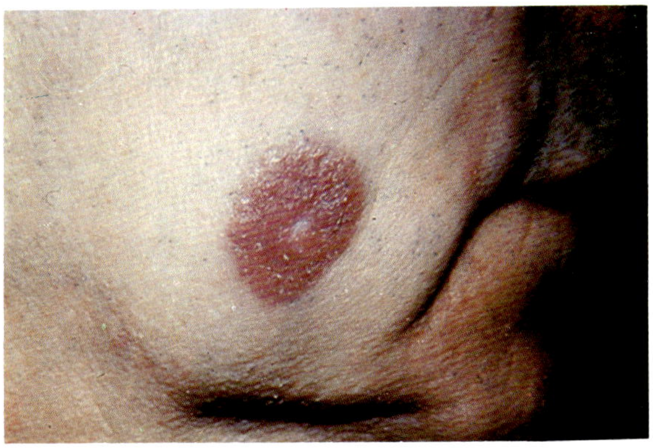

B

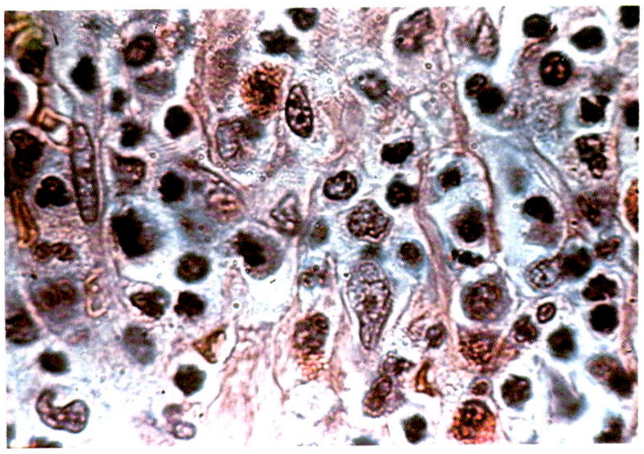

C
X1200

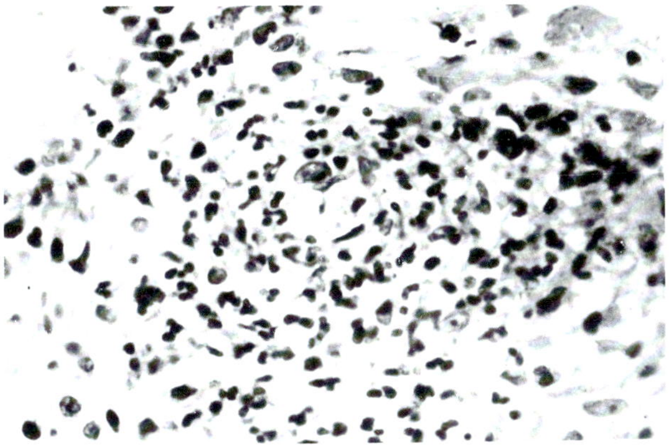

D
X520

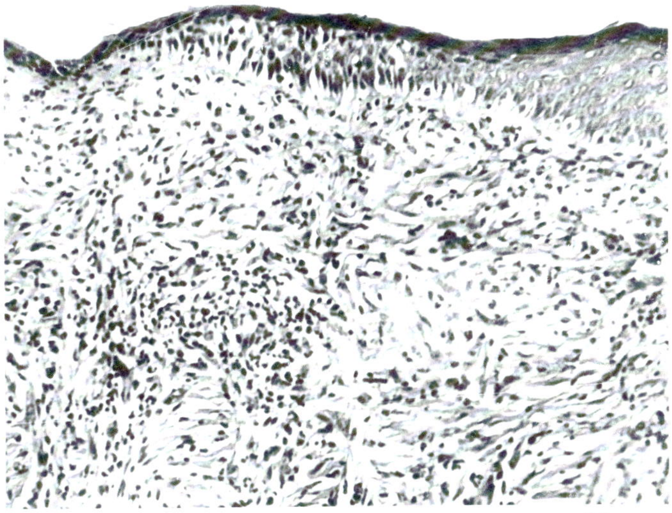

E X210

LEUKOCYTOCLASTIC VASCULITIS continued

Morphologically Distinctive Forms of Small Vessel Leukocytoclastic Vasculitis

ERYTHEMA ELEVATUM DIUTINUM

Erythema elevatum diutinum is a rare disorder of unknown origin. It is characterized by the presence of red to violaceous nodules and plaques, usually on the extremities. These occur principally on the extensor surfaces (especially the knuckles) (Fig. A), but also occasionally occur on the flexor surface (Fig. B). Bullae may be present in the early stages. Gyrate lesions may be seen. The course is variable, but chronicity is the rule.

Microscopic features

1. A dense inflammatory infiltrate is present in which neutrophils predominate, and in which there are varying numbers of lymphocytes, histiocytes, eosinophils, and plasma cells (Figs. C,D).
2. Leukocytoclastic vasculitis is a major component (Fig. E).
3. In some cases, there may be exocytosis, edema, and vesiculation of the epidermis which may be followed by necrosis.
4. As the lesions progress, fibrosis occurs.
5. Extracellular cholesterosis may be present.
6. Bullae, when present, are subepidermal.

Microscopic differential diagnosis (see granuloma faciale, p. 138).

Comment

Granuloma faciale and erythema elevatum diutinum have many features in common, and may be variants of the same basic process.

Sweet's syndrome (see p. 142) has a similar gross and microscopic morphology similar to erythema elevatum diutinum but has more widespread lesions and serious systemic manifestations, including fever and leukocytosis. Most patients are women.

ERYTHEMA ELEVATUM DIUTINUM

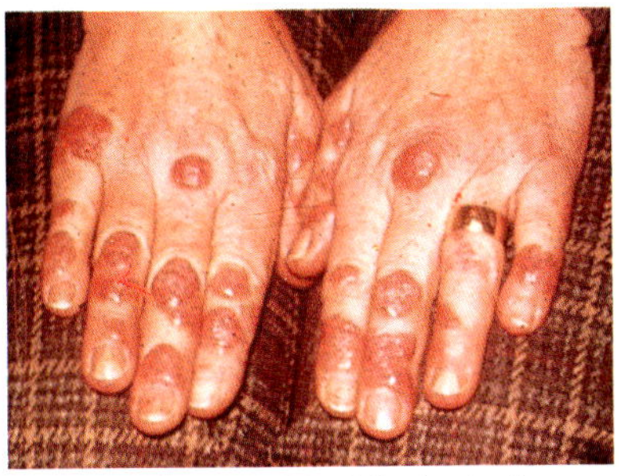

A Courtesy Dr. Martin Asch

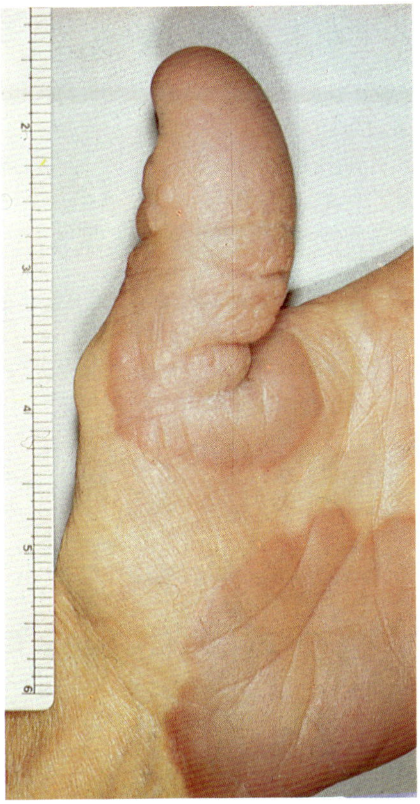

B Courtesy Dr. Don Flora

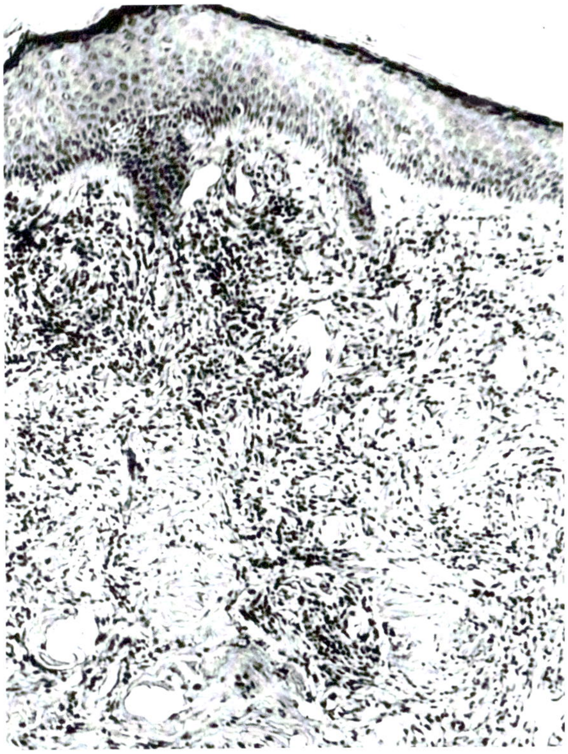

C
X250

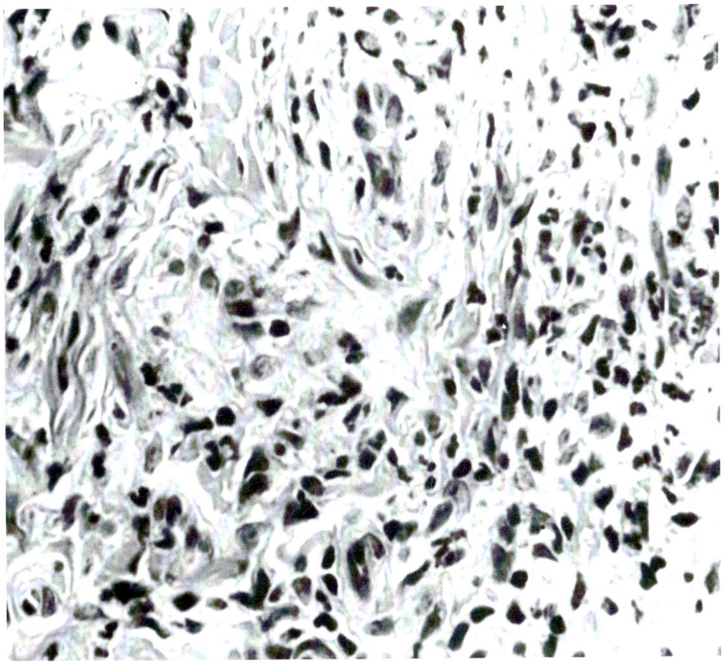

D
X730

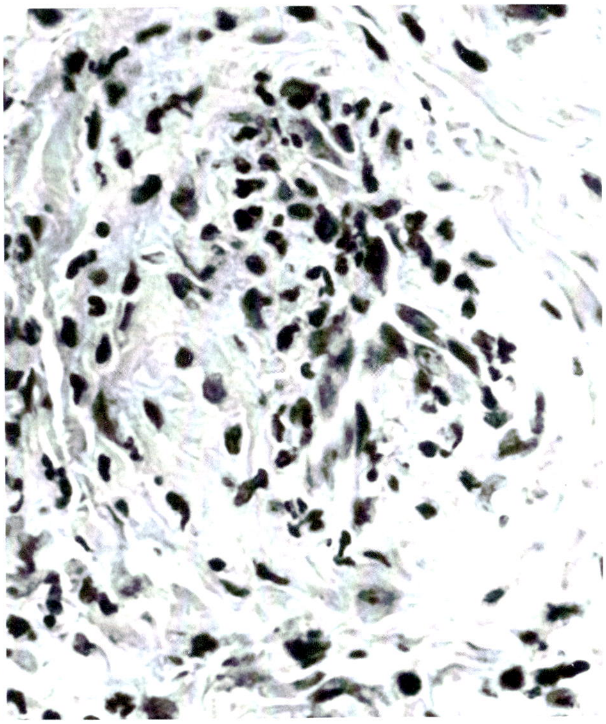

E
X1040

LEUKOCYTOCLASTIC VASCULITIS continued

Morphologically Distinctive Forms of Small Vessel Leukocytoclastic Vasculitis

ACUTE FEBRILE NEUTROPHILIC DERMATOSIS (SWEET'S SYNDROME)

Sweet's syndrome has gross and microscopic similarities to erythema elevatum diutinum, but differs by being an acute process with accompanying fever and leukocytosis. Lesions are usually located on the extremities, face, and neck. They are sharply marginated, raised plaques, which may have an annular configuration and crusting (Figs. A,B). There is a clinical similarity to halogen granulomas. Vesicles or pustules may be present. It is believed that Sweet's syndrome represents a hypersensitivity reaction. Some reported cases have followed upper respiratory infections. It has been suggested that other cases may have been induced by tumor antigens. An association with acute myelogenous leukemia has been reported.

Microscopic features

1. There is a massive infiltrate of neutrophils in the dermis (Fig. C).
2. The infiltrate is most pronounced around blood vessels (Figs. D,E). "Nuclear dust" is present (Figs. C,D,E) as well as scattered monocytes and eosinophils.
3. Endothelial swelling is usually visible (Figs. D,E), but hemorrhage and fibrin deposition are usually absent.
4. The epidermis may show spongiosis and crusting (Fig. C), and sometimes spongiotic vesicles are present.
5. Subepidermal edema is often pronounced (Fig. C), and this may lead to subepidermal bulla formation.

Comment

It is uncertain whether Sweet's syndrome is a specific disease entity or a reaction pattern to a variety of antigens.

SWEET'S SYNDROME

A

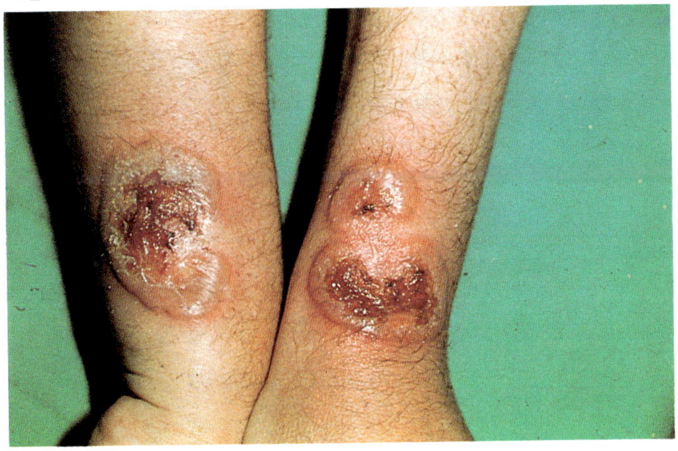

B

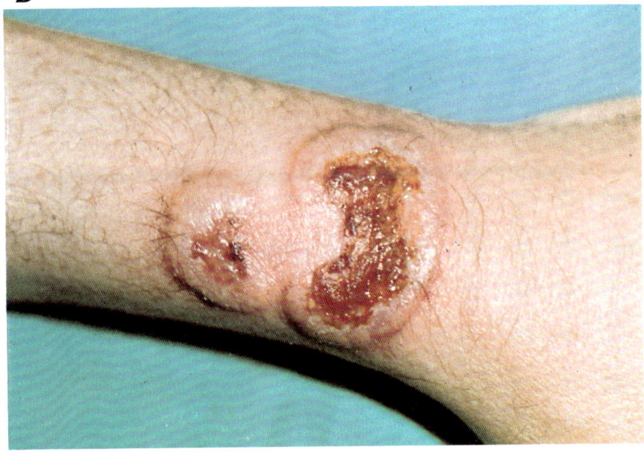

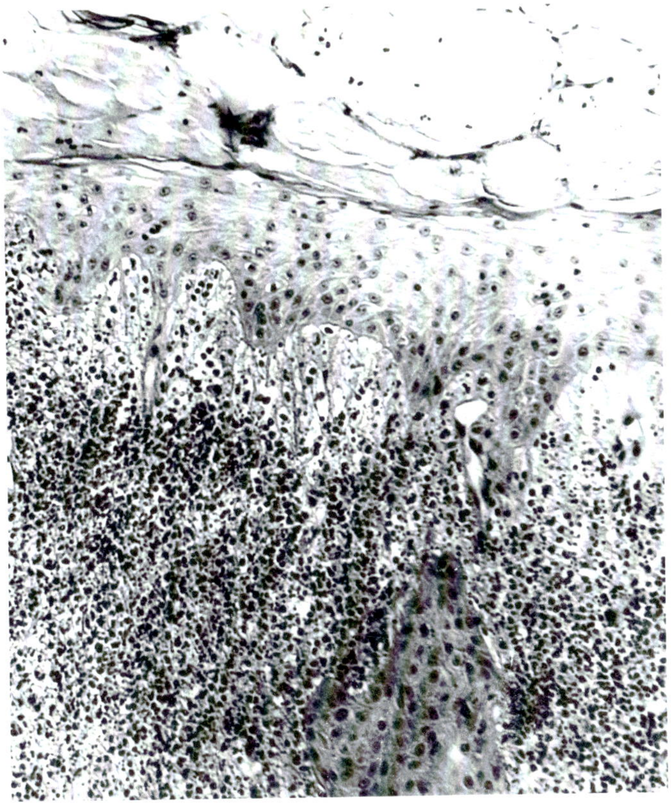

C
X290

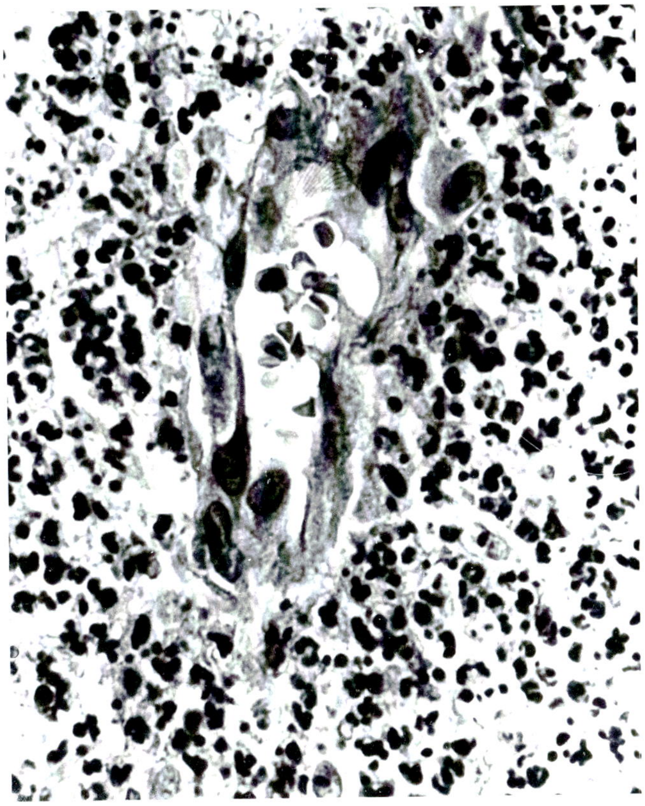

D
X720

Figs. A–E courtesy Dr. Kenneth Greer

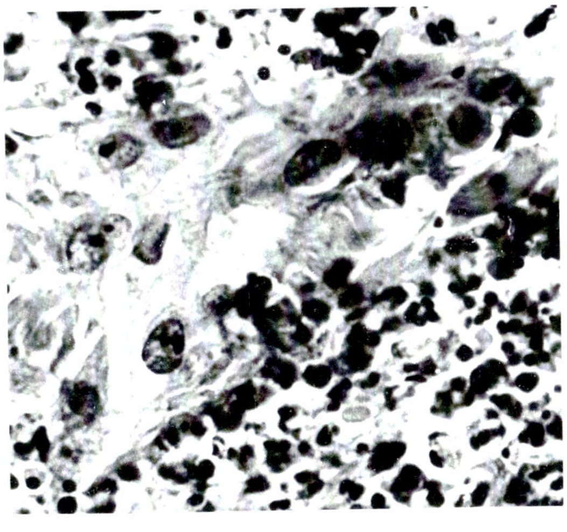

E
X720

LEUKOCYTOCLASTIC VASCULITIS continued

Leukocytoclastic Vasculitis of Large Vessels

PERIARTERITIS NODOSA (POLYARTERITIS NODOSA)

Periarteritis nodosa is a systemic, necrotizing panarteritis. Common clinical manifestations include fever, weakness, abdominal pain, hypertension, polyneuritis, and cardiac insufficiency. There may be renal involvement. Nodules develop along the course of cutaneous and subcutaneous arteries (Fig. A). The lower extremities are most frequently involved.

The spectrum of cutaneous lesions observed in small vessel leukocytoclastic vasculitis may be present (Fig. D), with hemorrhage and ulcerations. Livedo reticularis may be present, a pattern seen in a variety of vascular disorders.

Microscopic features of internal lesions of systemic periarteritis nodosa

1. Medium-sized and small arteries are involved.
2. The panarteritis has four stages:
   a. The first, or *degenerative stage* shows mucinous or fibrinoid necrosis in the media, and/or adventitia of the vessel wall which extends to involve the intima.
   b. In the second, or *inflammatory stage*, involved areas of the vessel wall show a dense inflammatory infiltrate consisting principally of neutrophils, but also with eosinophils, lymphoctyes, and later, histiocytes (Fig. E). This infiltrate eventually involves the entire vessel wall, with ultimate thrombosis (Figs. C,F).
   c. The third stage or *granulation stage* is characterized by the development of granulation tissue in the lesion, with ultimate fibrosis.
   d. The fourth stage or *fibrotic stage* is characterized by progressive replacement of the vessel wall by scar tissue.
3. Lesions occasionally contain giant cells (Fig. G), although this feature is more typical of granulomatous vasculitis.
4. Leukocytoclasis is always present (Fig. H).

Microscopic features of cutaneous lesions of systemic periarteritis nodosa

The picture is that of standard small vessel leukocytoclastic vasculitis (see p. 136). Biopsies of skin, nerves, or muscle cannot establish a diagnosis of systemic periarteritis nodosa.

Comment

1. Cutaneous periarteritis nodosa is a variant with predominantly cutaneous manifestations with musculoskeletal and neurological features. The histologic picture of cutaneous periarteritis nodosa corresponds to those of the internal lesions of systemic periarteritis nodosa: medium-sized and small arteries are involved; these may be at the junction of the dermis and subcutaneous fat (Fig. B). Vascular occlusion may produce a wedge-shaped infarct (Fig. B).
2. Periarteritis nodosa is by definition an idiopathic disorder. When the pattern of periarteritis nodosa is seen in association with other disorders, such as lupus erythematosus, rheumatoid arthritis, or hepatitis B infection, the term *systemic polyangiitis* is used.
3. There is an association of hepatitis B antigenemia with systemic periarteritis nodosa. It may also be associated with cutaneous periarteritis nodosa.

PERIARTERITIS NODOSA

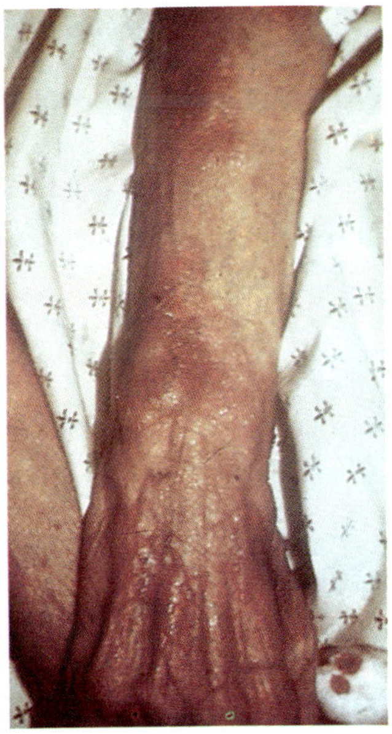

A

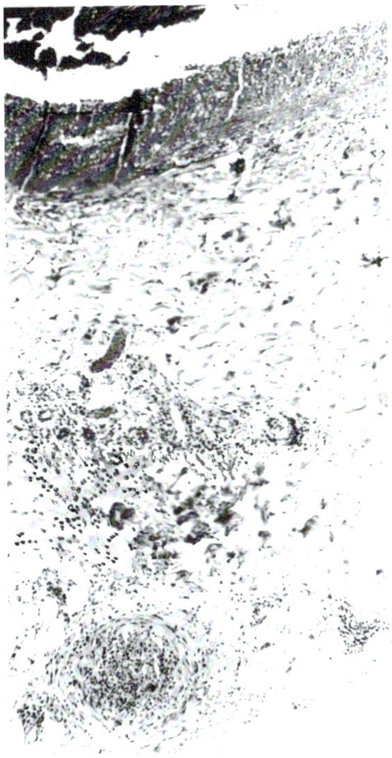

B
X49

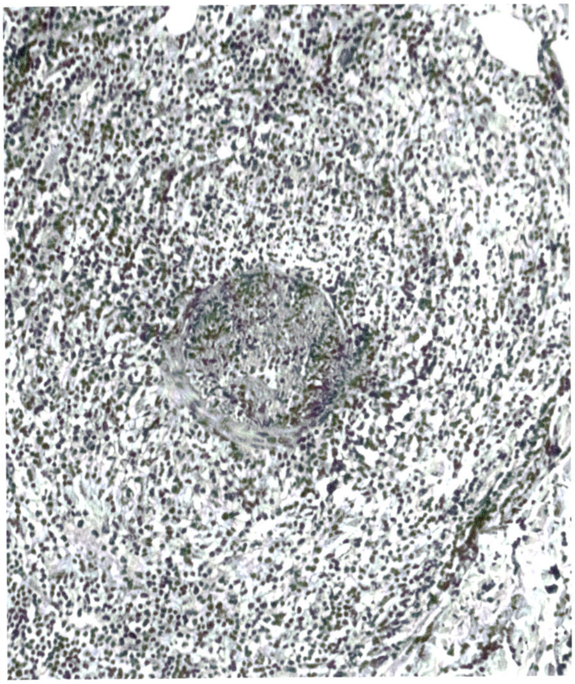

C
X200

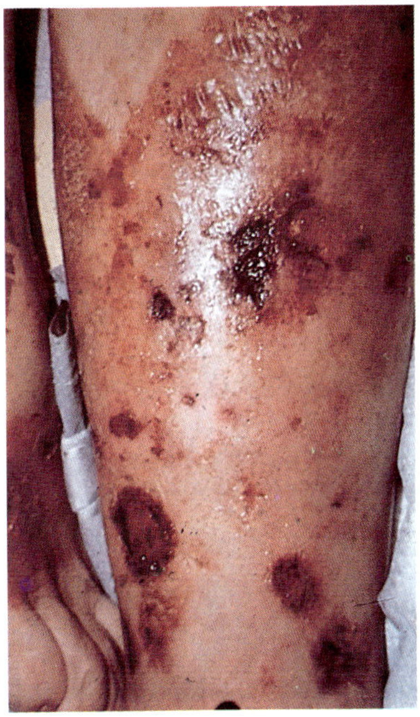

D Figs. A,D courtesy Dr. Juan Cordova

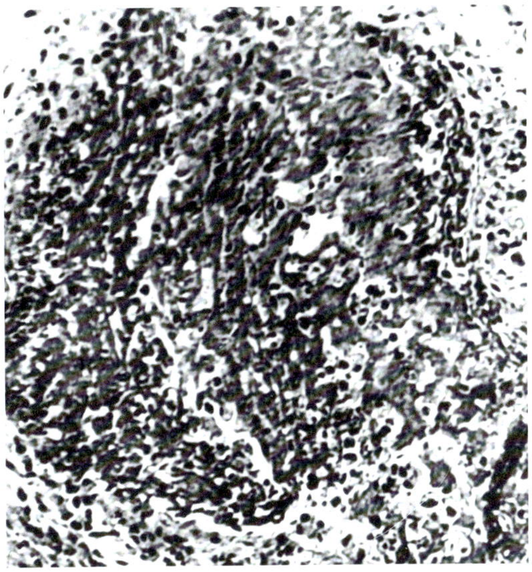

E
X260

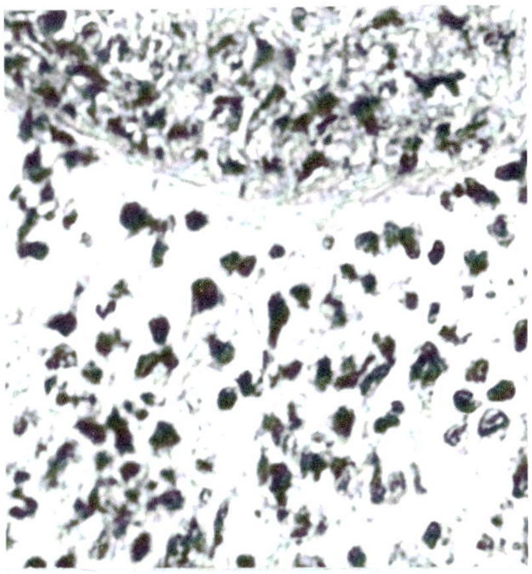

F
X780

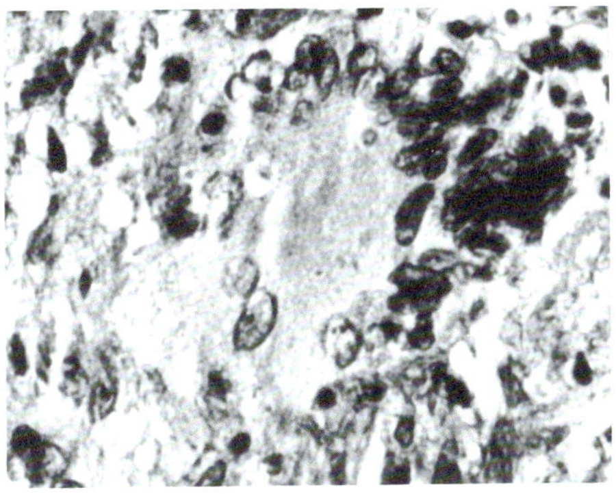

G
X630

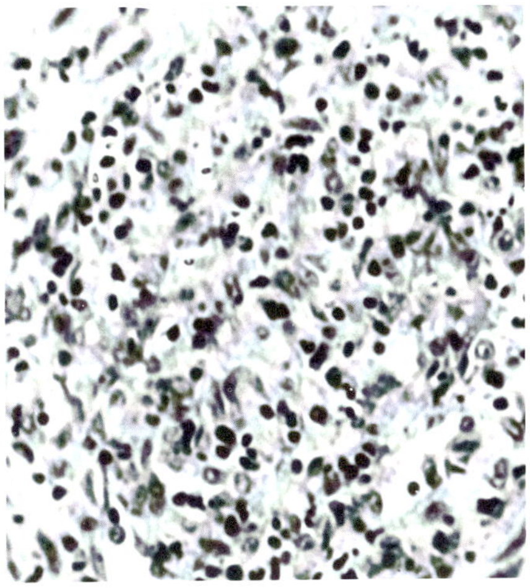

H
X280

Lymphocytic Vasculitis

Lymphocytic vasculitis is a lymphocytic inflammation of the small vessels of the upper dermis, resulting in vessel damage and hemorrhage.

There are two main idiopathic categories: pityriasis lichenoides and purpura pigmentosa chronica. Many other entities, including erythema multiforme and drug reactions, may show lymphocytic vasculitis.

PITYRIASIS LICHENOIDES

Pityriasis lichenoides is a generalized cutaneous eruption of unknown cause. It occurs in two forms: a more severe form, *pityriasis lichenoides et varioliformis acuta* (PLEVA) (Mucha-Habermann disease), and a milder form, *pityriasis lichenoides chronica*. In the acute form, the lesions are transient and occur in crops, but repeated attacks may extend over long periods of time. Pityriasis lichenoides et varioliformis acuta may gradually evolve into pityriasis lichenoides chronica, or the latter may develop *de novo*. Both forms are usually asymptomatic.

A microscopic variant of pityriasis lichenoides et varioliformis acuta, *lymphomatoid papulosis*, contains atypical cells, producing a resemblance to polymorphous lymphoma (see pp. 1323, 1329).

The lesions of pityriasis lichenoides et varioliformis acuta are sequentially macules, papules, vesicles, crusted ulcers (Fig. C) and, ultimately, varioliform scars. (Lymphomatoid papulosis has the identical clinical appearance.)

The lesions of pityriasis lichenoides chronica are small, scaling papules or patches. They do not ulcerate.

Microscopic features

Pityriasis lichenoides et varioliformis acuta (PLEVA)

1. There is a pronounced lymphocytic vasculitis characterized by invasion of the capillary walls by lymphocytes, along with edema of the endothelial cells and extravasation of red blood cells (Fig. E). In ulcerated lesions there may be a component of leukocytoclastic vasculitis.
2. Accumulations of lymphocytes and red blood cells are present at the epidermal-dermal junction, and there is infiltration of the epidermis by these cells (Figs. A,B).
3. The epidermis shows vesicles formed by intracellular and intercellular edema (Fig. A).
4. The vesiculation may progress to a stage of epidermal necrosis, with a crust composed of a mixture of fibrin, leukocytes, red blood cells, and parakeratotic epidermal cells (Fig. B).

Pityriasis lichenoides chronica

1. There is a mild lymphocytic vasculitis, with slight hemorrhage.
2. The epidermis shows moderate spongiosis and contains scattered lymphocytes and red blood cells (Fig. D). Hyperkeratosis and parakeratosis may be present.

Many other entities, including erythema multiforme and drug reactions, may show lymphocytic vasculitis.

PITYRIASIS LICHENOIDES ET VARIOLIFORMIS ACUTA

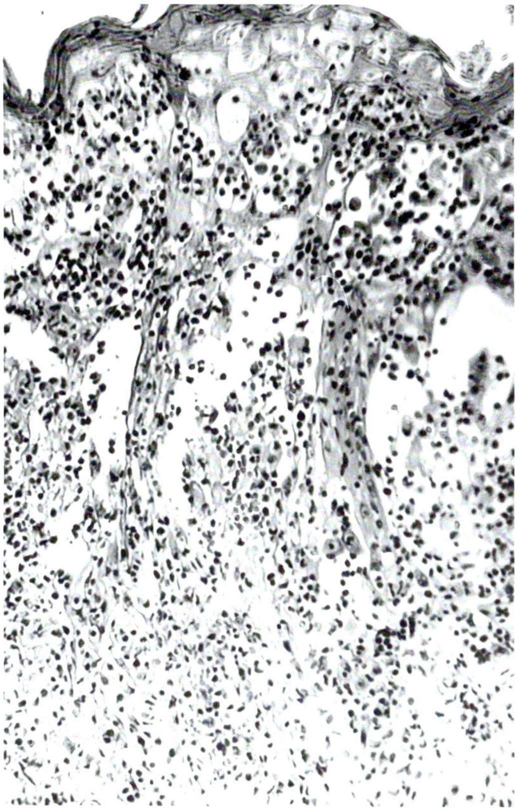

A X260

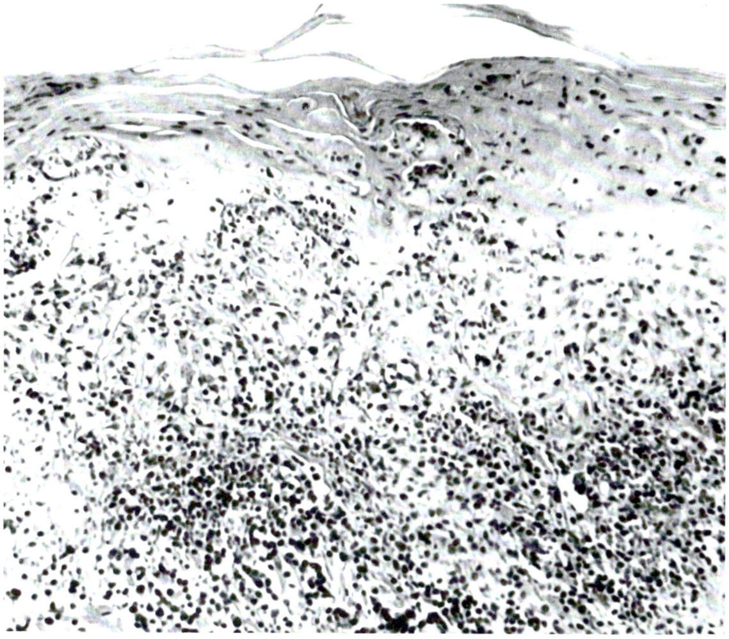

B X185

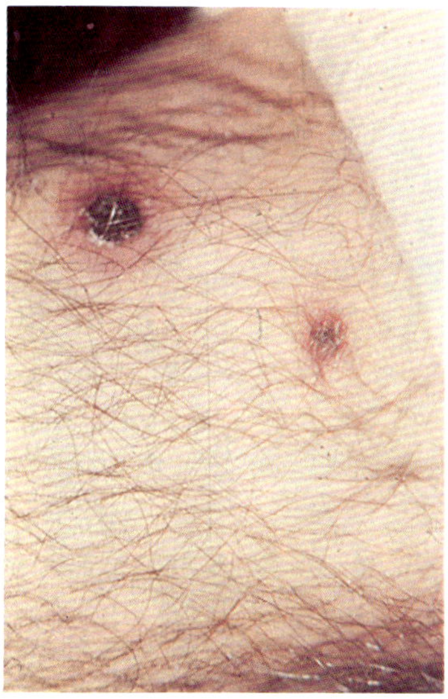

C

Courtesy Dr. Maury Tye

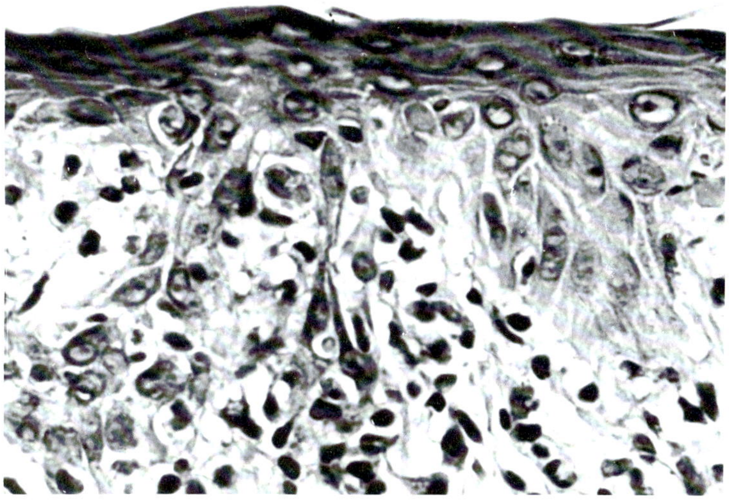

D X700

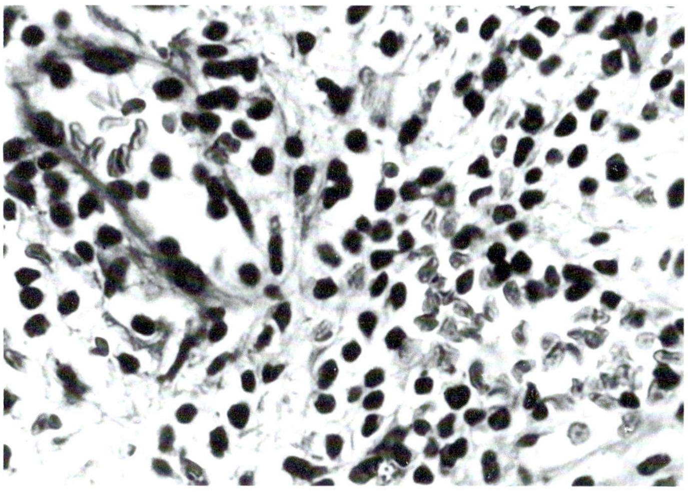

E X700

LYMPHOCYTIC VASCULITIS continued

PITYRIASIS LICHENOIDES

Microscopic differential diagnosis

1. The presence of epidermal changes helps differentiate pityriasis lichenoides chronica from purpura pigmentosa chronica (see below).
2. Differentiation from leukocytoclastic vasculitis is made on the basis of absence of leukocytoclasis, but overlapping can occur.
3. Erythema multiforme (see p. 570) may show a histologic resemblance to pityriasis lichenoides et varioliformis acuta, and may be impossible to differentiate without clinical data.

Comment

1. The lymphocytes involved are T lymphocytes.
2. The histologic picture of secondary syphilis may resemble PLEVA.

PURPURA PIGMENTOSA CHRONICA

This term encompasses a group of idiopathic disorders having as their common denominator grouped petechiae, most commonly present on the lower extremities. The variants include: *peculiar progressive pigmentary disease* or *progressive pigmentary dermatosis (Schamberg)* (Fig. A); *pigmented purpuric lichenoid dermatitis (Gougerot and Blum); purpura annularis telangiectoides (Majocchi)* (Fig. C); *eczematidlike purpura (Ducas, Kapetanakis); transitory pigmented purpuric eruption of the lower extremities (Osment); itching purpura (Loewenthal); disseminated pruriginous angiodermatitis (Mosto and Casala)*. In addition to petechiae, telangiectasia and hyperpigmentation may be present. A localized variant is *lichen aureus,* with closely aggregated, rust-colored papules on a reddish-brown background (Fig. E).

Microscopic features

1. There is a lymphocytic vasculitis involving small vessels of the upper dermis (Figs. B,D), characterized by endothelial edema, extravasation of red blood cells, and a lymphocytic infiltrate; histiocytes and neutrophils may occasionally be present.
2. Epidermal change is generally absent; occasionally acanthosis, intercellular edema, and exocytosis are present (Figs. B,D).
3. Older lesions show capillary dilation, endothelial proliferation, deposits of hemosiderin in the dermis, and a less pronounced lymphocytic infiltrate.

Microscopic differential diagnosis

1. The general absence of epidermal change helps differentiate purpura pigmentosa chronica from pityriasis lichenoides.
2. Purpura pigmentosa chronica can usually be differentiated from stasis dermatitis by the more superficial location of the inflammation and by the absence of dermal fibrosis and thickening of walls of vessels in the deeper dermis.

PURPURA PIGMENTOSA CHRONICA

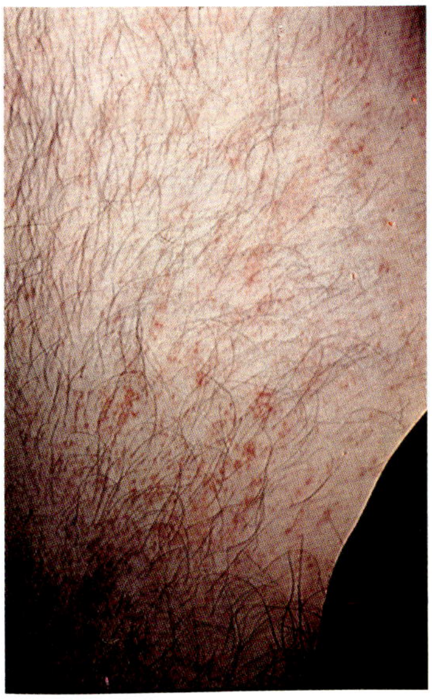
A

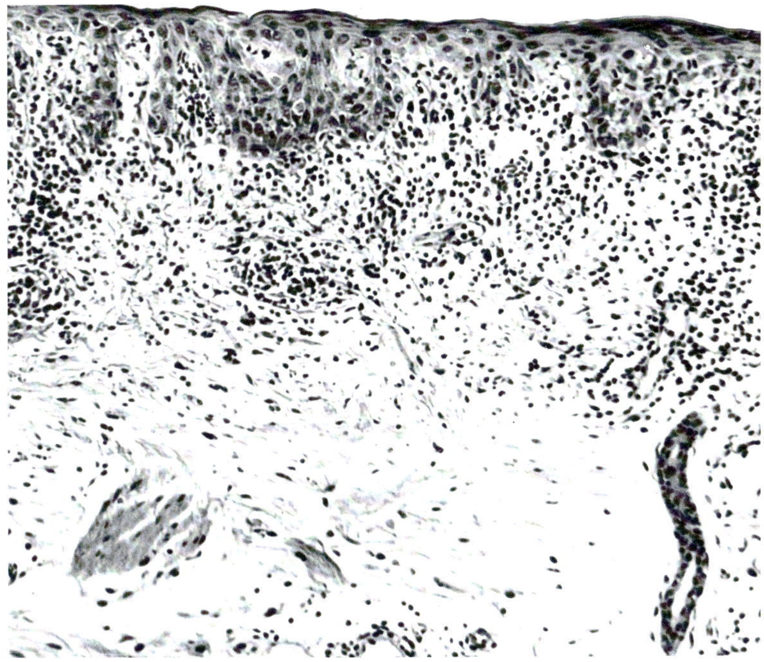
B
X185

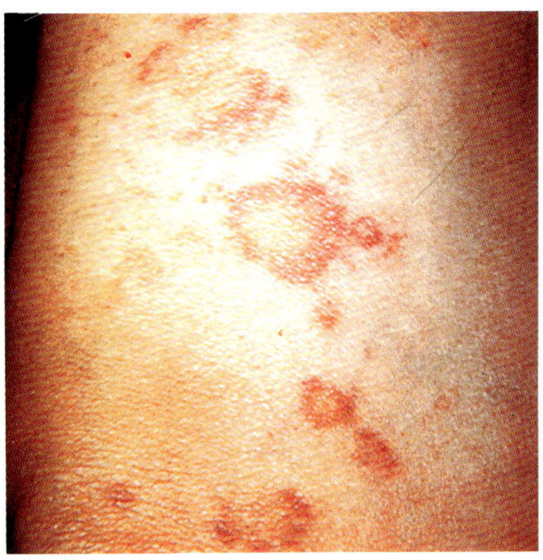
C

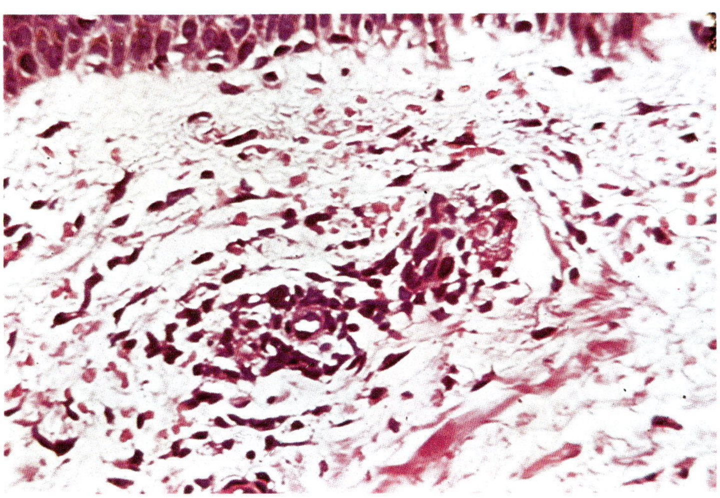
D
X720

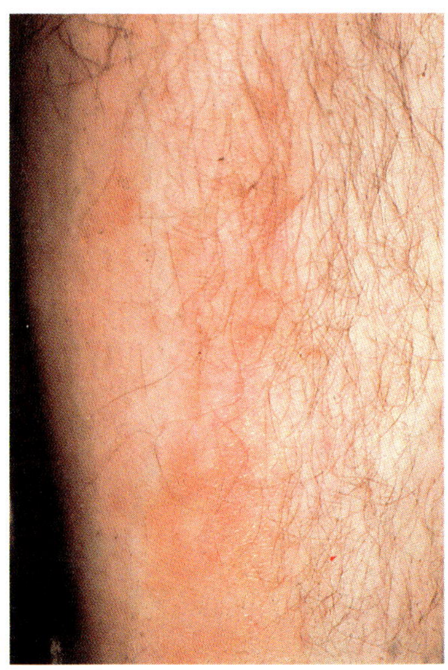
E

NONINFLAMMATORY PURPURA

Noninflammatory purpura is included in the section on inflammation because it must be differentiated from purpura associated with vasculitis. Causes of noninflammatory purpura include trauma, stasis, scurvy (Fig. C), senile alteration of connective tissue (Figs. A,B), bone marrow dysfunction, purpura fulminans, autoerythrocyte sensitization, idiopathic thrombocytopenic purpura (ITP), and thrombotic thrombocytopenic purpura (TTP). In senile purpura, hemorrhages (petechiae, purpura, and ecchymoses) are typically located on the dorsal surfaces of the forearms and hands (Figs. A,B). In scurvy (Fig. C) there are corkscrew hairs, and the hemorrhages tend to have a perifollicular distribution.

Microscopic features

1. The basic histologic change is extravasation of red blood cells into the dermis (Fig. D).
2. As the lesions age, hemosiderin accumulates in the dermis.
3. Certain types of noninflammatory purpura may have specific histologic features: a) in scurvy there is a characteristic perifollicular hemorrhage, which can be seen grossly in association with "corkscrew hairs" (Fig. C); b) in senile purpura there is solar elastosis in the upper dermis and atrophy of collagen fibers in the lower dermis; in the lower dermis, the collagen may be present as individual fibers rather than as bundles of fibers; c) in purpura fulminans there is extensive necrosis of the vessel walls, with or without leukotaxis.

NONINFLAMMATORY PURPURA

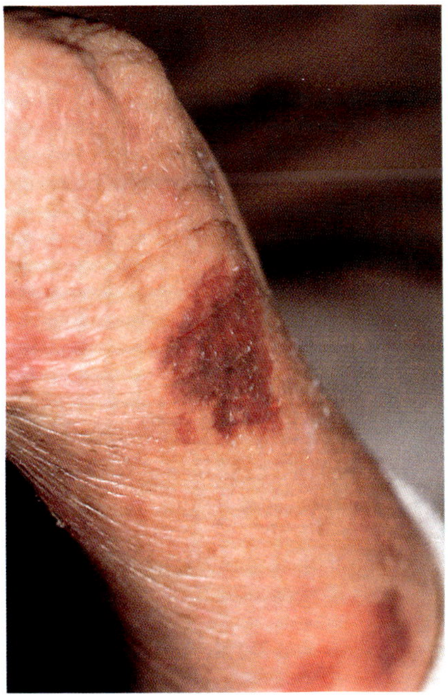

A

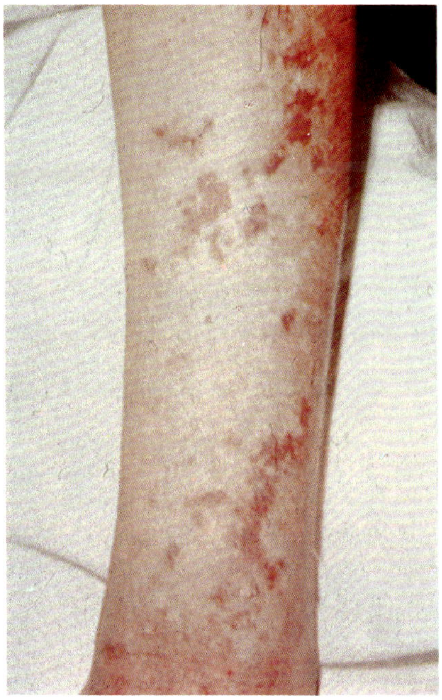

B

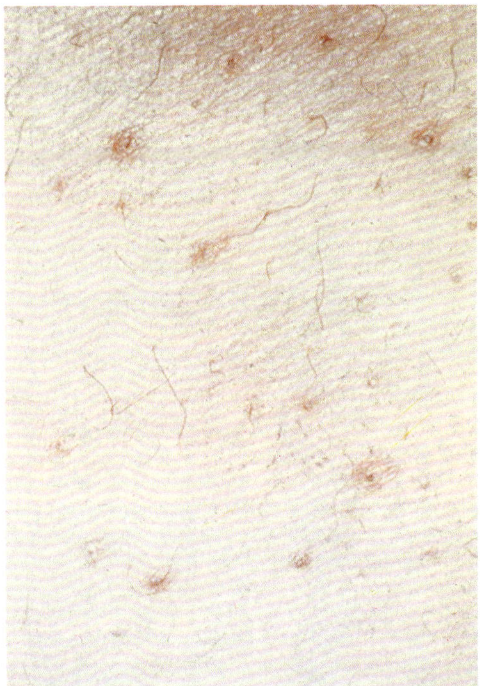

C

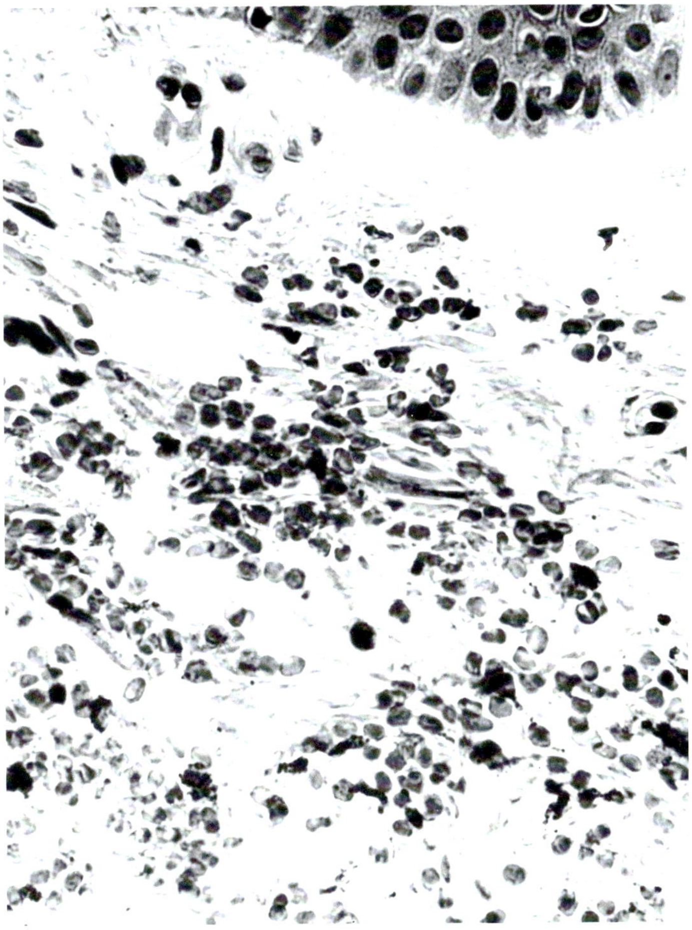

D
X650

Suggested Reading

Vasculitis

Leukocytoclastic Vasculitis

GENERAL REFERENCES

Copeman, P. Investigations into the pathogenesis of acute cutaneous angiitis. *Br. J. Dermatol.*, 82 (5, suppl.):51, 1970.

Copeman, P. and Ryan, T. The problems of classification of cutaneous angiitis with reference to histopathology and pathogenesis. *Br. J. Dermatol.*, 82 (5, suppl.):2, 1970.

Dixon, F. and Cochrane, C. The pathogenicity of antigen-antibody complexes. *Pathology Ann.*, 5:355, 1970.

Venkatachalam, M. and Cotran, R. Ultrastructure of the local Arthus phenomenon using horseradish peroxidase as antigen. *Lab. Invest.*, 23:129, 1970.

Winkelmann, R. and Ditto, W. Cutaneous and visceral syndromes of necrotizing or "allergic" angiitis: A study of 38 cases. *Medicine* (Baltimore), 43:59, 1964.

SMALL VESSEL VASCULITIS

Ansell, B. Henoch-Schönlein purpura with particular reference to the prognosis of the renal lesion. *Br. J. Dermatol.*, 82:211, 1970.

Baart de la Faille, K. et al. IgA-deposits in cutaneous blood-vessel walls and mesangium in Henoch-Schönlein syndrome. *Lancet*, 1:892, 1973.

Bard, I. and Winkelmann, R. Livedo vasculitis. *Arch. Dermatol.*, 96:489, 1967.

Bradford, W., Cook, C. and Vawter, G. Livedo reticularis: A form of allergic vasculitis: Report of 3 cases. *J. Pediatr.*, 60:266, 1962.

Callen, J. and Kalbfleisch, S. Urticarial vasculitis: A report of nine cases and review of the literature. *Br. J. Dermatol.*, 107:87, 1982.

Gray, H. et al. Atrophie blanche: Periodic painful ulcers of the lower extremities. *Arch. Dermatol.*, 93:187, 1966.

Knobler, H. et al. Urticarial vasculitis and recurrent pleural effusion: A systemic manifestation of urticarial vasculitis. *Dermatologica*, 172:120, 1986.

McCombs, R., Patterson, J. and MacMahon, H. Syndromes associated with "allergic" vasculitis. *N. Eng. J. Med.*, 255:251, 1956.

McDuffie, F. et al. Hypocomplementemia with cutaneous vasculitis and arthritis. *Mayo Clin. Proc.*, 48:340, 1973.

Mackel, S. and Jordon, R. Leukocytoclastic vasculitis. *Arch. Dermatol.*, 118:296, 1982.

Matarredona, J. et al. Systemic lupus erythematosus appearing as an urticarial vasculitis. *Internat. J. Dermatol.*, 25:446, 1986.

Monroe, E. et al. Vasculitis in chronic urticaria. *J. Invest. Dermatol.*, 76:103, 1981.

Norkin, S. and Wiener, J. Henoch-Schönlein syndrome: Review of pathology and report of two cases. *Am. J. Clin. Pathol.*, 35:55, 1960.

Pierard, J. and Geerts, M. Vascularite hyalisante segmentaire (livedo vasculitis). *Arch. Belg. Dermatol. Syph.*, 27:103, 1971.

Sams, W., Jr. Necrotizing vasculitis. (Review). *J. Am. Acad. Dermatol.*, 3:1, 1980.

Sanchez, N., Van Hale, H. and Su, D. Clinical and histopathologic spectrum of necrotizing vasculitis. *Arch. Dermatol.*, 121:220, 1985.

Schroeter, A. et al. Livedo vasculitis (the vasculitis of atrophie blanche): Immunohistopathologic study. *Arch. Dermatol.*, 111:118, 1975.

Soter, N. Chronic urticaria as a manifestation of necrotizing venulitis. *N. Eng. J. Med.*, 296:1440, 1977.

Zeek, P. Periarteritis nodosa and other forms of necrotizing angiitis. *N. Eng. J. Med.*, 248:764, 1953.

Granuloma Faciale

Johnson, W., Higdon, R. and Helwig, E. Granuloma faciale. *Arch. Dermatol.*, 79:42, 1959.
McCarthy, P. Granuloma faciale. *Arch. Dermatol.*, 77:458, 1958.
Okun, M., Bauman, L. and Minor, D. Granuloma faciale with lesions on the face and hands. *Arch. Dermatol.*, 92:78, 1965.
Pinkus, H. Granuloma faciale. *Dermatologica*, 105:85, 1952.
Rusin, L., Dubin, H. and Taylor, W. Disseminated granuloma faciale. *Arch. Dermatol.*, 112:1575, 1976.

Erythema Elevatum Diutinum

Cream, J., Levine, G. and Calnan, D. Erythema elevatum diutinum. *Br. J. Dermatol.*, 84:393, 1971.
Goldman, G. and Moschella, S. Acute febrile neutrophilic dermatosis (Sweet's Syndrome). *Arch. Dermatol.*, 103:654, 1971.
Haber, H. Erythema elevatum diutinum. *Br. J. Dermatol.*, 67:121, 1955.
Katz, S. et al. Erythema elevatum diutinum. *Medicine* (Baltimore), 56:443, 1977.
Ketron, L. Erythema elevatum diutinum. *Arch. Dermatol. Syph.*, 50:363, 1944.
Mraz, J. and Newcomer, V. Erythema elevatum diutinum: Presentation of a case and evaluation of laboratory and immunological status. *Arch. Dermatol.*, 96:235, 1967.
Raimer, S. and Duncan, C. Febrile neutrophilic dermatosis in acute myelogenous leukemia. *Arch. Dermatol.*, 114:413, 1978.

Sweet's Syndrome

Crow, K., Kerdel-Vegas, F. and Rook, A. Acute febrile neutrophilic dermatosis. Sweet's syndrome. *Dermatologica*, 139:123, 1969.
Evans, S. and Evans, C. Acute febrile neutrophilic dermatosis: Two cases. *Dermatologica*, 143:153, 1971.
Gisser, S. Acute febrile neutrophilic dermatosis (Sweet's Syndrome) in a patient with hairy-cell leukemia. *Am. J. Dermatopathol.*, 5:283, 1983.
Greer, K., Pruitt, J. and Bishop, G. Acute febrile neutrophilic dermatosis (Sweet's Syndrome). *Arch. Dermatol.*, 111:1461, 1975.
Mackie, R. Sweet's syndrome: A further case of acute febrile neutrophilic dermatosis. *Dermatologica*, 149:69, 1974.
Raimer, S. and Duncan, C. Febrile neutrophilic dermatosis in acute myelogenous leukemia. *Arch. Dermatol.*, 114:413, 1978.
Storer, J. et al. Sweet's syndrome. *Internat. J. Dermatol.*, 22:8, 1983.
Su, W. and Liu, H. Diagnostic criteria for Sweet's syndrome. *Cutis*, 37:167, 1986.
Sweet, R. An acute febrile neutrophilic dermatosis. *Br. J. Dermatol.*, 76:349, 1964.

Baum, E., Sams, M., Jr. and Payne, R. Giant cell arteritis: A systemic disease with rare cutaneous manifestations. *J. Am. Acad. Dermatol.*, 6:1081, 1982.

Borrie, P. Cutaneous polyarteritis nodosa. *Br. J. Dermatol.*, 87:87, 1972.

Cassan, S., Coles, D. and Harrison, E., Jr. The concept of limited forms of Wegener's granulomatosis. *Am. J. Med.*, 49:366, 1970.

Chumbley, L., Harrison, E., Jr. and Deremee, R. Allergic granulomatosis and angiitis (Churg-Strauss syndrome). Report and analysis of 30 cases. *Mayo Clin. Proc.*, 52:477, 1977.

Churg, J. and Strauss, L. Allergic granulomatosis, allergic angiitis, and periarteritis nodosa. *Am. J. Pathol.*, 27:277, 1951.

Cohen, R., Conn, D. and Ilstrup, D. Clinical features, prognosis, and response to treatment in polyarteritis. *Mayo Clin. Proc.*, 55:146, 1980.

Crissman, J. Midline malignant reticulosis and lymphomatoid granulomatosis. *Arch. Pathol.*, 103:561, 1979.

Crotty, C., Deremee, R. and Winkelmann, R. Cutaneous clinicopathologic correlation of allergic granulomatosis. *J. Am. Acad. Dermatol.*, 5:571, 1981.

Cupps, T. and Fauci, A. Wegener's granulomatosis. *Internat. J. Dermatol.*, 19:76, 1980.

DeOreo, G. Wegener's granulomatosis. *Arch. Dermatol.*, 81:169, 1960.

Deremee, R., Weiland, L. and McDonald, T. Polymorphic reticulosis, lymphomatoid granulomatosis: Two diseases or one? *Mayo Clin. Proc.*, 53:634, 1978.

Diaz-Perez, J., Schroeter, A. and Winkelmann, R. Cutaneous periarteritis nodosa. *Arch. Dermatol.*, 116:56, 1980.

Diaz-Perez, J. and Winkelmann, R. Cutaneous periarteritis nodosa. *Arch. Dermatol.*, 110:407, 1974.

Eichel, B. and Mabery, T. The enigma of the lethal midline granuloma. *Laryngoscope*, 78:1367, 1968.

Fauci, A. The spectrum of vasculitis. Ann. Int. Med., 89:660, 1978.

Fauci, A. and Wolff, S. Wegener's granulomatosis: Studies in eighteen patients and a review of the literature. *Medicine* (Baltimore), 52:535, 1973.

Fauci, A. et al. Lymphomatoid granulomatosis: Prospective clinical and therapeutic experience over 10 years. *N. Eng. J. Med.*, 306:68, 1982.

Foged, E. Chronische Ulzeration nach Biopsie der Arteria temporalis. *Hautarzt*, 32:647, 1981.

Frohnert, P. and Sheps, S. Long-term follow-up study of periarteritis nodosa. *Am. J. Med.*, 43:8, 1967.

Godman, G. and Churg, J. Wegener's granulomatosis: Pathology and review of the literature. *Arch. Pathol.*, 58:533, 1954.

Goodman, B., Jr. Temporal arteritis. (Review) *Am. J. Med.*, 67:839, 1979.

Henberg, R. The protracted superficial phenomenon in pathergic (Wegener's) granulomatosis. *Hum. Pathol.*, 12:458, 1981.

Hitch, J. Dermatologic manifestations of giant-cell (temporal, cranial) arteritis. *Arch. Dermatol.*, 101:409, 1970.

Hu, C., O'Laughlin, S. and Winkelmann, R. Cutaneous manifestations of Wegener's granulomatosis. *Arch. Dermatol.*, 113:175, 1977.

James, W., Odom, R. and Katzenstein, A. Cutaneous manifestations of lymphomatoid granulomatosis. *Arch. Dermatol.*, 117:196, 1981.

Kassel, S., Echevarria, R. and Guzzo, F. Midline malignant reticulosis (so-called lethal midline granuloma). *Cancer*, 23:920, 1969.

Katzenstein, A., Carringon, C. and Liebow, A. Lymphomatoid granulomatosis: A clinicopathologic study of 152 cases. *Cancer*, 43:360, 1979.

Kawasaki, T. et al. A new infantile acute febrile mucocutaneous lymph node syndrome (MLNS) prevailing in Japan. *Pediatrics*, 54:271, 1974.

Kinmont, P. and McCallum, D. The aetiology, pathology and course of giant-cell arteritis: The possible role of light sensitivity. *Br. J. Dermatol.*, 77:193, 1965.

——. Skin manifestations of giant-cell arteritis. *Br. J. Dermatol.*, 76:299, 1964.

Lober, C., Kaplan, R. and West, W. Midline granuloma. *Arch. Dermatol.*, 118:52, 1982.

Luger, A. and Wuketich, S. Kopfschwartennekrose bei temporaler Riesenzellarteriitis. *Dermatol. Wochenschr.*, 153:89, 1967.

Lyell, A. and Church, R. The cutaneous manifestations of polyarteritis nodosa. *Br. J. Dermatol.*, 66:335, 1954.

Meyrick, R. and Black M. The wide clinical spectrum of polyarteritis nodosa with cutaneous involvement. *Clin. Exp. Dermatol.*, 8:47, 1983.

Melish, M. et al. Mucocutaneous lymph node syndrome in the United States. *Am. J. Dis. Child.*, 130:599, 1976.
Minars, N., Kay, S. and Escobar, M. Lymphomatoid granulomatosis of the skin: A new clinicopathologic entity. *Arch. Dermatol.*, 111:493, 1975.
Parker, F. et al. Light and electron microscopic studies on human temporal arteries with special reference to alteration related to senescence, atherosclerosis, and giant-cell arteritis. *Am. J. Pathol.*, 79:57, 1975.
Reed, W. et al. The cutaneous manifestations in Wegener's granulomatosis. *Acta Derm. Venereol.*, 43:250, 1963.
Rosen, T. and Chernoski, M. Lymphomatoid granulomatosis. *Internat. J. Dermatol.*, 18:497, 1979.
Slinger, W. and Starck, V. Cutaneous form of polyarteritis nodosa: Report of a case. *Arch. Dermatol. Syph.*, 63:461, 1951.
Spear, G. and Walker W., Jr. Lethal midline granuloma (granuloma gangrenescens) at autopsy. *Bull. John Hopkins Hosp.*, 99:313, 1956.
Verbov, J. and Stanfeld, A. Cutaneous polyarteritis nodosa and Crohn's disease. *Trans. St. John's Hosp. Dermatol. Soc.*, 58:261, 1972.
Whittaker, S., Dover, J. and Greaves, M. Cutaneous polyarteritis nodosa associated with hepatitis B surface antigen. *J. Am. Acad. Dermatol.*, 15:1145, 1986.
Zeek, P. Periarteritis nodosa: A critical review. *Am. J. Clinical Pathol.*, 22:777, 1952.

Lymphocytic Vasculitis

PITYRIASIS LICHENOIDES ET VARIOLIFORMIS

Black, M. and Marks, R. The inflammatory reaction in pityriasis lichenoides. *Br. J. Dermatol.*, 87:533, 1972.

Burke, D., Adams, R. and Arundell, F. Febrile ulceronecrotic Mucha-Habermann's disease. *Arch. Dermatol.*, 100:200, 1969.

Clayton, R. and Haffenden, G. An immunofluourescence study of pityriasis lichenoides. *Br. J. Dermatol.*, 99:491, 1978.

Clayton, R. et al. Pityriasis lichenoides: An immune complex disease. *Br. J. Dermatol.*, 97:629, 1977.

Faber, W. and Van Joost, T. Pityriasis lichenoides: An immune complex disease. *Acta Derm. Venereol.* (Stockh.), 60:259, 1980.

Hayashi, T. Pityriasis lichenoides et varioliformis acuta: Immunohistopathologic study. *J. Dermatol.*, 4:173, 1977.

Hood, A. and Mark, E. Histopathologic diagnosis of pityriasis lichenoides et varioliformis acuta and its clinical correlation. *Arch. Dermatol.*, 118;478, 1982.

Marks, R., Black, M. and Wilson-Jones, E. Pityriasis lichenoides: A reappraisal. *Br. J. Dermatol.*, 86;215, 1972.

Muhlbauer, J. et al. Immunopathology of pityriasis lichenoides acuta. *J. Am. Acad. Dermatol.*, 10:783, 1984.

Muller, S. and Schulze, T., Jr. Mucha-Habermann disease mistaken for reticulum cell sarcoma. *Arch. Dermatol.*, 103:423, 1971.

Szymanski, F. Pityriasis lichenoides et varioliformis acuta: Histopathological evidence that it is an entity distinct from parapsoriasis. *Arch. Dermatol.*, 79:7, 1959.

PURPURA PIGMENTOSA CHRONICA

Baden, H. Familial Schamberg's disease. *Arch. Dermatol.*, 90:400, 1964.

Davis, M. and Lawler, J. Capillary alterations in pigmented purpuric disease of the skin. *Arch. Dermatol.*, 78:723, 1958.

Doucas, C. and Kapetanakis, J. Eczematid-like purpura. *Dermatologica,* 106:86, 1953.

Iwatsuki, K. et al. Immunofluorescence study in purpura pigmentosa chronica. *Acta Derm. Venereol.* (Stockh.), 60:341, 1980.

Loewenthal, L. Itching purpura. *Br. J. Dermatol.*, 66:95, 1954.

Mosto, S. and Casala, A. Disseminated pruriginous angiodermatitis (itching purpura). *Arch. Dermatol.*, 91:351, 1965.

Nichamin, S. and Brough, J. Chronic progressive pigmentary purpura. *Am. J. Dis. Child.*, 116:429, 1968.

Price, M. et al. Lichen aureus: A localized persistent form of pigmented purpuric dermatitis. *Br. J. Dermatol.*, 112: 307, 1985.

Randall, S., Kierland, R. and Montgomery, H. Pigmented purpuric eruptions. *Arch. Dermatol. Syph.*, 64:177, 1951.

Still, J. and Moyer, D. Schamberg's disease. *Arch. Dermatol.*, 94:626, 1966.

Waisman, M. and Waisman, M. Lichen aureus. *Arch. Dermatol.*, 112:696, 1976.

Bean, W. *Rare Diseases and Lesions. Springfield, IL, Thomas, 1967.*

Becker, F. and Buckley, R. Purpura fulminans associated with varicella. *Arch. Dermatol.*, 94:613, 1966.

Bithell, T. and Wintrobe, M. The purpuras. In: *Harrison's Principles of Internal Medicine.* Wintrobe, M. et al., eds., 6th Ed., New York, McGraw-Hill, 1970, p. 1646.

Bone, R. et al. Respiratory dysfunction in thrombotic thrombocytopenic purpura. *Am. J. Med.*, 65:262, 1978.

Bouhasin, J. Purpura fulminans. *Pediatrics,* 34:264, 1964.

Chambers, W., Holyoke, J. and Wilson, R. Purpura fulminans: Report of two cases following scarlet fever. *N. Eng. J. Med.*, 247:933, 1952.

Cram, D. and Soley, R. Purpura fulminans. *Br. J. Dermatol.*, 80:323, 1968.

Cream, J. Immunofluorescent studies of the skin in cryoglobulinaemic vasculitis. *Br. J. Dermatol.*, 84:48, 1971.

Dalldorf, G. The pathology of vitamin C deficiency. *JAMA,* 111:1376, 1938.

Dudgeon, D. et al. Purpura Fulminans. *Arch. Surg.*, 103:351, 1971.

Friedenberg, W. et al. Atypical purpura fulminans with benign monoclonal gammopathy. *Arch. Dermatol.*, 114:578, 1978.

Goldberg, L. and Barnett, E. Essential cryoglobulinemia. *Arch. Int. Med.*, 125:145, 1970.

Goldenfarb, P. and Finch, S. Thrombotic thrombocytopenic purpura. *JAMA,* 226:644, 1973.

Haim, S. et al. Disseminated intravascular coagulation presenting with cutaneous symptoms. *Dermatologica,* 141:239, 1970.

Handin, R. and Smith, A. Immunoidiopathic or immunogenic thrombocytopenic purpura. *N. Eng. J. Med.*, 268:720, 1970.

Horowitz, H. and Nachman, R. Drug purpura. *Seminars in Hematol.*, 2:287, 1965.

Koch-Weser, J. Coumarin necrosis. *Ann. Int. Med.*, 68:1365, 1968.

McMillan, R. Chronic idiopathic thrombocytopenic purpura. *N. Eng. J. Med.*, 304:1135, 1981.

Myers, T. et al. Thrombotic thrombocytopenic purpura: Combined treatment with plasmapheresis and antiplatelet agents. *Ann. Int. Med.*, 92:149, 1980.

Oei, S. et al. Abnormal circulating red blood cells in the painful bruising syndrome. *Arch. Dermatol. Res.*, 263:227, 1978.

Ratnoff, O. *Bleeding Syndromes.* Springfield, IL, Thomas, 1960.

Ratnoff, O. and Agle, D. Psychogenic purpura: A re-evaluation of the syndrome of autoerythrocyte sensitization. *Medicine,* 47:475, 1968.

Ridolfi, R. and Bell, W. Thrombotic thrombocytopenic purpura. (Review) *Medicine* (Baltimore), 60:413, 1981.

Spicer, T. and Rau, J. Purpura fulminans. *Am. J. Med.*, 61:566, 1976.

Stocker, W., McIntyre, O. and Clendenning, W. Psychogenic purpura. *Arch. Dermatol.*, 113:606, 1977.

Tattersall, R. and Seville, R. Senile purpura. *Q. J. Med.*, 19:151, 1950.

Walker, A. Chronic scurvy. *Br. J. Dermatol.*, 80:625, 1968.

Folliculitis

Folliculitis is an inflammatory process involving the pilar complex. The following is an outline of principal causes of folliculitis.

1. Infectious folliculitis
   - A. Bacterial
     - Ostio folliculitis (Bockhart's impetigo); sycosis barbae; acne necrotica (acne varioliformis); dissecting perifolliculitis.
   - B. Fungal
     - Inflammatory types of ringworm; Majocchi granuloma; pityrosporum folliculitis.
2. Folliculitis due to chemicals and drugs
   - A. Industrial contactants
     - Coal tar derivatives; chlorinated hydrocarbons; kerosene.
   - B. Drugs
     - Corticosteroids
3. Folliculitis of unknown or partially understood etiology
   - A. Acne vulgaris
   - B. Rosacea
   - C. Disseminate infundibulofolliculitis
   - D. Follicular occlusion triad
     - Hidradenitis suppurativa; acne conglobata; perifolliculitis capitis abscedens et suffodiens
   - E. Acute deep folliculitis
     - Furuncle
   - F. Chronic deep folliculitis
     - Folliculitis decalvans; folliculitis barbae; acne keloidalis.
4. Pseudofolliculitis of the beard
5. Folliculitis associated with AIDS

GENERAL CLINICAL CHARACTERISTICS OF FOLLICULITIS

1. Early lesions are papules, superficial and deep pustules, inflammatory cysts and abscesses.
2. Late changes due to deep folliculitis include retracted or hypertrophic scars.
3. Acneiform folliculitis may be associated with comedones and milia.

GENERAL MICROSCOPIC CHARACTERISTICS OF FOLLICULITIS

1. Mild forms of folliculitis are associated with a predominantly perifollicular lymphocytic infiltrate and perifollicular edema.
2. With more severe involvement there may be intrafollicular abscess formation.
3. Intercellular edema and breakdown of the outer root sheath may develop.
4. With rupture of the follicular wall, there is release of follicular contents into the surrounding dermis, producing foreign body granulomas and abscesses.
5. Perifollicular fibrosis follows rupture of the outer root sheath.

Folliculitis

The clinical and microscopic features of folliculitis can be approached by considering three types of folliculitis: acne vulgaris, rosacea, and disseminate infundibulofolliculitis.

ACNE VULGARIS

Acne vulgaris is a condition of adolescence and early adulthood involving sebaceous follicles (see p. 52). The face, upper chest, and back are the principal areas involved.

The cause of acne is not fully understood, but a key element is the interaction of androgens and sebaceous follicles. The role of *Proprionibacterium acnes,* a bacterium normally present, is uncertain.

Initially it is believed there is proliferation of epithelium of the lower part of the follicular infundibulum, with associated hyperkeratosis and the formation of open comedones (blackheads) or closed comedones (milia). Subsequent lesions can be papules, pustules, nodules, or cysts. Papules result from inflammation that develops, usually around closed comedones. (Some of the closed comedones can only be seen microscopically.) Pustules, nodules, and cysts develop after rupture of the follicular wall, with ensuing inflammatory and foreign body reaction.

Fig. D. shows open and closed comedones. Figs. A,B show papules, pustules, and milia of acne. It is not certain what causes the black color of blackheads. Some have suggested the black color represents melanin; others have proposed it is oxidized lipid.

Microscopic features

1. Comedones are characterized by follicular dilatation and hyperkeratotic plugging (Fig. E). The wall may be normal, atrophic, or hypertrophic.
2. Fig. C shows an acne pustule with neutrophils within the follicular canal. There is rupture of the follicle wall.
3. Perifolliculitis and granulomatous folliculitis are also common in acne.

ACNE VULGARIS

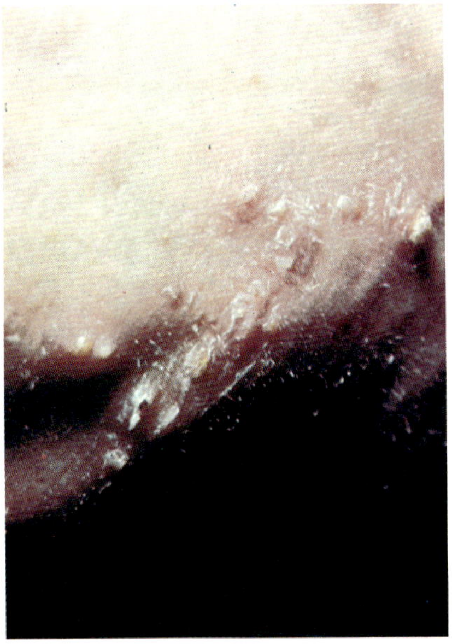

A

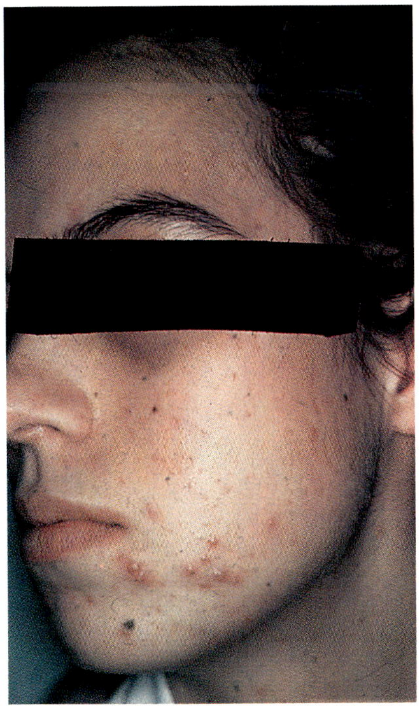

B

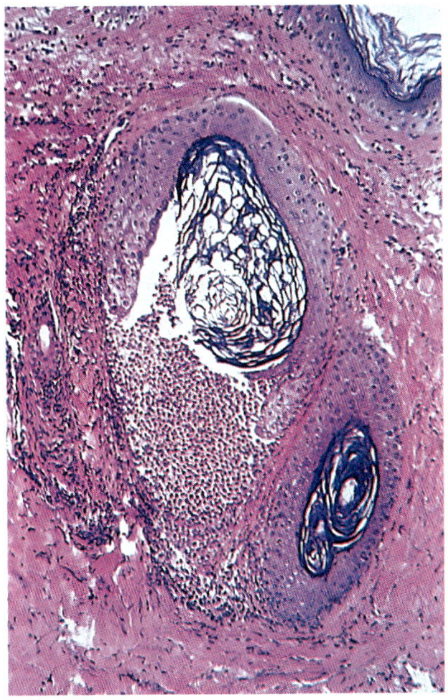

C
X100

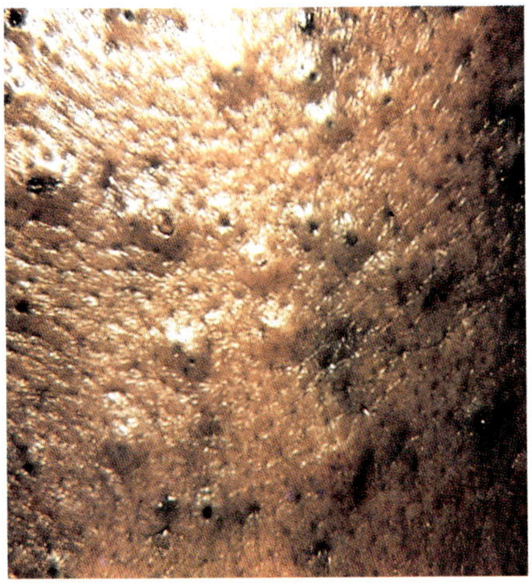

D

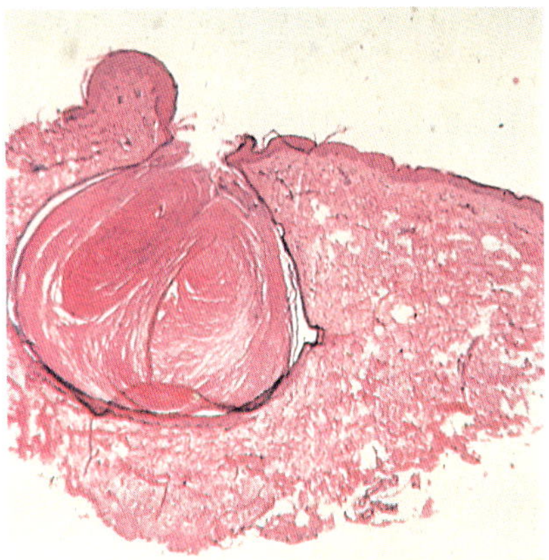

E
X20

ACNE continued ⇨

CYSTIC ACNE

Cystic acne is characterized by cystic inflammatory lesions which often result in hypertrophic and retracted scars (Fig. A).

Microscopic features

1. There is a greatly dilated, keratin-filled cyst (Fig. B) having the wall structure of an epidermal cyst.
2. Rupture of the wall (Fig. B) results in a surrounding zone of acute and chronic inflammation and foreign-body granuloma (Figs. B,C,D), including multinucleated foreign-body giant cells (Figs. C,D).
3. There is progressive fibrosis.

Comment

1. The term "follicular occlusion triad" has been used to describe *hidradenitis suppurativa, acne conglobata,* and *perifolliculitis capitis abscedens et suffodiens. Acne conglobata* is a severe form of acne involving the back, buttocks, and chest, with a tendency to form sinus tracts. Some authors consider acne conglobata to be distinct from acne vulgaris. Perifolliculitis capitis abscedens et suffodiens is acne conglobata involving the scalp. Hidradenitis suppurativa is a chronic inflammatory disorder of the apocrine areas (see p. 164).
2. Chronic deep folliculitis
   a. Acne keloidalis (folliculitis keloidalis nuchae) represents a chronic folliculitis of the nape of the neck, with tendency to form keloids (Fig. E).
   b. Folliculitis decalvans is a chronic folliculitis of the scalp or other hairy areas.
   c. Folliculitis barbae is a deep folliculitis of the beard area in men.
3. Pseudofolliculitis barbae is an inflammatory and foreign body reaction caused by ingrown hairs of the beard in men with curly hair, especially Blacks.
4. Acute folliculitis
   a. Superficial: Impetigo Bockhart, a staphylococcal infection with small, superficial follicular pustules.
   b. Deep: Furuncle; this is a necrotizing folliculitis.

CYSTIC ACNE; ACNE KELOIDALIS

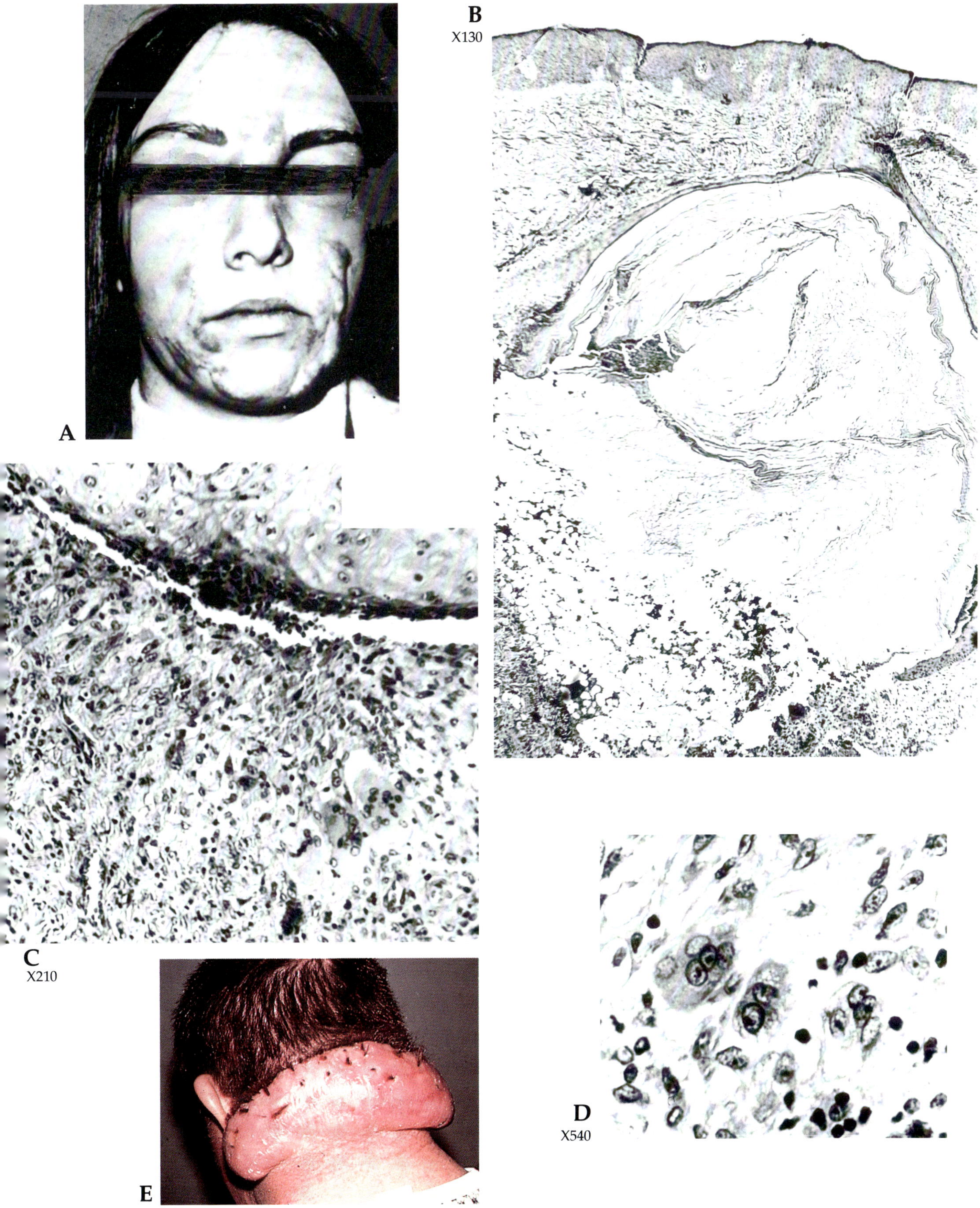

A

B X130

C X210

D X540

E

HIDRADENITIS SUPPURATIVA

Hidradenitis suppurativa is a chronic, purulent disorder of the apocrine areas, including the axillae, pubic, and perianal areas. The groin, abdomen, and inframammary areas may be involved. Initial abscesses are followed by the formation of sinus tracts having purulent drainage (Figs. A,B). Later stages show extensive deformity due to scar formation (Fig. A). The disorder does not occur before puberty, and it is rare in old age. It is widely believed that hidradenitis suppurativa represents a chronic, recurrent folliculitis, with secondary involvement of the apocrine glands. It is part of the follicular occlusion triad (see p. 162).

Microscopic features

1. In the early stages there is perifolliculitis.
2. This leads to endofolliculitis with pustule and abscess formation. Granulomatous folliculitis may be present, as well as granulation tissue with many plasma cells.
3. Ultimately, there is massive and deep inflammation (Figs. C,D), with secondary involvement of apocrine glands.
4. Keratin-filled sinus tracts lined by squamous epithelium may extend downward from the surface epidermis.
5. In late stages there is extensive fibrosis (Fig. E).

Comment

Squamous cell carcinoma may be a late sequel.

HIDRADENITIS SUPPURATIVA

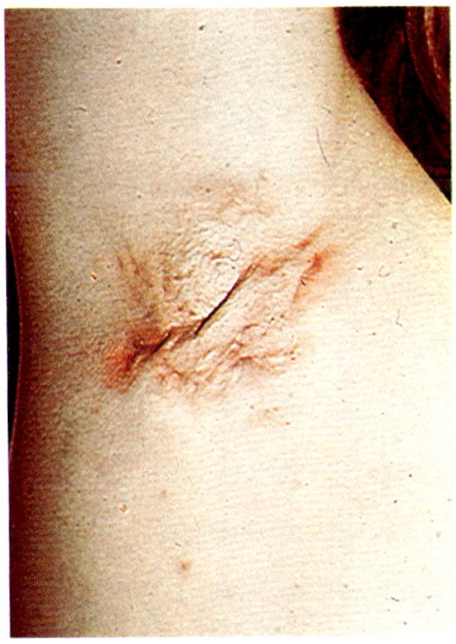

A

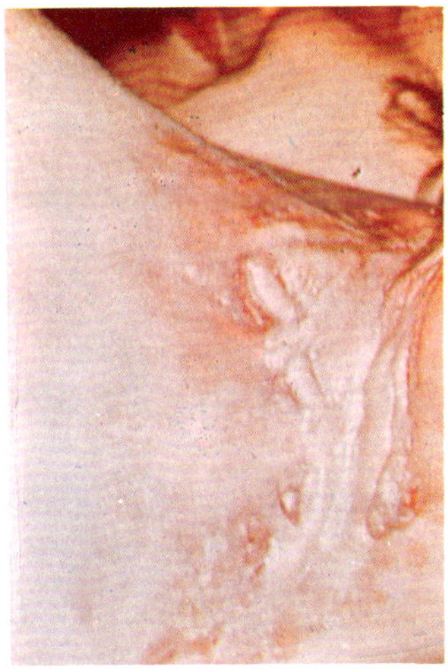

B

Courtesy Dr. Harvey Ansell

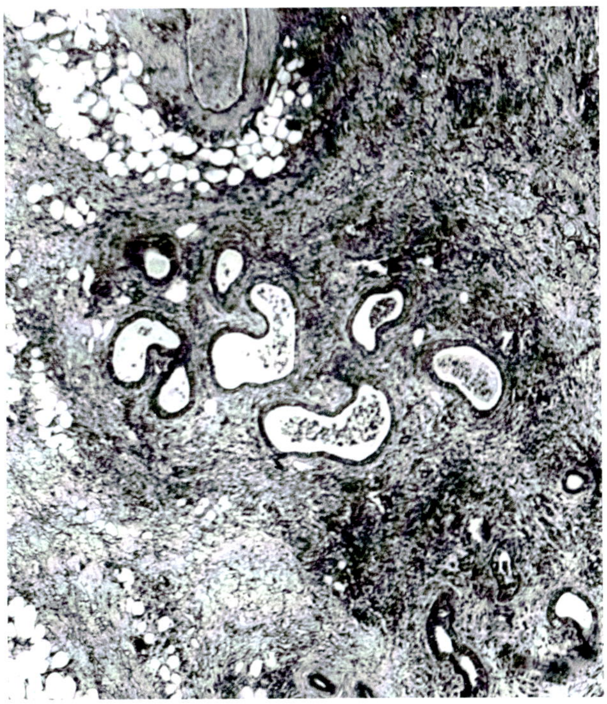

C
X45

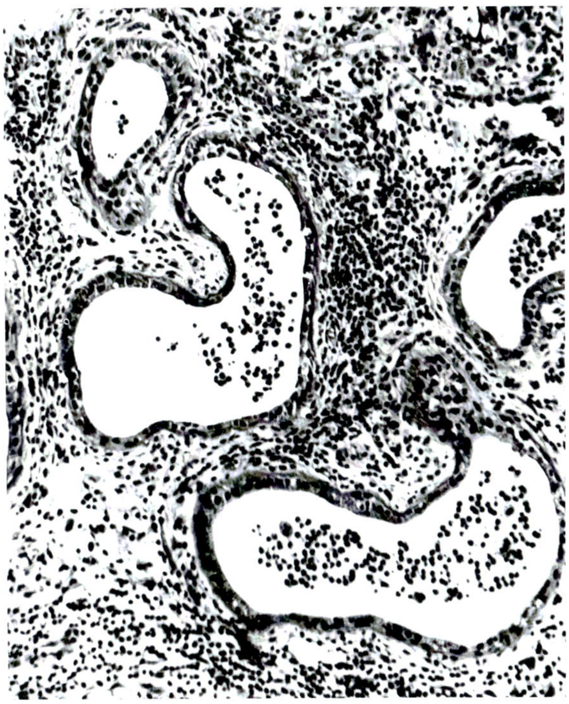

D
X180

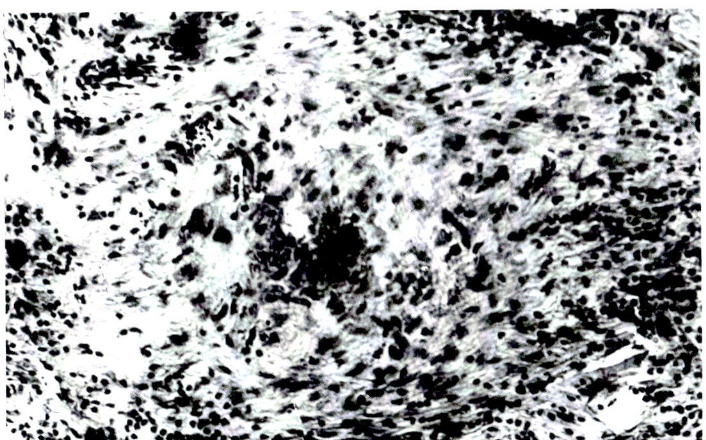

E
X220

ROSACEA (ACNE ROSACEA)

Rosacea is an idiopathic disorder involving pilosebaceous structures. It differs from acne vulgaris by its later onset (usually middle age) and absence of comedones, as well as by certain clinical and microscopic features.

The central area of the face is the main site of involvement. Clinical manifestations include flushing and telangiectasia (Fig. A), and papules and pustules (Fig. C). In addition, there may be a hyperplasia of sebaceous glands of the nose called *rhinophyma*. This tends to affect men more than women.

Microscopic features

1. There is a range of histologic features, depending on the type of lesion biopsied.
2. Perivasculitis and perifolliculitis may be present (Fig. B), as well as telangiectasia (Fig. D).
3. Epithelioid granulomas may be present (Fig. E). Caseation necrosis is usually absent.
4. Abscesses may be present in the dermis (Fig. F); there may be intrafollicular pustules.

Comment

1. A spectrum of ocular problems may accompany rosacea, including keratitis, iritis, blepharitis, conjunctivitis, and episcleritis. The blepharitis may be associated with seborrheic dermatitis, which is often observed in patients with rosacea.
2. *Perioral dermatitis,* a condition seen mainly in women of childbearing age, has a close resemblance to rosacea. It is characterized by clustered, erythematous, scaling papules and pustules, mainly in the central face, including the upper lip and chin. The proposal that it may represent a photosensitivity eruption has been largely abandoned. Some observers believe that topical corticosteroids, especially fluorinated corticosteroids, may aggravate or even cause perioral dermatitis. Perioral dermatitis shares responsiveness to tetracycline therapy with rosacea.

ROSACEA

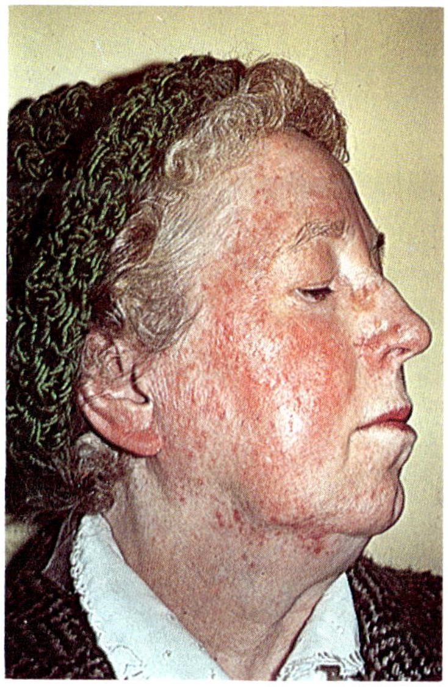

A

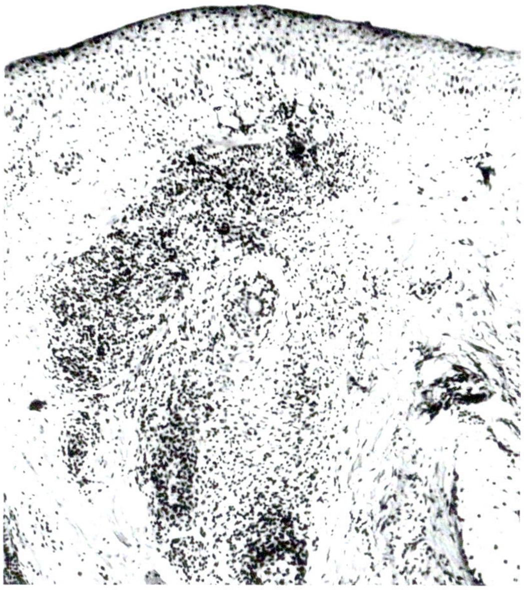

B
X165

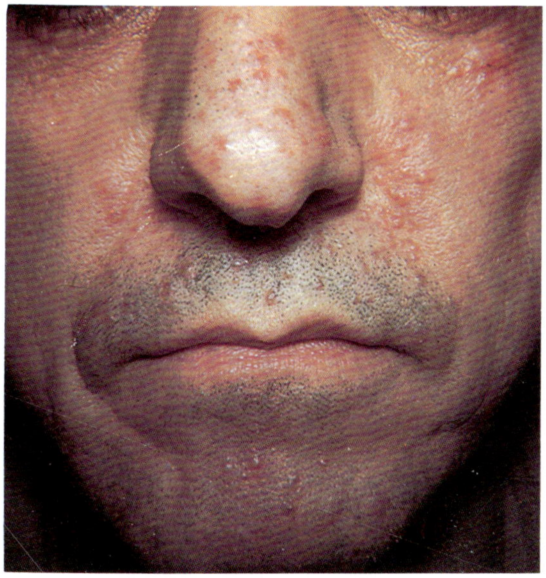

C

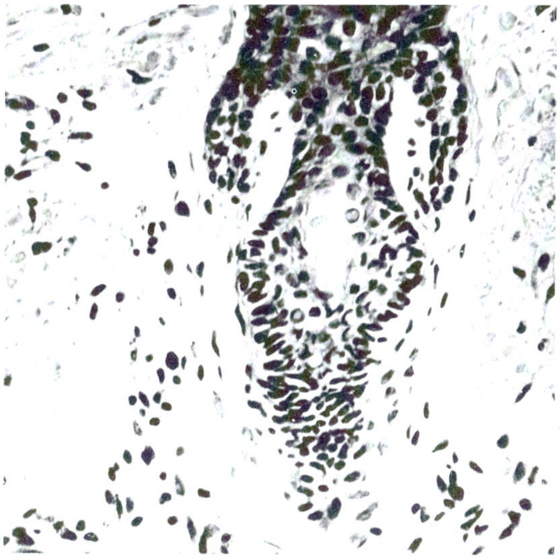

D
X350

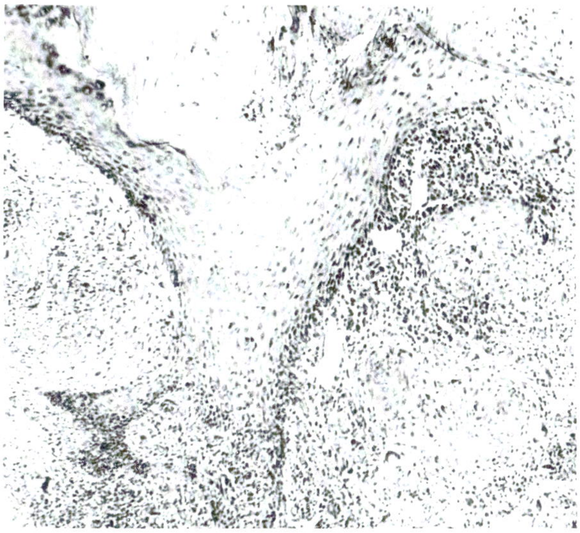

E
X180

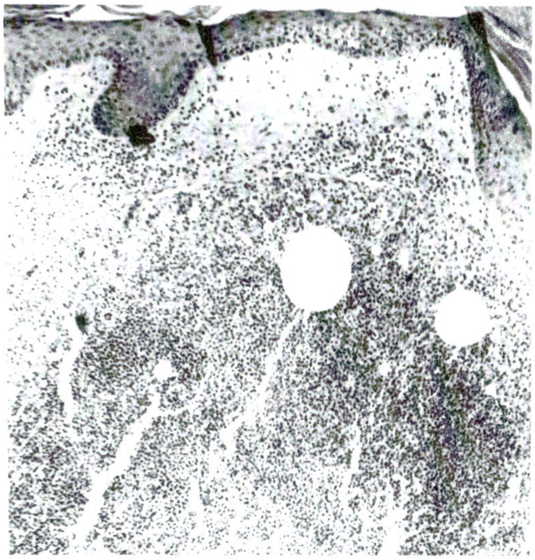

F
X160

ROSACEA continued

ROSACEA: LUPUS MILIARIS DISSEMINATUS FACIEI

Previously, many idiopathic granulomas, including granulomatous rosacea, were falsely attributed to tuberculosis.

Lupus miliaris disseminatus faciei is a condition characterized by papules on the face (Fig. A) made up of caseating granulomas. The eyelids and upper lip are common sites.

Often, but not always, there is associated rosacea. In the non-dermatologic literature, similar lesions have been considered pseudorheumatoid nodules. Lupus miliaris disseminatus faciei can be considered an idiopathic granuloma, sometimes associated with rosacea.

Microscopic features

There are large areas of central caseation necrosis surrounded by epithelioid granulomas (Fig. B). Acid fast bacilli cannot be demonstrated.

Comment

The histologic picture of rosacea, including granulomatous forms, is nonspecific. The granulomatous forms can resemble other granulomas histologically. Clinical data and other laboratory data are important in arriving at a correct diagnosis. PAS stain and Fite stain may be of value in identifying fungal and acid fast granulomas, but generally infectious granulomas with prominent epithelioid tubercles show few if any organisms.

ROSACEA: LUPUS MILIARIS DISSEMINATUS FACIEI

A
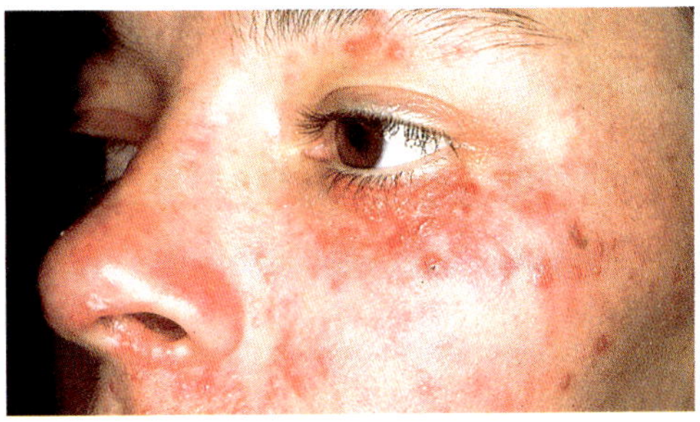

B
X62
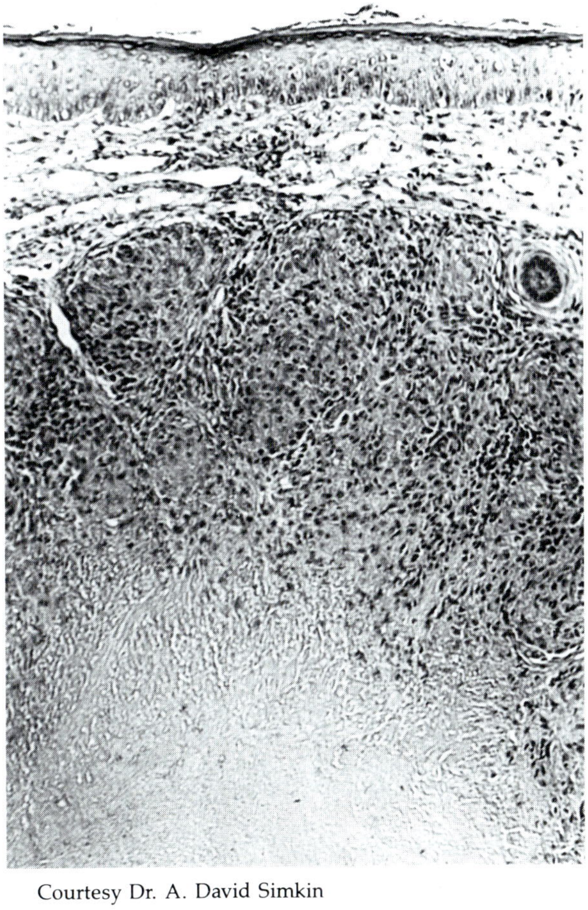

Courtesy Dr. A. David Simkin

ROSACEA continued

ROSACEA: RHINOPHYMA

Rhinophyma represents sebaceous gland hyperplasia of the nose which may accompany rosacea (Fig. A). It is more common in men than in women.

Microscopic features

1. There is lobular hyperplasia of sebaceous glands (Figs. B,C).
2. There is hyperkeratotic follicular plugging (Fig. B), as well as hyperkeratotic plugging of the sebaceous ducts (Fig. C).
3. Moderate chronic inflammation, capillary dilatation, and/or fibrosis may be present in the surrounding stroma (Figs. B,C).

ROSACEA: RHINOPHYMA

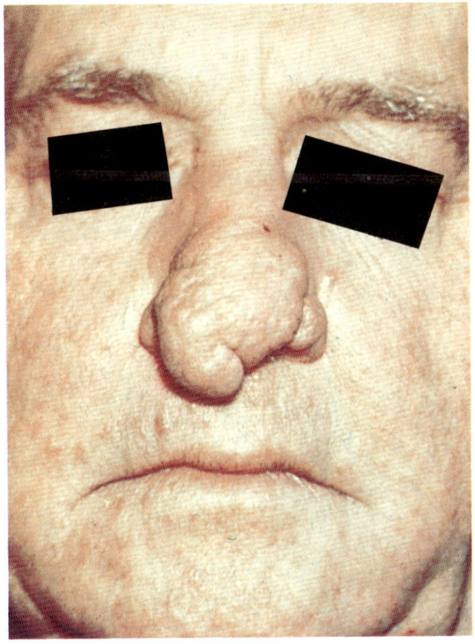

A

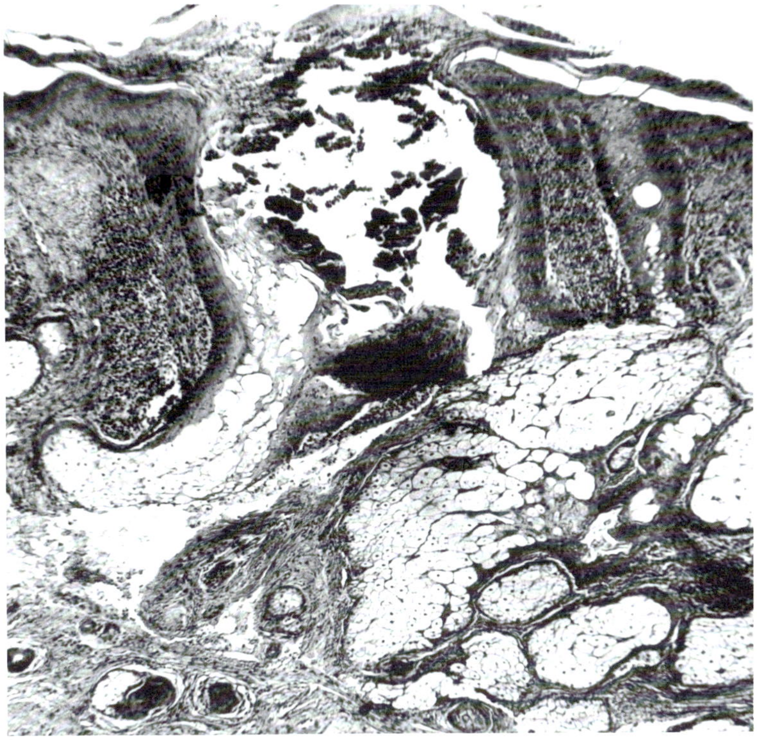

B
X135

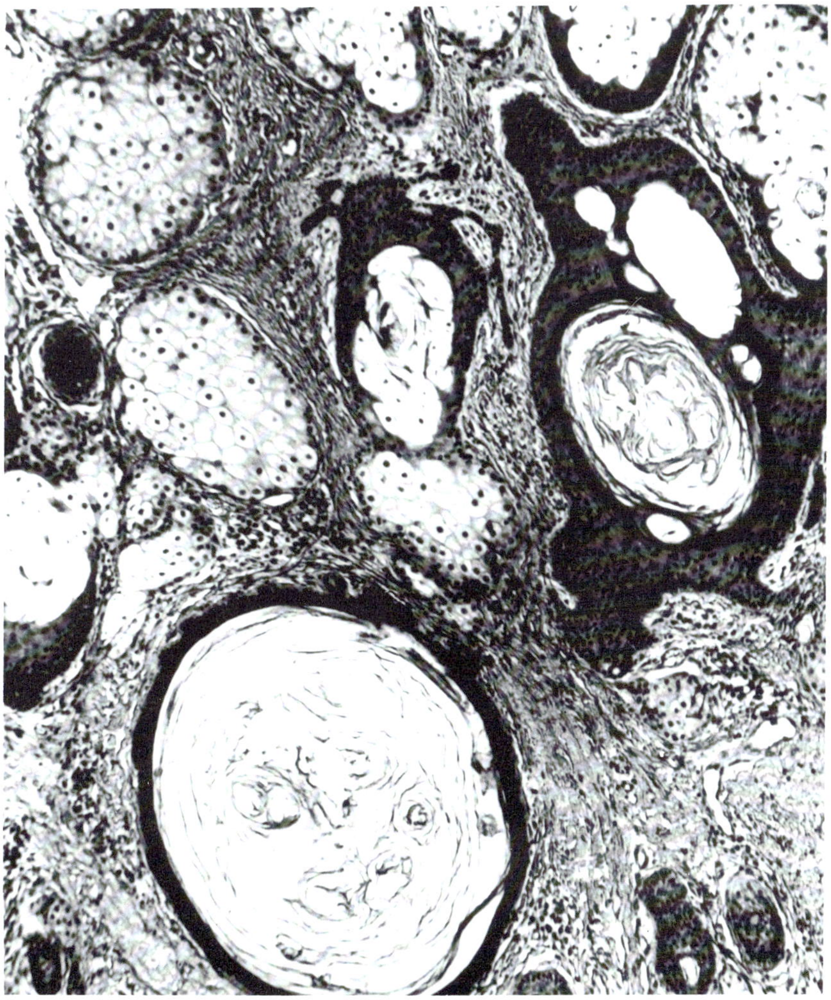

C
X190

DISSEMINATE INFUNDIBULOFOLLICULITIS

Infundibulofolliculitis is a recurrent and widely disseminated superficial folliculitis characterized by large numbers of uniform, minute, follicular papules ("goose flesh") (Fig. B). It occurs almost exclusively in Blacks. The trunk and proximal parts of the extremities are most commonly involved. The cause is unknown.

Disseminate infundibulofolliculitis is an example of superficial folliculitis with mild inflammation of the follicular infundibulum.

Microscopic features

1. There is mild intercellular and intracellular edema of the infundibular portion of the outer root sheaths (Figs. A,C).
2. A perifollicular and perivascular lymphocytic infiltrate is present (Figs. A,C).
3. Keratotic follicular plugging and suprafollicular parakeratosis may be present.

Comment

Eosinophilic pustular folliculitis is a rare condition, first described in Japan and subsequently in Europe. There are erythematous patches with papules and pustules that are largely follicular. Central clearing and peripheral extension tend to occur. The microscopic picture is characterized by an infiltrate in which eosinophils predominate. There may be intraepidermal eosinophil abscesses as well as spongiosis. In the dermis the infiltrate is perivascular. Hair follicles and sebaceous glands are penetrated by the infiltrate, sometimes with a degree of destruction. Leukocytosis and eosinophilia are often present. Eosinophilic pustular folliculitis may be associated with AIDS.

DISSEMINATE INFUNDIBULOFOLLICULITIS

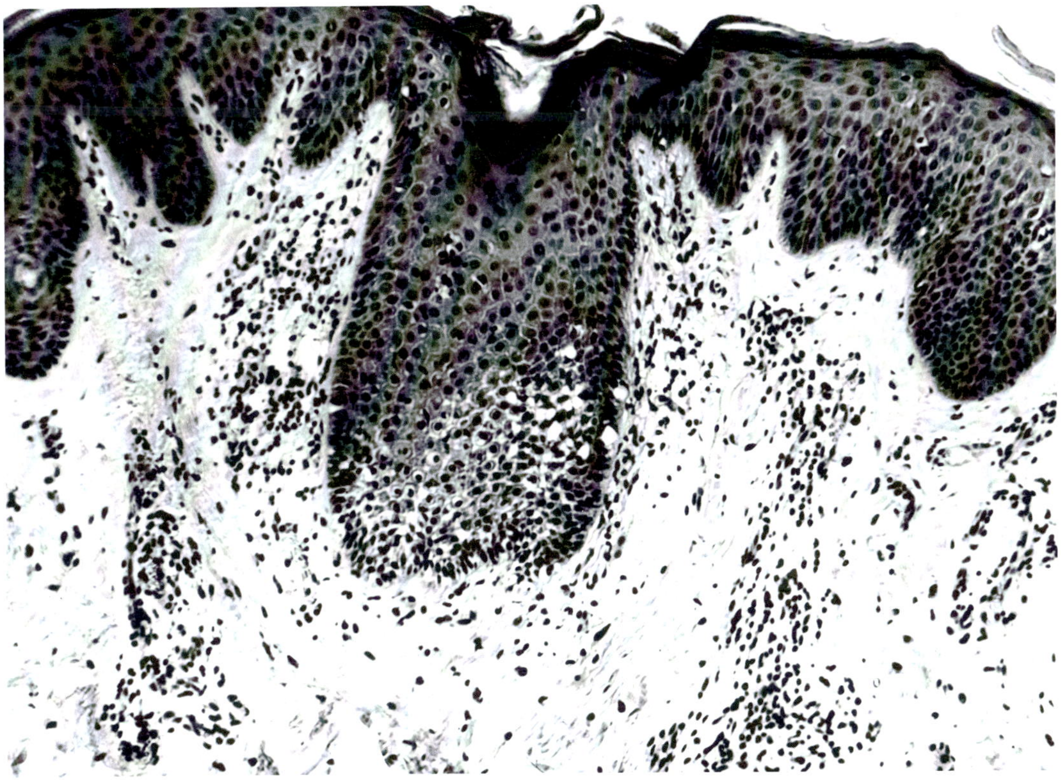

A
X190

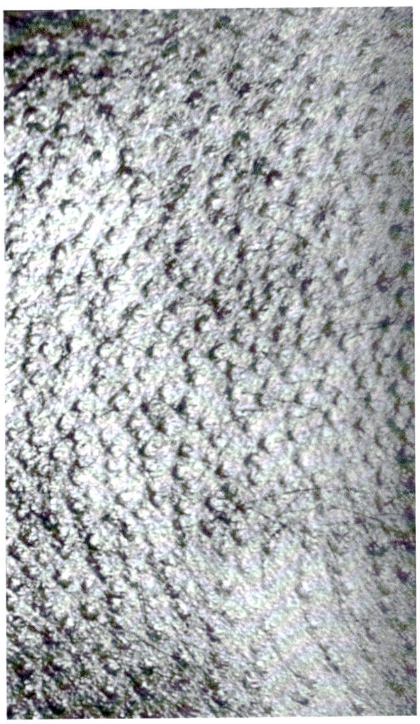

B

Courtesy Dr. William Tarnowski

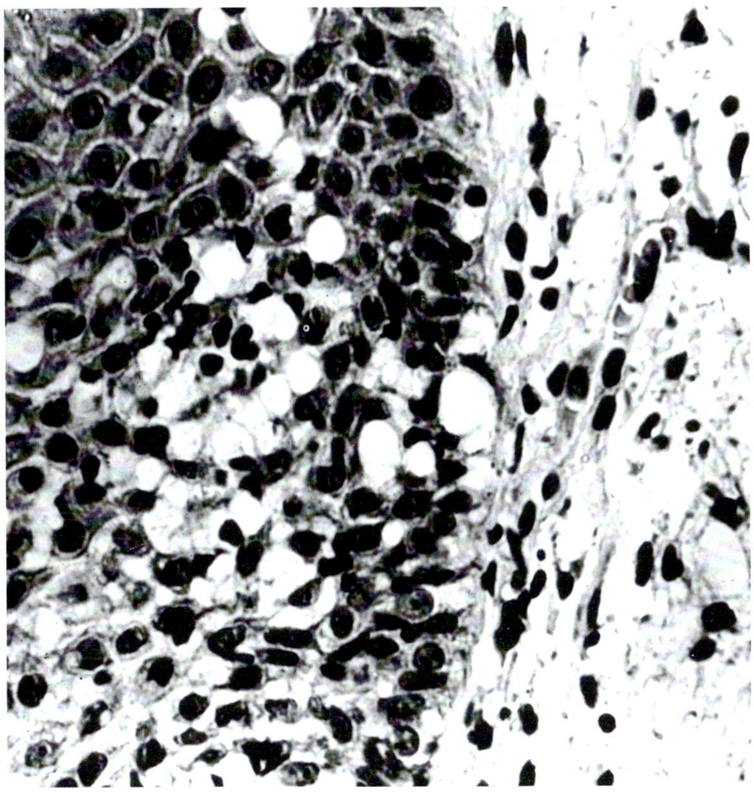

C
X700

Figs. A,C courtesy Dr. Herman Beerman
and Dr. Margaret Gray Wood

Suggested Reading

Folliculitis

General References

Brunner, M., Riddell, J., Jr. and Best, W. Cutaneous side effects of ACTH, cortisone and pregnenolone therapy. *J. Invest. Dermatol.*, 16:205, 1951.

Calnan, C. and O'Neill, D. Some observations on acne necrotica. *Trans. St. John's Hosp. Dermatol. Soc.*, 31:12, 1952.

Graham, J. et al. Tinea capitis. *Arch. Dermatol.*, 89:258, 1954.

Gross, K. Pseudofolliculitis barbae: Shaving bumps of blacks. *J. Assoc. Milit. Dermatol.*, 8:4, 1982.

Hitch, J. Acneiform eruptions induced by drugs and chemicals. *JAMA*, 200:879, 1967.

Laymon, C. and Murphy, R. The cicatricial alopecias. *J. Invest. Dermatol.*, 8:99, 1947.

McMullan, F. and Zeligman, I. Perifolliculitis capitis abscedens et suffodiens. *Arch. Dermatol.*, 73:256, 1956.

Maibach, H. Scalp pustules due to C. acnes. *Arch. Dermatol.*, 96:453, 1967.

Montgomery, H. Acne necrotica miliaris of the scalp. *Arch. Dermatol. Syph.*, 36:40, 1937.

Moschella, S., Klein, M. and Miller, R. Perifolliculitis abscedens et suffodiens. *Arch. Dermatol.*, 96:195, 1967.

Moyer, D. and Williams, R. Perifolliculitis capitis abscedens et suffodiens. *Arch. Dermatol. Syph.*, 85:378, 1962.

Scribner, M. Folliculitis decalvans. *Arch. Dermatol.*, 104:451, 1971.

Shelley, W. and Kligman, A. The experimental production of acne by penta- and hexachloronaphthalenes. *Arch. Dermatol.*, 75:689, 1957.

Smith, J. and Odom, R. Pseudofolliculitis capitis. *Arch. Dermatol.*, 113:328, 1977.

Sullivan, M. and Zeligman, I. Acneiform eruption due to corticotropin. *Arch. Dermatol.*, 73:133, 1956.

Suter, L. Folliculitis decalvans. *Hautarzt*, 32:429, 1981.

Wilson, J., Plunkett, O. and Gregersen, A. Nodular granulomatous perifolliculitis of the legs caused by T. rubrum. *Arch. Dermatol.*, 69:258, 1954.

Acne Vulgaris

Förström, L. The influence of sex hormones on acne. *Acta Derm. Venereol.* (Stockh.) 89 (suppl.):27, 1980.

Freinkel, R. Pathogenesis of acne vulgaris. *N. Eng. J. Med.*, 280:1161, 1969.

Ginsberg, G. et al. Androgen abnormalities in acne vulgaris. *Acta Derm. Venereol.* (Stockh.), 61:431, 1981.

Kaidbey, K. and Kligman, A. Pigmentation in comedones. *Arch. Dermatol.*, 109:60, 1974.

Kellum, R., Strangfeld, K. and Ray, L. Acne vulgaris: Studies in pathogenesis: Triglyceride hydrolysis by Corynebacterium acnes *in vitro. Arch. Dermatol.*, 101:41, 1970.

Kersey, P., Sussman, M. and Dahl, M. Delayed skin test reactivity to *Propionibacterium acnes* correlates with severity of inflammation in acne vulgaris. *Br. J. Dermatol.*, 103:651, 1980.

Kirshbaum, J. and Kligman, A. The pathogenic role of C. acnes in acne vulgaris. *Arch. Dermatol.*, 88:832, 1963.

Kligman, A. An overview of acne. *J. Invest. Dermatol.*, 62:268, 1974.

Lavker, R., Leyden J. and McGinley, K. The relationship between bacteria and the abnormal follicular keratinization in acne vulgaris. *J. Invest. Dermatol.*, 77:325, 1981.

Marples, R. The skin microflora in acne vulgaris. *J. Invest. Dermatol.*, 62:37, 1974.

Marynick, S. et al. Androgen excess in cystic acne. *N. Eng. J. Med.*, 308:981, 1983.

Mills, O. and Kligman, A. Acne aestivalis. *Arch. Dermatol.*, 111:891, 1975.

Plewig, G. Follicular keratinization. *J. Invest. Dermatol.*, 62:308, 1974.

——. Morphologic dynamics of acne vulgaris. *Acta Derm. Venereol.* (Stockh.) 89 (suppl.):9, 1980.

Plewig, G., Fulton, J. and Kligman, A. Cellular dynamics of comedone formation in acne vulgaris. *Arch. Dermatol. Forsch.*, 242:12, 1971.

Plewig, G. and Kligman, A. *Acne: Morphogenesis and Treatment.* Berlin, Springer-Verlag, 1975.

Pochi, P. Hormones and acne. *Semin. Dermatol.*, 1:265, 1982.

Puhvel, S. *Propionibacterium acnes* and acne vulgaris. *Semin. Dermatol.*, 1:293, 1982.

Puhvel, S. and Reisner, R. Effect of antibiotics on the lipases of Corynebacterium acnes *in vitro. Arch. Dermatol.*, 106:45, 1972.

Puhvel, S. and Sakamoto, M. A reevaluation of fatty acids as inflammatory agents in acne. *J. Invest. Dermatol.*, 68:93, 1977.

Sansone, G. and Reisner, R. Differential rates of conversion of testosterone to dihydrotestosterone in acne and in normal human skin: A possible pathogenic factor in acne. *J. Invest. Dermatol.*, 56:366, 1971.

Steinberger, E. et al. The menstrual cycle and plasma testosterone levels in women with acne. *J. Am. Acad. Dermatol.*, 4:54, 1981.

Strauss, J. and Kligman, A. The pathologic dynamics of acne vulgaris. *Arch. Dermatol.*, 82:779, 1960.

Strauss, J. and Pochi, P. Intracutaneous injection of sebum and comedones: Histological observations. *Arch. Dermatol.*, 92:443, 1965.

Van Scott, E. and MacCardle, R. Keratinization of the duct of the sebaceous gland and growth cycle of the hair follicle in the histogenesis of acne in human skin. *J. Invest. Dermatol.*, 27:405, 1956.

Webster, G. and Leyden, J. Characterization of serum independent polymorphonuclear leukocyte chemotactic factors produced by *Propionibacterium acnes. Inflammation*, 4:261, 1980.

——. Mechanisms of *Propionibacterium acnes*: Mediated inflammation in acne vulgaris. *Semin. Dermatol.*, 1:299, 1982.

Anderson, M., Jr. and Dockerty, M. Perianal hidradenitis suppurativa. *Dis. Colon Rectum*, 1:23, 1958.

Brunsting, H. Hidradenitis suppurativa: Abscess of the apocrine sweat glands: A study of the clinical and pathologic features, with a report of twenty-two cases and a review of the literature. *Arch. Dermatol. Syph.*, 39:108, 1939.

Humphrey, L., Playforth, H. and Leavell, U., Jr. Squamous cell carcinoma arising in hidradenitis suppurativa. *Arch. Dermatol.*, 100:59, 1969.

Hyland, C. and Kheir, S. Follicular occlusion disease with elimination of abnormal elastic tissue. *Arch. Dermatol.*, 116:925, 1980.

Knaysi, G., Jr., Cosman, B. and Crikelair, G. Hidradenitis suppurativa. *JAMA*, 203:19, 1968.

McMullan, F. and Zeligman, I. Perifolliculitis capitis abscedens et suffodiens. *Arch. Dermatol.*, 73:256, 1956.

Moschella, S., Klein, M. and Miller, R. Perifolliculitis abscedens et suffodiens. *Arch. Dermatol.*, 96:195, 1967.

Moyer, D. and Williams, R. Perifolliculitis capitis abscedens et suffodiens. *Arch. Dermatol. Syph.*, 85:378, 1962.

Paletta, F. Hidradenitis suppurativa: A pathologic study and use of skin flaps. *Plast. Reconstr. Surg.*, 31:307, 1963.

Pillsbury, D., Shelley, W. and Kligman, A. *Dermatology*, Philadelphia, Saunders, 1956, p. 481.

Shaughnessy, D. et al. Hidradenitis suppurativa. *JAMA*, 222:320, 1972.

Shelley, W. and Cahn, M. The pathogenesis of hidradenitis suppurativa in man: Experimental and histologic observations. *Arch. Dermatol.*, 72:562, 1955.

Warsaw, T. Conglobate acne vulgaris: Associated with low levels of serum gamma globulin. *J. Med. Soc. N.J.*, 62:218, 1967.

Windom, R., Sanford, J. and Ziff, M. Acne conglobata and arthritis. *Arthritis Rheum.*, 4:632, 1961.

Rosacea

Acker, D. and Helwig, E. Rhinophyma with carcinoma. *Arch. Dermatol.*, 95:250, 1967.

Borrie, P. The state of the blood vessels of the face in rosacea. *Br. J. Dermatol.*, 67:5, 1955.

Ecker, R. and Winkelmann, R. Demodex granuloma. *Arch. Dermatol.*, 115: 343, 1979.

Gajewska, M. Rosacea of common male baldness. *Br. J. Dermatol.*, 93:63, 1975.

Hewitt, M. Mites in the personal environment and their role in skin disorders. *Br. J. Dermatol.*, 89:401, 1973.

Hjorth, N. et al. Perioral dermatitis. *Br. J. Dermatol.*, 80:307, 1968.

Laymon, C. and Schoch, E., Jr. Micropapular tuberculid and rosacea. *Arch. Dermatol. Syph.*, 58:286, 1948.

Marks, R. and Harcourt-Webster, J. Histopathology of rosacea. *Arch. Dermatol.*, 100:683, 1969.

Mullanax, M. and Kierland, R. Granulomatous rosacea. *Arch. Dermatol.*, 101:206, 1970.

Pembroke, A. and Houang, E. Letter (subsequent to Cochran, R. and Thompson, J. Perioral dermatitis: A reappraisal). *J. Clin. Exp. Dermatol.*, 5:113, 1980.

Rao, N. and Font, R. Pseudorheumatoid nodules of the ocular adnexa. *Am. J. Ophthalmol.*, 79:471, 1975.

Rush, P. et al. Chronic arthritis following benign rheumatoid nodules of childhood. *Arthritis and Rheumatism*, 28:1175, 1985.

Sams, W. Rhinophyma: With unusual involvement of the chin. *Arch. Dermatol. Syph.*, 26:834, 1932.

Simon, N. Ist der Lupus miliaris disseminatus tuberkulöser Ätiololgie? *Hautarzt*, 26:625, 1975.

Spickett, S. Aetiology of rosacea. *Br. Med. J.*, 1:1625, 1962.

Wilkinson, D. et al. Perioral dermatitis. *Br. J. Dermatol.*, 101:245, 1979.

Eosinophilic Pustular Folliculitis

Guillaume, J. et al. Folliculite à éosinophiles (maladie d'Ofuji). *Ann. Dermatol. Venereol.*, 106:347, 1979.

Holst, R. Eosinophilic pustular folliculitis. *Br. J. Dermatol.*, 95:661, 1976.

Ishibashi, A. et al. Eosinophilic pustular folliculitis (Ofuji). *Dermatologica*, 149:240, 1974.

Ofuji, S. Eosinophilic pustular folliculitis. *Dermatologica*, 174:53, 1987.

Ofuji, S. et al. Eosinophilic pustular folliculitis. *Acta Derm. Venereol.* (Stockh.), 50:195, 1970.

Orfanos, C. and Sterry, W. Sterile eosinophile Pustulose. *Dermatologica*, 157:193, 1978.

Soeprono, F. and Schinella, R. Eosinophilic pustular folliculitis in patients with acquired immunodeficiency syndrome. *J. Am. Acad. Dermatol.*, 14:1020, 1986.

Disseminate Infundibulofolliculitis

Hitch, J. and Lund, H. Disseminate and recurrent infundibulofolliculitis. *Arch. Dermatol.*, 97:432, 1968.

——. Disseminate and recurrent infundibulofolliculitis. *Arch. Dermatol.*, 105:580, 1972.

Owen, W. and Wood, C. Disseminate and recurrent infundibulofolliculitis. *Arch. Dermatol.*, 115:174, 1979.

Wolf, M. and Tolmach, J. Disseminate and recurrent infundibulofolliculitis. *Arch. Dermatol.*, 103:552, 1971.

Inflammation of Sweat Glands

Inflammation of apocrine glands

FOX-FORDYCE DISEASE

The disorder usually affects young women. There is a pruritic eruption composed of follicular papules in the apocrine areas (Fig. A). Fox-Fordyce disease is considered to be an apocrine miliaria resulting from keratinous obstruction of the apocrine orifices.

Microscopic features

1. The principal pathologic change is considered to be a spongiotic vesicle forming around the terminal portion of the apocrine duct in the infundibulum of the hair follicle. This develops secondary to the formation of a keratotic plug in the hair follicle. Serial sections are usually required to demonstrate the spongiotic vesicle.
2. There may be dilatation and rupture of the walls of the dermal portions of the apocrine ducts, accompanied by dermal edema, inflammation, and deposition of neutral and acid mucopolysaccharides.
3. The dermis around the apocrine glands shows edema and a chronic inflammatory infiltrate (Fig. B).

FOX-FORDYCE DISEASE

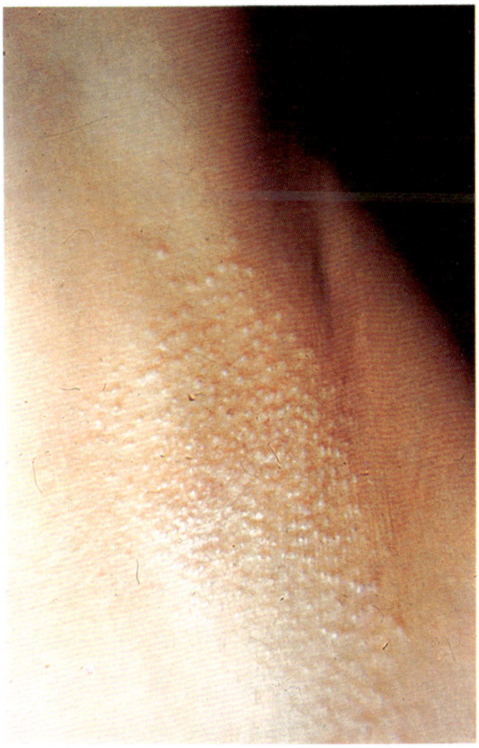

A

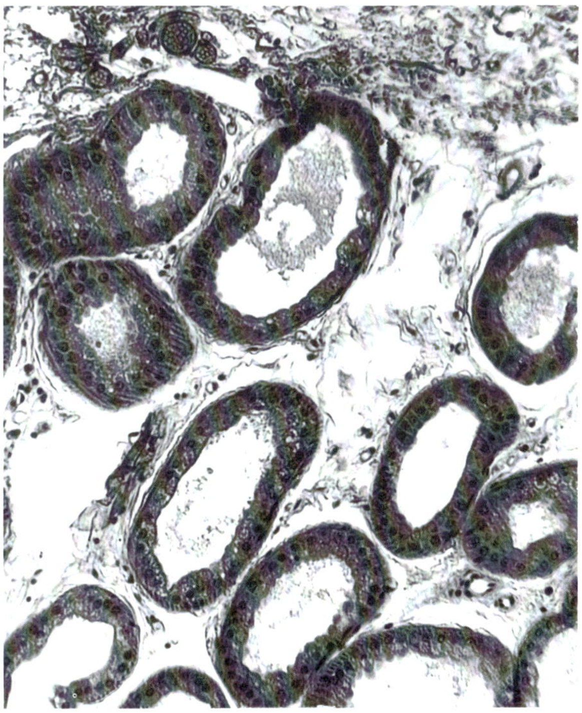

B
X155

Inflammation of eccrine glands

MILIARIA

Miliaria is an inflammatory disorder involving various portions of the eccrine duct; it is associated with excessive sweating and poral occlusion.

There are two principal types: *miliaria crystallina* and *miliaria rubra*. Both forms may coexist.

Miliaria crystallina is characterized by superficial, discrete, or confluent vesicles (Fig. A), often on the exposed areas. Miliaria crystallina may be associated with sunburn, febrile illness, or the use of occlusive dressings.

Miliaria rubra is characterized by the presence of erythematous papules, vesicles, and pustules (Fig. B), occurring principally on the covered areas of the body during periods of excessive sweating.

Miliaria pustulosa is a variant in which pustules predominate (Fig. C).

Microscopic features

1. Miliaria crystallina
   a. Vesicles are present within the stratum corneum, or just beneath it (Figs. D,E). These surround a ruptured terminal eccrine duct.
2. Miliaria rubra
   a. There is edema around the middle or lower portions of the terminal eccrine duct; the ruptured portion of the duct may be seen in serial sections.
   b. A chronic inflammatory infiltrate is present around the upper portion of the dermal eccrine duct, composed principally of lymphocytes (Fig. F).
   c. In *miliaria pustulosa* there are dense accumulations of neutrophils around the ruptured terminal portions of the eccrine duct (Fig. G).

Comment

Miliaria profunda is a rare disorder associated with anhidrosis. In this condition the vesicles are located in the deep portions of the epidermis and/or adjacent dermis.

MILIARIA

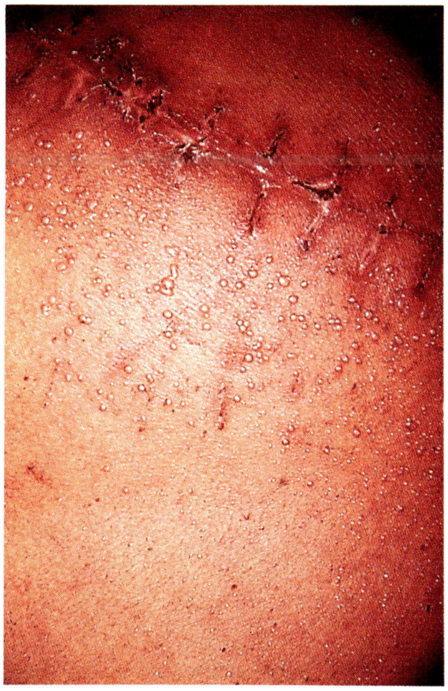

A

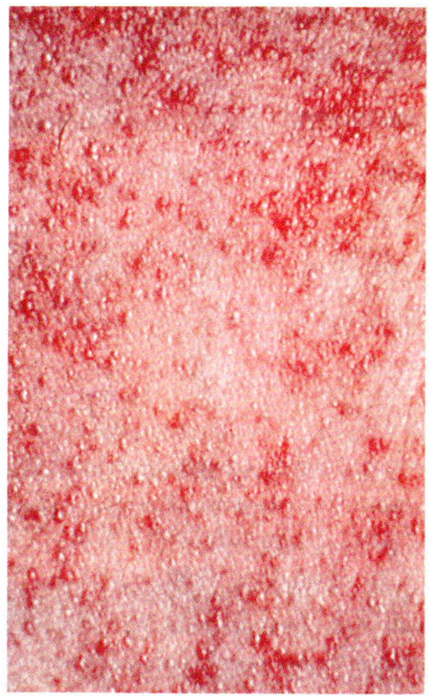

B

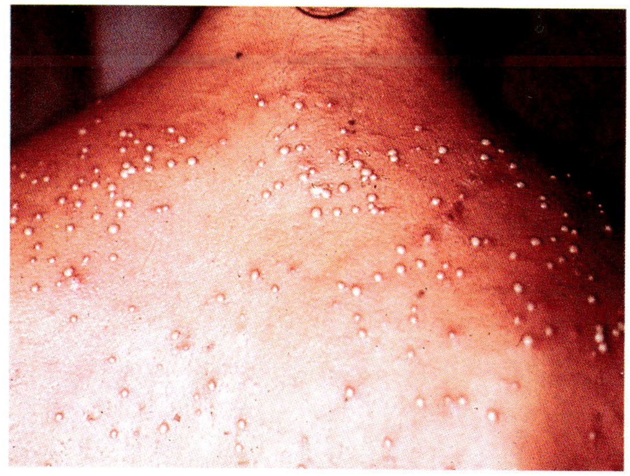

C

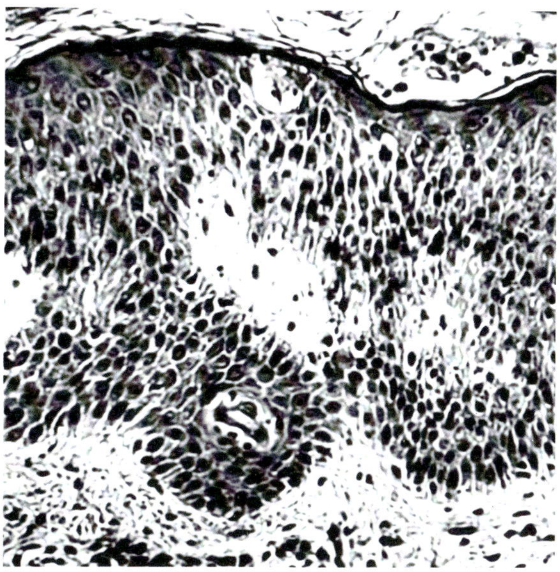

D
X280

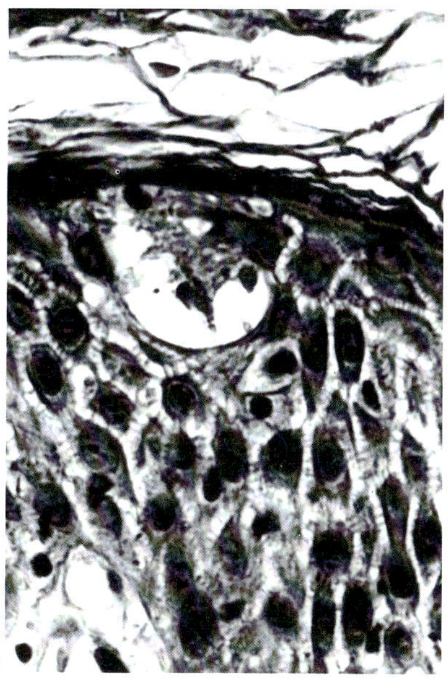

E
X720

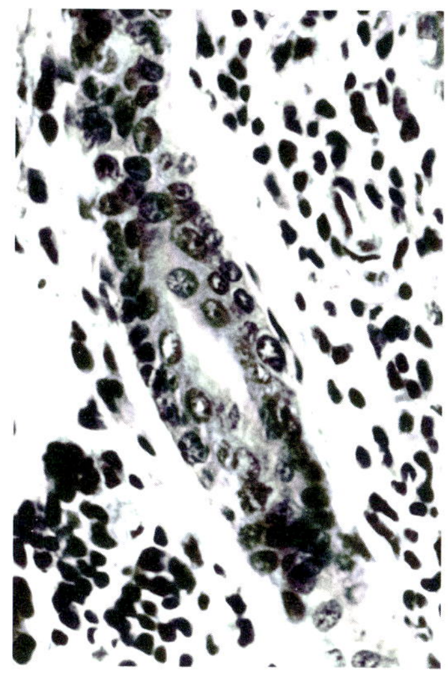

F
X520

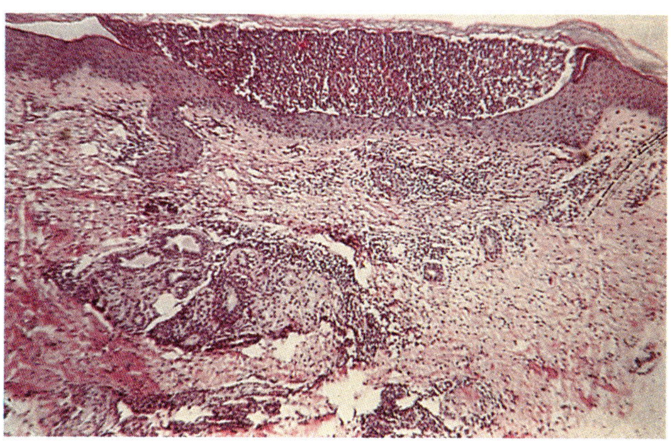

G
X120

Suggested Reading

Inflammation of Sweat Glands

Fox-Fordyce Disease

Cornbleet, T. Pregnancy and apocrine gland diseases: Hidradenitis, Fox-Fordyce disease. *Arch. Dermatol. Syph.*, 65:12, 1952.

Graham, J., Shafer, J. and Helwig, E. Fox-Fordyce disease in male identical twins. *Arch. Dermatol.*, 82:212, 1960.

Kronthal, H., Pomeranz, J. and Sitomer, G. Fox-Fordyce disease: Treatment with an oral contraceptive. *Arch. Dermatol.*, 91:243, 1965.

MacMillan, D. and Vickers, H. Fox-Fordyce disease. *Br. J. Dermatol.*, 84:181, 1971.

Mevorah, B., Duboff, G. and Wass, R. Fox-Fordyce disease in prepubescent girls. *Dermatologica*, 136:43, 1968.

Shelley, W. and Levy, E. Apocrine sweat retention in man. II. Fox-Fordyce disease (apocrine miliaria). *Arch. Dermatol.*, 73:38, 1956.

Spiller, R. and Knox, J. Fox-Fordyce disease with hidradenitis suppurativa. *J. Invest. Dermatol.*, 31:127, 1958.

Miliaria

Holzle, E. and Kligman, A. The pathogenesis of miliaria rubra: Role of the resident microflora. *Br. J. Dermatol.*, 99:117, 1978.

Loewenthal, L. The pathogenesis of miliaria: The role of sodium chloride. *Arch. Dermatol.*, 84:2, 1961.

Shelley, W. and Horvath, P. Experimental miliaria in man. II. Production of sweat retention anidrosis and miliaria crystallina by various kinds of injury. *J. Invest. Dermatol.*, 14:9, 1950.

——. Experimental miliaria in man. III. Production of miliaria rubra (prickly heat). *J. Invest. Dermatol.*, 14:193, 1950.

Sulzberger, M. and Harris, D. Miliaria and anhidrosis. III. Multiple small patches and the effects of different periods of occlusion. *Arch. Dermatol.*, 105:845, 1972.

Sulzberger, M. and Zimmerman, H. Studies on prickly heat. II. Experimental and histologic findings. *J. Invest. Dermatol.*, 7:61, 1946.

Panniculitis

Panniculitis is a component of a wide range of conditions. There is no universal agreement on its classification. Since entities are characterized by variable clinical and microscopic features, universal agreement is difficult.

Attempts to classify panniculitis on the basis of septal and lobular involvement and on the basis of presence or absence of vasculitis are of questionable value because of the variability within entities.

In this section we will discuss entities in which panniculitis is the sole or dominant manifestation.

ERYTHEMA NODOSUM

Erythema nodosum is a hypersensitivity response characterized by tender erythematous or violaceous nodules of short duration, most commonly located on the anterior aspects of the lower legs (Fig. A). The lesions often become ecchymotic and are often accompanied by fever. Individual lesions usually last for a few weeks. The overall process typically lasts for several months. There is a chronic form which may persist for years.

Causes include: infections (tuberculosis, streptococcal infections, and deep fungus infections), drugs (sulfonamides, halides, anovulatory agents, barbiturates, and antibiotics), immunopathies, and sarcoidosis. Internal malignancies may be associated with erythema nodosum. Some cases have no apparent cause.

Microscopic features.

1. The principal changes are in the subcutaneous fat. A chronic inflammatory infiltrate is present in the septa separating fat lobules and between the individual fat cells (Figs. B1,C,D,E). Septa may show edema and fibrinoid degeneration. The inflammatory process may be limited to the periphery of fat lobules.
2. In early lesions, there is a transient infiltrate of neutrophils. Later, the characteristic mixture of lymphocytes, histiocytes, and eosinophils appears.
3. The dermis shows a mild to moderate perivascular lymphocytic infiltrate (Fig. C).
4. Evolved lesions of classical erythema nodosum and lesions of chronic erythema nodosum (see below) show diffuse granuloma formation without caseation (Fig. B2).
5. Walls of vessels may show edema and infiltration by inflammatory cells (Figs. D,E,F).
6. Necrosis of fat does not occur.

Microscopic differential diagnosis (see table, p. 192)

Comment

1. *Chronic erythema nodosum* (nodular migratory panniculitis; erythema nodosum migrans) is a variant of erythema nodosum in which the lesions are few and are arranged around joints of the lower legs. The disease process may last a few years.
2. *Erythema nodosum leprosum* differs from erythema nodosum by the presence of leukocytoclastic vasculitis and lepra bacilli in the vessel walls. It is a form of reactional leprosy (see p. 320).

ERYTHEMA NODOSUM

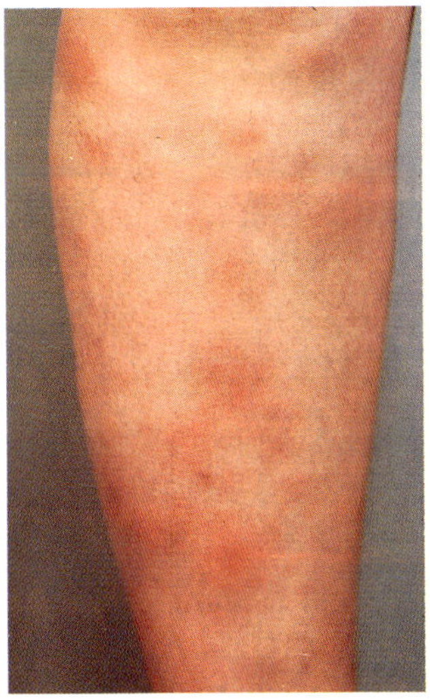

A

Courtesy Dr. K. Inaba

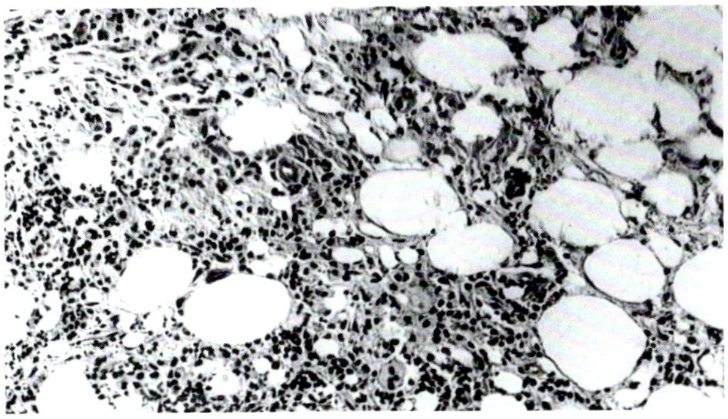

B1
X130

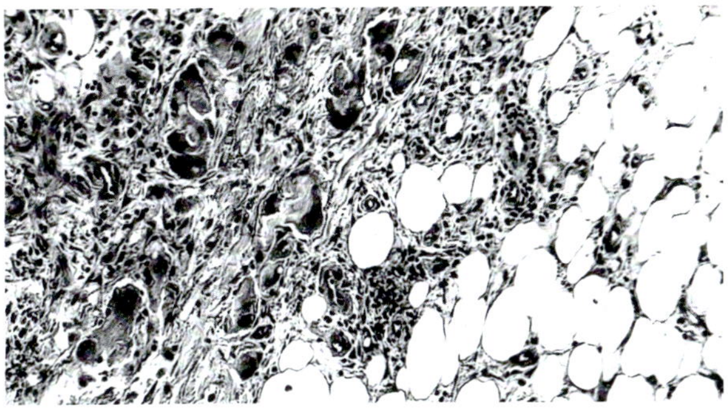

B2
X130

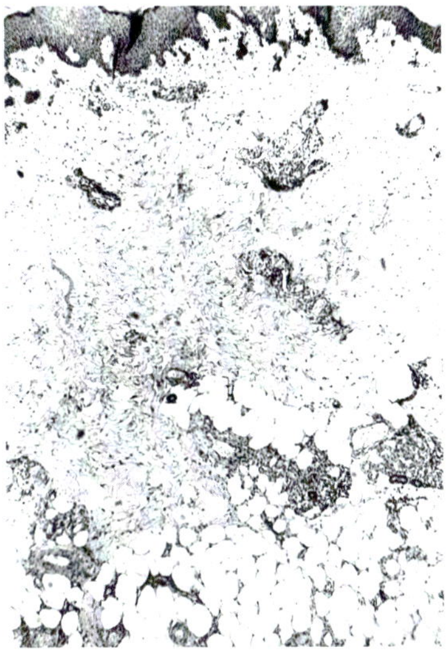

C
X30

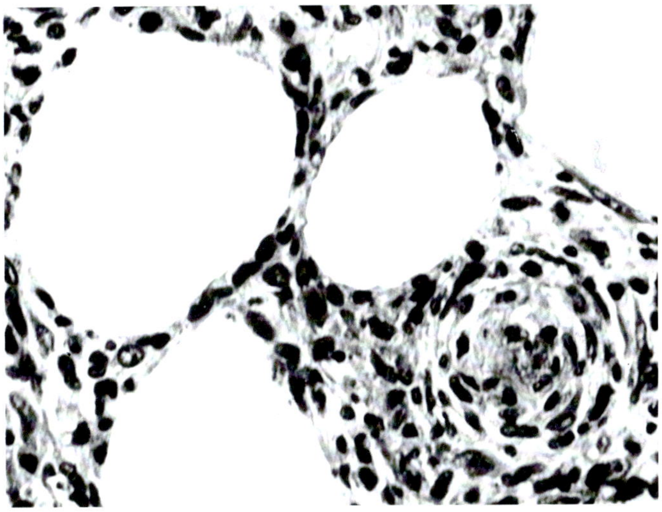

D
X800

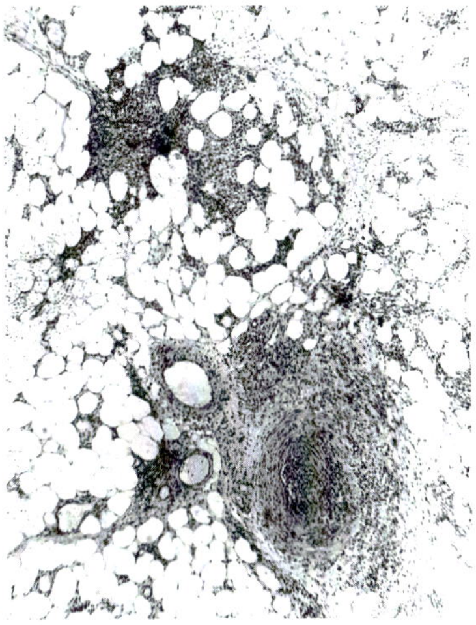

E
X80

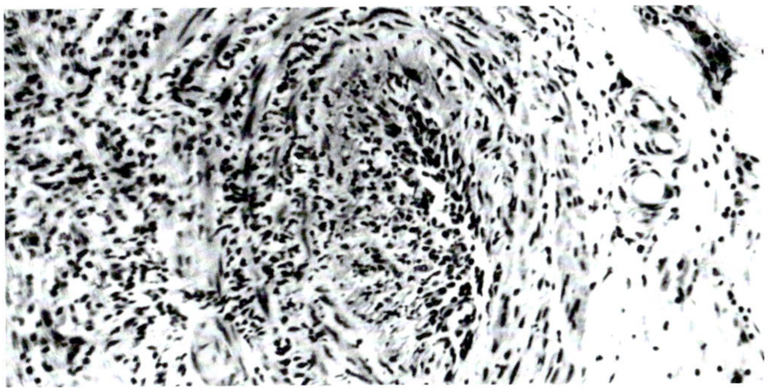

F
X180

PANNICULITIS continued ⇨

ERYTHEMA INDURATUM (BAZIN'S DISEASE)

Erythema induratum (Fig. A) is a chronic, recurrent disorder characterized by violaceous indurated areas and plaques, usually involving the posterior aspects of the legs. The lesions tend to ulcerate and form retracted scars. Erythema induratum has a predilection for women; recurrences may be precipitated by exposure to cold. An etiologic relationship to tuberculosis has not been substantiated. The prominence of vascular changes has led some authors to consider erythema induratum a form of granulomatous vasculitis. When vascular changes are particularly prominent, the process has been termed *nodular vasculitis*.

Microscopic features

1. The pathologic changes are generally confined to the subcutaneous fat, although there may be inflammatory changes in the dermis.
2. The infiltrate is ofen massive, replacing large areas of subcutaneous fat (Wucheratrophie) (Figs. B,D).
3. A chronic inflammatory infiltrate is intermingled with a tuberculoid granuloma (Figs. B,D,F). Many giant cells are usually present (Figs. B,D,E). Caseation frequently is present and often surrounds involved vessels (Fig. C).
4. Widespread and severe changes are present involving arteries and veins of all sizes. Vessel wall changes include edema, necrosis, infiltration with acute and chronic inflammatory cells; thrombosis (Fig. C) may develop.

Microscopic differential diagnosis (see table, p. 192)

Comment

Superficial migratory thrombophlebitis is characterized by tender, nonulcerating nodules of the legs. Medium-sized and small veins at the junction of the dermis and subcutaneous fat are thrombosed and show a chronic granulomatous phlebitis; there is a surrounding granulomatous panniculitis.

ERYTHEMA INDURATUM

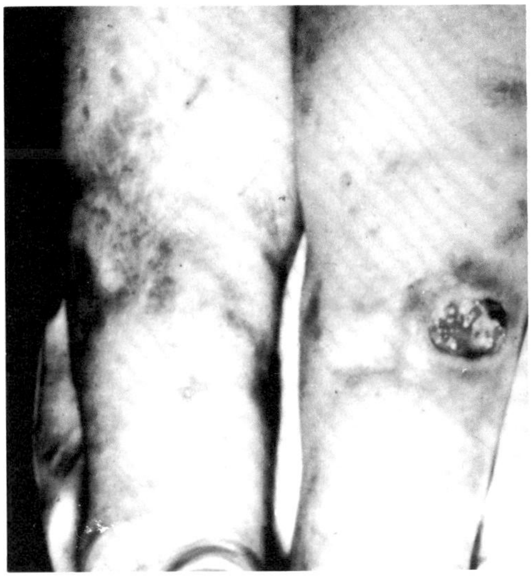

A

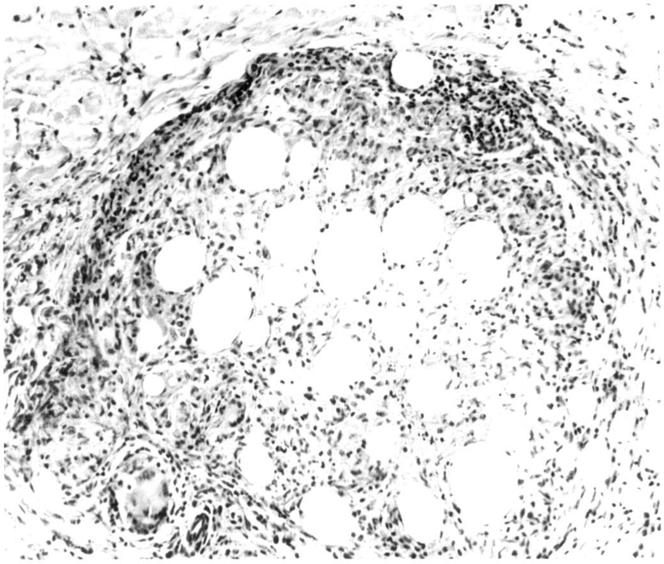

B X140

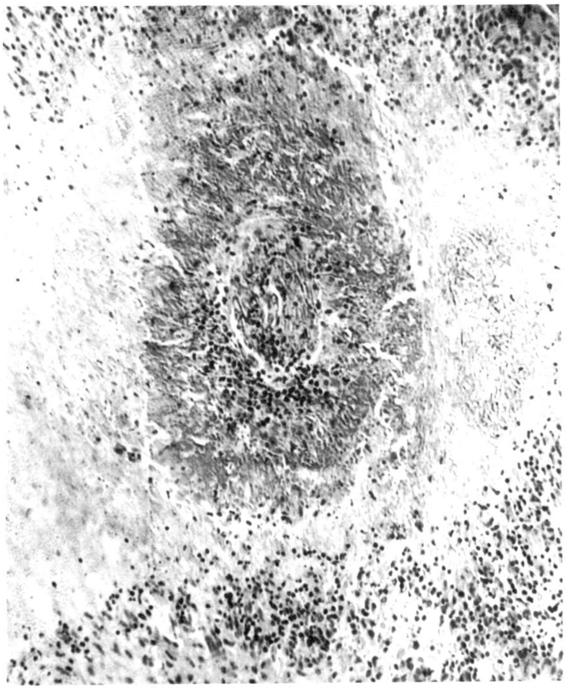

C X185

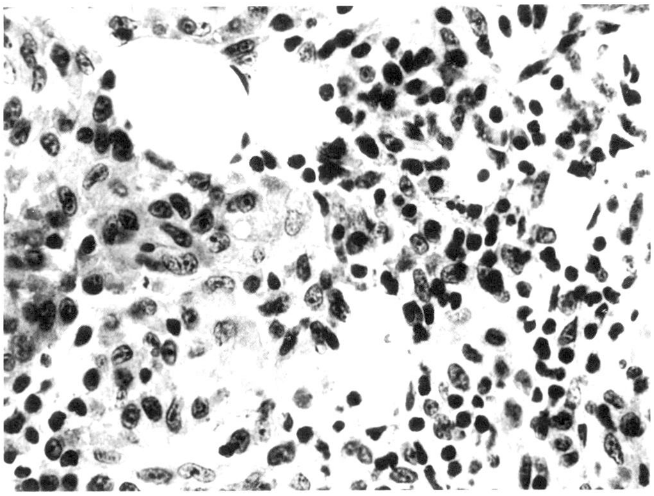

D X580

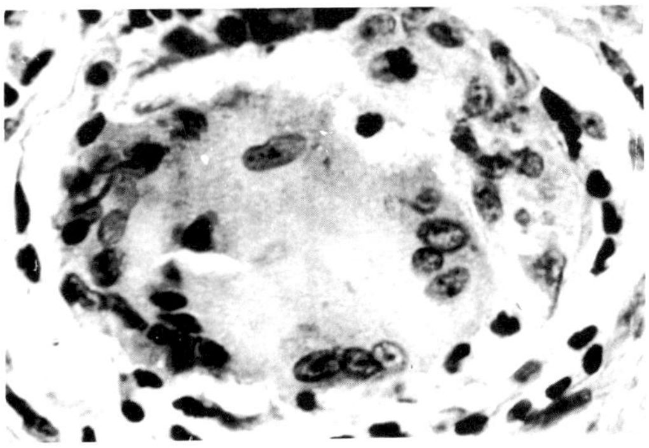

E X680

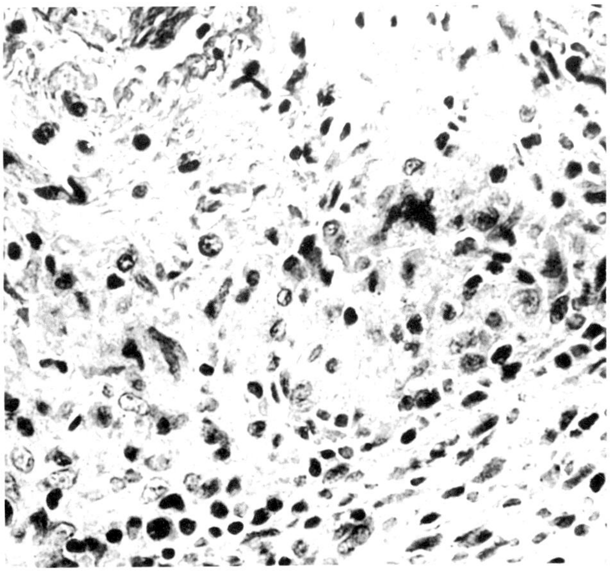

F X650

PANNICULITIS continued

WEBER-CHRISTIAN DISEASE (RELAPSING FEBRILE, NODULAR, NONSUPPURATIVE PANNICULITIS)

The disorder occurs predominantly in women and is characterized by crops of tender subcutaneous nodules (Fig. A) accompanied by fever. The buttocks and thighs are most commonly involved, but lesions may occur in other areas. In some instances there is a liquefying panniculitis, with breakdown of the surface epidermis. When the lesions heal, they leave flat, depressed scars. Rarely, Weber-Christian disease involves the visceral fat. Distinction from other types of panniculitis, particularly subcutaneous fat necrosis associated with pancreatic disease, may be difficult.

If systemic panniculitis occurs, there is a potentially fatal outcome.

Microscopic features

1. There are three stages:

Stage I

The subcutaneous fat contains a massive infiltrate composed mainly of neutrophils, with varying numbers of lymphocytes and histiocytes. There is focal degeneration of fat cells (Figs. B,C,D).

Stage II

The inflammatory infiltrate is replaced by large numbers of foam cells (Figs. E,F).

Foam cells may be so numerous that large areas of subcutaneous fat are almost completely replaced (Fig. E).

A chronic inflammatory infiltrate may be present.

Stage III

There is increasing fibrosis, with residual chronic inflammation.

Microscopic differential diagnosis (see table, p. 192)

Comment

1. In cases of Weber-Christian disease with liquefying panniculitis, large necrotic areas containing cellular debris are present.
2. The dermis and epidermis usually show no significant pathologic changes in Weber-Christian disease.
3. *Lipogranulomatosis subcutanea of Rothmann and Makai* has been described as a variant of Weber-Christian disease showing few cutaneous lesions, and no fever or visceral lesions. However, there is some reason to believe that cases described under this heading represented other types of panniculitis.
4. *Subcutaneous nodular fat necrosis associated with pancreatic disease* is due to the release of large amounts of lipase and possibly amylase and trypsin into the lymphatics. This is seen in some patients with pancreatitis or pancreatic carcinoma. Lesions are tender, erythematous nodules, generally on the legs. Periarticular and intraperitoneal fat necrosis may be present.

   The microscopic picture is dominated by extensive necrosis of the subcutaneous fat, with numerous "ghost-like" fat cells without nuclei, and basophilic calcium soaps. A granulomatous infiltrate usually surrounds areas of necrosis.

   The picture in the subcutaneous fat is identical to that of the peripancreatic fat in acute pancreatitis.

WEBER-CHRISTIAN DISEASE

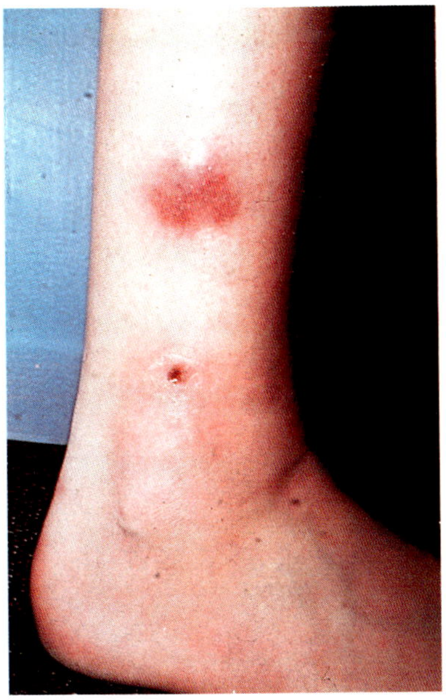

A

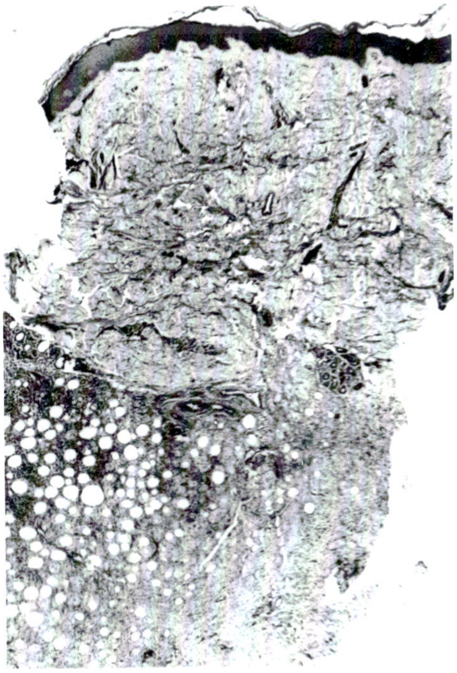

B
X28

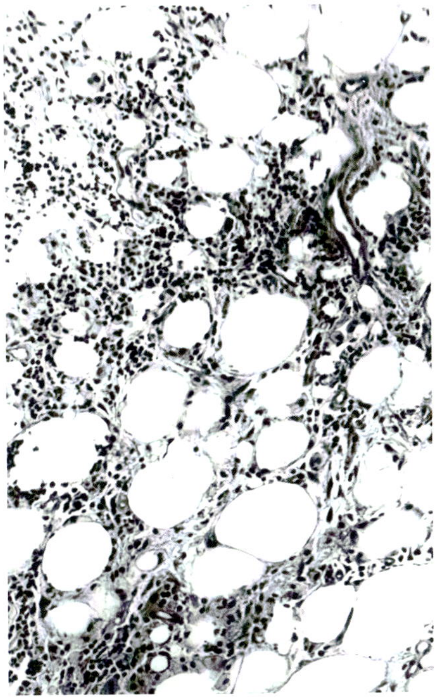

C
X180

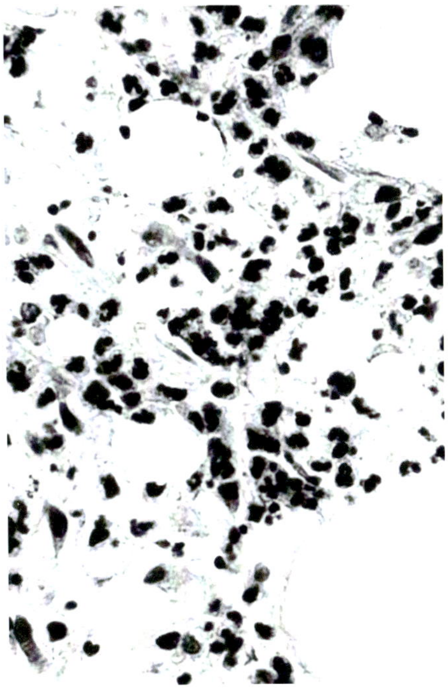

D
X520

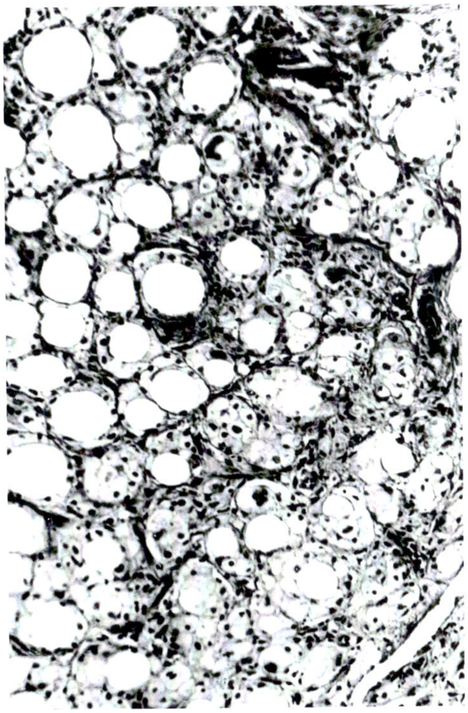

E
X160

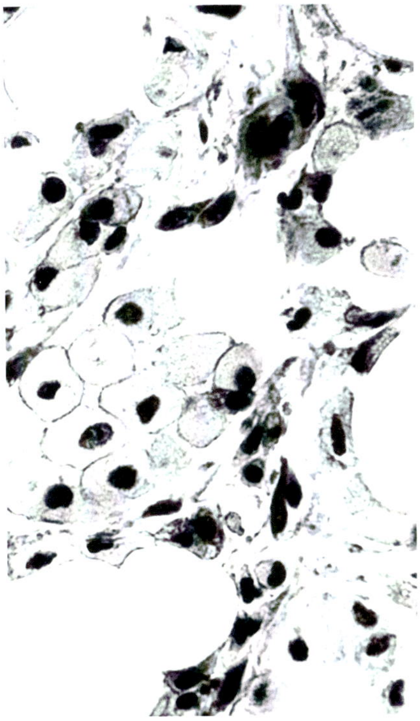

F
X650

PANNICULITIS continued ⇨

SUBCUTANEOUS FAT NECROSIS OF THE NEWBORN

Subcutaneous fat necrosis of the newborn is a disorder characterized by an accumulation of saturated fatty acids which crystallize with lowered environmental temperature, resulting in fat necrosis. There is a usually benign localized form and a potentially lethal generalized form (sclerema neonatorum). In the localized form there are varying numbers of circumscribed, indurated nodules (Fig. A). In the generalized form, the skin is diffusely hard and waxy. Visceral fat may be involved.

Microscopic features

1. The histologic changes in generalized and localized forms are similar. However, the granulomatous infiltrate (see below) and necrosis are more prominent in the localized form. The generalized form shows intersecting fibrous bands.
2. The characteristic feature is fat necrosis (Figs. B,F) and the presence of needle-like crystals in radial formation within degenerated fat cells (Fig. D). The crystals are smaller in the generalized form. With paraffin sections the crystals appear as empty spaces; with frozen sections the crystals are birefringent when examined with polarized light (Fig. E). In Fig. E, sections were stained with fat stain before polariscopic examination.
3. A chronic inflammatory infiltrate is present in the interlobular septa. In older lesions foreign-body giant cells may be present (Figs. B, C).
4. Calcification is often present and can be readily demonstrated with a calcium stain. (Fig. F).

Differential diagnosis (see table, p. 192)

Comment

1. Some authors consider subcutaneous fat necrosis of the newborn and sclerema neonatorum to be distinct entities.
2. *Cold panniculitis* is a transient form of panniculitis observed most commonly in infants. With direct application of cold materials, erythematous, tender nodules and plaques develop on the face or legs. Degeneration of fat cells may result in the formation of large cystic spaces.
3. *Progressive lipodystrophy* differs from *lipo-atrophic diabetes* by the localized rather than generalized loss of subcutaneous fat. Microscopically there is a complete absence of subcutaneous fat.

SUBCUTANEOUS FAT NECROSIS OF THE NEWBORN

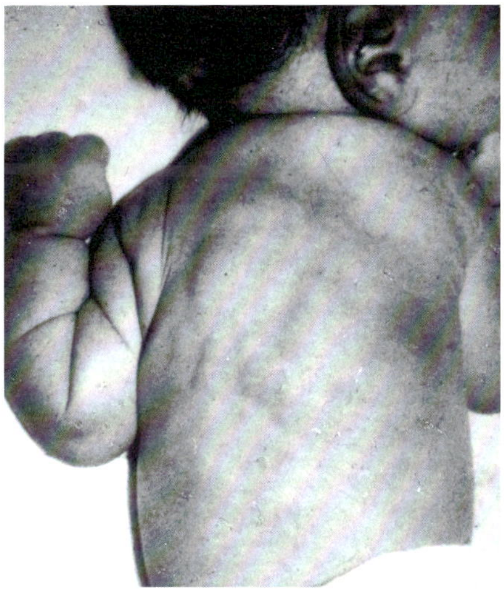

A

Figs. A,E courtesy Dr. David Fretzin

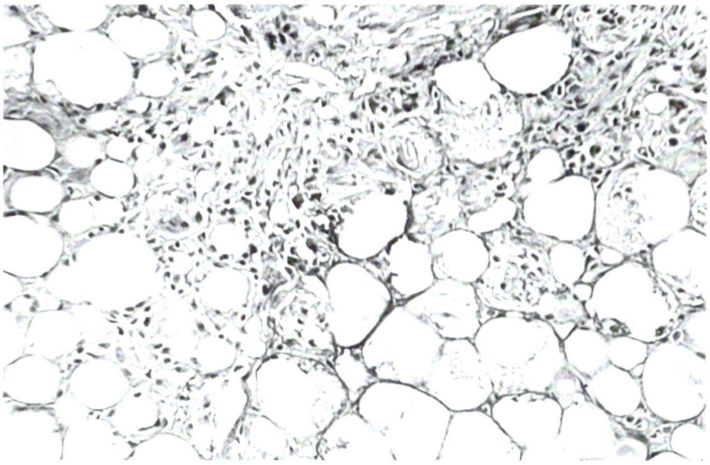

B
X270

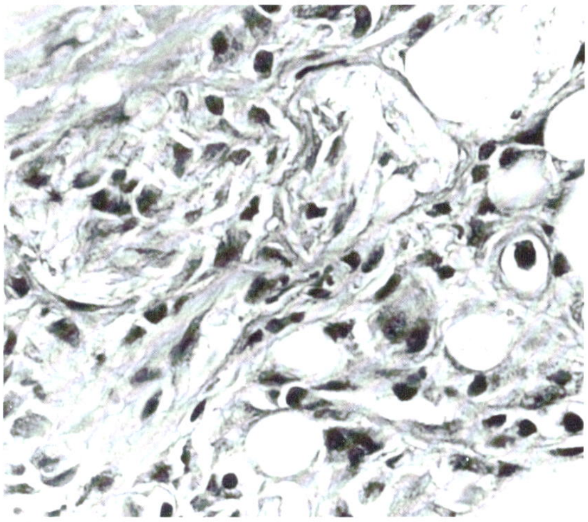

C
X530

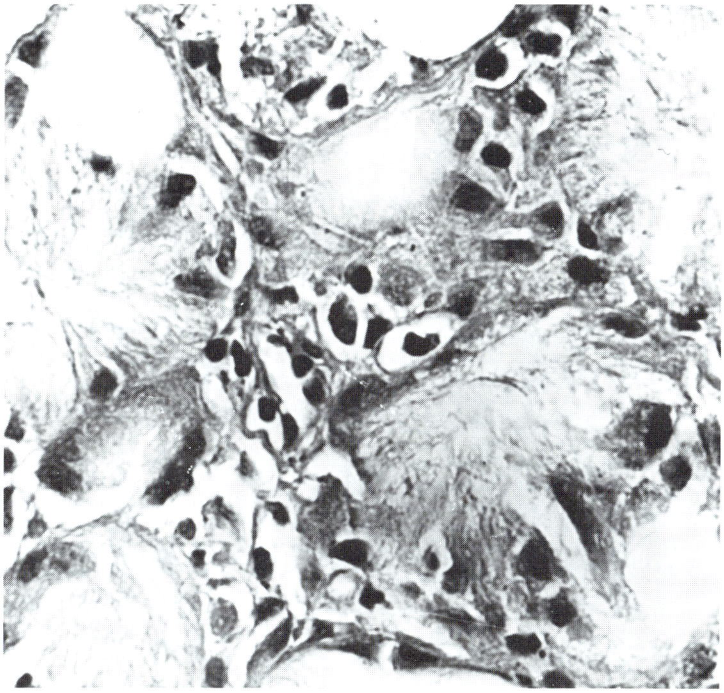

D
X680

OIL RED O STAIN:
POLARISCOPIC
EXAMINATION

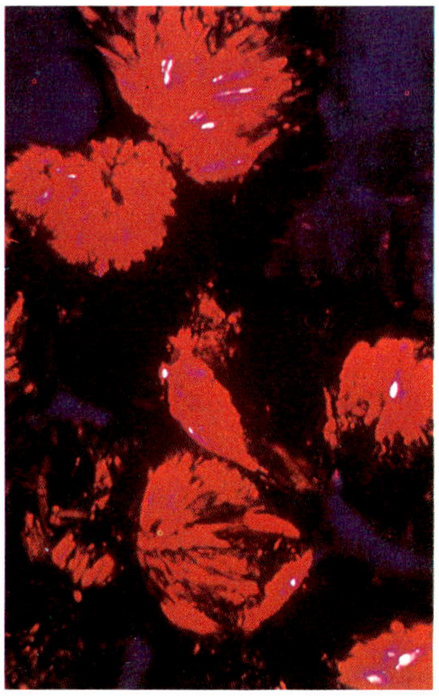

E
X530

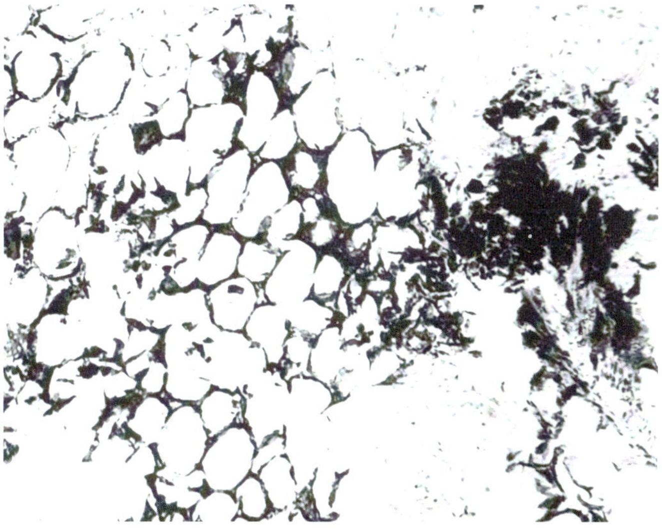

F
X180

VON KOSSA STAIN

PANNICULITIS continued

Panniculitis: Some Key Microscopic Differential Diagnostic Features

1. Erythema nodosum is typically a septitis with minimal degeneration of fat cells.
2. Erythema induratum is a caseating, granulomatous panniculitis.
3. The diagnostic hallmark of Weber-Christian disease is the presence of sheets of foam cells in stage II.
4. Crystals of abnormal lipid in radial arrangement characterize subcutaneous fat necrosis of the newborn.
5. Subcutaneous fat necrosis associated with pancreatic disease is characterized by the presence of calcium soaps.

Suggested Reading

Panniculitis

General References

Bondi, E. and Lazarus, G. Panniculitis. In: *Dermatology in General Medicine*. 3rd Edition. Fitzpatrick, T. et al. New York, McGraw-Hill, 1987, p. 1133.

Erythema Nodosum

Bäfverstedt, B. Erythema nodosum migrans. *Acta Derm. Venereol.*, 34:181, 1954.

Elizaga, F. Erythema nodosum and indomethacin. *Ann. Int. Med.*, 96:383, 1982.

Eng, A. and Aronson, I. Dermatopathology of panniculitis. *Semin. Dermatol.*, 3:1, 1984.

Favour, C. and Sosman, M. Erythema nodosum. *Arch. Int. Med.*, 80:435, 1947.

Fine, R. and Meltzer, H. Chronic erythema nodosum. *Arch. Dermatol.*, 100:33, 1969.

Förström, L. and Winkelmann, R. Granulomatous panniculitis in erythema nodosum. *Arch. Dermatol.*, 111:335, 1975.

Gordon, J. Erythema nodosum: A review of 115 cases. *Br. J. Dermatol.*, 73:393, 1961.

Jacobs, W. Erythema nodosum in inflammatory diseases of the bowel. *Gastroenterol.*, 37:286, 1959.

Lehman, C. Control of erythema nodosum with naproxen. *Cutis*, 26:66, 1980.

Löfgren, S. and Wahlgren, F. On the histopathology of erythema nodosum. *Acta Derm. Venereol.*, 29:1, 1949.

Macoul, K. Panniculitis, vasculitis, and a positive lupus erythematosus cell test. *JAMA*, 199:428, 1967.

Perry, H. and Winkelmann, R. Subacute nodular migratory panniculitis. *Arch. Dermatol.*, 89:170, 1964.

Rostas, A. Erythema nodosum migrans in a young woman. *Arch. Dermatol.*, 116:325, 1980.

Salvatore, M. and Lynch, P. Erythema nodosum, estrogens, and pregnancy. *Arch. Dermatol.*, 116:557, 1980.

Vilanova, X. and Piñol Aguadé, J. Subacute nodular migratory panniculitis. *Br. J. Dermatol.*, 71:45, 1959.

Erythema Induratum

Borrie, P. and Stansfeld, A. Cutaneous vasculitis. In: *Modern Trends in Dermatology*, Vol. 3. MacKenna, R., ed., London, Butterworths, 1966, p. 167.

Lebel, M. and Lassonde, M. Erythema induratum Bazin. *J. Am. Acad. Dermatol.*, 14:738, 1986.

Montgomery, H., O'Leary, P. and Barker, N. Nodular vascular diseases of the legs: Erythema induratum and allied conditions. *JAMA*, 128:335, 1945.

Wilkinson, D. The vascular basis of some nodular eruptions of the legs. *Br. J. Dermatol.*, 66:201, 1954.

Superficial Migratory Thrombophlebitis

Montgomery, H., O'Leary, P. and Barker, N. Nodular vascular disease of the legs: Erythema induratum and allied conditions. *JAMA*, 128:335, 1945.

Weber-Christian Disease

Achten, G. et al. Panniculite liquéfiante idiopathique à évolution fatale. *Ann. Dermatol. Venereol.*, 104:693, 1977.
Allen-Mersh, T. Weber-Christian panniculitis and auto-immune disease: A case report. *J. Clin. Pathol.*, 29:144, 1976.
Arnold, H. and Bainborough, A. Weber-Christian disease with visceral involvement: Case report and review of the literature. *Can. Med. Assoc. J.*, 89:1138, 1963.
Breit, S. et al. Familial occurrence of alpha-1 antitrypsin deficiency and Weber-Christian disease. *Arch. Dermatol.*, 119:198, 1983.
Christian, H. Relapsing febrile nodular nonsuppurative panniculitis. *Arch. Int. Med.*, 42:338, 1928.
Ciclitira, P., Wight, D. and Dick, A. Systemic Weber-Christian disease. *Br. J. Dermatol.*, 103:685, 1980.
Eravelly, J. and Waters, M. Thalidomide in Weber-Christian disease. *Lancet*, 1:251, 1977.
Förström, L. and Winkelmann, R. Acute generalized panniculitis with amylase and lipase in skin. *Arch. Dermatol.*, 111:497, 1975.
——. Acute panniculitis. *Arch. Dermatol.*, 113:909, 1977.
Hendricks, W., Ahmad, M. and Gratz, E. Weber-Christian syndrome in infancy. *Br. J. Dermatol.*, 98: 175, 1978.
Herrington, J., Jr., Edwards, W. and Grossman, L. Mesenteric manifestations of Weber-Christian disease. *Ann. Surg.*, 154:949, 1961.
Hotta, T. et al. Azathioprine-induced remission in Weber-Christian disease. *South. Med. J.*, 74:234, 1981.
Koorh, R. Weber-Christian's disease: A form of spontaneous panniculitis. *Dermatologica*, 101:332, 1950.
Lever, W. Nodular nonsuppurative panniculitis (Weber-Christian Disease): Report of a case in which an infiltrate of polymorphonuclear leukocytes represented the earliest lesion. *Arch. Dermatol. Syph.*, 59:31, 1949.
MacDonald, A. and Feiwel, M. A review of the concept of Weber-Christian panniculitis with a report of five cases. *Br. J. Dermatol.*, 80:355, 1968.
Martin, R. Cyclophosphamide induced remission in Weber-Christian disease. *Milit. Med.*, 142:158, 1977.
Olesk, A. and Panusch, R. Factitial Weber-Christian disease: A case report. *J. Rheumatol.*, 8:129, 1981.
Steinberg, B. Systemic nodular panniculitis. *Am. J. Pathol.*, 29:1059, 1953.
Weber, F. A case of relapsing nonsuppurative nodular panniculitis showing phagocytosis of subcutaneous fat-cells by macrophages. *Br. J. Dermatol.*, 37:301, 1925.

Lipogranulomatosis Subcutanea (Rothmann and Makai)

Laymon, C. and Peterson, W., Jr. Lipogranulomatosis subcutanea (Rothmann-Makai): An appraisal. *Arch. Dermatol.*, 90:288, 1964.
Rees, H. Sclerosing lipogranuloma. *Arch. Dermatol.*, 89:277, 1964.

Panniculitis Due to Pancreatitis

Bennett, R. and Petrozzi, J. Nodular subcutaneous fat necrosis. *Arch. Dermatol.*, 111:896, 1975.
Cannon, J., Pitha, J. and Everett, M. Subcutaneous fat necrosis in pancreatitis. *J. Cutan. Pathol.*, 6:501, 1979.
Hughes, P., Apisarnthanarax, P. and Mullins, J. Subcutaneous fat necrosis associated with pancreatic disease. *Arch. Dermatol.*, 111:506, 1975.
Levine, N. and Lazarus, G. Subcutaneous fat necrosis after paracentesis: Report of a case in a patient with acute pancreatitis. *Arch. Dermatol.*, 112:993, 1976.
Millns, J., Evans, H. and Winkelmann, R. Association of islet cell carcinoma of the pancreas with subcutaneous fat necrosis. *Am. J. Dermatopathol.*, 1:273, 1979.
Moore, S. The relation of pancreatic disease to Weber-Christian disease. *Can. Med. Assoc. J.*, 88:1238, 1963.

Mullin, G. et al. Arthritis and skin lesions resembling erythema nodosum in pancreatic disease. *Ann. Int. Med.*, 68:75, 1968.
Schrier, R., Melmon, K. and Fenster, L. Subcutaneous nodular fat necrosis in pancreatitis. *Arch. Int. Med.*, 116:832, 1965.
Szymanski, F. and Bluefarb, S. Nodular fat necrosis and pancreatic diseases. *Arch. Dermatol.*, 83:224, 1961.

Liquefying Panniculitis

Hoyos, N., Shaffer, B. and Beerman, H. Liquefying nodular panniculitis. *Arch. Dermatol.*, 94:436, 1966.
Shaffer, B. Liquefying nodular panniculitis: Report of a case. *Arch. Dermatol. Syph.*, 38:535, 1938.

Subcutaneous Fat Necrosis of the Newborn

Chen, T. et al. Subcutaneous fat necrosis of the newborn: A case report. *Arch. Dermatol.*, 117: 36, 1981.
Craig, W. An unusual case of subcutaneous fat necrosis in a newly born infant. *Arch. Dis. Child.*, 40:326, 1965.
Duhn, R., Shoen, E. and Siu, M. Subcutaneous fat necrosis with extensive calcification after hypothermia in two newborn infants. *Pediatrics*, 41:661, 1968.
Esterly, N. and Solomon, L. The skin. In: *Neonatal-Perinatal Medicine.* Fanaroff, A. and Martin, R., eds., St. Louis, CV Mosby, 1983, p. 939.
Fretzin, D. and Arias, A. Sclerema neonatorum and subcutaneous fat necrosis of the newborn. *Pediatr. Dermatol.*, 4:112, 1987.
Horsfield, G. and Yardley, H. Sclerema neonatorum. *J. Invest. Dermatol.*, 44:326, 1965.
Katz, D. et al. Subcutaneous fat necrosis of the newborn. *Arch. Dermatol.*, 120:1517, 1984.
Kellum, R., Ray, T. and Brown, F. Sclerema neonatorum: Report of a case and analysis of subcutaneous and epidermal-dermal lipids by chromatographic methods. *Arch. Dermatol.*, 97:372, 1968.
Noojin, R., Pace, B. and Davis, H. Subcutaneous fat necrosis of the newborn: Certain etiologic considerations. *J. Invest. Dermatol.*, 12:331, 1949.
Tsuji, T. Subcutaneous fat necrosis of the newborn: Light and electron microscopic studies. *Br. J. Dermatol.*, 95:407, 1976.
Zeek, P. and Madden, E. Sclerema adiposum neonatorum of both internal and external adipose tissue. *Arch. Pathol.*, 41:166, 1946.

Cold Panniculitis

Beacham, B. et al. Equestrian cold panniculitis in women. *Arch. Dermatol.*, 116:1025, 1980.
Duncan, W., Freeman, R. and Heaton, C. Cold panniculitis. *Arch. Dermatol.*, 94:722, 1966.
Epstein, E., Jr. and Oren, M. Popsicle panniculitis. *New Eng. J. Med.*, 282:966, 1970.
Surpure, J. Cold panniculitis of the cheeks in children. *Dermatol. Allergy*, 3:37, 1980.
Vickers, R. Equestrian cold panniculitis in women. *Arch. Dermatol.*, 117:315, 1981.

Progressive Lipodystrophy

Taylor, W. and Honeycutt, W. Progressive lipodystrophy and lipoatrophic diabetes. *Arch. Dermatol.*, 84:31, 1961.

Necrosis

General Considerations

Focal necrosis of the skin has many causes. Necrosis is generally followed by formation of granulation tissue and fibrosis (see section on regeneration). Causes of focal necrosis of the skin include ischemic and stasis ulcers, frostbite, burns, coumarin necrosis, Behçet's syndrome (Fig. B), aphthosis, pyoderma gangrenosum (Fig. A), and factitial injury. Conditions causing cutaneous necrosis with a relatively specific histologic picture include cryoglobulinemia and malignant atrophic papulosis (Degos disease).

Microscopic features

1. The epidermis is necrotic or absent, and there is necrosis of the connective tissue of the upper dermis and an infiltrate of acute and chronic inflammatory cells (Fig. C). Granulation tissue may be present, as well as fibrosis.
2. Undermining of the ulcer may be present (Fig. C). This is often pronounced in pyoderma gangrenosum.

Comment

1. Aphthosis and Behçet's syndrome are believed by some to represent autoimmune responses of the delayed hypersensitivity type. In addition to aphthosis, Behçet's syndrome includes genital ulceration and uveitis (triple syndrome), as well as involvement of other organ systems. In aphthosis the ulcers are preceded by invasion of the epithelium by lymphocytes and monocytes. Other cutaneous manifestations of Behçet's syndrome include pustules and leg lesions resembling erythema nodosum. There may be an element of vasculitis.
2. Pyoderma gangrenosum may be an autoimmune process. A variety of diseases have been associated with pyoderma gangrenosum. In some cases, pyoderma gangrenosum may not be associated with other diseases. Associated diseases include myelogenous leukemia, ulcerative colitis, regional enteritis, chronic rheumatoid polyarthritis, and IgA paraproteinemia. Cutaneous lesions begin as fluctuant nodules, which then ulcerate. Some authors have reported vascular changes.
3. Ulcerations from factitial injury often have bizarre shapes, with angular and straight components in the margins. Factitial lesions are often absent in areas that cannot be reached with the hands.
4. *Coumarin necrosis.* Patients on anticoagulant therapy may develop bullous, hemorrhagic necrosis between the third and tenth day of therapy. The condition is associated with venous thrombi.

NECROSIS

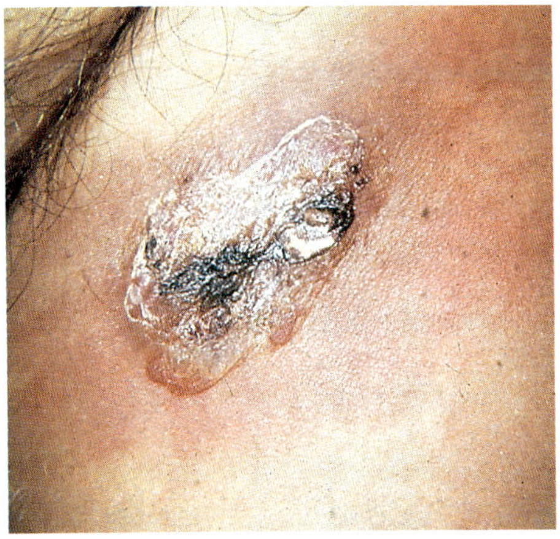

A

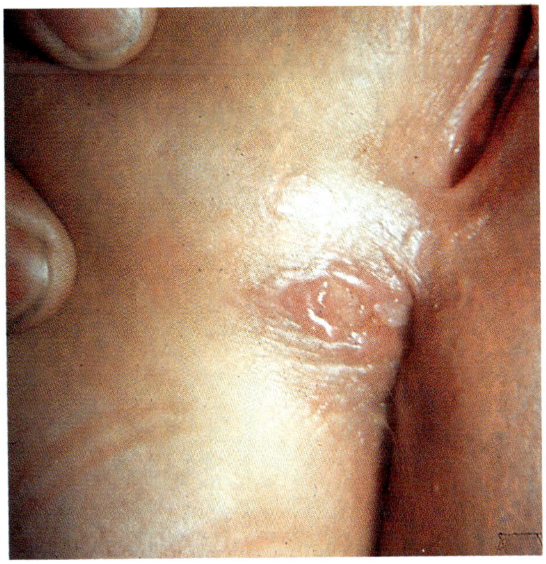

B

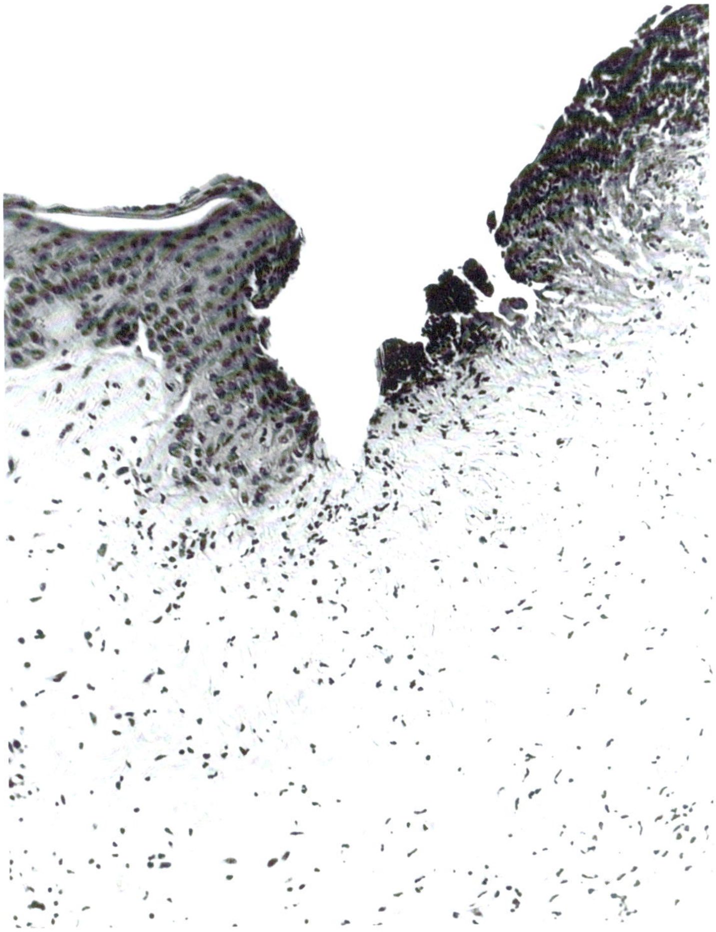

C
X170

NECROSIS continued ⇨

CRYOGLOBULINEMIA

Cryoglobulins are immunoglobulins that precipitate with cold temperatures and redissolve when the temperature is raised.

Cryoglobulinemia can be essential or associated with other diseases. It can be monoclonal or associated with two or three cryoglobulins (mixed cryoglobulinemia).

Monoclonal cryoglobulinemia may occur in multiple myeloma, Waldenström's macroglobulinemia, lymphoma, and lymphocytic leukemia.

Monoclonal cryoglobulinemia shows purpura and ulcerations that may be limited to the legs (Fig. A). There may be involvement of brain, kidneys, or lungs. Death may occur.

Microscopic features of monoclonal cryoglobulinemia

1. The key feature is the presence of an eosinophilic, PAS-positive material in the lumina of the dermal blood vessels (Figs. B,C).
2. Varying degrees of inflammation and hemorrhage may be present (Fig. B).
3. Cutaneous necrosis may occur secondary to the blocked vessels.

Comment

Cutaneous lesions of mixed cryoglobulinemia are characterized by leukocytoclastic vasculitis. Mixed cryoglobulinemia may occur in association with systemic lupus erythematosus, rheumatoid arthritis, Sjögren's syndrome, hepatitis B infection and leukocytoclastic vasculitis. The essential form of mixed cryoglobulinemia shows chronic dependent purpura, arthralgia, and occasionally diffuse proliferative glomerulonephritis.

CRYOGLOBULINEMIA

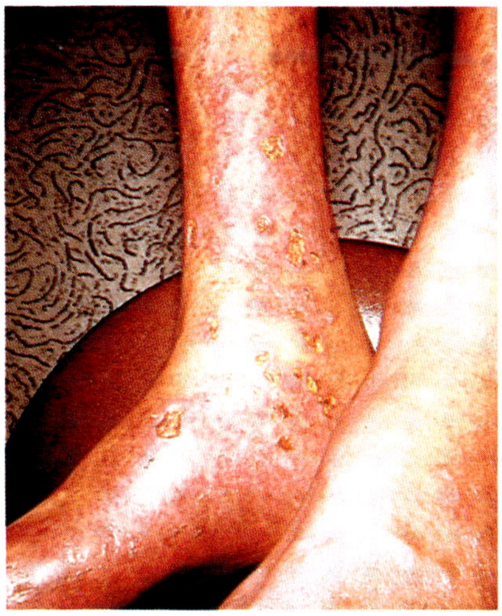
A

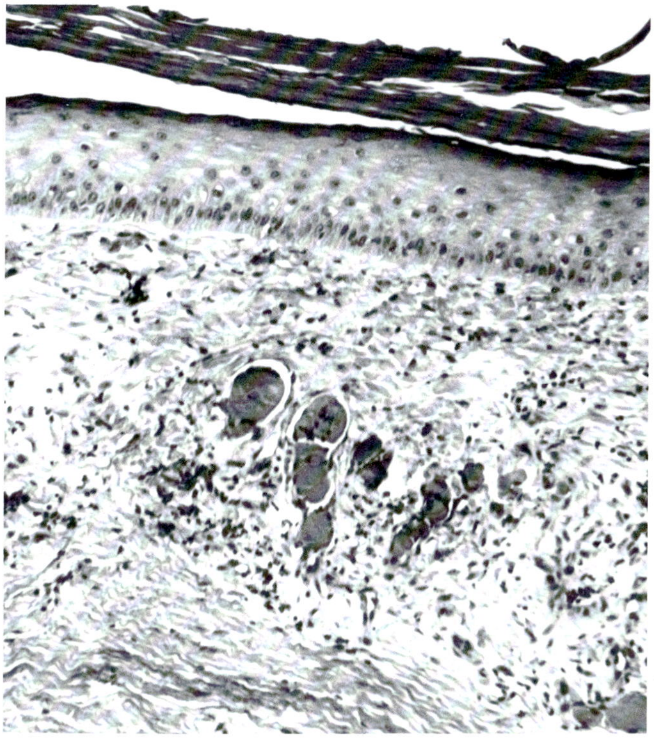
B
X190

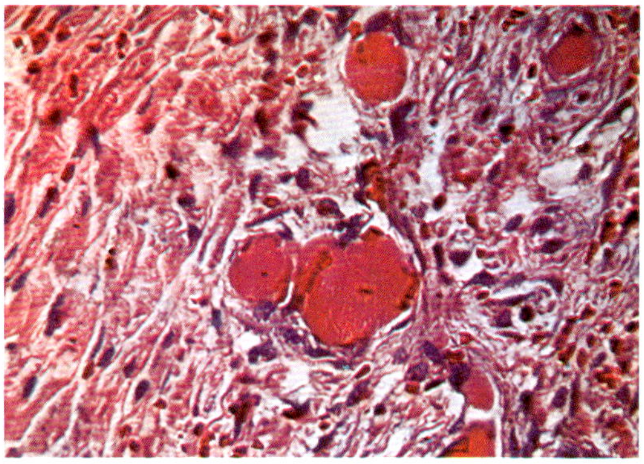
C
X620

NECROSIS continued ⇨

MALIGNANT ATROPHIC PAPULOSIS (DEGOS DISEASE)

This is a frequently lethal, infarctive disorder of unknown origin affecting the skin and mucous membranes, gastrointestinal tract (Fig. B), and occasionally the central nervous system. The cutaneous lesions are reddish-yellow papules which rapidly develop a central, porcelain-like atrophy (Fig. A).

Microscopic features

1. The cutaneous changes are those of an ischemic infarct.
2. The area of infarction is triangular with the base at the epidermis.
3. Early lesions show edema of collagen bundles and mucin deposition.
4. With progression, there is a decrease in fibroblasts and an increase in pale-staining, hyalinized collagen fibers (Figs. D,E). Capillaries are indistinct (Fig. C). An inflammatory infiltrate may be present around the zone of necrosis.
5. There is pronounced atrophy of the epidermis, often associated with hyperkeratosis (Figs. D,E).
6. The arterioles causing the infarction show endothelial proliferation, sometimes associated with deposition of PAS-positive material and thrombosis. They are located in the lower dermis or subcutaneous fat.

Comment

1. Lesions that resemble Degos disease, both clinically and microscopically, can occur in systemic lupus erythematosus. Therefore, systemic lupus erythematosus should be excluded before making a diagnosis of Degos disease.
2. There is no evidence that Degos disease has an autoimmune basis.

DEGOS DISEASE

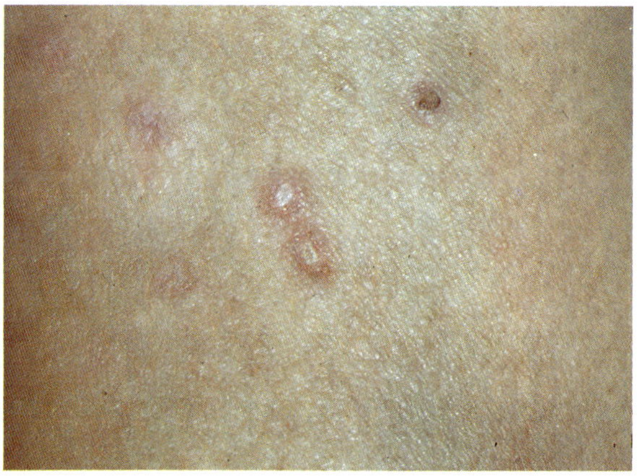

A

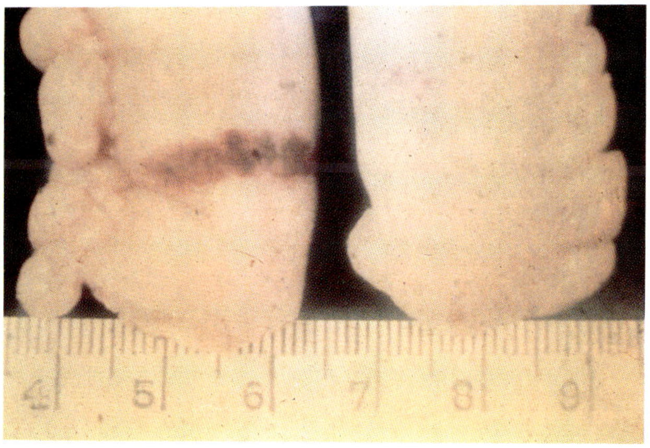

B

Figs. A,C,D courtesy Dr. Robert Degos

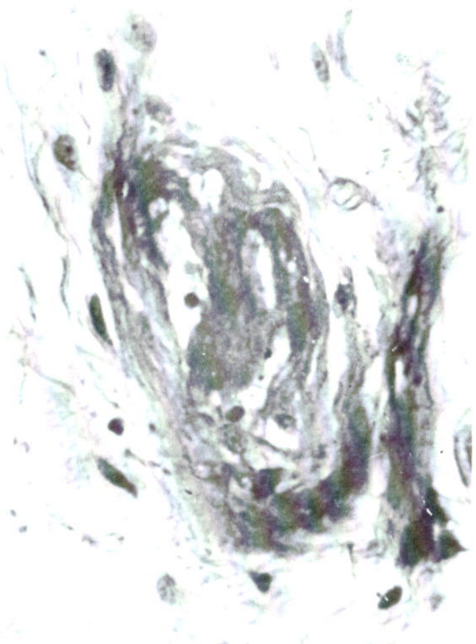

C
X300

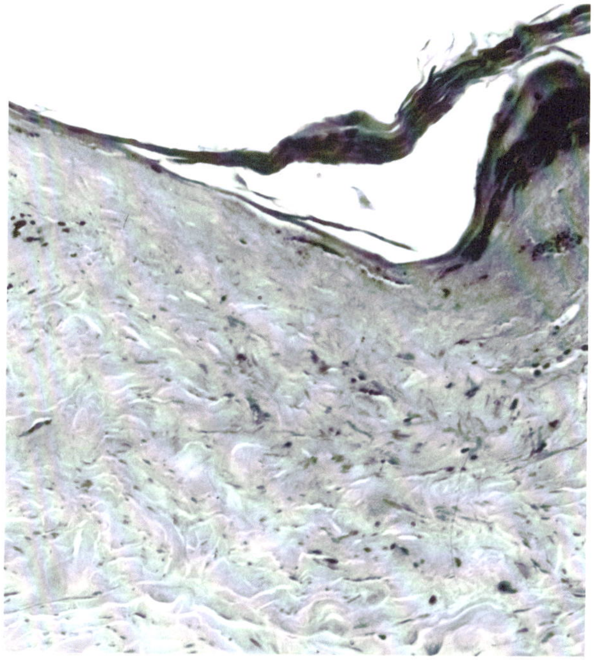

D
X195

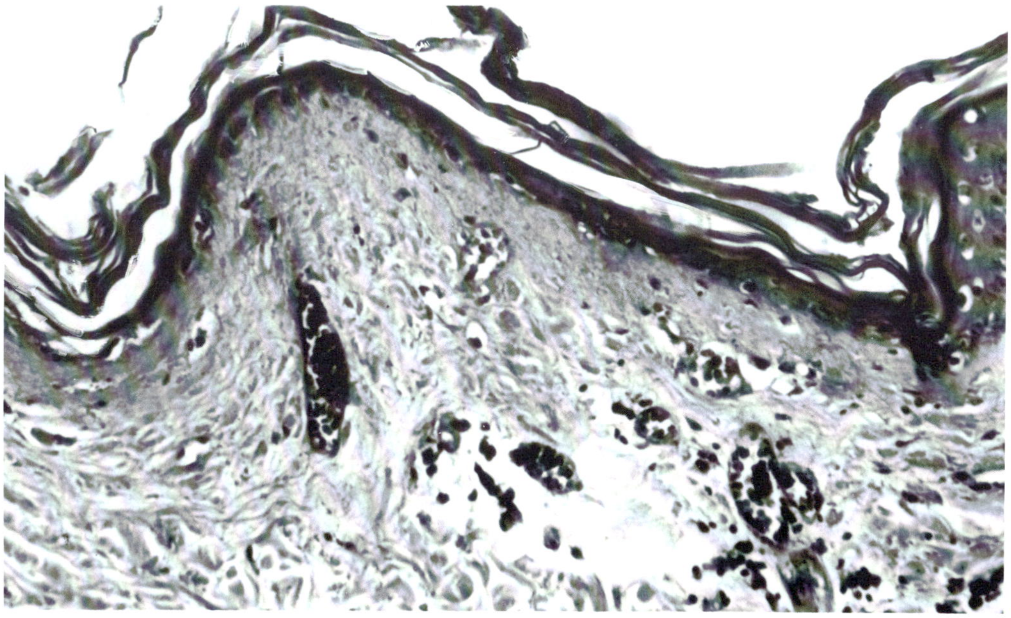

E
X260
Courtesy Dr. E. Feuerman

NECROSIS continued

ATROPHIE BLANCHE

Atrophie blanche is an idiopathic infarctive disorder involving the distal portions of the lower extremities, especially the ankles and dorsal surfaces of the feet. Women are more often affected than men. There are small, painful ulcers which may precede the development of whitish, atrophic areas. The atrophic areas may show hyperpigmentation and telangiectasia at their periphery (Fig. A). Livedo reticularis, a retiform violaceous eruption caused by spasm of mid- and deep dermal arterioles, may be present. Livedo reticularis is a reaction pattern associated with a variety of vascular problems.

Microscopic features

1. In early lesions, walls of vessels and lumina contain fibrinoid material, producing an infarction.
2. In atrophic areas, the walls of vessels show hyaline material (PAS-positive, diastase-resistant) and thickening of their intima (Fig. B). Vessels may be occluded with fibrinoid material. The epidermis is thin, and the dermis is sclerotic.

ATROPHIE BLANCHE

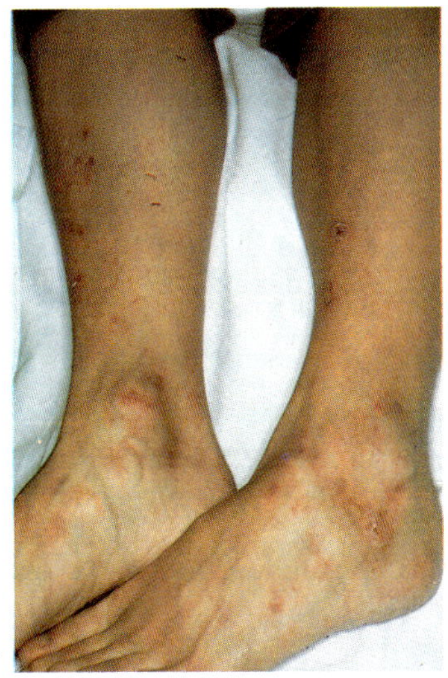

A

Figs. A,B courtesy Dept. of Dermatology
Boston University School of Medicine

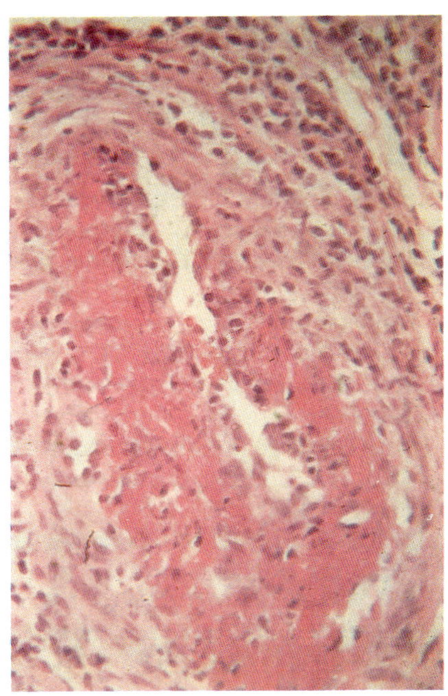

B
X180

Degos Disease

Black, M. and Hudson, P. Atrophie blanche lesions closely resembling malignant atrophic papulosis (Degos' disease) in systemic lupus erythematosus. *Br. J. Dermatol.*, 95:649, 1976.

Black, M. and Wilson-Jones, E. Malignant atrophic papulosis (Degos syndrome). *Br. J. Dermatol.*, 85:290, 1971.

Degos, R. Malignant atrophic papulosis. *Br. J. Dermatol.*, 100:21, 1979.

——. Malignant atrophic papulosis: A fatal cutaneo-intestinal syndrome. *Br. J. Dermatol.*, 66:304, 1954.

Feuerman, E., Dollberg, L. and Salvador, O. Malignant atrophic papulosis with mucin in the dermis. *Arch. Pathol.*, 90:310, 1970.

Hall-Smith, P. Malignant atrophic papulosis (Degos disease): Two cases occurring in the same family. *Br. J. Dermatol.*, 81:817, 1969.

Howsden, S. et al. Malignant atrophic papulosis of Degos. *Arch. Dermatol.*, 112:1582, 1976.

Mauss, J., Reichenberger, M. and Zambal, S. Papulosis atrophicans maligna (Degos): Vergleich der aus der Literatur bekannten Fälle, einschliesslich einer eigenen Beobachtung. *Hautarzt*, 20:389, 1969.

Metz, J., Amschler, A. and Henke, M. Morbus Degos (papulosis atrophicans maligna). *Hautarzt*, 31:108, 1980.

Muller, S. and Landry, M. Malignant atrophic papulosis (Degos disease). *Arch. Dermatol.*, 112:357, 1976.

Olmos, L. and Laugier, P. Ultrastructure de la maladie de Degos. (Review). *Ann. Dermatol. Venereol.*, 104:280, 1977.

Stahl, D., Thomsen, K. and Hou-Jensen, K. Malignant atrophic papulosis. *Arch. Dermatol.*, 114:1687, 1978.

Strole, W., Jr., Clark, W., Jr. and Isselbacher, K. Progressive arterial occlusive disease (Kohlmeier-Degos): A frequently fatal cutaneosystemic disorder. *N. Eng. J. Med.*, 276:195, 1967.

Su, D. et al. Clinical and histologic findings in Degos' syndrome (malignant atrophic papulosis). *Cutis*, 35:131, 1985.

Tribble, K. et al. Malignant atrophic papulosis: Absence of circulating immune complexes or vasculitis. *J. Am. Acad. Dermatol.*, 14:365, 1986.

Atrophie Blanche

Bard, I. and Winkelmann, R. Livedo vasculitis. *Arch. Dermatol.*, 96:489, 1967.

Gray, H. et al. Atrophie blanche: Periodic painful ulcers of the lower extremities. *Arch. Dermatol.*, 93:187, 1966.

Metz, J. and Sturm, G. Atrophie blanche (sog. Capillaritis alba). *Hautarzt*, 25:103, 1974.

Milian, G. Les atrophies cutanées syphilitiques. *Bull. Soc. Fr. Dermatol. Syph.*, 36:865, 1929.

Miura, T. and Torinuki, W. Clinical course of atrophie blanche. *J. Dermatol.*, 4:259, 1977.

Nelson, L. Atrophie blanche en plaque. *Arch. Dermatol.*, 72:242, 1955.

Posternak, F. et al. Livedoid vasculitis (vascularite hyalinisante segmentaire). *Ann. Dermatol. Venereol.*, 104:50, 1977.

Schroeter, A. et al. Livedo vasculitis (the vasculitis of atrophie blanche). *Arch. Dermatol.*, 111:188, 1976.

Stiefler, R. and Bergfeld, W. Atrophie blanche. (Review). *Internat. J. Dermatol.*, 21:1, 1982.

Van Hale, H. et al. Immunofluorescence microscopic studies of recurrent aphthous stomatitis. *Arch. Dermatol.*, 117:779, 1981.
Wong, R., Ellis, C. and Diaz, L. Behçet disease. *Internat. J. Dermatol.*, 23:25, 1984.

Pyoderma Gangrenosum

de Bast, C., Achten, G. and Moriame, G. Pyoderma gangrenosum. *Arch. Belg. Dermatol. Syph.*, 25:111, 1969.
Greenberg, S. et al. Pyoderma gangrenosum: Occurrence with altered cellular immunity and circulating serum factor. *Arch. Dermatol.*, 188:498, 1982.
Lazarus, G., Goldsmith, L. and Rocklin, R. Pyoderma gangrenosum, altered delayed hypersensitivity and polyarthritis. *Arch. Dermatol.*, 105:46, 1972.
Newell, L. and Malkinson, F. Commentary: Pyoderma gangrenosum. *Arch. Dermatol.*, 118:769, 1982.
Norris, D. et al. Pyoderma gangrenosum. *Arch. Dermatol.*, 114:906, 1978.
Powell, F. and Perry, H. Pyoderma gangrenosum in childhood. *Arch. Dermatol.*, 120:757, 1984.
Pye, R. and Choudhury, C. Bullous pyoderma as a presentation of acute leukemia. *Clin. Exp. Dermatol.*, 2:33, 1977.
Rook, A. and Goldin, D. Pyoderma gangrenosum. *Br. J. Dermatol.*, 93 (1, suppl.):31, 1975.
Schroeter, A. and Su, W. The vasculitis of pyoderma gangrenosum. (abstr.) *Arch. Dermatol.*, 116:1388, 1980.
Stathers, G., Abbott, L. and McGuinness, A. Pyoderma gangrenosum in association with regional enteritis. *Arch. Dermatol.*, 95:375, 1967.
Stolman, L. et al. Pyoderma gangrenosum and rheumatoid arthritis. *Arch. Dermatol.*, 111:1020, 1975.

Coumarin Necrosis

Altmeyer, P. et al. Zur Pathogenese der sogenannten Cumarin-Nekrose. *Akt. Dermatol.*, 2:65, 1976.
Jones, R. and Cunningham, J. Warfarin skin necrosis: The role of factor VII. *Br. J. Dermatol.*, 101:561, 1979.
Kahn, S. et al. Cutaneous and subcutaneous necrosis as a complication of coumarin-congener therapy. *Plast. Reconstr. Surg.*, 18:160, 1971.
Koch-Weser, J. Coumarin necrosis. *Ann. Int. Med.*, 68:1365, 1968.
Lacy, J. and Goodwin, R. Warfarin-induced necrosis of the skin. *Ann. Int. Med.*, 82:381, 1975.
Nalbandian, R. et al. Petechiae, ecchymoses and necrosis of skin induced by coumarin congeners. *JAMA*, 192:603, 1965.

Cryoglobulinemia

Ellis, F. The cutaneous manifestation of cryoglobulinemia. *Arch. Dermatol.*, 89:690, 1964.
James, K. et al. Studies on a unique diagnostic serum globulin in papular mucinosis (lichen myxedematosus). *Clin. Exp. Immunol.*, 2:153, 1967.
Koda, H. et al. Essential IgG cryoglobulinemia with purpura and cold urticaria. *Arch. Dermatol.*, 114:784, 1978.
McKenzie, W. et al. Essential cryoglobulinaemia. *Br. J. Dermatol.*, 73:22, 1961.
Moroz, L. and Rose, B. The cryopathies: In: *Immunological Diseases*. 3rd Edition. Vol. 1. Samter, M., ed., Boston, Little, Brown, 1978, p. 570.
Nir, M. et al. Mixed IgG-IgM cryoglobulinemia with follicular pustular purpura. *Arch. Dermatol.*, 109:539, 1974.
Waldenström, J. and Raiend, U. Plasmapheresis and cold sensitivity of immunoglobulin molecules. I. A study of hyperviscosity, cryoglobulinemia, euglobulinemia and macroglobulinemia vera. II. A study of macroglobulinemia polyclonalis spuria and immune complex disease. *Acta Med. Scand.*, 216:449, 1984.

Degos Disease

Black, M. and Hudson, P. Atrophie blanche lesions closely resembling malignant atrophic papulosis (Degos' disease) in systemic lupus erythematosus. *Br. J. Dermatol.*, 95:649, 1976.

Black, M. and Wilson-Jones, E. Malignant atrophic papulosis (Degos syndrome). *Br. J. Dermatol.*, 85:290, 1971.

Degos, R. Malignant atrophic papulosis. *Br. J. Dermatol.*, 100:21, 1979.

——. Malignant atrophic papulosis: A fatal cutaneo-intestinal syndrome. *Br. J. Dermatol.*, 66:304, 1954.

Feuerman, E., Dollberg, L. and Salvador, O. Malignant atrophic papulosis with mucin in the dermis. *Arch. Pathol.*, 90:310, 1970.

Hall-Smith, P. Malignant atrophic papulosis (Degos disease): Two cases occurring in the same family. *Br. J. Dermatol.*, 81:817, 1969.

Howsden, S. et al. Malignant atrophic papulosis of Degos. *Arch. Dermatol.*, 112:1582, 1976.

Mauss, J., Reichenberger, M. and Zambal, S. Papulosis atrophicans maligna (Degos): Vergleich der aus der Literatur bekannten Fälle, einschliesslich einer eigenen Beobachtung. *Hautarzt*, 20:389, 1969.

Metz, J., Amschler, A. and Henke, M. Morbus Degos (papulosis atrophicans maligna). *Hautarzt*, 31:108, 1980.

Muller, S. and Landry, M. Malignant atrophic papulosis (Degos disease). *Arch. Dermatol.*, 112:357, 1976.

Olmos, L. and Laugier, P. Ultrastructure de la maladie de Degos. (Review). *Ann. Dermatol. Venereol.*, 104:280, 1977.

Stahl, D., Thomsen, K. and Hou-Jensen, K. Malignant atrophic papulosis. *Arch. Dermatol.*, 114:1687, 1978.

Strole, W., Jr., Clark, W., Jr. and Isselbacher, K. Progressive arterial occlusive disease (Kohlmeier-Degos): A frequently fatal cutaneosystemic disorder. *N. Eng. J. Med.*, 276:195, 1967.

Su, D. et al. Clinical and histologic findings in Degos' syndrome (malignant atrophic papulosis). *Cutis*, 35:131, 1985.

Tribble, K. et al. Malignant atrophic papulosis: Absence of circulating immune complexes or vasculitis. *J. Am. Acad. Dermatol.*, 14:365, 1986.

Atrophie Blanche

Bard, I. and Winkelmann, R. Livedo vasculitis. *Arch. Dermatol.*, 96:489, 1967.

Gray, H. et al. Atrophie blanche: Periodic painful ulcers of the lower extremities. *Arch. Dermatol.*, 93:187, 1966.

Metz, J. and Sturm, G. Atrophie blanche (sog. Capillaritis alba). *Hautarzt*, 25:103, 1974.

Milian, G. Les atrophies cutanées syphilitiques. *Bull. Soc. Fr. Dermatol. Syph.*, 36:865, 1929.

Miura, T. and Torinuki, W. Clinical course of atrophie blanche. *J. Dermatol.*, 4:259, 1977.

Nelson, L. Atrophie blanche en plaque. *Arch. Dermatol.*, 72:242, 1955.

Posternak, F. et al. Livedoid vasculitis (vascularite hyalinisante segmentaire). *Ann. Dermatol. Venereol.*, 104:50, 1977.

Schroeter, A. et al. Livedo vasculitis (the vasculitis of atrophie blanche). *Arch. Dermatol.*, 111:188, 1976.

Stiefler, R. and Bergfeld, W. Atrophie blanche. (Review). *Internat. J. Dermatol.*, 21:1, 1982.

Regeneration

GRANULATION TISSUE

The connective tissue response to injury shows an early stage of inflammation and granulation tissue which progresses to a final stage of cicatrization.

Nonepithelialized granulation tissue is composed of numerous pink granules; epithelialized granulation tissue appears as soft, raised areas (Fig. A), which (in Caucasians) are erythematous.

Microscopic features

1. Granulation tissue is characterized by the proliferation of prominent endothelial cells, forming a rich network of capillaries within an edematous stroma (Figs. B,C). Fibroblasts as well as collagen fibers are present; these increase in number as granulation tissue develops into scar tissue. Granulation tissue is rich in contractile myofibroblasts.
2. There is an increase in interstitial mucopolysaccharides.
3. Inflammatory cells, including lymphocytes, plasma cells, histiocytes, and mast cells, are present (Figs. B,C). Hemorrhage may also be present (Fig. C).

Microscopic differential diagnosis

Granuloma pyogenicum may represent a distinctive form of granulation tissue with a polypoid architecture (see p. 1016).

GRANULATION TISSUE

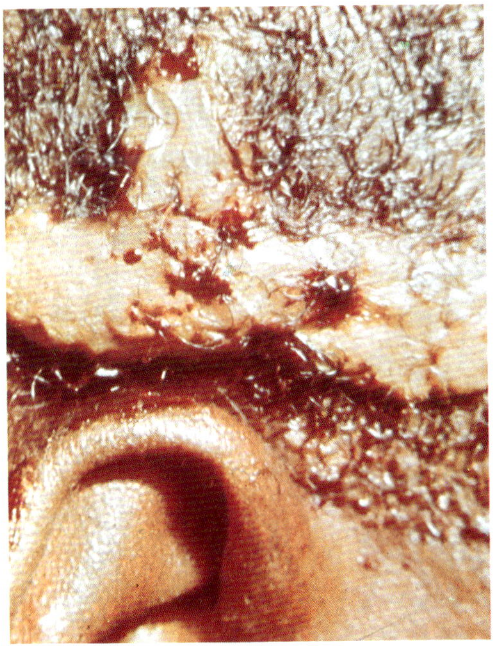

A

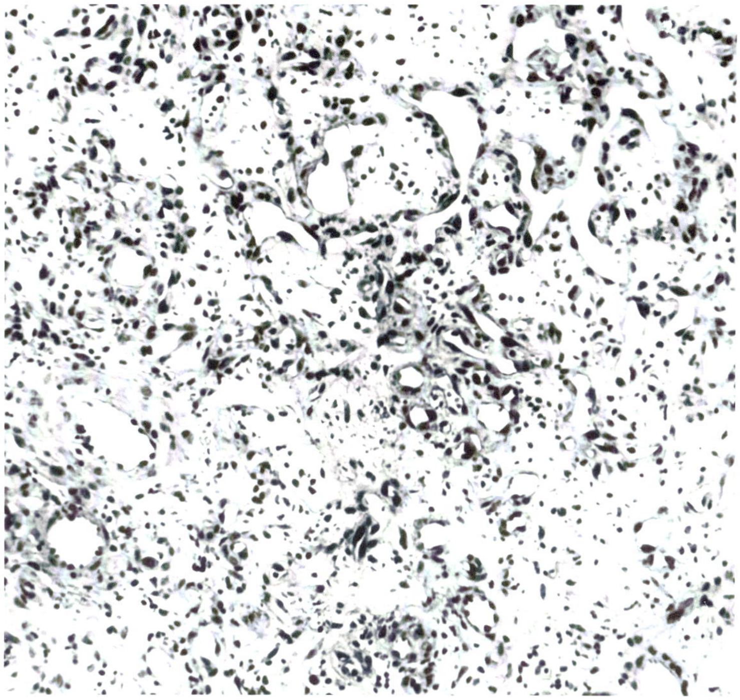

B
X200

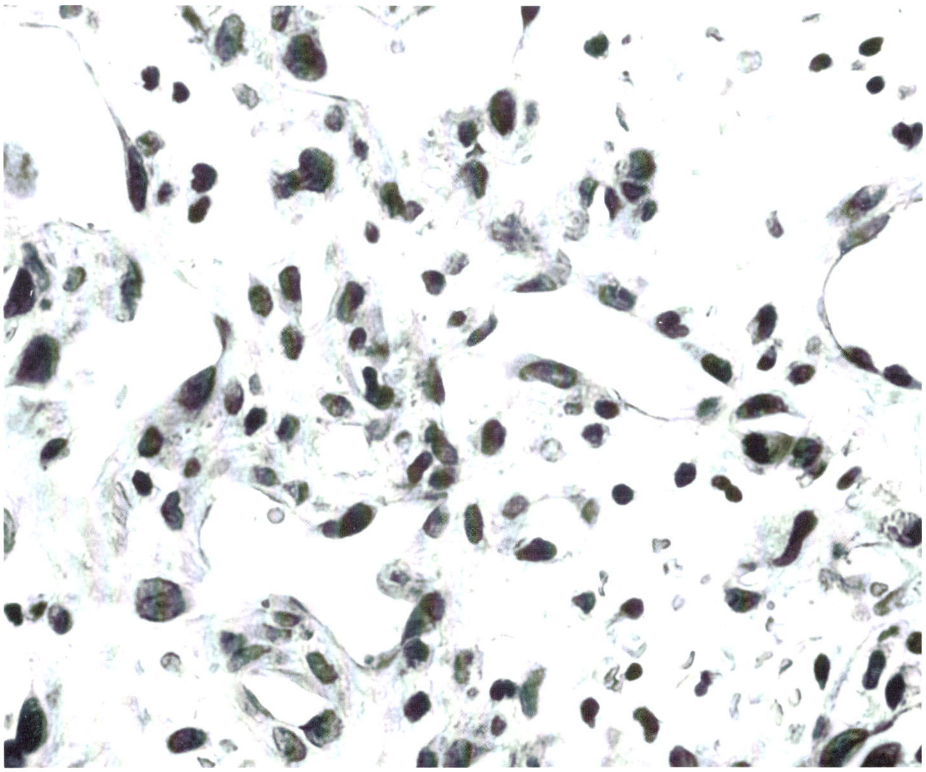

C
X680

SCARS

With increasing fibrosis, granulation tissue is transformed into scars. Scars are indurated areas which may be either retracted, or raised and hypertrophic. Keloids (Fig. A) are hypertrophic scars characterized by a prolonged phase of fibroblastic proliferation and a failure to regress. The upper back and presternal area are common sites of keloids. Blacks have a much greater predisposition to form keloids than whites.

Microscopic features

1. Early scars are characterized by the proliferation of elongated, spindle-shaped fibroblasts in dense parallel array (Figs. C,E).
2. With progression of fibrosis, there is decreased cellularity, and an increase in collagenization (Fig. D).
3. The final stage of scar formation is characterized by thickened, hyalinized collagen fibers (Fig. D). In normal wound healing, the hyalinized collagen fibers are relatively thin and are parallel to the skin surface. In hypertrophic scars and keloids the hyalinized collagen fibers are arranged in large bundles (Fig. D).

   In hypertrophic scars, the bundles gradually flatten out and become thinner, but this does not occur in keloids. Failure of keloids to shrink may be related to the paucity of myofibroblasts.
4. Scars may or may not (Fig. B) extend to the epidermis, which often is flattened (Fig. B).

Microscopic differential diagnosis

Scars and dermatofibromas (see p. 976) are both characterized by fibroblastic proliferation and may have a similar histologic appearance. However, certain features usually allow their differentiation:

1. Dermatofibromas usually show epidermal hyperplasia, which may resemble seborrheic keratosis or basal cell carcinoma (see p. 820). By contrast, scars show a normal or flattened epidermis.
2. In dermatofibromas, proliferating fibroblasts and young collagen are usually separated by normal, pre-existing collagen fibers. In scars, proliferating fibroblasts and newly-formed collagen fibers are densely aggregated.
3. In some cases, these microscopic criteria do not allow differentiation, and features of gross morphology and history must be considered.

SCARS

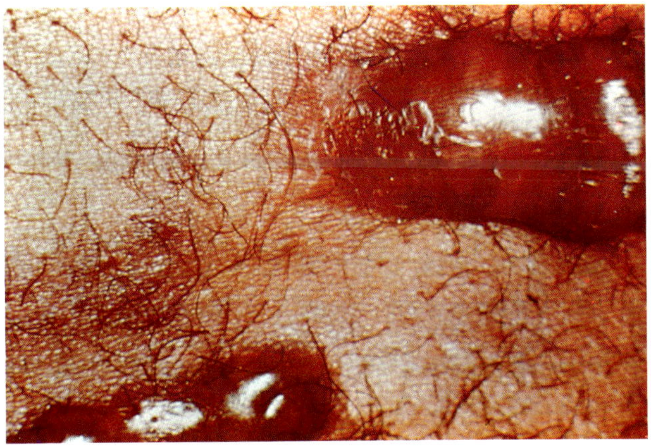

A

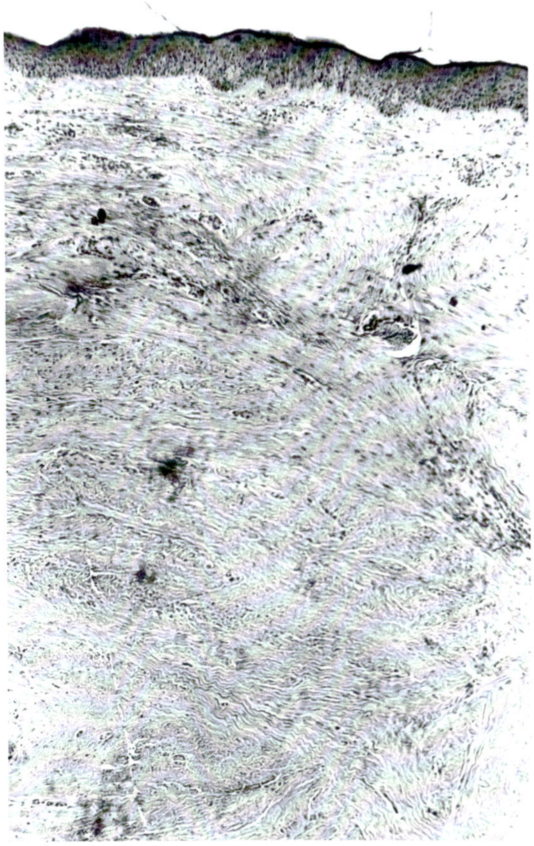

B
X90

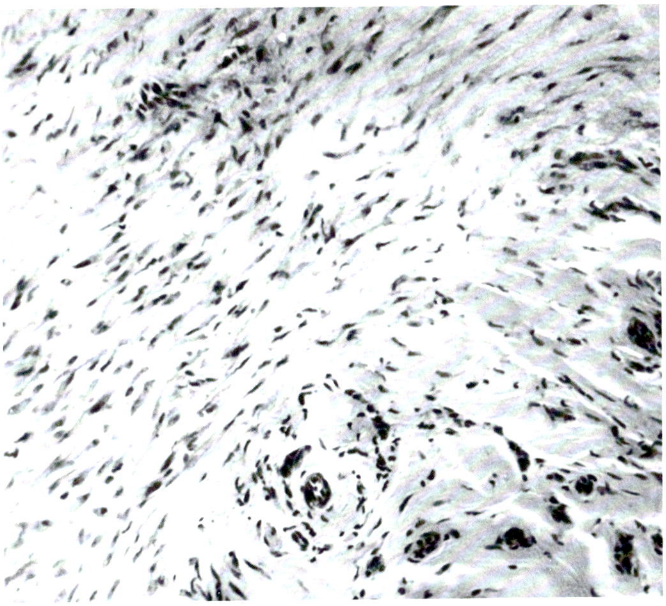

C
X180

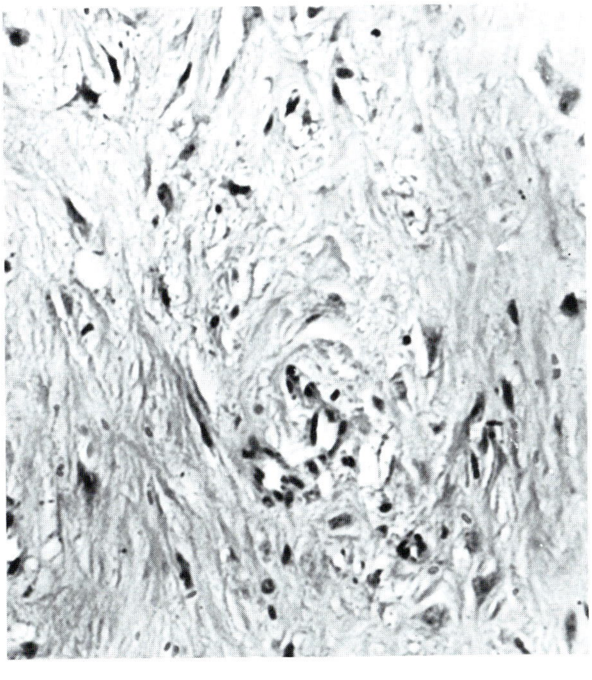

D
X540

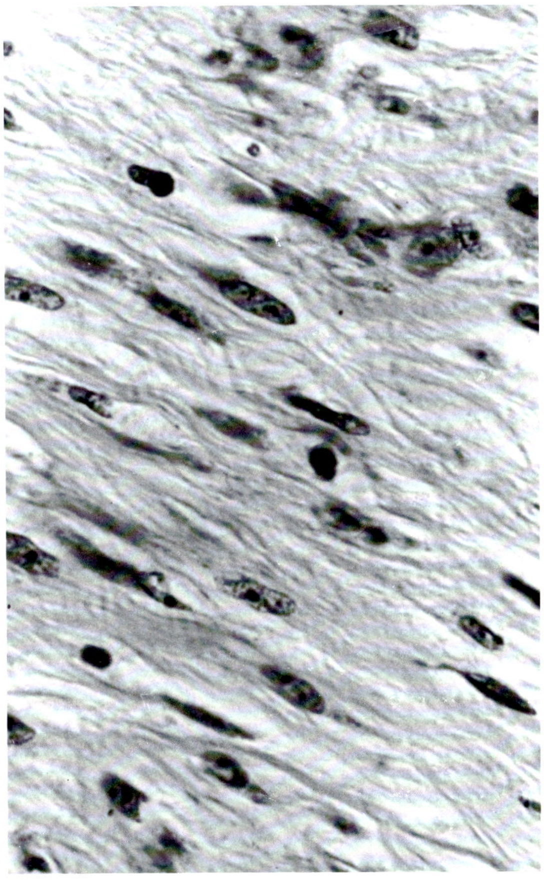

E
X730

EPITHELIAL REGENERATION

Regeneration of the surface epidermis takes place by proliferation of epithelial cells from the adjacent epidermis and from cutaneous appendages. Proliferating epithelial cells migrating into defects in the surface epidermis appear as elongated cells which parallel the skin surface. This is commonly observed in regenerating subepidermal bullae.

An exaggerated epidermal proliferation called *pseudoepitheliomatous hyperplasia* occurs at the edges of chronic ulcers, as well as in certain granulomas (bromide granuloma), blastomycosis, lupus vulgaris, and tumors (granular cell schwannoma).

Microscopic features (pseudoepitheliomatous hyperplasia)

1. There is an irregular downward proliferation of surface epidermis, either as a continuous mass or as separated islands of epithelium (Figs. A,B). This epithelium may penetrate deeply into the dermis.
2. Moderate dyskeratosis, and horn pearls (Figs. B,C), may be present.
3. Slight nuclear atypia may be present.
4. Inflammatory cells commonly migrate into the proliferating epithelium, with the formation of microabscesses containing neutrophils (Figs. A,D). These microabscesses are particularly common in blastomycosis and halide granulomas.

Microscopic differential diagnosis

1. Nuclear atypia and dyskeratosis are generally less severe in pseudoepitheliomatous hyperplasia than in well-differentiated squamous cell carcinoma. Blood vessel invasion and perineural invasion do not occur.
2. Microabscesses are more common in pseudoepitheliomatous hyperplasia than in well-differentiated squamous cell carcinoma.
3. Despite these differences, microscopic distinction cannot always be made. The occurrence of both squamous cell carcinoma and pseudoepitheliomatous hyperplasia at the edges of chronic ulcers provides added difficulty in their differentiation.

EPITHELIAL REGENERATION: PSEUDOEPITHELIOMATOUS HYPERPLASIA

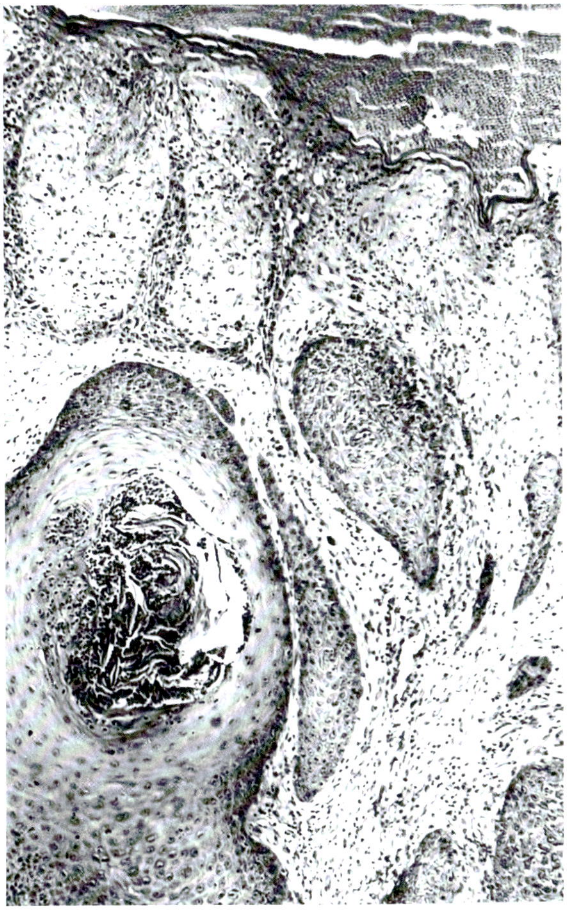

A
X70

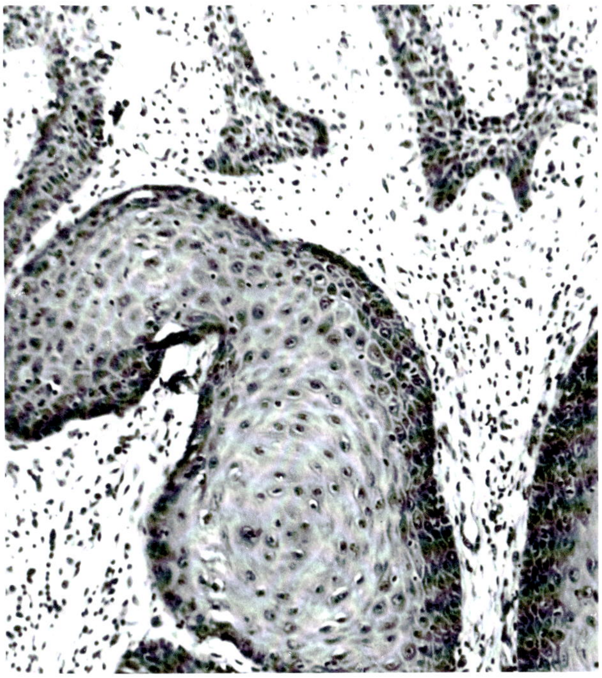

B
X150

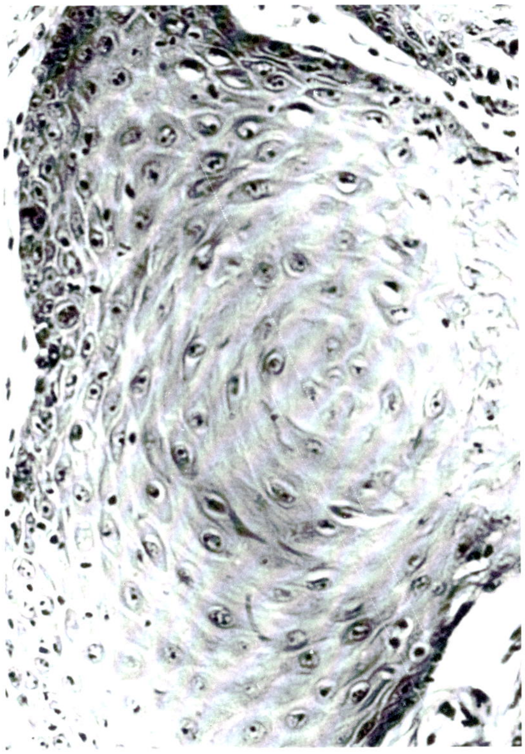

C
X320

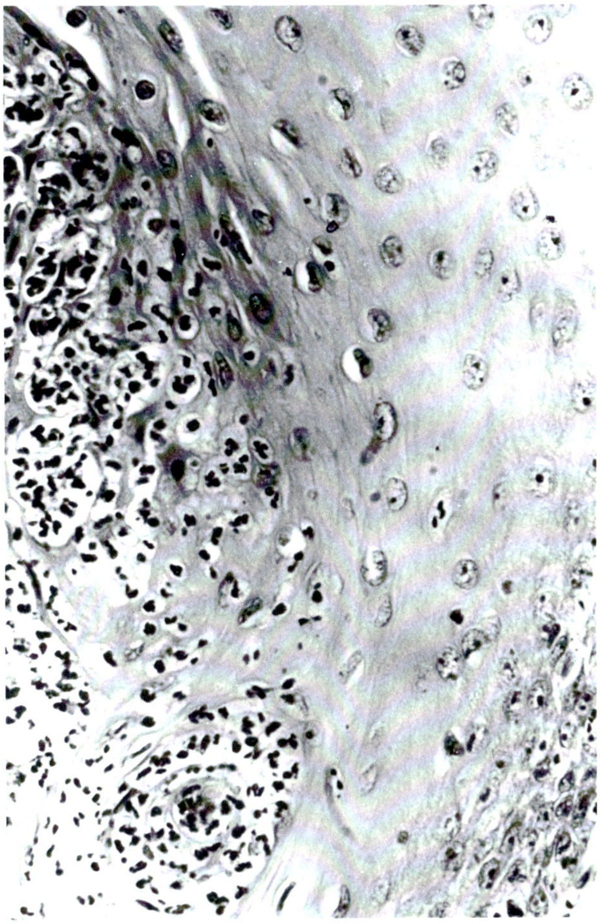

D
X320

EPITHELIAL REGENERATION: BEAU'S LINES

Beau's lines represent an interruption of nail matrix function with subsequent restoration; therefore they represent a regenerative phenomenon. They are transverse ridges (Fig. A) which migrate distally from the proximal part of the nail. Beau's lines are the result of a variety of systemic and local factors (systemic infection, childbirth, trauma, local inflammation).

BEAU'S LINES

A
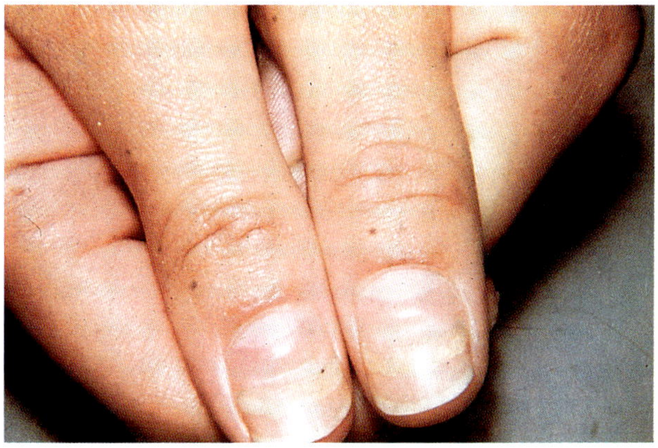

Suggested Reading

Regeneration

Granulation Tissue and Scar Formation

Allgöwer, M. *The Cellular Basis of Wound Repair.* Springfield, IL, Thomas, 1956.

Asboe-Hansen, G. Hypertrophic scars and keloids: Etiology, pathogenesis and dermatologic therapy. *Dermatologica,* 120:178, 1960.

Baur, P., Larson, D. and Stacey, T. The observation of myofibroblasts in hypertrophic scars. *Surg. Gynecol. Obstet.,* 141:22, 1975.

Billingham, R. and Russell, P. Studies on wound healing, with special reference to the phenomenon of contracture in experimental wounds in rabbits' skin. *Ann. Surg.,* 144:961, 1956.

Calnan, J. and Copenhagen, H. Autotransplantation of keloid in man. *Br. J. Surg.,* 54:330, 1967.

Craig, P. Collagenase activity in cutaneous scars. *Hand,* 5:239, 1973.

James, W., Besanceney, C. and Odom, R. The ultrastructure of a keloid. *J. Am. Acad. Dermatol.,* 3:50, 1980.

Kischer, C. et al. Perivascular myofibroblasts and microvascular occlusion in hypertrophic scars and keloids. *Human Pathol.,* 13:819, 1982.

Kurwa, A. Rubinstein-Taybi syndrome and spontaneous keloid. *Clin. Exp. Dermatol.,* 4:251, 1978.

Linares, H. and Larson, D. Early differential diagnosis between hypertrophic and non-hypertrophic healing. *J. Invest. Dermatol.,* 62:514, 1974.

Majno, G. et al. Contraction of granulation tissue *in vitro*: Similarity to smooth muscle. *Science,* 1973:548, 1971.

Mancini, R. and Quaife, J. Histogenesis of experimentally produced keloids. *J. Invest. Dermatol.,* 38:143, 1962.

Maximow, A. The morphology of the mesenchymal reactions. *Arch. Pathol. Lab. Med.,* 4:557, 1927.

Montagna, W. and Billingham, R. *Wound Healing.* In: *Advances in Biology of Skin.* Vol. 5, New York, Pergamon Press, 1964.

Moriguchi, T. and Fujimoto, D. Crosslink of collagen in hypertrophic scar. *J. Invest. Dermatol.,* 72:143, 1979.

Murray, J., Pollack, S. and Pinnel, S. Keloids: A review. *J. Am. Acad. Dermatol.,* 4:461, 1981.

Onwukwe, M. Classification of keloids. *J. Dermatol. Surg. Oncol.,* 4:534, 1978.

Ryan, G. et al. Myofibroblasts in human granulation tissue. *Human Pathol.,* 5:55, 1974.

Slome, D. *Wound Healing.* New York, Pergamon Press, 1961.

Epithelial Regeneration

Civatte, J. Pseudo-carcinomatous hyperplasia. *J. Cutan. Pathol.,* 12:214, 1985.

Freeman, R. On the pathogenesis of pseudoepitheliomatous hyperplasia *J. Cutan. Pathol.,* 1:231, 1974.

Ju, D. Pseudoepitheliomatous hyperplasia of the skin. *Dermatol. Internat.,* 6:82, 1967.

Sommerville, J. Pseudoepitheliomatous hyperplasia. *Acta Derm. Venereol.,* 33:236, 1953.

Su, W., Duncan, S. and Perry, H. Blastomycosis-like pyoderma. *Arch. Dermatol.,* 115:170, 1979.

Winer, L. Pseudoepitheliomatous hyperplasia. *Arch. Dermatol. Syph.,* 42:856, 1940.

Hyperkeratosis

Increase in thickness of the horny layer (hyperkeratosis) is a pathologic response of the skin associated with a variety of conditions. It is the result of increased production or decreased loss of keratinized cells. Hyperkeratosis, used in a generic sense, includes both orthohyperkeratosis, in which there is an increase in fully cornified cells, and parakeratosis, in which there is production of partially cornified cells (with retained pyknotic nuclei).

Apparent or relative hyperkeratosis exists when there is a decrease in epidermal thickness relative to the horny layer.

Hyperkeratosis may involve the glabrous skin (Figs. A,B) or hair follicles (Figs. C,D).

With rare exceptions (e.g., ichthyosis vulgaris), patterns of hyperkeratosis are not themselves diagnostic, but represent one area of multiple histologic features to be considered in making a diagnosis.

Scale is a clinical term referring to visible cornified cells on the skin surface.

Hyperkeratosis of glabrous skin

Examples

Friction: Corns (Fig. A) and calluses
Hereditary disorders: Ichthyosis, palmoplantar keratoderma (Fig. B)
Idiopathic papulosquamous disorders: Lichen planus
Tumors: Warts

Comment

Bazex syndrome is characterized by psoriasiform acral hyperkeratosis. It is usually associated with an occult squamous cell carcinoma of the upper digestive tract or upper respiratory tract that has metastasized to cervical lymph nodes.

Follicular hyperkeratosis

Examples

Idiopathic disorders:

1. Keratosis pilaris (a common disorder characterized by keratotic papules, principally on the extensor surfaces of the proximal parts of the extremities (Fig. C); an unusual variant is lichen spinulosus, with circumscribed groups of keratotic papules (Fig. D).
2. Pityriasis rubra pilaris (see page 460) is an idiopathic papulosquamous disorder in which follicular hyperkeratosis is an important feature.
3. Acne vulgaris (see p. 160) is a condition in which follicular hyperkeratosis is considered the primary event.

Vitamin deficiencies: In Vitamin A deficiency (phrynoderma) follicular hyperkeratosis is an important feature.

HYPERKERATOSIS

A 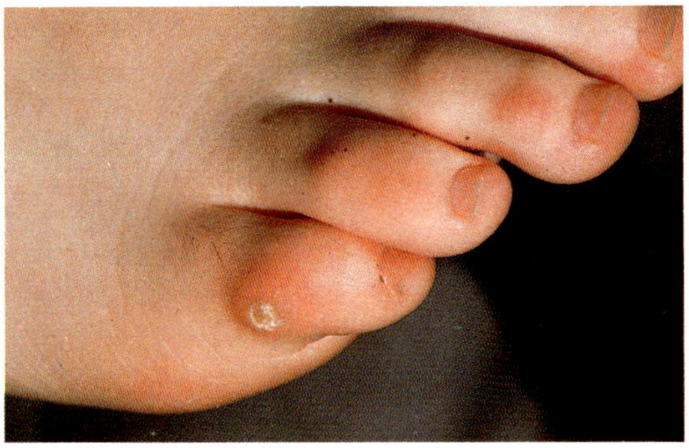

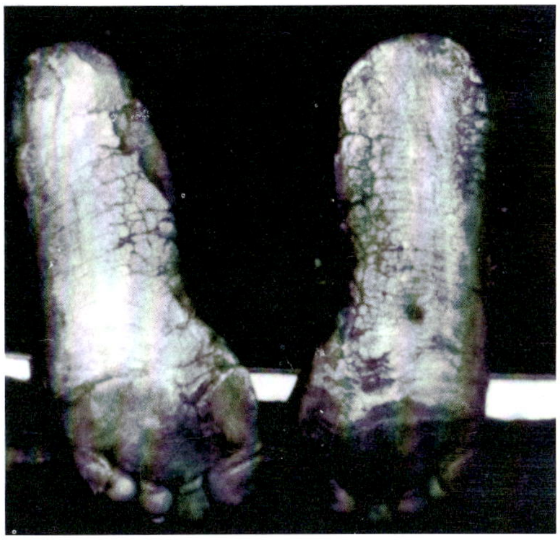 B

Courtesy Dr. Nur Or

C 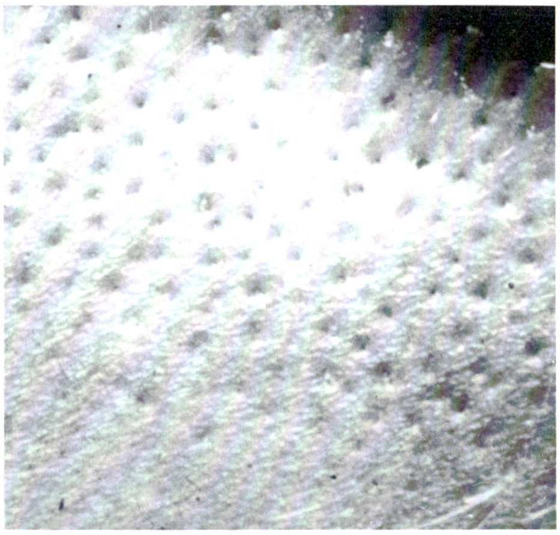

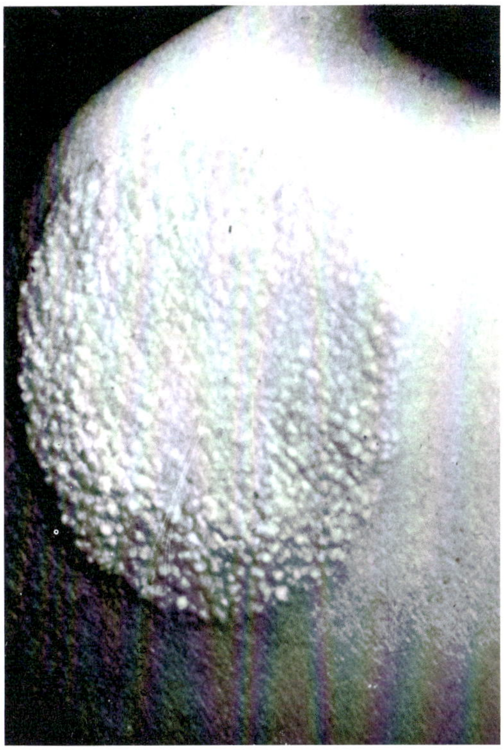 D

HYPERKERATOSIS continued

Hyperkeratosis

Microscopic features

1. Fig. A shows an example of orthohyperkeratosis of the glabrous skin. There is increased thickness of the horny layer due to an increased number of fully cornified cells. There is also an increase in the thickness of the granular layer; this usually parallels an increase in the thickness of the horny layer. Ichthyosis vulgaris is a notable exception.
2. Fig. B shows the microscopic picture of a corn. In addition to overall orthohyperkeratosis, there is a characteristic invagination filled with parakeratotic cells.

   There are many variants of palmoplantar keratoderma. Most of them show nonspecific orthohyperkeratosis. In palmoplantar keratoderma punctata, there are orthohyperkeratotic invaginations. Epidermolytic hyperkeratosis is occasionally observed in palmoplantar keratoderma.
3. Fig. C shows an example of follicular hyperkeratosis. There is an accumulation of cornified cells in the upper part of the follicular canal.

HYPERKERATOSIS

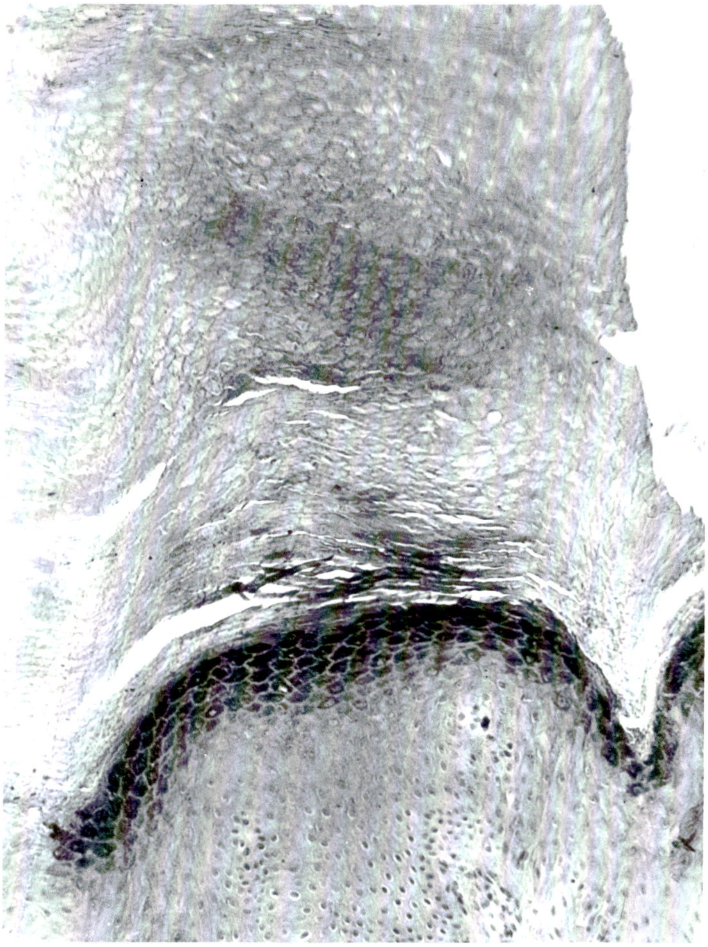

A
X185

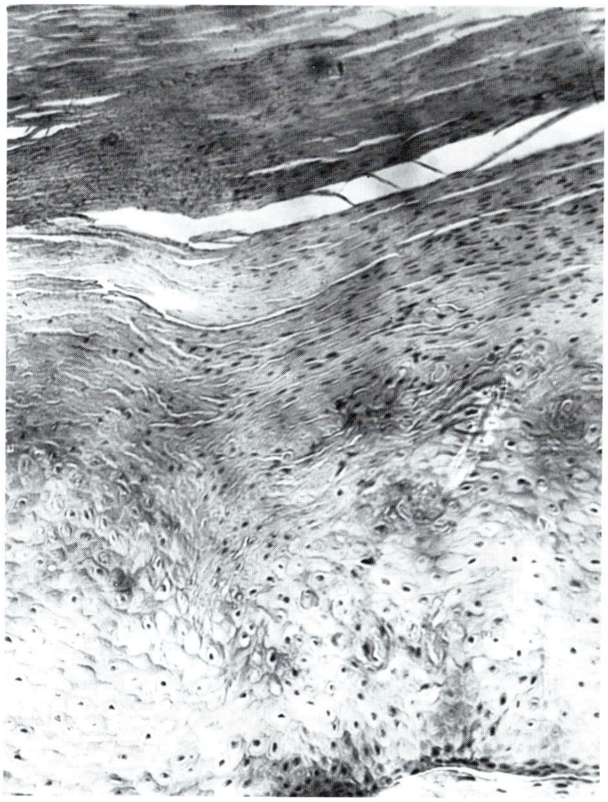

B
X144

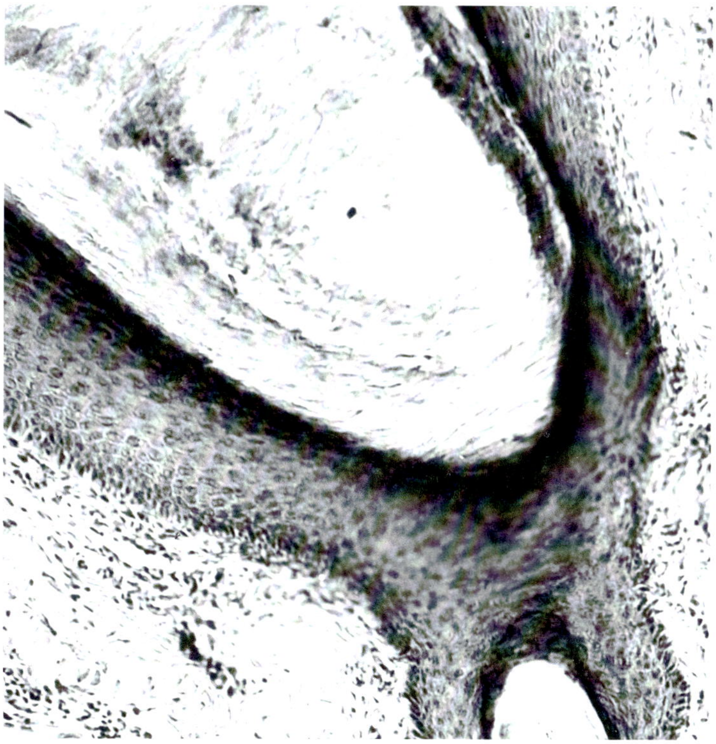

C
X160

Suggested Reading

Hyperkeratosis

Corns and Calluses

Allen, A. *The Skin: A Clinico-Pathological Treatise*, 2nd Ed. New York, Grune & Stratton, 1967, pp. 781, 784.

Montgomery, R. Corns, calluses, and warts: Differential diagnosis. *N. Y. State J. Med.*, 63:1532, 1963.

Palmoplantar Keratoderma

Ackerman, A. Histopathologic concept of epidermolytic hyperkeratosis. *Arch. Dermatol.*, 102:253, 1970.

Anderson, I. and Klintworth, G. Hypovitaminosis-A in a family with tylosis and syndactyly. *Br. Med. J.*, 1:1293, 1961.

Boudoulas, O. and Carnisa, C. Paraneoplastic acrokeratosis: Bazex syndrome. *Cutis*, 37:449, 1986.

Brown, F. Punctate keratoderma. *Arch. Dermatol.*, 104:682, 1971.

Buchanan, R., Jr. Keratosis punctata palmaris et plantaris. *Arch. Dermatol.*, 88:644, 1963.

Callan, N. Circumscribed palmoplantar keratoderma. *Austral. J. Dermatol.*, 11:76, 1970.

Camisa, C. and Williams, H. Epidermolytic variant of hereditary palmoplantar keratoderma. *Br. J. Dermatol.*, 112:221, 1985.

Cockayne, E. *Inherited Abnormalities of the Skin and Its Appendages*. London, Oxford Univ. Press, 1933.

Coupe, R. and Usher, B. Keratosis punctata palmaris et plantaris. *Arch. Dermatol.*, 87:91, 1963.

Fritsch, P., Hönigsmann, H. and Jaschke, E. Epidermolytic hereditary palmoplantar keratoderma. *Br. J. Dermatol.*, 99:561, 1978.

Greither, A. Keratosis extremitatum hereditaria progrediens mit dominantem Erbgang. *Hautarzt*, 3:198, 1952.

Haneke, E. The Papillon-Lefèvre syndrome: Keratosis palmoplantaris with periodontopathy: Report of a case and review of the cases in the literature. *Hum. Genet.*, 51:1, 1979.

Herman, P. Punctate porokeratotic keratoderma. *Dermatologica*, 147:206, 1973.

Klaus, S., Weinstein, G. and Frost, P. Localized epidermolytic hyperkeratosis: A form of keratoderma of the palms and soles. *Arch. Dermatol.*, 101:272, 1970.

Parnell, D. and Johnson, S. Tylosis palmaris et plantaris: Its occurrence with internal malignancy. *Arch. Dermatol.*, 100:7, 1969.

Follicular Hyperkeratosis

Bessey, O. and Wolbach, S. Vitamin A: Physiology and pathology. *JAMA*, 110:2072, 1938.

Fasal, P. Clinical manifestations of vitamin deficiencies as observed in the Federated Malay States. *Arch. Dermatol. Syph.*, 50:160, 1944.

Forman, L. Keratosis pilaris. *Br. J. Dermatol.*, 66:279, 1954.

Frazier, C. and Mu, C. Nature and distribution according to age of cutaneous manifestations of vitamin A deficiency: A study of two hundred and seven cases. *Arch. Dermatol. Syph.*, 33:825, 1936.

Stannus, H. Vitamin A and the Skin. *Proc. R. Soc. Med.*, 38:337, 1945.

Wechsler, H. Vitamin A deficiency following small-bowel bypass surgery for obesity. *Arch. Dermatol.*, 115:73, 1979.

Alopecia

There are many causes of alopecia, but relatively few which are amenable to histopathologic analysis. Alopecia is broadly divided into scarring and nonscarring alopecia. A special type of alopecia, characterized by mucinous changes in the hair follicle [alopecia mucinosa (follicular mucinosis)] is discussed on p. 670.

Microscopic analysis of alopecia is not easy and is dependent on obtaining an adequate biopsy sample and on correlation with clinical information.

Nonscarring alopecia

PATTERN ALOPECIA (ANDROGENETIC ALOPECIA)

This is dependent on androgenic stimulus and heredity and is far more common in males than females. In males, onset is usually in adolescence or early adult life. In females, onset is usually later and the degree of hair loss is usually less. Androgenetic alopecia in females may be a sign of endocrine abnormality. In male pattern alopecia, hair loss typically progresses from the frontotemporal and crown regions (Fig. A). In females, the hair loss is often diffuse. Microscopically, there is an increase in the proportion of vellus hairs and a decrease in the proportion of terminal hair follicles. Ultimately, no hairs remain. Recently, it has been noted that a ladder-like stack of Arao-Perkins bodies (the cluster of elastic tissue at the necks of hair papillae) remain as the hairs get progressively smaller in pattern alopecia.

ALOPECIA AREATA

Alopecia areata is characterized by sharply circumscribed areas of hair loss (Fig. B). "Exclamation point" hairs are often present at the borders of the patches. Such attenuation of hair shafts reflects regression of follicles. The cause is unknown, but there is evidence for an autoimmune mechanism. The scalp is most often involved, but any hair-bearing area can be affected. Progression to large areas of hair loss may occur. *Alopecia totalis* refers to complete loss of scalp hair. *Alopecia universalis* (Fig. C) refers to complete loss of all hair. Regrowth of hair is the rule in cases with limited hair loss. Vitiligo, pernicious anemia, thyroid disease, Addison's disease, Down's syndrome, nail changes, and cataracts have been reported to be associated with alopecia areata. Alopecia areata can be part of the Vogt-Koyanagi-Harada syndrome, in which there is aseptic meningitis followed by dysacousia and uveitis. Vitiligo may be present.

Microscopic features

1. The key feature is the presence of miniature anagen (Fig. D) or telogen hairs showing dystrophic hair shafts.
2. The connective tissue sheaths of the affected hair follicles extend down to the level of the previously normal hair follicle (Fig. D).
3. A usually sparse inflammatory infiltrate is present (Figs. D,E) around the affected pilosebaceous structures ("swarm of bees"). Inflammatory cells may penetrate the follicle itself.
4. Sebaceous glands may be normal or atrophic.

Comment

It has been suggested that the initial event in alopecia areata is the premature entry of anagen follicles into telogen, followed by re-entry into anagen with growth halted in anagen III.

ALOPECIA AREATA

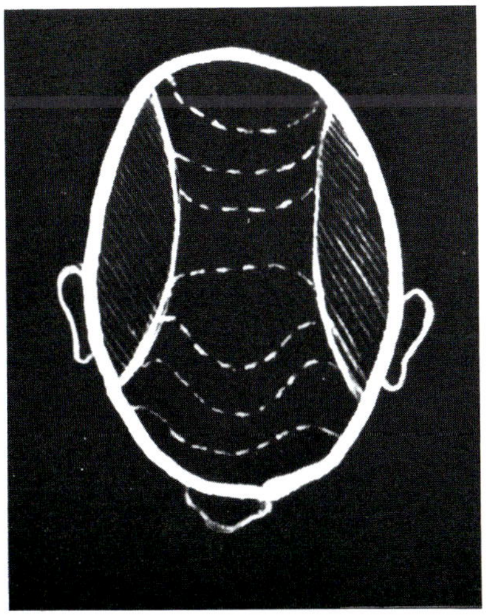

A

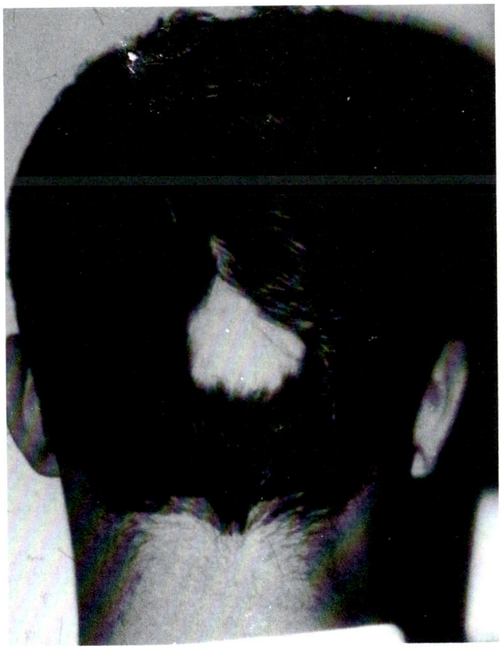

B

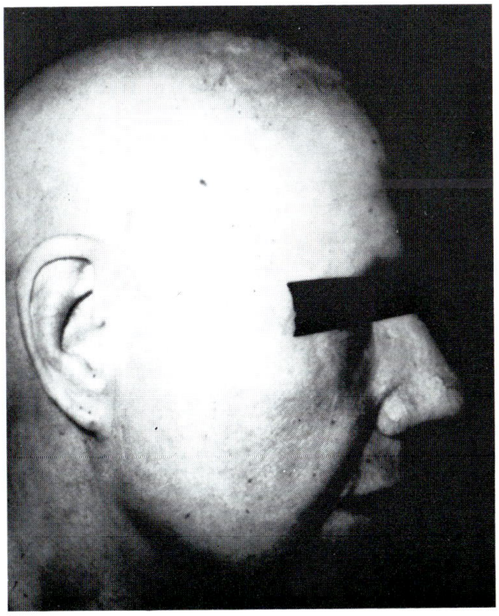

C

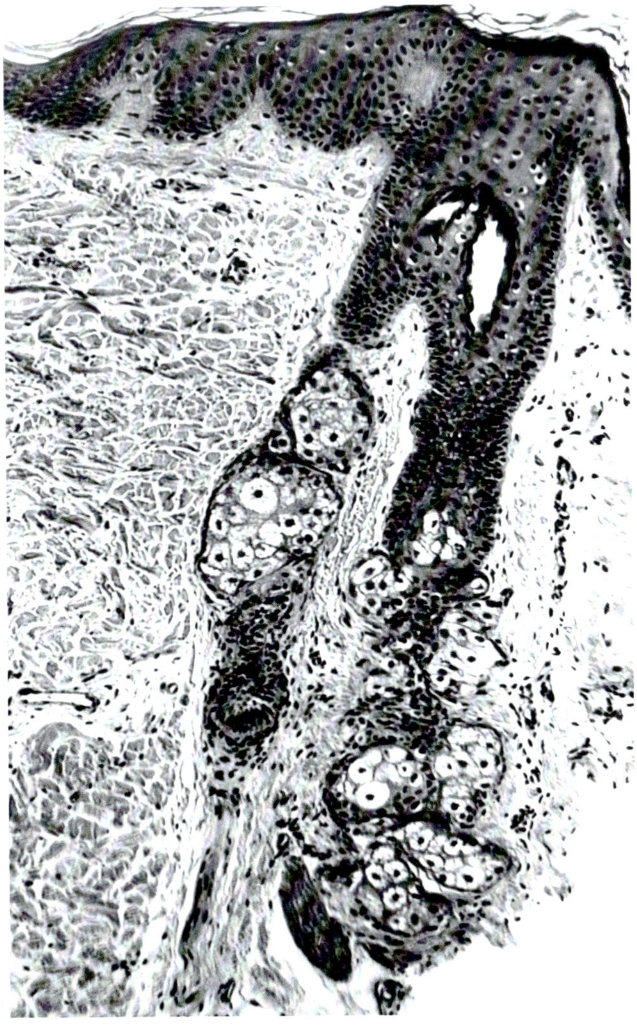

D
X260

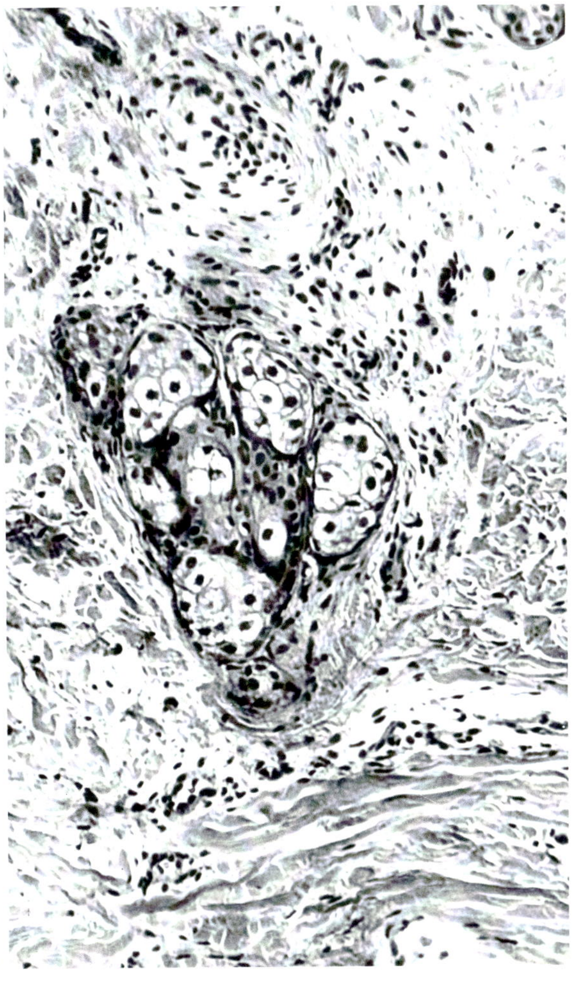

E
X230

ALOPECIA continued

TELOGEN EFFLUVIUM

Telogen effluvium is transient alopecia in which the hair follicles are arrested in telogen. Causes include acute febrile illnesses and endocrine changes following pregnancy. Discontinuation of certain drugs or birth control pills may cause telogen effluvium.

ANAGEN EFFLUVIUM

This is a diffuse hair loss with hairs arrested in anagen. Causes include cancer chemotherapy, coumarin, thallium, and the post-partum state.

TRICHOTILLOMANIA

Compulsive pulling of hair can produce a temporary alopecia resembling alopecia areata clinically. Hair loss is not as complete as in alopecia areata. Microscopically there can be evidence of trauma, such as clefts in the hair matrix, hemorrhage, and separation of the follicular epithelium from the connective tissue sheath. Many hair follicles without hair shafts may be present, and there may be evidence of transformation to the catagen stage.

Scarring alopecia

Scarring alopecia is the result of any deep, destructive process, terminating in fibrosis and the permanent loss of hair follicles. Causes include infections, neoplasms, burns, and specific cutaneous disorders, such as lupus erythematosus, scleroderma (morphea), lichen planopilaris, sarcoidosis, aplasia cutis congenita, and pseudopelade of Brocq.

Pseudopelade of Brocq (alopecia cicatrisata) is a disorder of middle age, characterized by confluent patches of alopecia associated with atrophic scarring. Usually there are scattered persistent hairs within the affected area (Fig. A).

Microscopic features

1. The cause of the scarring alopecia can sometimes be identified by histologic features of the underlying disease (see discussion under pertinent entities). In longstanding lesions, specific features are absent and there is only fibrosis and a decrease in the number of hair follicles.
2. Pseudopelade of Brocq does not have a specific microscopic appearance. It progresses from an inflammatory stage, in which an inflammatory infiltrate surrounds and penetrates the upper two thirds of the follicles, to a late fibrotic stage in which there is a decrease in hair follicles associated with fibrosis (Figs. B,C). The fibrous areas contain much elastic tissue. Occasional remaining hairs (Figs. B,C) show intense perifollicular fibrosis.

Comment

Justification for considering pseudopelade of Brocq as an entity has been questioned. It has been suggested that this disease is a late stage of lichen planopilaris, lupus erythematosus, folliculitis decalvans, or scleroderma.

Some authors believe that pseudopelade of Brocq is a distinct entity.

PSEUDOPELADE OF BROCQ

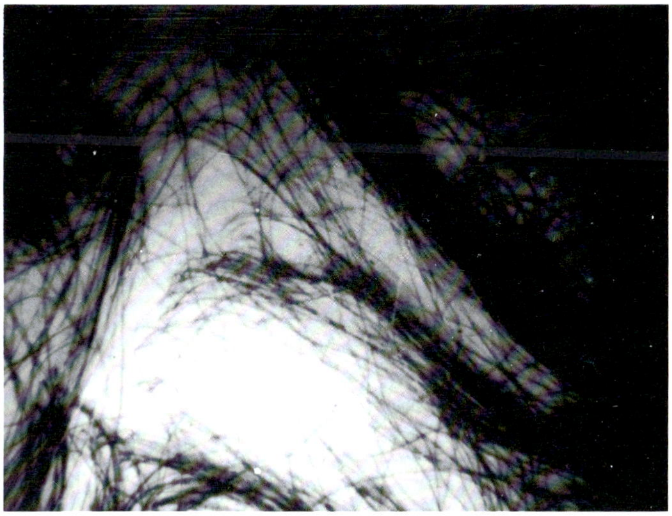

A

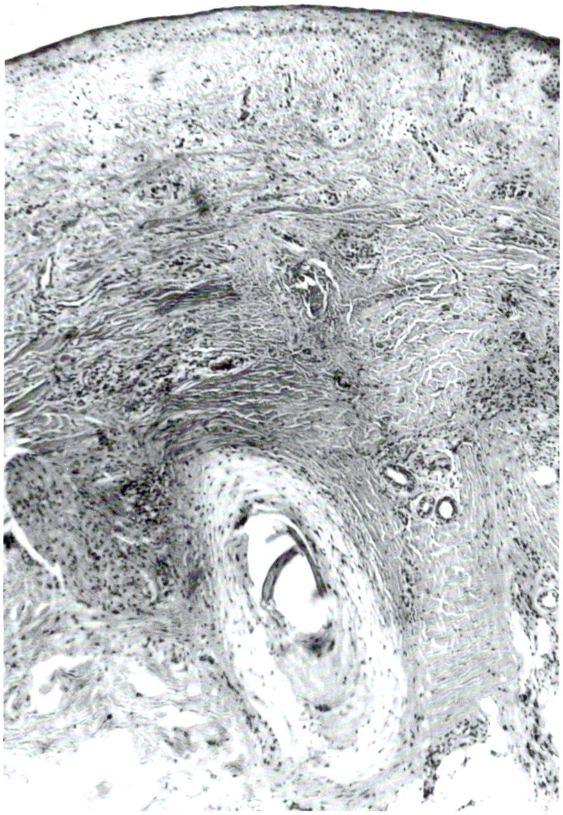

B
X52

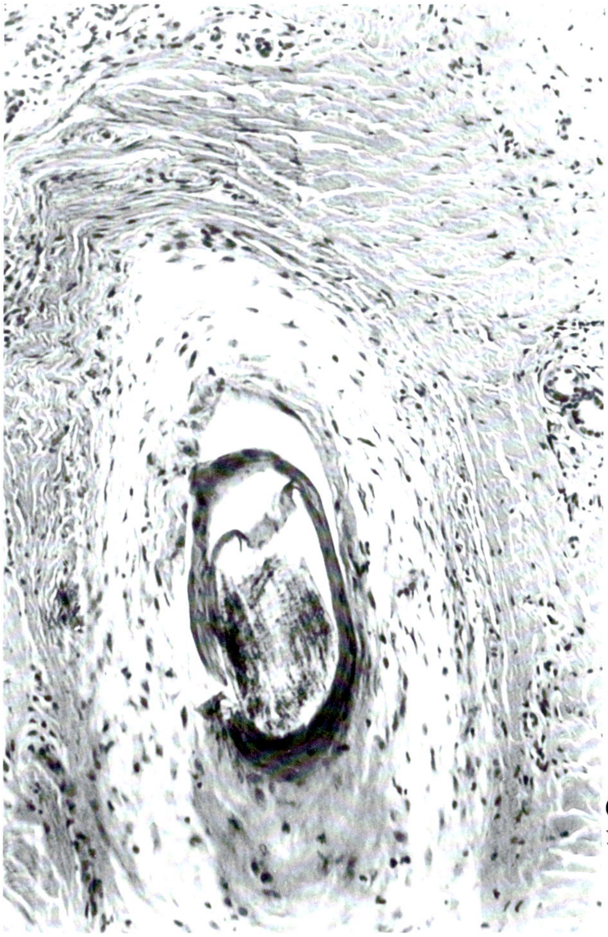

C
X155

Suggested Reading

Alopecia

Male Pattern Baldness

Ellis, R. Aging of the human male scalp. In: *The Biology of Hair Growth*. Montagna, W. and Ellis, R., eds., New York, Academic Press, 1958, p. 469.

Hamilton, J. Male hormone stimulation is prerequisite and an incitement in common baldness. *Am. J. Anat.*, 71:451, 1942.

Kasick, J. et al. Adrenal androgenetic female-pattern alopecia: Sex hormones and the balding woman. *Cleve. Clin. Q.*, 50:111, 1983.

Lattanand, A. and Johnson, W. Male pattern alopecia: A histopathologic and histochemical study. *J. Cutan. Pathol.*, 2:58, 1975.

Ludwig, E. Classification of the types of androgenetic alopecia (common baldness) arising in the female sex. *Br. J. Dermatol.*, 97:249, 1977.

Maguire, H., Jr. and Kligman, A. The histopathology of common male baldness. In: *Proceedings of the XII International Congress of Dermatology*. Pillsbury, D. and Livingood, C. eds., Amsterdam, Excerpta Medica, 1963, p. 1438.

Maguire, H., Jr. and Kligman, A. Common baldness in women. *Geriatrics*, 18:329, 1963.

Smith, M. and Wells, R. Male-type alopecia, alopecia areata, and normal hair in women. *Arch. Dermatol.*, 89:95, 1964.

Anagen Effluvium

Lattanand, A. and Johnson, W. Male pattern alopecia: A histopathologic and histochemical study. *J. Cutan. Pathol.*, 2:58, 1975.

Maguire, H., Jr. and Kligman, A. Common baldness in women. *Geriatrics*, 18:329, 1963.

Telogen Effluvium

Kligman, A. Pathologic dynamics of human hair loss. I. Telogen effluvium. *Arch. Dermatol.*, 83:175, 1961.

Lynfield, Y. Effect of pregnancy on the human hair cycle. *J. Invest. Dermatol.*, 35:323, 1960.

Schiff, B. and Kern, A. Study of postpartum alopecia. *Arch. Dermatol.*, 87:609, 1963.

Alopecia Areata

Brown, A., Olkowski, Z. and McLaren, J. Thymus lymphocytes of the peripheral blood in patients with alopecia areata. *Arch. Dermatol.*, 113:688, 1977.

Burton, J. and Marshall, A. Hypertrichosis due to minoxidil. *Br. J. Dermatol.*, 101:593, 1979.

Eckert, J., Church, R. and Ebling, F. The pathogenesis of alopecia areata. *Br. J. Dermatol.*, 80:203, 1968.

Goos, M. Zur Histopathologie der Alopecia Areata. *Arch. Derm. Forsch.* 240:160, 1971.

Juhlin, L. Reactions to infusion of a histamine liberator: Effects of compound 48/80 on eosinophil and basophil leukocytes in patients with atopic dermatitis, urticaria, and alopecia areata. *Arch. Dermatol.*, 88:771, 1963.

Kopf, A. and Orentreich, N. Alkaline phosphatase in alopecia areata. *Arch. Dermatol.*, 76:288, 1957.

Messenger, A., Slater, D. and Bleehen, S. Alopecia areata: Alterations in the hair growth cycle and correlation with the follicular pathology. *Br. J. Dermatol.*, 114:337, 1986.

Perret, C., Wiesner-Menzel, L. and Happle, R. Immunohistochemical analysis of T-cell subsets in the peribulbar and intrabulbar infiltrates of alopecia areata. *Acta Derm. Venereol.* (Stockh.), 64:26, 1984.

Sauder, D. et al. Alopecia areata: An inherited autoimmune disease. In: *Hair, Trace Elements and Human Illness*. Brown, A. and Crounse, R., eds., New York, Prager, 1980, p. 343.

Schenk, E. et al. Autoantibodies in alopecia and vitiligo. In: *Hair, Trace Elements and Human Illness*. Brown, A. and Crounse, R., eds., New York, Prager, 1980, p. 343.

Tago, H. A stereohistomorphological study of alopecia areata. *Jpn. J. Dermatol.*, (Ser. B) 78:80, 1968.

Tan, R. and Delaney, T. Circular regrowth in alopecia areata. *Br. J. Dermatol.*, 92:233, 1975.

Todes-Taylor, N. et al. T cell subpopulations in alopecia areata. *J. Am. Acad. Dermatol.*, 11:216, 1984.

Van Scott, E. Morphologic changes in pilosebaceous units and anagen hairs in alopecia areata. *J. Invest. Dermatol.*, 31:35, 1958.

Alopecia Cicatrisata

Braun-Falco, O. et al. Pseudopelade of Brocq. *Dermatologica*, 172:18, 1986.

Laymon, C. The Cicatricial Alopecias: A historical and clinical review and a histologic investigation. *J. Invest. Dermatol.*, 8:99, 1947.

Male, O. Über die ulzerös-atrophisierende Form des Lichen ruber planus *Z. Haut.*, 45:17, 1970.

Miescher, G. and Lenggenhager, R. Über Pseudopelade Brocq. *Dermatologica*, 94:122, 1947.

Pinkus, H. Differential patterns of elastic fibers in scarring and non-scarring alopecias. *J. Cutan. Pathol.*, 5:93, 1978.

Prieto, J. Pseudopelade of Brocq: Its relationship to some forms of cicatricial alopecias and to lichen planus. *J. Invest. Dermatol.*, 24:323, 1955.

Chapter 4
Genodermatoses

There are numerous hereditary dermatoses. In this chapter we will discuss some hereditary dermatoses having histopathologic interest and importance. Not all of the hereditary dermatoses included in the book are in this chapter. Some are in other chapters because of their morphologic relationship to nonhereditary dermatoses. For example, Darier's disease and epidermolysis bullosa are in the chapter on bullous dermatoses.

Ichthyosis

Ichthyosis refers to a group of genodermatoses characterized by a disorder of keratinization leading to the accumulation of coarse scales ("fish scales").

The chart (p. 239) gives classification and essential clinical and microscopic features of the ichthyoses.

ICHTHYOSIS VULGARIS (see chart, p. 239)

Ichthyosis vulgaris is an autosomal dominant inherited disorder beginning in infancy or childhood. Fine, light-colored scales are present, which spare the flexural areas (Figs. A,B,C). The scales accumulate because of the increased adhesiveness of the cornified cells. Palmar and plantar hyperkeratosis may be present.

Microscopic features

There is hyperkeratosis and a decreased to absent granular layer (Fig. D). Follicular hyperkeratosis is often present.

Comment

1. Ichthyosis vulgaris has a statistically significant association with atopic dermatitis and keratosis pilaris.
2. Acquired icthyosiform changes may be associated with visceral malignancy or immunodeficiency states.
3. The increased adhesiveness of the cornified cells is believed to result from a delay in dissolution of the desmosomes.
4. *X-linked ichthyosis* is recessively inherited. Female heterozygotes have a mild form of the disorder. Males have a more severe form. It affects flexor as well as extensor surfaces and shows a visible granular layer with light microscopy. As in ichthyosis vulgaris, there is retention hyperkeratosis due to increased adhesiveness of the cornified cells. Corneal opacities may be present.
5. *Pityriasis rotunda* is characterized by round or oval scaling patches. It tends to occur in dark-skinned races and may represent a localized variant of acquired ichthyosis. It is often associated with debilitating or malignant disease. Histologic findings are consistent with ichthyosis vulgaris.

ICHTHYOSIS VULGARIS

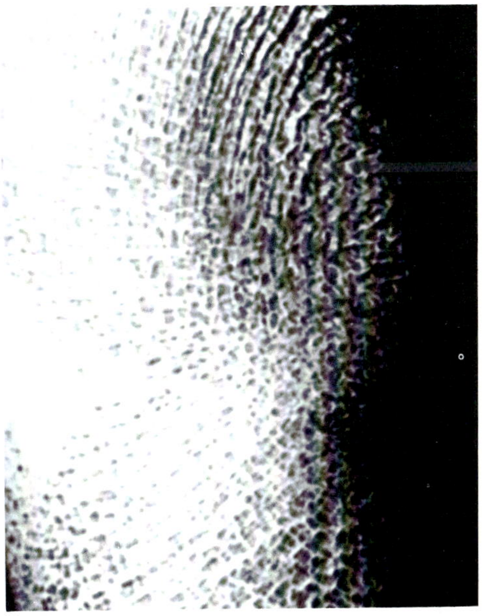

A

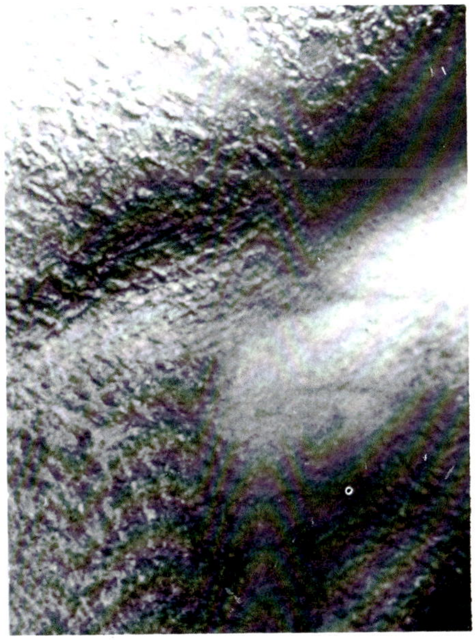

B

Courtesy Dr. Harvey Ansell

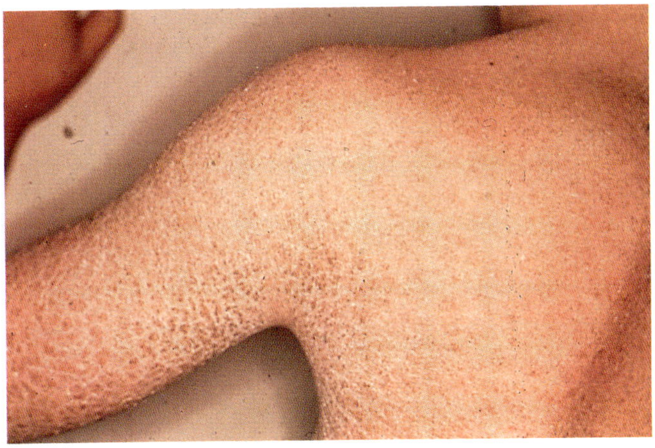

C

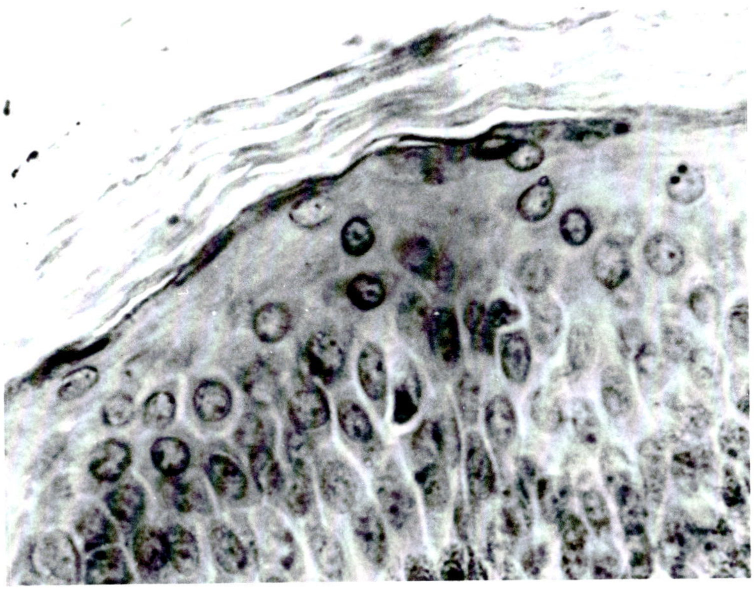

D
X720

ICHTHYOSIS continued ⇨

LAMELLAR ICHTHYOSIS (NONBULLOUS ICHTHYOSIFORM ERYTHRODERMA) (see chart p. 239)

Lamellar ichthyosis is an autosomal recessive inherited disorder. It is usually present at birth. "Collodion baby" (Fig. B) has parchment-like skin.

When the collodion-like horny layer detaches, the skin shows diffuse erythema and scaling, with involvement of the flexor as well as the extensor surfaces. The scales are large and rhomboidal (Fig. A). Ectropion is frequent. Erythema with scaling may persist throughout life. In milder cases, the erythema may subside.

Microscopic features

Changes are nonspecific (see chart, p. 239)

Comment

1. There is an increased incidence of clear cell acanthoma in patients with lamellar ichthyosis.
2. *Harlequin fetus* (harlequin ichthyosis) is a very rare autosomal recessive disorder, formerly considered a variant of collodion baby. The skin has a thick, fissured, horny layer. Ears are rudimentary or absent; there is ectropion and eclabium. Death within days usually occurs. Histologically, there is massive hyperkeratosis. The granular layer is diminished or absent.
3. Collodion baby can also be seen in X-linked ichthyosis and epidermolytic hyperkeratosis.

LAMELLAR ICHTHYOSIS

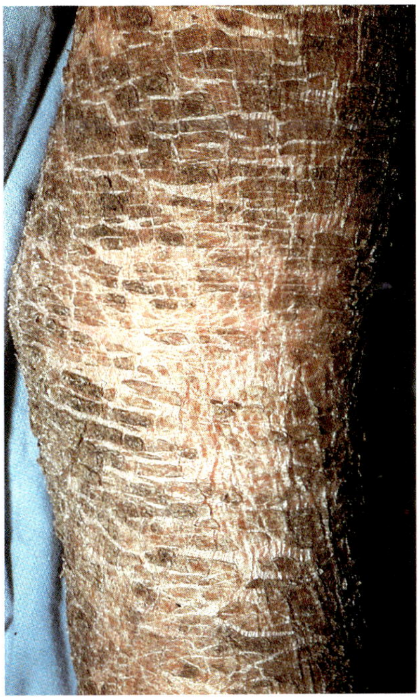

A

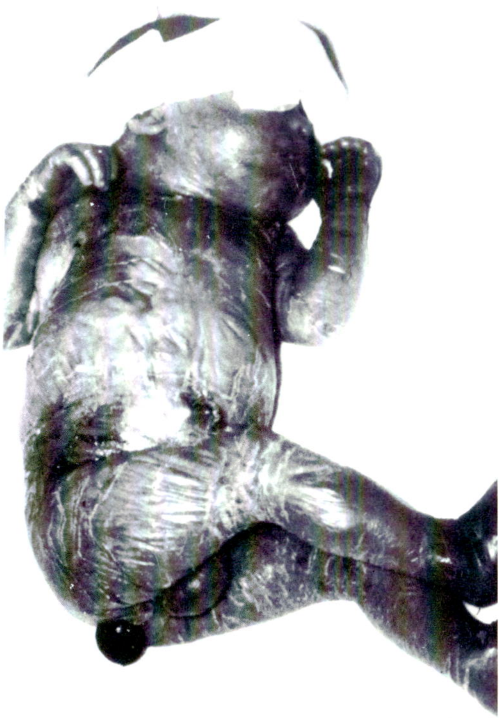

B

ICHTHYOSIS continued

EPIDERMOLYTIC HYPERKERATOSIS (BULLOUS CONGENITAL ICHTHYOSIFORM ERYTHRODERMA) (see chart, p. 239).

This is an autosomal dominant disorder. There is generalized erythema, present at birth. Within a few days after birth verrucous lesions develop. Vesicles and bullae are present only in early childhood. The verrucous lesions are most pronounced in the flexural areas (Figs. A,B). Fig. B, in addition, shows several erosions, representing ruptured bullae.

Microscopic features

1. There is hyperkeratosis (Figs. C,D), without parakeratosis.
2. Keratinocytes of the stratum granulosum and upper stratum Malpighii show apparent intracellular edema (vacuolar degeneration) (Figs. C,D). Vacuoles may coalesce to form vesicles. The cell walls are indistinct (Figs. C,D). When bullae form, they form intraepidermally.
3. Many cells in the area of vacuolar degeneration show pyknotic nuclei (Figs. C,D).
4. Clumped keratohyaline-like granules are present in the upper epidermis (Figs. C,D).
5. A moderate chronic inflammatory infiltrate is present in the papillary dermis (Fig. C); lymphocytes predominate.

Comment

1. With electron microscopy, actual vacuolization of the keratinocytes is not observed. There is an excess of tonofilaments, which are aggregated around the nuclei of the cells. Prematurely formed keratohyaline granules are enmeshed in the clumped tonofilaments. There is an altered association of desmosomes with tonofilaments, resulting in acantholysis.
2. Although the histologic picture of epidermolytic hyperkeratosis distinguishes it from the other types of ichthyosis, the picture is not specific. It can be seen in epidermal nevus, other benign papillomas, palmoplantar keratoderma, and as a coincidental finding in a variety of conditions (see p. 218).

EPIDERMOLYTIC HYPERKERATOSIS

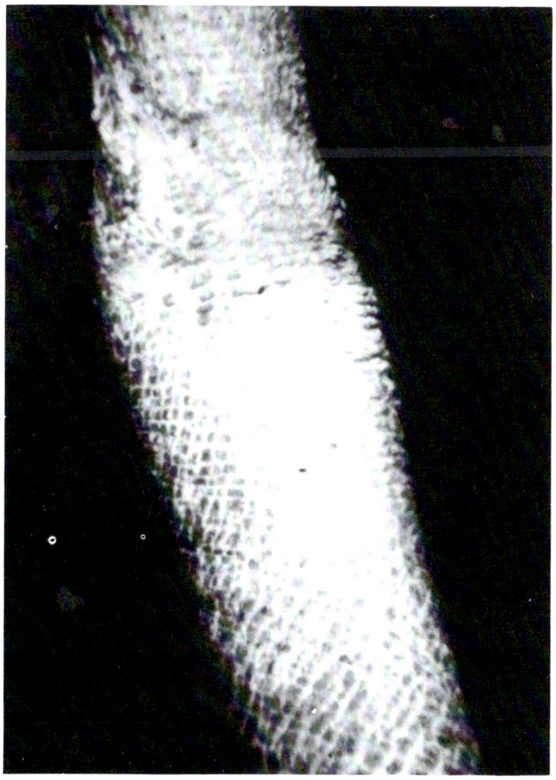

A

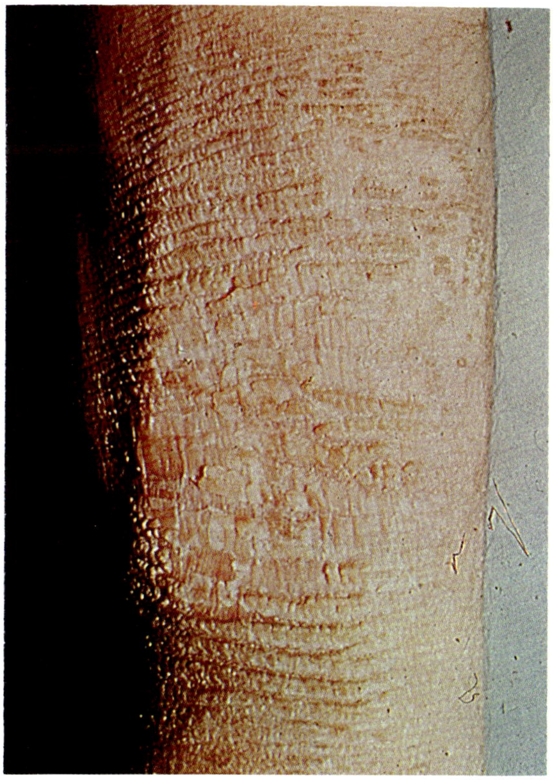

B

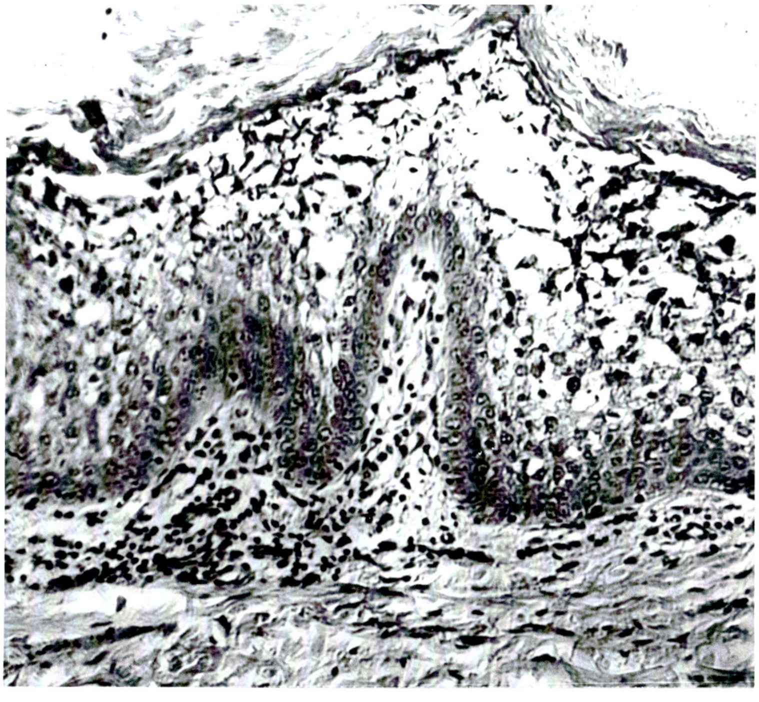

C X230

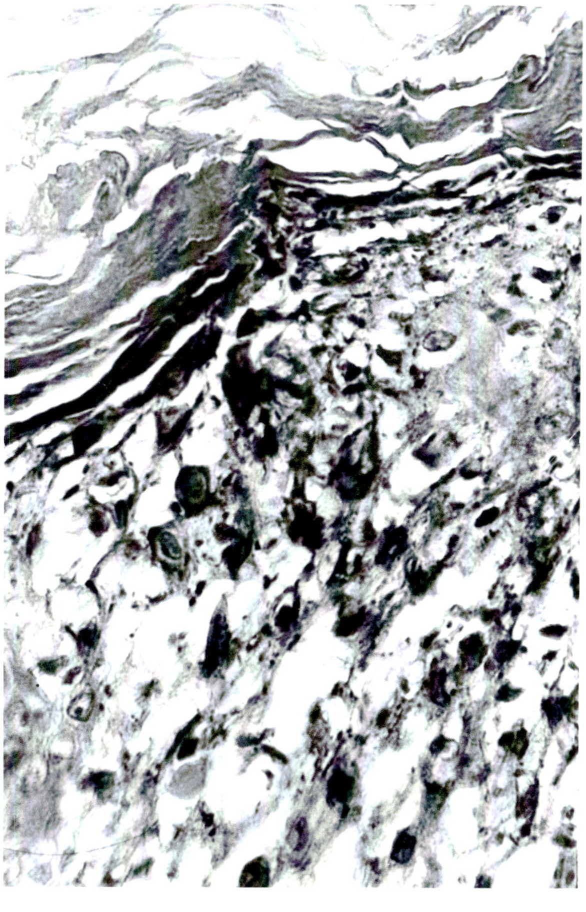

D X520

Microscopic differential diagnosis of ichthyosiform dermatoses

1. A minimal or absent granular layer is diagnostic of ichthyosis vulgaris.
2. The acanthosis and hyperkeratosis of X-linked ichthyosis and lamellar ichthyosis are nonspecific.
3. Changes identical to those of epidermolytic hyperkeratosis occasionally can be seen in solar keratoses, linear epidermal nevus, ichthyosis hystrix, palmoplantar keratodermas, seborrheic keratoses, and squamous cell carcinoma.
4. Verruca plana resembles epidermolytic hyperkeratosis, but shows less degeneration and less hypergranulosis.

Comment

1. An increased rate of transepidermal water loss is a pathophysiologic abnormality common to the ichthyoses.
2. Some syndromes are associated with ichthyosis:
   a. Rud's syndrome—ichthyosis vulgaris with infantilism and epilepsy.
   b. Refsum's syndrome—ichthyosis vulgaris with ataxia, progressive paresis of the extremities, and retinitis pigmentosa. The underlying metabolic defect is an inability to degrade exogenous phytanic acid. Epidermal cells show lipid-containing vacuoles.
   c. Sjögren-Larsen syndrome—congenital ichthyosiform erythroderma with mental retardation and spastic paresis.
   d. Netherton's syndrome—ichthyosis linearis circumflexa (see below) or lamellar ichthyosis with bamboo hairs.
   e. Conradi's syndrome: Whorled ichthyosis is associated with skeletal and ocular abnormalities.
3. Two rare forms of ichthyosis are the dominantly inherited *erythrokeratoderma variabilis* and recessively inherited *ichthyosis linearis circumflexa*. The former is characterized by figurate erythema and hyperkeratotic plaques. The latter is characterized by migratory polycyclic erythema and scales with double-edged margins. Neither of these disorders has a specific histologic picture.

ICHTHYOSIS

	Ichthyosis vulgaris	*X-linked ichthyosis*	*Lamellar ichthyosis*	*Epidermolytic hyperkeratosis*
Synonyms			Some consider it to be the dry form of congenital ichthyosiform erythroderma	Bullous form of congenital ichthyosiform erythroderma
Inheritance	Autosomal dominant	X-linked recessive	Autosomal recessive	Autosomal dominant
Age of onset	Early infancy or childhood	Birth or early infancy	Birth	Birth
Gross features	Coarse scales or fine, light-colored scales sparing flexural areas	Large, dark scales; head, neck and trunk often involved. Flexural areas may be involved	Large, coarse scales—generalized. Palms and soles involved. Often seen as the "collodion baby" at birth	First week—generalized bullae and erythema, followed by development of verrucous lesions. Flexural areas most heavily involved
Microscopic features	Hyperkeratosis with minimal or absent granular layer	Hyperkeratosis; normal or increased granular layer	Hyperkeratosis; normal or increased granular layer; acanthosis with increased mitotic index	Hyperkeratosis; vacuolization of keratinocytes of granular layer and upper malpighian layer; clumped keratohyaline-like granules (granular degeneration)

Porokeratosis

Porokeratosis is a disorder of keratinization characterized by crateriform hyperkeratotic lesions. The lesions have atrophic centers and raised margins. Five types of porokeratosis are now recognized:

a) *Plaque type (Mibelli)*: There are one or several large lesions;
b) *Linear type*: Lesions may be localized or widely disseminated. They resemble linear epidermal nevus;
c) *Disseminated type*: There are widely distributed small shallow lesions; these typically involve the trunk and the palms and soles. The oral mucosa may be involved.
d) *Disseminated superficial actinic porokeratosis type*: There are lesions resembling the superficial disseminated type, but with a distribution limited to the sun-exposed areas.
e) *Punctate type*: This is a rare form with limited distribution. Lesions on the palms and soles can resemble punctate palmoplantar keratoderma.

Porokeratosis is transmitted as an autosomal dominant trait, with the exception of the linear type, whose mode of inheritance is uncertain. Sporadic cases without apparent hereditary pattern also occur.

Squamous cell carcinoma or Bowen's disease may develop in lesions of porokeratosis.

POROKERATOSIS–PLAQUE TYPE

The head, neck, and extremities are preferentially affected. The primary lesions are small keratotic papules which progress to crateriform lesions (Figs. A,B) with hyperkeratotic margins and atrophic, hypopigmented, hairless centers.

Microscopic features

1. The principal feature is the *cornoid lamella*: a tier of parakeratotic cells extending upward from a groove in the malpighian layer (Figs. C,D). The cornoid lamella, together with adjacent hyperkeratosis (Fig. C), form the raised, hyperkeratotic margin of the lesion seen grossly. Dyskeratotic cells are present (Fig. D) beneath the cornoid lamella.
2. The name "porokeratosis" is misleading. The cornoid lamellae are not limited to the sweat pores; however, they can be present in sweat pores and follicular openings.
3. The epidermis beneath the cornoid lamella has an absent granular layer, but the granular layer is prominent elsewhere in the invagination (Figs. C,D).
4. The epidermis in the center of the lesion is usually atrophic (Fig. C, right), but occasionally may be hyperkeratotic and acanthotic.
5. A predominantly lymphocytic infiltrate may be present in the dermis.
6. The cornoid lamella is not entirely pathognomonic for porokeratosis. It has been also reported to occur in a variety of inflammatory and neoplastic disorders.

Comment

The microscopic features of the other types of porokeratosis parallel those of the plaque type, but are usually less pronounced.

POROKERATOSIS—PLAQUE TYPE

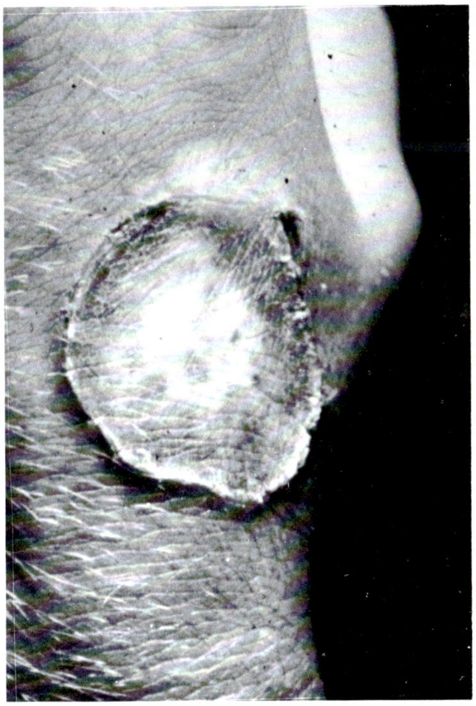

A

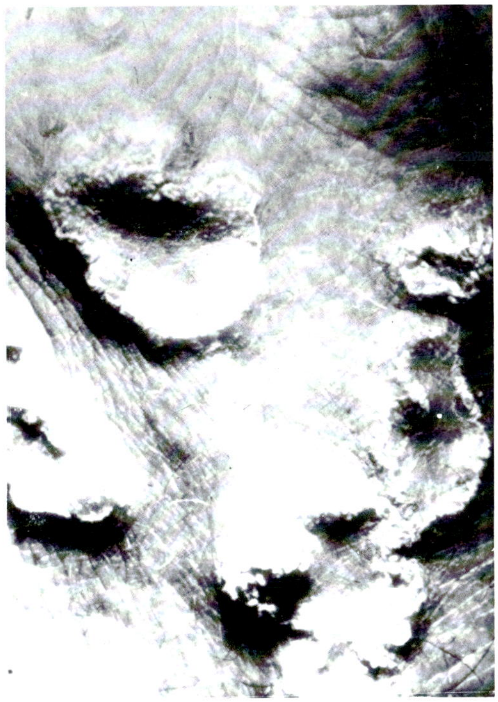

B

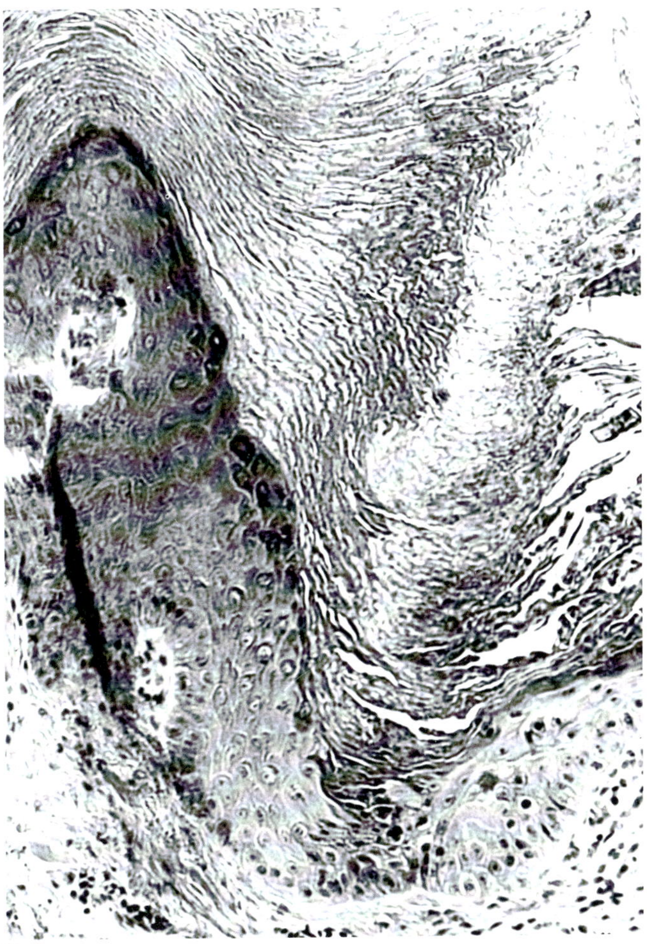

C
X240

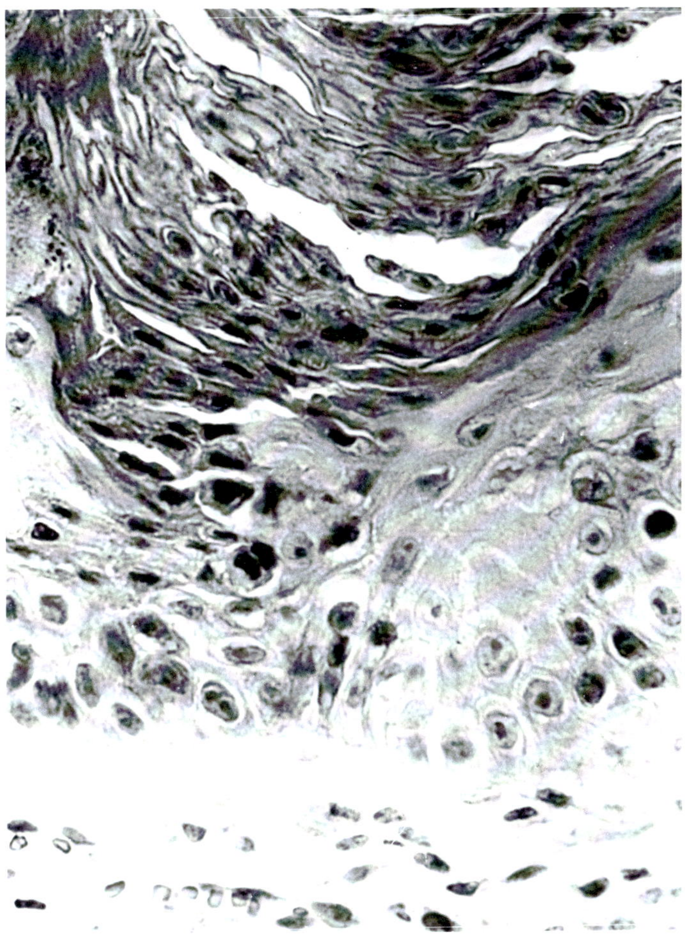

D
X720

POROKERATOSIS continued ⇨

DISSEMINATED SUPERFICIAL ACTINIC POROKERATOSIS (DSAP)

Lesions of DSAP are smaller than those of porokeratosis of the plaque type and have less pronounced hyperkeratotic margins (Fig. A). They may resemble solar keratoses. DSAP can coexist with other types of porokeratosis.

Microscopic features

Histologic features of DSAP differ from those of porokeratosis of the plaque type only in degree. The microscopic changes are less pronounced (Fig. B) (see p. 240).

DISSEMINATED SUPERFICIAL ACTINIC POROKERATOSIS

A

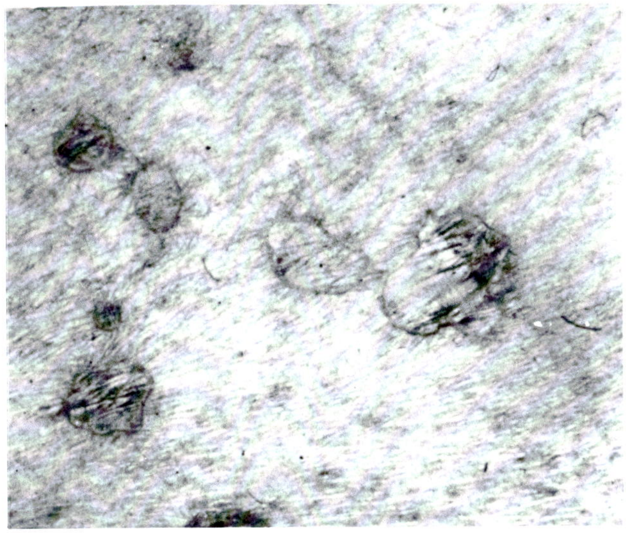

Courtesy Dr. William Tarnowski

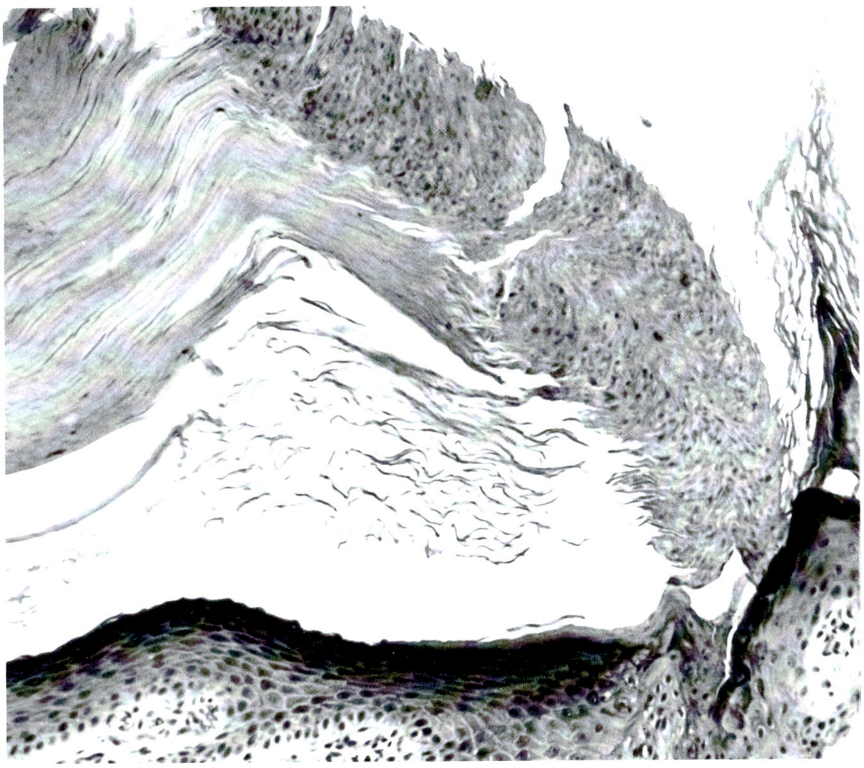

B
X190

XERODERMA PIGMENTOSUM

Xeroderma pigmentosum is an autosomal recessive disorder characterized by premature solar aging of the skin and a severe intolerance to sunlight. Initially, the skin shows mottled erythema and pigmentation, followed by the development of poikilodermatous changes similar to those seen in chronic radiodermatits or solar degeneration in adults (Fig. A). Ultimately, the affected exposed areas develop basal cell and squamous cell carcinomas (Fig. A), keratoacanthomas, malignant melanomas, and rarely fibrosarcomas. Some patients have progressive neurological degeneration.

Microscopic features

1. There are no specific microscopic features.
2. Early stages are characterized by epidermal atrophy and a subepidermal non-specific inflammatory infiltrate. Increased melanization may be present in the basal layer of the epidermis and "melanophages" may be present in the upper dermis.
3. In the next stage, basophilic degeneration of collagen and telangiectasia (Fig. B) develop, with or without solar keratoses. These changes are indistinguishable from solar changes occurring in adults.
4. Squamous cell or basal cell carcinomas (Figs. C,D), (and melanomas) when present, have their characteristic histologic appearance.

Comment

1. Fibroblasts cultured from the skin of some patients with xeroderma pigmentosum show a deficiency of the endonuclease of repair (excision enzyme) which repairs ultraviolet damage to DNA. This biochemical abnormality may have a role in the pathogenesis of the disorder.

   In the XP variant, conversion from low to high molecular weight DNA is defective (postreplication repair).
2. In a variant called *DeSanctis-Cacchione syndrome*, retarded growth, neurologic manifestations, microcephaly, and cerebellar ataxia are observed.
3. Eye changes may occur in xeroderma pigmentosum, including photophobia and conjunctival injection. There may be keratitis with corneal injection. Squamous cell carcinomas or malignant melanomas may occur in sun-exposed portions of the eyes.

XERODERMA PIGMENTOSUM

A

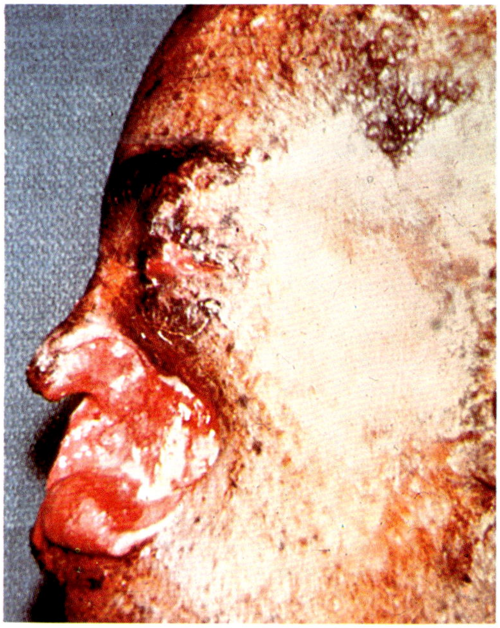

Courtesy Dr. John Knox

B X180

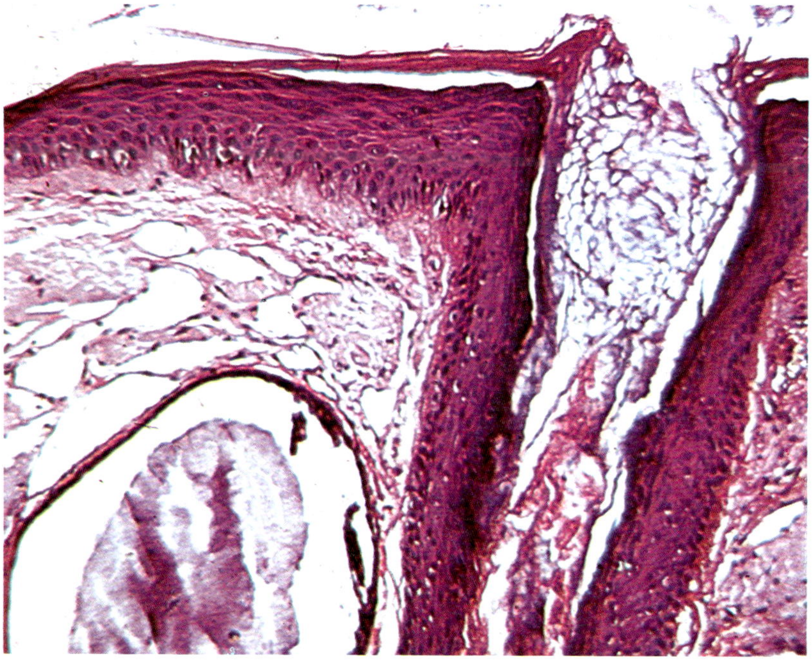

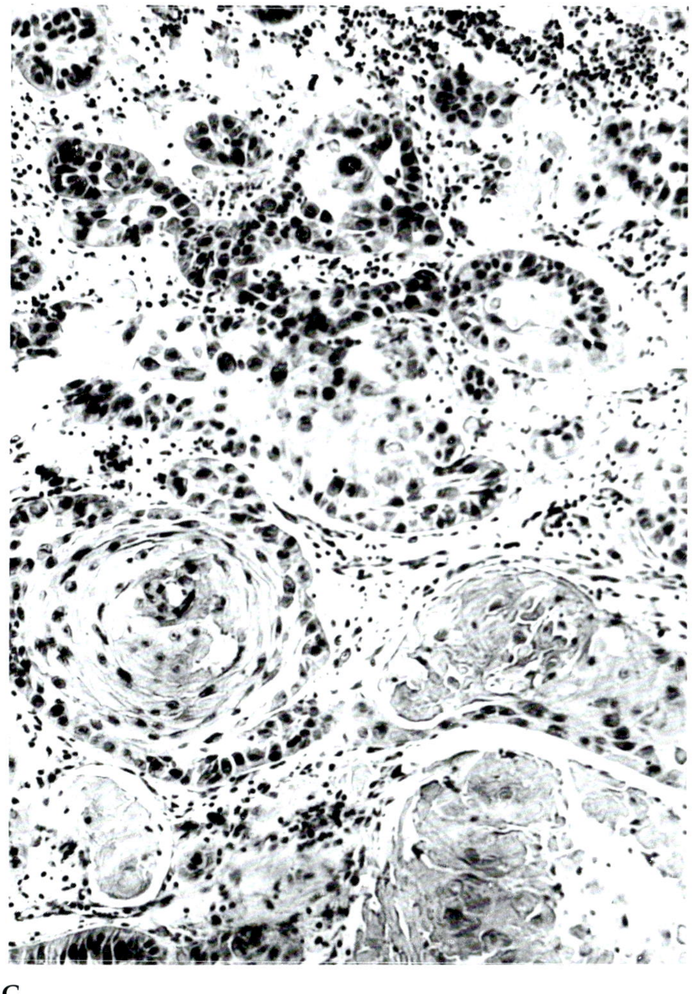

C
X360

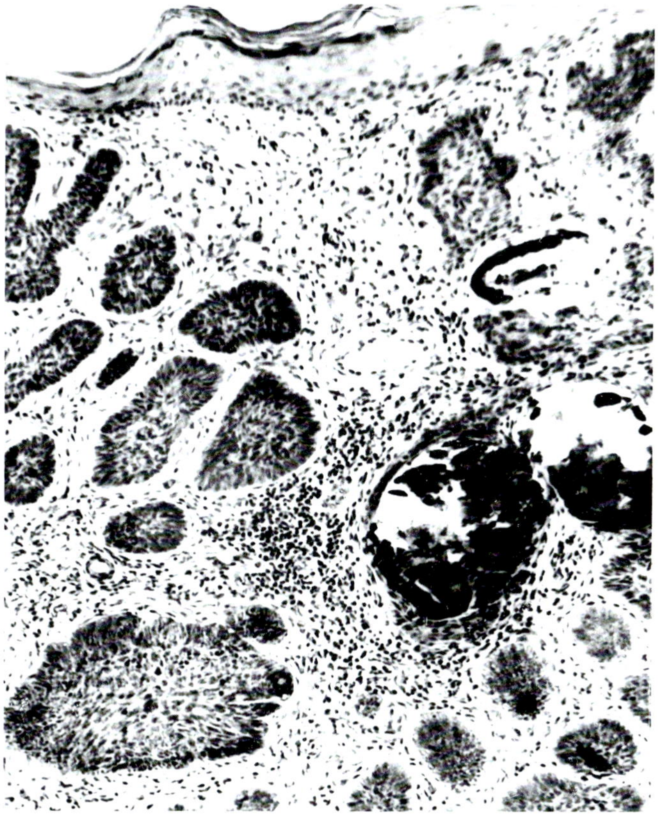

D
X180

PSEUDOXANTHOMA ELASTICUM (PXE)

Pseudoxanthoma elasticum is a hereditary disorder characterized by alterations in elastic fibers with a tendency towards calcification. Lesions can occur in the skin, arteries, and retina. Gastric arteries, coronary arteries, and large peripheral arteries are commonly involved. There are four variants: The classic type of PXE is recessive type 1. In the dominant type 1 form, the picture parallels that of recessive type 1, but there is greater severity; in the dominant type 2 form, the changes are less severe. The rare recessive type 2 form shows only cutaneous lesions, which are quite extensive. Cutaneous lesions of PXE are usually first seen in the second or third decades and increase in severity and extent with time. They resemble lesions of solar elastosis (see p. 608); the skin is typically lax and wrinkled, with clustered soft yellow papules (Fig. A). Telangiectasia may be present. Lesions commonly occur on the sides of the neck (Fig. A), as well as the axillary folds, umbilical area, inguinal areas, and antecubital areas.

Microscopic features

1. The basic changes are fragmentation, clumping, curling (Figs. B,C,D,E), and calcification (Figs. B,D) of elastic fibers.
2. With H&E stain, the affected elastic fibers are deeply basophilic and are observed in the middle and lower thirds of the reticular dermis (Figs. B,D).
3. The affected fibers take elastic tissue stains (Figs. C,E) and calcium stains.
4. Deposits of acid mucopolysaccharides or foreign body granulomas may be observed in the vicinity of degenerated elastic fibers.

Comment

1. Important non-cutaneous changes in PXE include alterations in Bruch's membrane of the retina, resulting in angioid streaks (Fig. F). These are seen as grayish lines in the fundus.
2. Vascular changes may result in gastrointestinal hemorrhage, occlusive peripheral vascular disease, coronary artery disease, cerebral vascular accidents, or aneurysms of the major arteries.
3. On occasion, there is an association between PXE and elastosis perforans serpiginosa. Some of the reported cases of elastosis perforans serpiginosa associated with PXE were actually calcific elastosis.
4. *Calcific elastosis* has been referred to as periumbilical perforating pseudoxanthoma elasticum, but it is not a variant of pseudoxanthoma elasticum. Calcific elastosis is one of the perforating dermatoses. It is observed in multiparous, middle-aged women, and appears as a pigmented periumbilical patch that may contain hyperkeratotic papules, verrucous areas, or a verrucous border. The histologic picture is similar to that of PXE, except that the altered, calcified elastic fibers are extruded through a transepidermal canal containing a hyperkeratotic plug.
5. *Connective tissue nevus* is a hamartoma with increased amounts of collagen fibers and variable changes of elastic tissue. Lesions are nodules or plaques. Connective tissue nevi may have no associated abnormalities or may occur in association with tuberous sclerosis or osteopoikilosis.

PSEUDOXANTHOMA ELASTICUM

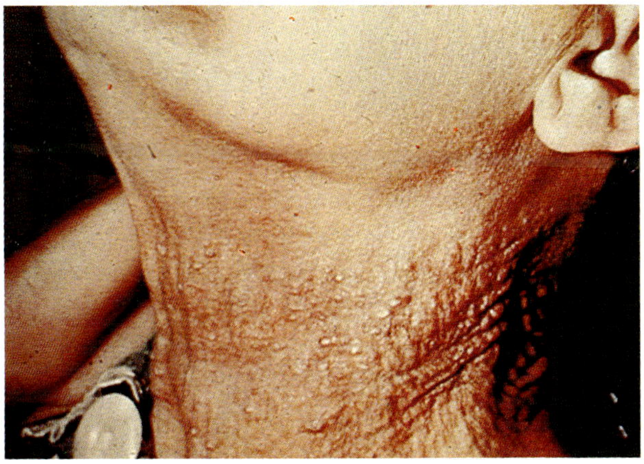

A

Courtesy Dr. John Knox

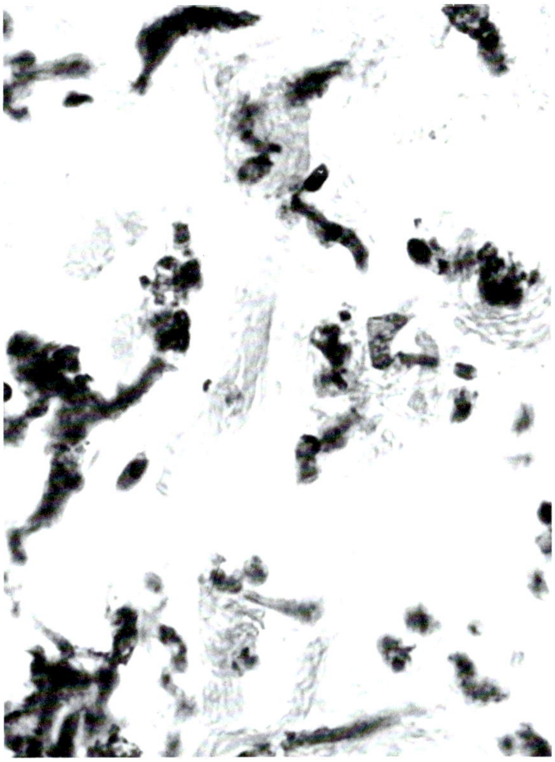

B
X700

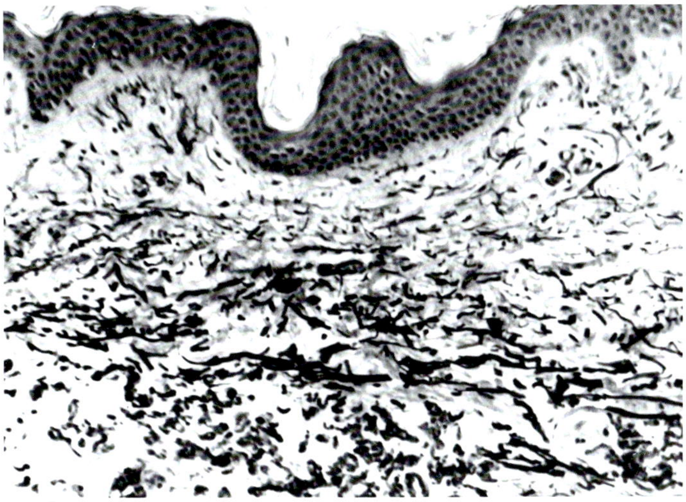

C
X190

ACID ORCEIN GIEMSA STAIN

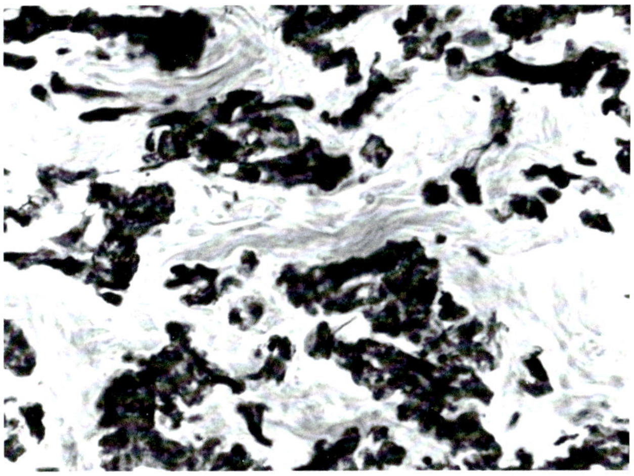

E
X520

ACID ORCEIN GIEMSA STAIN

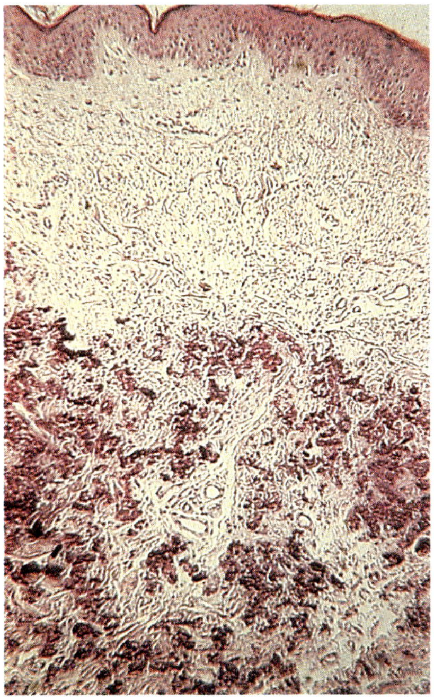

D
X60

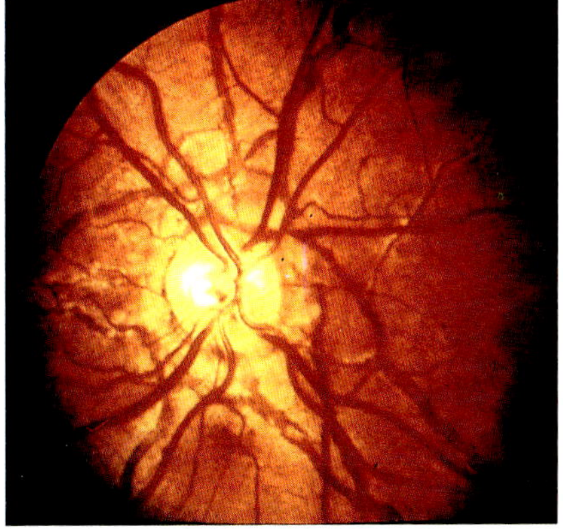

F

Courtesy Dr. Jean Braun

PSEUDOXANTHOMA ELASTICUM (PXE)

Microscopic differential diagnosis of PXE

	Area Involved	*Pathologic Changes*	*Calcification*
PXE	middle & lower third of dermis	curling, clumping, & fragmentation of elastic fibers	present
Solar elastosis	upper third of dermis	fragmented fibers and amorphous elastotic material	absent
Cutis laxa	entire dermis	absent elastic tissue fibers in upper dermis; granular degeneration of elastic fibers elsewhere	absent
Connective tissue nevus	entire dermis	increase, decrease, or no change in the number of normal-appearing elastic fibers	absent
Elastosis perforans serpiginosa	dermal papillae and epidermis	coarse, clumped elastic fibers; transepidermal canal	absent
Ehlers-Danlos syndrome		no alteration in elastic fibers	absent
Calcific elastosis	middle and lower third of dermis with extension to surface canal	curling, clumping, and fragmentation of elastic fibers; transepidermal canal	present

GENODERMATOSES continued

EHLERS-DANLOS SYNDROME (CUTIS HYPERELASTICA)

Ehlers-Danlos syndrome is an inherited spectrum of disorders. In some types there are alterations in collagen fibers. The key clinical features include hyperextensibility of the skin (Fig. A), increased mobility of the joints (with possible dislocation) (Fig. B), and increased fragility of the skin with impaired wound healing and possible atrophic scars. Occasionally raisin-like pseudotumors (Figs. A,C) are present at sites of traumatic hematomas. Spheroid subcutaneous nodules due to fat necrosis may occur.

At least 11 types of Ehlers-Danlos syndrome are now recognized. Types I, II and III are transmitted as an autosomal dominant trait and are the most common forms of the disorder. They vary only in degree, with type I being the most severe.

The other types vary in mode of inheritance and biochemical abnormality, and include additional manifestations, such as arterial weakness with rupture, periodontitis, clotting abnormalities, scoliosis, and eye abnormalities.

Microscopic features

1. Usually no distinct abnormalities are observed. The dermis is thinner than normal.
2. Raisin-like pseudotumors may show a proliferation of connective tissue and capillaries, or occasionally a foreign body granuloma.
3. Subcutaneous nodules show fat necrosis with calcification, surrounded by dense collagen.

Comment

Cutis laxa is a rare group of disorders characterized by loose skin which tends to hang in folds (Fig. D). Hereditary types show varying modes of transmission. Associated features include vascular abnormalities, hernias, diverticula of the G-I and G-U tracts, and emphysema. There is an acquired type. Sometimes the acquired type shows an eruption of erythematous plaques or vesicular lesions.

Microscopically, changes are limited to the elastic fibers. Initially, elastic fibers are diminished and show abnormalities in appearance—including thickening of their midportion and tapering of their ends. Borders of fibers may be indistinct and staining may be uneven. In advanced lesions, only dust-like orceinophilic granules may remain. There is an increase in mucopolysaccharides.

The inflammatory reaction that may accompany the acquired type of cutis laxa shows a nonspecific inflammatory infiltrate. Vesicles, when present, show a subepidermal mode of formation and may be accompanied by papillary microabscesses with neutrophils and eosinophils, resembling microabscesses seen in dermatitis herpetiformis or bullous pemphigoid.

EHLERS-DANLOS SYNDROME; CUTIS LAXA

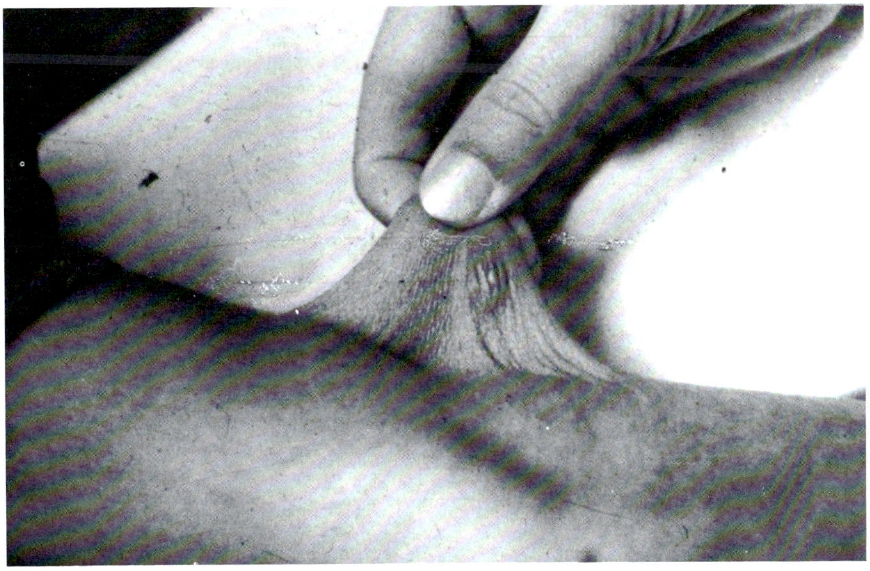

A

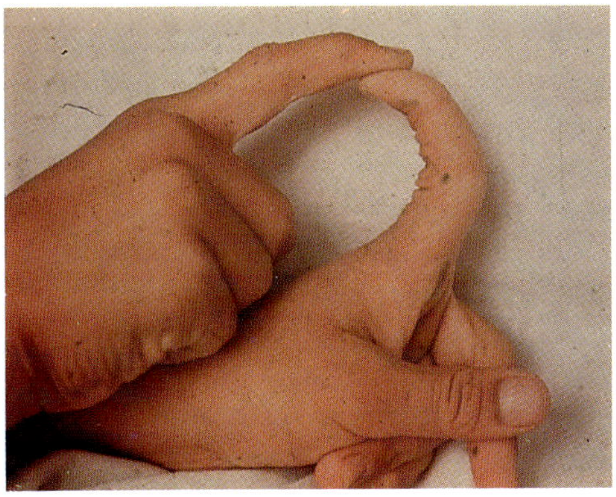

B

Figs. A,B,C courtesy Dr. Nur Or

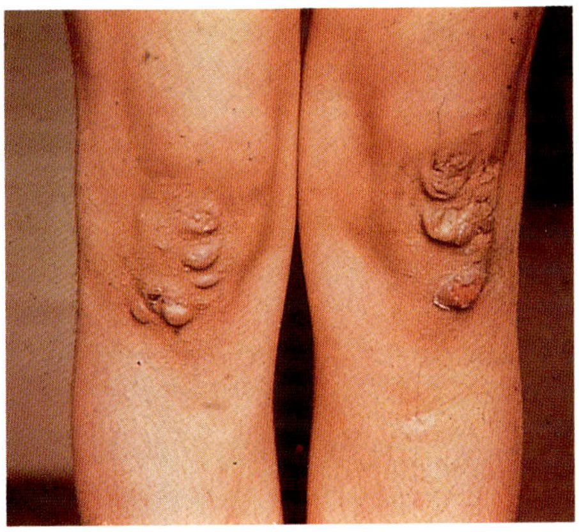

C

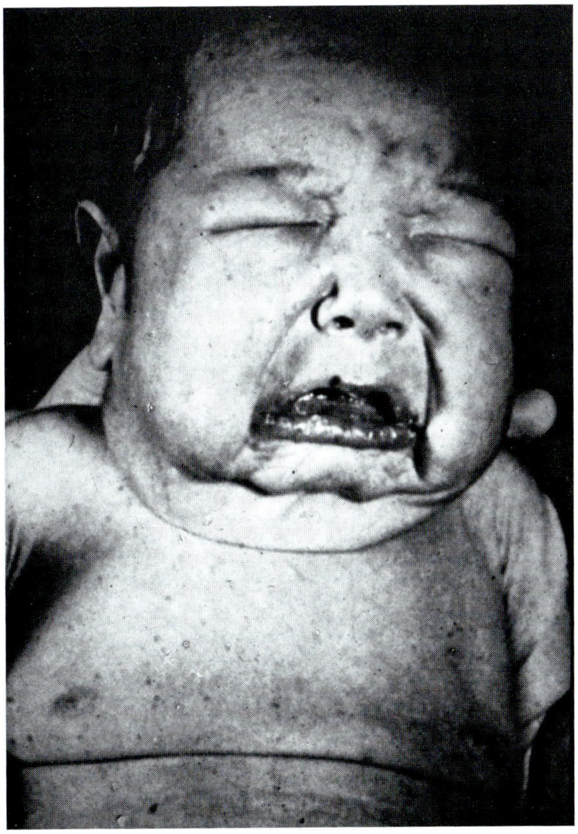

D

INCONTINENTIA PIGMENTI (BLOCH-SULZBERGER SYNDROME)

Incontinentia pigmenti (Bloch-Sulzberger syndrome) is a cutaneous disorder with associated developmental defects, including defects of the eyes, skeletal system, teeth, and central nervous system. Partial alopecia of the vertex of the scalp may be observed. There is usually a dominantly inherited X-linked mode of inheritance; occasionally there is an X-linked recessive mode of inheritance. The disorder is usually lethal in the male. The cutaneous lesions appear immediately after birth and are characterized by three sequential stages: 1. vesiculobullous stage; 2. lichenoid stage; 3. hyperpigmented stage.

VESICULOBULLOUS STAGE

Illustrated are erythematous vesiculobullous lesions of the first stage (vesiculobullous stage). The grouped clear vesicles tend to have a linear arrangement and have some resemblance to plant dermatitis (Fig. A).

Microscopic features

1. Spongiotic vesicles containing large numbers of eosinophils (Figs. B,C) are present. Eosinophils are also scattered diffusely throughout the epidermis (Figs. B,C).
2. The dermis shows an infiltrate composed principally of eosinophils and histiocytes (Fig. B).
3. Dyskeratosis with horn pearl formation may be present (Fig. D).

Comment

Often there is leukocytosis with eosinophilia (with values up to 65%).

INCONTINENTIA PIGMENTI

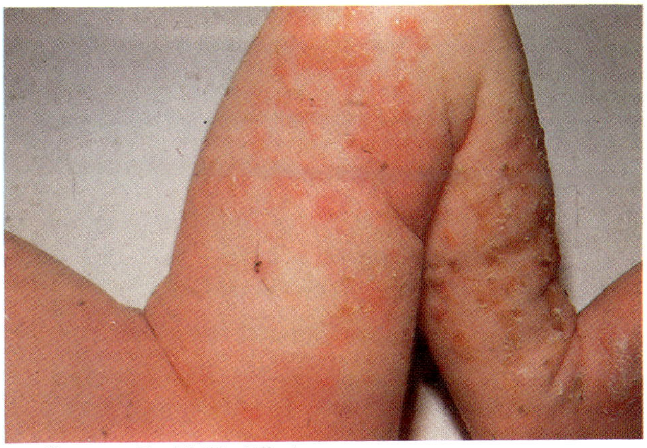

A

Courtesy Dr. Phillip Ellerin

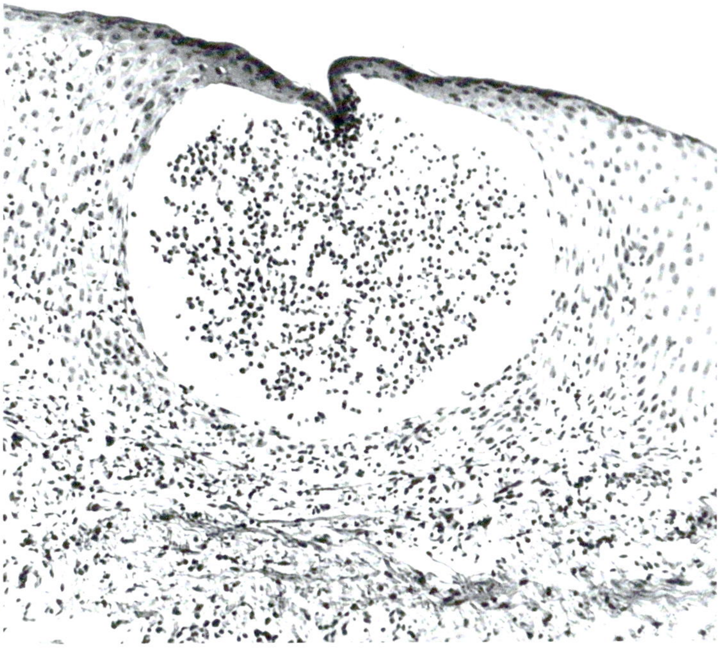

B
X160

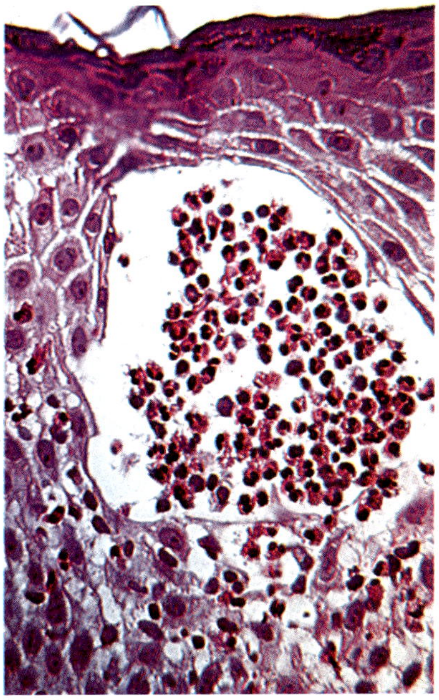

C
X620

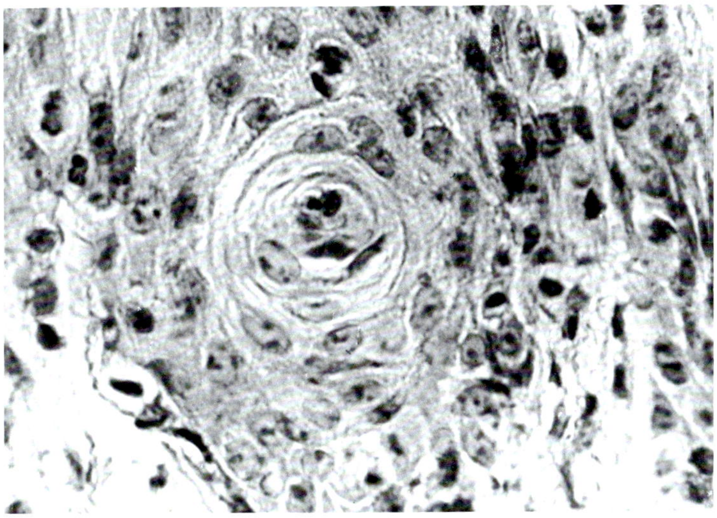

D
X720

INCONTINENTIA PIGMENTI continued ⇨

INCONTINENTIA PIGMENTI

LICHENOID STAGE

Linear, violaceous, papular lesions develop at the sites of the resolving vesicles (Fig. A).

Microscopic features

1. Hyperkeratosis, acanthosis (Fig. B), and papillomatosis are present. Horn pearls and dyskeratotic cells may be observed.
2. The dermis contains a chronic inflammatory infiltrate in which eosinophils are few or absent (Fig. B).

HYPERPIGMENTED STAGE

Macular, hyperpigmented whorls are present (Fig. C), usually on the trunk.

Microscopic features

Numerous "melanophages" are present in the upper dermis (Fig. D).

Microscopic differential diagnosis of incontinentia pigmenti

1. The vesicular stage can be distinguished from pemphigus vegetans by the absence of acantholysis, and from bullous pemphigoid and dermatitis herpetiformis by the intraepidermal position of the vesicles. In erythema toxicum neonatorum accumulations of eosinophils are not intraepidermal and are present at the follicular orifices. (Erythema toxicum neonatorum is a benign, transient, macular erythema of the newborn.)
2. The lichenoid stage cannot be distinguished from chronic dermatitis and/or benign papillomas.
3. The hyperpigmented stage is indistinguishable from post-inflammatory hyperpigmentation or the late stages of fixed drug eruption. Erythema dyschromicum perstans, lichen planus, lupus erythematosus, and poikiloderma vasculare atrophicans show dermal "melanophages", but have distinct hydropic degeneration of the basal layer.

Comment

Hypomelanosis of Ito was formerly called incontinentia pigmenti achromians, since the pattern of hypopigmentation seen in this condition has a resemblance to the pattern of hyperpigmentation in incontinentia pigmenti. However, there is no pigmentary "incontinence" in hypomelanosis of Ito. There are two forms, both with autosomal dominant inheritance: 1. The more common cutaneous form has pigmentary loss in late childhood, with repigmentation in early adulthood; 2. the neurocutaneous form develops pigmentary loss in infancy and is accompanied by central nervous system dysfunction and bone abnormalities. Microscopically, there is a loss of epidermal melanin with decrease in size and dopa oxidase activity of epidermal melanocytes. Other abnormalities may be present.

INCONTINENTIA PIGMENTI

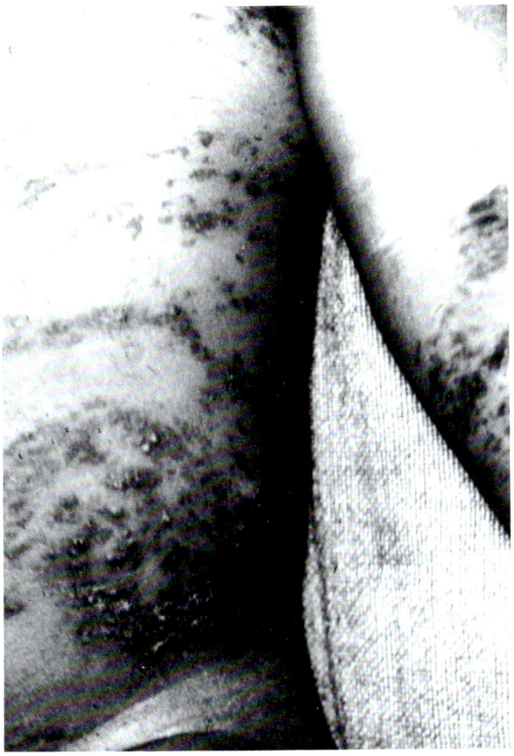

A

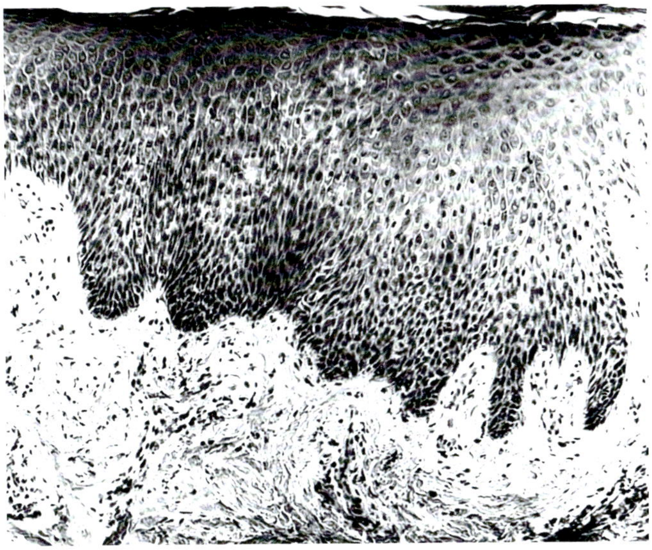

B
X130

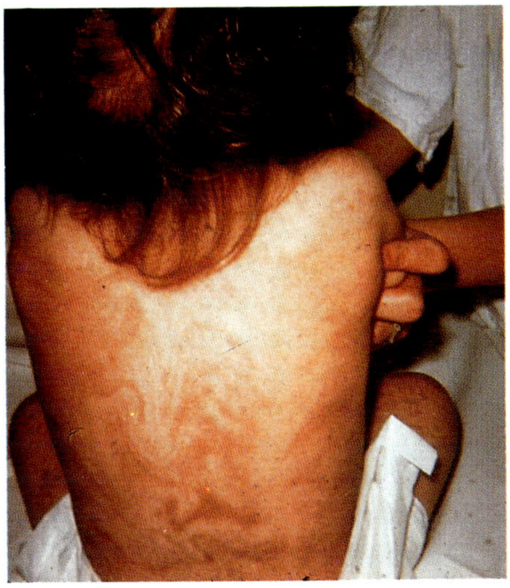

C

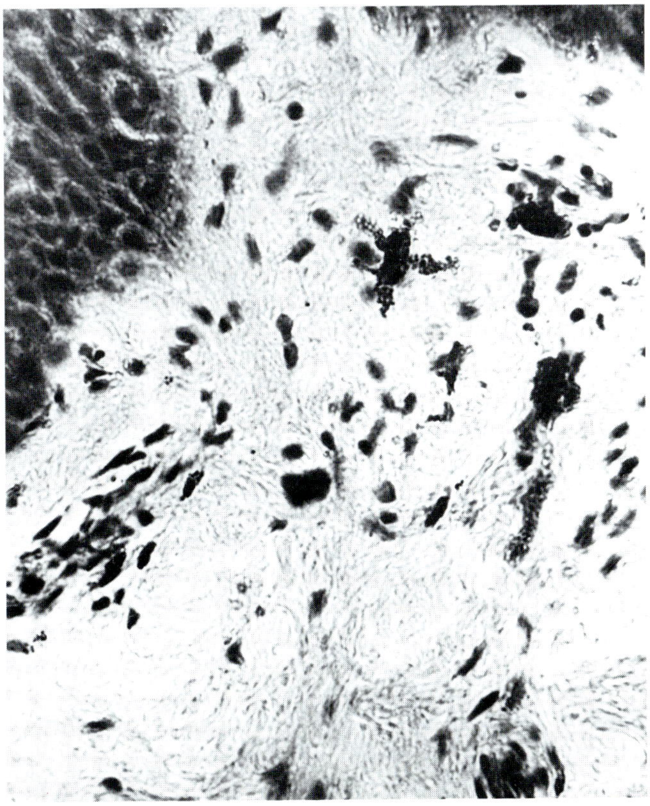

D
X680

NEUROFIBROMATOSIS (VON RECKLINGHAUSEN'S DISEASE)

Neurofibromas may be solitary or multiple. When multiple lesions are present, there usually are accompanying pigmented spots, and the condition is called neurofibromatosis (Von Recklinghausen's disease). Solitary neurofibromas are sometimes called neural nevi (see p. 1134). Neurofibromatosis may have an autosomal dominant mode of transmission, but a large percentage of cases have no family history and are regarded as arising by spontaneous mutation. In neurofibromatosis, tumors may be present at various sites throughout the body. Neurofibromatosis and phaeochromocytoma are commonly associated.

Skin lesions are multiple, soft, tan, or violaceous tumors, which are sometimes pedunculated (Fig. A). Large pendulous tumors (plexiform neuromas) and subcutaneous nodules also occur. The light brown spots which may accompany the tumors are called café-au-lait spots (Fig. B). Axillary freckling is common (Fig. C).

Multiple symptoms and signs attributable to neural involvement at various sites may occur. Central nervous system abnormalities, including glial tumors, may be present. There may be syndromes due to cranial nerve involvement. Precocious puberty, mental deficiency, or seizures may occur. Bony abnormalities are common in neurofibromatosis.

Microscopic features

Neurofibromas are composed of Schwann cells, endoneurial cells, and perineurial cells, with occasional axons.

1. There are whorls of loosely arranged, moderately cellular fibrillar tissue (Figs. D,E). Verocay bodies may be present, but they are usually not as well-developed as in neurilemmoma (see. p. 1100).
2. The tumors are usually circumscribed but not encapsulated, and are moderately vascular (Figs. D,E). Subcutaneous neurofibromas are encapsulated, with the perineurium of the involved nerve forming the capsule of the tumor.
3. The tumors are often raised and are generally covered by a normal epidermis (Fig. D). Tumor cells are usually absent in the papillary dermis (Figs. D,E).

NEUROFIBROMATOSIS

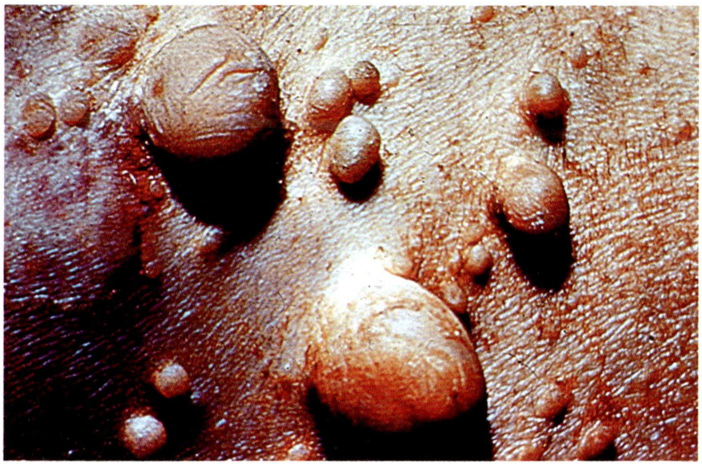

A

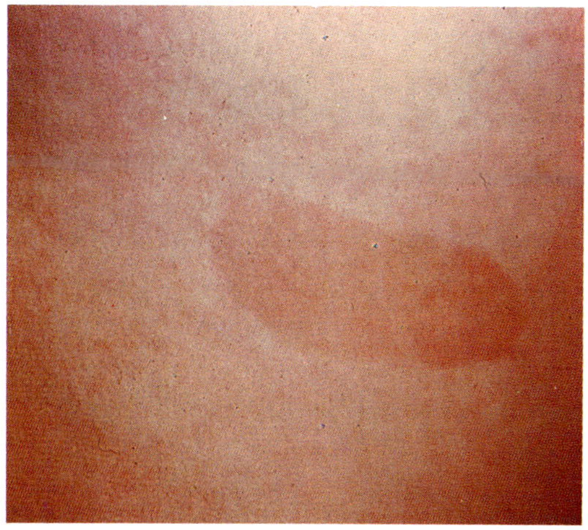

B

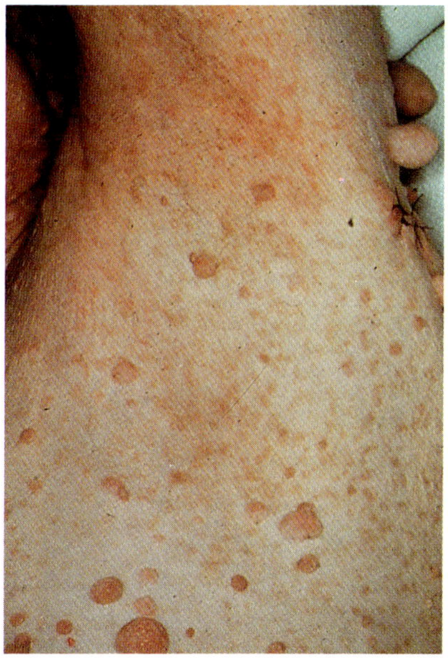

C

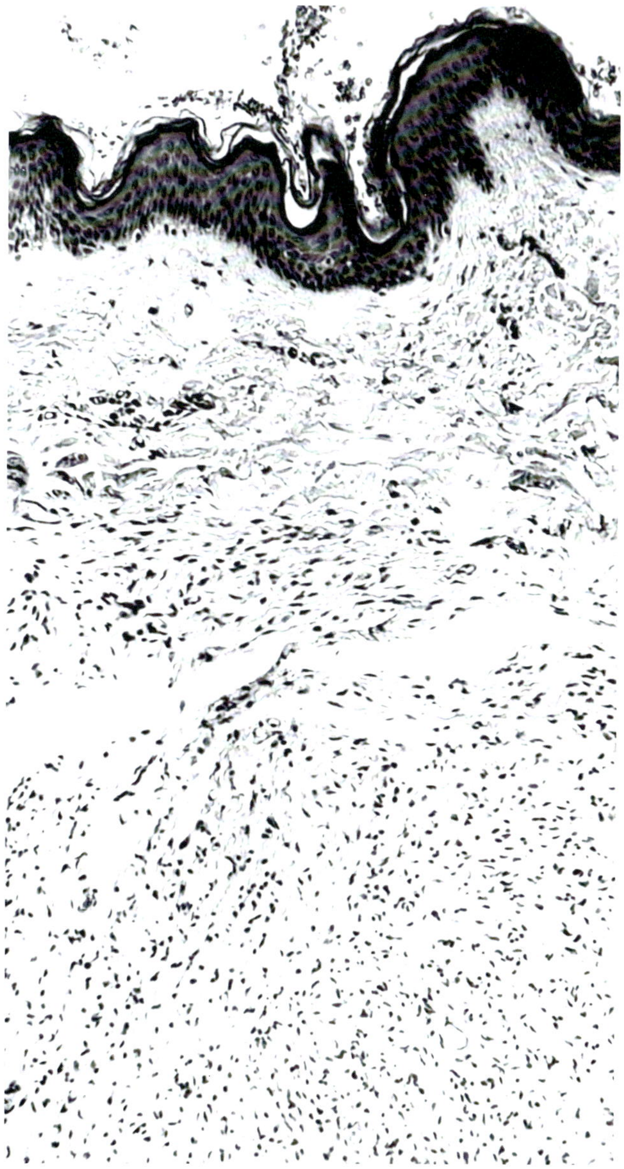

E
X190

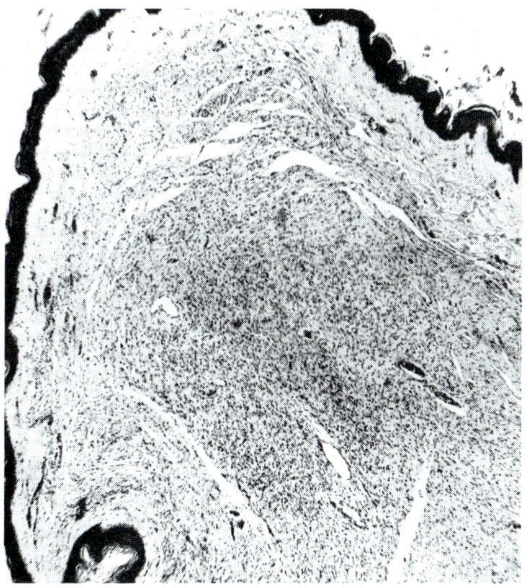

D
X50

NEUROFIBROMATOSIS continued ⇨

NEUROFIBROMATOSIS

Microscopic features

4. With higher magnification, fibers have the appearance of loosely arranged, wavy, young collagen containing oval or somewhat elongated nuclei (Fig. A). With H&E stain, these fibers often have a bluish appearance characteristic of immature collagen. However, in some areas of the tumor, more mature, eosinophilic collagen fibers may be present. Old lesions may be composed principally of mature collagen.
5. Mucin deposition is common (Fig. B).
6. The wavy fibers of neurofibroma stain red with Masson's trichrome stain or Mallory aniline blue stain, and yellow with Van Gieson stain.
7. Elastic fibers are reduced in number or absent; reticulum fibers are significantly increased.
8. Giemsa stain or other stains for sulfated acid mucopolysaccharides reveal the presence of mast cells, often in large numbers.
9. Bodian stain or other similar stains demonstrate nerve fibers within most of the tumors.
10. Café-au-lait spots show an increase in melanin in the basal cells. These may contain abnormally large melanosomes visible by light or electron microscopy. There may be increased numbers of melanocytes and increased dopa oxidase activity.

    The large melanosomes are called *giant melanosomes*. They may be present in a variety of other pigmentary conditions. These include melanotic macules of Albright's syndrome, nevocellular nevi, nevus spilus, and multiple lentiginosis syndrome. They can even occur in normal epidermis.

Microscopic differential diagnosis

1. Neurofibromas may resemble dermatofibromas or leiomyomas. Differential diagnostic features: a) neurofibromas lack epidermal proliferation typical of dermatofibromas (see p. 976); b) early lesions of neurofibroma lack large, mature collagen fibers typical of dermatofibromas; c) the wavy pattern of fibrils of neurofibroma contrast with the straight or arciform pattern of smooth muscle fibers of leiomyoma; d) the nuclei of leiomyomas are more elongated than nuclei of neurofibromas, and have blunt ends.
2. Special stains are not of great value in distinguishing these three lesions. Neurofibromas, leiomyomas, and immature collagen of dermatofibromas have similar staining characteristics (e.g., fibers stain red with Masson trichrome stain); on the other hand, mature collagen fibers in each category also stain similarly (e.g., blue with Masson trichrome stain).

Comment

Malignant change rarely occurs in lesions of neurofibromatosis. The highest incidence of malignant transformation is in tumors of the large nerve trunks. Malignant neurofibromas (also called malignant schwannomas) can show features ranging from minimal evidence of malignancy—with slight nuclear pleomorphism and a few mitotic figures, to a picture indistinguishable from fibrosarcoma. The presence of even minimal mitotic activity raises the possibility of malignancy. Malignant schwannoma has a serious prognosis.

MAST CELLS, MELANOCYTES, AND MELANOGENESIS

Morphologic, cytochemical, and ultrastructural parallels between mast cells and melanocytes have been demonstrated in our laboratory, which suggest that melanocytes and mast cells have a common connective tissue stem cell, and that, under some circumstances, mast cells represent a transitional phase in the differentiation of melanocytes. Embryological evidence that much connective tissue is of neural crest origin has provided a developmental basis for this hypothesis. Other studies in our laboratory have indicated that mammalian melanogenesis in melanocytes is based on the synergistic action of peroxidase and copper-dependent, aerobic dopa oxidase (incorrectly called "tyrosinase").

The peroxidase is responsible for the hydroxylation of tyrosine, as well as the oxidation of dopa to melanin, whereas the aerobic dopa oxidase has no ability to hydroxylate tyrosine. Mast cell granules contain peroxidase, but no aerobic dopa oxidase. Studies of other investigators and studies in our laboratory have shown preformed melanin in mast cells, and EM studies have shown that this melanin is often in mast cell granules. It is likely that this preformed melanin is the result of the enzymatic activity of peroxidase. It is of related interest that another peroxidase-active granular cell, the eosinophil, universally contains preformed melanin. This was shown in a study in our laboratory.

The hyperpigmentation observed in lesions of mastocytosis is due to an increase in melanin in the basal layer of the epidermis, as well as to melanin in dermal "melanophages" and in some mast cells.

MASTOCYTOSIS (URTICARIA PIGMENTOSA)

Mastocytosis is a disorder characterized by an abnormal infiltration of mast cells in the skin and other organs. Most cases are sporadic, although some cases of familial mastocytosis have been described, with autosomal dominant inheritance. Mastocytosis arising in infancy or early childhood has a tendency to improve or resolve at puberty, and systemic lesions are absent or minimal. Mastocytosis arising in adolescence or adult life does not have a tendency to regress and has a higher incidence of systemic lesions. Systemic mast cell disease may involve the bones, gastrointestinal tract, liver, spleen, or meninges. Progressive systemic mastocytosis with fatal termination is infrequent. Rarely, mast cell leukemia may occur.

Cutaneous lesions of mastocytosis tend to be copper-colored and urticate on stroking (Darier's sign). The cutaneous lesions fall into two principal categories: the maculopapular type (Fig. A) and the nodular type. Both types occur in the infantile and adult forms of mastocytosis. Less frequent are the solitary type, diffuse erythrodermic type, and a type called *telangiectasia macularis eruptiva perstans*. The first two are usually observed in the infantile form of mastocytosis, and the last is usually observed in the adult form. Solitary lesions are plaques (Fig. B) that tend to form bullae on stroking. The diffuse erythrodermic type shows a copper-colored, diffusely infiltrated skin (Fig. C). Bullae may also form on stroking with this type (Fig. E), and rapidly become denuded. Telangiectasia macularis eruptiva perstans is characterized by macular lesions with fine telangiectasia (Fig. D). Lesions may be unilateral. Nodular mastocytosis (Fig. F) is characterized by papules and nodules, often with a reddish-brown color. The lesions can resemble dermal nevi or neurofibromas.

Patients with extensive mast cell infiltration may have attacks of flushing, diarrhea, and palpitation due to histamine release.

MASTOCYTOSIS

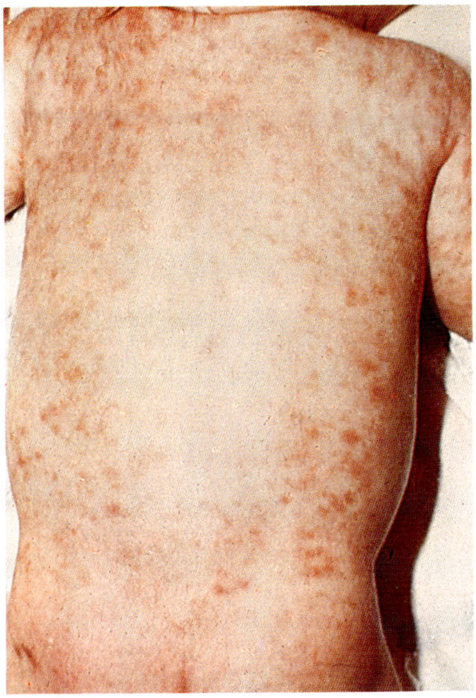

A

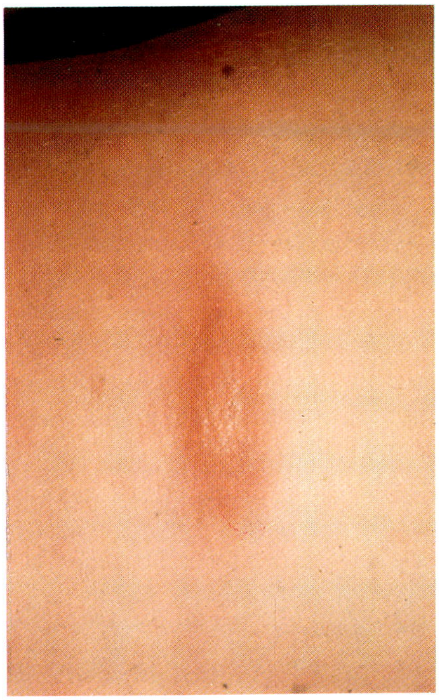

B Courtesy Dr. Douglas Wooldridge

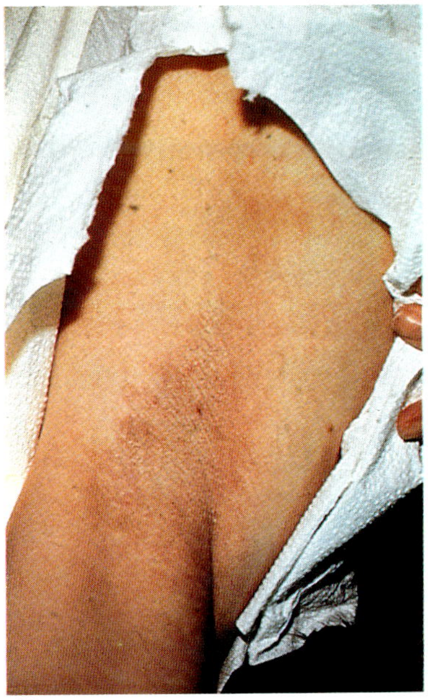

C Courtesy Dr. Daniel Clarke

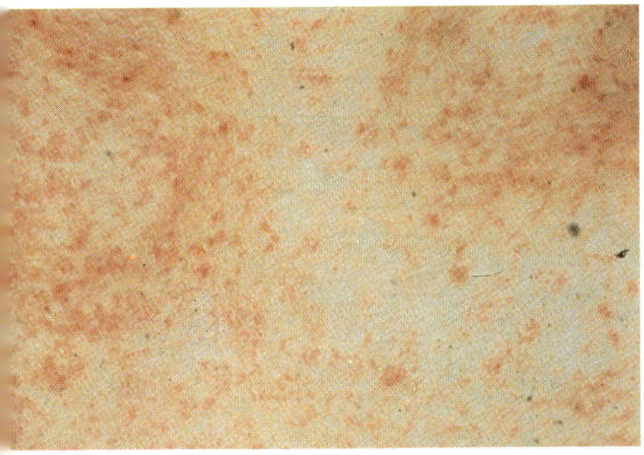

D

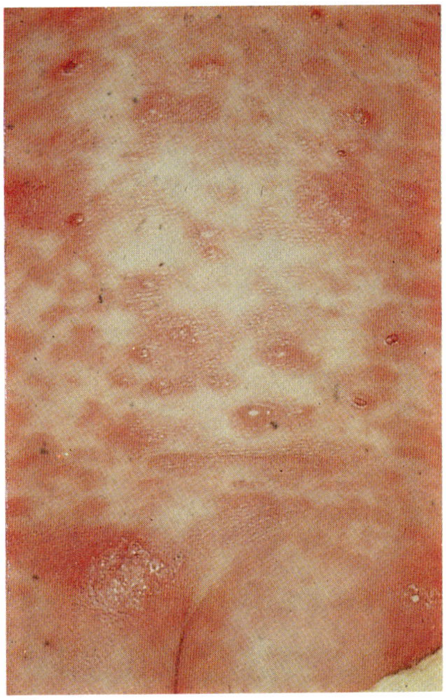

E

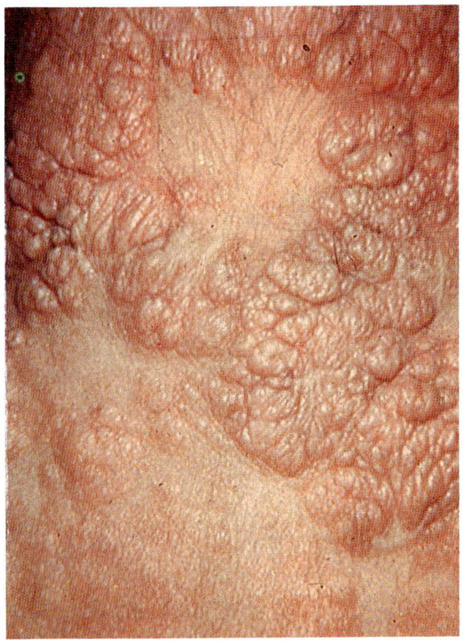

F

MASTOCYTOSIS continued ⇨

MASTOCYTOSIS

Microscopic features (maculopapular form and telangiectasia macularis eruptiva perstans)

1. There is an aggregation of mast cells in the upper dermis (Figs. A,B).
2. Most of the mast cells are elongated or bipolar (Figs. A,B) rather than cuboidal and may not be recognizable with routine stains. With Giemsa stain or other stains with metachromatic dyes, mast cells stain metachromatically (violet or purple) (Fig. B) and can be easily recognized. Mast cells tend to be numerous in loose connective tissue, such as perivascular tissue.
3. Varying numbers of eosinophils are usually present.
4. In telangiectasia macularis eruptiva perstans, there is telangiectasia, and mast cells are relatively sparse. Histologic diagnosis can be difficult.

Microscopic features (diffuse erythrodermic lesions and bullous lesions)

1. In diffuse erythrodermic lesions, there is a dense, band-like infiltrate of mast cells having a rather uniform appearance.
2. In bullous mastocytosis (Fig. C), there is subepidermal bulla formation, in addition to the mast cell infiltrate. The bulla cavity usually contains numerous mast cells and some eosinophils. When there is regeneration, bullae may be intraepidermal.

MASTOCYTOSIS

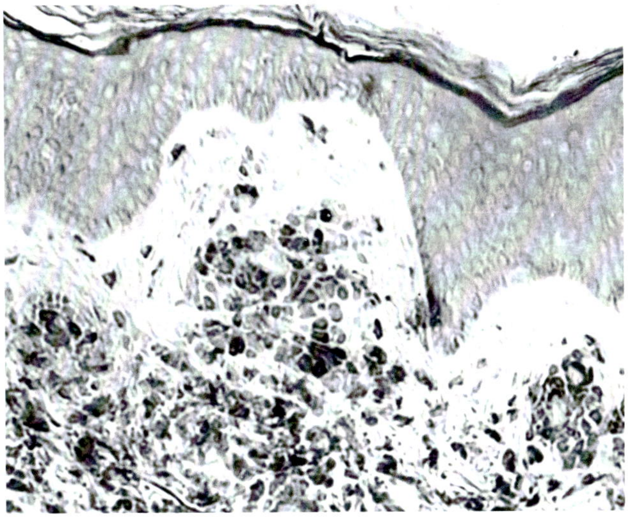

A
X260
GIEMSA STAIN

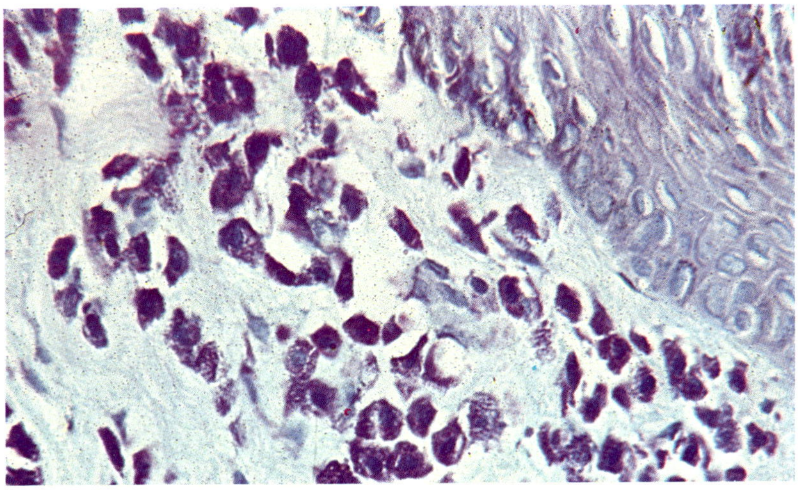

B
X500
GIEMSA
STAIN

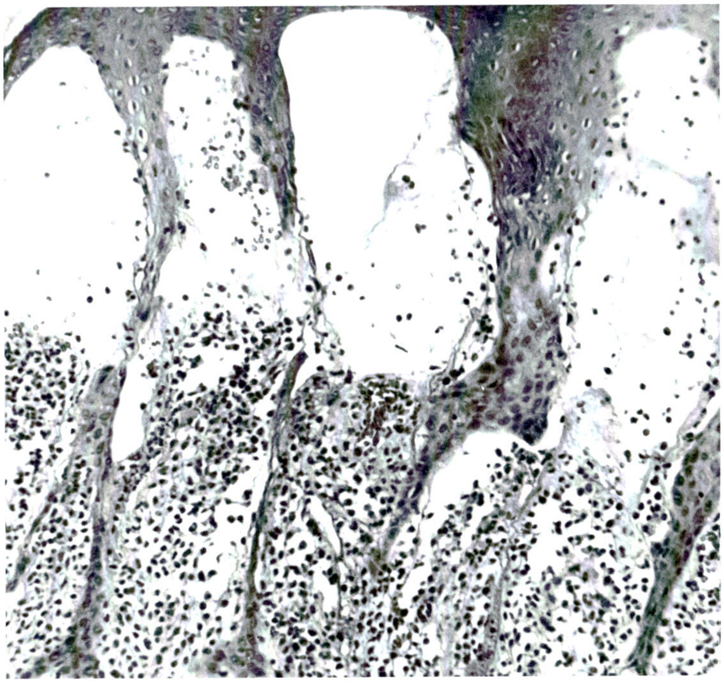

C
X175

MASTOCYTOSIS continued

NODULAR MASTOCYTOSIS

Microscopic features

1. Aggregates of mast cells involve wide areas of the dermis (Fig. A) and subcutaneous fat.
2. Mast cells, for the most part, are cuboidal with an eosinophilic cytoplasm and a small, centrally placed nucleus (Fig. B). With Giemsa stain the granules are metachromatic (Fig. C). Eosinophils are usually present.
3. Dilated capillaries and edema are common.
4. In some cases of nodular mastocytosis, the mast cells are spindle shaped (Fig. D).

NODULAR MASTOCYTOSIS

A X165

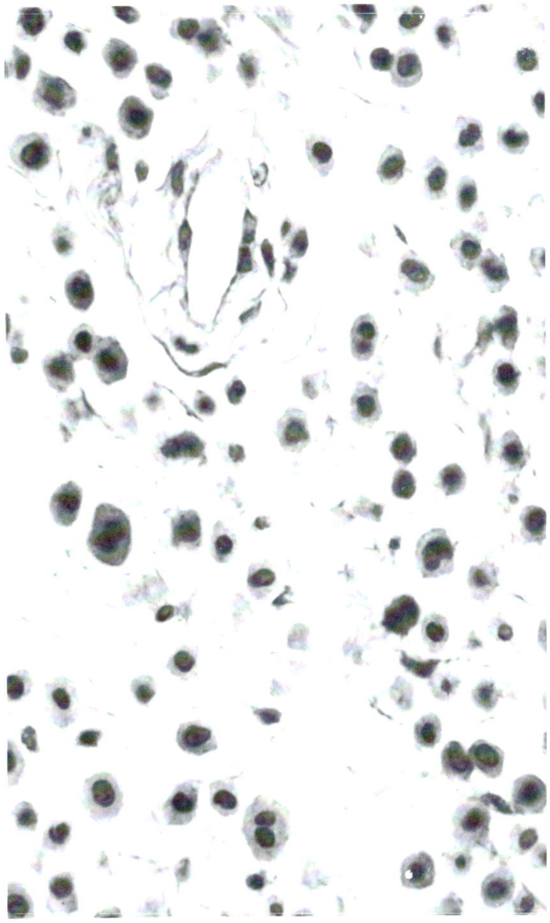

B X760

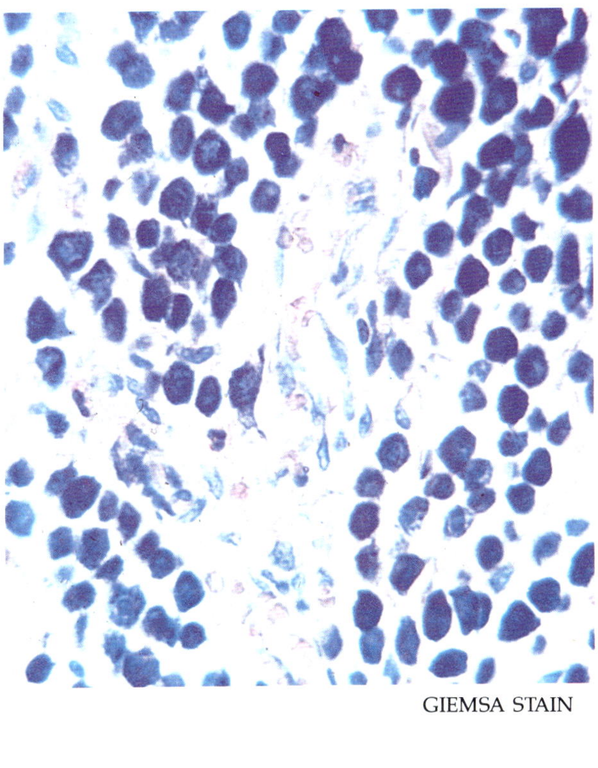

C X760

GIEMSA STAIN

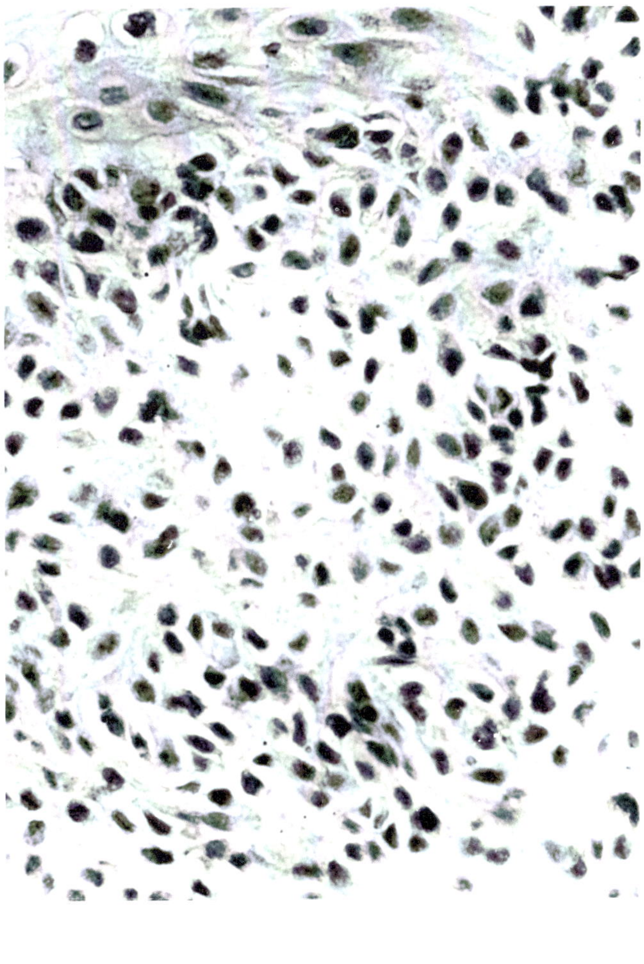

D X620

TUBEROUS SCLEROSIS (ADENOMA SEBACEUM; EPILOIA; PRINGLE'S DISEASE)

Tuberous sclerosis is a protean developmental disorder transmitted by an autosomal dominant gene showing variability of expression. The triad of facial angiofibromas (Figs. A,B), mental deficiency, and epilepsy constitute the most common clinical pattern. Facial angiofibromas are multiple small, reddish papules (Figs. A,B) distributed symmetrically on the face, particularly the nasolabial folds, cheeks, and chin. The cutaneous lesions include: periungual fibromata (Koenen's tumors), hard fibrous plaques of the forehead and scalp, pedunculated fibromas of the neck and axillae, hyperpigmented macules (café-au-lait spots), and hypopigmented macules (ash-leaf spots). A connective tissue nevus (shagreen patch) is often present and frequently involves the presacral area.

Benign tumors of the kidneys, heart (rhabdomyoma), testes, retina, gastrointestinal tract, thyroid, or central nervous system, as well as cysts in the lungs and bones, may be present.

Microscopic features

1. The basic change is a fibroblastic proliferation accompanying a proliferation of telangiectatic capillaries (Figs. C,D). The fibroblasts sometimes have a stellate ("glial") appearance. Elastic fibers may be absent. In the fibrous plaques and pedunculated fibromas, the vascular component is less prominent than in the angiofibromas.
2. Sebaceous glands undergo atrophy, rather than hyperplasia, as the fibrosis progresses. Fibrous tissue is often arranged concentrically around the pilosebaceous units.

TUBEROUS SCLEROSIS

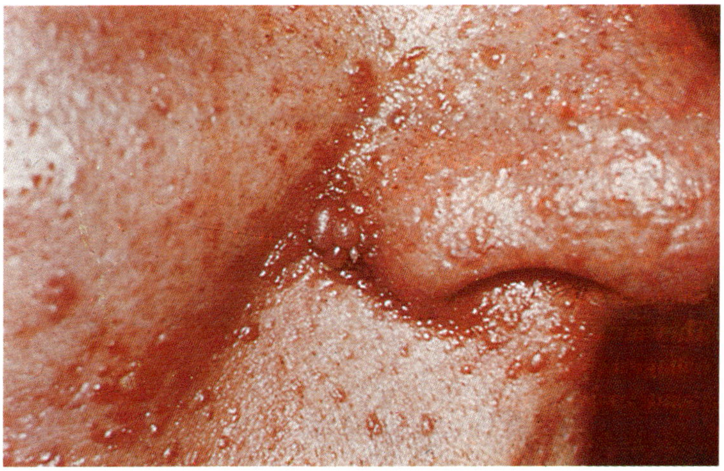

A

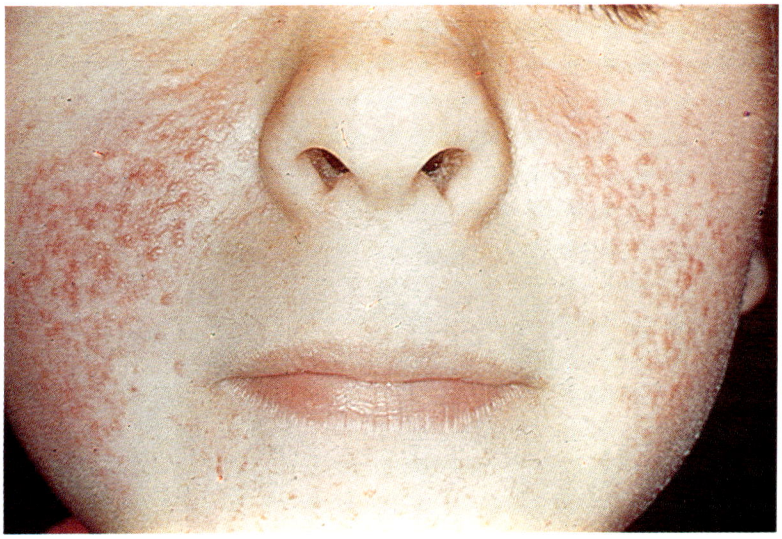

B

Courtesy Dr. Harvey Ansell

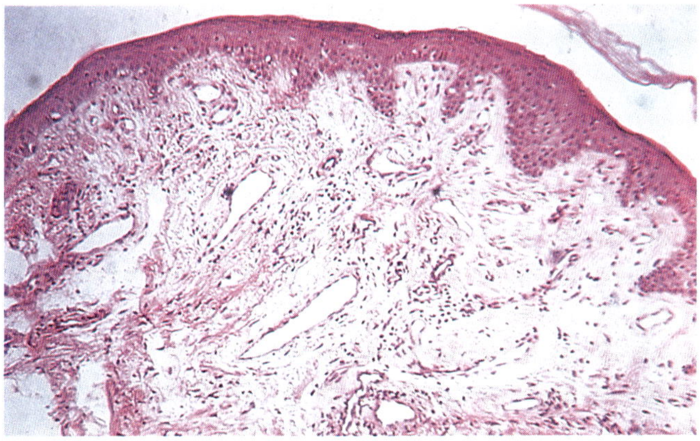

C
X80

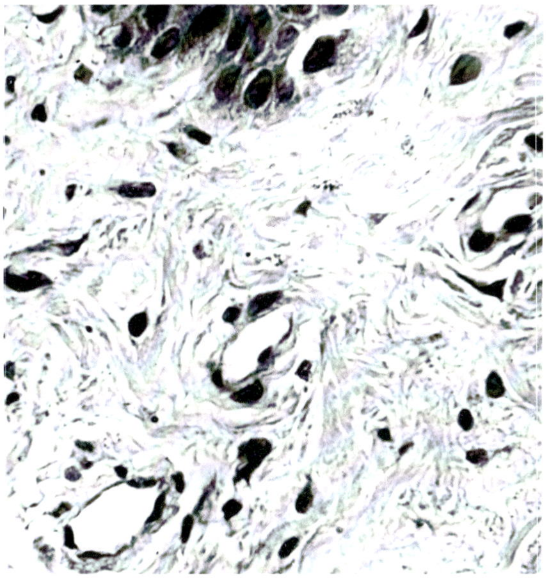

D
X520

TUBEROUS SCLEROSIS continued

TUBEROUS SCLEROSIS

Periungual fibromas are reddish-brown, firm tumors clustered in and around the nail bed. They may be pedunculated (Fig. A).

Microscopic features

1. Microscopic changes are similar to those of the facial angiofibromas, differing by the presence of fine collagen fibrils embedded in a hyaline matrix (Fig. B).
2. *Ash leaf spots* are oval areas of hypopigmentation (Fig. C) with no significant microscopic features in routine sections.
3. *Shagreen patches* are soft plaques with a rippled, cobblestone surface (Fig. D). They are a form of connective tissue nevus. There may be an increase in normal collagen in the reticular dermis producing a resemblance to morphea. Elastic tissue may be reduced in amount.

Microscopic differential diagnosis

Angiofibromas resemble vascularized scars. Clinical data may be required to make the distinction. Solitary angiofibromas of the face (fibrous papules) have a histologic picture indistinguishable from angiofibromas of tuberous sclerosis.

Comment

Focal dermal hypoplasia (Goltz syndrome) (Fig. E) represents the antithesis of a connective tissue nevus, with areas of decrease or absence of the dermis. It is found mainly in females, since it is transmitted as an X-linked dominant gene, usually lethal in homozygous males. Manifestations include areas of dermal hypoplasia resembling striae distensae, papillomas of the mucous membranes and periorificial areas, ulcerations, soft yellow nodules ("pseudotumors"), absence of digits, syndactyly, agenesis of an eye, colobomata of the eyes, microphthalmia, and hypoplasia of the hair, nails, or teeth. The key microscopic feature is a decrease or absence of dermis with abnormally high location of fat.

Vertical striations of the metaphysis of long bones (osteopathia striata) constitute a reliable marker of Goltz syndrome.

Illustrated is an example of Goltz syndrome.

TUBEROUS SCLEROSIS; FOCAL DERMAL HYPOPLASIA

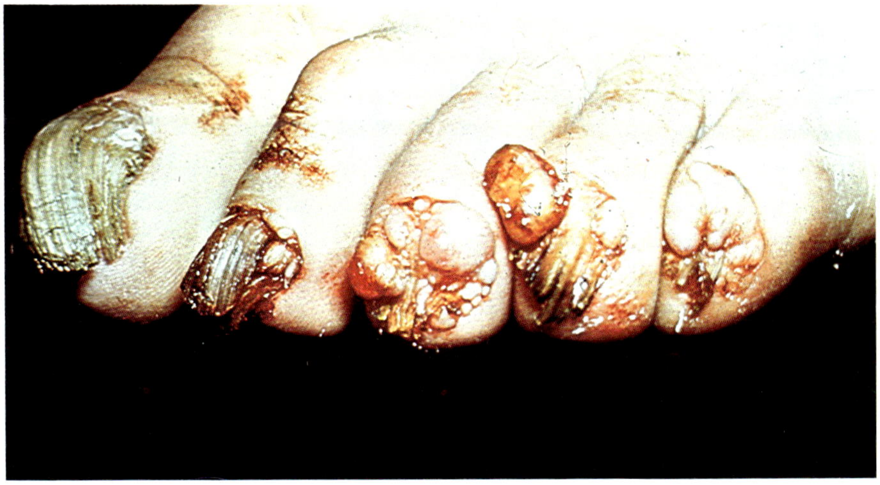

A

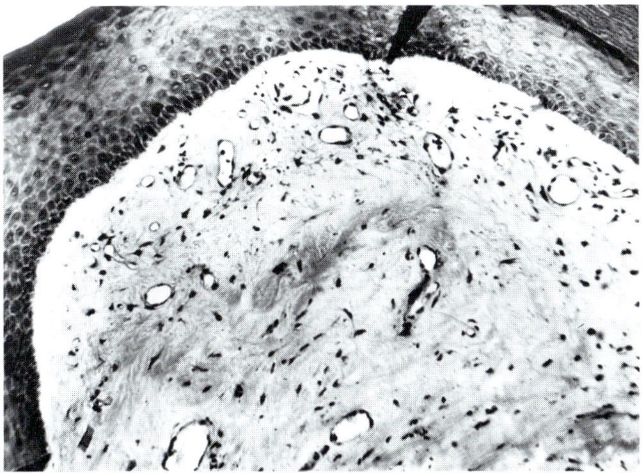

B
X175

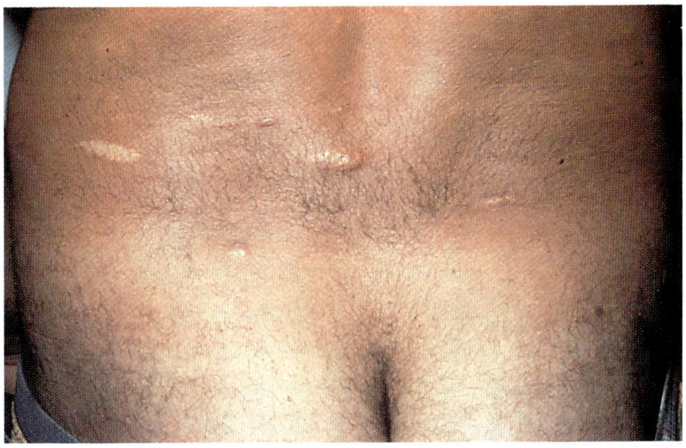

C

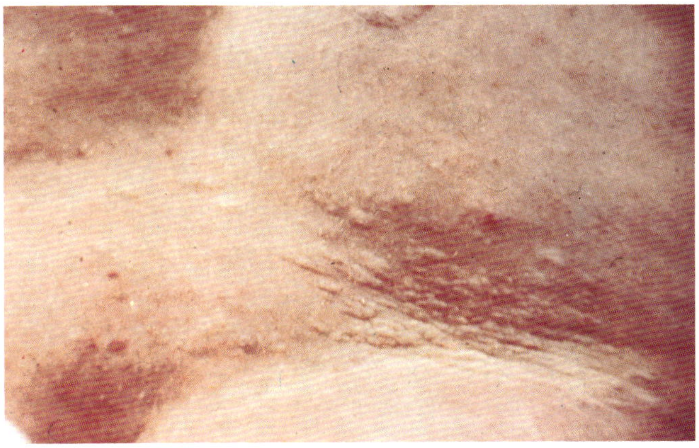

D

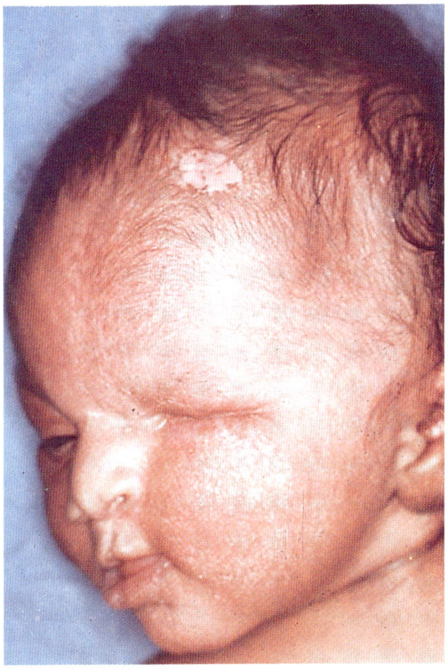

E

Suggested Reading

Genodermatoses

General References

Butterworth, T. *Manual of Dermatologic Syndromes.* 2nd Ed., Philadelphia, Lippincott, 1972.
Butterworth, T. and Strean, L. *Clinical Genodermatology.* Baltimore, Williams & Wilkins, 1962.
Font, R. and Ferry, A. The phakomatoses. *Internat. Ophthalmol. Clin.*, 12:1, 1972.
Jacobs, A. Symposium on pediatric dermatology. *Pediatr. Clin. N. Amer.*, 18:713, 1971.
Korting, G. *Diseases of the Skin in Children and Adolescents.* American Ed. translated by Curth, W. and Curth, H. Philadelphia, W. B. Saunders, 1970.
Leider, M. *Practical Pediatric Dermatology.* 2nd Ed., St. Louis, Mosby, 1961.
McKusick, V. *Heritable Disorders of Connective Tissue.* 4th Ed., St. Louis, Mosby, 1972.
Moynahan, E. Genetic disorders of the skin. *Practitioner.* 208:633, 1972.
Perlman, H. *Pediatric Dermatology.* Chicago, Yearbook Medical Publishers, 1960.
Solomon, L. and Esterly, N. *Neonatal Dermatology.* Philadelphia, W. B. Saunders, 1973.
——. Neonatal dermatology. I. The newborn skin. *J. Pediatr.*, 77:888, 1970.

Ichthyosiform Dermatoses

Ackerman, A. Histopathologic concept of epidermolytic hyperkeratosis. *Arch. Dermatol.*, 102:253, 1970.
Ackerman, A. and Goldman, G. Combined epidermolytic hyperkeratosis and focal acantholytic dyskeratosis. *Arch. Dermatol.*, 109:385, 1974.
Anton-Lamprecht, I. and Schnyder, U. Ultrastructure in inborn errors of keratinization. *Arch. Dermatol. Forsch.*, 250:207, 1974.
Baden, H. et al. Keratinization in the harlequin fetus. *Arch. Dermatol.*, 118:14, 1982.
Baden, H. et al. Sulfatase activity of keratinizing tissues in X-linked ichthyosis. *Pediatr. Res.*, 14:1347, 1980.
Bloom, D. and Goodfried, M. Lamellar ichthyosis of the newborn. The "collodion baby": A clinical and genetic entity: Report of a case and review of the literature with special consideration of pathogenesis and classification. *Arch. Dermatol.*, 86:336, 1962.
Davies, M. et al. Epidermal abnormalities in Refsum's disease. *Br. J. Dermatol.*, 97:401, 1977.
Edidin, D. et al. Chondrodysplasia punctata: Conradi-Hünermann syndrome. *Arch. Dermatol.*, 113:1431, 1977.
Epstein, E., Jr., Williams, M. and Elias, P. Editorial: Steroid sulfatase, X-linked ichthyosis, and stratum corneum cohesion. *Arch. Dermatol.*, 117:761, 1981.
Epstein, E. et al. X-linked ichthyosis: Increased blood cholesterol sulfate and electrophoretic mobility of low density lipoprotein. *Science*, 214:659, 1981.
Esterly, N. The ichthyosiform dermatoses. *Pediatrics*, 42:990, 1968.
Esterly, N. and Solomon, L. Neonatal dermatology. II. Blistering and scaling dermatoses. *J. Pediatr.*, 77:1075, 1970.
Feinstein, A., Ackerman, A. and Ziprkowski, L. Histology of autosomal dominant ichthyosis vulgaris and X-linked ichthyosis. *Arch. Dermatol.*, 101:524, 1970.
Finley, A. et al. The "dry" non-eczematous skin associated with atopic eczema. *Br. J. Dermatol.*, 103:249, 1980.
Fritsch, P., Hönigsmann, H. and Jaschke, E. Epidermolytic hereditary palmoplantar keratoderma. *Br. J. Dermatol.*, 99:561, 1978.
Frost, P. and Van Scott, E. Ichthyosiform dermatoses: Classification based on anatomic and biometric observations. *Arch. Dermatol.*, 94:113, 1966.
Frost, P., Weinstein, G. and Van Scott, E. The ichthyosiform dermatoses. II. Autoradiographic studies of epidermal proliferation. *J. Invest. Dermatol.*, 47:561, 1966.
Frost, P. et al. Ichthyosiform dermatoses. III. Studies of transepidermal water loss. *Arch. Dermatol.*, 98:230, 1968.
Greither, A. Keratosis extremitatum hereditaria progrediens mit dominantem Erbgang. *Hautarzt*, 3:198, 1952.

Jorizzo, J., Crounse, R. and Wheeler, C., Jr. Lamellar ichthyosis, dwarfism, mental retardation, and hair shaft anomalies. *J. Am. Acad. Dermatol.*, 2:309, 1980.
Kansky, A. and Arzensek, J. Is palmoplantar keratoderma of Greither's type a separate nosologic entity? *Dermatologica*, 158:244, 1979.
Lentz, C. and Altman, J. Lamellar ichthyosis: The natural clinical course of collodion baby. *Arch. Dermatol.*, 97:3, 1968.
McCurdy, J. and Beare, J. Congenital bullous ichthyosiform erythroderma. *Br. J. Dermatol.*, 79:294, 1967.
Niizuma, K. Isolated epidermolytic acanthoma. *Dermatologica*, 159:30, 1979.
Rand, R. and Baden, H. The ichthyoses: A review. *J. Am. Acad. Dermatol.*, 8:285, 1983.
Reed, W. and Heijer, A. Ichthyosiform dermatoses with neurological complications. *Cutis*, 4:1223, 1968.
Reed, W. et al. Lamellar ichthyosis of the newborn. *Arch. Dermatol.*, 105:394, 1972.
Rubin, M. and Mathes, B. Pityriasis rotunda: Two cases in black Americans. *J. Am. Acad. Dermatol.*, 14:74, 1987.
Schnyder, U. Inherited ichthyoses. *Arch. Dermatol.*, 102:240, 1970.
Shapiro, L. et al. X-linked ichthyosis due to steroid-sulphatase deficiency. *Lancet*, 1:70, 1978.
Vandersteen, P. and Muller, S. Lamellar ichthyosis: An enzyme histochemical, light and electron microscope study. *Arch. Dermatol.*, 106:694, 1972.
van Dijk, E. Ichthyosiform atrophy of the skin associated with internal malignant diseases. *Dermatologica*, 127:413, 1963.
Waisman, M. Pityriasis rotunda. *Cutis*, 38:247, 1986.
Wells, R. and Jennings, M. X-linked ichthyosis and ichthyosis vulgaris. *JAMA*, 202:485, 1967.
Wells, R. and Kerr, C. Genetic classification of ichthyosis. *Arch. Dermatol.*, 92:1, 1965.
Williams, M. and Elias, P. X-linked ichthyosis: Elevated cholesterol sulfate in pathological stratum corneum. (abstr.). *J. Invest. Dermatol.*, 76:312, 1981.

Incidental Acantholytic Dyskeratosis and Epidermolytic Hyperkeratosis

Ackerman, A. Focal acantholytic dyskeratosis. *Arch. Dermatol.*, 106:702, 1972.
——. Histopathologic concept of epidermolytic hyperkeratosis. *Arch. Dermatol.*, 102:253, 1970.
Ackerman, A. and Reed, R. Epidermolytic variant of solar keratosis. *Arch. Dermatol.*, 107:104, 1973.
Botet, M. and Sánchez, J. Vesiculation of focal acantholytic dyskeratosis in acral lentiginous malignant melnoma. *J. Dermatol. Surg. Oncol.*, 5:798, 1979.
Gebhart, W. and Kidd, R. Das solitäre epidermolytische Akanthom. *Z. Haut.*, 47:1, 1972.
Hirone, T. and Fukushiro, R. Disseminated epidermolytic acanthoma. *Acta Derm. Venereol.* (Stockh.), 53:393, 1973.
Mehregan, A. Epidermolytic hyperkeratosis. *J. Cutan. Pathol.*, 5:76, 1978.
Miyamoto, Y. et al. Disseminated epidermolytic acanthoma. *J. Cutan. Pathol.*, 6:272, 1979.
Nagashima, M. and Matsuoka, S. So-called granular degeneration as incidental histopathological finding. *Jpn. J. Dermatol.* (Series B), 81:494, 1971.
Niizuma, K. Isolated epidermolytic acanthoma. *Dermatologica*, 159:30, 1979.
Shapiro, L. and Baraf, C. Isolated epidermolytic acanthoma. *Arch. Dermatol.*, 101:220, 1970.
Stern, J., Wolf, J., Jr. and Rosen, T. Focal acantholytic dyskeratosis in pityriasis rosea. *Arch. Dermatol.*, 115:497, 1979.

Porokeratosis

Anderson, D. and Chernosky, M. Disseminated superficial actinic porokeratosis (DSAP): Genetic aspects. *Arch. Dermatol.*, 99:408, 1969.
Bloom, D. and Abramowitz, E. Porokeratosis Mibelli: Report of three cases in one family: Histologic studies. *Arch. Dermatol. Syph.*,47:1, 1943.
Braun-Falco, O. and Balsa, R. Zur Histochemie der cornoiden Lamelle. *Hautarzt*, 20:543, 1969.
Chernosky, M. and Anderson, D. Disseminated superficial actinic porokeratosis (DSAP): Clinical studies and experimental production of lesions. *Arch. Dermatol.*, 99:401, 1969.

Chernosky, M. and Freeman, R. Disseminated superficial actinic porokeratosis (DSAP). *Arch. Dermatol.*, 96:611, 1967.
Dover, J. et al. Disseminated superficial actinic porokeratosis: Co-existence with other porokeratotic variants. *Arch. Dermatol.*, 122:890, 1986.
Goldner, R. Zosteriform porokeratosis of Mibelli. *Arch. Dermatol.*, 104:425, 1971.
Guss, S., Osbourn, R. and Lutzner, M. Porokeratosis plantaris, palmaris et disseminata. *Arch. Dermatol.*, 104:366, 1971.
Inamoto, N. et al. Porokeratosis of Mibelli: Benzylhydrochlorothiazide-induced new lesions accompanied by eosinophilic spongiosis. *J. Am. Acad. Dermatol.*, 11:357, 1984.
James, W. and Rodman, O. Squamous cell carcinoma arising in porokeratosis of Mibelli. *Internat. J. Dermatol.*, 25:389, 1987.
Mann, P. et al. Ultrastructural studies on two cases of porokeratosis of Mibelli. *Br. J. Dermatol.*, 90:697, 1974.
Mehregan, A., Khalili, H. and Fazel, Z. Mibelli's porokeratosis of the face. *J. Am. Acad. Dermatol.*, 3:394, 1980.
Mikhail, G. and Wertheimer, F. Clinical variants of porokeratosis (Mibelli). *Arch. Dermatol.*, 98:124, 1968.
Nabai, H. and Mehregan, A. Porokeratosis of Mibelli: A report of two unusual cases. *Dermatologica*, 159:325, 1979.
Rahbari, H., Cordero, A. and Mehregan, A. Linear porokeratosis: A distinctive clinical variant of porokeratosis of Mibelli. *Arch. Dermatol.*, 109:526, 1974.
Rahbari, H., Cordero, A. and Mehregan, A. Punctate porokeratosis: A clinical variant of porokeratosis of Mibelli. *J. Cutan. Pathol.*, 4:338, 1977.
Reed, R. and Leone, P. Porokeratosis: A mutant clonal keratosis of the epidermis. *Arch. Dermatol.*, 101:340, 1970.
Sato, A., Anton-Lamprecht, I. and Schnyder, U. Ultrastructure of inborn errors of keratinization. VII. Porokeratosis Mibelli and disseminated superficial actinic porokeratosis. *Arch. Dermatol. Res.*, 255:271, 1976.
Saunders, T. Porokeratosis: A disease of epidermal eccrine sweat-duct units. *Arch. Dermatol.*, 84:890, 1961.
Schwarz, T., Seiser, A. and Gschnait, F. Disseminated superficial "actinic" porokeratosis. *J. Am. Acad. Dermatol.*, 11:724, 1984.
Taylor, A. Chromosomal instability associated with susceptibility to malignant disease in patients with porokeratosis Mibelli. *J. Natl. Cancer Inst.*, 51:371, 1973.
Wade, T. and Ackerman, A. Cornoid lamellation: A histologic reaction pattern. *Am. J. Dermatopathol.*, 2:5, 1980.
Wilkin, J., Rosenberg, E. and Kanzaki, T. Cornoid Lamella in Pachyonychia Congenita. *Arch. Dermatol.*, 114:1795, 1979.

Xeroderma Pigmentosum

Bell, E. and Rothnem, T. Xeroderma pigmentosum with carcinoma of the lower lip in 2 brothers aged 16 and 13 years. *Am. J. Cancer*, 30:574, 1937.
Cleaver, J. Defective repair replication of DNA in xeroderma pigmentosum. *Nature*, 218:652, 1968.
——. DNA damage and repair in light-sensitive human skin disease. *J. Invest. Dermatol.*, 54:181, 1970.
——. Xeroderma pigmentosum: Genetic and environmental influences in skin carcinogenesis. *Internat. J. Dermatol.*, 17:435, 1978.
——. Xeroderma pigmentosum: Variants with normal DNA repair and normal sensitivity to ultraviolet light. *J. Invest. Dermatol.*, 38:124, 1972.
Friedberg, E. Recent studies on the DNA repair defects. *Arch. Pathol.*, 102:3, 1978.
Guerrier, C. et al. An electron microscopical study of the skin in 18 cases of xeroderma pigmentosum. *Dermatologica*, 146:211, 1973.
Kraemer, K. Xeroderma pigmentosum. In: *Clinical Dermatology*. Vol. 4. Demis, D. et al., eds., Hagerstown, Harper & Row, 1980, p. 1.
Kraemer, K., Lee, M. and Scotto, J. Xeroderma pigmentosum: Cutaneous, ocular and neurologic abnormalities in 830 published cases. *Arch. Dermatol.*, 123:241, 1987.
Lynch, H., Frichot, B., III and Lynch, J. Cancer control in xeroderma pigmentosum. *Arch. Dermatol.*, 113:193, 1977.
Montgomery, H. and Reuter, M. Xeroderma pigmentosum: Report of a mild case with histopathologic studies. *Arch. Dermatol. Syph.*, 26:256, 1932.

Reed, W., Sugarman, G. and Mathis, R. DeSanctis-Cacchione syndrome. *Arch. Dermatol.*, 113:1561, 1977.
Reed, W. et al. Xeroderma pigmentosum: Clinical and laboratory investigation of its basic defect. *JAMA*, 207:2073, 1969.
Robbins, J., Kraemer, K. and Flaxman, B. DNA repair in tumor cells from the variant of xeroderma pigmentosum. *J. Invest. Dermatol.*, 64:150, 1975.
Ronchese, F. Melanomata: Pathologically malignant, clinically nonmalignant, in a case of xeroderma pigmentosum. *Arch. Dermatol. Syph.*, 68:355, 1953.
Setlow, R. Repair deficient human disorders and cancer. *Nature*, 271:713, 1978.

Pseudoxanthoma Elasticum

Caro, I., Sher, M. and Rippey, J. Pseudoxanthoma elasticum and elastosis perforans serpignosa: Report of 2 cases. *Dermatologica*, 150:36, 1975.
Christensen, O. An exogenous variety of pseudoxanthoma elasticum in old farmers. *Acta Derm. Venereol.* (Stockh.), 58:319, 1978.
Danielsen, L. and Kobayasi, T. Pseudoxanthoma elasticum. *Acta Derm. Venereol.*, 54:121, 1974.
Eddy, D. and Farber, E. Pseudoxanthoma elasticum. Internal manifestations: A report of cases and a statistical review of the literature. *Arch. Dermatol.*, 86:729, 1962.
Flatley, F., Atwell, M. and McEvoy, R. Pseudoxanthoma elasticum with gastric hemorrhage. *Arch. Int. Med.*, 112:352, 1963.
Goodman, R. et al. Pseudoxanthoma elasticum: A clinical and histopathological study. *Medicine*, 42:297, 1963.
Huang, S. et al. Ultrastructural changes of elastic fibers in pseudoxanthoma elasticum: A study of histogenesis. *Arch. Pathol.*, 83:108, 1967.
Loria, P. et al. Pseudoxanthoma elasticum (Grönblad-Strandberg syndrome): A clinical, light and electron microscopic study. *Arch. Dermatol.*, 76:609, 1957.
McKee, P. et al. A study of four cases of pseudoxanthoma elasticum. *J. Cutan. Pathol.*, 4:146, 1977.
Mendelsohn, G., Bulkley, B. and Hutchins, G. Cardiovascular manifestations of pseudoxanthoma elasticum. *Arch. Pathol.*, 102:298, 1978.
Neldner, K. and Martinez-Hernandez, A. Localized acquired cutaneous pseudoxanthoma elasticum. *J. Am. Acad. Dermatol.*, 1:523, 1979.
Pasquali-Ronchetti, T. et al. Pseudoxanthoma elasticum: Chemical and ultrastructural studies. *Dermatologica*, 163:307, 1981.
Pope, F. Autosomal dominant pseudoxanthoma elasticum. *J. Med. Genet.*, 11:152, 1974.
——. Historical evidence for the genetic heterogeneity of pseudoxanthoma elasticum. *Br. J. Dermatol.*, 92:493, 1975.
——. Two types of autosomal recessive pseudoxanthoma elasticum. *Arch. Dermatol.*, 110:209, 1974.
Reeve, E. et al. Development of calcification of skin lesions in thirty-nine patients with pseudoxanthoma elasticum. *Clin. Exp. Dermatol.*, 4:291, 1979.
Smith, J. et al. Pseudoxanthoma elasticum: Histochemical and biochemical alterations. *Arch. Dermatol.*, 86:741, 1962.
Verhoeff, F. Histological findings in a case of angioid streaks. Br. J. Ophthalmol., 32:531, 1948.
Whitcomb, F., Jr. and Brown, C. Pseudoxanthoma elasticum: Report of twelve cases. *Ann. Int. Med.*, 56:834, 1962.
Yamamura, T. and Sano, S. Ultrastructural and histochemical analysis of thready material in pseudoxanthoma elasticum. *J. Cutan. Pathol.*, 11:282, 1984.

Ehlers-Danlos Syndrome

Arneson, M. et al. A new form of Ehlers-Danlos syndrome. *JAMA*, 244:144, 1980.
Barabas, A. Heterogeneity of the Ehlers-Danlos syndrome: Description of 3 clinical types and a hypothesis to explain the basic defects. *Br. Med. J.*, 2:612, 1967.
Beighton, P. *The Ehlers-Danlos Syndrome*. London, Heinemann, 1970.
Bruno, M. and Narasimhan, P. The Ehlers-Danlos syndrome: A report of four cases in two generations of a Negro family. *N. Eng. J. Med.*, 264:274, 1961.

Byers, P. et al. Altered secretion of type III procollagen in a form of type IV Ehlers-Danlos syndrome. *Lab. Invest.*, 44:336, 1981.
Holbrook, K. and Byers, P. Ultrastructural characteristics of the skin in a form of the Ehlers-Danlos syndrome type IV: Storage in the rough endoplasmic reticulum. *Lab. Invest.*, 44:342, 1981.
Hult, A., Goltz, R. and Midtgaard, K. The dermal elastic fibers in cutis hyperelastica (Ehlers-Danlos syndrome) and in cutis laxa (generalized elastolysis) *Acta Derm. Venereol.*, 44:415, 1964.
Imahori, S. et al. Ehlers-Danlos syndrome with multiple arterial lesions. *Am. J. Med.*, 47:967, 1969.
Jansen, L. The structure of the connective tissue: An explanation of the symptoms of the Ehlers-Danlos syndrome. *Dermatologica*, 110:108, 1955.
Johnson, S. and Falls, H. Ehlers-Danlos syndrome. *Arch. Dermatol. Syph.*, 60:82, 1949.
McFarland, W. and Fuller, D. Mortality in Ehlers-Danlos syndrome due to spontaneous rupture of large arteries. *N. Eng. J. Med.*, 271:1309, 1964.
Nelson, D. and King, R. Ehlers-Danlos syndrome type VIII. *J. Am. Acad. Dermatol.*, 5:297, 1981.
Nordschow, C. and Marsolais, E. Ehlers-Danlos syndrome: Some recent biophysical observations. *Arch. Pathol.*, 88:65, 1969.
Pierard, G., Pierard-Franchimont, C. and Lapiere, C. Histopathological aid at the diagnosis of the Ehlers-Danlos syndrome, gravis and mitis types. *Internat. J. Dermatol.*, 22:300, 1983.
Pinnell, S. Molecular defects in the Ehlers-Danlos syndrome. *J. Invest. Dermatol.*, 79:90, 1982.
Pinnell, S. et al. Ehlers-Danlos syndrome: A heritable disorder of connective tissue. *N. Eng. J. Med.*, 286:1011, 1972.
Scarpelli, D. and Goodman, R. Observations on the fine structure of the fibroblast from a case of Ehlers-Danlos syndrome with the Marfan's syndrome. *J. Invest. Dermatol.*, 50:214, 1968.
Sevenich, M., Schultz-Ehrenburg, U. and Orfanos, C. Ehlers-Danlos Syndrom: Eine Fibroblasten- und Kollagenkrankheit. *Arch. Dermatol. Res.*, 267:237, 1980.
Steinmann, B. et al. Evidence for a structural mutation of procollagen type I in a patient with Ehlers-Danlos syndrome type VII. *J. Biol. Chem.*, 255:8887, 1980.
Strause, B. and Tojaratchi, N. Biochemical abnormalities in Ehlers-Danlos syndrome. *Arch. Int. Med.*, 118:461, 1966.
Sulica, V. et al. Cutaneous histologic features in Ehlers-Danlos syndrome. *Arch. Dermatol.*, 115:40, 1979.
Uitto, J. and Lichtenstein, J. Defects in the biochemistry of collagen in diseases of connective tissue. (Review). *J. Invest. Dermatol.*, 66:59, 1976.
Wechsler, H. and Fisher, E. Ehlers-Danlos syndrome. *Arch. Pathol.*, 77:613, 1964.
——. Ehlers-Danlos syndrome: Pathologic, histochemical, and electron microscopic observations. *Arch. Pathol.*, 77:613, 1964.

Cutis Laxa

Beighton, P. The dominant and recessive forms of cutis laxa. *J. Med. Genet.*,9:216, 1972.
Byers, P. et al. X-linked cutis laxa. Defective cross-link formation in collagen due to decreased lysyl oxidase activity. *N. Eng. J. Med.*, 303:61, 1980.
Chadfield, H. and North, J. Cutis laxa. *Trans. St. John's Hosp. Dermatol. Soc.*, 57:181, 1971.
Goltz, R. et al. Cutis laxa: A manifestation of generalized elastolysis. *Arch. Dermatol.*, 92:373, 1965.
Harris, R., Heapy, M. and Perry, H. Generalized elastolysis (cutis laxa). *Am. J. Med.*, 65:815, 1979.
Hashimoto, K. and Kanzaki, T. Cutis laxa. *Arch. Dermatol.*, 111:861, 1975.
Kerl, H., Burg, G. and Hashimoto, K. Fatal penicillin induced, generalized postinflammatory elastolysis (cutis laxa). *Am. J. Dermatopathol.*, 5:267, 1983.
Koch, S. and Williams, M. Acquired cutis laxa: Case report and review of disorders of elastolysis. *Pediat. Dermatol.*, 2:282, 1985.
Lambert, D. et al. Cutis laxa généralisée congenitale. *Ann. Dermatol. Venereol.*, 110:129, 1983.
Ledoux-Corbusier, M. Cutis laxa, congenital form with pulmonary emphysema: An ultrastructural study. *J. Cutan. Pathol.*, 10:340, 1983.
Lewis, E. Cutis laxa. *Proc. R. Soc. Med.*, 41:864, 1948.

Mehregan, A., Lee, S. and Nabai, H. Cutis laxa (generalized elastolysis). *J. Cutan. Pathol.*, 5:116, 1978.
Nanko, H. et al. Acquired cutis laxa (generalized elastolysis). *Acta Derm. Venereol.* (Stockh.), 59:315, 1979.
Randle, H. and Muller, S. Generalized elastolysis associated with systemic lupus erythematosus. *J. Am. Acad. Dermatol.*, 8:869, 1983.
Reed, W., Horowitz, R. and Beighton, P. Acquired cutis laxa: Primary generalized elastolysis. *Arch. Dermatol.*, 103:661, 1971.
Robinson, H., Jr. and and Ellis, F. Cutis laxa. *Arch. Dermatol.*, 77:656, 1958.
Schreiber, M. and Tilley, J. Cutis laxa. *Arch. Dermatol.*, 84:266, 1961.
Scott, M., Kauh, Y. and Luscombe, H. Acquired cutis laxa associated with multiple myeloma. *Arch. Dermatol.*, 112:853, 1976.
Sestak, Z. Ehlers-Danlos syndrome and cutis laxa: An account of families in the Oxford area. *Ann. Hum. Genet.*, 25:313, 1962.

Incontinentia Pigmenti

Caputo, R., Gianotti, F. and Innocenti, M. Ultrastructural findings in incontinentia pigmenti. *Internat. J. Dermatol.*, 14:46, 1975.
Carney, R. Incontinentia pigmenti. *Arch. Dermatol.*, 112:535, 1976.
Carney, R. and Carney, R., Jr. Incontinentia pigmenti. *Arch. Dermatol.*, 102:157, 1970.
Emeret, I. et al. Incontinentia pigmenti: Chromosomal study of a family. *Ann. Dermatol. Venereol.*, 105:119, 1978.
Epstein, S., Vedder, J. and Pinkus, H. Bullous variety of incontinentia pigmenti (Bloch-Sulzberger). *Arch. Dermatol. Syph.*, 65:557, 1952.
Gordon, H. and Gordon, W. Incontinentia pigmenti: Clinical and genetic studies of two familial cases. *Dermatologica*, 140:150, 1970.
Haber, H. The Bloch-Sulzberger syndrome (incontinentia pigmenti). *Br. J. Dermatol.*, 64:129, 1952.
Kelly, T. et al. Incontinentia pigmenti: A chromosomal breakage syndrome. *J. Hered.*, 67:171, 1976.
McPherson, A. and Auth, T. Bloch-Sulzberger syndrome (incontinentia pigmenti): Report of a case with prominent neurological features. *Arch. Neurol.*, 8:332, 1963.
Morgan, J. Incontinentia pigmenti (Bloch-Sulzberger syndrome). *Am. J. Dis. Child.*, 122:294, 1971.
Rubin, L. and Becker, S., Jr. Pigmentation in the Bloch-Sulzberger syndrome (incontinentia pigmenti). *Arch. Dermatol.*, 74:263, 1956.
Schaumburg-Lever, G. and Lever, W. Electron microscopy of incontinentia pigmenti. *J. Invest. Dermatol.*, 61:151, 1973.
Sulzberger, M. Incontinentia Pigmenti (Bloch-Sulzberger): Report of an additional case with comment on possible relation to a new syndrome of familial and congenital anomalies. *Arch. Dermatol. Syph.*, 38:57, 1938.
Wiklund, D. and Weston, W. Incontinentia pigmenti: A four generation study. *Arch. Dermatol.*, 116:701, 1980.

Erythema Toxicum Neonatorum

Freeman, R., Spiller, R. and Knox, J. Histopathology of erythema toxicum neonatorum. *Arch. Dermatol.*, 82:586, 1960.
Pohlandt, F. et al. Zum Bild des Erythema toxicum neonatorum. *Hautarzt*, 28:469, 1977.

Hypomelanosis of Ito

Aram, H. Incontinentia pigmenti achromians (Ito). *Cutis*, 6:197, 1970.
Carney, R. Incontinentia pigmenti. *Arch. Dermatol.*, 112:535, 1976.
Griffiths, A. and Payne, C. Incontinentia pigmenti achromians. *Arch. Dermatol.*, 111:751, 1975.
Grosshans, E. et al. Incontinentia pigmenti achromians (Ito). *Dermatologica*, 142:65, 1971.
Hamada, T. et al. Incontinentia pigmenti achromians (Ito). *Arch. Dermatol.*, 96:673, 1967.

Hellgren, L. Incontinentia pigmenti achromians (Ito). *Acta Derm. Venereol.*, 55:237, 1975.
——. Incontinentia pigmenti achromians (Ito). *Acta Derm. Venereol.* (Stockh.), 55:237, 1975.
Jelinek, J. et al. Hypomelanosis of Ito: Incontinentia pigmenti achromians: Report of three cases and review of the literature. *Arch. Dermatol.*, 107:596, 1973.
Kato, T. et al. Incontinentia pigmenti achromians. *Jpn. J. Dermatol. Urol.*, 8:214, 1954.
Morohashi, M. et al. Ultrastructural studies of vitiligo, Vogt-Koyanagi syndrome, and incontinentia pigmenti achromians. *Arch. Dermatol.*, 113:755, 1977.
Nohara, N. and Tasaka, S. Incontinentia pigmenti achromians. *Jpn. J. Dermatol.*, 56:130, 1961.
Nordlund, J., Klaus, S. and Gino, J. Hypomelanosis of Ito. *Acta Derm. Venereol.* (Stockh.), 57:261, 1977.
Piñol-Aguade, J. et al. Incontinentia pigmenti achromians (Ito). *Med. Cutan. Iber. Lat. Am.*, 3:287, 1968.
Rubin, M. Incontinentia pigmenti achromians. *Arch. Dermatol.*, 105:424, 1972.
Stoebner, P. and Grosshans, E. Incontinentia pigmenti achromians (Ito). Étude ultrastructural. *Arch. Klin. Exp. Dermatol.*, 239:227, 1970.
Takematsu, H. et al. Incontinentia pigmenti achromians. *Arch. Dermatol.*, 119:391, 1983.

Neurofibromatosis

Benedict, P. et al. Melanotic macules in Albright's syndrome and in neurofibromatosis. *JAMA*, 205:618, 1968.
Brasfield, R. and Das Gupta, T. Von Recklinghausen's disease: A clinicopathologic study. *Ann. Surg.*, 175:86, 1972.
Crowe, F. Axillary freckling as a diagnostic aid in neurofibromatosis. *Ann. Int. Med.*, 61:1142, 1964.
Crowe, F., Schull, W. and Neel, J. *A Clinical, Pathological and Genetic Study of Multiple Neurofibromatosis*. Springfield, Il., Thomas, 1956.
D'Agostino, A., Soule, E. and Miller, R. Sarcomas of the peripheral nerves and somatic soft tissues associated with multiple neurofibromatosis (von Recklinghausen's disease). *Cancer*, 16:1015, 1963.
Fienman, N. and Yakovac, W. Neurofibromatosis in childhood. *J. Pediatr.*, 76:339, 1970.
Foot, N. Histology of tumors of the peripheral nerves. *Arch. Pathol.*, 30:772, 1940.
Griffith, B. et al. Von Recklinghausen's disease in children. *Plast. Reconstr. Surg.*, 49:647, 1972.
Jimbow, K., Szabo, G. and Fitzpatrick, T. Ultrastructure of giant pigment granules (macromelanosomes) in the cutaneous pigmented macules of neurofibromatosis. *J. Invest. Dermatol.*, 61:300, 1973.
Johnson, B. and Charneco, D. Café-au-lait spot in neurofibromatosis and in normal individuals. *Arch. Dermatol.*, 102:442, 1970.
Klaus, S. and Winkelmann, R. Cholinesterase activity in neurofibromas *in vitro*. *J. Invest. Dermatol.*, 41:301, 1963.
Knight, W., III, Murphy, W. and Gottlieb, J. Neurofibromatosis associated with malignant neurofibrosarcomas. *Arch. Dermatol.*, 107:747, 1973.
McNairy, D. and Montgomery, H. Cutaneous tumors of von Recklinghausen's disease (neurofibromatosis), *Arch. Dermatol. Syph.*, 51:384, 1945.
Miller, R. and Sparks, R. Segmental neurofibromatosis. *Arch. Dermatol.*, 113:837, 1977.
Reed, R. Cutaneous manifestations of neural crest disorders (neurocristopathies). (Review). *Internat. J. Dermatol.*, 16:807, 1977.
Riccardi, V. Von Recklinghausen neurofibromatosis. (Review). *N. Eng. J. Med.*, 305:1617, 1981.
Rosman, N. and Pearce, J. The brain in neurofibromatosis (von Recklinghausen's disease): A suggested neuropathological basis for the associated mental defect. *Brain*, 90:829, 1967.
Santa Cruz, D. and Yates, A. Pigmented storiform neurofibroma. *J. Cutan. Pathol.*, 4:9, 1977.
Schenkein, I. et al. Increased nerve-growth-stimulating activity in disseminated neurofibromatosis. *N. Eng. J. Med.*, 290:613, 1974.
Shelley, W. and Arthur, R. Nerve fibers: A neglected component of intradermal cellular nevi. *J. Invest. Dermatol.*, 34:59, 1960.
Silvers, D., Greenwood, R. and Helwig, E. Café-au-lait spots without giant pigment granules. *Arch. Dermatol.*, 110:87, 1974.

Sordillo, P. et al. Malignant schwannoma: Clinical characteristics, survival, and response to therapy. *Cancer*, 47:2503, 1981.
Stein, K., Shmunes, E. and Thew, M. Neurofibromatosis presenting as the epidermal nevus syndrome. *Arch. Dermatol.*, 105:229, 1972.
Storm, F. et al. Neurofibrosarcoma. *Cancer*, 45:126, 1980.
Taxy, J. et al. Electron microscopy in the diagnosis of malignant schwannoma. *Cancer*, 48:1381, 1981.
Trojanowski, J., Kleinman, G. and Proppe, K. Malignant tumors of nerve sheath origin. *Cancer*, 46:1202, 1980.
Wachstein, M. and Wolf, E. General neurofibromatosis (von Recklinghausen's disease) with local sarcomatous change and metastasis to regional lymph nodes. *Arch. Pathol.*, 37:331, 1944.
Weber, K. and Braun-Falco, O. Zur Ultrastruktur der Neurofibromatose. *Hautarzt*, 23:116, 1972.
Winkelmann, R. and Johnson, L. Cholinesterases in neurofibromas. *Arch. Dermatol.*, 85:106, 1962.
Winkelmann, R., Neldner, K. and Muller, S. Neurofibromatous dermal nevus. *Arch. Dermatol.*, 87:334, 1963.

Mastocytosis

Asboe-Hansen, G. The mast cell in health and disease. *Acta Derm. Venereol.*, 53 (73, suppl.): 139, 1973.
——. Urticaria pigmentosa with generalized tissue mastocytosis and blood basophilia. *Arch. Dermatol.*, 81:198, 1960.
Baraf, C. and Shapiro, L. Solitary mastocytoma. *Arch. Dermatol.*, 99:589, 1969.
Benditt, E. and Lagunoff, D. The mast cell: Its structure and function. *Progr. Allerg.*, 8:195, 1964.
Bowdler, A. and Tullett, G. Urticaria pigmentosa and polycythaemia vera: A case report. *Br. Med. J.*, 1:396, 1960.
Brodeur, P. and Gardner, L. Urticaria pigmentosa as a problem in diagnosis: Report of two cases, one with systemic involvement. *N. Eng. J. Med.*, 254:1165, 1956.
Burgoon, C., Graham, J. and McCaffree, D. Mast cell disease. *Arch. Dermatol.*, 98:590, 1968.
Caplan, R. The natural course of urticaria pigmentosa: Analysis and follow-up of 112 cases. *Arch. Dermatol.*, 87:146, 1963.
Cramer, H. Telangiectasia macularis eruptiva perstans, eine Sonderform der Urticaria pigmentosa. *Hautarzt*, 15:370, 1964.
Dewar, W. and Milne, J. Bullous urticaria pigmentosa: Summary of literature and report of two cases. *Arch. Dermatol. Syph.*, 71:717, 1955.
Diamond, J. and Gross, L. Urticaria pigmentosa complicated by polycythemia vera: Report of a case. *Blood*, 27:253, 1966.
Drennan, J. The mast cells in urticaria pigmentosa. *J. Pathol. Bacteriol.*, 63:513, 1951.
Drennan, J. and Beare, J. Solitary mast-cell naevus. *J. Pathol. Bacteriol.*, 68:345, 1954.
Efrati, P., Klajman, A. and Spitz, H. Mast cell leukemia? Malignant mastocytosis with leukemia-like manifestations. *Blood*, 12:869, 1957.
Ellis, J. Urticaria pigmentosa. *Arch. Pathol.*, 48:426, 1949.
Fowler, J., Jr., Parsley, W. and Cotter, P. Familial urticaria pigmentosa. *Arch. Dermatol.*, 122:80, 1986.
Freeman, R. Diffuse urticaria pigmentosa. *Am. J. Clin. Pathol.*, 48:187, 1967.
Fried, S. and Lynfield, Y. Unilateral telangiectasia macularis eruptiva perstans. *J. Am. Acad. Dermatol.*, 16:250, 1987.
Friedman, B. et al. Tissue mast cell leukemia. *Blood*, 13:70, 1958.
Gonnella, J. and Lipsey, A. Mastocytosis manifested by hepatosplenomegaly: Report of a case. *N. Eng. J. Med.*, 271:533, 1964.
Johnson, W. and Helwig, E. Solitary mastocytosis (urticaria pigmentosa). *Arch. Dermatol.*, 84:806, 1961.
Kilburn, H. Solitary mastocytoma of infancy. *Clin. Pediatr.*, 13:60, 1974.
Klaus, S. and Winkelmann, R. The clinical spectrum of urticaria pigmentosa. *Proc. Mayo Clin.*, 40:923, 1965.
——. Course of urticaria pigmentosa in children. *Arch. Dermatol.*, 86:68, 1962.
Leder, L. Subtle clues to diagnosis by histochemistry in mast cell disease. *Am. J. Dermatopathol.*, 1:261, 1979.

Lennert, K. and Parwaresch, M. Mast cell neoplasia: A review. *Histopathology,* 3:349, 1979.
Lucaya, J. et al. Mastocytosis with skeletal and gastrointestinal involvement in infancy. *Pediatr. Radiol.,* 131:363, 1979.
Mikhail, G. and Miller-Milinska, A. Mast cell population in human skin. *J. Invest. Dermatol.,* 43:249, 1964.
Miller, R. and Shapiro, L. Bullous urticaria pigmentosa in infancy. *Arch. Dermatol.,* 91:595, 1965.
Monheit, G., Murad, T. and Conrad, M. Systemic mastocytosis and the mastocytosis syndrome. *J. Cutan. Pathol.,* 6:42, 1979.
Okun, M. Histogenesis of melanocytes. *J. Invest. Dermatol.,* 44:285, 1965.
Okun, M. and Bhawan, J. Combined melanocytoma-mastocytoma in a case of nodular mastocytosis. *J. Am. Acad. Dermatol.,* 1:338, 1979.
Okun, M. and Chorzelski, T. Metachromatic granules in dendritic cells within epithelial structures in alopecia mucinosa. *J. Invest. Dermatol.,* 45:129, 1965.
Okun, M. and Donnellan, B. Ultrastructural relationship of melanocytes to mast cells and "melanophages" in a lesion of alopecia mucinosa. *J. Invest. Dermatol.,* 59:211, 1972.
Okun, M. and Zook, B. Histologic parallels between mastocytoma and melanoma. *Arch. Dermatol.,* 95:275, 1967.
Okun, M. et al. Latency of the dopa reaction in mast cells. *Histochemie,* 25:1, 1971.
Reilly, E., Shintani, J. and Goodman, J. Systemic mast-cell disease with urticaria pigmentosa. *Arch. Dermatol. Syph.,* 71:561, 1955.
Roberts, L., II et al. Mastocytosis without urticaria pigmentosa: A frequently unrecognized cause of recurrent syncope. *Trans. Assoc. Am. Physicians,* 95:36, 1982.
Rodermund, O., Klingmüller, G. and Rohner, H. Interne Befunde bei Mastozytose. *Hautarzt,* 31:175, 1980.
Sagher, F. and Even-Paz, Z. *Mastocytosis and the Mast Cell.* Chicago, Yearbook Medical Publishers, 1967.
Selyé, H. *The Mast Cells.* London, Butterworth, 1965.
Sostre, S. and Handler, H. Bony lesions in systemic mastocytosis. *Arch. Dermatol.,* 113:1245, 1977.
Szweda, J. et al. Systemic mast cell disease: A review and report of three cases: Massive gastrointestinal hemorrhage in one patient. *Am. J. Med.,* 32:227, 1962.
Waters, W. and Larson, P. Mast cell leukemia presenting as urticaria pigmentosa: Report of a case. *Pediatrics,* 19:1033, 1957.

Tuberous Sclerosis

Burkhart, C. and El-Shaar, A. Computerized axial tomography in the early diagnosis of tuberous sclerosis. *J. Am. Acad. Dermatol.,* 4:59, 1981.
Butterworth, T. and Wilson, M., Jr. Dermatologic aspects of tuberous sclerosis. *Arch. Dermatol. Syph.,* 43:1, 1941.
Elliott, G. and McGeachy, W. The monster Purkinje-cell nature of so-called "congenital rhabdomyoma of heart": A forme fruste of tuberous sclerosis. *Am. Heart J.,* 63:636, 1962.
Fitzpatrick, T. et al. White leaf-shaped macules: Earliest visible sign of tuberous sclerosis. *Arch. Dermatol.,* 98:1, 1968.
Font, R. and Ferry, A. The phakomatoses. *Internat. Ophthalmol. Clin.,* 12:1, 1972.
Gold, A. and Freeman, J. Depigmented nevi: The earliest sign of tuberous sclerosis. *Pediatrics,* 35:1003, 1965.
Gomez, M. *Tuberous Sclerosis.* New York, Raven Press, 1979, p. 246.
Hurwitz, S. and Braverman, I. White spots in tuberous sclerosis. *J. Pediatr.,* 77:587, 1970.
Lagos, J. and Gomez, M. Tuberous sclerosis: Reappraisal of a clinical entity. *Mayo Clin. Proc.,* 42:26, 1967.
Nickel, W. and Reed, W. Tuberous sclerosis: Special reference to the microscopic alterations in the cutaneous hamartomas. *Arch. Dermatol.,* 85:209, 1962.
Price, E., Jr. and Mostofi, F. Symptomatic angiomyolipoma of the kidney. *Cancer,* 18:761, 1965.
Reed, W., Nickel, W. and Campion, G. Internal manifestations of tuberous sclerosis. *Arch. Dermatol.,* 87:715, 1963.
Sareen, C. et al. Tuberous sclerosis: Clinical, endocrine, and metabolic studies. *Am. J. Dis. Child.,* 123:34, 1972.
Scheig, R. and Bornstein, P. Tuberous sclerosis in the adult: An unusual case without mental deficiency or epilepsy. *Arch. Int. Med.,* 108:789, 1961.

Connective Tissue Nevus

Danielsen, L., Kobayasi, T. and Jacobsen, G. Ultrastructural changes in disseminated connective tissue nevi. *Acta Derm. Venereol.* (Stockh.), 57:93, 1977.

Hegedus, S. and Schorr, W. Familial cutaneous collagenoma. *Cutis*, 10:283, 1972.

Moriguchi, T. and Fujimoto, D. Crosslink of collagen in hypertrophic scar. *J. Invest. Dermatol.*, 72:143, 1979.

Morrison, J., Wilson-Jones, E. and MacDonald, D. Juvenile elastoma (the Buschke-Ollendorff syndrome). *Br. J. Dermatol.*, 97:417, 1977.

Prakken, J. Connective tissue naevi. *Br. J. Dermatol.*, 64:87, 1952.

Rocha, G. and Winkelmann, R. Connective tissue nevus. *Arch. Dermatol.*, 85:722, 1962.

Smith, A. and Waisman, M. Connective tissue nevi: Familial occurrence and association with osteopoikilosis. *Arch. Dermatol.*, 81:249, 1960.

Smith, L. and Bernstein, B. Eruptive collagenoma. *Arch. Dermatol.*, 114:1710, 1978.

Sosis, A. and Johnson, W. Connective tissue nevus. *Dermatologica*, 144:57, 1972.

Starrico, R. and Mehregan, A. Nevus elasticus and nevus elasticus vascularis. *Arch. Dermatol.*, 84:943, 1961.

Uitto, J., Santa-Cruz, J. and Eisen, A. Famial cutaneous collagenoma: Genetic studies on a family. *Br. J. Dermatol.*, 101:185, 1979.

Verbov, J. Buschke-Ollendorff syndrome (disseminated dermatofibrosis with osteopoikilosis). *Br. J. Dermatol.*, 96:87, 1977.

Weidmann, F., Anderson, N. and Ayres, S., Jr., Juvenile elastoma. *Arch. Dermatol. Syph.*, 28:182, 1933.

Focal Dermal Hypoplasia

Goltz, R. et al. Focal dermal hypoplasia. *Arch. Dermatol.*, 86:708, 1962.

Goltz, R. et al. Focal dermal hypoplasia syndrome. *Arch. Dermatol.*, 101:1, 1970.

Gorlin, R. et al. Focal dermal hypoplasia syndrome. *Acta Derm. Venereol.*, 43:421, 1963.

Happle, R. and Lenz, W. Striation of bone in focal dermal hypoplasia: Manifestation of functional mosaicism. *Br. J. Dermatol.*, 96:133, 1977.

Howell, J. and Reynolds, J. Osteopathia striata. *Trans. St. John's Hosp. Dermatol. Soc.*, 60:178, 1974.

Ishibashi, A. and Kurihara, Y. Goltz's syndrome: Focal dermal hypoplasia syndrome. *Dermatologica*, 144:156, 1972.

Chapter 5
Infectious Diseases

Infectious Diseases: Bacterial

IMPETIGO

Impetigo is a superficial skin infection caused by group A beta-hemolytic streptococci, coagulase-positive staphylococci, or a combination of these organisms. There are two main types of impetigo. *Nonbullous impetigo* (impetigo contagiosa) is caused by group A streptococci. *Bullous impetigo* is usually caused by phage group II staphylococci. Impetigo contagiosa is seen mainly in preschool age children, sometimes in epidemics. It is characterized by transient vesiculopustules (Fig. A), which rupture to form yellowish crusts, which are sometimes confluent (Fig. B). These crusts may have a circinate arrangement, producing a resemblance to a granuloma, such as a granuloma of North American blastomycosis (Fig. C). Acute glomerulonephritis is an occasional sequel of impetigo contagiosa. Bullous impetigo is typically observed in the newborn, in infants, and in young children. When it occurs in adults, it tends to be associated with a deficiency in cell-mediated immunity. Lesions are vesicles that evolve into flaccid bullae. The flaccid bullae may become generalized and resemble staphylococcal scalded skin syndrome (a special type of bullous impetigo). Staphylococcal scalded skin syndrome (Ritter's disease) is almost entirely limited to the newborn and infants. Initially, there is widespread erythema, followed by the development of large, flaccid bullae, which rupture and leave large sheets of exfoliating superficial epidermis. It has been said that staphylococcal scalded skin syndrome differs from bullous impetigo by the inability to grow phage group II staphylococci from intact bullae. Staphylococcal scalded skin syndrome differs from the erythema multiforme type of scalded skin syndrome (see p. 574) by exfoliation of the stratum corneum rather than sheets of whole epidermis. The bullae of staphylococcal scalded skin syndrome are caused by *exfoliatin,* a staphylococcal toxin. Staphylococcal scalded skin syndrome in adults has a much poorer prognosis than in infants. Impetigo of Bockhart is impetigo involving follicular orifices.

Impaired cellular immunity or coexisting disease are predisposing factors in adults.

IMPETIGO

A 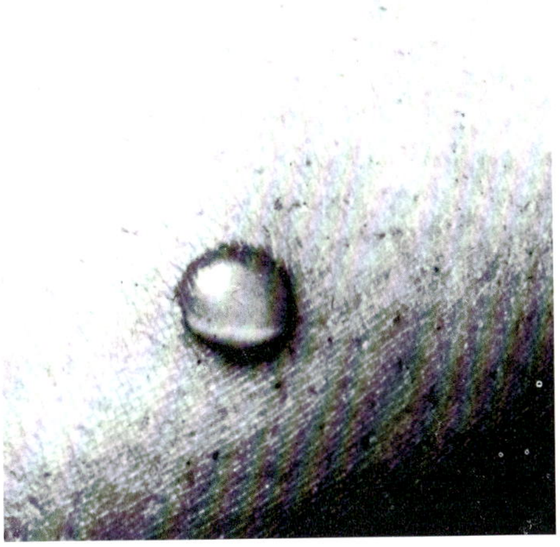

B 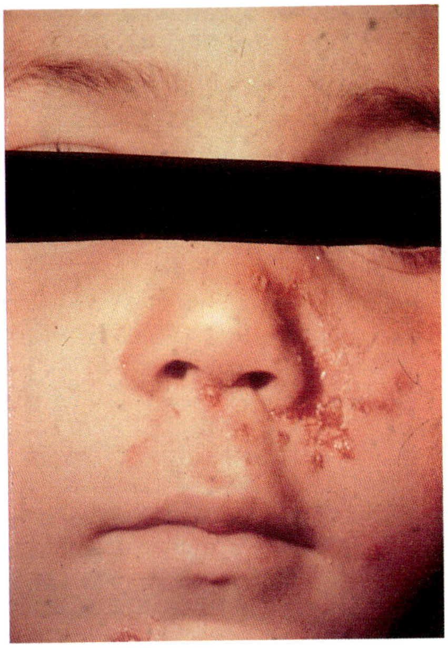

C 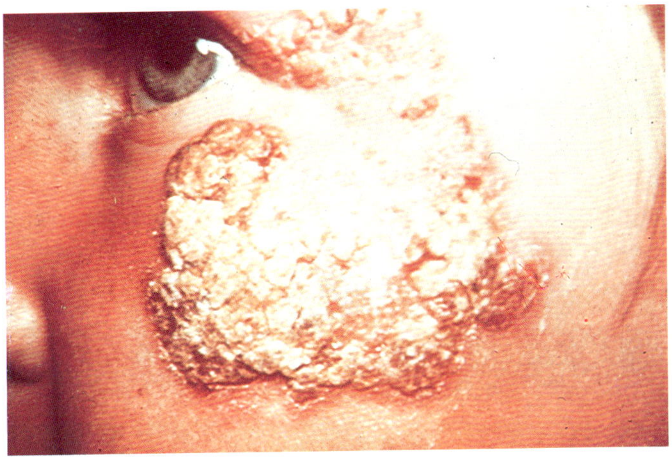

IMPETIGO continued ⇨

IMPETIGO

Microscopic features

1. In all forms of impetigo, the vesiculopustule forms beneath the stratum corneum and contains many neutrophils (Figs. A,B). Enlargement of the vesiculopustule results in bulla formation. In bullous impetigo and staphylococcal scalded skin syndrome, inflammatory cells in the bulla cavity may be few or absent.
2. A few acantholytic cells may be present within the pustule (Fig. B).
3. The epidermis beneath the pustule shows spongiosis and migration of neutrophils through the epidermis (Fig. B).
4. The upper dermis shows a nonspecific inflammatory infiltrate, primarily perivascular (Fig. A).
5. Ruptured pustules show an absence of the stratum corneum and a crust composed of cellular debris.
6. The causative organisms are occasionally demonstrable with Gram stain.

Microscopic differential diagnosis

1. With H&E stain, impetigo is histologically indistinguishable from subcorneal pustular dermatosis of Sneddon and Wilkinson (see p. 588).
2. Microscopic features of impetigo may resemble those of pemphigus foliaceus (see p. 540), but can usually be distinguished by the following:
   a. acantholytic cells are much more numerous in pemphigus foliaceus;
   b. neutrophils are usually scant or absent in pemphigus foliaceus;
   c. dyskeratosis is absent in impetigo.
3. The subcorneal pustule of erythema toxicum neonatorum resembles the pustule of impetigo of Bockhart (see p. 159), but differs by the presence of eosinophils rather than neutrophils in the pustule cavity.
4. The histologic picture is identical to that of acropustulosis of infancy, an idiopathic pustular eruption of the distal portions of the extremities which clears spontaneously.

Comment

1. *Ecthyma* is an ulcerating variant of impetigo.
2. *Blastomycosis-like pyoderma* is a condition resembling blastomycosis clinically, found in debilitated individuals. It is believed to be secondary to bacterial invaders. Except for the organisms, the microscopic picture resembles that of blastomycosis (see p. 358).

IMPETIGO

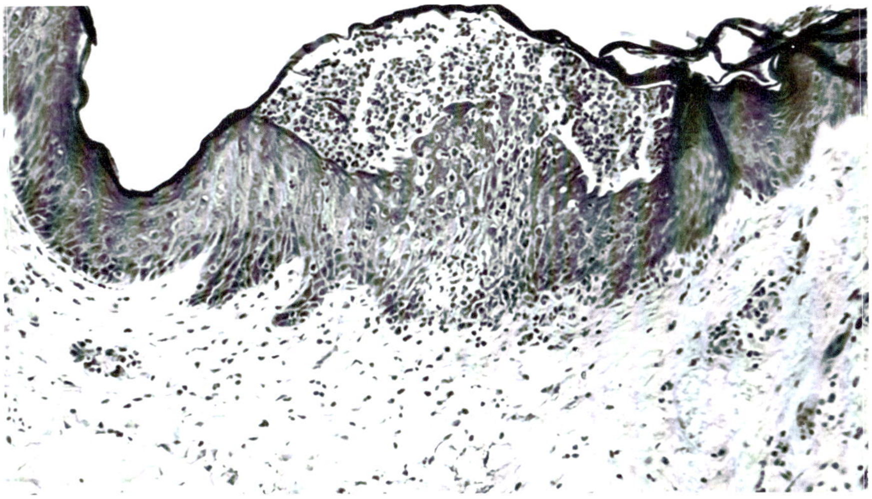

A
X195

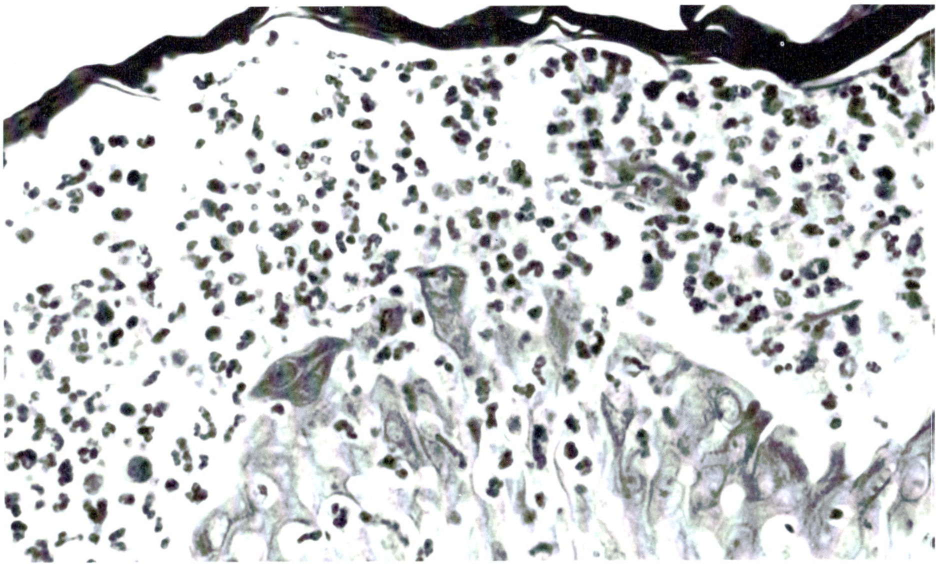

B
X530

ERYSIPELAS

Erysipelas is an acute superficial cellulitis caused by group A streptococci. Lesions are well-demarcated reddish areas of swelling (Fig. A). The face is the most common location, followed by the extremities. Repeated attacks of cellulitis of the extremities or penis may cause chronic lymphedema (elephantiasis).

Microscopic features

1. The basic feature is perivasculitis, with an inflammatory infiltrate around blood and lymph vessels throughout the dermis.
2. The inflammatory infiltrate, which may be sparse, is composed mainly of neutrophils.
3. With Giemsa or Gram stain, streptococci can be demonstrated in connective tissue or lymphatics.

ERYSIPELAS

A

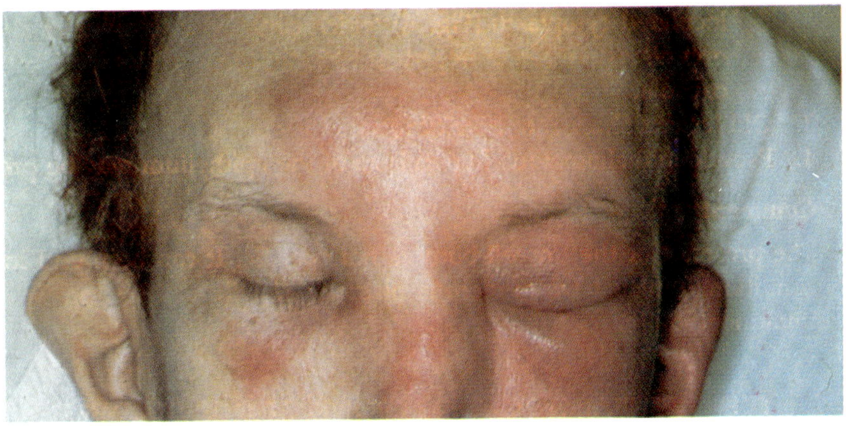

RHINOSCLEROMA

Rhinoscleroma is a chronic infectious disease believed to be due to the Frisch bacillus (*Klebsiella rhinoscleromatis*). The disease involves the upper respiratory tract and adjacent skin, and produces extensive granulomatous masses, particularly in the nose and on the upper lip (Figs. A,B).

Microscopic features

1. There is a chronic inflammatory infiltrate in which plasma cells predominate (Figs. C,D).
2. The infiltrate contains two special cells:
   a. The *Russell body* derives from the plasma cell. It is about twice the diameter of a plasma cell, and has a refractile eosinophilic cytoplasm (Fig. D).
   b. The *Mikulicz cell*. This cell has a diameter averaging 100 microns and a loculated cytoplasm (Fig. E) which contains numerous organisms. These organisms are Gram-negative, PAS-positive rods which have a gelatinous capsule.
3. Old lesions show extensive fibrosis.
4. Pseudoepitheliomatous hyperplasia of the epithelium may be present.

Comment

The presence of the Russell body is not specific. It can be found in many other conditions which have numerous plasma cells. Russell bodies are composed of immunoglobulins.

DIFFERENTIAL DIAGNOSIS OF INFECTIOUS DISEASES WITH HISTIOCYTIC INCLUSIONS

	Key histologic features	*Appearance of Organism*
Granuloma inguinale	Scattered abscesses composed of neutrophils. Numerous infected histiocytes.	Encapsulated ovoid bodies, 1–2 microns in diameter. Organism is Gram-negative and appears red with Giemsa stain; capsule does not stain. With silver stain, the organism has a bipolar appearance.
Rhinoscleroma	Very large infected histiocytes (Mikulicz cells). Russell bodies.	Encapsulated ovoid bodies, 2–5 microns in diameter. Organism is Gram-negative and PAS-positive.
Histoplasmosis	Foci of necrosis. Numerous infected histiocytes.	Ovoid bodies 2–4 microns in diameter, with PAS-positive cell wall; organism is surrounded by a halo representing a lysosomal vacuole.
Leishmaniasis	Numerous infected histiocytes. Tuberculoid infiltrates in late lesions.	The organism is not encapsulated; it shows a nucleus and kineteplast which stain red with Giemsa stain.

RHINOSCLEROMA

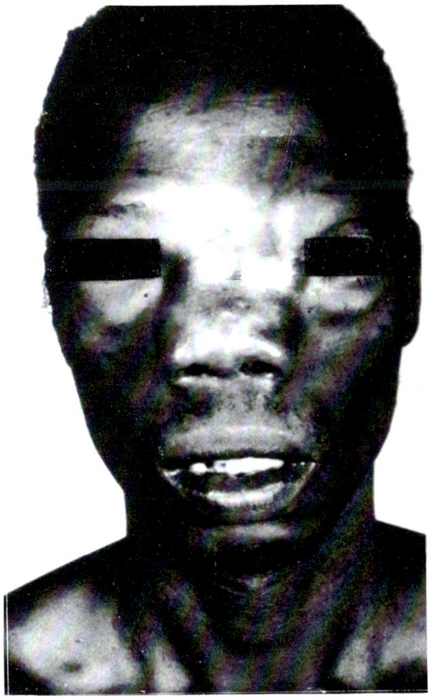

A

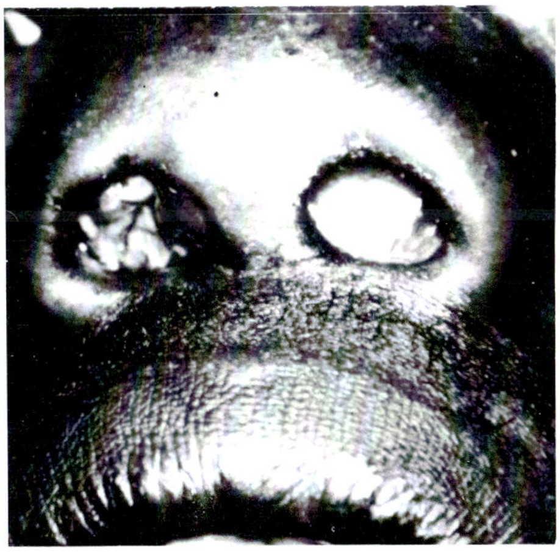

B

Figs. A,B courtesy Dr. S. Templeton

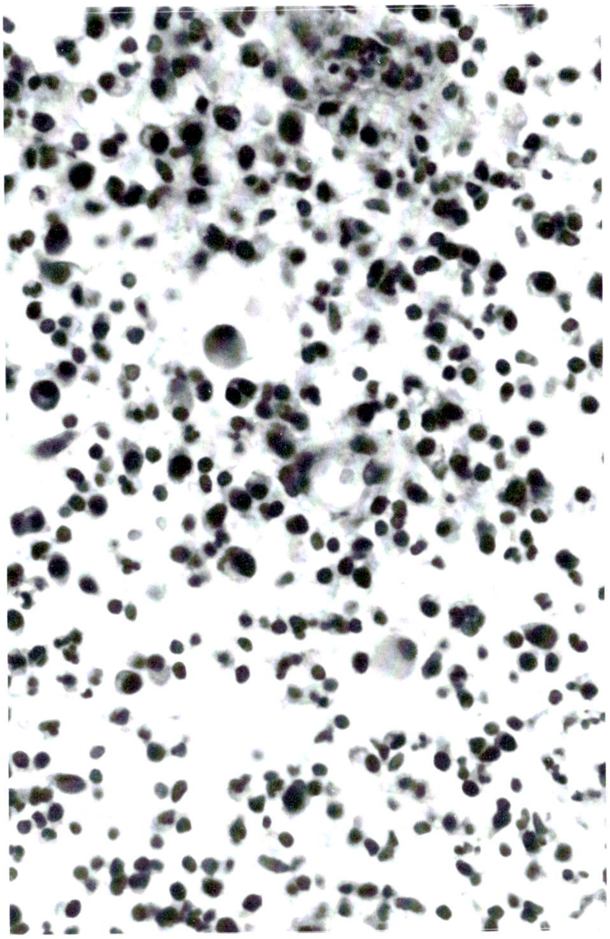

C
X720

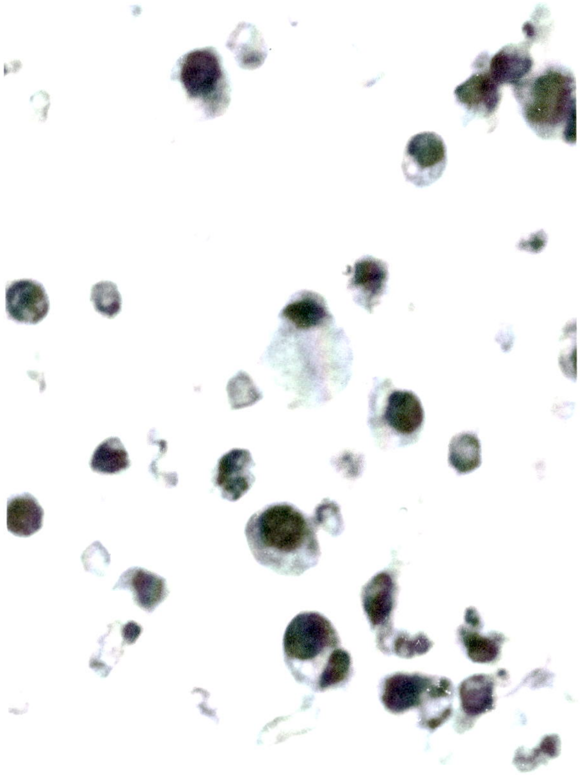

D
X1200

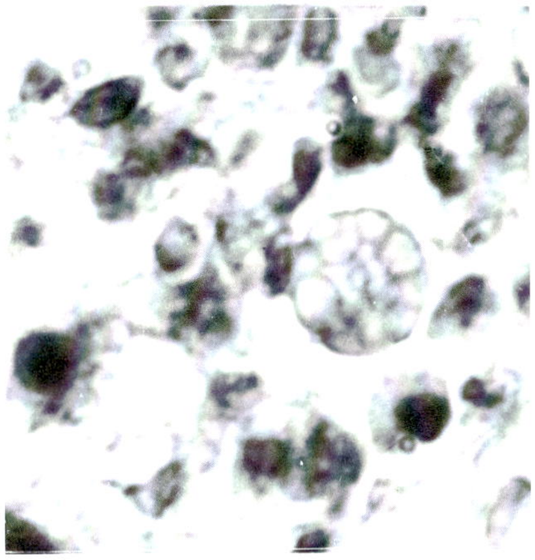

E
X1200

Figs. C,D,E courtesy Dr. John Knox

Some Bacterial Diseases of Minor Histologic Importance

ANTHRAX

Anthrax is caused by a Gram-positive bacillus (*Bacillus anthracis*) and is transmitted to man by infected animal materials (e.g., wool, hides). Lesions start as papules and enlarge with progressive necrosis, resulting in an ulceration covered by a black crust (eschar). Edema and sometimes vesiculation or erythema surround the lesion.

The microscopic picture is that of a nonspecific ulceration, with pronounced dermal edema and hemorrhage. Vascular necrosis may be present. Diagnosis is based on the presence of large numbers of the organism in the lesion. With Gram stain, the anthrax bacillus is large, distinctly rectangular and is surrounded by a capsule. Organisms are not found intracellularly.

STREPTOCOCCAL CELLULITIS

Streptococcal cellulitis, including erysipelas (a well-demarcated form of superficial cellulitis) has the nonspecific histologic pattern of perivasculitis with extensive dermal edema. Neutrophils are typically present. Organisms can be demonstrated in tissue spaces with Gram stain or Giemsa stain, sometimes with difficulty.

INFECTIOUS DISEASES CAUSING VASCULITIS

Acute septicemia due to meningococcus or gonococcus is characterized by leukocytoclastic vasculitis. Diagnosis is based on identification of the organisms with Gram stain, immunofluorescent tests, and bacterial culture. Chronic forms show less severe microscopic changes than acute forms. Rickettsial diseases also show a leukocytoclastic vasculitis. In Rocky Mountain spotted fever (a rickettsial disease) organisms are too small to be demonstrated with light microscopy; they can be demonstrated with direct immunofluorescence. *Ecthyma gangrenosum* is a result of pseudomonas septicemia. The infection usually occurs in debilitated individuals. Lesions are punched-out ulcers. Bacilli invade the walls of veins and superficial vessels. In overwhelming infection, there is no inflammatory response. Septic emboli with gangrene may occur.

ERYTHRASMA

Erythrasma is a superficial infection caused by *Corynebacterium minutissimum*. Lesions are sharply-marginated, reddish-brown patches in the intertrigenous areas which fluoresce with a coral-red color under Wood's lamp. Microscopically, Gram-positive rods are observed in the stratum corneum. Organisms are PAS-positive and diastase-resistant.

CHANCROID

Chancroid ("soft chancre") is a venereal disease caused by the Ducrey bacillus (*Hemophilus ducreyi*). Chancroid is characterized by one or more painful ulcers in the genital region (Fig. A). The ulcers are usually nonindurated and occur in greater numbers than the chancres of primary syphilis. Soft chancres also differ from the chancres of primary syphilis by their jagged, undermined margins. Regional nodes are painful and tender. Suppuration and drainage may occur.

Microscopic features

1. Histologic changes are not diagnostic, and resemble those of the luetic chancre. However, plasma cells may not be as abundant (Figs. B,C). Rarely the Gram-negative coccobacilli are visible in the upper portions of the lesion.
2. The organisms also stain with Giemsa stain. Fluorescent antibody staining of smears is a reliable method for confirming the diagnosis. In the absence of indentification of the organism, genital herpes simplex is sometimes misdiagnosed as chancroid.

CHANCROID

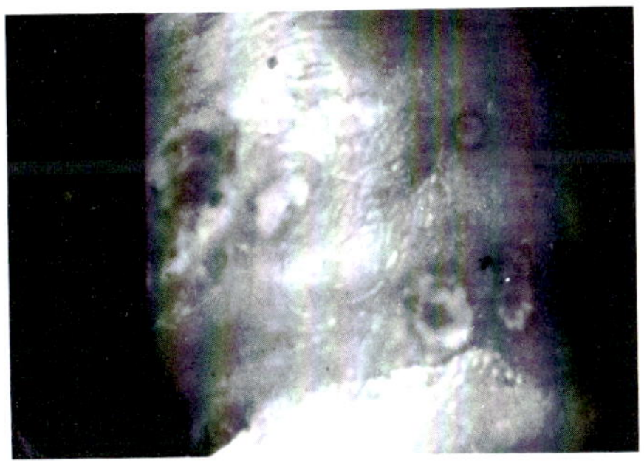

A

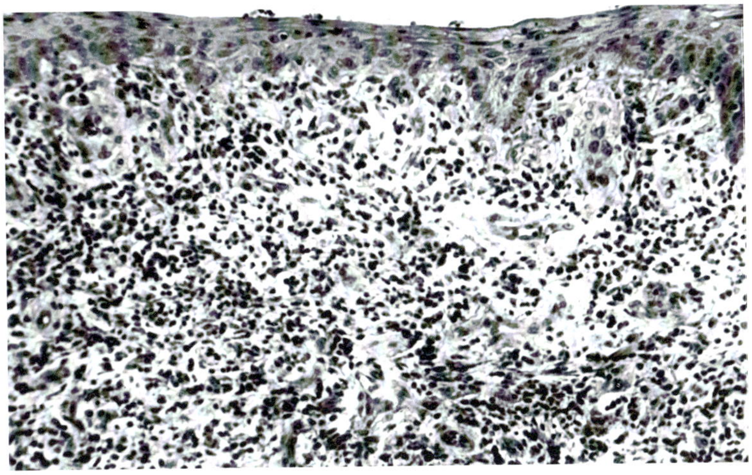

B
X180

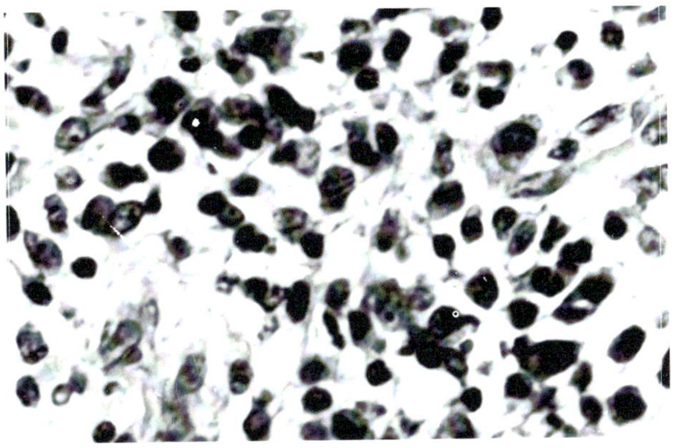

C
X670

SYPHILIS

Syphilis is a treponematosis caused by *Treponema pallidum*. It can be acquired by sexual contact, or it can be congenital. Early syphilis includes primary and secondary stages. Late syphilis is called tertiary syphilis. There is also a latent stage (early and late). Organisms are usually not demonstrable in lesions of late syphilis.

Cutaneous lesions of congenital syphilis are the same as those of acquired secondary or tertiary syphilis, except that bullous lesions occur and juxta-articular nodes do not occur.

The basic pathologic change in syphilis is proliferation and endothelial swelling of capillaries accompanied by a perivascular lymphoid and plasma cell infiltrate. The late stages have the additional feature of granuloma formation, with or without caseation necrosis.

Although histologic patterns may suggest a diagnosis of syphilis, they are not specific enough to establish the diagnosis. The diagnosis of syphilis is made by serologic tests or by direct demonstration of the organism.

PRIMARY SYPHILIS

Primary syphilis is characterized by single or multiple, painless, eroded papules at the site of contact which progress to form indurated, well-defined ulcers (chancres) (Fig. A). Chancres are accompanied by regional lymphadenopathy without drainage.

Microscopic features

1. There is a dense, usually confluent dermal infiltrate, composed principally of lymphocytes and plasma cells. Occasionally, in early lesions, neutrophils and lymphocytes predominate. Where the infiltrate is less dense, it generally has a perivascular distribution. (Figs. B,C).
2. Endothelial proliferation and edema may be present. Some vessels may show inflammatory cells within their walls.
3. Special stains, such as the Levaditi silver stain (Fig. D) reveal spirochetes extracellularly and intracellularly in the lesions. Spirochetes are numerous in endothelial cells and in the perivascular areas. Currently, fluorescent antibody techniques (Fig. E) can be used to demonstrate spirochetes in frozen sections.
4. The involved regional lymph nodes show a nonspecific inflammatory reaction, occasionally accompanied by granuloma formation. Spirochetes are present.

PRIMARY SYPHILIS

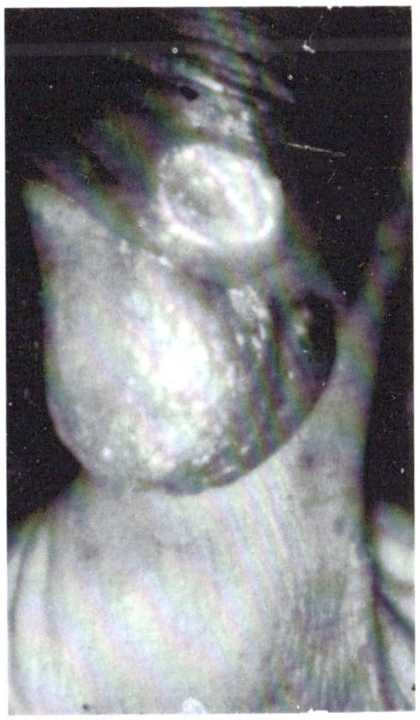

A

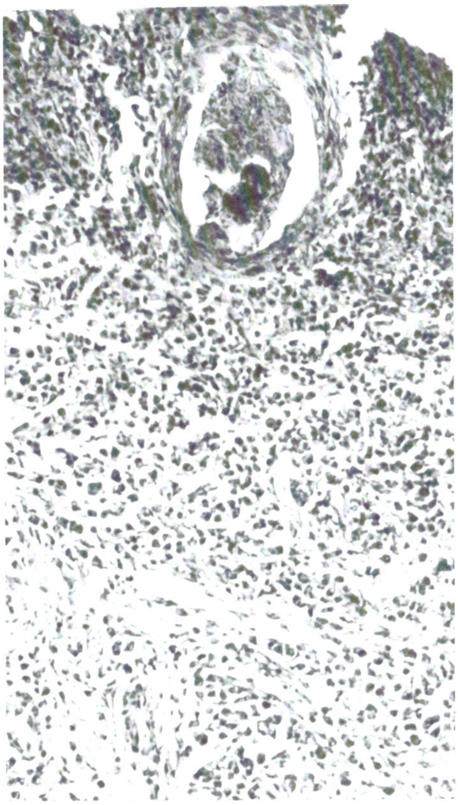

B
X230

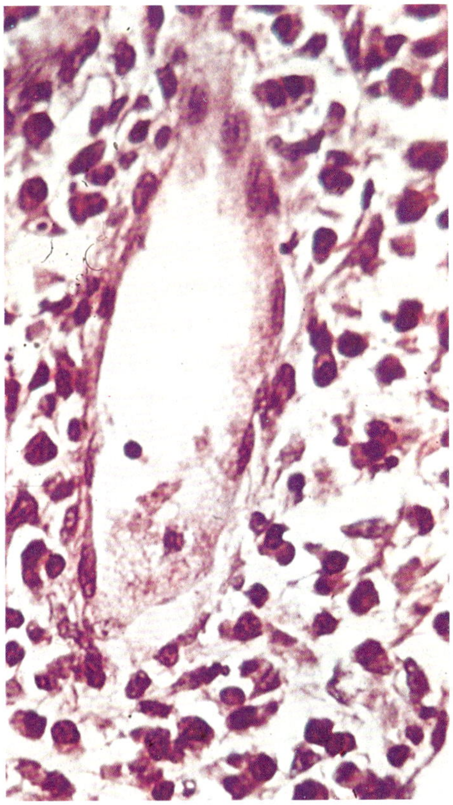

C
X840

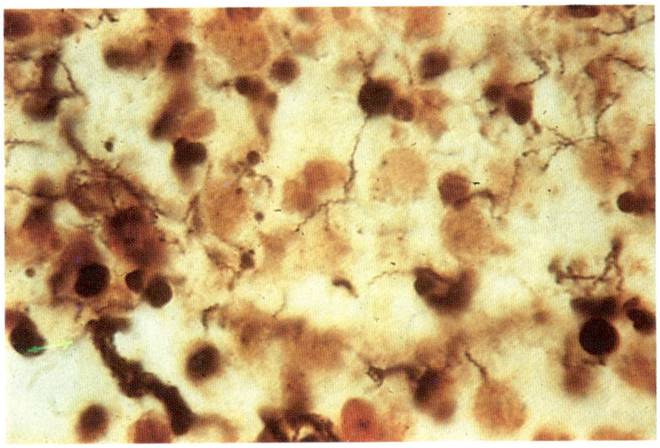

D
X1000

Figs. D,E courtesy Dr. Nicholas Fiumara

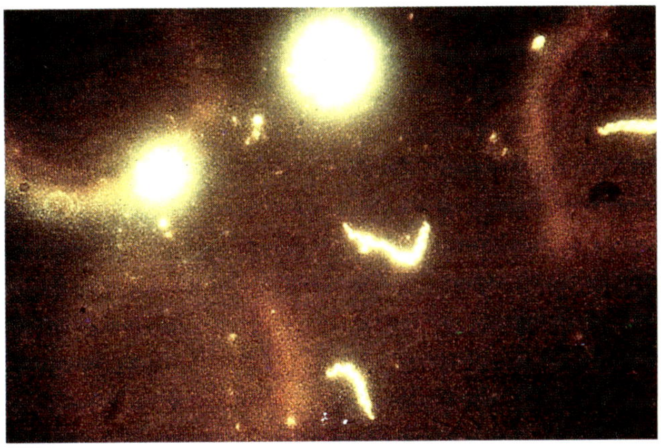

E
X1000

SYPHILIS continued

SECONDARY SYPHILIS

Secondary syphilis represents a stage of spirochetemia, with widespread dissemination of organisms and constitutional symptoms. Occasionally, there is a benign self-limited hepatitis. Less frequently, glomerulonephritis or nephrosis occur. Cutaneous lesions show great variability in appearance and number. Macular lesions resemble viral or bacterial exanthems, but may have a rather distinctive coppery color (Fig. A). Papulosquamous lesions are common. Some resemble psoriasis (Fig. B), and others show a peripheral scale (collarette) (Figs. C,D). The palms, soles, and perioral area are often involved. Pustules occur, and when they rupture there is an accumulation of scale and crust (Fig. E). Ulcerating lesions occur in the rare lues maligna.

The early exanthem seen in AIDS before seroconversion may be clinically indistinguishable from early secondary syphilis.

SECONDARY SYPHILIS

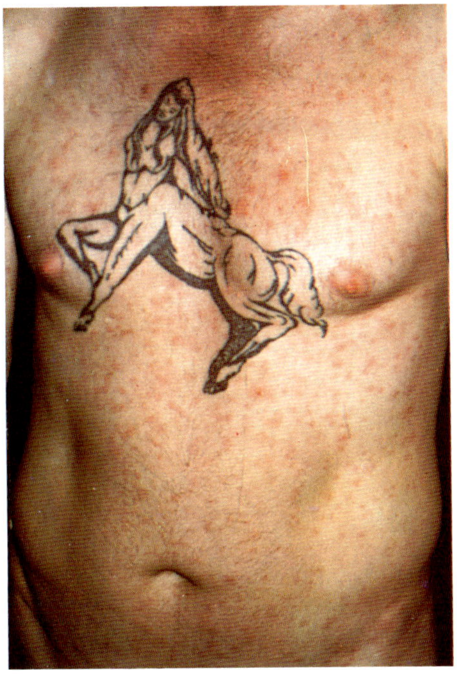

A

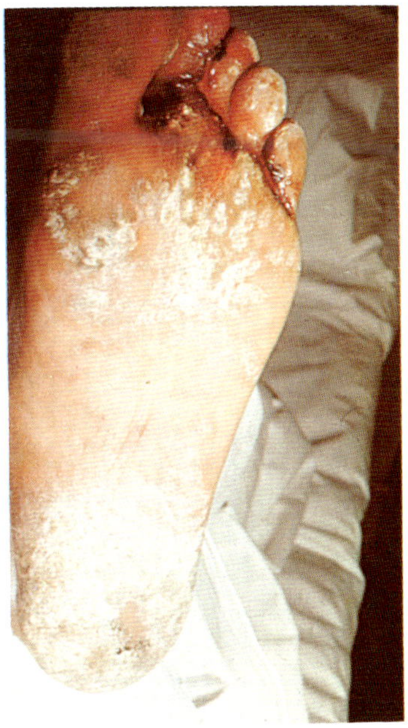

B

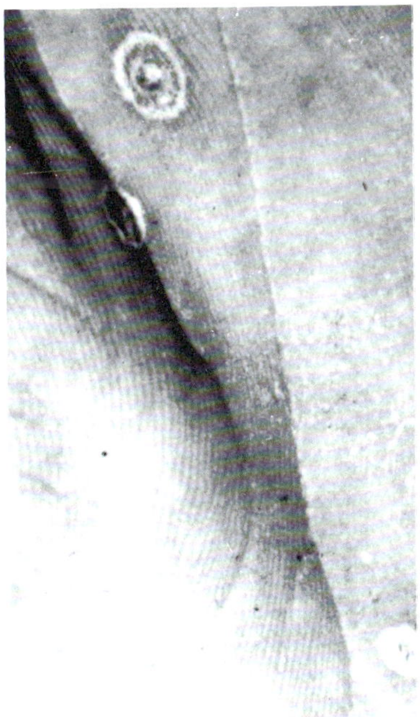

C

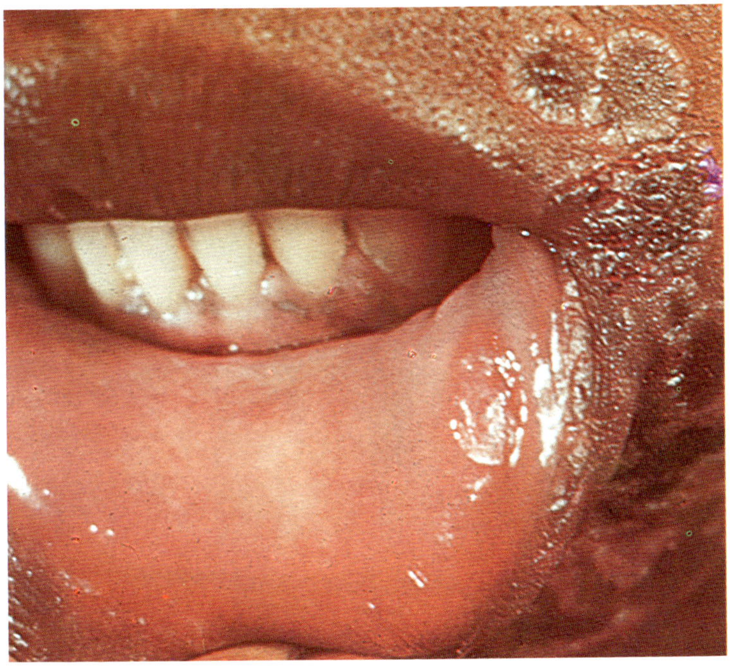

D

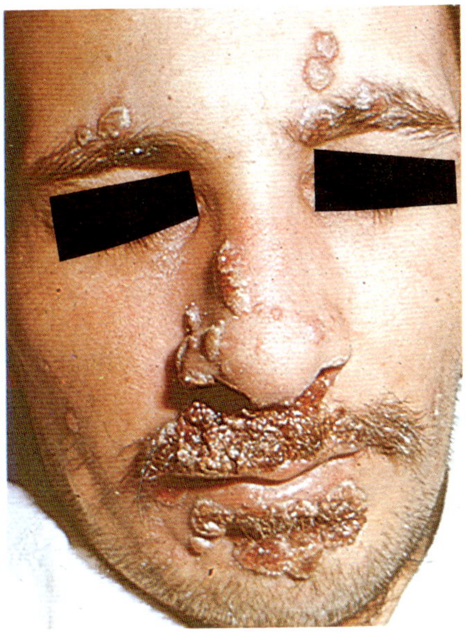

E

SYPHILIS continued ⇨

SECONDARY SYPHILIS

Lesions of late secondary syphilis may be nodular (Fig. A) and resemble nodules of lymphoma, both clinically and histologically. Moist, eroded papules of the intertriginous areas and mucocutaneous junctions are called *condylomata lata* (Fig. B). Superficial, necrotic areas of the mucous membranes may develop. These are called *mucous patches* (Figs. C,D,E).

A moth-eaten alopecia may occur.

SECONDARY SYPHILIS

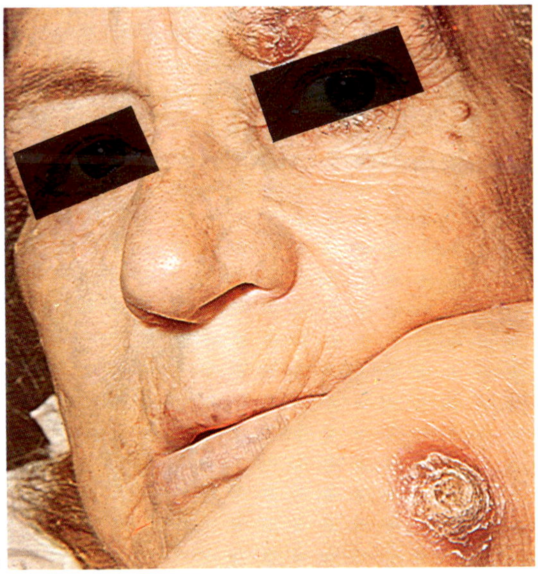

A

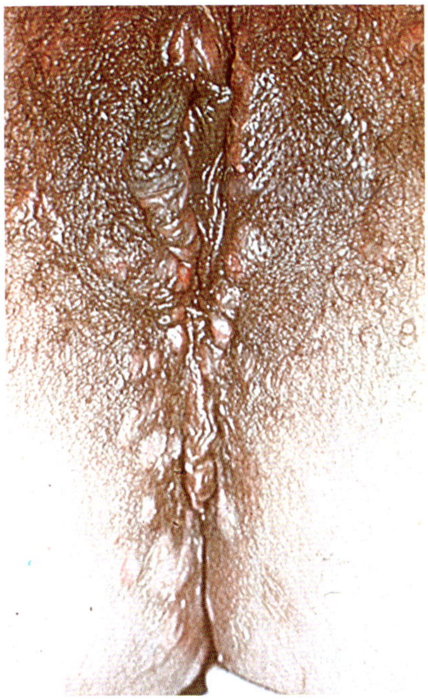

B

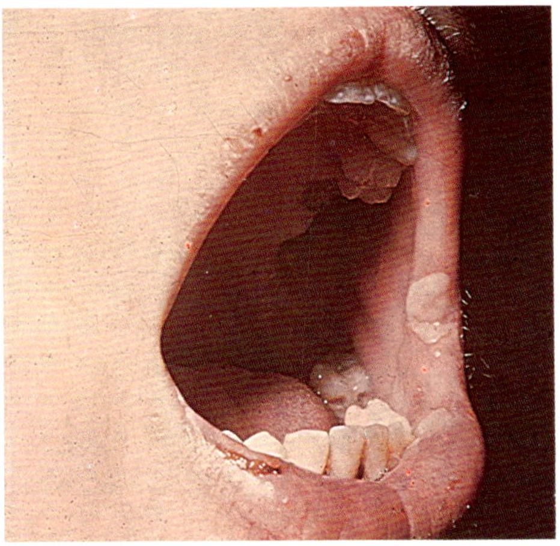

C

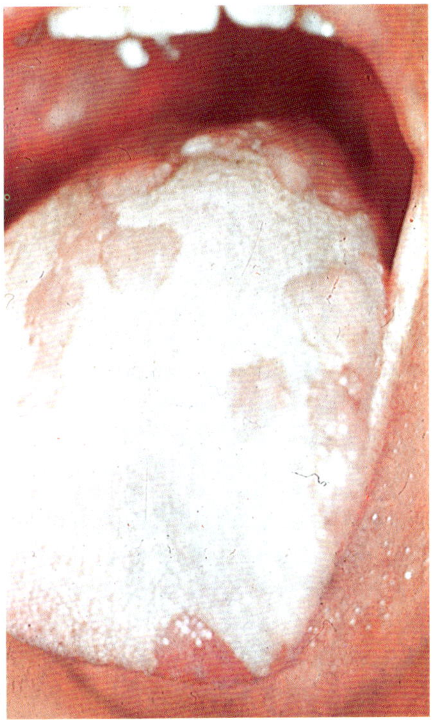

D

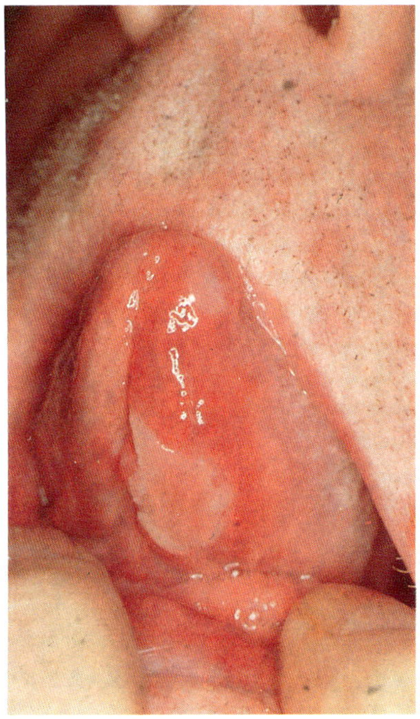

E

SYPHILIS continued

SECONDARY SYPHILIS

Microscopic features

1. Lesions show endothelial swelling (Fig. B), sometimes accompanied by endothelial proliferation and an inflammatory infiltrate.
2. There is a sharply marginated, patchy, perivascular infiltrate ("coat-sleeve") composed principally of plasma cells (Figs. A,B). Occasionally lymphocytes and neutrophils may predominate. In macular lesions the infiltrate is often minimal and nonspecific. A leukocytoclastic vasculitis is rarely present.
3. Irregular acanthosis is often present in crusted lesions, and the epidermis is frequently infiltrated by neutrophils. Papulosquamous lesions can show a picture resembling psoriasis, with clubbing acanthosis, Munro microabscesses, and spongiform pustules.
4. Ulcerative lesions may occur due to the endarteritis ("lues maligna").
5. Condylomata lata show epidermal erosions, with acanthosis and intercellular edema of the adjacent epidermis, in addition to the inflammatory changes cited above.
6. The Levaditi stain or immunofluorescence staining may show varying numbers of spirochetes. These are most numerous in lesions involving mucous membrane and mucocutaneous junctions. Spirochetes are sparse in morbilliform lesions.
7. Luetic alopecia shows a nonspecific perifolliculitis with large numbers of plasma cells and occasional giant cells.
8. In late lesions of secondary syphilis, granulomas may occur, making distinction from tertiary syphilis difficult.
9. Follicular papulopustular secondary syphilis shows a perifollicular arrangement of sarcoidal granulomas, as well as the usual inflammatory infiltrate of secondary syphilis.

SECONDARY SYPHILIS

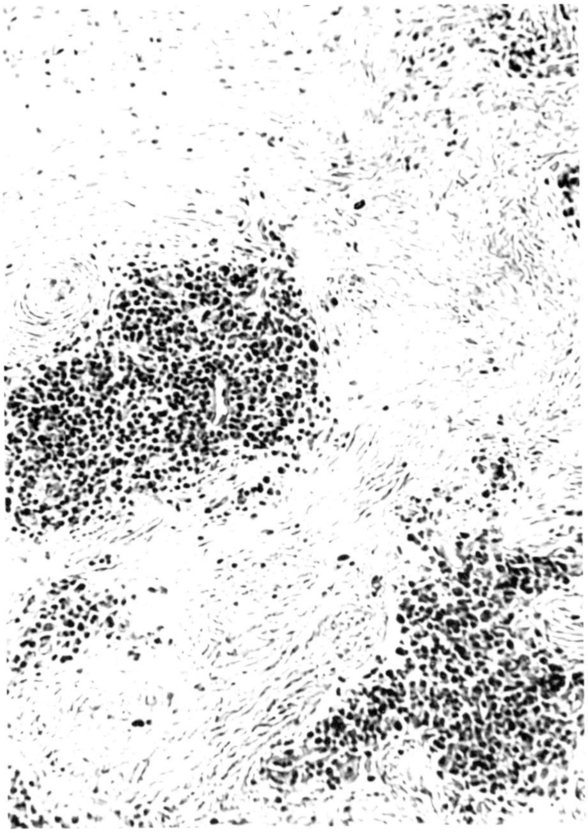

A
X220

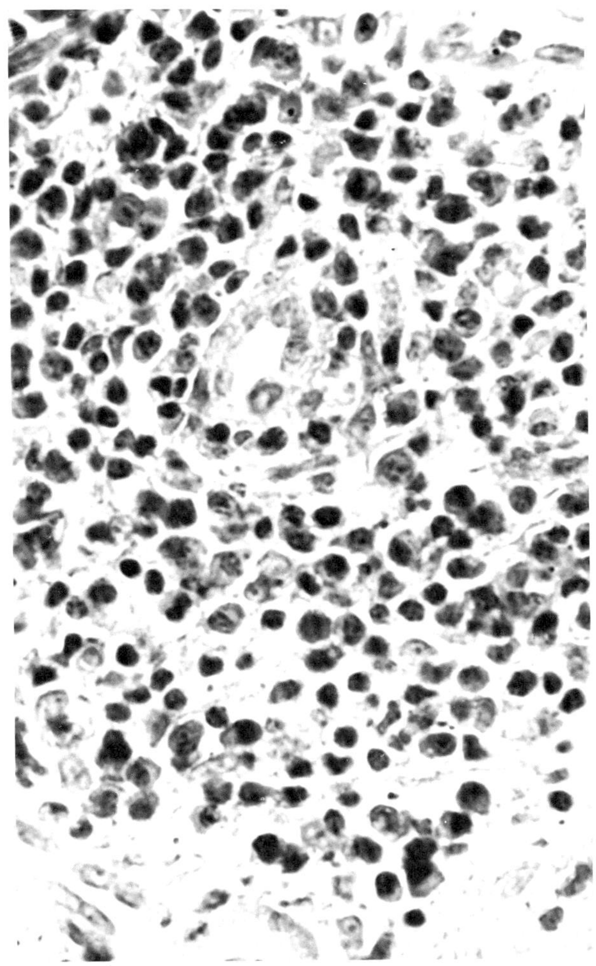

B
X780

SYPHILIS continued

SECONDARY SYPHILIS

Microscopic differential diagnosis

1. The patchy infiltrate of secondary syphilis has a resemblance to cutaneous lymphoma. Differentiation can sometimes be made on the basis of vascular changes in secondary syphilis and the presence of cellular atypicality in lymphoma. However, atypical nuclei have been reported in secondary syphilis. Conversely, cellular atypicality may be absent in well-differentiated lymphoma.
2. Lupus erythematosus may have a patchy dermal infiltrate, but usually can be distinguished from secondary syphilis by the characteristic epidermal changes and by the absence or sparsity of plasma cells.
3. The distinct perivascular cuffing of the infiltrate of erythema annulare centrifugum (see p. 122) results in a resemblance to typical secondary syphilis under low power. However, erythema annulare centrifugum usually lacks an endarteritis and significant plasma cell component.
4. It is important to remember that the histologic picture in secondary syphilis is variable, and at best can be considered suggestive, but not diagnostic. The histologic picture can resemble a variety of inflammatory conditions already cited. In addition, there can be a resemblance to PLEVA (see p. 146). However, when a pattern of PLEVA is seen together with many plasma cells, secondary syphilis must be suspected.

SYPHILIS continued

TERTIARY CUTANEOUS SYPHILIS

Cutaneous lesions of tertiary syphilis occur in a superficial nodular form and in a deeper form (gumma). The nodular lesions may become confluent and form an expanding arcuate margin (Figs. A,B). Superficial ulcerations may develop in such lesions.

Infrequently, asymptomatic subcutaneous nodules called *juxta-articular nodes* develop in patients with cutaneous tertiary syphilis. They are often symmetrically arranged in the vicinity of joints.

Microscopic features (nodular tertiary syphilis)

1. In tertiary syphilis, vascular changes similar to those described in secondary syphilis are usually present.
2. Frequently, a granulomatous infiltrate composed of lymphoid cells, plasma cells, histiocytes, fibroblasts, epithelioid cells, and giant cells is also present (Figs. C,D). Some of these giant cells may be of the Langhans type (Fig. C). Caseation is seen less frequently in the nodular form than in the gummatous form.
3. In nodular tertiary syphilis the pathologic process is more superficial than in gummatous tertiary syphilis and is limited to the dermis. Granuloma formation may be minimal in nodular tertiary syphilis, resulting in a histologic similarity to late secondary syphilis.
4. In late lesions of tertiary syphilis, fibrosis may be present.

Comment

Spirochetes are difficult to demonstrate in cutaneous lesions of tertiary syphilis.

TERTIARY SYPHILIS (NODULAR FORM)

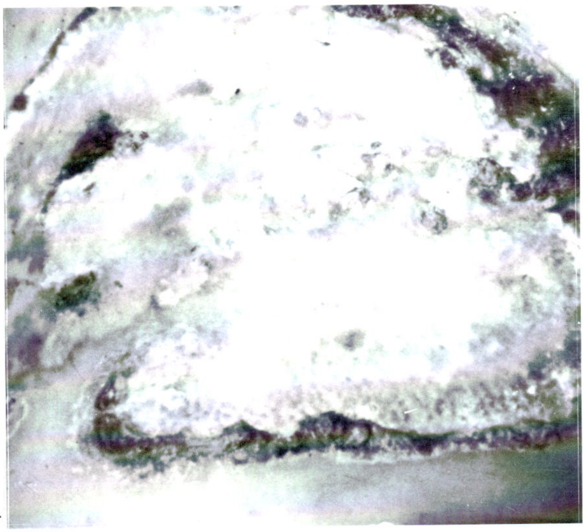

A

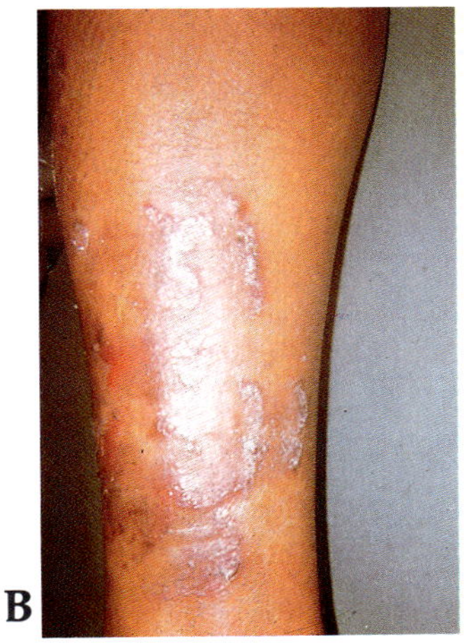

B

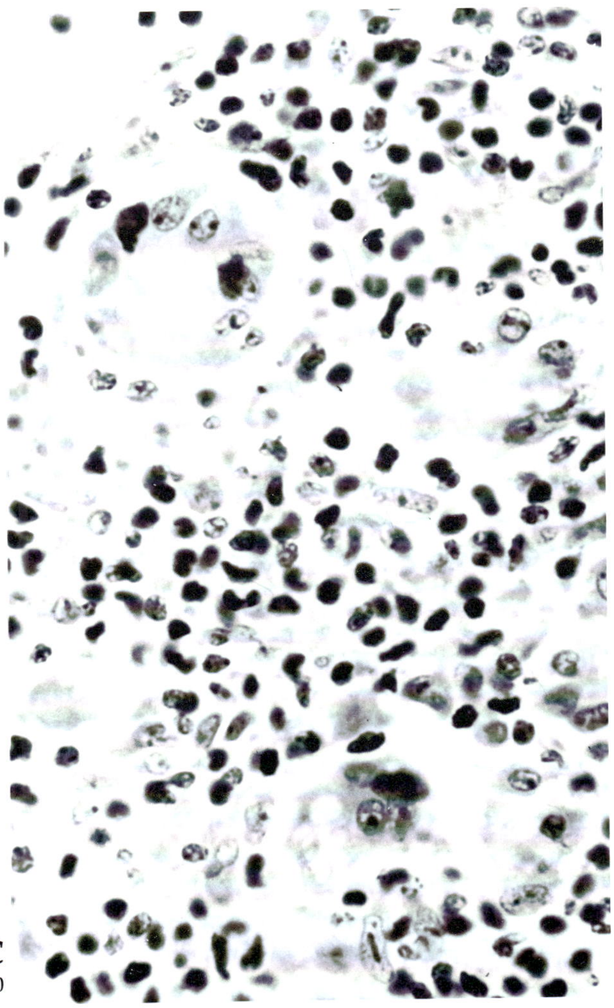

C
X810

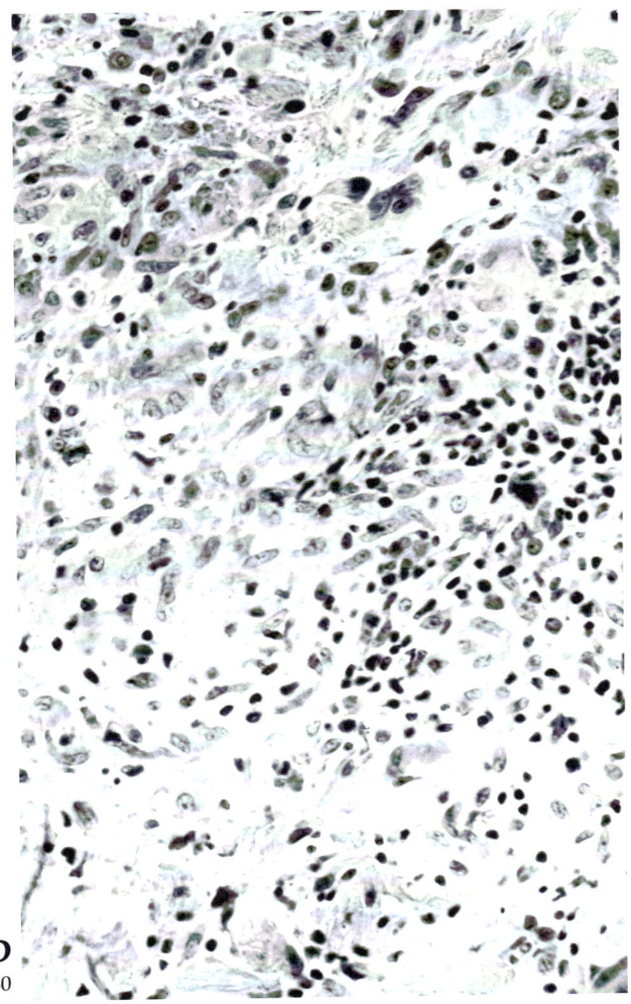

D
X380

SYPHILIS continued ⇨

TERTIARY CUTANEOUS SYPHILIS

Gummas are ulcerating granulomatous lesions, with extensive necrosis involving the dermis and subcutaneous tissue (Fig. A).

Microscopic features

1. Lesions show a granulomatous pattern similar to that of nodular tertiary syphilis (Fig. B), but have a greater degree of caseation (Fig. C). The infiltrate of lymphoid cells around the granulomas may be very dense (Figs. B,C).
2. Unlike nodular tertiary syphilis, the deeper dermis and subcutaneous fat are often involved.

Microscopic differential diagnosis of tertiary cutaneous syphilis

1. Unequivocal differentiation from other infectious and noninfectious granulomas is not possible.
2. Nodular tertiary syphilis greatly resembles lupus vulgaris; gummatous tertiary syphilis greatly resembles scrofuloderma and erythema induratum.
3. The presence of vascular changes and significant numbers of plasma cells favors a diagnosis of tertiary syphilis.

Comment

1. Juxta-articular nodes show varying degrees of inflammation, granuloma formation, and fibrosis. Late lesions show extensive fibrosis with thickened, hyalinized collagen fibers.
2. *Granuloma inguinale* is a chronic venereal infection involving the anogenital and/or inguinal areas. It is caused by a Gram-negative bacterium, *Calymmatobacterium granulomatis*. Fully developed lesions are sharply demarcated, confluent, granulating ulcers with raised margins. Squamous cell carcinoma may develop in longstanding lesions.

   The histologic picture shows an ulceration with a dense infiltrate composed principally of histiocytes and plasma cells. Scattered abscesses are present within the infiltrate. Large vacuolated histiocytes contain the organism (Donovan bodies); these are bright red with Giemsa stain and have a bipolar configuration. The bipolar configuration is easily demonstrated with silver stains. The capsule around the organism does not stain (see chart, p. 290).

   Organisms can be readily demonstrated in smears and thin sections.
3. *Yaws* and *pinta* are nonvenereal treponematoses caused by organisms which are morphologically identical to *T. pallidum*. Yaws is endemic to many tropical areas, and pinta is endemic to central America. The disorders have certain clinical and microscopic parallels to syphilis.
4. *Lyme disease* (erythema chronicum migrans) is a spirochetal infection transmitted by ticks of the genus *Ixodes*. An expanding erythematous ring forms around the tick bite. There may be late atrophic changes resembling morphea or acrodermatitis chronica atrophicans. Nonspecific inflammation is seen histologically, but the spirochete can be demonstrated with Levaditi stain or Warthin-Starry stain. Systemic symptoms can be present, as well as arthritis, cardiac abnormalities, and neurologic abnormalities. Lyme disease was first described in Europe. Initial cases in the United States were first observed in the Lyme, Connecticut area, with subsequent spread to other areas.

TERTIARY SYPHILIS (GUMMATOUS FORM)

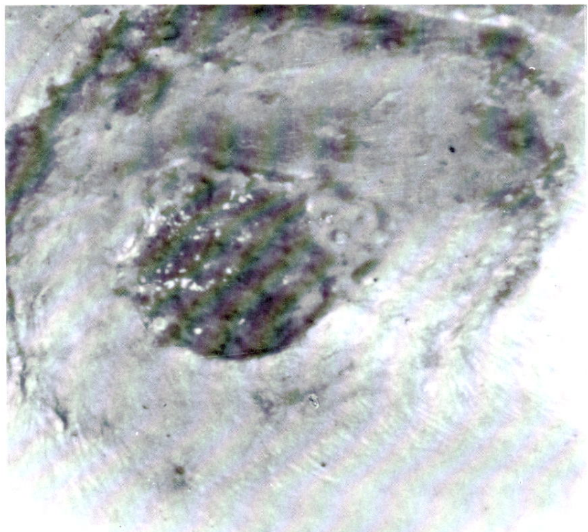

A

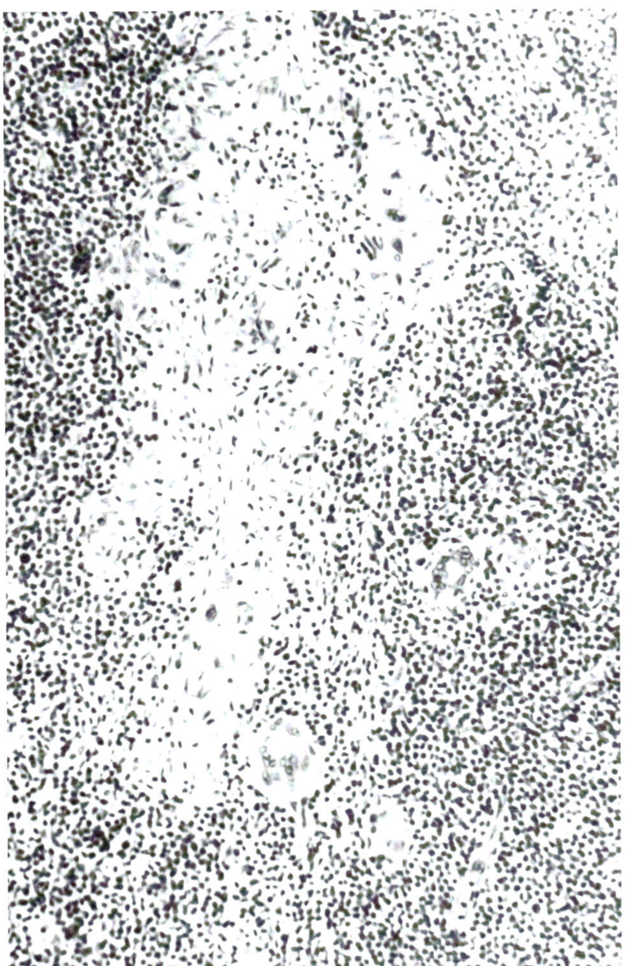

B PHLOXINE METHYLENE BLUE STAIN
X190

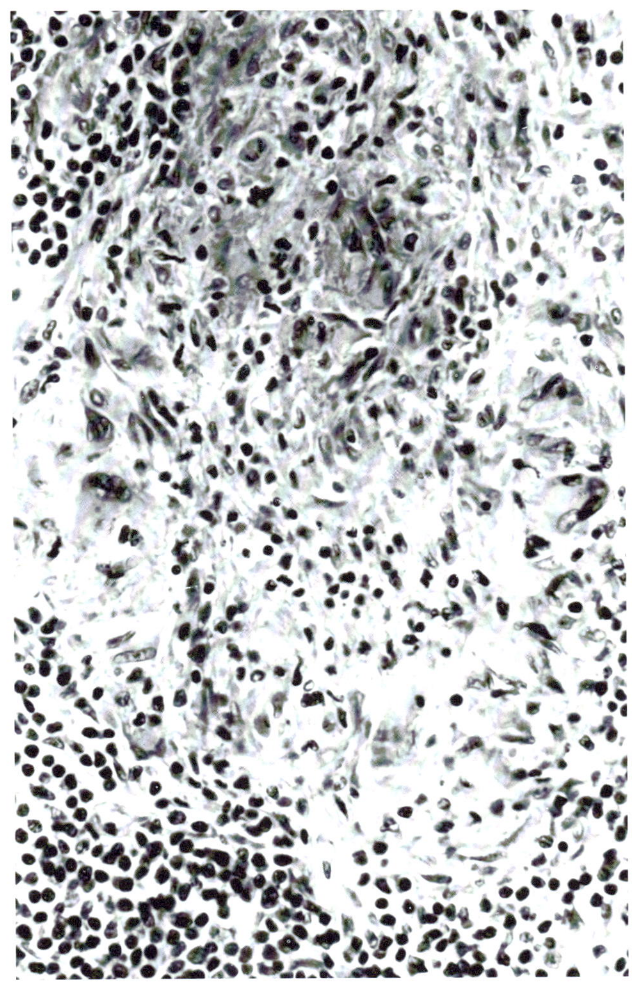

C PHLOXINE METHYLENE BLUE STAIN
X450

CUTANEOUS TUBERCULOSIS

Cutaneous tuberculosis is a granulomatous infectious disease caused by the acid-fast bacillus, *Mycobacterium tuberculosis*. There are two principal types: primary inoculation tuberculosis and reinfection tuberculosis. Primary inoculation tuberculosis of the skin is uncommon. The primary complex of the skin consists of a tuberculous chancre and the affected regional lymph nodes. Miliary tuberculosis represents generalized primary tuberculosis resulting from hematogenous dissemination in patients without significant immune response. It occurs most frequently in infants. The skin lesions are very small macules, papules, or purpuric areas on an erythematous base, which become vesicular and necrotic. Reinfection tuberculosis (secondary tuberculosis) occurs in individuals who have partial immunity. There are five cutaneous forms:

a. *Lupus vulgaris* is the most common form of cutaneous tuberculosis. It most frequently involves the head and neck, particularly the earlobes (Fig. A), nose, and cheeks (Fig. B). Initial lesions are soft, reddish-brown maculopapules which become confluent. Lesions progressively enlarge, ulcerate, and develop areas of atrophy and hypertrophic scarring (Fig. B). Involvement of underlying structures may result in mutilation. Squamous cell carcinoma may develop within areas of scarring.
b. *Tuberculosis verrucosa cutis* is a rare form of tuberculosis characterized by warty plaques. The extremities (Fig. C), particularly the dorsal surfaces of the hands and fingers, are most frequently involved. The clinical picture resembles that of blastomycosis and other deep mycoses.
c. *Scrofuloderma* results from tuberculous infection of the skin overlying deeper structures, such as lymph nodes, bones, and joints. A common site is the temporomandibular area. Initial lesions are subcutaneous nodules which break down to form draining ulcerations, fistulae, and sinus tracts (Figs. D,E), and ultimately granulation tissue and scars.
d. *Tuberculous gumma* (tuberculosis colliquativa) arises by hematogenous spread rather than by extension from underlying structures.
e. *Orificial tuberculosis* is a rare form of tuberculosis occurring in mucous membranes and adjacent skin by dissemination of organisms from involved viscera. The lesions are nodules which break down to form ulcers.

TUBERCULOSIS

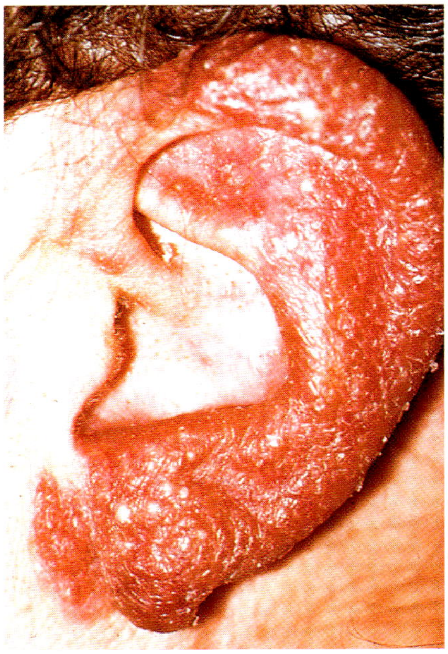
A

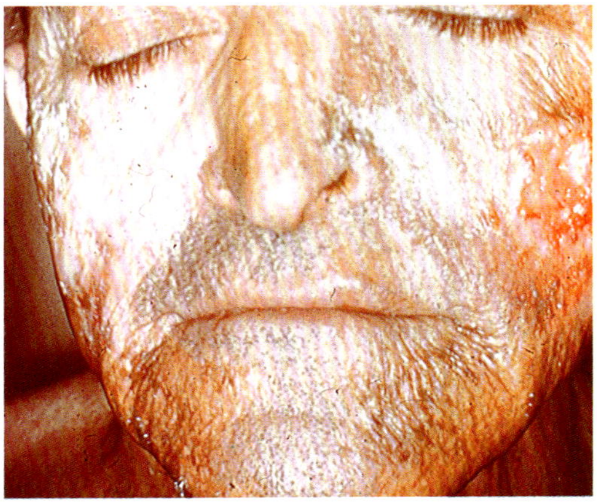
B

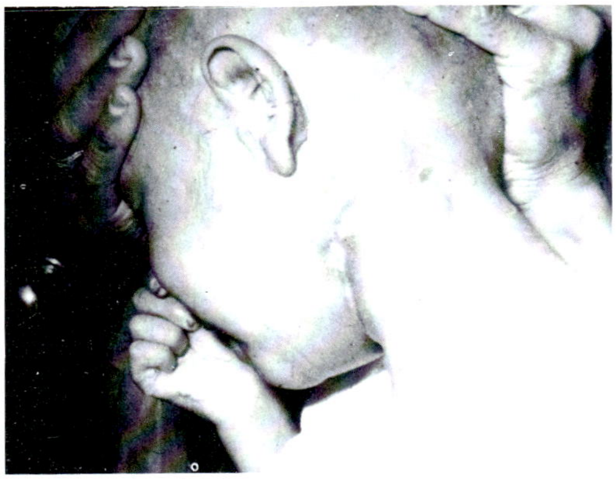
D

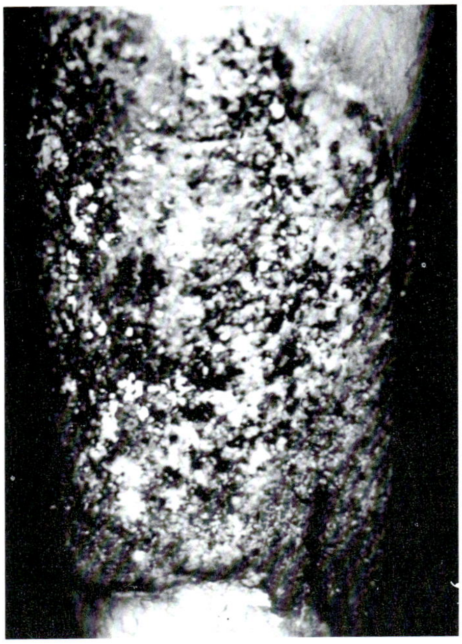
C

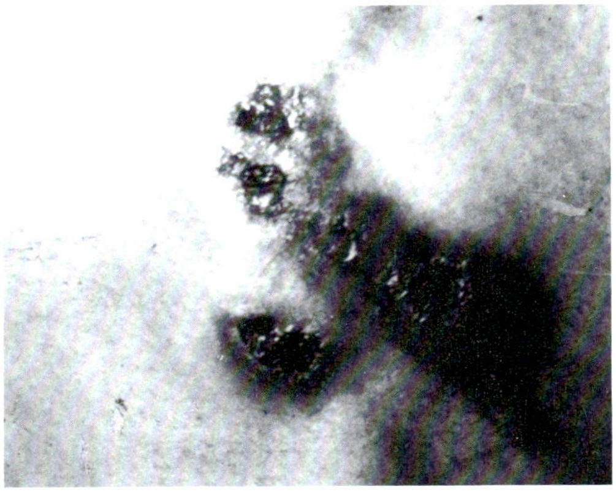
E

TUBERCULOSIS continued

CUTANEOUS TUBERCULOSIS

Microscopic features

1. Infection with *Mycobacterium tuberculosis* results in accumulations of macrophages which are transformed into epithelioid cells after they have phagocytosed organisms. This transformation was believed to be produced by an immunologic response to the lipoprotein in the organism.
2. Tuberculous infiltrates consist of discrete accumulations of epithelioid cells and Langhans giant cells (tubercles), surrounded by a ring of lymphoid cells (Figs. A,C,D). Caseation necrosis (which is believed to result from the degeneration of macrophages) (Fig. A) is frequently present in the centers of the tubercles. In some instances the epithelioid cells are more diffusely arranged.
3. All cutaneous forms of tuberculosis include these basic features.
4. In primary tuberculosis there is a transient early stage characterized by acute inflammation, necrosis, and ulceration. Many tubercle bacilli are present at this stage, and can be demonstrated with acid fast stain. Within 3 to 6 weeks a tuberculous infiltrate forms. The involved regional lymph nodes show the same pathologic changes as the cutaneous lesions.
5. In lupus vulgaris, the classical tuberculous infiltrate (tuberculoid infiltrate) is present (Figs. A,B,C,D) (usually in the upper dermis). Caseation necrosis may be pronounced (Figs. A,B) but is usually minimal (Fig. C). Tubercle bacilli are present in such small numbers that they are difficult to demonstrate histologically or even with culture. Late lesions show extensive fibrosis. Epidermal changes vary, but include atrophy, acanthosis, papillomatosis, and erosion. The infiltrate may cause loss of epidermal appendages. Margins of ulcers may show pseudocarcinomatous hyperplasia. In rare instances, squamous cell carcinoma may develop at the margins.
6. In tuberculosis verrucosa cutis, there is pronounced hyperkeratosis, papillomatosis, and acanthosis, along with the classical tuberculous infiltrate. Bacilli may be observed. An acute inflammatory infiltrate may be present in the upper dermis, and abscesses may be present in the upper dermis and epidermis.
7. In scrofuloderma and tuberculous gumma, the centers or superficial portions of the lesions show abscess formation, resulting in ulcerations or sinus tracts. Peripheral or deeper portions of lesions show a typical tuberculous infiltrate with pronounced caseation necrosis. Organisms are fairly numerous.
8. Orificial tuberculosis shows nonspecific inflammatory changes and/or the standard tuberculous infiltrate, with easily demonstrable tubercle bacilli. Tubercle bacilli are deep in the dermis. There is extensive necrosis.
9. Miliary tuberculosis has a nonspecific microscopic picture consisting of a perivasculitis with neutrophils, macrophages, and considerable necrosis; rarely, hemorrhage is present. Organisms are numerous.

TUBERCULOSIS

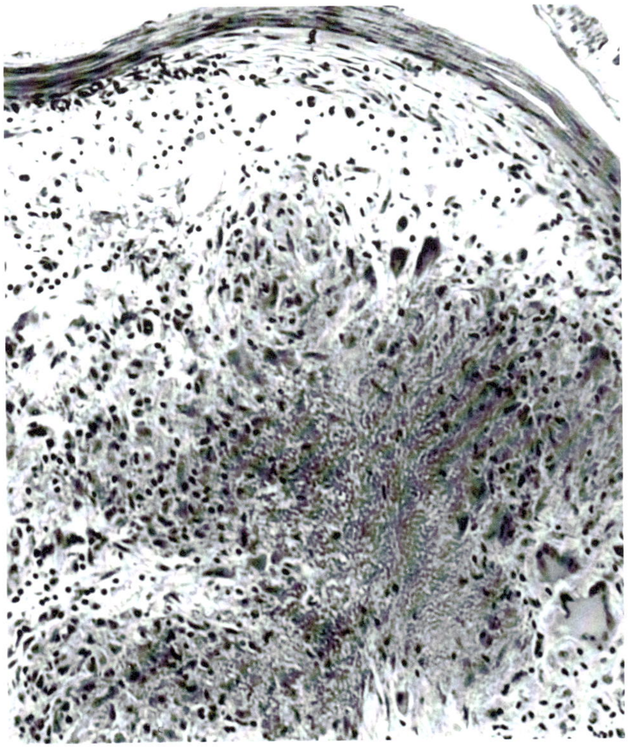

A
X260

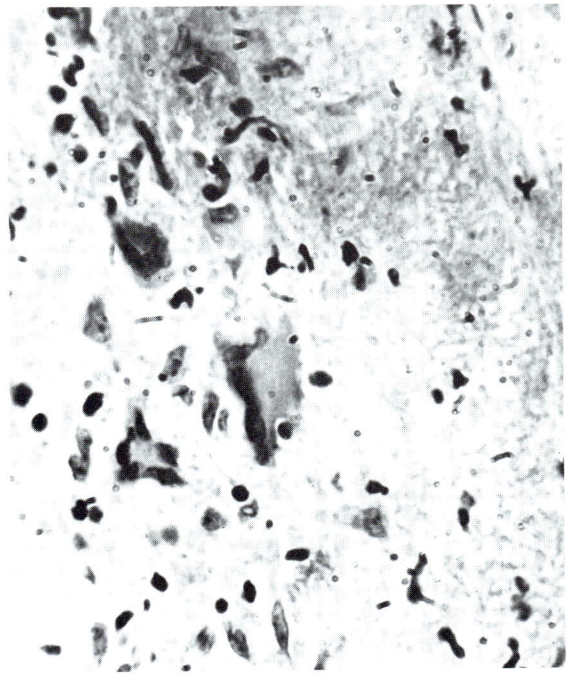

B
X550

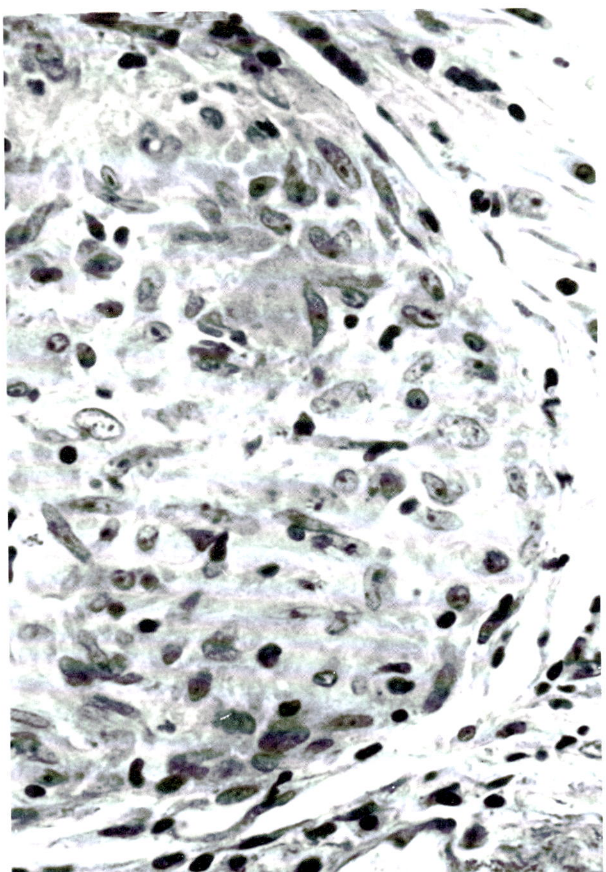

C
X730

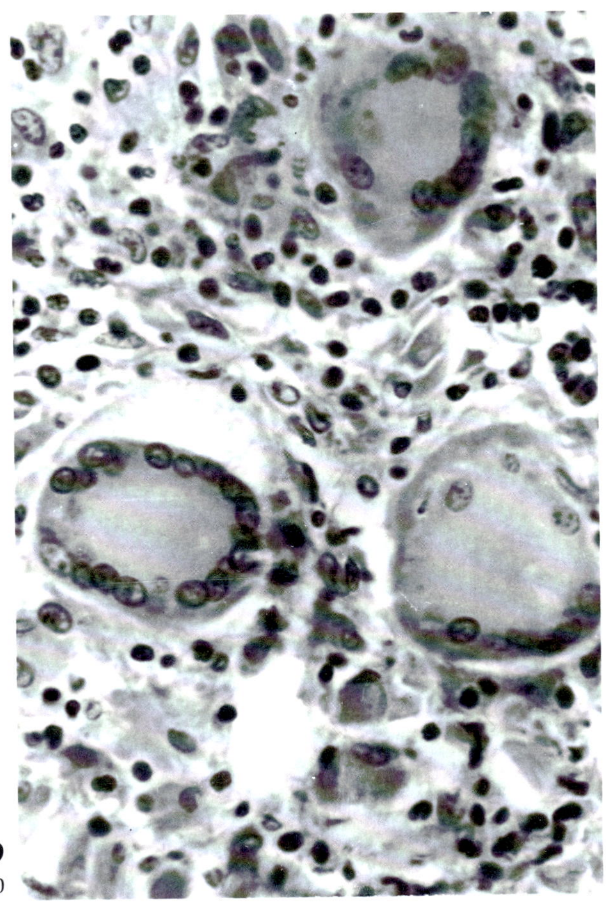

D
X720

TUBERCULOSIS continued ⇨

CUTANEOUS TUBERCULOSIS

Microscopic differential diagnosis

Like tertiary syphilis, the microscopic picture of tuberculosis is not specific and resembles that of many other infectious and non-infectious granulomas. Diagnosis depends on demonstration of the organism, either directly or by culture. Tubercle bacilli have classically been demonstrated in sections with acid fast stains. Newer methods, such as fluorescent staining with auramine on rhodamine can give results superior to those with acid fast stains.

Comment

1. In the past, many cutaneous granulomas were falsely believed to represent tuberculosis and were called *tuberculids*. Included in this category were erythema induratum (a form of panniculitis), lupus miliaris disseminatus faciei (a variant of rosacea), papulonecrotic tuberculid (possibly a variant of lymphocytic vasculitis), and lichen scrofulosorum (possibly representing either sarcoidosis or granuloma annulare).
2. Recent immunofluorescence studies have shown that the lymphoid cells at the periphery of tubercles are monocytes.

Atypical Mycobacterial infections

SWIMMING POOL GRANULOMA

Cutaneous granulomas which may heal spontaneously over a period of months are produced by infection with *Mycobacterium marinum (M. balnei). M. marinum* is an acid-fast bacillus with transverse bands; it is longer and broader than the tubercle bacillus and is cultured at 31° C. Infections with atypical mycobacteria other than *M. marinum* are rare.

The organism enters via abrasions sustained in swimming pools, fish tanks, oceans, or lakes. Initial lesions are soft papules and nodules, which tend to form crusted erosions (Figs. A,B). Common sites are the extensor aspects of the extremities, particularly hands, feet, elbows, and knees. Most lesions are solitary. Occasionally, a primary verrucous lesion at the distal end of an extremity is followed by satellite papules or ascending subcutaneous nodules (a picture resembling sporotrichosis).

Microscopic features

1. Early lesions show a nonspecific, mixed inflammatory infiltrate (Figs. C,D) in which acid fast organisms (Fig. E) may be demonstrated in small numbers within histiocytes.
2. With further development of the lesions, a diffuse granulomatous infiltrate forms. Caseation is usually minimal or absent. Organisms are difficult to find at this stage. Diagnosis can be established by culture or animal inoculation.
3. The epidermis may show erosions or reactive hyperplasia.

Microscopic differential diagnosis

Lesions most closely resemble tuberculosis verrucosa cutis; differentiation can be made by bacteriological studies.

Comment

1. Other atypical mycobacteria can produce lesions resembling swimming pool granuloma.
2. *Buruli ulceration* is a disorder endemic to central Africa and other tropical areas, caused by *M. ulcerans*. Exposed parts of the skin show a large, solitary ulceration. Acid-fast organisms are found in great numbers in necrotic tissue, which does not exhibit a significiant inflammatory response.
3. Atypical mycobacterial infections may occur in immunosuppressed individuals, including persons with AIDS.

SWIMMING POOL GRANULOMA

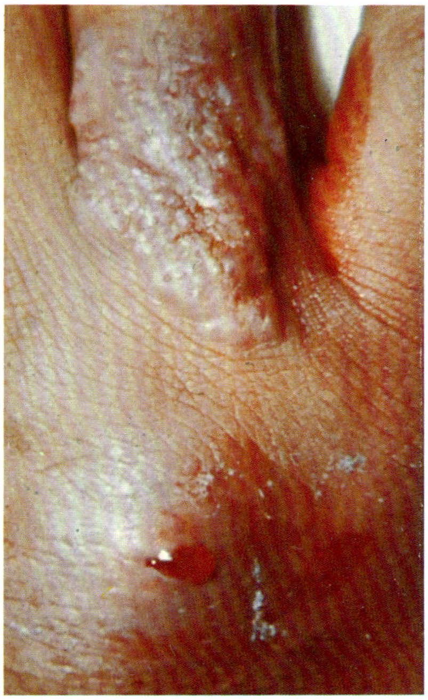

A

Figs. A,C,D courtesy Dr. John Knox

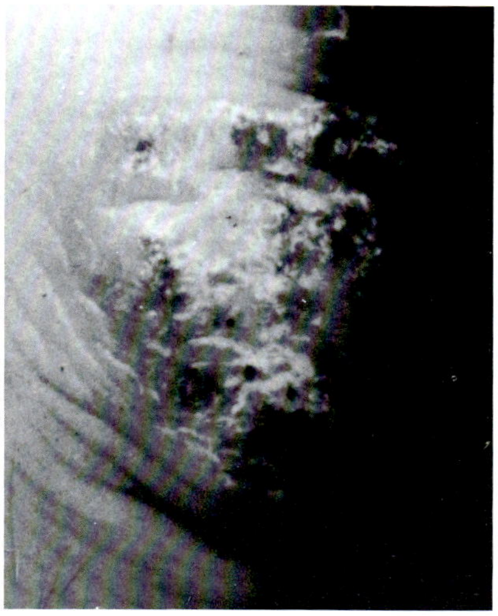

B

Courtesy Dr. Arthur Daily

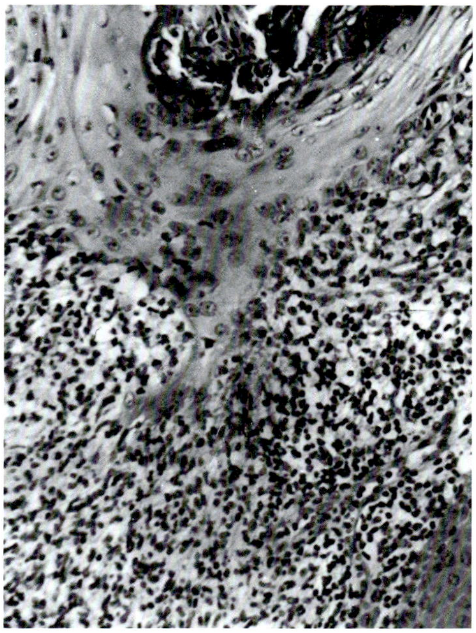

C

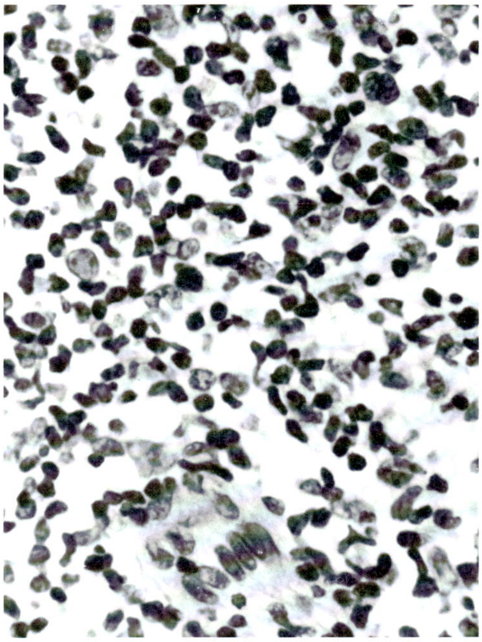

D
X720

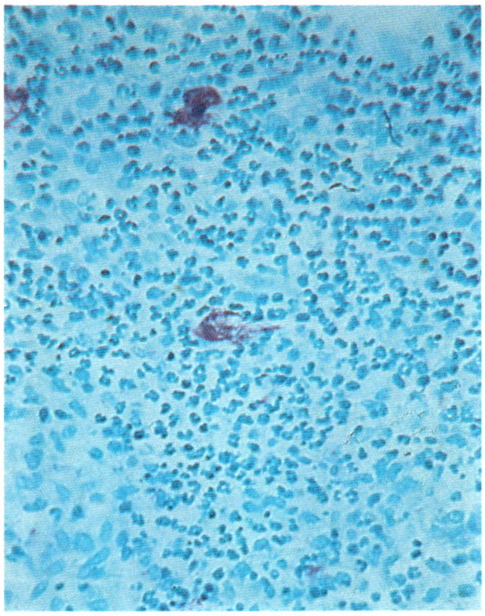

E
X500

LEPROSY (HANSEN'S DISEASE)

Leprosy is a chronic granulomatous disease due to *Mycobacterium leprae*. There is a predilection for the skin, peripheral nerves, and upper respiratory tract. The clinical manifestations vary with the host response; the severity of the disease is in inverse ratio to the immunological response, as indicated by the lepromin test.

Many cases are at either end of the host response spectrum: a) lepromatous leprosy—having the least host response; b) tuberculoid leprosy—having the greatest host response. In the middle of the spectrum are a range of forms with intermediate clinical, microscopic, and immunologic manifestations. *Indeterminate leprosy* refers to early erythematous or hypopigmented macules which may heal spontaneously or evolve into other forms of leprosy. Indeterminate leprosy shows a scattered nonspecific inflammatory infiltrate in the dermis.

LEPROMATOUS LEPROSY

Lepromatous leprosy most commonly affects the skin, mucous membranes, and peripheral nerves. Viscera (especially the liver and spleen) may be involved as the disease progresses. The eyes and testes may be involved.

Cutaneous lesions are usually symmetrical and begin as poorly defined macules with variable hypopigmentation. With progression, papules, nodules, and plaques appear (Fig. A). Extensive infiltrative lesions of the face result in leonine facies (Fig. A); this is often accompanied by loss of eyebrows and eyelashes (madarosis).

Early lesions of lepromatous leprosy have unimpaired sensory function and sweating. Eventually peripheral nerves become involved, with resulting sensory and autonomic impairment, trophic ulcers, atrophy, and paralysis.

Microscopic features

1. Lepra bacilli are slender rods about 5 microns in length. They are less acid-fast than tubercle bacilli. For this reason precautions must be taken against excessive decolorization during the acid-fast staining procedure. The Fite-Faracco stain is a good method for demonstrating lepra bacilli. Lepra bacilli have a tendency to be grouped in clumps or masses called *globi* (they resemble a pack of cigars) (Fig. E). The number of organisms present is in inverse ratio to the degree of immunity; in lepromatous leprosy, therefore, they are quite numerous.
2. The characteristic dermal infiltrate consists of numerous lipidized histiocytes called *lepra cells*. These are present in small groups or larger masses (Figs. B,C,D). The infiltrate is usually separated from the epidermis by an uninvolved zone (grenz zone).
3. Plasma cells and lymphoid cells may be present in the infiltrate, usually in very small numbers; they are present in greatest numbers in the perineurium.
4. In older lesions, there is destruction of the cutaneous appendages.
5. Large peripheral nerves are generally more severely involved than the small cutaneous nerves, and show invasion of Schwann cells by numerous lepra bacilli; in late stages the nerves become thickened and hyalinized.

Comment

The lepromin test is not a diagnostic test for leprosy. It is used as a prognostic indicator in patients with the disease to determine tissue response to the organism. The lepromin test may be positive or negative in persons without leprosy.

LEPROMATOUS LEPROSY

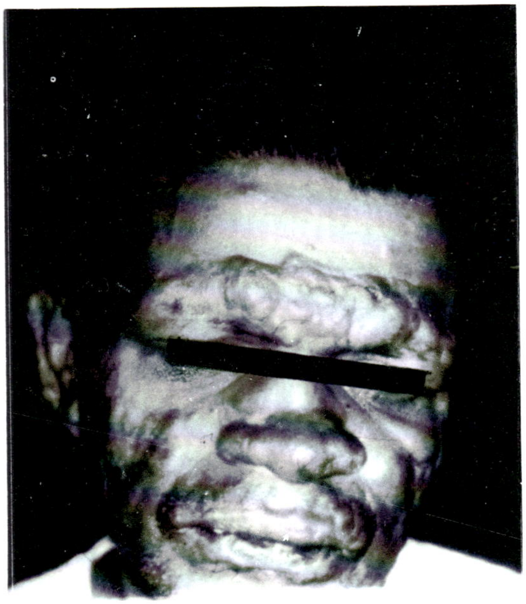

A

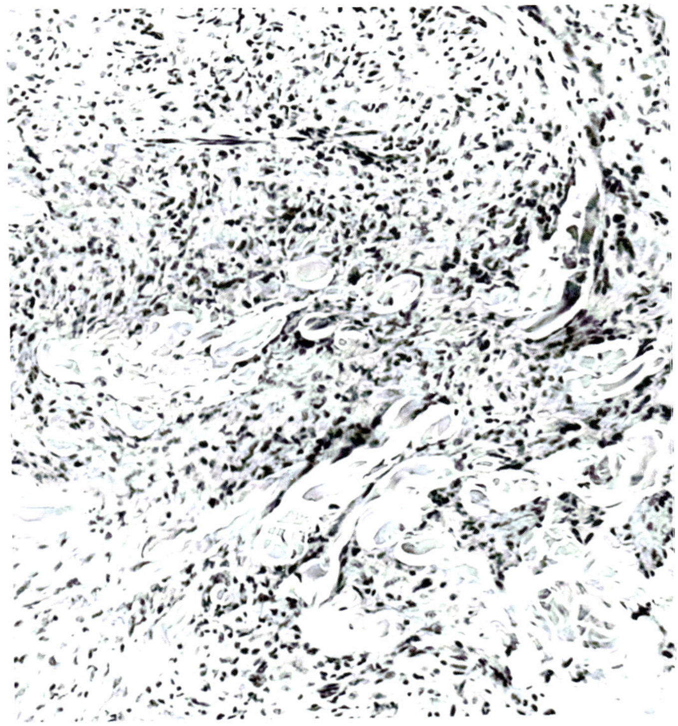

B
X260

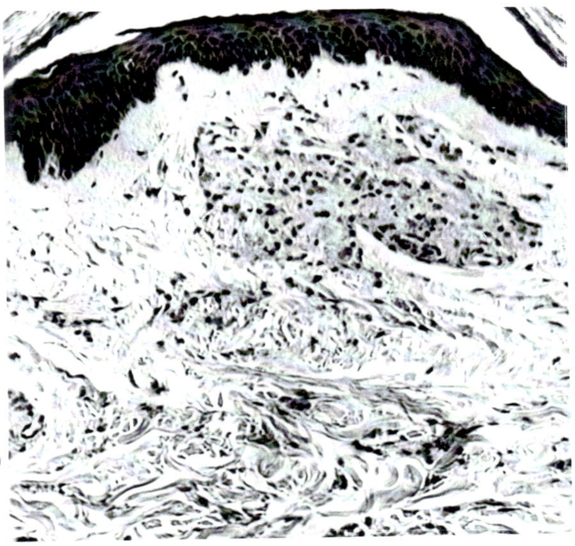

C
X260

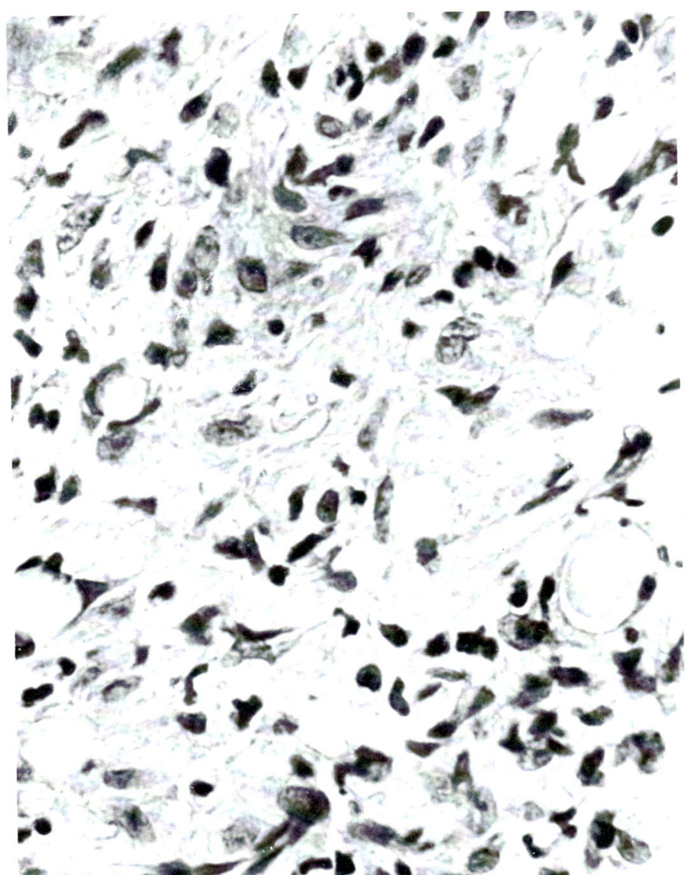

D
X760

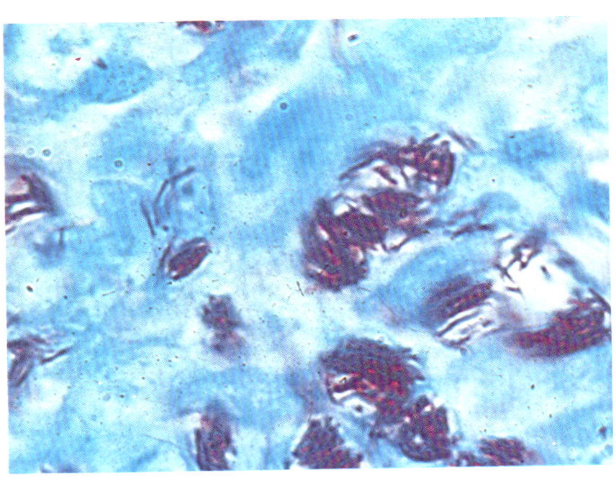

E FITE STAIN X1200

LEPROSY continued ⇨

REACTIONAL LEPROSY

Reactional leprosy refers to leprosy undergoing a shift in its immunologic status. Included in this category are three types of reaction: erythema nodosum leprosum, the Lucio phenomenon, and the lepra reaction.

Erythema nodosum leprosum usually occurs as a result of the destruction of large numbers of lepra bacilli in patients who are undergoing therapy. Erythema nodosum leprosum, unrelated to therapy, may occur. Systemic manifestations of fever, malaise, and arthralgia are accompanied by plaques and nodules (Figs. A,B), and by vesicles and purpuric lesions. Lesions are not limited to the legs.

The Lucio phenomenon occurs in patients with lepromatous leprosy of the diffusely infiltrated type. Lesions are cutaneous hemorrhagic infarcts. The Lucio phenomenon is usually observed in patients who have received little or no treatment.

The most common type of reactional leprosy (the lepra reaction) occurs in non-polar cases, and consists of constitutional symptoms and swelling of existing skin and nerve lesions. When it occurs with treatment, there usually is a shift towards tuberculoid leprosy; when it occurs without treatment, there usually is a shift towards lepromatous leprosy.

Microscopic features

1. Erythema nodosum leprosum is a necrotizing angiitis in which large numbers of degenerating lepra bacilli are present in macrophages and in the walls and lumina of blood vessels.
2. The Lucio phenomenon shows a microscopic picture similar to that of erythema nodosum leprosum, but the angiitis is usually more severe and may involve larger blood vessels as well as capillaries.

ERYTHEMA NODOSUM LEPROSUM

A

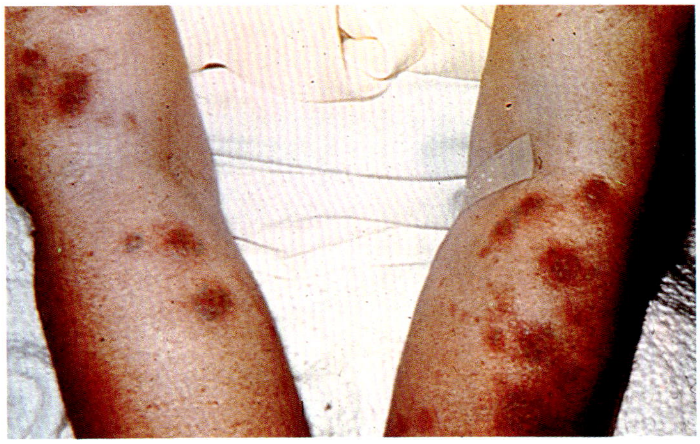

Figs. A,B courtesy USPHS Hospital, Carville, LA

B

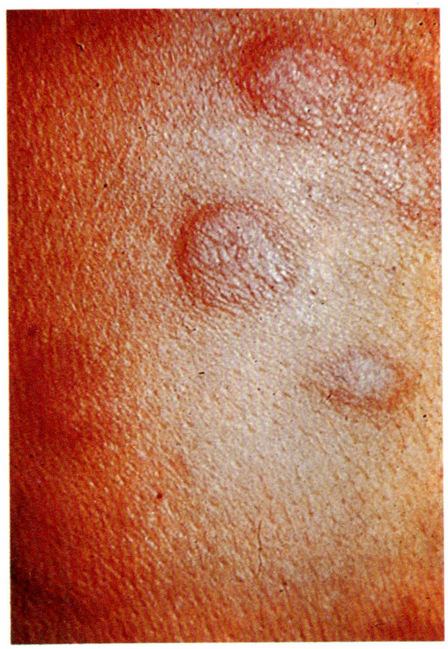

LEPROSY continued

TUBERCULOID LEPROSY

Tuberculoid leprosy is limited to the skin and nerves or to nerves alone. Nerve involvement may result in sensory and/or motor impairment.

Cutaneous lesions are solitary or few in number and appear as well-defined, asymmetrical erythematous or hypopigmented macules. These lesions may develop a raised margin (Fig. A). Hyperpigmented plaques with hypopigmented centers may develop (Fig. C). Lesions may be accompanied by anesthesia, anhidrosis, and hair loss. Nerve damage is manifested by enlarged, sometimes palpable nerves (Fig. A).

Microscopic features

1. The cutaneous lesions of tuberculoid leprosy are characterized by the presence on non-caseating, or slightly caseating epithelioid tubercles having an admixture of lymphoid cells and occasional giant cells. The tubercles resemble those of sarcoidosis (Fig. B).
2. In contrast to lepromatous leprosy, the infiltrate may extend to, or penetrate, the epidermis.
3. Lepra bacilli are usually absent, but can occasionally be found in small numbers at the active margins of the lesions.
4. The granulomatous infiltrate involves the nerves of the dermis and subcutaneous tissue. Necrotic nerve tissue may be found in the centers of granulomas. Intact nerves may be hard to find.

TUBERCULOID LEPROSY

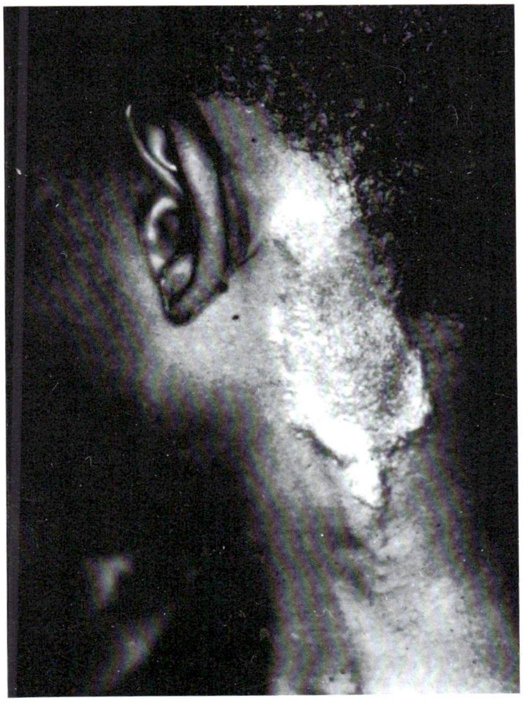

A

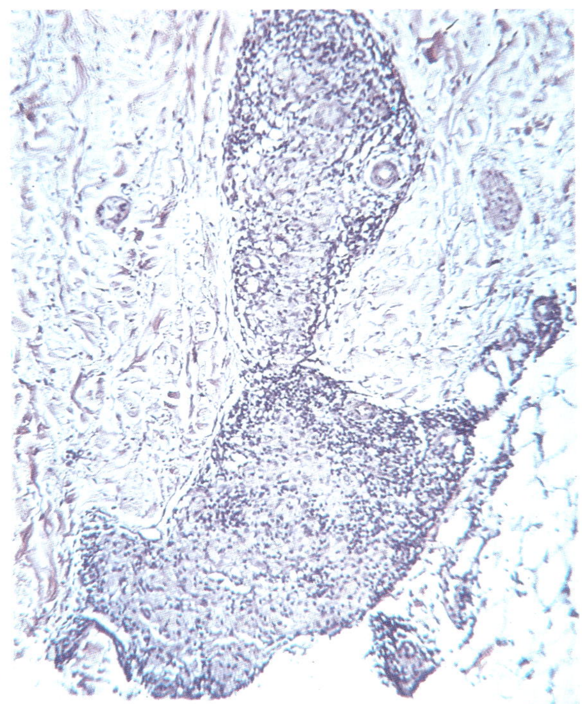

B
X100

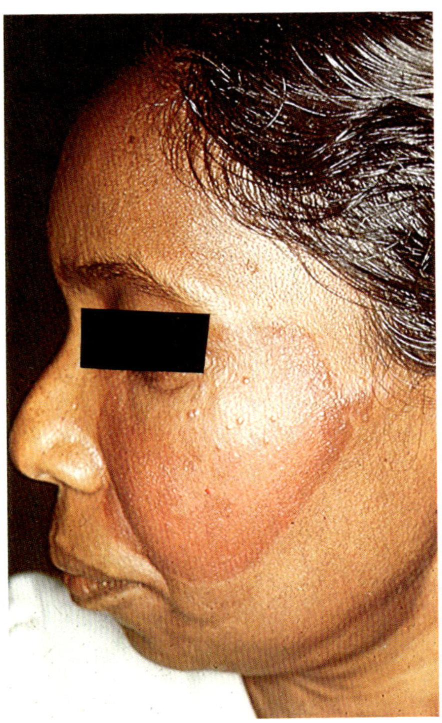

C

Suggested Reading

Infectious Diseases: Bacterial

Impetigo

Allen, A., Taplin, D. and Twigg, L. Cutaneous streptococcal infections in Vietnam. *Arch. Dermatol.*, 104:271, 1971.

Connor, B. Impetigo contagiosa in the United Kingdom. *Br. J. Dermatol.*, 86 (8, suppl.):48, 1972.

Dajani, A., Ferrieri, P. and Wannamaker, L. Endemic superficial pyoderma in children. *Arch. Dermatol.*, 108:517, 1973.

——. Natural history of impetigo. II. Etiologic agents and bacterial interactions. *J. Clin. Invest.*, 51:2863, 1972.

Dillon, H., Jr. Impetigo contagiosa: Suppurative and non-suppurative complications. *Am. J. Dis. Child.*, 115:530, 1968.

Dimond, R. and Wuepper, K. Das staphylogene Lyell-Syndrom. *Hautarzt*, 28:447, 1977.

Elias, P., Fritsch, P. and Epstein, E., Jr. Staphylococcal scalded skin syndrome. (Review). *Arch. Dermatol.*, 113:207, 1977.

Elias, P. and Levy, S. Bullous impetigo: Occurrence of localized scalded skin syndrome in an adult. *Arch. Dermatol.*, 112:856, 1976.

El Zawahry, M., Aziz, A. and Soliman, M. The etiology of impetigo contagiosa. *Br. J. Dermatol.*, 87:420, 1972.

Epstein, S. Staphylococcic impetigo contagiosa. *Arch. Dermatol. Syph.*, 42:840, 1940.

Ferrieri, P. et al. Natural history of impetigo. I. Site, sequence of acquisition and familial patterns of spread of cutaneous streptococci. *J. Clin. Invest.*, 51:2851, 1972.

Fox, W. On impetigo contagiosa, or porrigo. *Br. Med. J.*, 1:467, 1864.

Kahn, G. and Rywlin, A. Acropustulosis of infancy. *Arch. Dermatol.*, 115:831, 1979.

Kelly, C., Taplin, D. and Allen, A. Streptococcal ecthyma. *Arch. Dermatol.*, 103:306, 1971.

Lyell, A. A review of toxic epidermal necrolysis in Britain. *Br. J. Dermatol.*, 79:662, 1967.

Markowitz, M. et al. The bacteriologic findings, streptococcal immune response and renal complications in children with impetigo. *Pediatrics*, 35:393, 1965.

Melish, M. and Glasgow, L. The staphylococcal scalded skin syndrome. *N. Eng. J. Med.*, 282:1114, 1970.

Peter, G. and Smith, A. Group A streptococcal infections of the skin and pharynx. *N. Eng. J. Med.*, 297:311, 1977.

Poon-King, T. et al. Recurrent epidemic nephritis in South Trinidad. *N. Eng. J. Med.*, 277:728, 1967.

Reid, L., Weston, W. and Humbert, J. Staphylococcal scalded skin syndrome. *Arch. Dermatol.*, 109:239, 1974.

Van Toorn, M. On the staphylococcal and streptococcal etiology of impetigo. *Dermatologica*, 123:391, 1961.

Blastomycosis-like Pyoderma (Pyoderma Vegetans)

Brunsting, L. and Underwood, L. Pyoderma vegetans in association with chronic ulcerative colitis. *Arch. Dermatol. Syph.*, 60:161, 1949.

Djawari, D. and Hornstein, O. *In vitro* studies on macrophage functions in chronic pyoderma vegetans. *Arch. Dermatol. Res.*, 263:97, 1978.

Forman, L. Pemphigus vegetans of Hallopeau. *Arch. Dermatol.*, 114:627, 1978.

Getlik, A. et al. Pyoderma vegetans bei zellulärer Immunitätsdefizienz. *Dermatol. Monatsschr.*, 166:645, 1980.

Ruzicka, T. and Goerz, G. Beobachtungen bei der Pyodermite végétante Hallopeau. *Z. Haut.*, 54:24, 1979.

Su, W., Duncan, S. and Perry, H. Blastomycosis-like pyoderma. *Arch. Dermatol.*, 115:170, 1979.

Williams, H., Jr. and Stone, O. Blastomycosis-like pyoderma. *Arch. Dermatol.*, 93:226, 1966.

Erysipelas

Tappeiner, J. and Pfleger, L. Zur Histopathologie cutaner Lymphgefässe beim chronisch-rezidivierenden Erysipel der unteren Extremitäten. *Hautarzt,* 15:517, 1970.

Rhinoscleroma

Convit, J., Kerdel-Vegas, F. and Gordon, B. Rhinoscleroma: Review and presentation of a case. *Arch. Dermatol.,* 84:55, 1961.

Erlach, E., Gebhart, W. and Niebauer, G. Ultrastructural investigations on the morphogenesis of Russell bodies. *J. Cutan. Pathol.,* 3:145, 1976.

Fisher, E. and Dimling, C. Rhinoscleroma: Light and electron microscopic studies. *Arch. Pathol.,* 78:501, 1964.

Hoffmann, E., Loose, L. and Markin, J. The Mikulicz cell in rhinoscleroma. *Am. J. Pathol.,* 73:47, 1973.

Kline, P. and Brody, E. Scleroma: Review of literature and first report of multiple familial occurrence in the United States. *Arch. Dermatol. Syph.,* 59:606, 1949.

Anthrax

Gold, H. Anthrax: A report of one hundred seventeen cases. *Arch. Int. Med.,* 96:387, 1955.

Kohout, E., Sehat, A. and Ashraf, M. Anthrax: A continuous problem in southwest Iran. *Am. J. Med. Sci.,* 247:565, 1964.

Lamb, R. Anthrax. *Br. Med. J.,* 1:57, 1973.

Lebowich, R., McKillip, B. and Conboy, J. Cutaneous anthrax: A pathologic study with clinical correlation. *Am. J. Clin. Pathol.,* 13:505, 1943.

Matz, M. and Brugsch, H. Anthrax in Massachusetts, 1943 through 1962. *JAMA,* 188:635, 1964.

Stein, C. Anthrax in animals and its relationship to the disease in man. *Ann. N. Y. Acad. Sci.,*48:507, 1947.

Streptococcal Cellulitis

Amrew, D., Anderson, A. and Wannamaker, L. Perianal cellulitis associated with group A streptococci. *Am. J. Dis. Child,* 112:546, 1966.

Böszörményi, J. et al. The erysipelas problem. *Acta Med. Acad. Scientiarum Hungaricae,* 23:337, 1967.

Noble, W. An epidemic of streptococcal infection in a skin hospital. *Br. J. Dermatol.,* 81:259, 1969.

Tappeiner, J. and Pfleger, L. Zur Histopathologie cutaner Lymphgefässe beim chronisch-rezidivierenden Erysipel der unteren Extremitäten. *Hautarzt,* 15:218, 1964.

Gonococcemia

Abu-Nassar, H. et al. Cutaneous manifestations of gonococcemia: A review of 14 cases. *Arch. Int. Med.,* 112:731, 1963.

Ackerman, A. Hemorrhagic bullae in gonococcemia. *N. Eng. J. Med.,* 282:793, 1970.

Ackerman, A., Miller, R. and Shapiro, L. Gonococcemia and its cutaneous manifestations. *Arch. Dermatol.,* 91:227, 1965.

Bjornberg, A. Benign gonococcal sepsis. *Acta Derm. Venereol.,* 50:313, 1970.

Glicksman, J. et al. Gonococcal skin lesions: Report of a case of gonococcal ecthyma. *Arch. Dermatol.,* 96:74, 1967.

Holmes, K., Counts, G. and Beaty, H. Disseminated gonococcal infection. *Ann. Int. Med.,* 74:979, 1971.

Kahn, G. and Danielsson, D. Septic gonococcal dermatitis: Demonstration of gonococci and gonococcal antigens in skin lesions by immunofluorescence. *Arch. Dermatol.,* 99:421, 1969.

Schoolnik, G. et al. Gonococci causing disseminated gonococcal infection are resistant to the bactericidal action of normal human sera. *J. Clin. Invest.*, 58:163, 1976.

Shapiro, L., Teisch, J. and Brownstein, M. Dermatohistopathology of chronic gonococcal sepsis. *Arch. Dermatol.*, 107:403, 1973.

Thayer, J. and Garson, W. The gonococcus. In: *Bacterial and Mycotic Infections of Man*, 4th Ed. Dubos, R. and Hirsch, J., eds., Philadelphia, Lippincott, 1965, p. 451.

Meningococcemia

Band, J. et al. Trends in meningococcal disease in the United States, 1975–1980. *J. Infect. Dis.*, 148:754, 1983.

Benoit, F. Chronic meningococcemia: Case report and review of the literature. *Am. J. Med.*, 35:103, 1963.

Dalldorf, F. and Jennette, J. Fatal meningococcal septicemia. *Arch. Pathol.*, 101:6, 1977.

Ferguson, J. and Chapman, O. Fulminating meningococcic infections and the so-called Waterhouse-Friderichsen syndrome. *Am. J. Pathol.*, 24:763, 1948.

Gibbons, R. and Van Houte, J. Adherence in oral microbial ecology. *Ann. Rev. Microbiol.*, 29:19, 1975.

Hill, W. and Kinney, T. The cutaneous lesions in acute meningococcemia: A clinical and pathologic study. *JAMA*, 134:513, 1947.

McGehee, W., Rapaport, S. and Hjort, P. Intravascular coagulation in fulminant meningococcemia. *Ann. Int. Med.*, 67:250, 1967.

Ognibene, A. and Dito, W. Chronic meningococcemia: Further comments on the pathogenesis of associated skin lesions. *Arch. Int. Med.*, 114:29, 1964.

Ross, S. and Densen, P. Complement deficiency states and infection: Epidemiology, pathogenesis and consequences of neisserial and other infections in an immune deficiency. *Medicine* (Baltimore), 63:243, 1984.

Sotto, M. et al. Pathogenesis of cutaneous lesions in acute meningococcemia in humans: Light, immunofluorescent, and electron microscopic studies of skin biopsy specimens. *J. Infect. Dis.*, 133:506, 1976.

Tompkins, V. The diagnostic value of smears from purpuric lesions of the skin in meningococcic disease. *JAMA*, 123:31, 1943.

Pseudomonas Septicemia

Curtin, J., Petersdorf, R. and Bennet, I., Jr. Pseudomonas bacteremia: A review of 91 cases. *Ann. Int. Med.*, 54:1077, 1961.

Dorff, G. et al. Pseudomonas septicemia: Illustrated evolution of its skin lesion. *Arch. Int. Med.*, 128:591, 1971.

Hall, J. et al. Pseudomonas aeruginosa in dermatology. *Arch. Dermatol.*, 97:312, 1968.

Heffner, R. and Smith, M. Ecthyma gangrenosum in pseudomonas septicemia. *Am. J. Dis. Child.*, 99:524, 1960.

Rapaport, S. et al. Pseudomonas septicemia with intravascular clotting leading to the generalized Shwartzman reaction. *N. Eng. J. Med.*, 271:80, 1964.

Erythrasma

Montes, L., Black, S. and McBride, M. Bacterial invasion of the stratum corneum in erythrasma. I. Ultrastructural evidence for a keratolytic action exerted by Corynebacterium minutissimum. *J. Invest. Dermatol.*, 49:474, 1967.

Montes, L. et al. Erythrasma and diabetes mellitus. *Arch. Dermatol.*, 99:674, 1969.

Munro-Ashman, D., Wells, R. and Clayton, Y. Erythrasma in adolescence. *Br. J. Dermatol.*, 75:401, 1963.

Sarkany, I., Taplin, D. and Blank, H. Incidence and bacteriology of erythrasma. *Arch. Dermatol.*, 85:578, 1962.

Somerville, D. Erythrasma in normal young adults. *J. Med. Microbiol.*, 3:57, 1970.

——. A quantitative study of erythrasma lesions. *Br. J. Dermatol.*, 87:130, 1972.

Somerville, D. et al. Erythrasma in a hospital for the mentally subnormal. *Br. J. Dermatol.*, 82:355, 1970.

Temple, D. and Boardman, C. The incidence of erythrasma of the toewebs. *Arch. Dermatol.*, 86:518, 1962.

Chancroid

Borchardt, K. and Hoke, A. Simplified laboratory technique for diagnosis of a chancroid. *Arch. Dermatol.*, 102:188, 1970.
Centers for Disease Control. Chancroid-California. *MMWR*, 31:173, 1982.
Denys, G. et al. An indirect fluorescent antibody technique for *Haemophilus ducreyi. Health Lab. Sci.*, 15:128, 1978.
Felman, Y. and Nikitas, J. Chancroid. *Cutis*, 26:464, 1980.
Fitzpatrick, J. and Aeling, S. Chancroid: A review with emphasis on recent changes in incidence and treatment. *J. Assoc. Milit. Dermatol.*, 8:31, 1982.
Hadley, A. Chancroid. *Am. Fam. Physician*, 20:83, 1979.
Hammond, G. et al. Comparison of specimen collection and laboratory techniques for isolation of *Haemophilus ducreyi. J. Clin. Microbiol.*, 7:39, 1978.
Heyman, A., Beeson, P. and Sheldon, W. Diagnosis of chancroid: The relative efficiency of biopsies, cultures, smears, autoinoculations and skin tests. *JAMA*, 129:935, 1945.
Kraus, S. et al. Pseudogranuloma inguinale caused by *Haemophilus ducreyi. Arch. Dermatol.*, 118:494, 1982.
Lykke-Olesen, L. et al. Epidemic of chancroid in Greenland. *Lancet*, 1:654, 1979.
Margolis, R. and Hood, A. Chancroid: Diagnosis and treatment. *J. Am. Acad. Dermatol.*, 6:493, 1982.
Marsch, W., Haas, N. and Stüttgen, G. Ultrastructural detection of *Haemophilus ducreyi* in biopsies of chancroid. *Arch. Dermatol. Res.*, 263:153, 1978.
Nayyar, K. et al. Rising incidence of chancroid in Rotterdam: Epidemiological, clinical, diagnostic, and therapeutic aspects. *Br. J. Vener. Dis.*, 55:439, 1979.
Olansky, S. and Lucas, J. Chancroid. In: *Communicable and Infectious Diseases*. Top, F. and Wehrle, P., eds, 7th Ed., St. Louis, Mosby, 1972, p. 128.
Pund, E., Greenblatt, R. and Huie, G. The role of biopsy in diagnosis of venereal diseases: Histologic differentiation of venereal granuloma, lymphogranuloma and chancroid. *Am. J. Syph.*, 22:495, 1938.
Rajan, V. and Pang, R. Treatment of chancroid with Bactrim. *Ann. Acad. Med. Singapore*, 8:63, 1979.
Sheldon, W. and Heyman, A. Studies on chancroid. I. Observations on the histology with an evaluation of biopsy as a diagnostic procedure. *Am. J. Pathol.*, 22:415, 1946.
Sottnek, F. et al. Isolation and identification of *Haemophilus ducreyi* in a clinical study. *J. Clin. Microbiol.*, 12:170, 1980.

Syphilis

Abell, E., Marks, R. and Wilson Jones, E. Secondary syphilis: A clinico-pathological review. *Br. J. Dermatol.*, 93:53, 1975.
Ackerman, A., Goldfaden, G. and Cosmides, J. Acquired syphilis in early childhood. *Arch. Dermatol.*, 106:92, 1972.
Azar, H., Pham, T. and Kurban, A. An electron microscopic study of a syphilitic chancre. *Arch. Pathol.*, 90:143, 1970.
Baum, E. et al. Secondary syphilis: Still the great imitator. *JAMA*, 249:3069, 1983.
Beckett, J. and Bigbee, J. Immunoperoxidase localization of *Treponema pallidum. Arch. Pathol.*, 103:135, 1979.
Bos, J. et al. T-lymphoid cells in primary syphilis: Quantitative studies. *Br. J. Vener. Dis.*, 56:74, 1980.
Brown, W. et al. *Syphilis and Other Venereal Diseases.* London, Oxford Univ. Press, 1970.
Bulova, S., Schwartz, E. and Harrer, W. Hydrops fetalis and congenital syphilis. *Pediatrics*, 49:285, 1972.
Chapel, T. The signs and symptoms of secondary syphilis. *Sex. Transm. Dis.*, 7:161, 1980.
Chapel, T. et al. How reliable is the morphological diagnosis of penile ulcerations? *Sex. Transm. Dis.*, 4:150, 1977.
Cochran, R. et al. Histology simulating reticulosis in secondary syphilis. *Br. J. Dermatol.*, 95:251, 1976.

Communicable Disease Center. *World Forum on Syphilis and Other Treponematoses*. US Dept. HEW, 1964.

Drusin, L. et al. Infectious syphilis mimicking neoplastic disease. *Arch. Int. Med.*, 137:156, 1977.

Ferris, H. and Turner, T. Comparative histology of yaws and syphilis in Jamaica. *Arch. Pathol.*, 24:703, 1937.

Fisher, D., Chang, L. and Tuffanelli, D. Lues maligna. *Arch. Dermatol.*, 99:70, 1979.

Freeman, H. Juxta-articular nodules, tertiary syphilis with aortic insufficiency and dermatitis due to mercupurin. *Arch. Dermatol. Syph.*, 43:206, 1941.

Graham, W. and Duvic, M. Nodular secondary syphilis. *Arch. Dermatol.*, 118:205, 1982.

Grimble, A. *Diagnosis and Treatment of Venereal Disease*. Edinburgh, Livingstone, 1969.

Handsfield, H. et al. Demonstration of *Treponema pallidum* in a cutaneous gumma by indirect immunofluorescence. *Arch. Dermatol.*, 119:677, 1983.

Hartsock, R., Halling, L. and King, F. Luetic lymphadenitis. *Am. J. Clin. Pathol.*, 53:304, 1970.

Hasegawa, T. Electron microscopic observations on the lesions of condyloma latum. *Br. J. Dermatol.*, 81:367, 1969.

Holtzmann, H. and Hassenpflug, K. Tertiärsyphilitische Lymphknotenbeteiligung von granulierendem Typ bei einem Kranken mit plattenartigen Gummen der Haut. *Arch. Klin. Exp. Dermatol.*, 215:230, 1962.

Hu, C. et al. Isolation of virulent Treponema pallidum from human aorta thirty-two hours after death from cardiovascular syphilis. *Am. J. Med.*, 1:301, 1946.

Jeerapaet, P. and Ackerman, A. Histologic patterns of secondary syphilis. *Arch. Dermatol.*, 104:373, 1973.

Jensen, J. and From, E. Alterations in T lymphocytes and T-lymphocyte subpopulations in patients with syphilis. *Br. J. Vener. Dis.*, 58:18, 1982.

Kahn, L. and Gordon, W. Sarcoid-like granulomas in secondary syphilis. *Arch. Pathol.*, 92:334, 1971.

Kalz, F. and Newton, B. Syphilitic juxta-articular nodules. *Arch. Dermatol. Syph.*, 46:626, 1943.

Kerdel-Vegas, F., Kopf, A. and Tolmach, J. Keratoderma punctatum syphiliticum: Report of a case. *Br. J. Dermatol.*, 66:449, 1954.

Lambert, W. et al. Pustular acneiform secondary syphilis. *Cutis*, 37:69, 1986.

Lantis, L., Petrozzi, J. and Hurley, H. Sarcoid granuloma in secondary syphilis. *Arch. Dermatol.*, 99:748, 1969.

Lauderdale, V. and Goldman, J. Serial ultrathin sectioning demonstrating intracellularity of Treponema pallidum: An electron microscopic study. *Br. J. Venereal. Dis.*, 48:87, 1972.

Lochner, J. and Pomeranz, J. Lichenoid secondary syphilis. *Arch. Dermatol.*, 109:81, 1974.

Longstreth, P., Hoke, A. and McElroy, C. Hepatitis and bone destruction as uncommon manifestation of early syphilis. *Arch. Dermatol.*, 112:1451, 1976.

Matsuda-John, S. et al. Nodular late syphilis. *J. Am. Acad. Dermatol.*, 9:269, 1983.

Mikhail, G. and Chapel, T. Follicular papulopustular syphilid. *Arch. Dermatol.*, 100:471, 1969.

Paterou, M. et al. Histologie de la syphilis secondaire. *Ann. Dermatol. Venereol.*, 106:923, 1979.

Pembroke, A., Michell, P. and McKee, P. Nodulo-squamous tertiary syphilide. *Clin. Exp. Dermatol.*, 5:361, 1980.

Petrozzi, J., Lockshin, N. and Berger, B. Malignant syphilis. *Arch. Dermatol.*, 109:387, 1974.

Schofield, C. *Sexually Transmitted Diseases*. Edinburgh, Livingstone, 1972.

Sullivan, W. Syphilitic gumma misdiagnosed midline granuloma. *Arch. Int. Med.*, 114:336, 1964.

Tuta, J. and Coombs, R. Symmetric syphilitic granulomas of the elbows. *Arch. Dermatol. Syph.*, 46:375, 1942.

Vander Ploeg, D. and Stagnone, J. Eyebrow alopecia in secondary syphilis. *Arch. Dermatol.*, 90:172, 1964.

Wecke, J., Bartunek, J. and Stüttgen, G. *Treponema pallidum* in early syphilitic lesions in humans during high-dosage penicillin therapy: An electron microscopical study. *Arch. Dermatol. Res.*, 257:1, 1976.

Wilcox, R. *Textbook of Venereal Diseases and Treponematoses*. London, Heinemann, 1964.

Wilcox, R. and Gunthe, T. *Treponema pallidum*: A bibliographical reveiw of the morphology, culture and survival of *T. pallidum* and associated organisms. *Bull. WHO* 35 (suppl.), 1966.

Wile, U. and Belote, G. Syphilitic alopecia: Its relation to neurosyphilis. *Arch. Dermatol. Syph.*, 13:495, 1926.

Willcox, J. An atypical case of secondary syphilis. *Br. J. Vener. Dis.*, 57:30, 1981.

Granuloma Inguinale

Alexander, L. and Schoch, A. Granuloma inguinale: The successful use of Giemsa stain to demonstrate typical pathologic findings. *Am. J. Syph.*, 24:180, 1940.

Alexander, L. and Shields, T. Squamous cell carcinoma of the vulva secondary to granuloma inguinale. *Arch. Dermatol. Syph.*, 67:395, 1953.

Beerman, H. and Sonck, C. The epithelial changes in granuloma inguinale. *Am. J. Syph.*, 36:501, 1952.

Davis, C. Granuloma inguinale. *JAMA*, 211:632, 1970.

Davis, C. and Collins, C. Granuloma inguinale: An ultrastructural study of Calymmatobacterium granulomatis. *J. Invest. Dermatol.*, 53:315, 1969.

Dodson, R., Fritz, G. and Hubler, W., Jr. Donovanosis: A morphological study. *J. Invest. Dermatol.*, 62:611, 1974.

Goldberg, J., Weaver, R. and Packer, H. Studies on granuloma inguinale. I. Bacteriologic behavior of Donovania granulomatis. *Am. J. Syph.*, 37:60, 1953.

Kuberski, T. Granuloma inguinale (donovanosis). *Sex. Transm. Dis.*, 7:29, 1980.

Olansky, S. and Prentz, D. Granuloma inguinale. In: *Communicable and Infectious Diseases.* Top, F. and Wehrle, P., eds., 7th Ed., St. Louis, Mosby, 1972, p. 281.

Pund, E. and Greenblatt, R. Specific histology of granuloma inguinale. *Arch. Pathol.*, 23:224, 1937.

Rao, M. et al. Oral lesions of granuloma inguinale. *J. Oral. Surg.*, 34:1112, 1976.

Torpin, R., Greenblatt, R. and Pund, E. Granuloma inguinale (venereum) in the female. *Am. J. Surg.*, 44:551, 1939.

Lyme Disease

Berger, B., Clemmensen, O. and Ackerman, A. Lyme disease is a spirochetosis: A review of the disease and evidence for its cause. *Am. J. Derm. Pathol.*, 5:111, 1983.

Gross, G. et al. Erythema chronicum migrans with purpura and polymorphonuclear infiltrates. *Arch. Dermatol.*, 115:873, 1979.

Mast, W. and Burrows, W. Erythema chronicum migrans in the United States. *JAMA*, 236:859, 1976.

Naversen, D. and Gardner, L. Erythema chronicum migrans in America. *Arch. Dermatol.*, 114:253, 1978.

Park, H., Jones, B. and Barbour, A. Erythema chronicum migrans of Lyme disease: Diagnosis by monoclonal antibodies. *J. Am. Acad. Dermatol.*, 15:406, 1986.

Scrimenti, R. Erythema chronicum migrans. *Arch. Dermatol.*, 102:104, 1970.

Smith, L. et al. Erythema chronicum migrans. *Cutis*, 17:962, 1976.

Sonck, C. Erythema chronicum migrans with multiple lesions. *Acta Derm. Venereol.* (Stockh.), 45:34, 1965.

Steere, A. and Malawista, S. Cases of Lyme disease in the United States: Locations correlated with distribution of *Ixodes dammini*. *Ann. Int. Med.*, 91:730, 1979.

Tuberculosis

Beyt, B. et al. Cutaneous mycobacteriosis: Analysis of 34 cases with a new classification of the disease. *Medicine* (Baltimore), 60:95, 1980.

Blumenthal, F. Cutaneous tuberculosis: Its relation to the immune allergic state. *Arch. Dermatol. Syph.*, 35:1037, 1937.

Brown, F. et al. Cutaneous tuberculosis. *J. Am. Acad. Dermatol.*, 6:101, 1982.

Brunsgaard, E. The so-called "primary complex" of tuberculosis in the skin. *Br. J. Dermatol.*, 46:113, 1934.

Bryant, J. Oral tuberculosis. *Am. Rev. Tuberc.*, 39:738, 1939.

Clark, B. *Causes and Prevention of Tuberculosis*, Edinburgh, Livingstone, 1952.

Clasen, K. and Horwitz, O. The morbidity from pulmonary tuberculosis in patients suffering from extrapulmonary tuberculosis disease; lupus vulgaris cutis. *Adv. Tuberc. Res.*, 10:237, 1960.

Editorial: New tuberculosis. *Lancet*, 1:199, 1984.

Fethke, N. and Anderson, R. Chemistry of the lipids of tubercle bacilli: A contribution to the study of acid-fastness. *Am. Rev. Tuberc.*, 57:294, 1948.

Fisher, J. Miliary tuberculosis with unusual cutaneous manifestations. *JAMA*, 238:241, 1977.

Francis, J. *Tuberculosis in Animals and Man*. London, Cassell, 1958.

Goethe, D., Jacobson, K. and Doty, R. Primary inoculation tuberculosis of the skin. *Arch. Dermatol.*, 114:567, 1978.

Graham-Brown, R. and Sarkany, I. Lichen scrofulosorum with tuberculous dactylitis. *Br. J. Dermatol.*, 103:561, 1980.

Hart, V. and Weedon, D. Lupus vulgaris and *Mycobacterium bovis*. *Aust. J. Dermatol.*, 18:86, 1977.

Heilman, K. and Muschenheim, C. Primary cutaneous tuberculosis resulting from mouth-to-mouth respiration: Report of a case. *N. Eng. J. Med.*, 273:1035, 1965.

Hill, L. and Kelly, D. Tuberculosis in children. *J. Pediatr.*, 14:815, 1939.

Horwitz, O. The localization of lupus vulgaris of the skin. *Acta Tuberc. Scand.* (47, suppl.):175, 1959.

——. Lupus vulgaris cutis in Denmark 1895–1954: Its relation to the epidemiology of other forms of tuberculosis. *Acta Tuberc. Scand.* (49, suppl.):1, 1960.

Iden, D., Rogers, R., III and Schroeter, A. Papulonecrotic tuberculid secondary to *Mycobacterium bovis*. *Arch. Dermatol.*, 114:564, 1978.

Lurie, M. *Resistance to Tuberculosis*. Cambridge, Harvard Univ. Press, 1964.

McCarthy, L. The chronic specific inflammations of the skin. In: *Histopathology of Skin Diseases*. St. Louis, Mosby, 1931, p. 239.

McCray, M. and Esterly, N. Cutaneous eruptions in congenital tuberculosis. *Arch. Dermatol.*, 117:460, 1981.

Marcussen, P. Lupus vulgaris following BCG vaccination. *Br. J. Dermatol.*, 66:121, 1954.

Michelson, H. The primary complex of tuberculosis of the skin. *Arch. Dermatol. Syph.*, 32:589, 1935.

——. Scrofuloderma gummosa (tuberculosis colliquativa). *Arch. Dermatol. Syph.*, 10:565, 1924.

Michelson, H. and Winer, L. Tuberculodermas of the face. *Arch. Dermatol. Syph.*, 29:251, 1934.

Miller, F. Recognition of primary tuberculosis infection of the skin and mucosae. *Lancet*, 1:5, 1953.

Minkowitz, S. et al. "Prosector's wart" (cutaneous tuberculosis) in a medical student. *Am. J. Clin. Pathol.*, 51:261, 1969.

Mitchell, P. Tuberculosis verrucosa cutis among Chinese in Hong Kong. *Br. J. Dermatol.*, 66:444, 1954.

Montgomery, H. Histopathology of various types of cutaneous tuberculosis. *Arch. Dermatol. Syph.*, 35:698, 1937.

Myers, J. *Tuberculosis and Other Communicable Diseases*. Springfield, IL, Thomas, 1959.

O'Leary, P. and Harrison, M. Inoculation tuberculosis. *Arch. Dermatol. Syph.*, 44:371, 1941.

Pandhi, R. et al. Cutaneous tuberculosis: A clinical and investigative study. *Indian. J. Dermatol.*, 22:99, 1977.

Papadimitriou, J. and Spector, W. The origin, properties and fate of epithelioid cells. *J. Pathol.*, 105:187, 1971.

Platou, R. and Lennox, R. Tuberculous cutaneous complexes in children. *Am. Rev. Tuberc.*, 74 (2, pt. 2):160, 1956.

Regan, W. and Harley, W. Orificial and pulmonary tuberculosis: Report of a case. *Aust. J. Dermatol.*, 20:88, 1979.

Satenstein, D. Tuberculosis of the skin: Histologic consideration. *Arch. Dermatol. Syph.*, 23:309, 1931.

Schermer, D. et al. Tuberculosis cutis miliaris acuta generalisata. *Arch. Dermatol.*, 99:64, 1969.

Sheingold, M. and Sheingold, H. Oral tuberculosis. *Oral Surg.*, 4:239, 1951.

Shima, K., Dannenberg, A., Jr. and Ando, M. Macrophage accumulation, division, maturation and digestive and microbicidal capacities in tuberculous lesions. *Am. J. Pathol.*, 67:159, 1972.

Simpson, C. Fungating lymphatic tuberculosis or sporotrichial type of skin tuberculosis. *South Med. J.*, 21:789, 1928.

Stokes, J. Tuberculous paronychia: Report of a case with unusual features. *Arch. Dermatol. Syph.*, 8:44, 1923.

Sulzberger, M. and Goodman, J. Tuberculoderms. *Med. Clin. No. Am.*, 20:995, 1936.

Terplan, K. Anatomical Studies on Human Tuberculosis. In: *The American Review of Tuberculosis*. Pinner, M., ed., New York, National Tuberculosis Assoc., 1940.

Tileston, W. Disseminated miliary tuberculosis of the skin: An important sign in general miliary tuberculosis of infancy. *Arch. Int. Med.*, 4:21, 1909.

van der Lugt, L. Some remarks about tuberculosis of the skin and tuberculids. *Dermatologica,* 131:266, 1965.

Warin, A. and Wilson-Jones, E. Cutaneous tuberculosis of the nose with unusual clinical and histological features leading to a delay in the diagnosis. *Clin. Exp. Dermatol.,* 2:235, 1977.

Wilner, G. et al. Fluorescent staining for mycobacteria in sarcoid and tuberculous granulomas. *Am. J. Clin. Pathol.,* 51:584, 1969.

Wong, K., Lee, K. and Chiu, S. Tuberculosis of the skin in Hong Kong (A review of 160 cases). *Br. J. Dermatol.,* 80:424, 1968.

Yegian, D. and Vanderlinde, R. The nature of acid-fastness. *J. Bacteriol.,*54:777, 1947.

Atypical Mycobacterial Infections

Adams, R. et al. Tropical fish aquariums: A source of *Mycobacterium marinum* infections resembling sporotrichosis. *JAMA,* 211:457, 1970.

Bolivar, R., Satterwhite, T. and Floyd, M. Cutaneous lesions due to *M. kansasii. Arch. Dermatol.,* 116:207, 1980.

Brock, J., Kennedy, C. and Clark, W., Jr. Cutaneous infection with an atypical mycobacterium. *Arch. Dermatol.,* 82:918, 1960.

Chapman, J. *The Atypical Mycobacteria and Human Mycobacteriosis.* New York, Plenum Press, 1977.

Christiansen, J. Lupus vulgaris gigantea caused by Mycobacterium avium. In: *Proceedings of the 13th International Congress of Dermatology,* Vol. 2, Jadassohn, W. and Shirren, C., eds., Springer, 1968, p. 1319.

Cole, G. and Gebhard, J. *Mycobacterium avium* infection of the skin resembling lepromatous leprosy. *Br. J. Dermatol.,* 101:71, 1979.

Connor, D. and Lunn, H. Buruli ulceration. *Arch. Pathol.,* 81:183, 1966.

Cott, R., Carter, D. and Sall, T. Cutaneous disease caused by atypical mycobacteria: Report of two chromogen infections and review of the subject. *Arch. Dermatol.,* 95:259, 1967.

Cox, S. and Stransbough, L. Chronic cutaneous infection caused by *Mycobacterium intracellulare. Arch. Dermatol.,* 117:794, 1981.

Dickey, R. Sporotrichoid mycobacteriosis caused by *M. marinum (balnei), Arch. Dermatol.,* 98:385, 1968.

Dore, N., Collins, J. and Mankiewicz, E. A sporotrichoid-like *Mycobacterium kansasii* infection of the skin treated with minocycline hydrochloride. *Br. J. Dermatol.,* 101:75, 1979.

Even-Paz, Z. et al. *Mycobacterium marinum* skin infections mimicking cutaneous leishmaniasis. *Br. J. Dermatol.,* 94:435, 1976.

Fainstein, V. et al. Disseminated infection due to *Mycobacterium avium-intracellulare* in a homosexual man with Kaposi's sarcoma. *J. Infect. Dis.,* 145:586, 1982.

Fenske, N. and Millns, J. Resistant cutaneous infection caused by *Mycobacterium chelonei. Arch. Dermatol.,* 117:151, 1981.

Getzler, N., Linton, W. and Jegyud, A. Atypical cutaneous tuberculosis. *Arch. Dermatol.,* 84:439, 1961.

Gombert, M. et al. Disseminated *Mycobacterium marinum* infection after renal transplantation. *Ann. Int. Med.,* 94:486, 1981.

Greer, K., Gross, G. and Martensen, S. Sporotrichoid cutaneous infection due to *Mycobacterium chelonei. Arch. Dermatol.,* 115:738, 1979.

Hirsh, F. and Saffold, O. *Mycobacterium kansasii* infection with dermatologic manifestations. *Arch. Dermatol.,* 112:706, 1976.

Hoffman, P. et al. Two outbreaks of sternal wound infections due to organisms of the *Mycobacterium fortuitum* complex. *J. Infect. Dis.,* 143:533, 1981.

Izumi, A., Hanke, C. and Higaki, M. *Mycobacterium marinum* infections treated with tetracycline. *Arch. Dermatol.,* 113:1067, 1977.

Jänner, M. et al. Infektion mit *Mycobacterium marinum* aus einem Aquarium. *Hautarzt,* 34:635, 1983.

Jolly, H., Jr. and Seabury, J. Infections with *Mycobacterium marinum. Arch. Dermatol.,* 106:32, 1972.

King, A. et al. Disseminated cutaneous *Mycobacterium marinum* infection. *Arch. Dermatol.,* 119:268, 1983.

Knox, J. et al. Atypical acid-fast organism infection of the skin. *Arch. Dermatol.,* 84:386, 1961.

Mansson, T. et al. Aquariumborne infection with *Mycobacterium marinum. Acta Derm. Venereol.,* 50:119, 1970.

Mezo, A. et al. Unusual mycobacteria in 5 cases of opportunistic infection. *Pathology*, 11:277, 1979.
Philpott, J., Jr. et al. Swimming pool granuloma: A study of 290 cases. *Arch. Dermatol.*, 88:158, 1963.
Rees, R. and Bennett, J. Granuloma following swimming pool abrasion. *JAMA*, 152:1606, 1953.
Robicsek, F. et al. *Mycobacterium fortuitum* epidemics after openheart surgery. *J. Thorac. Cardiovasc. Surg.*, 75:91, 1978.
Saxe, N. Mycobacterial skin infections. *J. Cutan. Pathol.*, 12:300, 1985.
Schaefer, W. and Davis, C. A bacteriologic and histopathologic study of skin granulomas due to *Mycobacterium balnei*. *Am. Rev. Respir. Dis.*, 84:837, 1961.
Sommer, A., Williams, R. and Mandel, A. *Mycobacterium balnei* infection: Report of two cases. *Arch. Dermatol.*, 86:316, 1962.
Sybert, A. et al. Cutaneous infection due to *Mycobacterium szulgai*. *Am. Rev. Respir. Dis.*, 115:695, 1977.
Wallace, R. et al. Spectrum of disease due to rapidly growing mycobacteria. *Rev. Infect. Dis.*, 5:657, 1983.
Yip, S. et al. Tuberculoid cutaneous infection due to a niacin-positive *Mycobacterium chelonei*. *Br. J. Dermatol.*, 101:63, 1979.
Zeligman, I. *Mycobacterium marinum* granuloma. *Arch. Dermatol.*, 106:26, 1972.

Leprosy

Azulay, R. Histopathology of skin lesions in leprosy. *Internat. J. Lepr.*, 39:244, 1971.
Browne, S. The variegated clinical pattern of leprosy. *Internat. J. Lepr.*, 33:400, 1965.
Cochrane, R. and Davey, T. *Leprosy in Theory and Practice*, 2nd Ed., Baltimore, Williams and Wilkins, 1964.
Convit, J. and Ulrich, M. Recent advances in the immunology of leprosy. *Internat. J. Dermatol.*, 15:157, 1976.
Cowdry, E. Cytological studies on globi in leprosy. *Am. J. Pathol.*, 16:103, 1940.
Desikan, K. and Job, C. A review of postmortem findings in 37 cases of leprosy. *Internat. J. Lepr.*, 36:32, 1968.
Donner, R. and Shively, J. The "Lucio phenomenon" in diffuse leprosy. *Ann. Int. Med.*, 67:831, 1967.
Fields, J. Leprosy. *Arch. Dermatol.*, 100:650, 1969.
Fite, G. Leprosy from the histologic point of view. *Arch. Pathol.*, 35:611, 1943.
——. The vascular lesions of leprosy. *Internat. J. Lepr.*, 9:193, 1941.
Hansen, G. and Looft, C. *Leprosy: In its clinical and pathological aspects.* London, Simpkin and Marshall, 1895.
Imaeda, T. Electron microscopy of leprosy lesions. *Dermatol. Internat.*, 7:116, 1968.
Job, C. *Mycobacterium leprae* in nerve lesions of lepromatous leprosy. *Arch. Pathol.*, 89:195, 1970.
Job, C. and Desikan, K. Pathologic changes and their distribution in peripheral nerves in lepromatous leprosy. *Internat. J. Lepr.*, 36:257, 1968.
Jolliffe, D. Leprosy reactional states and their treatment. (Review). *Br. J. Dermatol.*, 97:345, 1977.
Jopling, W. and Harman, R. Leprosy. In: *Textbook of Dermatology*, Vol. I, Book, A., Wilkinson, D. and Ebling, F., eds., London, Blackwell, 1972, p. 680.
Khanolkar, V. Pathology of leprosy. In: Cochrane, R. and Davey, T., eds., *Leprosy in Theory and Practice*, 2nd Ed., Baltimore, Williams and Wilkins, 1964, p. 125.
Kuper, S. The lepromin reaction. In: Cochrane, R. and Davey, T., eds., *Leprosy in Theory and Practice*, 2nd Ed., Baltimore, Williams and Wilkins, 1964, p. 183.
Kwittken, J. and Peck, S. Borderline leprosy. *Arch. Dermatol.*, 95:50, 1967.
Mabalay, M. et al. The histopathology and histochemistry of erythema nodosum leprosum. *Internat. J. Lepr.*, 33:28, 1965.
Mitsuda, K. The significance of the vacuole in the Virchow lepra cells, and the distribution of lepra cells in certain organs. *Internat. J. Lepr.*, 4:491, 1936.
Moschella, S. A current review of leprosy. *Cutis*, 10:27, 1972.
Powell, C. and Swan, L. Leprosy: Pathologic changes observed in fifty consecutive necropsies. *Am. J. Pathol.*, 31:1131, 1955.
Pursley, T., Jacobson, R. and Apisarnthanarax, P. Lucio's phenomenon. *Arch. Dermatol.*, 116:201, 1980.

Rea, T. and Levan, N. Current concepts in the immunology of leprosy. (Review). *Arch. Dermatol.*, 113:345, 1977.

——. Lucio's phenomenon and diffuse nonnodular lepromatous leprosy. *Arch. Dermatol.*, 114:1023, 1978.

Rea, T. et al. Immunologic responses in patients with lepromatous leprosy. *Arch. Dermatol.*, 112:791, 1976.

Rees, R. New prospects for the study of leprosy in the laboratory. *Bull. WHO*, 40:785, 1969.

Ridley, D. *Skin Biopsy in Leprosy*. Basel, Ciba-Geigy, 1977.

Ridley, D. and Jopling, W. Classification of leprosy according to immunity: A five group system. *Internat. J. Lepr.*, 34:255, 1966.

Ridley, D. and Wise, M. Reaction of the dermis in leprosy. *Internat. J. Lepr.*, 32:24, 1964.

Sanchez, N. et al. Erythema nodosum leprosum: An immune complex mediated necrotizing vasculitis. (abstr.). *J. Invest. Dermatol.*, 75:461, 1980.

Sehgal, V. et al. Application of clinical and histopathological classification of leprosy. *Dermatologica*, 161:93, 1980.

Wemambu, S. et al. Erythema nodosum leprosum: A clinical manifestation of Arthus phenomenon. *Lancet*, 2:933, 1969.

Wiersma, J. and Binford, C. The identification of leprosy among epithelioid cell granulomas of the skin. *Internat. J. Lepr.*, 40:10, 1972.

Wolstenholme, G. and O'Connor, M. *Pathogenesis of Leprosy*, Boston, Little, Brown, 1963 (CIBA Foundation Study Group No. 15).

Infectious Diseases: Fungal

Fungus infections can be loosely divided into three main categories:

1. *Dermatophyte infections.* These are limited to keratinous areas of the hair, skin, and nails.
2. *Intermediate fungus infections.* One organism, *Candida albicans*, produces infections in this category. Infections can involve skin, mucous membranes, and under certain circumstances, viscera.
3. *Deep fungus infections.* These can involve any portion of the body.

COMMON DERMATOPHYTE INFECTIONS

Type	Area Involved	Clinical Appearance of Lesions	Common Causative Organisms
Tinea corporis	Trunk, limbs, nonhairy areas of the face	Lesions are circinate with papulovesicular, raised borders and clearing centers; scaling is common; clinical appearance varies with species; *T. rubrum* and *T. verrucosum* may be associated with folliculitis.	*Microsporum canis; Trichophyton mentagrophytes; Trichophyton rubrum; Trichophyton verrucosum*
Tinea versicolor	Trunk	There are scaling oval lesions, which have a tendency to become confluent; hyperpigmentation and hypopigmentation are common.	*Pityrosporum orbiculare (Malassezia furfur)*
Pityrosporum folliculitis	Chest and back	Follicular papules and pustules.	*Pityrosporum orbiculare*
Tinea capitis	Scalp	Patches of broken scalp hairs are present. Boggy folliculitis (kerion) may occur with *M. canis* infections and *T. tonsurans* infections.	*M. audouini; M. canis; T. tonsurans*
Tinea barbae	Beard area	Boggy folliculitis is present.	*T. mentagrophytes; T. verrucosum*
Nodular perifolliculitis (Majocchi's granuloma)	Often on the legs of women, especially with shaved legs. It is commonly associated with fungus infection of the soles.	Erythematous nodules.	*T. rubrum; T. verrucosum*
Favus	Scalp	The infection is characterized by perifollicular crusts (scutula) with scarring.	*T. schoenleini*
Tinea cruris	Upper, inner surface of thighs	Lesions are confluent, with erythematous, scaling areas and raised papular or vesicular border.	*Epidermophyton floccosum; T. rubrum*
Tinea pedis and tinea manum	Palms, soles, interdigital areas	Diffuse erythema and scaling are present, vesiculation and maceration are frequent with *T. mentagrophytes* infection.	*T. rubrum; T. mentagrophytes*
Tinea unguium (onychomycosis)	Nails	Yellowish subungual hyperkeratosis; changes in nail plate.	*T. rubrum*

HISTOLOGIC FEATURES OF DERMATOPHYTE INFECTIONS

Histologic changes are those of nonspecific inflammation; organisms are best visualized in sections with PAS stain, since their walls contain diastase-resistant neutral polysaccharides. The organisms appear as filaments (hyphae or mycelia) and oval or round spores.

Tinea of glabrous skin	Acute, subacute, or chronic dermatitis may be present; organisms are present in varying numbers in the stratum corneum. Trichophyton and Microsporum infections show only hyphae; *Epidermophyton floccosum* infections show spores and hyphae; *P. orbiculare* infections show large numbers of spores and hyphae.
T. rubrum granuloma* nodular perifolliculitis; Majocchi's granuloma	When folliculitis is present, the picture is that of a granulomatous folliculitis, with the organisms present in hairs, and occasionally in the dermal infiltrate.
Tinea capitis Tinea barbae	There is a perifolliculitis, with or without giant cells; PAS-positive fungi penetrate the hair to a level 30 microns above the keratogenous zone.
Favus	The perifollicular crust (scutulum) consists of hyperkeratotic and parakeratotic material, fibrin, and inflammatory cells. It contains many hyphae and a few spores, some of which show degeneration. Many hyphae and a few spores are present in the adjacent stratum corneum and within and around hairs. The dermis shows a dense inflammatory reaction with many plasma cells and occasional giant cells. Late lesions show fibrosis and loss of appendages.

***T. verrucosum* can also cause a folliculitis, but it is usually nongranulomatous. Unlike *T. rubrum* granuloma, organisms are not generally found in the dermal infiltrate.

FUNGUS INFECTIONS continued ⇨

DERMATOPHYTE FUNGUS INFECTIONS OF THE GLABROUS SKIN

Tinea versicolor is characterized by violet or tan oval lesions with a fine scale (Fig. A). Lesions tend to become confluent and appear hypopigmented after sun exposure (Fig. B). The trunk is the usual site.

Tinea corporis due to M. canis is characterized by circinate lesions with an erythematous, scaling border (Fig. C). Some authors designate tinea corporis of the face as *tinea faciei*.

Tinea corporis due to T. rubrum is characterized by numerous circinate lesions, which tend to become confluent, producing a polycyclic border (Fig. D).

Tinea cruris shows confluent, erythematous areas with variable scaling, and raised papular or vesicular borders (Fig. E).

Tinea pedis and tinea manum lesions range from diffuse erythema and scaling to areas of vesiculation. Maceration is commonly present in intertriginous tinea pedis (Fig. F).

Comment

The fungus that causes tinea versicolor is normally present on the skin in its yeast form as a commensal organism. It is believed that transformation of this fungus into its dimorphous form (spores and hyphae) is correlated with the development of tinea versicolor. Pityrosporum folliculitis, however, typically involving the chest and back, shows only the yeast form of the organism. It is usually present in the upper part of dilated, keratin-filled follicular canals.

FUNGUS INFECTIONS OF THE GLABROUS SKIN

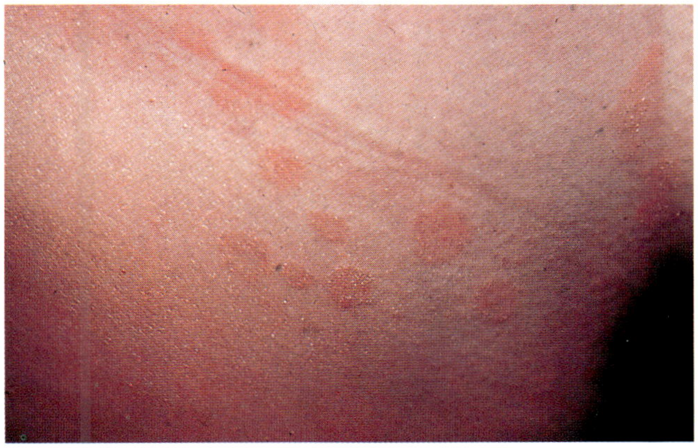

A

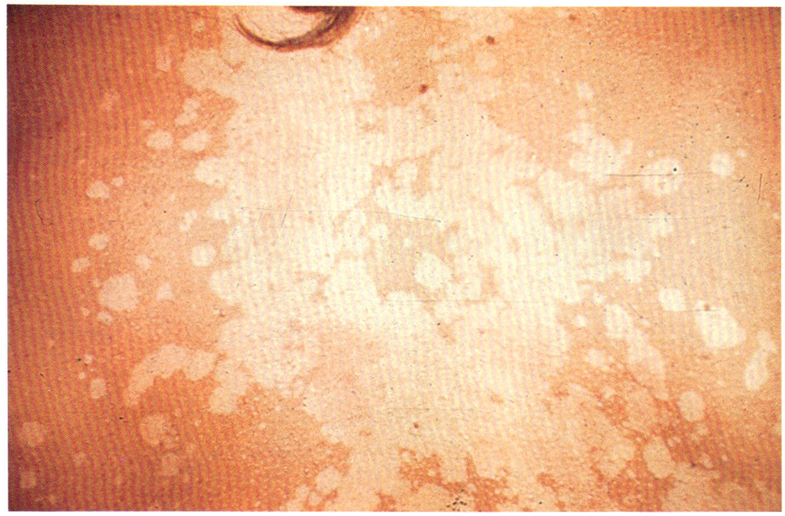

B

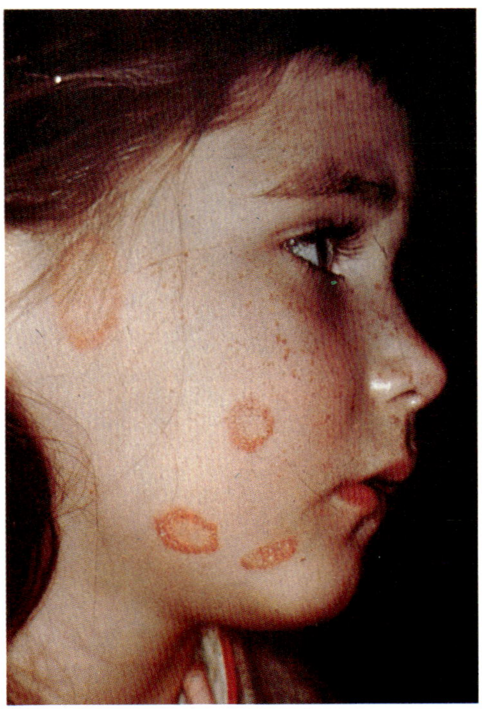

C

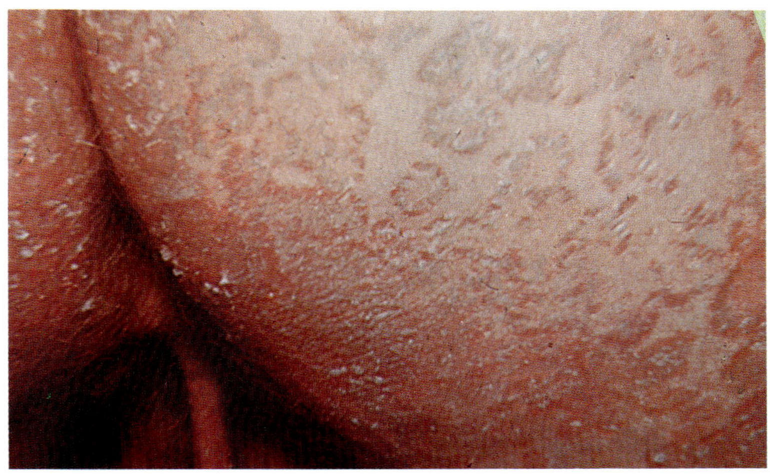

D

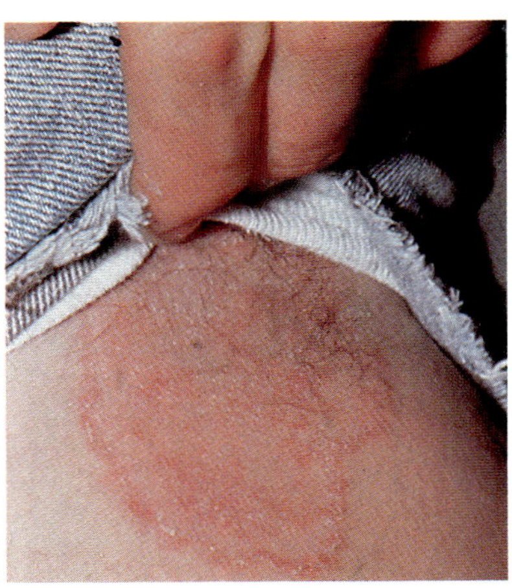

E

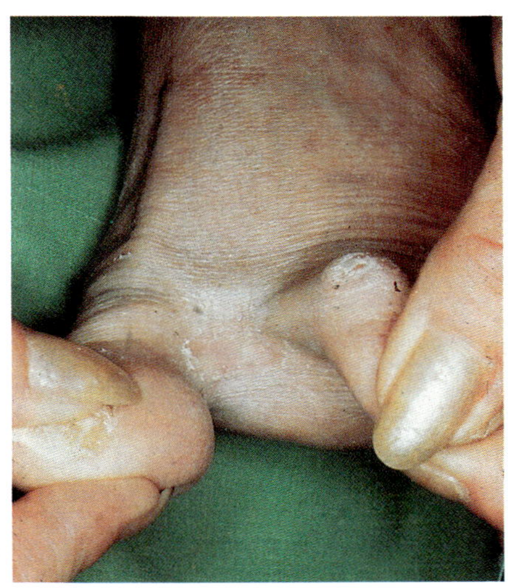

F

FUNGUS INFECTIONS continued

DERMATOPHYTE FUNGUS INFECTIONS OF THE GLABROUS SKIN

Microscopic features

1. The microscopic picture is similar in all types of dermatophytosis. With H&E stain the picture is that of dermatitis, usually subacute to chronic. With special stains, such as PAS stain, spores and hyphae in varying proportions are observed in the stratum corneum (Figs. A,B). In tinea versicolor (Fig. A), the percentage of spores is higher than in other dermatophyte infections.
2. Spores and hyphae can be demonstrated in unstained scrapings of scales in potassium hydroxide solution (KOH preparation [Fig. C]).

Comment

The methenamine silver stain can also be used to demonstrate fungi. With this stain, fungi appear black.

FUNGUS INFECTIONS OF THE GLABROUS SKIN

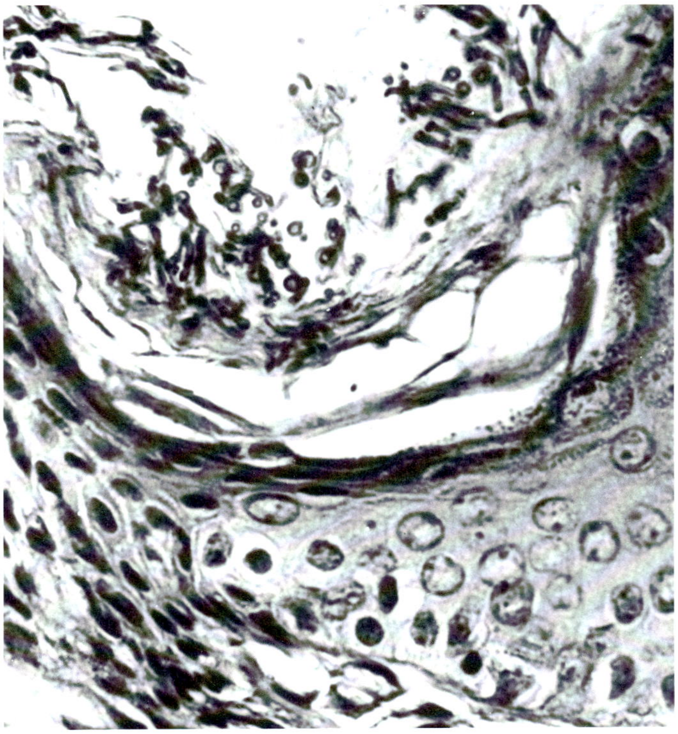

A
X720

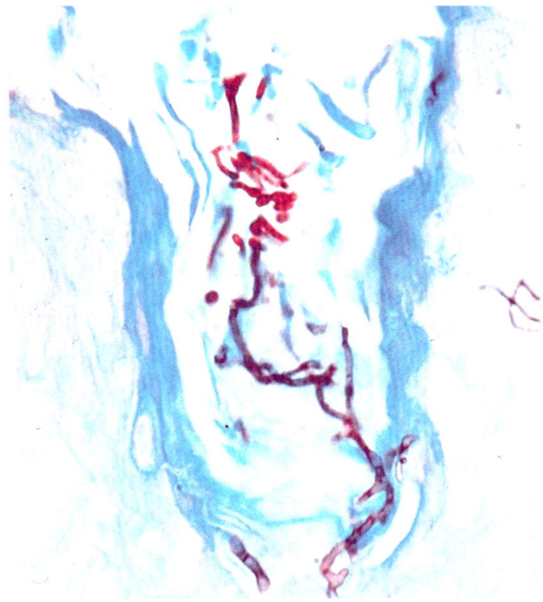

B
X720

PAS STAIN

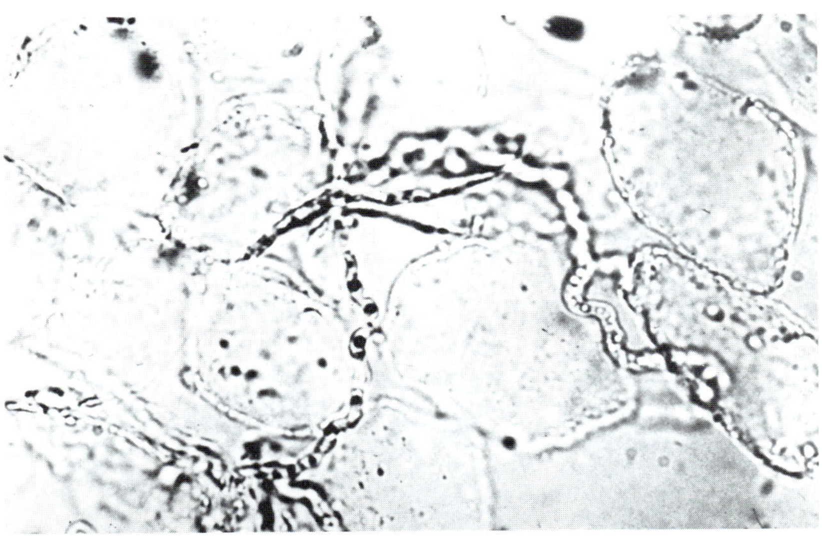

C
X800

FUNGUS INFECTIONS continued ⇨

TINEA CAPITIS

Tinea capitis is characterized by breaking off of scalp hairs near the level of the scalp and by varying degrees of scaling and inflammation of the skin of the scalp. Follicular papules may be present. Pronounced inflammation with boggy folliculitis, diffuse edema, and crusting is called a *kerion*.

Prior to 1960, most cases of tinea capitis in the United States were caused by *Microsporum canis* or *Microsporum audouini*. Since then *Trichophyton tonsurans* has become the dominant organism. Infections with *Microsporum* are limited to prepubertal children. Infections with *Trichophyton* organisms can occur in children or adults. Most hairs infected with *Microsporum* organisms fluoresce a metallic green with Wood's light; hairs infected with *Trichophyton* organisms do not fluoresce.

Infections with *M. audouini* show areas of broken off hairs with moderate scaling (Fig. A). Infections with *M. canis* or *T. tonsurans* tend to show more inflammation, which in its extreme form is a kerion (Fig. B). *T. tonsurans* infection, with only scaling and broken off scalp hairs, is called *black dot ringworm*.

Favus is a fungus infection of the scalp with considerable inflammation, perifollicular crusts and scarring (Fig. C). It is rare in the United States. The causative organism is *Trichophyton schoenleini*.

Microscopic features

1. Fungi (spores and hyphae) can usually be demonstrated in sections with special stains, such as PAS stain (Fig. D). The organism is present in and around hair shafts. Fungi also usually can be observed without staining in KOH whole mounts of affected hairs (Fig. E).
2. When inflammation is present, it is represented by perifolliculitis, with or without granuloma formation and sometimes by follicular pustules, depending on the intensity of the inflammatory reaction.
3. In favus the crusts and scales contain many hyphae and few spores. The dermis shows an inflammatory reaction and ultimately, fibrosis.

TINEA CAPITIS

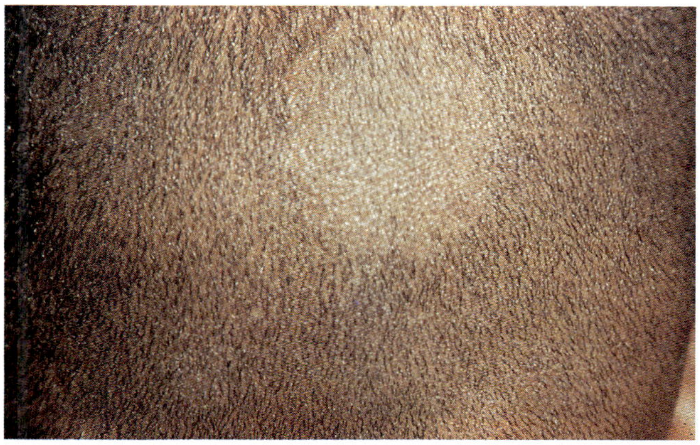

A

B

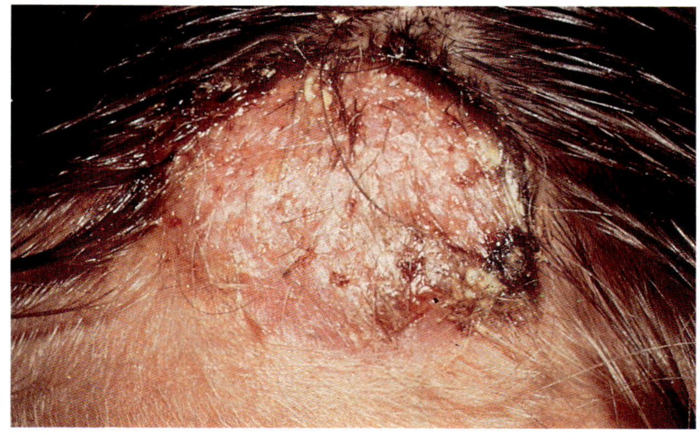

C

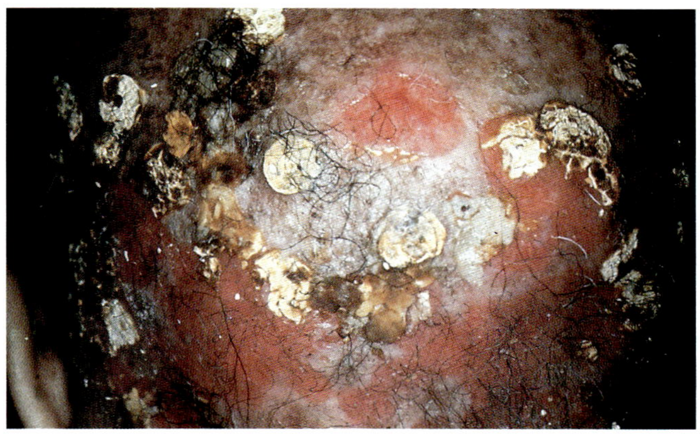

D

X500

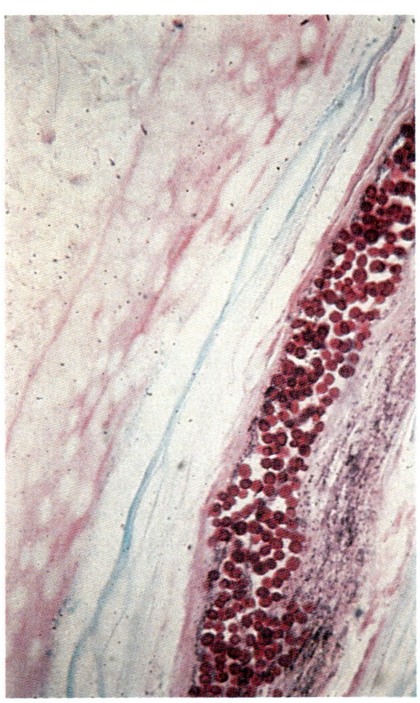

PAS STAIN

E

X500

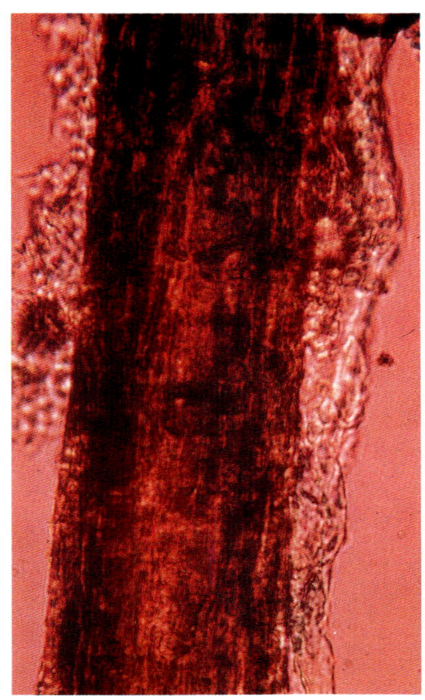

KOH WHOLE MOUNT

FUNGUS INFECTIONS continued ⇨

TRICHOPHYTON RUBRUM GRANULOMA (MAJOCCHI GRANULOMA)

T. rubrum or *T. verrucosum* may produce a nodular, granulomatous perifolliculitis (Fig. A), often on the legs of women who shave. There is often an associated fungus infection of the soles.

Microscopic features

1. There are varying degrees of folliculitis. The follicular wall may be penetrated by inflammatory cells (Fig. B). Spores may be seen at the periphery of hair shafts. A granulomatous component or suppuration may be present.
2. With PAS stain (Fig. C) or with silver methenamine stain (Fig. D), hyphae can be demonstrated within the hair shafts and occasionally in the dermis.

T. RUBRUM GRANULOMA

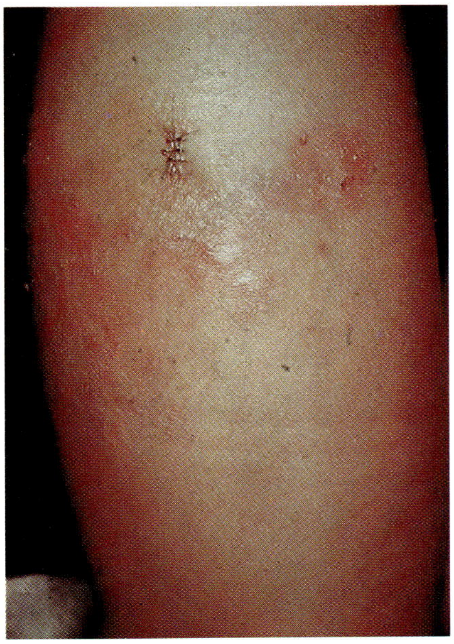

A

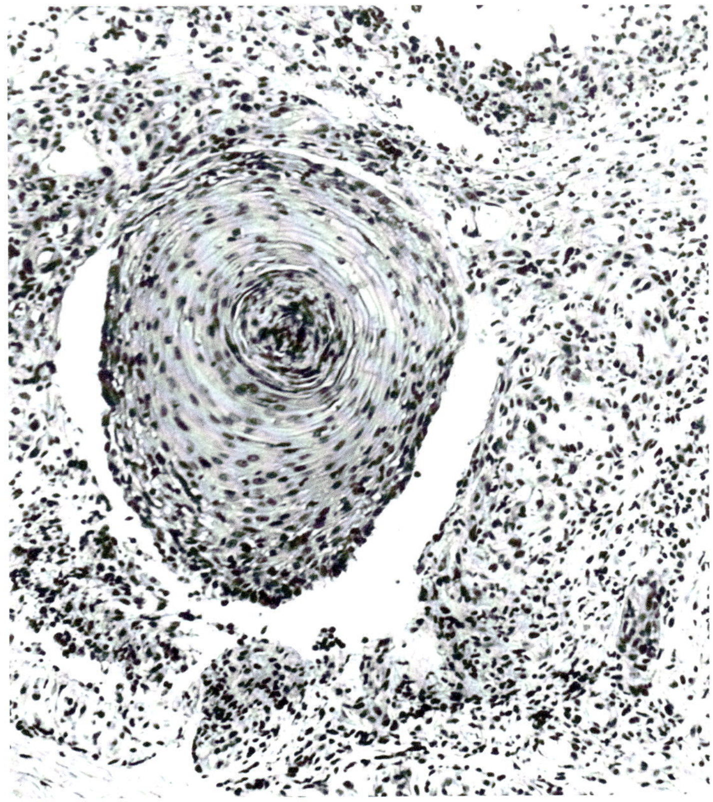

B
X175

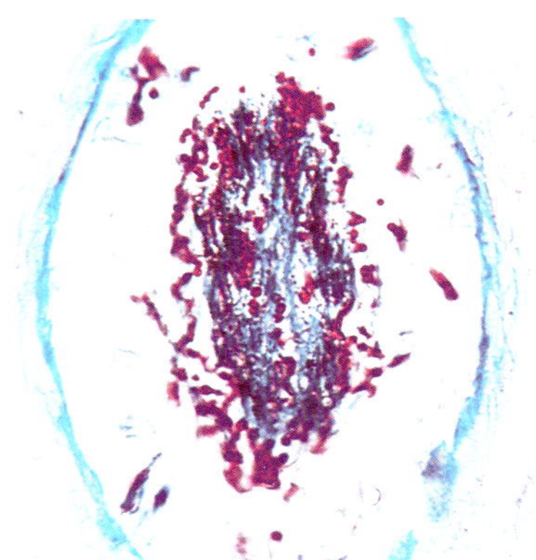

C
X720

PAS STAIN

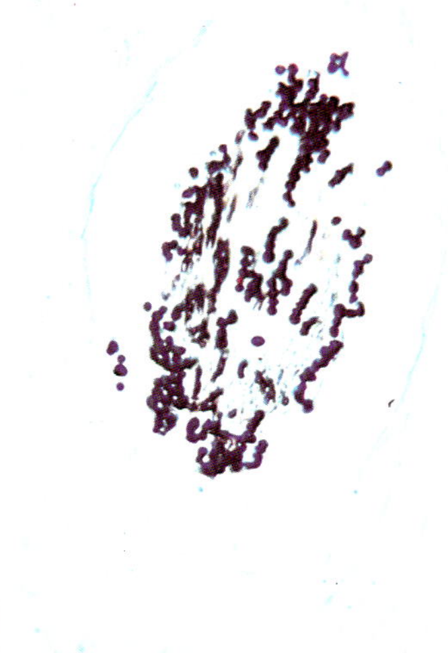

D
X720

SILVER METHENAMINE STAIN

FUNGUS INFECTIONS continued ⇨

ONYCHOMYCOSIS (TINEA UNGUIUM)

Dermatologists generally consider both of these terms to represent infection of the nails with dermatophyte fungi. Some mycologists have restricted the term *onychomycosis* to represent infection with yeasts and nondermatophyte fungi.

When there is dermatophyte infection of the nails, the nail plate may show various degrees of distortion (including pitting and ridging and various degrees of dissolution). Subungual hyperkeratosis is typically present, resulting in a yellowish zone, extending inward from the free edge (Fig. A). Clear-cut distinction of onychomycosis from psoriasis of the nails on clinical grounds is not possible (see p. 450).

Microscopic features

With special stains, such as PAS stain, hyphae and spores can be demonstrated in the nail plate and beneath it (Fig. B).

ONYCHOMYCOSIS

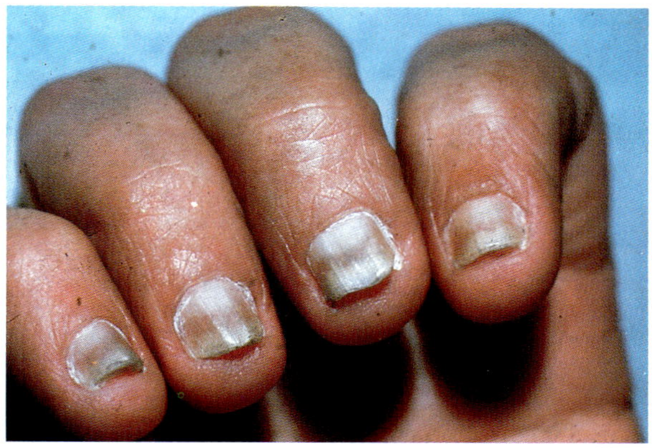

A

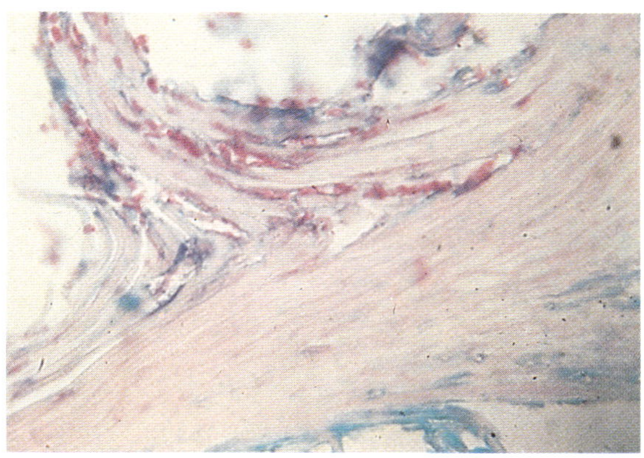

B

X500

PAS STAIN

FUNGUS INFECTIONS continued

Intermediate Fungus Infections: Candidiasis

Candida species are part of the normal flora of the mouth and gastrointestinal tract. The organisms are opportunistic. Local factors favoring infection include moisture and friction (as in intertriginous areas); systemic factors include diabetes and other endocrine diseases, pregnancy, broad spectrum antibiotic therapy, use of immunosuppressive drugs, and neoplastic disorders. Candidiasis is commonly observed in AIDS and ARC.

Candidiasis can be divided into acute and chronic mucocutaneous forms and systemic forms.

Candida albicans, the causative organism, is dimorphous, showing both yeast and filamentous forms in skin lesions.

ACUTE MUCOCUTANEOUS CANDIDIASIS

Acute mucocutaneous candidiasis often involves intertriginous areas of the skin, including the interdigital areas (Fig. A), groin (Fig. B), mucous membranes (including mouth [Fig. D] and vulvovaginal area), and fingernails (paronychia or onychia). In infants, candidiasis is often a component of diaper rash (Fig. C).

Cutaneous lesions of acute mucocutaneous candidiasis are vesiculopustules in their early stage. Later, the lesions are confluent, erythematous, or weeping areas (Figs. B,C). In such areas satellite lesions occur (Fig. B). *Erosio interdigitalis blastomycetica* refers to erosions caused by Candida in the interdigital webs (Fig. A).

CANDIDIASIS

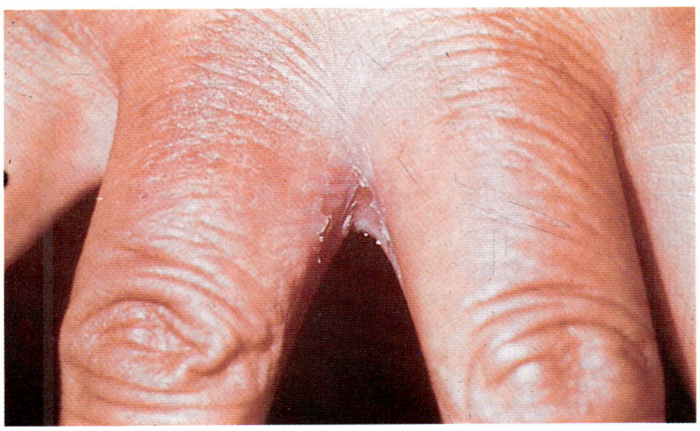

A

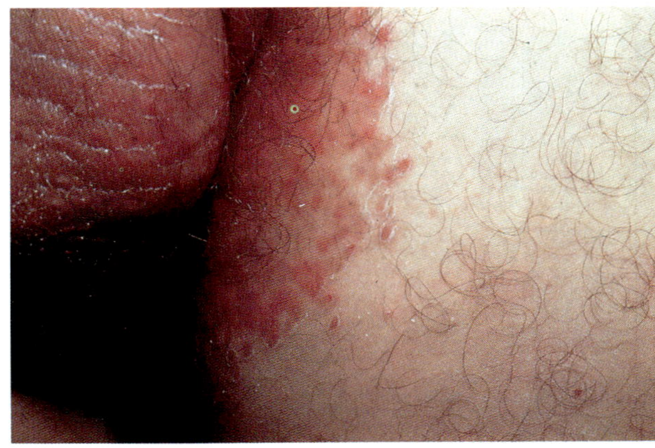

B

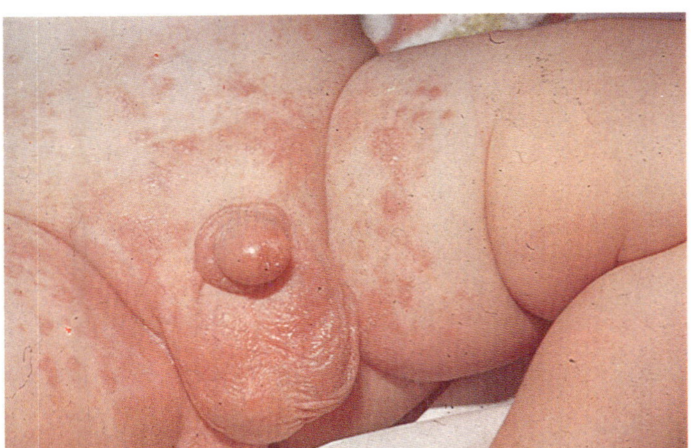

C

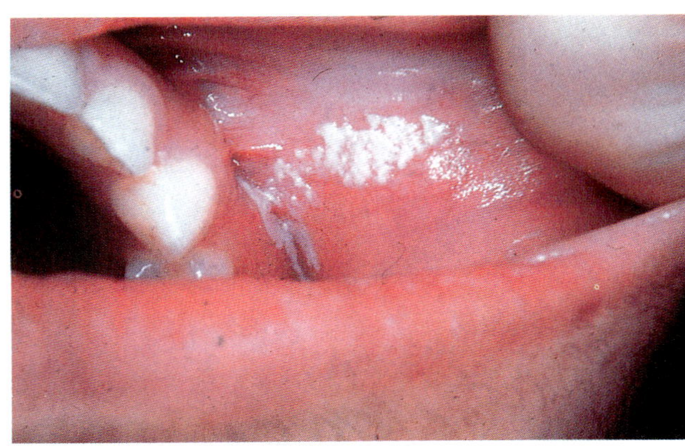

D

FUNGUS INFECTIONS continued ⇨

ACUTE MUCOCUTANEOUS CANDIDIASIS

Microscopic features

1. The initial lesion of superficial cutaneous candidiasis is a subcorneal pustule, similar to that of impetigo (Figs. A,B). Spongiform pustules may be present (Fig. B) (see p. 456).
2. Small numbers of PAS-positive organisms are present in the stratum corneum. These consist of oval blastospores and septate, branching hyphae (Fig C.)

Comment

1. *Chronic mucocutaneous candidiasis* is associated with a spectrum of congenital defects, immunological disorders, and endocrine disorders. Histologic findings parallel those of acute mucocutaneous candidiasis except in candidal granuloma, which shows a granulomatous tissue reaction.
2. *Systemic candidiasis* is a serious and potentially fatal disorder associated with an impaired immune system. Therapy with corticosteroids, chemotherapy, and hematologic malignancies are examples of factors that predispose to systemic candidiasis. Systemic candidiasis may involve the blood and a variety of organs. Skin lesions may be present; they are typically red or purple papulonodules. Histopathological examination with PAS stain or silver methenamine stain may show budding spores and hyphae in areas of vessel damage.
3. *Acrodermatitis enteropathica* is an autosomal recessive inherited disorder with an underlying zinc deficiency. It is characterized by retarded growth, diffuse alopecia, and diarrhea. The mucocutaneous lesions resemble those of candidiasis. *Candida albicans* can often be recovered from these lesions; it has been proposed that this disease is associated with an inherited susceptibility to Candida albicans. Cutaneous lesions tend to be periorificial and acral. Paronychia is common. The histologic pattern of acrodermatitis enteropathica is that of subacute or chronic dermatitis.
4. *Granuloma gluteale infantum* is a nodular eruption of the buttocks, usually observed in infants. It is believed to be related to diaper dermatitis and to topical application of corticosteroids. Granuloma gluteale infantum may be associated with secondary Candida infection.
5. *Candida folliculitis* has been described in heroin addicts, possibly related to hematogenous dissemination of the organism.

CANDIDIASIS

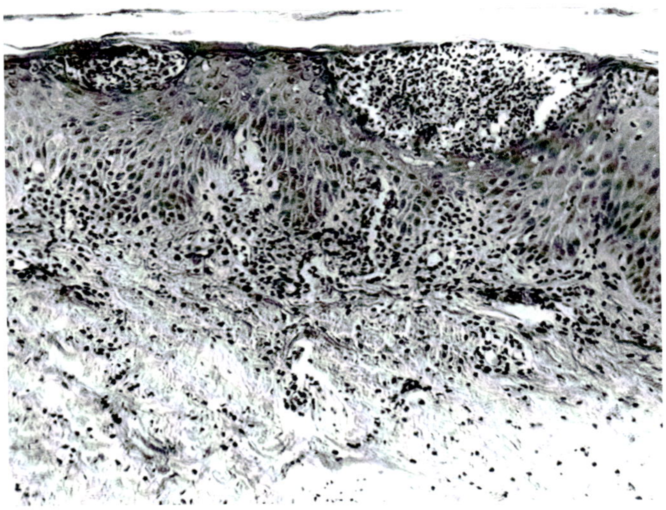

A
X200

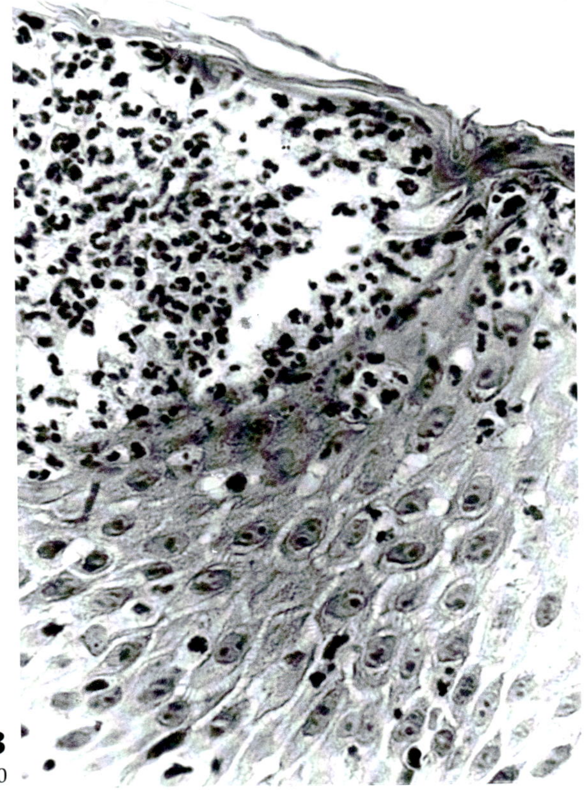

B
X690

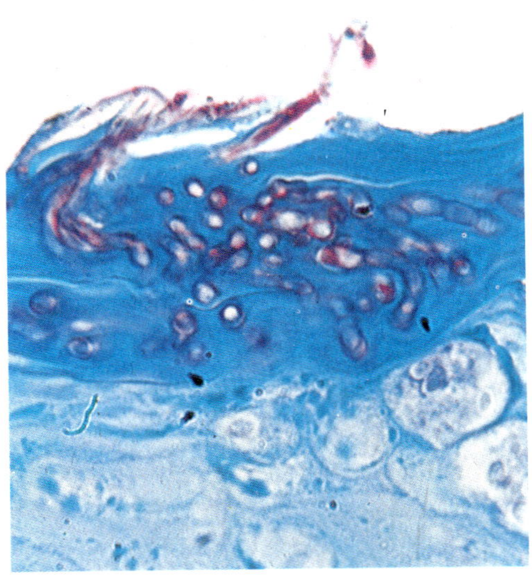

C
X1200

PAS STAIN

FUNGUS INFECTIONS continued

Deep Fungus Infections

Deep fungus infection refers to disorders caused by organisms that are not limited to keratinous areas and can invade a variety of tissues. There are two principal groups: true pathogenic fungi and opportunistic fungi. The first group includes *Blastomyces, Coccidioides, Paracoccidioides,* and *Histoplasma*. The second group includes *Mucor* and *Cryptococcus*. *Candida* can be included in this category, but is discussed elsewhere due to its ability to produce superficial localized disease in normal individuals. Deep fungus infections commonly affect patients with AIDS.

Opportunistic fungus infections are caused by organisms of low virulence, which cause disease in individuals with low host resistance due to other diseases or therapeutic agents.

Some pathogenic fungi are of relatively limited virulence and usually cause cutaneous or subcutaneous disease at the site of implantation; *Sporotrichum* and species causing chromomycosis are in this group.

Most infections with the true pathogenic fungi are either asymptomatic or of relatively short duration. Rapid development of cell-mediated immunity with a granulomatous response is the rule. Deep fungus infections often have limited geographical distribution. Adult, dark-skinned males are most susceptible.

Systemic disease due to the true pathogenic fungi usually has a pulmonary portal of entry, with subsequent disseminated granulomatous lesions.

The histologic picture of deep fungus infection is often characterized by reactive epidermal hyperplasia and by a granulomatous infiltrate with foci of abscess formation. The most common clinical pattern is the formation of verrucous, granulomatous cutaneous lesions at the site of inoculation.

Actinomycosis is included in this section even though the causative organism is now considered a bacterium. The organism resembles a fungus, and in the past it was so considered. *Mycetoma* is also caused by organisms now considered to be bacteria, but is included for similar reasons.

Deep Fungus Infections

HISTOLOGIC FEATURES OF DEEP FUNGUS INFECTIONS

Suppurative granulomas are the hallmark of deep fungus infections.

North American blastomycosis	1. Organisms appear in tissue as PAS-positive, solitary spores with single buds; the spores are approximately 10 microns in diameter. 2. There is pseudoepitheliomatous hyperplasia with intraepidermal abscesses and Langhans giant cells. 3. The dermis contains a mixed infiltrate with many neutrophils which form small abscesses. Langhans giant cells and noncaseating granulomas are present. 4. Spores are located in giant cells or are free in the dermis; with H&E stain they appear as "punched-out" areas in giant cells. 5. The histologic pattern resembles bromide granuloma.
South American blastomycosis	1. The organisms appear in tissue as PAS-positive spores, 60 microns in diameter, and often show multiple buds ("pilot-wheel" appearance). 2. The dermis shows a granulomatous infiltrate with foreign-body and Langhans giant cells. Acute inflammatory cells and abscesses are present. 3. The organisms are present both in giant cells and free in tissue, particularly in areas of abscess formation.
Chromomycosis	1. Organisms appear in tissue as thick-walled brown spores with an average diameter of 12 microns; cross-walls may be present. Spores are often present in clusters or chains. 2. The histologic pattern of the verrucous nodules and plaques is similar to that of North American blastomycosis. Organisms are in giant cells or in the intercellular spaces. 3. Subcutaneous abscesses are enclosed by a granulomatous zone and a fibrous tissue capsule. The picture resembles scrofuloderma.
Coccidioidomycosis	1. Organisms appear in tissue as PAS-positive spherules as large as 80 microns in diameter. Endospores may be present. 2. Verrucous lesions of disseminated coccidioidomycosis have a histologic pattern similar to that of North American blastomycosis and differ by the occasional presence of caseation necrosis and fewer abscesses. 3. Subcutaneous abscesses show a picture similar to that of chromomycosis.
Sporotrichosis	1. Organisms are only rarely visualized in tissue, and are best demonstrated by PAS stain after diastase digestion. They appear as round or oval spores 5 microns in diameter or as cigar-shaped structures 6 microns in length. Spores with radiating projections (asteroid bodies) are rare except in cases of sporotrichosis originating in S. Africa. 2. The early chancre shows a nonspecific mixed infiltrate. 3. Verrucous lesions show a picture similar to that of North American blastomycosis. 4. Lymphatic nodules show central abscesses surrounded by a tuberculoid infiltrate and a zone of lymphocytes and plasma cells. The histologic picture resembles that of lymphopathia venereum or cat scratch fever.
Cryptococcosis	1. Organisms appear in tissue as PAS-positive spherical spores with a diameter ranging from 5 to 20 microns. Budding may be present. Spores have a gelatinous capsule which take stains for acid mucopolysaccharides. 2. There are two types of histologic patterns: a. *gelatinous*—groups of organisms are present with little tissue reaction; b. *granulomatous*—there is a dense infiltrate composed of histiocytes, giant cells, lymphocytes, and fibroblasts, with foci of necrosis. Organisms are in histiocytes and giant cells and in the intercellular spaces.
Histoplasmosis (see chart p. 290)	1. Organisms appear in tissue as PAS-positive spores averaging 3 microns in diameter. With H&E stain, the spores appear to be surrounded by a ring or pseudocapsule. 2. In primary histoplasmosis, disseminated histoplasmosis, or localized histoplasmosis there is a nonspecific inflammatory infiltrate with areas of necrosis and occasional giant cells. The spores are present within large histiocytes. Regional lymph nodes also show spores within histiocytes. Granulomas can be present in less fulminating forms.
Actinomycosis	1. Organisms are present in draining purulent material in clumps called *sulfur granules* which are lobulated groups of filaments with club-shaped free ends. Sulfur granules are PAS-positive and Gram-positive. 2. Large abscesses surrounded by granulation tissue and fibrosis are present.
Mycetoma-Maduromycosis	The histologic picture is similar to that of actinomycosis. In actinomycetoma the granules are composed of filamentous bacteria. In eumycetoma the granules are composed of thick-walled true fungi.

FUNGUS INFECTIONS continued ⇨

CHROMOMYCOSIS

Chromomycosis is usually limited to the skin, but rarely can have cystic subcutaneous or cerebral involvement. The infection is caused by species of *Fonsecaea, Phialophora,* or *Cladosporium*. These are saprophytes that can be found in soil or decaying vegetation. Cerebral chromomycosis is caused by *Cladosporium trichoides*.

The primary lesion is believed to develop after traumatic implantation of the organism into the skin. The lower extremities are sites of predilection. Lesions consist of verrucous nodules and plaques (Fig. A).

Microscopic features

1. The organisms appear as thick-walled brown spores having an average diameter of 12 microns (Fig. B). They are usually present in clusters. Reproduction is by fission, resulting in septations. No buds are observed.
2. The histologic picture generally corresponds to that of disseminated cutaneous lesions of North American blastomycosis (see p. 358). Subcutaneous lesions are abscesses surrounded by a granulomatous zone and a zone of fibrosis.

CHROMOMYCOSIS

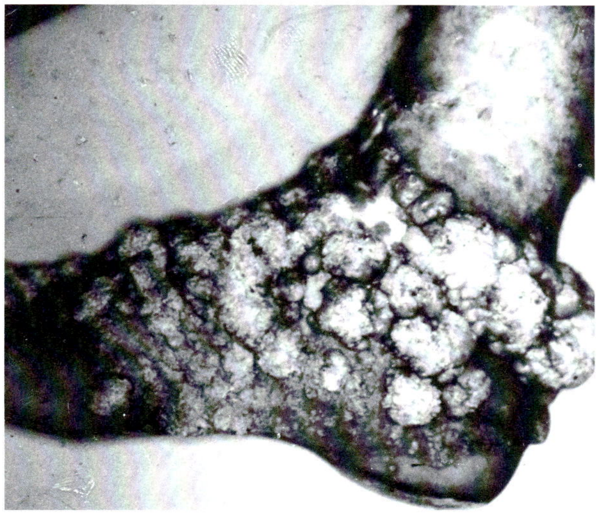

A

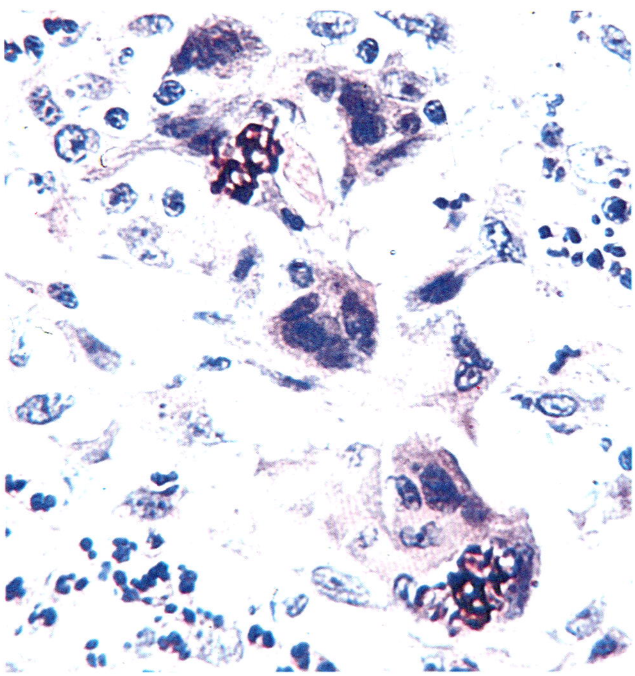

B
X1000

Courtesy Center for Disease Control

FUNGUS INFECTIONS continued ⇨

SPOROTRICHOSIS

The causative organism, *Sporotrix schenkii* is found in soil and decaying vegetation. The most common form of the infection is primary inoculation sporotrichosis. This usually is expressed as lymphocutaneous lesions. Initially, a papule forms, which then ulcerates. Subsequently, nodules form along lymph vessels, and these may suppurate and ulcerate (Fig. A). Primary sporotrichosis may also be expressed as the fixed cutaneous form—a plaque with ulcerative, crusted, or verrucous surface, typically on the face or on an arm. Lesions of sporotrichosis can resemble pyoderma gangrenosum.

There is an asymptomatic pulmonary form of sporotrichosis as well as unifocal and multifocal systemic forms. The systemic form may be associated with depression of the immune system.

Microscopic features

1. The organisms only rarely can be observed in the tissues. With PAS stain they appear as oval to round budding spores, averaging 5 microns in greatest diameter (Fig. D). To localize organisms in sections it is helpful to remove glycogen with diastase before staining with PAS stain. Asteroid bodies (spores with radiating projections) are rarely seen in cases originating in the United States, but are frequently seen in cases originating in South Africa, Japan, and Australia. Asteroid bodies are eosinophilic with H&E stain (Fig. E).
2. Early primary lesions and lymphatic nodules show a nonspecific infiltrate composed of neutrophils, plasma cells, lymphocytes, and histiocytes. As lesions progress, characteristic stellate abscesses form (Figs. B,C). These show a central abscess (Figs. B,C), surrounded by a tuberculoid infiltrate and an outermost zone of chronic inflammatory cells (Fig. B). Lesions which have progressed to the verrucous stage show a picture resembling that of North American blastomycosis.

Microscopic differential diagnosis

1. The histologic picture resembles that of lymphogranuloma venereum and cat scratch disease (see p. 396), and microscopic differentiation may be impossible.
2. North American blastomycosis can be differentiated from the verrucous stage of sporotrichosis by the presence of characteristic blastospores of *Blastomyces dermatitidis*.

SPOROTRICHOSIS

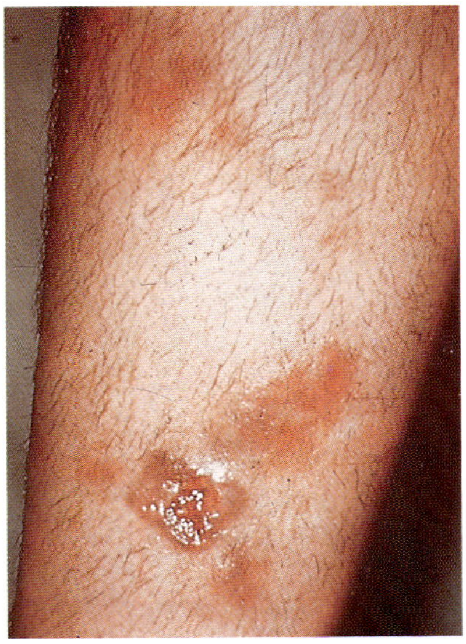

A

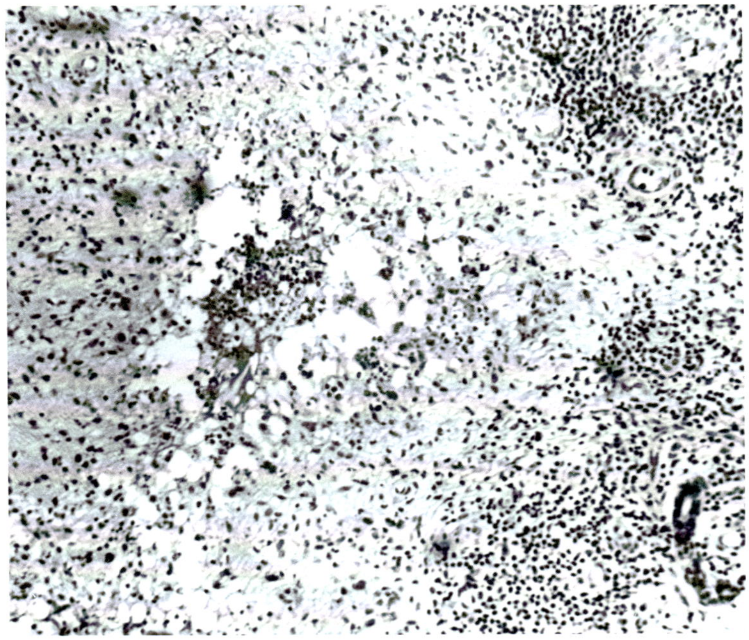

B
X250

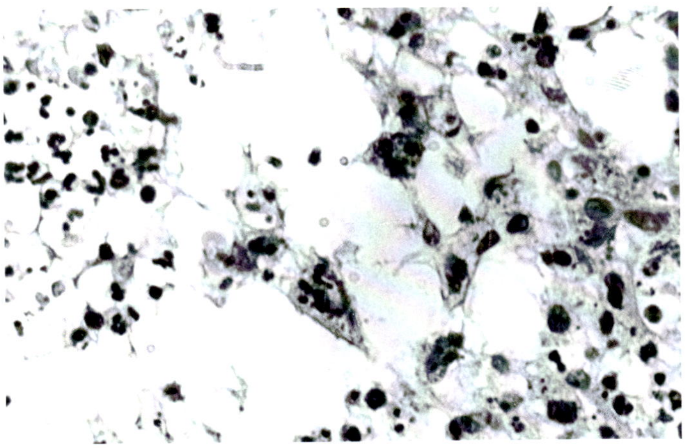

C
X530

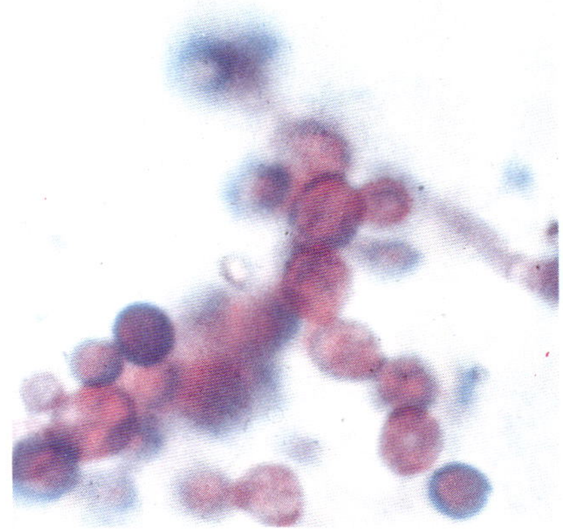

D
X1300
Courtesy Dr. Herbert Mescon PAS STAIN

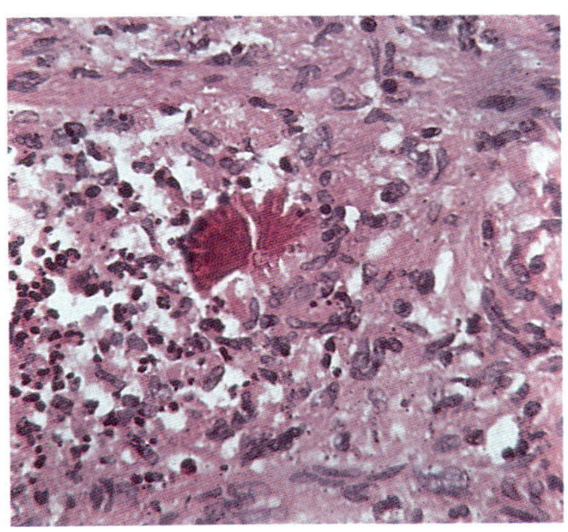

E
X500
Courtesy Center for Disease Control

FUNGUS INFECTIONS continued

NORTH AMERICAN BLASTOMYCOSIS

North American blastomycosis is a deep fungus infection due to the dimorphic organism *Blastomyces dermatitidis*. The primary focus is usually in the lungs; this may be followed by pulmonary disease. A primary cutaneous chancre is rare; it is accompanied by lymphadenitis and lymphadenopathy. Disseminated lesions from the primary pulmonary focus commonly involve the skin, bones, central nervous system, and genitalia. Cutaneous blastomycosis is the most common form of extrapulmonary disease. Papules, pustules, or erosions develop into verrucous areas with sharply defined margins (Figs. A,B). There may be involvement of the oral or nasal mucosa.

Microscopic features

1. Organisms appear in tissues as thick-walled spores (with single buds) averaging 10 microns in diameter. They can be demonstrated with silver methenamine stain (Fig. C) or PAS stain. The spores may lie free in tissue or they may be within phagocytes, especially giant cells.
2. The verrucous lesions of disseminated cutaneous blastomycosis typically show pseudoepitheliomatous hyperplasia (Figs. D,E). Intraepidermal abscesses are common (Figs. D,E); scattered Langhans giant cells (Figs. D,E) and non-caseating tuberculoid granulomas may be present. The dermis contains a mixed inflammatory infiltrate with many neutrophils and occasional abscesses.

   Laryngeal involvement may produce pseudoepitheliomatous hyperplasia, causing confusion with squamous cell carcinoma.

NORTH AMERICAN BLASTOMYCOSIS

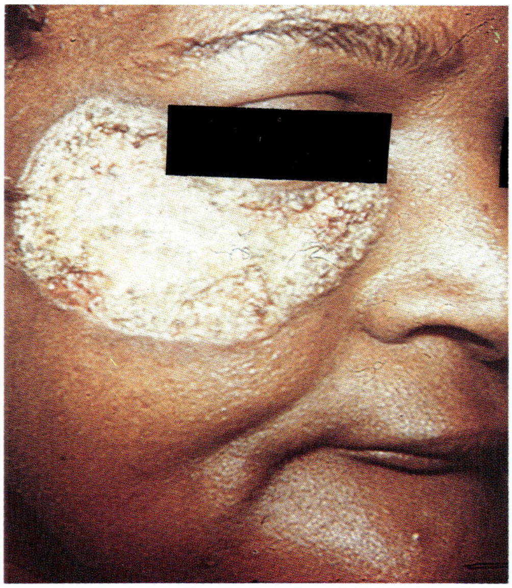

A

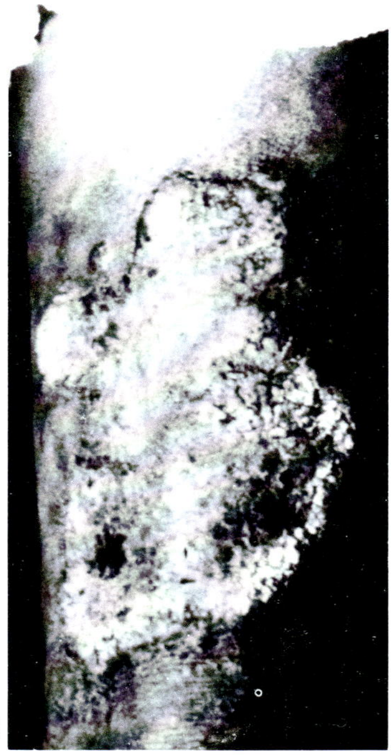

B

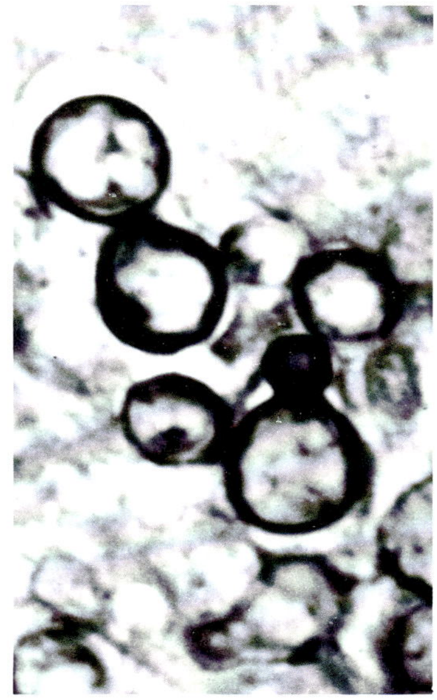

C
X2400

SILVER METHENAMINE STAIN

Courtesy Center for Disease Control

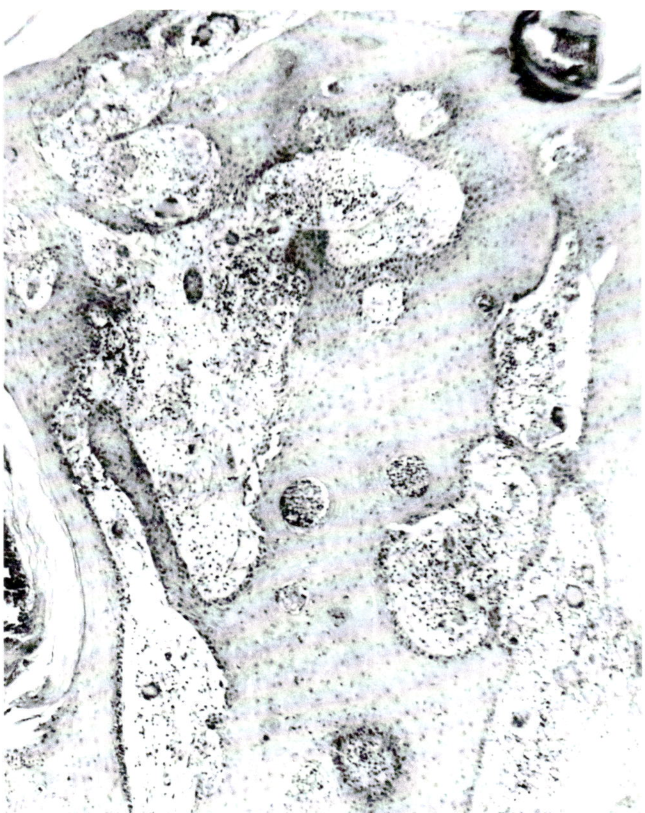

D
X48

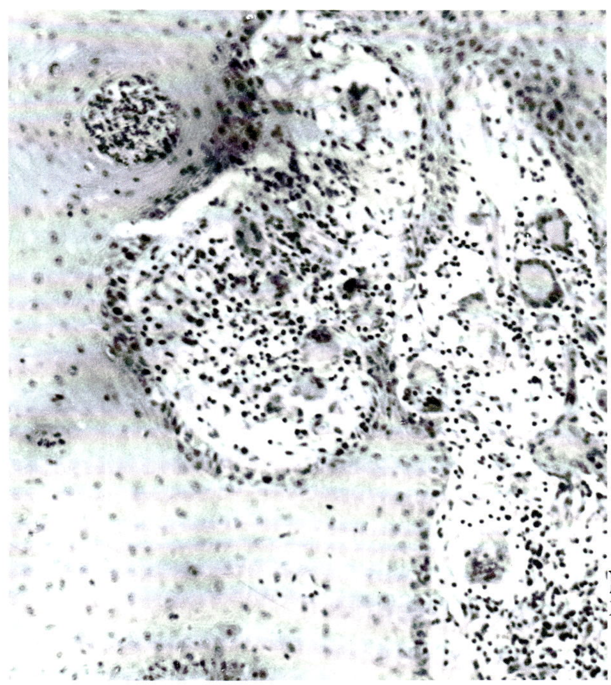

E
X120

FUNGUS INFECTIONS continued

NORTH AMERICAN BLASTOMYCOSIS

Microscopic features

3. In some areas organisms are interspersed among masses of histiocytes (Fig. A).
4. Spores are often located in Langhans giant cells (Figs. B,C); with H&E they appear as punched-out areas (Fig. B); with PAS stain they appear bright red (Fig. C).
5. In primary cutaneous blastomycosis there is a nonspecific infiltrate containing numerous organisms. Regional lymph nodes show a granulomatous infiltrate.

NORTH AMERICAN BLASTOMYCOSIS

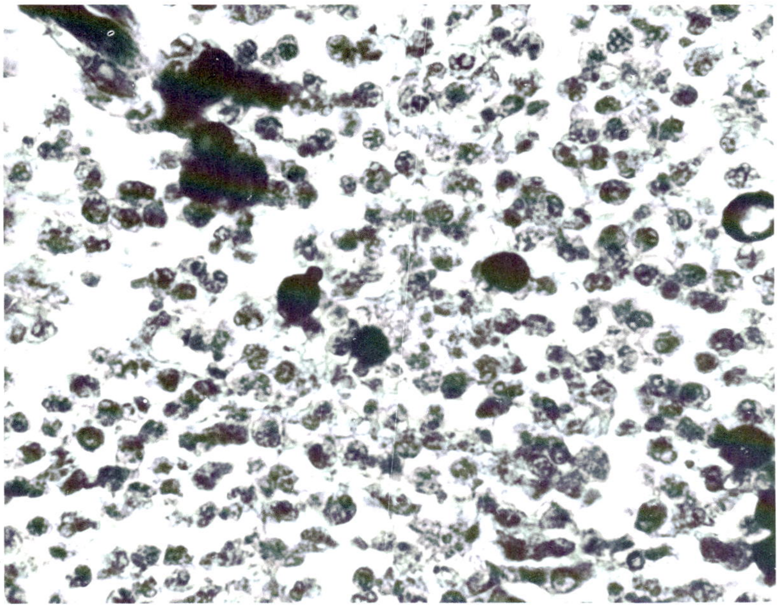

A
X1350
SILVER METHENAMINE
STAIN

Courtesy Center for Disease Control

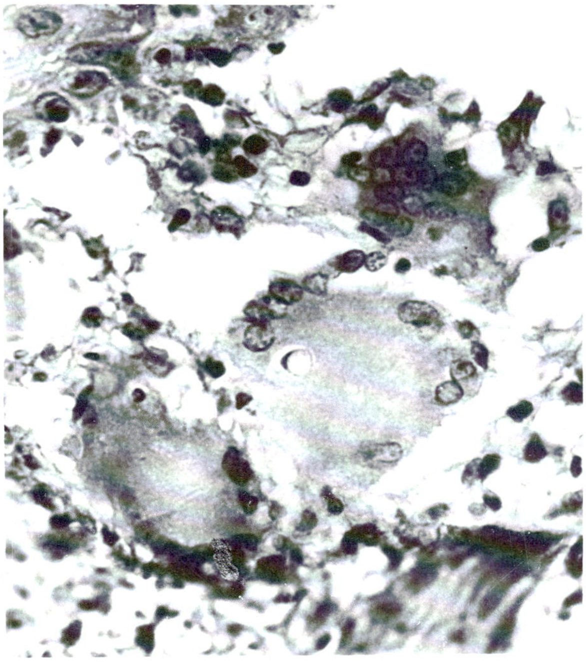

B
X580

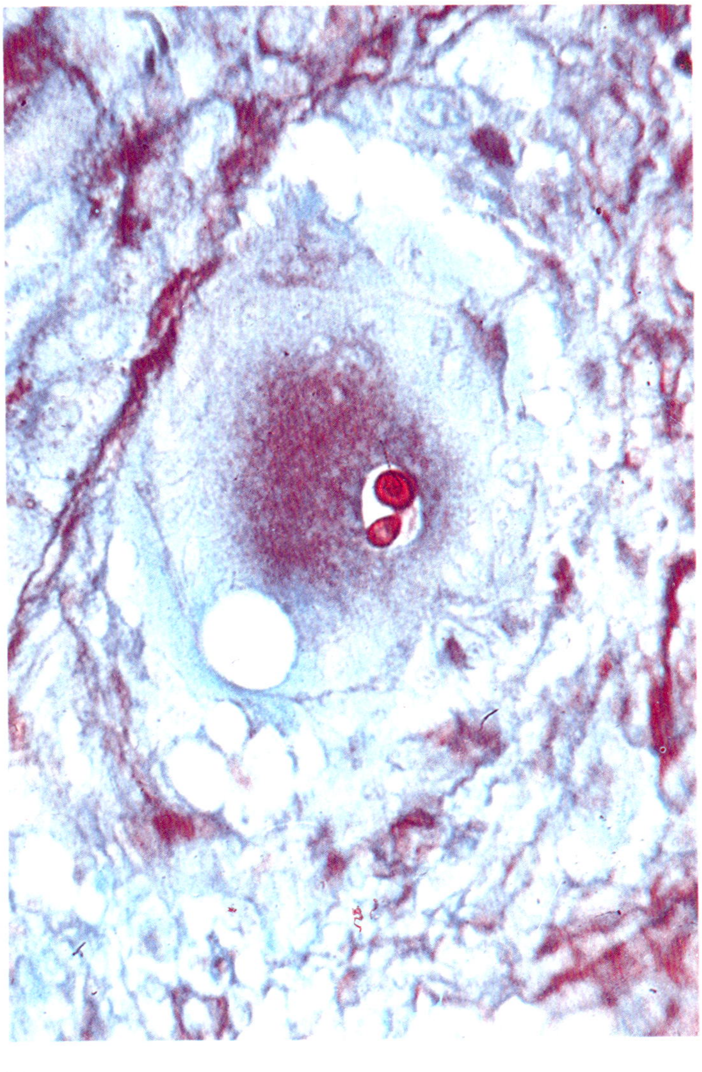

C
X800
PAS
STAIN

FUNGUS INFECTIONS continued ⇨

SOUTH AMERICAN BLASTOMYCOSIS (PARACOCCIDIOIDOMYCOSIS)

Paracoccidioidomycosis (South American blastomycosis) is caused by *Paracoccidioides brasiliensis* and is endemic to Central and South America. The disease pattern parallels that of North American blastomycosis.

The primary focus is usually in the lungs. Symptomatic or asymptomatic pulmonary disease may be followed by disseminated disease. About 50% of the patients with disseminated disease develop ulcerated, granulomatous lesions of the skin (Fig. A) or upper respiratory tract. Regional lymphadenopathy is common. Visceral involvement may include lesions of the intestinal tract or adrenals.

Microscopic features

1. With silver methenamine stain (Fig. B) or PAS stain, spores with multiple buds ("pilot's wheel" pattern) can be demonstrated. The average diameter of the spores is 60 microns. The configuration of the spores is diagnostic. Spores with single buds are also present.
2. The overall histologic picture of disseminated cutaneous lesions corresponds to that of North American blastomycosis (see p. 358).

Comment

Lobomycosis is a granulomatous cutaneous fungus infection observed in parts of Central and South America. Organisms are believed to enter the skin after injury. Lesions are keloidal nodules and plaques. The organism (*Loboa loboi*) is a spore, which tends to form chains. Single buds may be present.

SOUTH AMERICAN BLASTOMYCOSIS

A
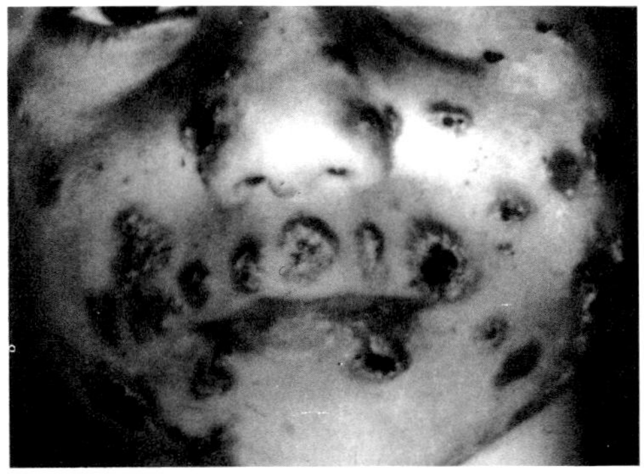

Courtesy Center for Disease Control

B
X520
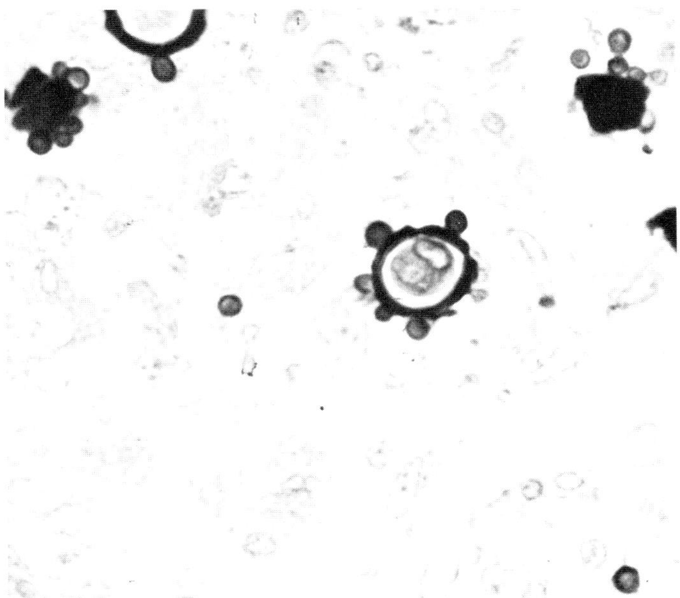

SILVER METHENAMINE STAIN

COCCIDIOIDOMYCOSIS

Coccidioidomycosis is another deep fungus infection whose disease pattern parallels that of North American blastomycosis. It is caused by *Coccidioides immitis*, an organism found in the soil. Coccidioidomycosis is endemic to southwestern United States and northern Mexico. Primary inoculation coccidioidomycosis is rare. The usual portal of entry is the lungs. Pulmonary disease is often accompanied by erythema nodosum. Asymptomatic or symptomatic pulmonary disease may follow. Asymptomatic pulmonary disease may be activated by immunosuppressive therapy. In 0.1% of the cases, disseminated disease develops. Cutaneous lesions are verrucous granulomas, nodules (Fig. A), or subcutaneous abscesses, which may break through the surface and drain.

Microscopic features

1. The organism appears as a thick-walled spherule ranging in size from 10 to 80 microns. It contains numerous endospores (Fig. B). In the primary inoculation form, hyphae may be present.
2. The histologic picture of disseminated disease corresponds in overall picture to that of the disseminated cutaneous lesions of North American blastomycosis (see p. 358). Caseation necrosis is occasionally present. When subcutaneous abscesses are present, the histologic picture resembles that of scrofuloderma.

COCCIDIOIDOMYCOSIS

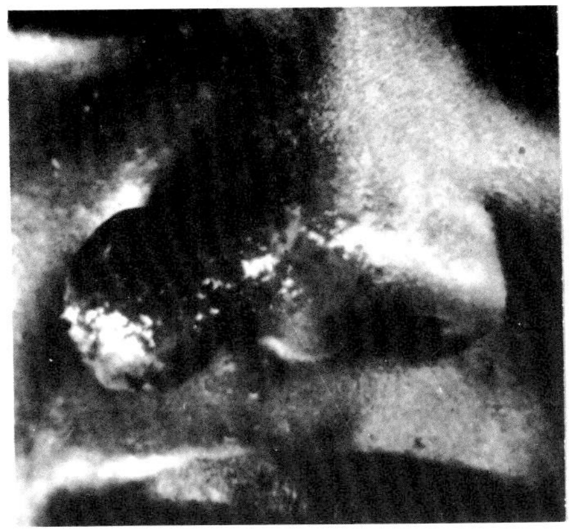

A

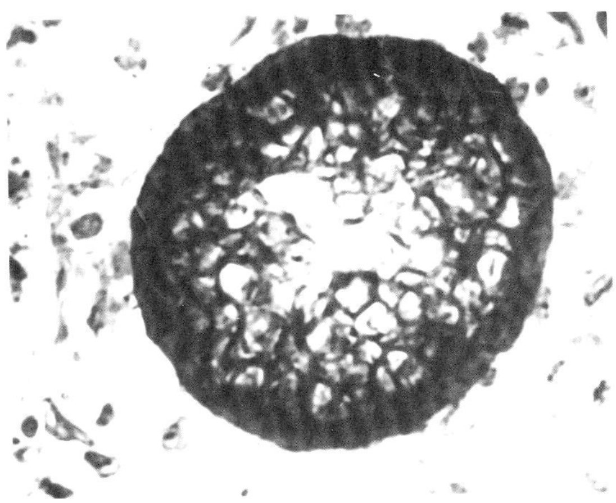

B
X1200

SILVER METHENAMINE STAIN

FUNGUS INFECTIONS continued

HISTOPLASMOSIS

Histoplasmosis is another disease whose pattern parallels that of North American blastomycosis. The causative organism is the dimorphous fungus *Histoplasma capsulatum*, which is found in the soil. The disease has worldwide distribution; it is endemic to central-eastern United States. Histoplasmosis is usually acquired by inhalation. The majority of cases have asymptomatic pulmonary infection, but acute or chronic pulmonary disease may occur. In a very small percentage of cases, disseminated disease may develop, with widespread lesions. The reticuloendothelial system and adrenals are often involved. About 50% of the cases develop lesions of the oral mucosa. Cutaneous lesions are not common. They are often indurated ulcers (Fig. A). Sinus tracts may develop, particularly in the penis (Fig. C), resulting in a "watering can" appearance. Cutaneous lesions may occasionally be associated with a disseminated erythroderma.

Microscopic features

1. The key feature is the presence of numerous spores within the cytoplasm of macrophages (histiocytes). They can be seen with H&E stain as well as with special stains, such as PAS or methenamine silver. The spores average 3 microns in diameter and are surrounded by a clear space called a pseudocapsule (Fig. B). This clear space has been shown with electron microscopy to represent the matrix of a secondary lysosome containing the organism. Budding spores can be demonstrated (Fig. D). Giant cells may be present.
2. There is usually ulceration and necrosis, sometimes accompanied by pseudocarcinomatous hyperplasia.
3. More chronic lesions can show epithelioid tubercles (Fig. E).

Microscopic differential diagnosis

(see chart, p. 290.)

HISTOPLASMOSIS

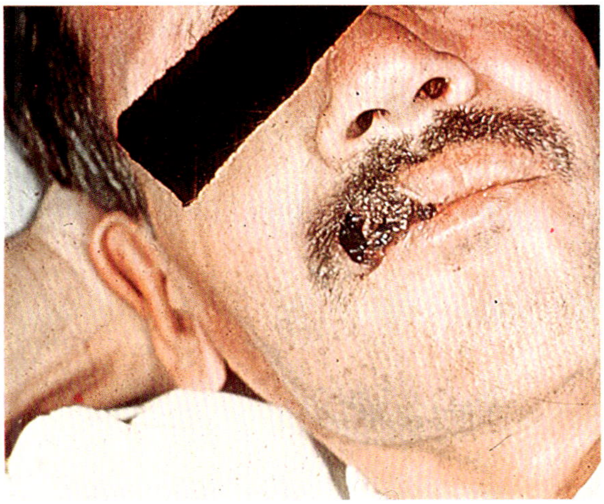

A

Figs. A,C,D courtesy Center for Disease Control

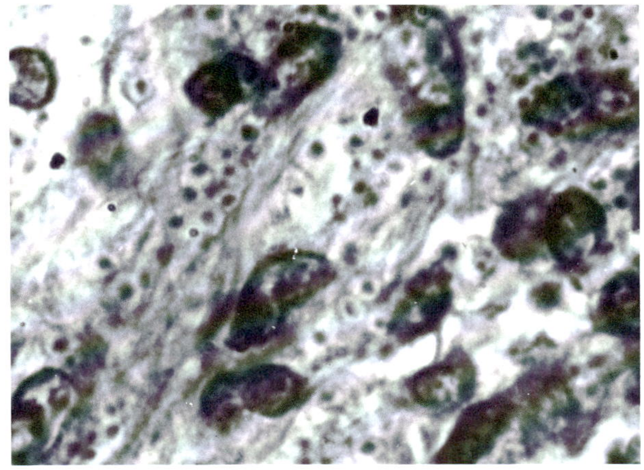

B
X1000

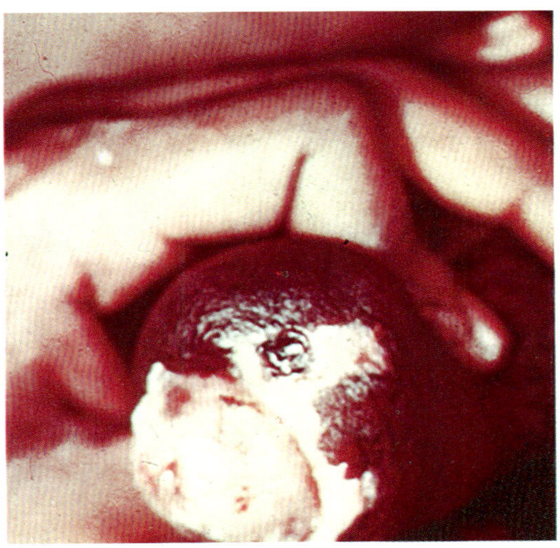

C

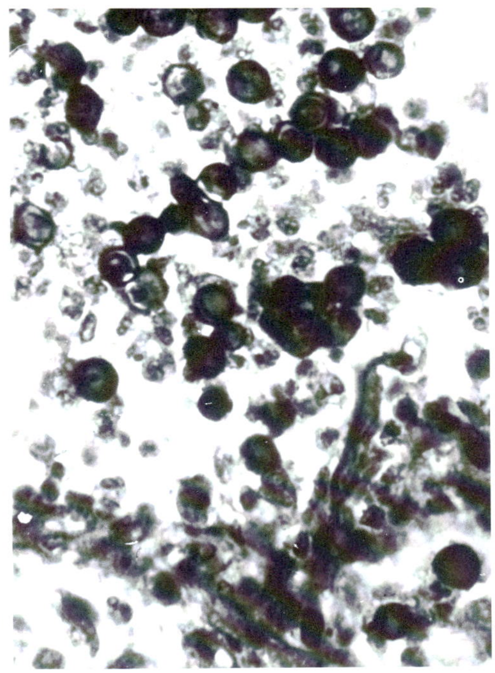

D
X3300

SILVER METHENAMINE STAIN

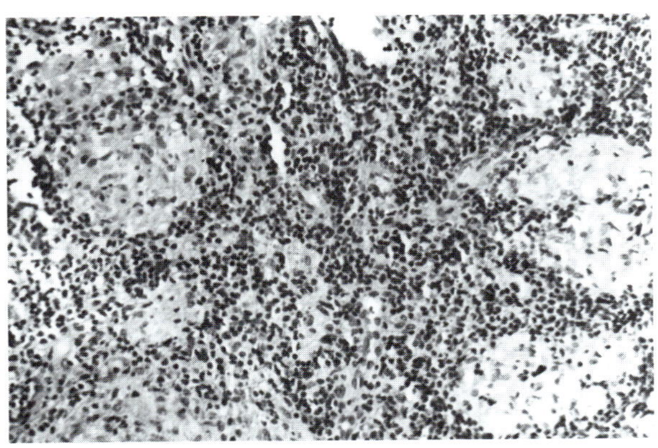

E
X130

FUNGUS INFECTIONS continued

CRYPTOCOCCOSIS (TORULOSIS)

Cryptococcosis is a chronic infectious disease caused by *Cryptococcus neoformans*, an organism found in soil and avian excreta. The primary focus is in the respiratory tract. Most often dissemination is to the meninges and occasionally to the skin and kidneys. Some authors believe that a primary cutaneous form exists. Cryptococcosis generally occurs in individuals having some debilitating factor, such as lymphoma, diabetes, AIDS, or prolonged immunosuppressive therapy. Cutaneous lesions are varied and may appear as papules, nodules with a ring of erythema, pustules, plaques, ulcers (Fig. A), or abscesses.

Microscopic features

1. The organism is readily visualized with PAS stain (Fig. B). It appears in tissue as a spherical or oval spore with a diameter of 2 to 12 microns; budding may be present. Spores are generally surrounded by a gelatinous capsule which does not stain with H&E or PAS stain (Fig. B), but which accepts stains for acid mucopolysaccharides. When the capsule is lacking, the organism is hard to distinguish from *Blastomyces dermatitidis*.
2. Two types of histologic patterns are observed: a) *gelatinous pattern* with numerous organisms and little tissue reaction; b) *granulomatous pattern* with infiltrates composed of lymphocytes, histiocytes, giant cells, and fibroblasts. Granulomatous areas may show foci of necrosis, with organisms principally within histiocytes and giant cells. Both patterns may coexist in the same lesion.

Comment

Rapid diagnosis of cryptococcosis can be made by India ink preparations, which outline the capsule of the organism.

RHINOSPORIDIOSIS

Rhinosporidiosis is a chronic granulomatous disease of mucous membranes which produces large polypoid lesions. It is endemic to India. The mucous membrane of the nose is the most common site. The cause is *Rhinosporidium seeberi*.

Microscopic features

The polypoid lesions show a nonspecific chronic inflammatory infiltrate and numerous thick-walled sporangia containing endospores (Figs. C,D). These may attain a maximum diameter of 0.5 mm.

CRYPTOCOCCOSIS

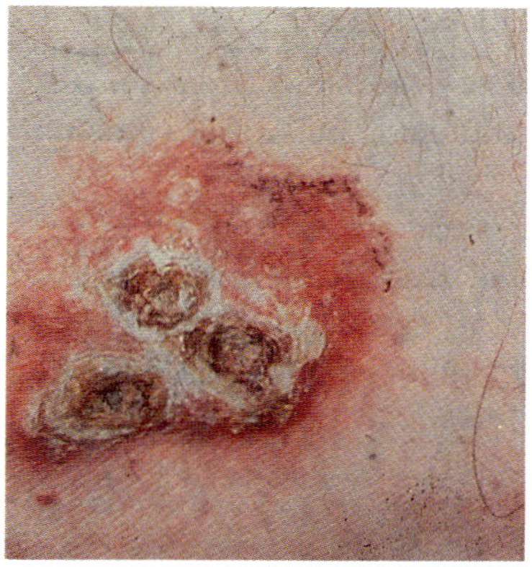

A

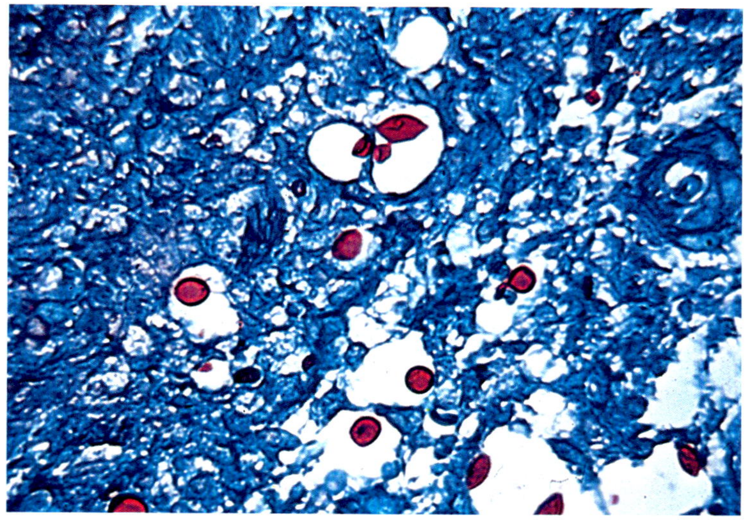

B
X1000

PAS STAIN

RHINOSPORIDIOSIS

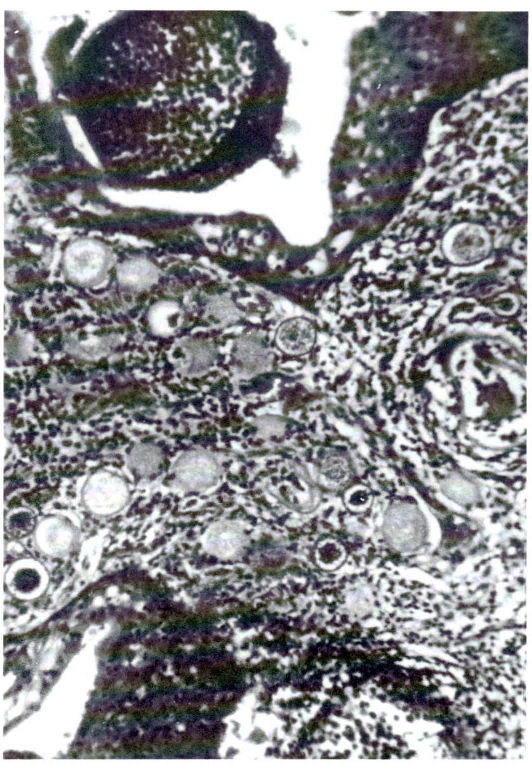

C
X130

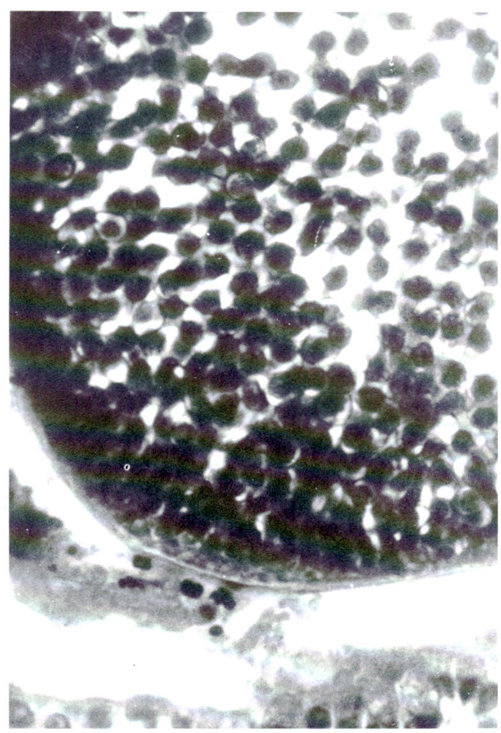

D
X530

Figs. C,D courtesy Dr. Jag Bhawan

FUNGUS INFECTIONS continued ⇨

PHYCOMYCOSIS

Phycomycosis is caused by several members of the class *Phycomycetes* (true fungi): *Rhizopus, Mucor, Absidia, Mortierella,* and *Basidiobolus*. The organisms are opportunistic and may cause systemic disease in debilitated patients, including patients with severe burns, uncontrolled diabetes mellitus, leukemia, and impairment of the immune system. The paranasal sinuses are commonly involved, and the infection may spread rapidly to the orbit, brain, and gastrointestinal tract. Involvement of the paranasal sinuses may produce severe periorbital edema (Fig. A).

Cutaneous forms have been described in healthy persons—pustules and ulcers from contaminated adhesive tape, and subcutaneous lesions in tropical zones.

Microscopic features

1. The organisms have large, nonseptate, branching hyphae, which can be observed with H&E stain in areas of necrosis or granulation tissue (Fig. B). In cross-section, the organisms appear as large rings, up to 30 microns in diameter (Fig. C).

Comment

Aspergillus is another opportunistic organism. It produces subcutaneous abscesses, pustules, ulcers, or areas of cellulitis.

Systemic infection may occur, with skin involvement being secondary.

Histologically, granulomatous inflammation is often seen. Organisms have thick, septate hyphae with terminal dilatations branching at an acute angle (60°). There may be invasion of blood vessels.

PHYCOMYCOSIS

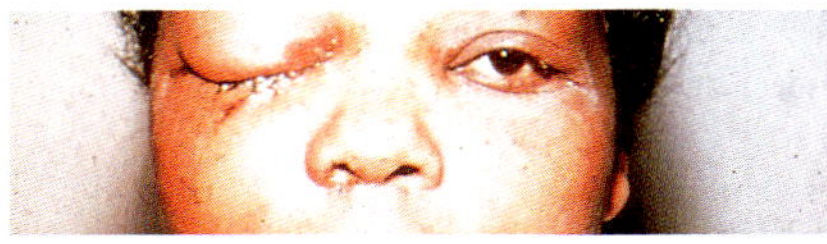

A

B1
X500

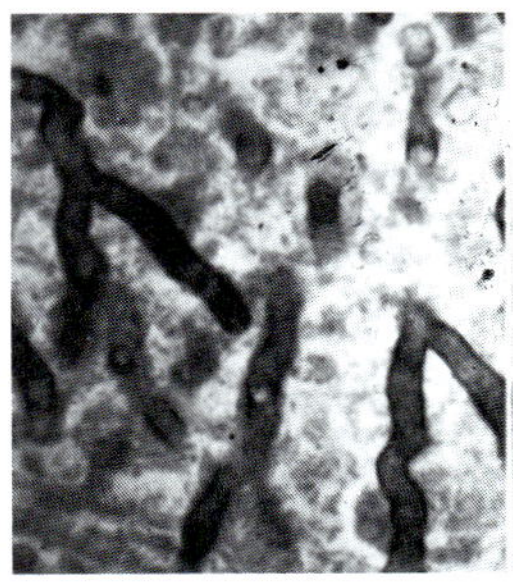

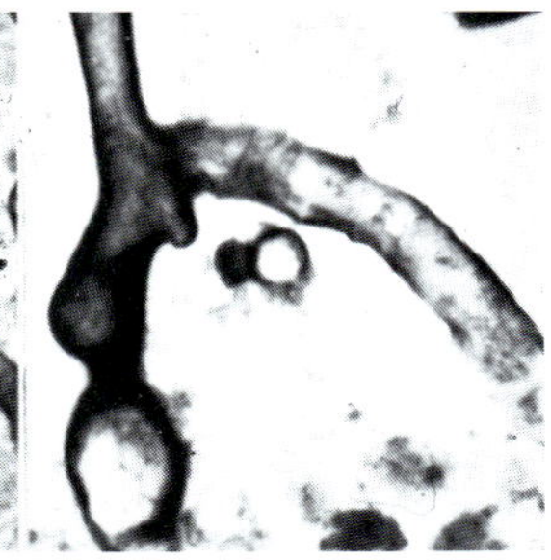

B2
X1000

Courtesy Emmons, C.W., et al.; Medical Mycology.
Lea and Febiger, Philadelphia, 1977.

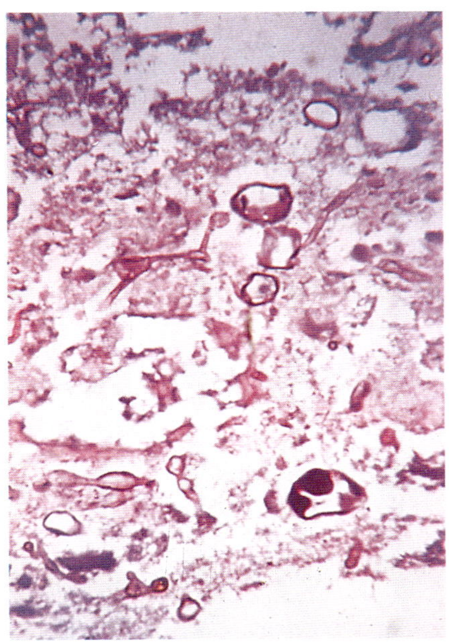

C
X200

FUNGUS INFECTIONS continued ⇨

MYCETOMA

Actinomycetoma is caused by filamentous bacteria (aerobic and anaerobic actinomycetes). Eumycetoma is caused by true fungi (species of *Allescheria* and *Madurella*). The clinical picture is the same in actinomycetoma and eumycetoma. Large vegetating masses and sinus tracts are present. The skin, subcutaneous tissue, and bones of the foot (Figs. A,B) are involved.

Microscopic features

1. Abscesses, surrounded by granulation tissue and fibrosis, are present.
2. Organisms are present in clumps called *granules* (Fig. C). The morphology of the granules varies with the type of organism. *Nocardia brasiliensis* is characterized by branching, mildly acid-fast filaments. *Madurella grisea* is characterized by round or lobate granules with hyperpigmented thick-walled, septate hyphae at the periphery.
3. A Gram stain and PAS stain may be of value in distinguishing actinomycetoma from eumycetoma. The granules of actinomycetoma are composed of Gram-positive filaments, and those of eumycetoma are composed of PAS-positive hyphae. The distinction is important since therapy is different.

ACTINOMYCOSIS

Actinomycosis is caused by the anaerobic organism, *Actinomyces israelii*. It is a chronic disease characterized by fibrosing sinus tracts in the cervicofacial (Figs. D,E), thoracic, or abdominal areas. Pulmonary actinomycosis affects the skin by extension from the lung; abdominal actinomycosis affects the skin by extension from the intestinal tract.

Microscopic features

1. The organism is generally found in draining, purulent material, grouped in basophilic, lobate clumps (Fig. F) called *sulfur granules*. Sulfur granules are composed of filaments having club-shaped free ends (Fig. G). The organisms are Gram-positive and PAS-positive.
2. The abscesses are surrounded by granulation tissue, and in longstanding lesions, by areas of fibrosis.

Comment

1. *Botryomycosis* represents a chronic, localized bacterial infection with sinus tracts. The granulation tissue with foci of suppuration contains basophilic grains composed of bacteria embedded in homogeneous, amorphous material. The bacteria are usually *Staphylococcus aureus*, but sometimes are *Pseudomonas aeruginosa*.
2. *Nocardia asteroides* can produce infection mimicking sporotrichosis.

MYCETOMA

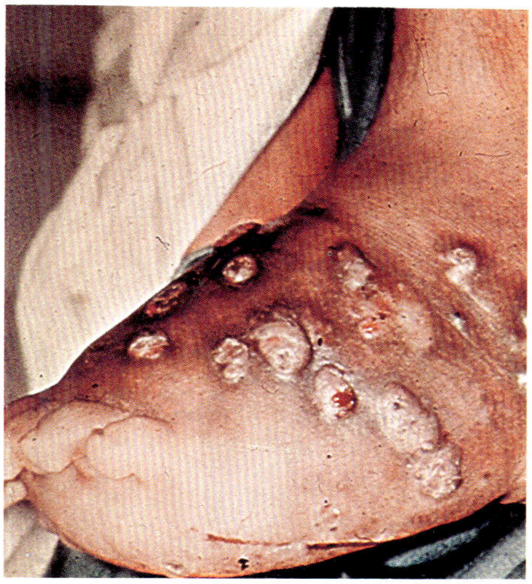
A Courtesy Dr. John Knox

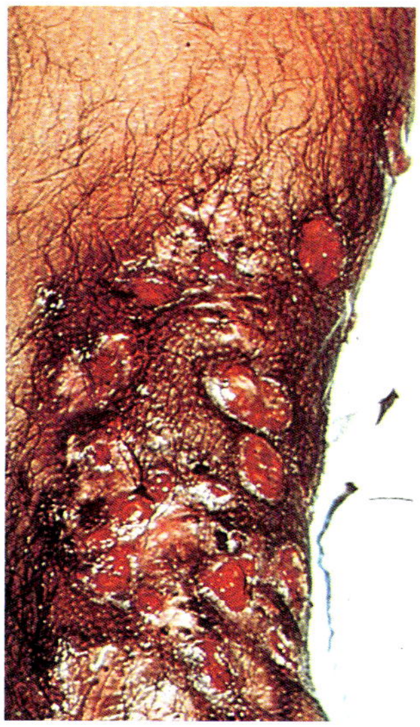
B

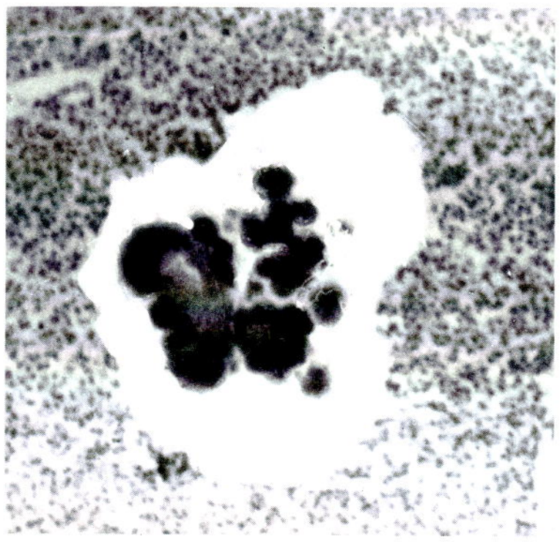
C
X110

ACTINOMYCOSIS

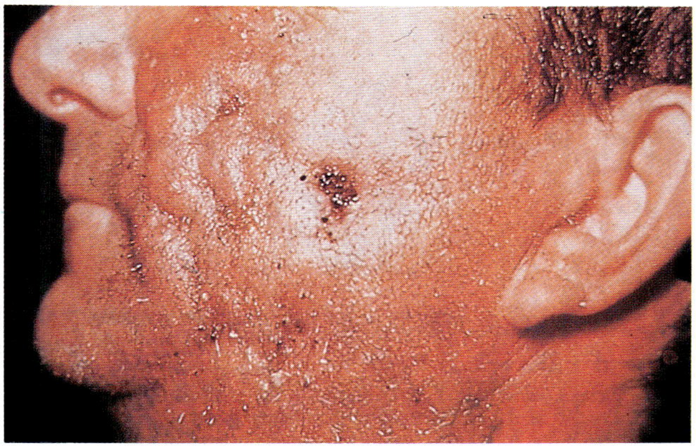
D

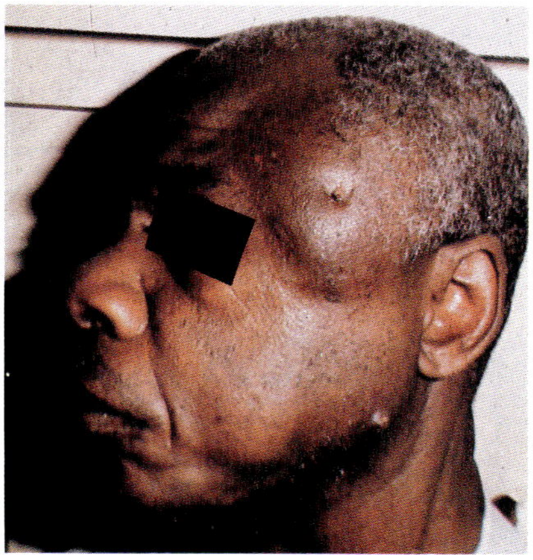
E

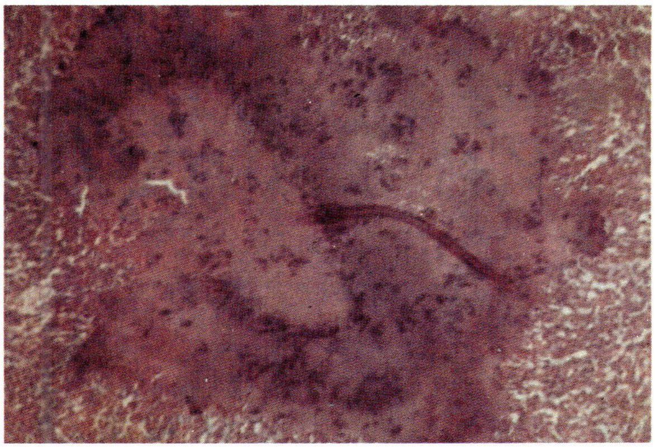
F
X210

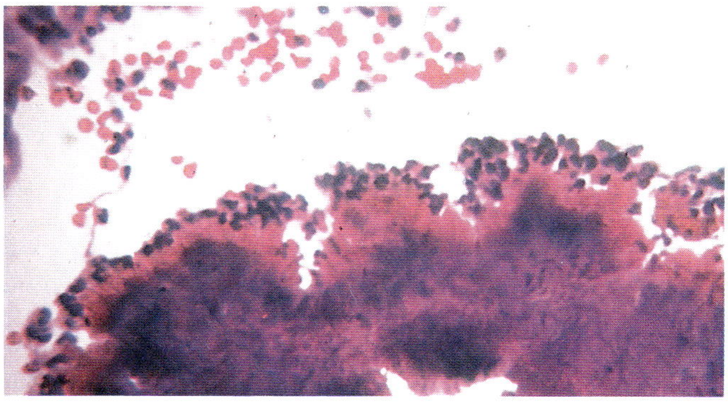
G
X540

Suggested Reading

Infectious Diseases: Fungal

General References

Ajello, L. *Laboratory Manual for Medical Mycology*. Atlanta, U.S.P.H.S. Pub. #994, 1963.
Baker, R. *The Pathologic Anatomy of Mycoses: Human Infection with Fungi, Actinomycetes, and Algae*. New York, Springer-Verlag, 1971.
Beneke, E. and Rogers, A. *Medical Mycology Manual*. 3rd Ed., Minneapolis, Burgess, 1970.
Conant, N. et al. *Manual of Clinical Mycology*. 3rd Ed., Philadelphia, W. B. Saunders, 1971.
Emmons, L., Binford, C. and Utz, J. *Medical Mycology*. 2nd Ed., Philadelphia, Lea & Febiger, 1970.
Ferguson, E. and Rothman, S. Fungus Infections of the Skin. *Pediatr. Clin. N. Am.*, 3:555, 1956.
Hildick-Smith, G., Blank, H. and Sarkany, I. *Fungus Diseases and Their Treatment*. Boston, Little, Brown, 1964.
Kaplan, W. and Kraft, D. Demonstration of pathogenic fungi in formalin-fixed tissues by immunofluorescence. *Am. J. Clin. Pathol*, 52:420, 1969.
Kligman, A., Mescon, H. and Delamater, E. The Hotchkiss-McManus stain for histopathologic diagnosis of fungus diseases. *Am. J. Clin. Pathol.*, 21:86, 1951.
Rebell, G. and Taplin, D. *Dermatophytes: Their Recognition and Identification*. Coral Gables, FL, Univ. of Miami Press, 1970.
Rippon, J. *Medical Mycology*: The Pathogenic Fungi and the Pathogenic Actinomycetes. Philadelphia, W. B. Saunders, 1974.
Sinski, J. *Dermatophytes in Human Skin, Hair and Nails*. Springfield, IL, Thomas, 1974.
Wilson, J. and Plunkett, O. *The Fungus Diseases of Man*. Berkeley, Univ. Calif. Press, 1965.

Superficial Fungal Diseases

Allen, H., Charles, C. and Johnson, B. Hyperpigmented tinea versicolor. *Arch. Dermatol.*, 112:1110, 1976.
Alteras, I. and Feuerman, E. Atypical cases of *Microsporum canis* infection in the adult. *Mycopathologica*, 74:181, 1981.
Alteras, I. et al. The high incidence of tinea pedis and unguium in patients with Kaposi's sarcoma. *Mycopathologica*, 74:177, 1981.
Berretty, P. et al. Follikulitis, verursacht durch Pityrosporum. *Hautarzt*, 31:613, 1980.
Berretty, P. et al. *Pityrosporum* folliculitis: Is it a real entity? *Br. J. Dermatol.*, 103:565, 1980.
Blank, F. and Mann, S. *Trichophyton rubrum* infections according to age, anatomical distribution and sex. *Br. J. Dermatol.*, 92:171, 1975.
Burgoon, C. et al. Mycetoma formation in Trichophyton rubrum infection. *Br. J. Dermatol.*, 90:155, 1974.
Catterall, M. Tinea versicolor: A reappraisal. *Internat. J. Dermatol.*, 19:84, 1980.
Dvoretzky, I. et al. Favus. *Internat. J. Dermatol.*, 19:89, 1980.
Feuerman, E. et al. Kerion-like tinea capitis and barbae caused by *Microsporum gypseum* in Israel. *Mycopathologica*, 58:165, 1976.
Graham, J. et al. Tinea capitis: A histopathological and histochemical study. *Arch. Dermatol.*, 89:528, 1964.
Hay, R. Chronic dermatophyte infections. I. Clinical and mycological features. *Br. J. Dermatol.*, 106:1, 1982.
Heid, E. et al. Folliculites pityrosporiques. *Ann. Dermatol. Venereol.*, 105:133, 1978.
Hernandez, A. An approach to the diagnosis and therapy of dermatophytosis. *Internat. J. Dermatol.*, 19:540, 1980.
Jung, E. and Bohnert, E. Mechanism of depigmentation in pityriasis versicolor alba. *Arch. Dermatol. Res.*, 256:333, 1976.
Keddie, F. A novel cellular reaction caused by tinea versicolor: Extracellular glycogen deposits. *J. Invest. Dermatol.*, 53:363, 1969.

Kligman, A. The pathogenesis of tinea capitis due to *Microsporum audouini* and *Microsporum canis*. I. Gross observations following the inoculation of humans. *J. Invest. Dermatol.*, 18:231, 1952.

——. Tinea capitis due to *Microsporum audouini* and *Microsporum canis*. II. Dynamics of the host-parasite relationship. *Arch. Dermatol. Syph.*, 71:313, 1955.

McGinley, K., Lantis, L. and Marples, R. Microbiology of tinea versicolor. *Arch. Dermatol.*, 102:168, 1970.

Michalowski, R. and Rodziewicz, H. Pityriasis versicolor in the aged. *Br. J. Dermatol.*, 77:388, 1965.

Mikhail, G. *Trichophyton rubrum* granuloma. *Internat. J. Dermatol.*, 9:41, 1970.

Mitchell, J. Ringworm of hands and feet: Historical review. *JAMA*, 146:541, 1951.

Onsberg, P. The fungal flora of normal and diseased nails. *Curr. Ther. Res.*, 22:20, 1977.

Otcenasek, M. Ecology of the dermatophytes. *Mycopathologica*, 65:67, 1978.

Philpot, C. Geographical distribution of the dermatophytes: A review. *J. Hyg.* (London), 80:301, 1978.

Piéard, J. and Dockx, P. The ultrastructure of tinea versicolor and Malassezia furfur. *Internat. J. Dermatol.*, 11:116, 1972.

Porro, M. et al. Induction of hyphae in cultures of *Pityrosporum* by cholesterol and cholesterol esters. *J. Invest. Dermatol.*, 69:531, 1977.

Pravda, D. and Pugliese, M. Tinea faciei. *Arch. Dermatol.*, 114:250, 1978.

Rippon, J. *The Pathogenic Fungi and the Pathogenic Actinomycetes*. Philadelphia, W. B. Saunders, 1982, p. 145.

Roberts, S. Pityriasis versicolor: A clinical and mycological investigation. *Br. J. Dermatol.*, 81:315, 1969.

——. Pityrosporum orbiculare: Incidence and distribution on clinically normal skin. *Br. J. Dermatol.*, 81:264, 1969.

Rudolph, A. The clinical recognition of tinea capitis from *Trichophyton tonsurans*. *JAMA*, 242:1770, 1979.

Shelley, W. and Wood, M. New technic for instant visualization of fungi in hair. *J. Am. Acad. Dermatol.*, 2:69, 1980.

——. The white spot target for microscopic examination of nails for fungi. *J. Am. Acad. Dermatol.*, 6:92, 1982.

Tuzun, Y. *Microsporum* infections of the nails. *Arch. Dermatol.*, 116:620, 1980.

Weary, P. and Canby, C. Keratinolytic activity of *Trichophyton schoenleini, Trichophyton rubrum* and *Trichophyton mentagrophytes*. *J. Invest. Dermatol.*, 48:240, 1967.

Whiting, D. and Bisset, E. The investigation of superficial fungal infections by skin surface biopsy. *Br. J. Dermatol.*, 91:57, 1974.

Wilson, J., Plunkett, O. and Gregersen, A. Nodular granulomatous perifolliculitis of the legs caused by *Trichophyton rubrum*. *Arch. Dermatol. Syph.*, 69:258, 1954.

Wyre, H. and Johnson, W. Neonatal pityriasis versicolor. *Arch. Dermatol.*, 117:752, 1981.

Yu, R., Harmon, S. and Blank, H. Hair digestion by a keratinase of *Trichophyton mentagrophytes*. *J. Invest. Dermatol.*, 53:166, 1969.

Zaias, N., Oertel, I. and Elliot, D. Fungi in toenails. *J. Invest. Dermatol.*, 53:140, 1969.

Zaslow, L. and Derbes, V. The immunologic nature of kerion celsi formation. *Dermatol. Internat.*, 8:1, 1971.

Candidiasis

Balandran, L. et al. Cutaneous manifestations of systemic candidiasis. *Ann. Int. Med.*, 78:400, 1973.

Beare, J., Cheeseman, E. and MacKenzie, D. The association between *Candida albicans* and lesions of seborrheic eczema. *Br. J. Dermatol.*, 80:675, 1968.

Bodey, G. and Fainstein, V. Systemic candidiasis. In: *Candidiasis*. Bodey, G. and Fainstein, V., eds., New York, Raven Press, 1985, p. 135.

Burgoon, C., Jr., Urbach, F. and Grover, W. Diaper dermatitis. *Pediatr. Clin. N. Am.*, 8:835, 1961.

Catterall, R. *Candida albicans* and the contraceptive pill. *Lancet*, 2:830, 1966.

Chapel, T. et al. Congenital cutaneous candidiasis. *J. Am Acad. Dermatol.*, 6:926, 1982.

Chesney, R. et al. *Candida* endocrinopathy syndrome with membranoproliferative glomerulonephritis: Demonstration of glomerular *Candida* antigen. *Clin. Nephrol.*, 5:232, 1976.

Craig, J., Schiff, L. and Boone, J. Chronic moniliasis associated with Addison's disease. *Am. J. Dis. Child.*, 89:669, 1955.

Delaplane, D. et al. Congenital mucocutaneous candidiasis following diagnostic amniocentesis. *Am. J. Obstet. Gynecol.*, 147:342, 1983.
Dreizen, S. Oral candidiasis. *Am. J. Med.*, 77(4D):28, 1984.
Drouhet, E. Pathology, diagnosis and treatment of moniliasis. *Irish J. Med. Sci.*, 378:242, 1957.
Epstein, J. et al. Oral candidiasis: Pathogenesis and host defense. *Rev. Infect. Dis.*, 6:96, 1984.
Grossman, M., Silvers, D. and Walther, R. Cutaneous manifestations of disseminated candidiasis. *J. Am. Acad. Dermatol.*, 2:111, 1980.
Hauser, F. and Rothman, S. Monilial granuloma. *Arch. Dermatol. Syph.*, 61:297, 1950.
Higgs, J. and Wells, R. Chronic mucocutaneous candidiasis: Associated abnormalities of iron metabolism. *Br. J. Dermatol.*, 86 (8, suppl.):88, 1972.
Horsmanheimo, M. et al. Immunologic features of chronic granulomatous mucocutaneous candidiasis before and after treatment with transfer factor. *Arch. Dermatol.*, 115:180, 1979.
Jacobs, M., Magid, M. and Jarowski, C. Disseminated candidiasis. *Arch. Dermatol.*, 116:1277, 1980.
Jarowski, C. et al. Fever, rash and muscle tenderness: A distinctive clinical presentation of disseminated candidiasis. *Arch. Int. Med.*, 138:544, 1978.
Jorizzo, J. The spectrum of mucosal and cutaneous candidosis. *Dermatologic Clinics*, 2:19, 1984.
Juljulian, H. and Kurban, A. Acantholysis: A feature of acrodermatitis enteropathica. *Arch. Dermatol.*, 103:105, 1971.
Kirkpatrick, C. and Sohnle, P. Chronic mucocutaneous candidiasis. In: *Immunodermatology*. Safai, B. and Good, R., eds., New York, Plenum Press, 1981, p. 495.
Kirkpatrick, C. and Windhorst, D. Mucocutaneous candidiasis and thymoma. *Am. J. Med.*, 66:939, 1979.
Klein, R. et al. Oral candidiasis in high-risk patients as the initial manifestation of the acquired immunodeficiency syndrome. *N. Eng. J. Med.*, 311:354, 1984.
Klotz, S. et al. *Pityrosporum* folliculitis: Its potential for confusion with skin lesions of systemic candidiasis. *Arch. Int. Med.*, 142:2126, 1982.
Kozinn, P., Taschdjian, C. and Weiner, H. Incidence and pathogenesis of neonatal candidiasis. *Pediatrics*, 21:421, 1958.
Kressel, B., Szewczyk, C. and Tuazon, C. Early clinical recognition of disseminated candidiasis by muscle and skin biopsy. *Arch. Int. Med.*, 138:429, 1978.
Leclerc, G. et al. Candida folliculitis in heroin addicts. *Internat. J. Dermatol.*, 25:100, 1986.
McCarthy, P. and Shklar, G. *Diseases of the Oral Mucosa*. Philadelphia, Lea & Febiger, 1980, p. 88.
Maize, J. and Lynch, P. Chronic mucocutaneous candidiasis in the adult. *Arch. Dermatol.*, 105:96, 1972.
Meech, R. et al. Pathogenic mechanisms in recurrent genital candidosis in women. *N. Z. Med. J.*, 98:1, 1985.
Montes, L. and Wilborn, W. Fungus-host relationship in candidiasis: A brief review. *Arch. Dermatol.*, 121:119, 1985.
Montes, L. et al. Chronic mucocutaneous candidiasis: Influence of thyroid status. *JAMA*, 221:156, 1972.
Myerowitz, R. et al. Disseminated candidiasis: Changes in incidence, underlying diseases, and pathology. *Am. J. Clin. Pathol.*, 68:29, 1977.
Ray, T. and Wuepper, K. Recent advances in cutaneous candidiasis. *Internat. J. Dermatol.*, 17:683, 1978.
Rebora, A. and Leyden, J. Napkin (diaper) dermatitis and gastrointestinal carriage of *Candida albicans*. *Br. J. Dermatol.*, 105:551, 1981.
Rebora, A., Marples, R. and Kligman, A. Erosio interdigitalis blastomycetica. *Arch. Dermatol.*, 108:66, 1973.
Richman, R. et al. Candidiasis and multiple endocrinopathy. *Arch. Dermatol.*, 111:625, 1975.
Rockoff, A. Chronic mucocutaneous candidiasis. *Arch. Dermatol.*, 115:322, 1979.
Schoch, E., Jr. Thymic conversion of *Candida albicans* from commensalism to pathogenism. *Arch. Dermatol.*, 103:311, 1971.
Smith, C. Candidiasis: Pathogenesis, host resistance, and predisposing factors. In: *Candidiasis*. Bodey, G. and Fainstein, V., eds., New York, Raven Press, 1985, p. 53.
Sobel, J. Vulvovaginal candidiasis: What we do and do not know. *Ann. Int. Med.*, 101:390, 1984.
Tappeiner, J. and Pfleger, L. Granuloma gluteale infantum. *Hautarzt*, 22:383, 1971.
Taschdjian, C. and Kozinn, P. Laboratory and clinical studies on candidiasis in the newborn infant. *J. Pediatr.*, 50:426, 1957.

Waugh, M. Clinical presentation of candidal balanitis: Its differential diagnosis and treatment. *Chemotherapy*, 28 (1, suppl.):56, 1982.
Winner, H. and Hurley, R. *Candida albicans*. London, Churchill, 1964.

Granuloma Gluteale Infantum

Altmeyer, P. Die Bedeutung fluorierter Glucocorticoide in der Aetiopathogenese des Granuloma glutaeale infantum (Tappeiner und Pfleger). *Z. Haut.*, 48:621, 1973.
Bonifazi, E. et al. Granuloma gluteale infantum with atrophic scars: Clinical and histological observations in eleven cases. *Clin. Exp. Dermatol.*, 6:23, 1981.
Delacrétaz, J. et al. Candidose nodulaire de la région inguino-génitale et des fesses (granuloma glutaeale infantum). *Dermatologica*, 144:144, 1972.
Simmons, I. Granuloma gluteale infantum. *Aust. J. Dermatol.*, 18:20, 1977.
Maekaway, Y., Sakazaki, Y. and Hayashibara, T. Diaper area granuloma of the aged. *Arch. Dermatol.*, 114:382, 1978.
Tappeiner, J. and Pfleger, L. Granuloma glutaeale infantum. *Hautarzt*, 22:383, 1971.
Uyeda, K., Nakayasu, K. and Takaishi, Y. Kaposi sarcoma-like granuloma on diaper dermatitis. *Arch. Dermatol.*, 107:605, 1973.

Deep Fungus Diseases

CHROMOMYCOSIS

Azulay, R. and Serruya, J. Hematogenous dissemination in chromoblastomycosis. *Arch. Dermatol.*, 95:57, 1967.
Batres, E. et al. Transepithelial elimination of cutaneous chromomycosis. *Arch. Dermatol.*, 114:1231, 1978.
Caplan, R. Epidermoid carcinoma arising in extensive chromoblastomycosis. *Arch. Dermatol.*, 97:38, 1968.
Carrion, A. Chromoblastomycosis and related infections: New concepts, differential diagnosis and nomenclatorial implications. *Internat. J. Dermatol.*, 14:27, 1975.
Derbes, V. and Friedman, L. Chromoblastomycosis. *Dermatol. Trop.*, 3:201, 1964.
French, A. and Russell, S. Chromoblastomycosis: Report of first case recognized in Michigan, apparently contracted in South Carolina. *Arch. Dermatol. Syph.*, 67:129, 1953.
Greer, K. et al. Cystic chromomycosis due to *Wangiella dermatitidis*. *Arch. Dermatol.*, 115:1433, 1979.
McGinnis, M. Chromoblastomycosis and phaeohyphomycosis: New concepts, diagnosis, and mycology. *J. Am. Acad. Dermatol.*, 8:1, 1983.
Moore, M., Cooper, Z. and Weiss, R. Chromomycosis (chromoblastomycosis). *JAMA*, 122:1237, 1943.
Nsanzumuhire, H., Vollum, D. and Poltera, A. Chromomycosis due to *Cladosporium trichoides* treated with 5-fluorocytosine: A case report. *Am. J. Clin. Pathol.*, 61:257, 1974.
Pardo-Castello, V., Leon, E. and Trespalacios, F. Chromoblastomycosis in Cuba. *Arch. Dermatol. Syph.*, 45:119, 1942.
Vollum, D. Chromomycosis: A review. *Br. J. Dermatol.*, 96:454, 1977.
Watson, K. Cerebral chromoblastomycosis. *J. Pathol. Bacteriol.*, 84:233, 1962.
Zaias, N. Chromomycosis. *J. Cutan. Pathol.*, 5:155, 1978.

SPOROTRICHOSIS

Auld, J. and Beardsmore, G. Sporotrichosis in Queensland: A review of 37 cases at the Royal Brisbane Hospital. *Aust. J. Dermatol.*, 20:14, 1979.
Carr, R. et al. Extensive verrucous sporotrichosis of long duration: Report of a case resembling cutaneous blastomycosis. *Arch. Dermatol.*, 89:124, 1964.
Cawley, E. Sporotrichosis, a protean disease: With report of a disseminated subcutaneous gummatous case of the disease. *Ann. Int. Med.*, 30:1287, 1949.
Collins, W. Disseminated ulcerating sporotrichosis with widespread visceral involvement: Report of a case. *Arch. Dermatol. Syph.*, 56:523, 1947.
Dellatorre, D. et al. Fixed cutaneous sporotrichosis of the face. *J. Am. Acad. Dermatol.*, 6:97, 1982.
Dolezal, J. Blastomycoid sporotrichosis. *J. Am. Acad. Dermatol.*, 4:523, 1981.

Fetter, B. Human cutaneous sporotrichosis due to *Sporotrichum schenckii*: Technique for demonstration of organisms in tissues. *Arch. Pathol.*, 71:416, 1961.

Fetter, B. and Tindall, J. Cutaneous sporotrichosis: Clinical study of nine cases utilizing an improved technique for demonstration of organisms. *Arch. Pathol.*, 78:613, 1964.

Kariya, H. and Iwatsu, T. Statistical survey of 100 cases of sporotrichosis. *J. Dermatol.*, 6:211, 1979.

Lurie, H. Histopathology of sporotrichosis: Notes on the nature of the asteroid body. *Arch. Pathol.*, 75:421, 1963.

Lynch, P. and Botero, F. Sporotrichosis in children. *Am. J. Dis. Child.*, 122:325, 1971.

Lynch, P., Voorhees, J. and Harrell, E. Systemic sporotrichosis. *Ann. Int. Med.*, 73:23, 1970.

Maberry, J., Mullins, J. and Stone, O. Sporotrichosis with demonstration of hyphae in human tissue. *Arch. Dermatol.*, 93:65, 1966.

Pinkus, H. and Grekin, J. Sporotrichosis with asteroid tissue forms. *Arch. Dermatol. Syph.*, 61:813, 1950.

Segal, R. and Jacobs, P. Sporotrichosis. *Internat. J. Dermatol.*, 18:639, 1979.

Smith, P. et al. Disseminated cutaneous sporotrichosis. *Arch. Dermatol.*, 117:143, 1981.

Spiers, E. et al. Sporotrichosis masquerading as pyoderma gangrenosum. *Arch. Dermatol.*, 122:691, 1987.

Stroud, J. Sporotrichosis presenting as pyoderma gangrenosum. *Arch. Dermatol.*, 97:667, 1968.

NORTH AMERICAN BLASTOMYCOSIS

Berger, R. and Kraman, S. Acute miliary blastomycosis after "short-course" corticosteroid treatment. *Arch. Int. Med.*, 141:1223, 1981.

Harrell, E. and Curtis, A. North American blastomycosis. *Am. J. Med.*, 27:750, 1959.

Hashimoto, K. et al. Pustular blastomycosis. *Internat. J. Dermatol.*, 16:277, 1977.

Hughs, W., Franco, S. and Oh, M. Systemic blastomycosis in childhood. *Clin. Pediatr.*, 8:597, 1969.

Klapman, M., Superfon, N. and Solomon, L. North American blastomycosis. *Arch. Dermatol.*, 101:653, 1970.

Sarosi, G. and Davies, S. Blastomycosis. *Am. Rev. Resp. Dis.*, 120:911, 1979.

Schwarz, J. and Baum, G. Blastomycosis. *Am. J. Clin. Pathol.*, 21:999, 1951.

Smith, J., Jr. et al. An epidemic of North American blastomycosis. *JAMA*, 158:641, 1955.

Su, D., Duncan, S. and Perry, H. Blastomycosis-like pyoderma. *Arch. Dermatol.*, 115:170, 1979.

Wilson, J. et al. Primary cutaneous North American blastomycosis. *Arch. Dermatol. Syph.*, 71:39, 1955.

Witorsch, P. and Utz, J. North American blastomycosis: A study of 40 patients. *Medicine*, 47:169, 1968.

SOUTH AMERICAN BLASTOMYCOSIS

Furtado, T. Infection versus disease in South American blastomycosis. *Internat. J. Dermatol.*, 14:117, 1975.

Furtado, T., Wilson, J. and Plunkett, O. South American blastomycosis or paracoccidioidomycosis: The mycosis of Lutz, Splendore and Almeida. *Arch. Dermatol. Syph.*, 70:166, 1954.

Londero, A. and Ramos, C. Paracoccidioidomycosis. *Am. J. Med.*, 52:771, 1972.

Murray, H., Littman, M. and Roberts, R. Disseminated paracoccidioidomycosis (South American blastomycosis). *Am. J. Med.*, 56:209, 1974.

Perry, H., Weed, L. and Kierland, R. South American blastomycosis: Report of a case and review of laboratory features. *Arch. Dermatol. Syph.*, 70:477, 1954.

LOBOMYCOSIS

Azulay, R. et al. Keloidal blastomycosis (Lobo's disease) with lymphatic involvement. *Internat. J. Dermatol.*, 15:40, 1976.

Bhawan, J. et al. Lobomycosis. *J. Cutan. Pathol.*, 3:5, 1976.

Jaramillo, D. et al. Lobomycosis. *J. Cutan. Pathol.*, 3:180, 1976.

Tapia, A., Torres-Calcindo, A. and Arosemena, R. Keloidal blastomycosis (Lobo's disease) in Panama. *Internat. J. Dermatol.*, 17:572, 1978.

COCCIDIOIDOMYCOSIS

Carroll, G., Haley, L. and Brown, J. Primary cutaneous coccidioidomycosis. *Arch. Dermatol.*, 113:933, 1977.

Feigin, R. et al. Subcutaneous abscess due to *Coccidioides immitis*. *Am. J. Dis. Child.*, 124:734, 1972.

Fiese, M. *Coccidioidomycosis*. Springfield, IL, Thomas, 1958.

Harell, E. and Honeycutt, W. Coccidioidomycosis: A traveling fungus disease. *Arch. Dermatol.*, 87:188, 1963.

Levan, N. and Huntington, R., Jr. Primary cutaneous coccidioidomycosis in agricultural workers. *Arch. Dermatol.*, 92:215, 1965.

Overholt, E. and Hornick, R. Primary cutaneous coccidioidomycosis. *Arch. Int. Med.*, 114:149, 1964.

Schwartz, R. and Lamberts, R. Isolated nodular cutaneous coccidioidomycosis: Initial manifestation of disseminated disease. *J. Am. Acad. Dermatol.*, 4:38, 1981.

Stevens, D. *Coccidioidomycosis*. New York, Plenum Press, 1980.

Trimble, J. and Doucette, J. Primary cutaneous coccidioidomycosis: Report of a case of laboratory infection. *Arch. Dermatol.*, 74:405, 1956.

Werner, S. et al. An epidemic of coccidioidomycosis among archeology students in Northern California. *N. Eng. J. Med.*, 286:507, 1972.

Wilson, J. Factors which may increase the severity of coccidioidomycosis. *Lab. Invest.*, 11:1146, 1962.

Wilson, J., Smith, C. and Plunkett, O. Primary cutaneous coccidioidomycosis: The criteria for diagnosis and a report of a case. *Calif. Med.*, 79:233, 1953.

Winer, L. Histopathology of the nodose lesion of acute coccidioidomycosis. *Arch. Dermatol. Syph.*, 61:1010, 1950.

Winn, W. Primary cutaneous coccidioidomycosis: Re-evaluation of its potentiality based on a study of three new cases. *Arch. Dermatol.*, 92:221, 1965.

HISTOPLASMOSIS

Baum, G. et al. Mucocutaneous histoplasmosis. *Arch. Dermatol.*, 76:4, 1957.

Curtis, A. and Cawley, E. Genital histoplasmosis. *J. Urol.*, 57:781, 1947.

Curtis, A. and Grekin, J. Histoplasmosis: A review of the cutaneous and adjacent mucous membrane manifestations with a report of three cases. *JAMA*, 134:1217, 1947.

Dumont, A. and Piche, C. Electron microscopic study of human histoplasmosis. *Arch. Pathol.*, 87:168, 1969.

Flegel, H., Knaben, U. and Westphal, H. Afrikanische Histoplasmose. *Hautarzt*, 31:50, 1980.

Goodwin, R., Jr. and Des Prez, R. Histoplasmosis. *Am. Rev. Respir. Dis.*, 117:929, 1978.

Goodwin, R., Jr. et al. Chronic pulmonary histoplasmosis. *Medicine* (Baltimore), 55:413, 1976.

Goodwin, R., Jr. et al. Disseminated histoplasmosis: Clinical and pathologic correlations. (Review). *Medicine* (Baltimore), 59:1, 1980.

Hay, R. The skin and systemic fungal infection. *Clin. Exp. Dermatol.*, 4:365, 1979.

Jacobsen, E. and Strauss, S. Reevaluation of diagnostic histoplasma serology. *Am. J. Med. Sci.*, 281:143, 1981.

Kauffman, C. et al. Histoplasmosis in immunosuppressed patients. *Am. J. Med.*, 64:923, 1978.

Lucas, A. Cutaneous manifestations of African histoplasmosis. *Br. J. Dermatol.*, 82:435, 1970.

Miller, H. et al. Histoplasmosis: Cutaneous and mucomembranous lesions, mycologic and pathologic observations. *Arch. Dermatol. Syph.*, 56:715, 1947.

Nethercott, J. et al. Histoplasmosis due to *Histoplasma capsulatum var* duboisii in a Canadian immigrant. *Arch. Dermatol.*, 114:595, 1978.

Reddy, P. et al. Progressive disseminated histoplasmosis as seen in adults. *Am. J. Med.*, 48:629, 1970.

Shulz, D. Histoplasmosis: A statistical morphologic study. *Am. J. Clin. Pathol.*, 24:11, 1954.

Silverman, F. et al. Histoplasmosis. *Am. J. Med.*, 19:410, 1955.

Soo-Hoo, T., Adams, B. and Yusof, D. Disseminated primary cutaneous histoplasmosis. *Aust. J. Dermatol.*, 21:105, 1980.

Straub, M. and Schwarz, J. The healed primary complex in histoplasmosis. *Am. J. Clin. Pathol.*, 25:727, 1955.

Sweany, H. *Histoplasmosis*. Springfield, IL, Thomas, 1960.

Symmers, W. Localized cutaneous histoplasmosis. *Br. Med. J.*, 2:790, 1956.

Tesh, R. et al. Histoplasmosis in children. *Pediatrics*, 33:894, 1964.

Tosh, F. et al. Primary cutaneous histoplasmosis: Report of a case. *Arch. Int. Med.*, 114:118, 1964.

Wheat, L. et al. A large urban outbreak of histoplasmosis: Clinical features. *Ann. Int. Med.*, 94:331, 1982.

CRYPTOCOCCOSIS

Baker, R. and Haugen, R. Tissue changes and tissue diagnosis in cryptococcosis: A study of 26 cases. *Am. J. Clin. Pathol.*, 25:14, 1955.

Brier, R., Mopper, C. and Stone, J. Cutaneous cryptococcosis: Presentation of a case and a review of previously reported cases. *Arch. Dermatol.*, 75:262, 1957.

Cawley, E., Grekin, R. and Curtis, A. Torulosis: A review of the cutaneous and adjoining mucous membrane manifestations. *J. Invest. Dermatol.*, 14:327, 1950.

Chu, A., Hay, R. and MacDonald, D. Cutaneous cryptococcosis. *Br. J. Dermatol.*, 103:95, 1980.

De Wyte, C. et al. Cryptococcal meningitis: A review of 32 years' experience. *J. Neurol. Sci.*, 53:283, 1982.

Gandy, W. Primary cutaneous cryptococcosis. *Arch. Dermatol. Syph.*, 62:97, 1950.

Gendel, B., Ende, M. and Norman, S. Cryptococcosis: A review with special reference to apparent association with Hodgkin's disease. *Am. J. Med.*, 9:343, 1950.

Godwin, J. et al. Fatal pneumocystis pneumonia, cryptococcosis, and Kaposi's sarcoma in a homosexual man. *AJR*, 138:580, 1982.

Kerkering, T. et al. The evolution of pulmonary cryptococcosis: Clinical implications from a study of 41 patients with and without compromising host factors. *Ann. Int. Med.*, 94:611, 1981.

Littman, M. and Walter, J. Cryptococcosis: Current status. *Am. J. Med.*, 45:922, 1968.

Littman, M. and Zimmerman, L. *Cryptococcosis: Torulosis or European Blastomycosis*. New York, Grune & Stratton, 1956.

Moore, M. Cryptococcosis with cutaneous manifestations: Four cases with a review of published reports. *J. Invest. Dermatol.*, 28:159, 1957.

Noble, R. and Fajardo, L. Primary cutaneous cryptococcosis. *Am. J. Clin. Pathol.*, 57:13, 1972.

Rook, A. and Woods, B. Cutaneous cryptococcosis. *Br. J. Dermatol.*, 74:43, 1962.

Ruiter, M. and Ensink, G. Acute primary cutaneous cryptococcosis. *Dermatologica*, 128:185, 1964.

Sarosi, G., Silberfarb, P. and Toh, F. Cutaneous cryptococcosis: A sentinel of disseminated disease. *Arch. Dermatol.*, 104:1, 1971.

Saúl, A., Lavalle, P. and Rodríguez, G. Cutaneous cryptococcosis. *Internat. J. Dermatol.*, 19:457, 1980.

Schupbach, C. et al. Cutaneous manifestations of disseminated cryptococcosis. *Arch. Dermatol.*, 112:1734, 1976.

RHINOSPORIDIOSIS

Agarwal, S., Sharma, K. and Srivastava, J. Generalized rhinosporidiosis with visceral involvement. *Arch. Dermatol.*, 80:22, 1959.

Jain, S. Etiology and incidence of rhinosporidiosis. *Indian J. Otolaryngol.*, 19:1, 1967.

Karunaratne, W. *Rhinosporidiosis in Man*. London, Athlone Press, 1964.

Reddy, D. Rhinosporidiosis: A review based on the study of 150 biopsies. *Antisepsis*, 51:702, 1954.

PHYCOMYCOSIS (MUCORMYCOSIS)

Gartenberg, G. et; al. Hospital-acquired mucormycosis (*Rhizopus rhizopodiformis*) of the skin and subcutaneous tissue. *N. Eng. J. Med.*, 299:1115, 1978.

Hammond, D. and Winkelmann, R. Cutaneous phycomycosis. *Arch. Dermatol.*, 115:990, 1979.

Herstoff, J., Bogaars, H. and McDonald, C. Rhinophycomycosis entomophthorae. *Arch. Dermatol.*, 114:1674, 1978.

Kramer, B. et al. Cutaneous infarction: Manifestation of disseminated mucormycosis. *Arch. Dermatol.*, 113:1075, 1977.

Lehrer, R. et al. Mucormycosis. *Ann. Int. Med.*, 93:93, 1980.

Meyer, R. et al. Cutaneous lesions in disseminated mucormycosis. *JAMA*, 225:737, 1973.

Rabin, E., Lundberg, G. and Mitchell, E. Mucormycosis in severely burned patients. *N. Eng. J. Med.*, 264:1286, 1961.

Roberts, H. Cutaneous mucormycosis. *Arch. Int. Med.*, 110:108, 1962.

Veliath, A. et al. Cutaneous phycomycosis (mucormycosis) with fatal pulmonary dissemination. *Arch. Dermatol.*, 112:509, 1976.

ASPERGILLOSIS

Bruck, H. et al. Opportunistic fungal infection of the burn wound with phycomycetes and *Aspergillus*. *Arch. Surg.*, 102:476, 1971.
Cahill, K., El Mofty, A. and Kawaguchi, T. Primary cutaneous aspergillosis. *Arch. Dermatol.*, 96:545, 1967.
Carlile, J. et al. Primary cutaneous aspergillosis in a leukemic child. *Arch. Dermatol.*, 114:78, 1978.
Caro, I. and Dogliotti, M. Aspergillosis of the skin. *Dermatologica*, 146:244, 1973.
Cawley, E. Aspergillosis and the aspergilli. *Arch. Int. Med.*, 80:423, 1947.
Cheetham, H. Subcutaneous infection due to *Aspergillus terreus*. *J. Clin. Pathol.*, 17:251, 1964.
Estes, S. et al. Primary cutaneous aspergillosis. *J. Am. Acad. Dermatol.*, 3:397, 1980.
Gurwith, M., Stinson, E. and Remington, J. *Aspergillus* infection complicating cardiac transplantation. *Arch. Int. Med.*, 128:541, 1971.
Panke, T., McManus, A. and Spebar, M. Infection of a burn wound by *Aspergillus niger*. *Am. J. Clin. Pathol.*, 72:230, 1979.
Young, R., Bennett, J. and Vogel, C. Aspergillosis. *Medicine*, 49:147, 1970.

MYCETOMA

Ballenger, C., Jr. and Goldring, D. Nocardiosis in childhood. *J. Pediatr.*, 50:145, 1957.
Barnetson, R. and Milne, L. Mycetoma. (Review). *Br. J. Dermatol.*, 99:227, 1978.
Butz, W. and Ajello, L. Black grain mycetoma. *Arch. Dermatol.*, 104:197, 1971.
Curry, W. Human nocardiosis: A clinical review with selected case reports. *Arch. Int. Med.*, 140:818, 1980.
Mahvi, T. Disseminated nocardiosis caused by *Nocardia brasiliensis*: First case report in the United States. *Arch. Dermatol.*, 89:426, 1964.
Montes, L., Freeman, R. and McClarin, W. Maduromycosis due to *Madurella grisea*. *Arch. Dermatol.*, 99:74, 1969.
Robboy, S. and Vickery, A., Jr. Tinctorial and morphological properties distinguishing actinomycosis and nocardiosis. *N. Eng. J. Med.*, 282:593, 1970.
Taralakshmi, V. et al. Mycetoma caused by *Madurella mycetomii* in Madras. *Aust. J. Dermatol.*, 19:125, 1978.
Winslow, D. and Steen, F. Considerations in the histologic diagnosis of mycetoma. *Am. J. Clin. Pathol.*, 42:164, 1964.
Zaias, N., Taplin, D. and Rebell, G. Mycetoma. *Arch. Dermatol.*, 99:215, 1969.
Ziprkowski, L. et al. Mycetoma pedis. *Arch. Dermatol.*, 75:855, 1957.

ACTINOMYCOSIS

Caron, G. and Sarkany, I. Cervico-facial actinomycosis. *Br. J. Dermatol.*, 76:421, 1964.
Cope, Z. *Actinomycosis*. London, Oxford Univ. Press, 1938.
Graybill, J. Sulfur granules. *Arch. Int. Med.*, 123:430, 1969.
McQuown, A. Actinomycosis and nocardiosis. *Am. J. Clin. Pathol.*, 25:2, 1965.
Montgomery, R. and Welton, W. Primary actinomycosis of the upper extremity. *Arch. Dermatol.*, 79:578, 1959.
Tsuboi, R. et al. Lymphocutaneous nocardiosis caused by Nocardia asteroides. *Arch. Dermatol.*, 122:1183, 1986.

Infectious Diseases: Viral

Viruses have a range of sizes, but individual viruses are generally too small to be visualized individually with the light microscope. However, groups of viruses or intracellular remnants of these groups, called *inclusion bodies*, can be visualized with light microscopy.

In this section the discussion will cover vesicular viral diseases, cat-scratch disease, lymphogranuloma venereum, and molluscum contagiosum. Verruca vulgaris, caused by a human papillomavirus, is discussed under benign tumors of the surface epidermis. The viral exanthems usually do not produce a specific microscopic picture in the skin, and the picture they produce can be described as perivasculitis.

Herpes simplex, varicella, herpes zoster, variola, vaccinia, and hand-foot-and-mouth disease have vesicular cutaneous lesions. Herpes zoster represents reinfection with the *herpesvirus varicellae* or activation of latent infection.

Kaposi's varicelliform eruption is a widespread infection caused either by the herpes simplex virus or by the vaccinia virus. (Vaccinia infections have almost disappeared.) Kaposi's varicelliform eruption occurs in individuals with a severe pre-existing dermatosis, such as atopic dermatitis or Darier's disease.

CAUSATIVE ORGANISMS OF VESICULAR VIRAL INFECTIONS OF THE SKIN

Herpes simplex	*Herpesvirus hominis* types 1 and 2 (HSV 1 and HSV 2). (Genital infections are usually caused by type 2)
Varicella	*Herpesvirus varicellae*
Herpes zoster	*Herpesvirus varicellae*
Variola	*Poxvirus variolae*
Vaccinia	*Poxvirus vaccinae*
Hand-foot-and-mouth disease	*coxsackievirus type A16* (rarely other types of coxsackie virus)

The vesicular viral diseases have similar histologic features. The histologic features of vesicular viral diseases will be discussed together.

Cat-scratch disease and lymphogranuloma venereum are believed to be caused by chlamydiae, now regarded as bacteria-like organisms. They are included in this chapter because of previous views that they were of viral origin.

CLINICAL FEATURES OF HERPES SIMPLEX, HERPES ZOSTER, VARICELLA, VARIOLA, VACCINIA, AND HAND-FOOT-AND-MOUTH DISEASE

	Skin and mucous membrane lesions	*Other involvement*
Varicella	A generalized eruption of skin and mucous membranes is present. Lesions have papular, vesicular, and crusted stages. The typical lesion is a vesicle on an erythematous base. At any given time, lesions are present in all stages, in contrast to smallpox.	Occasionally pneumonitis, or meningoencephalitis may develop. Disseminated varicella is rare.
Herpes zoster	Lesions are grouped vesicles, usually with a unilateral dermatomal distribution. Lesions commonly are hemorrhagic or necrotic. Occasionally the cutaneous eruption is generalized; there may be mucous membrane involvement.	There is infection of the dorsal root ganglion and sensory nerves; the central nervous system and eye are occasionally involved. Systemic dissemination may occur, particularly in patients with immunologic defects.
Primary herpes simplex	Clinical manifestations include stomatitis, vaginitis, or keratoconjunctivitis; rarely, there is a generalized cutaneous eruption. Most infections are subclinical.	Meningoencephalitis may occasionally occur; viremia and disseminated disease may occur in the newborn.
Recurrent herpes simplex	Lesions are grouped vesicles on an erythematous base which become crusted. The lips and genitalia are most often involved; herpetic folliculitis has been reported in the beard area; occasionally the cornea is infected. Erythema multiforme may follow herpes simplex infection.	Meningoencephalitis or pneumonia may occur. Systemic herpes simplex with viremia may occur in the newborn.
Kaposi's varicelliform eruption (caused by the herpes simplex or vaccinia virus)	Typical vesicles are umbilicated and resemble lesions of smallpox. Lesions develop at sites of dermatoses, particularly atopic dermatitis.	Meningoencephalitis may occur.
Variola	The generalized cutaneous eruption shows uniform lesions at any given time. Lesions have papular, vesicular, and pustular stages. The typical lesion is an umbilicated pustule. Hemorrhage is common. Scarring is often severe.	Encephalitis may develop.
Hand-foot-and-mouth disease	There are ulcers in the mouth, and vesicles on the palms, soles, and digits.	

HERPES SIMPLEX

Herpes simplex is a very common infection caused by *Herpesvirus hominis,* a DNA virus with two antigenic strains. Type 1 usually is the cause of herpes labialis and infection of other nongenital areas; type 2 is usually the cause of genital herpes simplex.

Herpes simplex infection has a primary stage and a recurrent stage. The majority of primary infections with type 1 virus occur in childhood and are subclinical. Primary infections with type 2 virus are transmitted sexually, and therefore occur after the onset of sexual activity.

Clinically evident primary infections tend to be severe and can involve the oral cavity, genitals, lungs, cornea, or brain. Rarely, the primary infection is expressed as disseminated disease.

Recurrent herpes simplex is believed to be caused by reactivation of latent virus in nerves, salivary glands, and lachrymal glands. Triggering factors include exposure to sunlight, febrile illness, menses, and trauma. Sometimes there is no apparent triggering factor. A striking feature of recurrent herpes simplex is its tendency to recur at the same site.

The lips are by far the most common site of recurrent type 1 herpes infection. Visible lesions may be preceded by burning and itching. Initial lesions are clustered vesicles on an inflamed base (Fig. A); vesicles readily rupture to form yellowish crusts (Fig. B). The average duration of lesions is one week.

Herpes simplex can involve the cornea and can produce dendritic ulcers. Other notable forms of recurrent herpes simplex are herpetic folliculitis of the beard area and herpetic whitlow, involving the volar or paronychial areas of the distal phalanx.

Recurrent herpes simplex of the genitals and adjoining areas is usually caused by type 2 virus, but some cases are caused by type 1 virus. Lesions are clustered vesicles (Fig. C), which readily rupture to form erosions (Fig. D). Genital erosions make up the usual presenting clinical picture. This stage of genital herpes simplex is sometimes misdiagnosed as chancroid.

Kaposi's varicelliform eruption is a widespread infection with either the herpes simplex virus or with the vaccinia virus; it occurs in individuals with certain predisposing skin diseases, usually atopic dermatitis (but sometimes Darier's disease, pemphigus foliaceus, and others).

Lesions of Kaposi's varicelliform eruption are umbilicated vesicles and pustules (Fig. E) which tend to rupture and form denuded areas and crusts.

Kaposi's varicelliform eruption can represent primary or recurrent herpes simplex infection (with either type 1 or type 2 virus). The primary form tends to be more severe, with systemic symptoms and possible internal organ involvement. The recurrent form tends to be limited to the skin, except in immunocompromised individuals.

Pneumonitis and meningoencephalitis are serious and potentially fatal forms of herpes simplex infection.

Erythema multiforme is a common concomitant of herpes simplex infection.

Microscopic features (see p. 388)

HERPES SIMPLEX

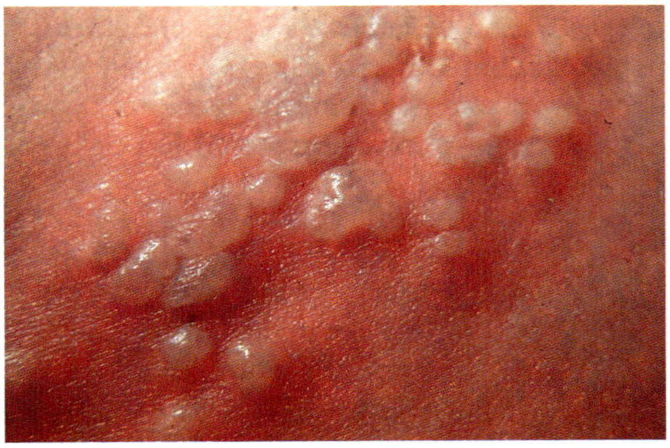

A

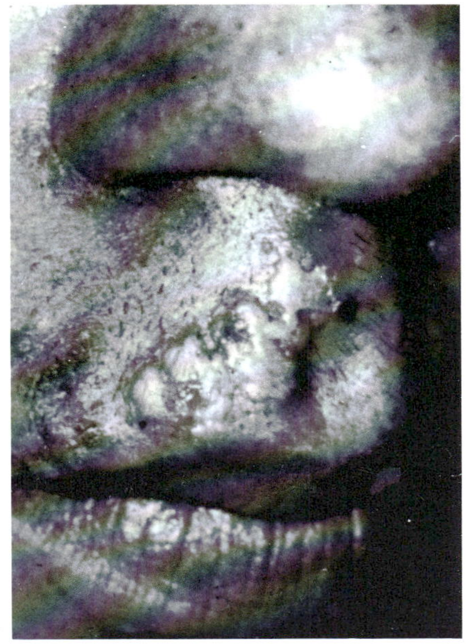

B

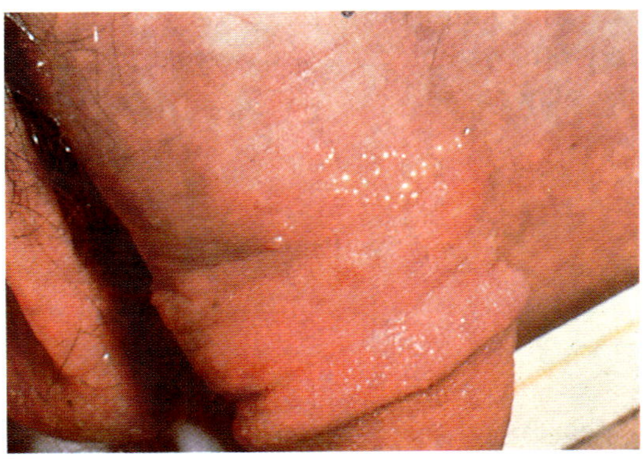

C

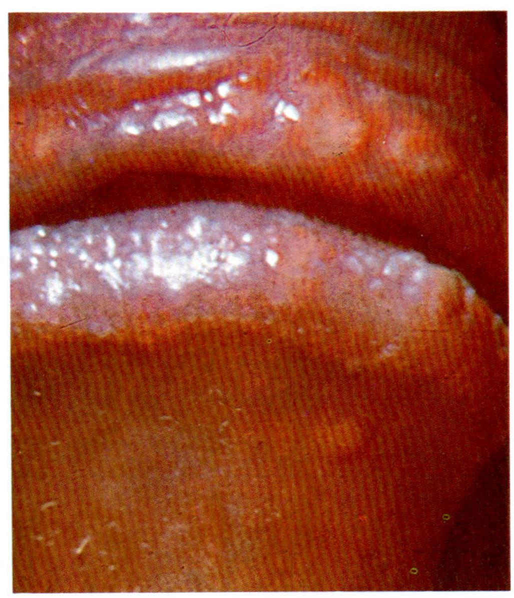

D

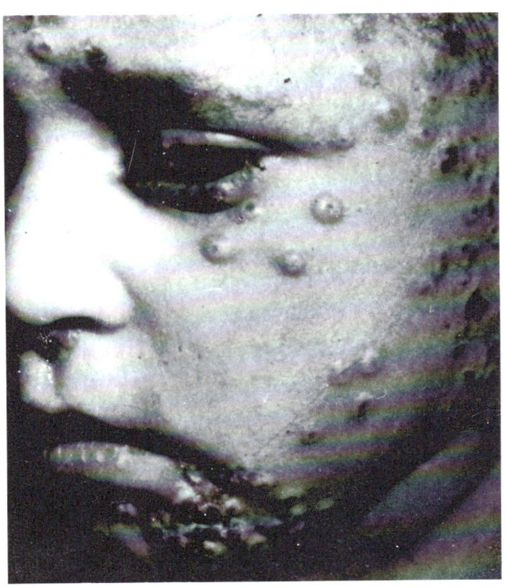

E

VESICULAR VIRAL DISEASES continued

VARICELLA AND HERPES ZOSTER

Varicella and herpes zoster are caused by the same DNA virus, *Herpesvirus varicellae*. Varicella (chickenpox) represents infection of a nonimmune host (initial infection). Herpes zoster generally represents reactivation of latent infection via viruses in sensory nerves, deposited during hematogenous dissemination in varicella. Rarely does herpes zoster develop by exposure of partially immune hosts to cases of herpes zoster or varicella. Varicella can develop by exposure to varicella or herpes zoster.

Varicella

Most patients are children. After an incubation period that averages two weeks, there is fever and malaise followed by widespread papules that evolve into vesicles and crusts. The classic picture of a chickenpox lesion is a vesicle on an erythematous base ("dewdrop on a rose petal" [Fig. A]). In contrast to variola (smallpox), lesions usually are in different stages at a given time. However, relative uniformity of lesions may be observed in varicella (Fig. B).

Serious possible complications of varicella include varicella pneumonia, disseminated varicella, and Reye's syndrome, a rare, fatal condition occurring in infants and children with varicella and other viral diseases. Reye's syndrome involves the liver and brain; aspirin may play a role.

Herpes zoster

In herpes zoster there is a spread of the virus from dorsal root ganglia to corresponding sensory nerves and to the skin supplied by these nerves. Pain and hyperesthesia are followed days later by clusters of papules and vesicles on an inflamed base (Figs. C,D,E). The eruption is almost always unilateral, although scattered individual lesions and sometimes a widespread eruption may be observed beyond the unilateral, segmental confines. Vesicles evolve into pustules and crusts, and sometimes into necrotic areas (Fig. F).

When there is involvement of the nasociliary nerve, there may be vesicles on the lateral aspect of the nose and keratitis.

The incidence and severity of herpes zoster increase in immunocompromised patients, such as those on chemotherapy or those with hematologic malignancy. Pneumonia and encephalitis are possible complications.

Neuralgia, after clearing of the cutaneous eruption, may last for months or years (postherpetic neuralgia).

In persons at risk for AIDS, the occurrence of herpes zoster may herald the marked depression of cellular immunity associated with AIDS or ARC.

Microscopic features (see p. 388)

VARICELLA AND HERPES ZOSTER

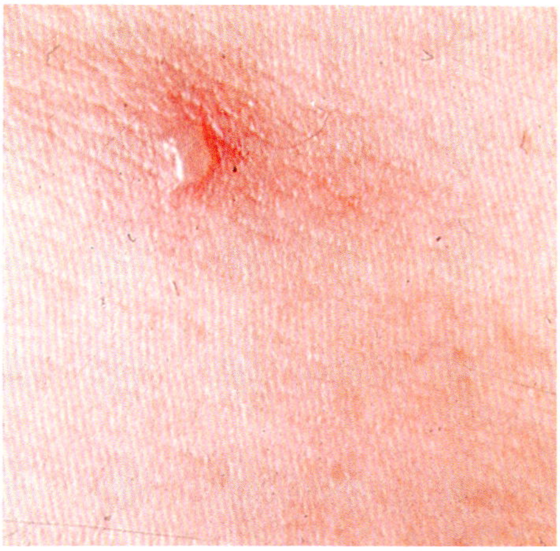
A

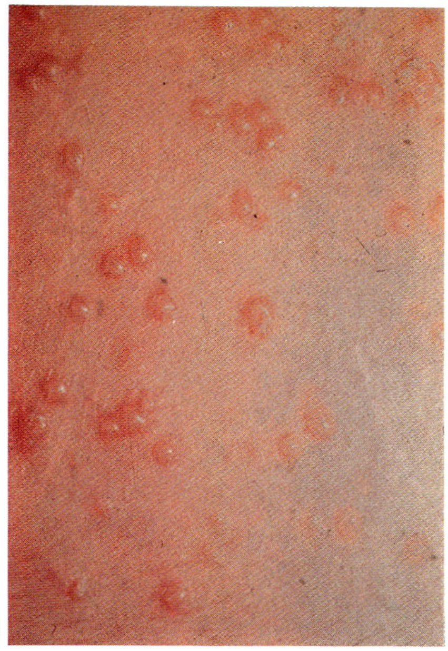
B

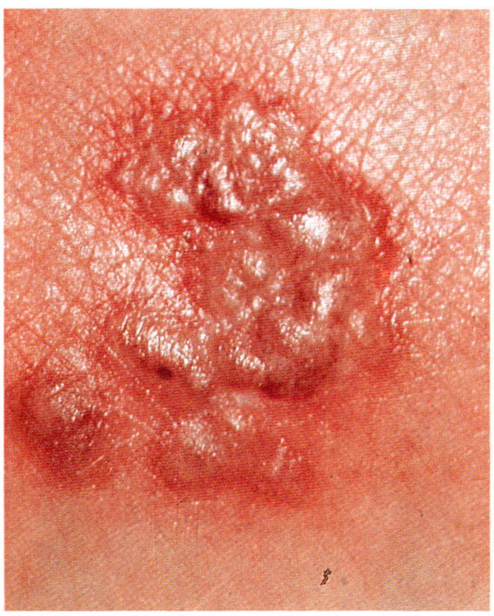
C

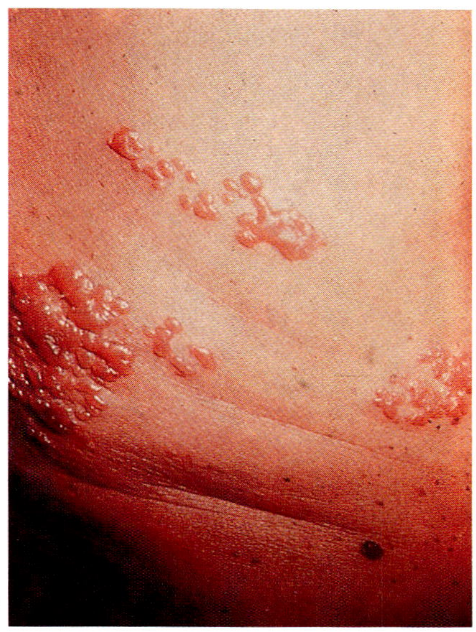
D

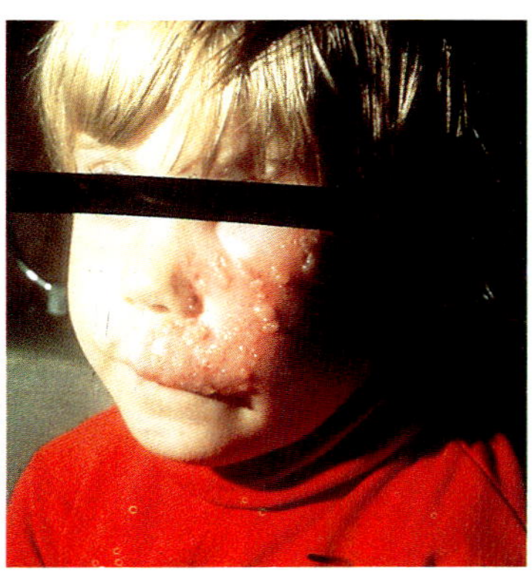
E

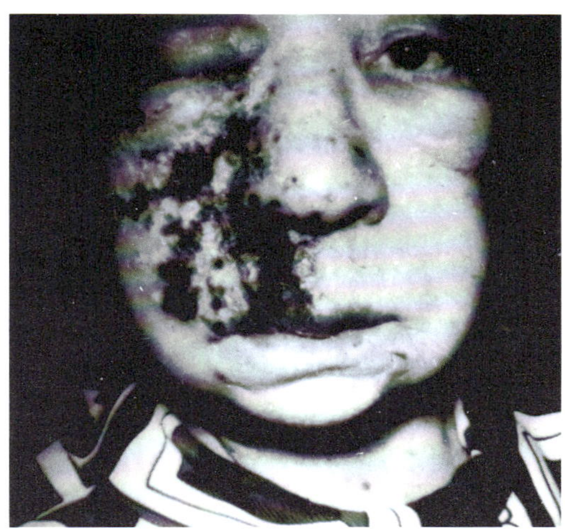
F

VESICULAR VIRAL DISEASES continued

Microscopic features of vesicular viral diseases

1. The microscopic features of herpes simplex, varicella, and herpes zoster are identical; variola and vaccinia have somewhat different features.
2. All of these diseases are characterized by intraepidermal vesicles (Fig. A) which form by two principal mechanisms: ballooning degeneration and reticular degeneration. In late lesions, the separation may appear subepidermal.

Ballooning degeneration

This is characterized by enlargement of the epidermal cells and loss of intercellular bridges (acantholysis) (Figs. A,B,C,D) with separation of the cells. Balloon cell formation is most pronounced in herpes simplex, varicella, and herpes zoster and less pronounced in variola and vaccinia. In all of these diseases except variola and vaccinia, the balloon cells are often multinucleated (Fig. C).

Early lesions of ballooning degeneration show little or no separation of epidermal cells and therefore no frank vesiculation (Fig. E).

VESICULAR VIRAL DISEASES

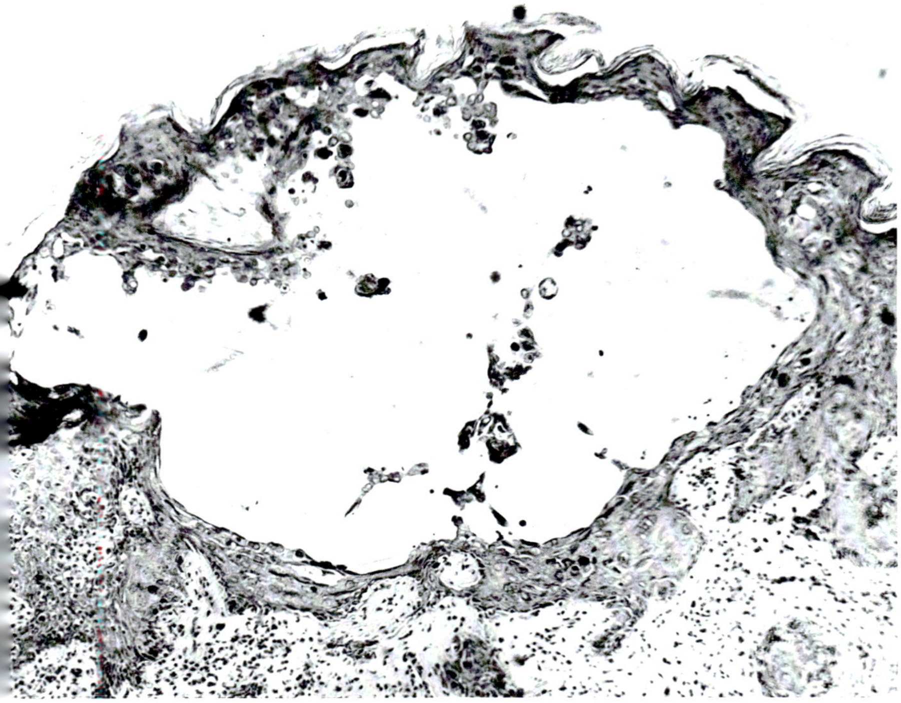

A
X120

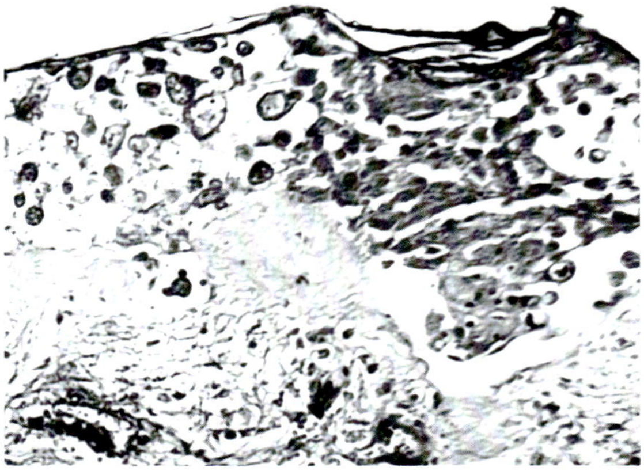

B
X210

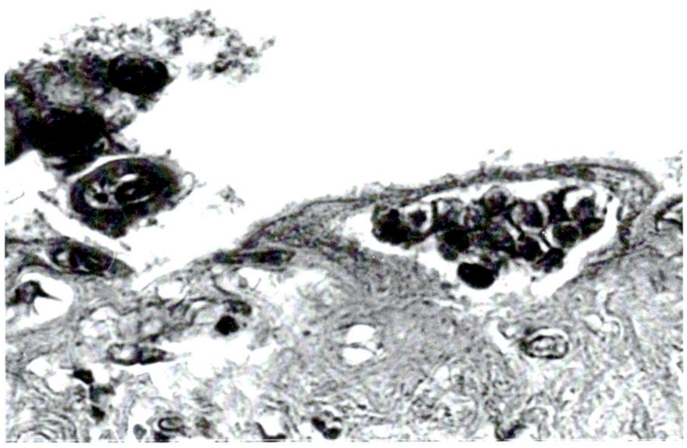

C
X780

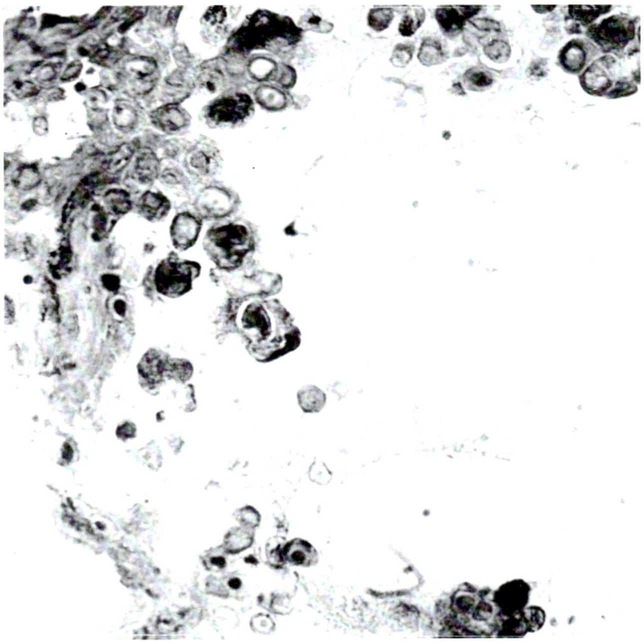

D
X1040

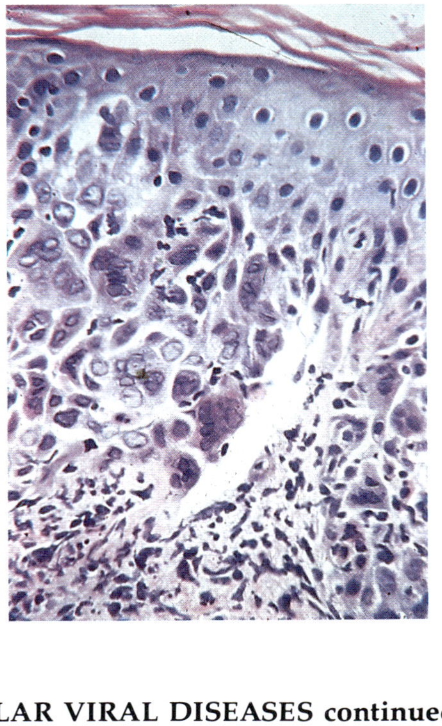

E
X540

VESICULAR VIRAL DISEASES continued

Microscopic features of vesicular viral diseases

Ballooning degeneration

Balloon cells have a homogeneous eosinophilic cytoplasm and single or multiple nuclei (Figs. A,B). Ballooning degeneration occurs principally at the base of the viral vesicles (Fig. A), and may also involve sebaceous glands and hair follicles.

The diagnosis of viral vesicle can sometimes be made by a cytologic technique called the *Tzanck smear*. Scrapings from the base of a vesicle are smeared on a slide, air-dried, fixed with alcohol, and are stained with Wright's stain, Giemsa stain, or Papanicolaou stain. Balloon cells indicate a viral vesicle (Fig. D).

Eosinophilic inclusion bodies (5 to 10 microns in diameter), surrounded by a halo, are present (Figs. A,B). In herpes simplex, varicella, and herpes zoster they are intranuclear (Figs. A,B); in vaccinia they are intracytoplasmic; in variola they are principally intracytoplasmic and occasionally intranuclear. Inclusion bodies of herpes simplex, varicella, and herpes zoster are generally Feulgen-negative (since they generally no longer contain the virus); those of variola and vaccinia are Feulgen-positive. Inclusion bodies are more easily demonstrable with Papanicolaou stain than with H&E.

The dermis shows an inflammatory infiltrate of varying intensity (Fig. C). In severe cases, there may be an inflammatory purpura.

Reticular degeneration (severe hydropic degeneration)

Reticular degeneration is characterized by rupture of epidermal cells due to severe intracellular edema and formation of multilocular vesicles bordered by the residual cell walls (Fig. C). As lesions age, coalescence of the subdivisions results in the formation of unilocular vesicles. Reticular degeneration is usually most pronounced in the superficial and peripheral parts of the vesicles. It is more pronounced in variola and vaccinia than in herpes simplex, varicella, or herpes zoster.

Microscopic differential diagnosis (see chart on bullous diseases, p. 528)

Viral vesicles can generally be differentiated from spongiotic vesicles of acute dermatitis by the presence of balloon cells and inclusion bodies.

VESICULAR VIRAL DISEASES

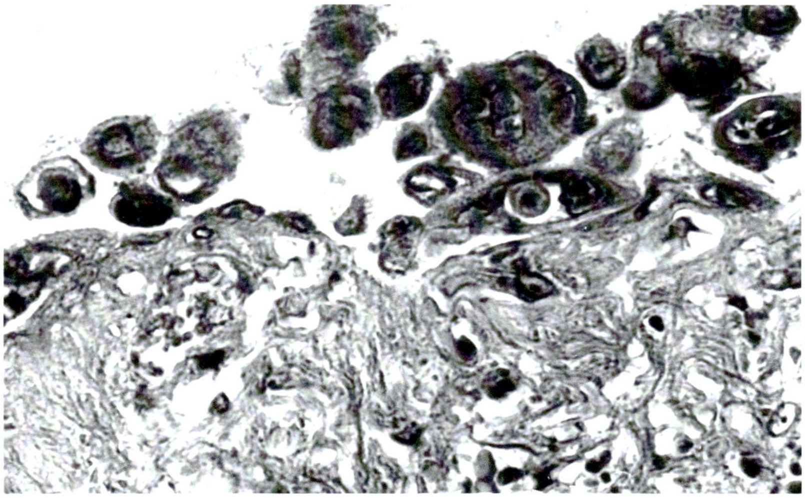

A
X730

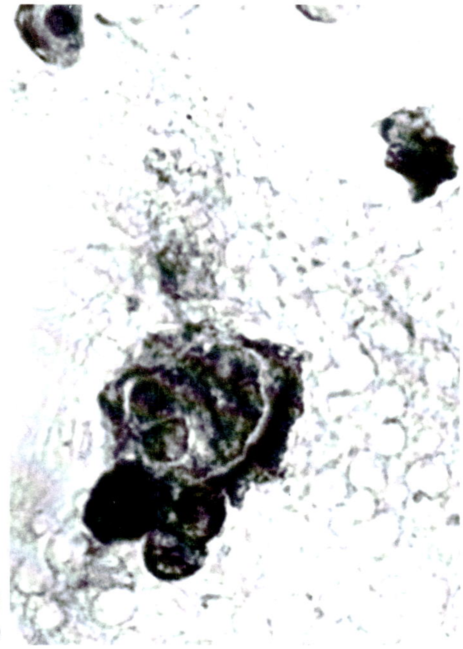

B
X720

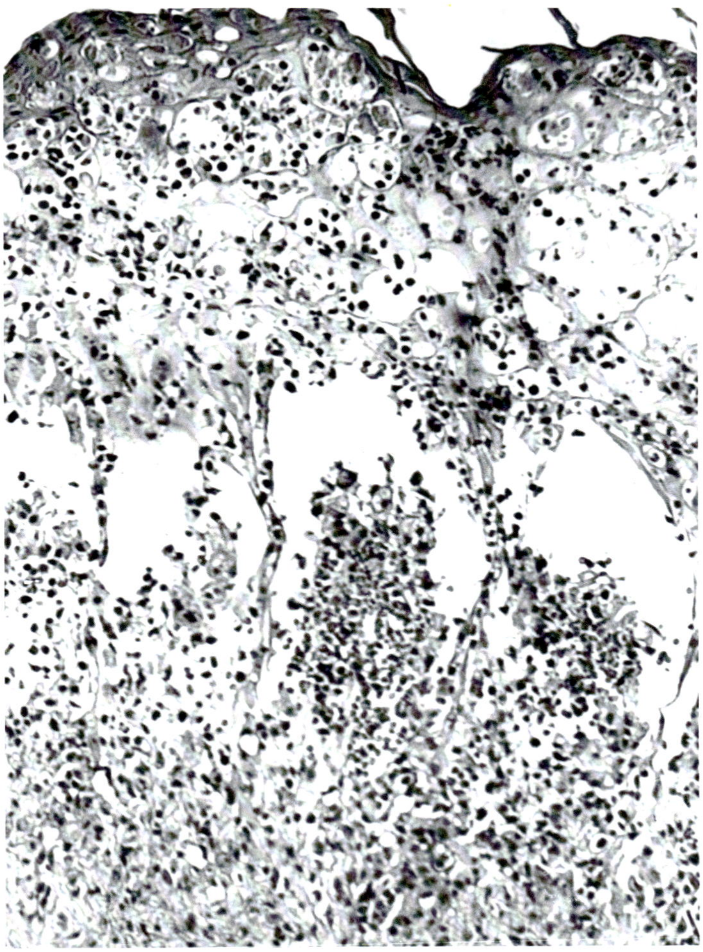

C
X260

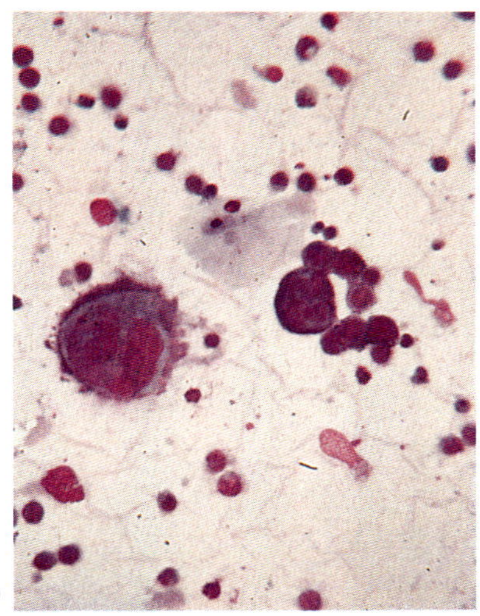

D
X1000

GIEMSA STAIN

VESICULAR VIRAL DISEASES continued ⇨

Comment

1. *Milkers' nodules* are transmitted by cows infected with paravaccinia. The nodules occur on the fingers and have a violaceous color. The histologic picture is that of dermatitis with reactive hyperplasia of the epidermis and multilocular vesicles. Intracytoplasmic and occasionally intranuclear eosinophilic inclusion bodies can be found within vacuolated epidermal cells.
2. *Ecthyma contagiosum (orf)* is a papulovesicular viral eruption acquired by handling sheep.

   The histologic picture is usually similar to that of milker's nodule.
3. *Variola* (smallpox) has largely been eradicated. It is caused by a pox virus. Vesicles evolve into pustules. Lesions are at the same stage at any given time. Histologically, ballooning degeneration and reticular degeneration occur; ballooning degeneration is not prominent. There are intracytoplasmic inclusion bodies.
4. *Hand-foot-and-mouth disease* is a mild infection caused by a coxsackie virus. It affects mainly children and young adults. Lesions may be confined to the mouth (vesicles which tend to ulcerate). Vesicles may occur on the hands and feet. Reticular degeneration dominates the microscopic picture. Ballooning degeneration may occur. Inclusion bodies and multinucleated balloon cells are not found. Late vesicles may be subepidermal.

VESICULAR VIRAL DISEASES continued

MOLLUSCUM CONTAGIOSUM

Molluscum contagiosum is caused by a virus of the pox family. It is characterized by small, waxy, umbilicated papules of the skin (Figs. A,B) and mucous membranes; lesions may show a linear arrangement (Fig. B), and usually contain "cheesy" material.

Eventual spontaneous involution is the rule. Numerous lesions may be present in patients with AIDS and in other immunosuppressed individuals.

Microscopic features

1. There is a central crater, beneath which the epidermis shows pronounced downward growth (Fig. C) with "pear-shaped" lobules.
2. Intracytoplasmic inclusion bodies (molluscum bodies) appear in the cells of the lower malpighian layer and occupy increasing portions of the cellular cytoplasm as the infected cells approach the surface (Fig. C). Ultimately, molluscum bodies occupy most of the keratinocyte, with the remnants of the cytoplasm and nucleus compressed into a crescent-shaped mass against the cell wall (Fig. D). The eosinophilic inclusion bodies in the lower part of the lesion become basophilic and increasingly Feulgen-positive as the granular layer is reached. The horny layer contains numerous basophilic inclusion bodies between the keratin fibers. The inclusion bodies are released and accumulate in the central crater (Fig. C).
3. Dermal inflammation is usually minimal, except when a foreign-body reaction results from release of molluscum bodies into the dermis.

MOLLUSCUM CONTAGIOSUM

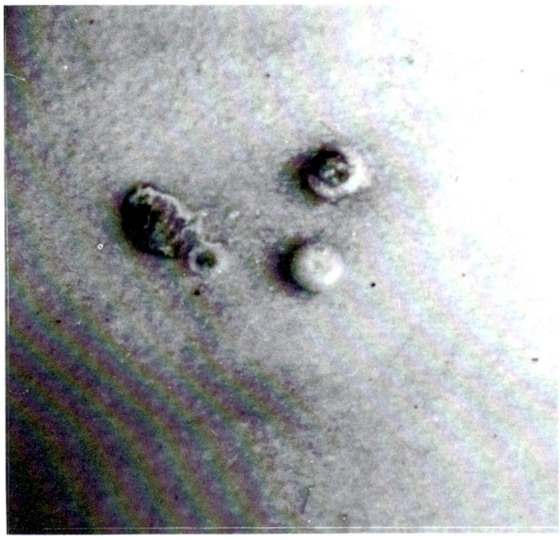

A

Courtesy Dr. K. Inaba

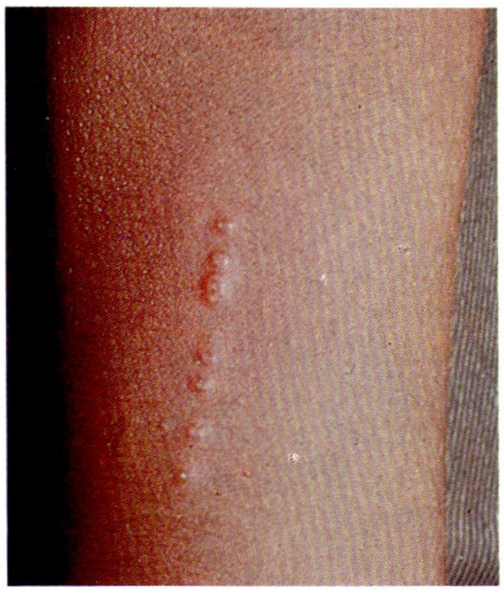

B

Courtesy Dr. Harvey Ansell

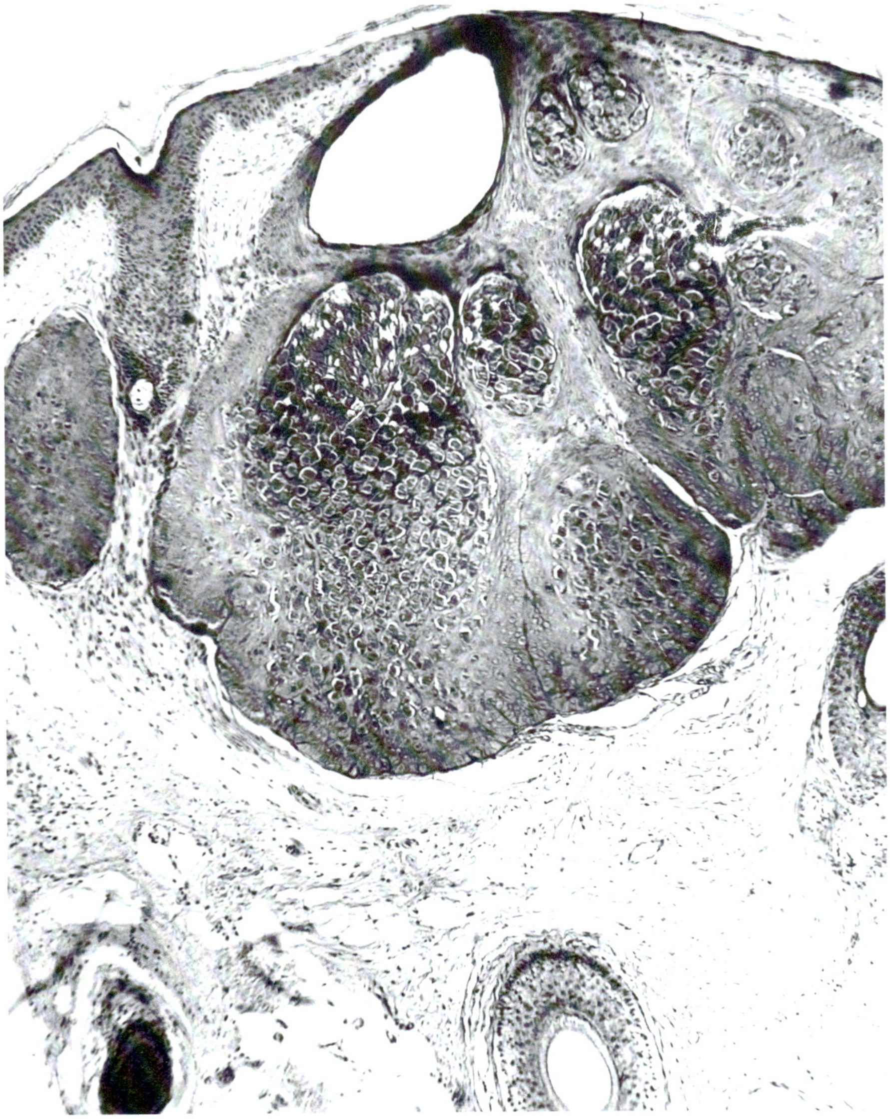

C
X60

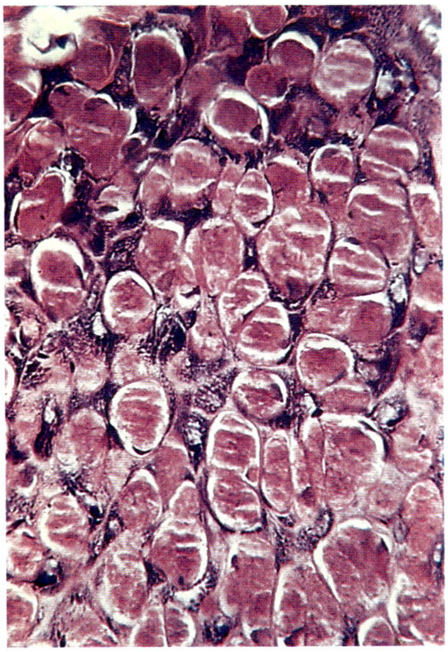

D
X500

CAT-SCRATCH DISEASE

Cat-scratch disease may show one or more primary crusted papules and regional adenitis. The causative agent is believed to be an organism (Chlamydiae) related to the organism causing lymphogranuloma venereum.

Chlamydiae are no longer considered viruses. They are considered to be bacteria-like organisms closely related to rickettsiae. Therefore, inclusion of cat-scratch disease and lymphogranuloma venereum in this section is an accommodation to tradition rather than microbiological accuracy.

Microscopic features

Both the primary lesion and involved lymph nodes show central stellate necrosis (Figs. A,C) surrounded by a zone of histiocytes and epithelioid cells (Figs. A,C) and an outermost zone of lymphoid cells (Figs. A,B,C). Lymphoid hyperplasia resembling lymphoma (Fig. C) is usually present. In the lymph nodes there is abscess formation.

Microscopic differential diagnosis

The microscopic pattern resembles that of lymphogranuloma venereum and sporotrichosis.

LYMPHOGRANULOMA VENEREUM

Lymphogranuloma venereum is caused by an organism in the lymphogranuloma-psittacosis group (Chlamydia [see above]). It is transmitted by sexual contact. The primary lesion is a papule, vesicle, or erosion appearing on the penis, vaginal wall, or cervix. This is transient and is followed by enlargement of lymph nodes, including those in the inguinal, iliac, and anorectal regions. Inguinal lymph nodes are involved in affected heterosexual men. In women whose infection begins in the lower vagina, anorectal and iliac lymph nodes are involved. Nodes become confluent and develop draining sinuses. Rectal stricture and perineal ulcerations are possible sequelae in women. Genital elephantiasis or penile ulcerations are rare complications in men. The microscopic pattern in lymph nodes is similar to that of cat-scratch disease or sporotrichosis.

CAT-SCRATCH DISEASE

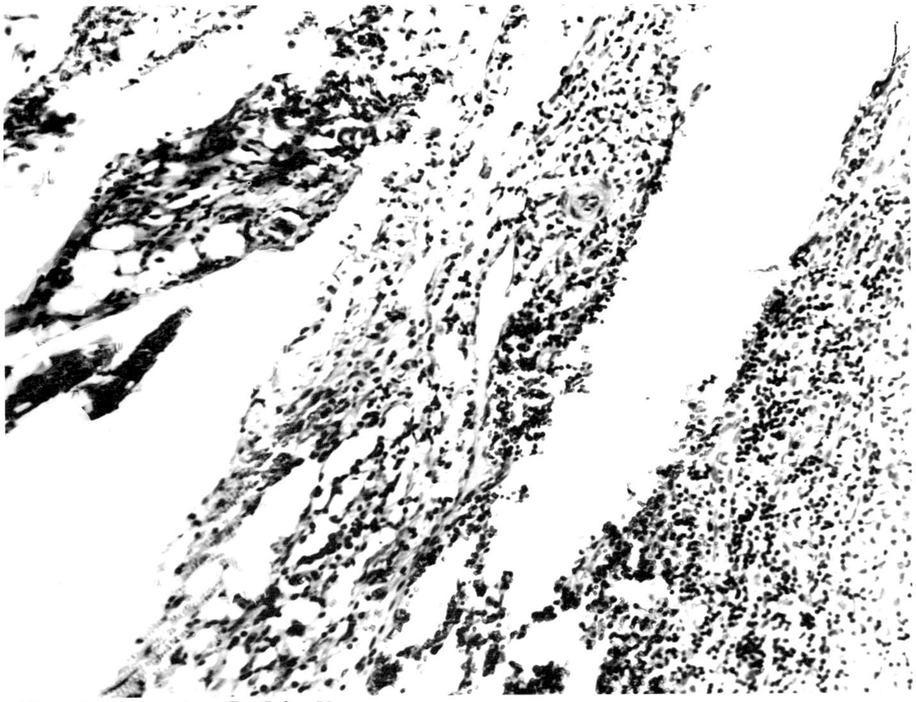

A
X130

Figs. A,B,C courtesy Dr. John Knox

B X130

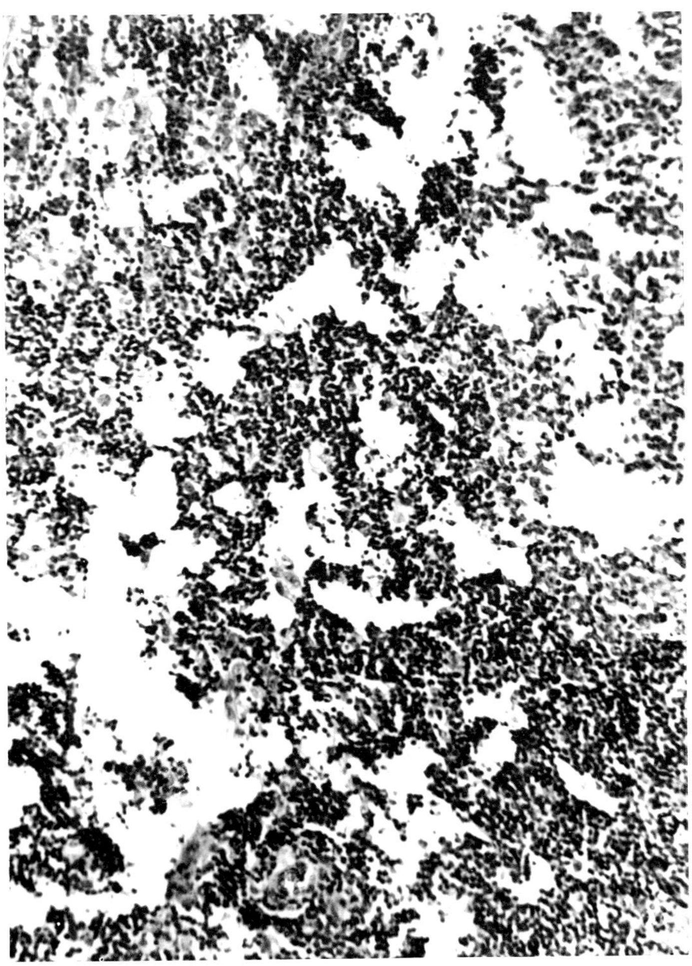

C X45

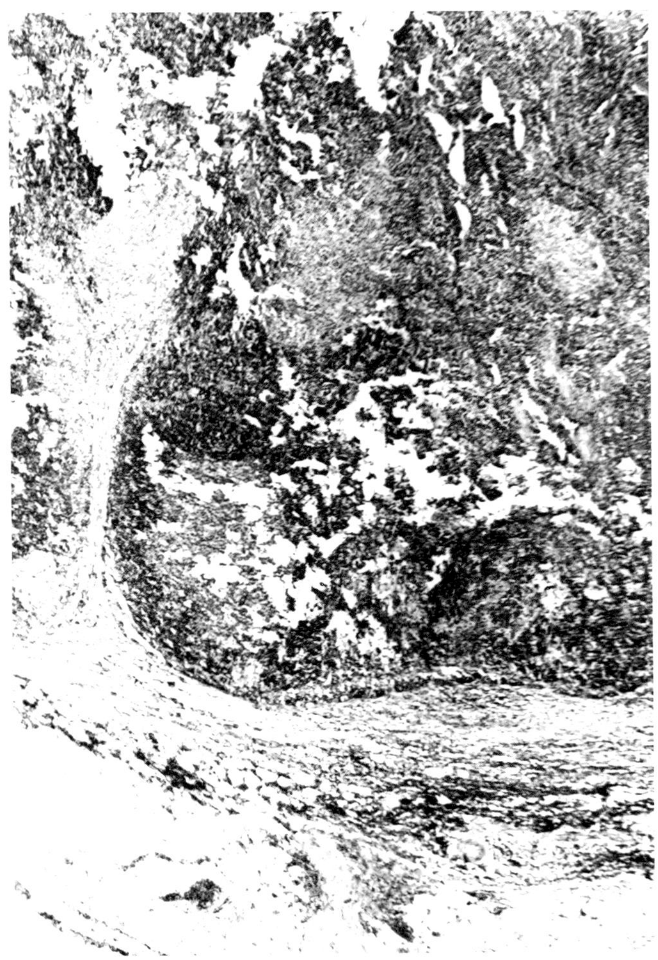

Suggested Reading

Infectious Diseases: Viral

General References

Behbehani, A. *Human Viral, Bedsonial, and Rickettsial Diseases*. Springfield, IL, Thomas, 1972.

Cohen, A. *Textbook of Medical Virology*. Oxford, Blackwell, 1969.

Higgins, P. Virus Infections of the Skin and Mucous Membranes. In: *Current Problems in Clinical Virology*. Edinburgh, Churchill Livingstone, 1971.

Horsfall, F. and Tamm, I. *Viral and Rickettsial Infections of Man*. 4th Ed., Philadelphia, Lippincott, 1965.

Koprowski, C. and Koprowski, H. *Viruses and Immunity*. New York, Academic Press, 1975.

Robinson, W. and Fox, C. *Mechanisms of Virus Disease*. Menlo Park, CA, Benjamin Press, 1974.

White, D. Viral infections of the skin. *Austral. J. Dermatol.*, 11:5, 1970.

Herpes Simplex, Herpes Zoster, and Varicella

Allen, D. and Cole, P. Viruses and human cancer. *N. Eng. J. Med.*, 286:70, 1972.

Asano, Y. et al. Viremia is present in incubation period in nonimmunocompromised children with varicella. *J. Pediatr.*, 106:69, 1985.

Bader, C. et al. The natural history of recurrent facial-oral infection with herpes simplex virus. *J. Infect. Dis.*, 138:897, 1978.

Barr, R. et al. Rapid method for Tzanck preparations. *JAMA*, 237:1119, 1977.

Bastian, F. et al. Herpesvirus hominis: Isolation from human trigeminal ganglion. *Science*, 178:306, 1972.

Bastian, F. et al. Herpesvirus varicellae. *Arch. Pathol.*, 97:331, 1974.

Blank, H. Herpetism. *Arch. Dermatol.*, 115:1440, 1979.

Blank, H. and Haines, H. Viral diseases of the skin, 1975: A 25-year perspective. *J. Invest. Dermatol.*, 67:169, 1976.

Blank, H. and Rake, G. *Viral and Rickettsial Diseases of the Skin, Eye and Mucous Membranes of Man*. Boston, Little, Brown, 1955.

Brehmer-Andersson, E. Diagnostic importance of punch biopsy and cytologic examination in herpes zoster and herpes simplex. *Acta Derm. Venereol.*, 45:262, 1965.

Brunnell, P. and Kotchmar, G. Zoster in infancy: Failure to maintain virus latency following intrauterine infection. *J. Pediatr.*, 98:71, 1981.

Catalano, L., Jr. et al. Disseminated herpesvirus infection in a newborn infant: Virologic, serologic, coagulation, and interferon studies. *J. Pediatr.*, 79:393, 1971.

Centers for Disease Control: Reye syndrome: United States, 1984. *MMWR*, 34:13, 1985.

Chang, T., Fiumara, N. and Weinstein, L. Genital herpes. *JAMA*, 229:544, 1974.

Cheatham, W. et al. Varicella: Report of two fatal cases with necropsy, virus isolation, and serologic studies. *Am. J. Pathol.*, 32:1015, 1956.

Corey, L. et al. Genital herpes simplex virus infections: Clinical manifestations, course and complications. *Ann. Int. Med.*, 98:958, 1983.

Crouse, H. et al. Cytochemical studies on the intranuclear inclusion of herpes simplex. *J. Immunol.*, 65:119, 1950.

Denny-Brown, D., Adams, R. and Fitzgerald, P. Pathologic features of herpes zoster: A note on "geniculate herpes." *Arch. Neurol. Psych.*, 51:216, 1944.

Dolin, R. et al. Herpes zoster-varicella infections in immunosuppressed patients. *Ann. Int. Med.*, 89:375, 1978.

Elliot, W. et al. Herpes simplex type 1 hepatitis in renal transplantation. *Arch. Int. Med.*, 140:1656, 1980.

Ey, J. et al. Varicella hepatitis without neurologic symptoms or findings. *Pediatrics*, 67:285, 1981.

Feldman, S. et al. A viremic phase for herpes zoster in children with cancer. *Pediatrics*, 91:597, 1977.

Foley, F. et al. Herpes virus infection in burned patients. *N. Eng. J. Med.*, 282:652, 1970.

Friedman-Keim, A. et al. Herpes zoster: A possible early clinical sign for development of acquired immunodeficiency syndrome in high-risk individuals. *JAAD*, 14:1023, 1986.
Fulginiti, V. et al. Aspirin and Reye syndrome. *Pediatrics*, 69:810, 1982.
Gershon, A. et al. IgM to varicella-zoster virus: Demonstration in patients with and without clinical zoster. *Pediatr. Infect. Dis.*, 1:164, 1982.
Gershon , A. et al. Varicella-zoster-associated encephalitis: Detection of specific antibody in cerebrospinal fluid. *J. Clin. Microbiol.*, 12:764, 1980.
Golden, B., Bell, W. and McKee, A. Disseminated herpes simplex with encephalitis in a newborn. *JAMA*, 209:1219, 1969.
Goldstein, L. et al. Monoclonal antibodies to herpes simplex viruses: Use in antigenic typing and rapid diagnosis. *J. Infect. Dis.*, 147:829, 1983.
Haburchak, D. Recurrent herpetic whitlow due to herpes simplex virus type 2. *Arch. Int. Med.*, 138:1418, 1978.
Hasegawa, T. Further electron microscopic observations of herpes zoster virus. *Arch. Dermatol.*, 103:45, 1971.
Higgins, P. Virus Infections of the Skin and Mucous Membranes. In: *Current Problems in Clinical Virology*. Edinburgh, Churchill Livingstone, 1971.
Izumi, A., Kim, R. and Arnold, H., Jr. Herpes sycosis. *Arch. Dermatol.*, 106:372, 1972.
Jeansson, S. and Molin, L. Genital Herpes virus hominis infection: A venereal disease. *Lancet*, 1:1064, 1970.
Jemsek, J. et al. Herpes zoster-associated encephalitis: Clinicopathologic report of 12 cases and review of the literature. *Medicine* (Baltimore), 62:81, 1983.
Juel-Jensen, B. Some current problems in infections of the skin with the virus of herpes simplex and varicella zoster. *Public Health* (London), 83:169, 1969.
Juel-Jensen, B. and MacCallum, F. *Herpes simplex, Varicella and Zoster*. London, Heinemann, 1972.
Kamiya, H. et al. Diagnostic skin test reaction with varicella virus antigen and clinical application of the test. *J. Infect. Dis.*, 136:784, 1977.
Komorous, J. et al. Intrauterine herpes simplex infections. *Arch. Dermatol.*, 113:918, 1977.
Lichtenstein, P. et al. Grade 1 Reye's syndrome: A frequent cause of vomiting and liver dysfunction after varicella and upper-respiratory-tract infection. *N. Eng. J. Med.*, 309:133, 1983.
Logan, W., Tindall, J. and Elson, M. Chronic cutaneous Herpes simplex. *Arch. Dermatol.*, 103:606, 1971.
Long, J., Wheeler, C., Jr. and Briggaman, R. Varicella-like infection due to herpes simplex. *Arch. Dermatol.*, 114:406, 1978.
Lopyan, L., Young, A., Jr. and Menegus, M. Generalized acute mucocutaneous herpes simplex type 2 with fatal outcome. *Arch. Dermatol.*, 113:816, 1977.
Luby, J. Varicella-zoster virus. *J. Invest. Dermatol.*, 61:212, 1973.
Luby, J. et al. A longitudinal study of varicella-zoster virus infections in renal transplant recipients. *J. Infect. Dis.*, 135:659, 1977.
Lutzner, M. Molluscum contagiosum, verruca and zoster viruses: Electron microscopic studies in the skin. *Arch. Dermatol.*, 87:436, 1963.
Merselis, J., Jr., Kaye, D. and Hook, E. Disseminated herpes zoster: A report of 17 cases. *Arch. Int. Med.*, 113:679, 1964.
Morecki, R. and Becker, N. Human herpes virus infection: Its fine structure identification in paraffin-embedded tissue. *Arch. Pathol.*, 86:292, 1968.
Muller, S., Herrmann, E., Jr. and Winkelmann, R. Herpes simplex infections in hematologic malignancies. *Am. J. Med.*, 52:102, 1972.
Muller, S. and Winkelmann, R. Cutaneous nerve changes in zoster. *J. Invest. Dermatol.*, 52:71, 1969.
Myers, M. Viremia caused by varicella-zoster virus: Association with malignant progressive varicella. *J. Infect. Dis.*, 140:229, 1979.
Nahmias, A., Visentine, A. and Josey, W. Cesarean section and genital herpes. *N. Eng. J. Med.*, 296:1359, 1977.
Nahmias, A. et al. and the Collaborative Antiviral Study Group. Herpes simplex virus encephalitis: Laboratory evaluations and their diagnostic significance. *J. Infect. Dis.*, 145:829, 1982.
O'Donnell, P. et al. Recurrent herpes zoster encephalitis. *Arch. Neurol.*, 38:49, 1981.
Pettay, O. et al. Herpes simplex virus infection in the newborn. *Arch. Dis. Child.*, 47:97, 1972.
Pinkerton, H. Rickettsial, chlamydial, and viral diseases. In: *Pathology*. 7th Ed., Vol. 1, Anderson, W. and Kissane, J., eds., St. Louis, CV Mosby, 1977, p. 452.

Rado, J. et al. Herpes zoster house epidemic in steroid-treated patients: A clinical and viral study. *Arch. Int. Med.*, 116:329, 1965.
Ragozzino, M. et al. Population-based study of herpes zoster and its sequelae. *Medicine* (Baltimore), 61:310, 1982.
Ragozzino, M. et al. Risk of cancer after herpes zoster. A population-based study. *N. Eng. J. Med.*, 307:393, 1982.
Ramsay, A. Herpes simplex virus infections. *Postgrad. Med. J.*, 43:110, 1967.
Ramsey, P. et al. Herpes simplex virus pneumonia: Clinical, virologic and pathologic features in 20 patients. *Ann. Int. Med.*, 97:813, 1982.
Reboul, F., Donaldson, S. and Kaplan, H. Herpes zoster and varicella infections in children with Hodgkin's disease. *Cancer*, 41:95, 1978.
Reeves, W. et al. Risk of recurrence after first episodes of genital herpes. *N. Eng. J. Med.*, 305:315, 1981.
Richman, D. et al. Rapid viral diagnosis. *J. Infect. Dis.*, 149:298, 1984.
Rogers, R., III and Tindall, J. Herpes zoster in children. *Arch. Dermatol.*, 106:204, 1972.
Ruckdeschel, J. et al. Herpes zoster and impaired cell-associated immunity to the varicella-zoster virus in patients with Hodgkin's disease. *Am. J. Med.*, 62:77, 1977.
Schimpff, S. et al. Varicella-zoster infection in patients with cancer. *Ann. Int. Med.*, 76:241, 1972.
Schmidt, N. et al. Direct immunofluorescence staining for detection of herpes simplex and varicella-zoster virus antigens in vesicular lesions and certain tissue specimens. *J. Clin. Microbiol.*, 12:651, 1980.
Shneidman, D., Barr, R. and Graham, J. Chronic cutaneous herpes simplex. *JAMA*, 241:592, 1979.
Siegel, F. et al. Severe acquired immunodeficiency in male homosexuals, manifested by chronic perianal ulcerative herpes simplex lesions. *N. Eng. J. Med.*, 305:1439, 1981.
Sokal, J. and Firat, D. Varicella-zoster infection in Hodgkin's disease: Clinical and epidemiological aspects. *Am. J. Med.*, 39:452, 1965.
Southam, J., Colley, I. and Clarke, N. Oral herpetic infection in adults. *Br. J. Dermatol.*, 80:248, 1968.
Stern, H. et al. Herpetic whitlow: A form of cross-infection in hospitals. *Lancet*, 2:871, 1959.
Takashima, S. and Becker, L. Neuropathology of fatal varicella. *Arch. Pathol.*, 103:209, 1979.
Torphy, D. et al. Herpes simplex virus infection in infants: A spectrum of disease. *J. Pediatr.*, 76:405, 1970.
Vonderheid, E. et al. Chronic herpes simplex: Infection in cutaneous T-cell lymphoma. *Arch. Dermatol.*, 116:1018, 1980.
Weller, T. Varicella and herpes zoster: Changing concepts of the natural history, control, and importance of a not-so-benign virus. *N. Eng. J. Med.*, 309:1362, 1983.
Wheeler, C. and Huffines, W. Primary disseminated herpes simplex of the newborn. *JAMA*, 191:455, 1965.
White, J. Fulminating infection with herpex-simplex virus in premature and newborn infants. *N. Eng. J. Med.*, 269:455, 1963.
Womack, L. and Liesegang, T. Complications of herpes zoster ophthalmicus. *Arch. Ophthalmol.*, 101:42, 1983.
Wukelich, S. Primary herpes simplex infection of the finger: Report of a case. *J. Can. Dent. Assoc.*, 38:39, 1972.

Eczema Vaccinatum—Herpeticum

Barton, R. and Brunsting, L. Kaposi's varicelliform eruption: Review of the literature and report of two cases of its occurrence in adults. *Arch. Dermatol. Syph.*, 50:99, 1944.
Blank, H. and Haines, H. Viral diseases of the skin, 1975: A 25-year perspective. *J. Invest. Dermatol.*, 67:169, 1976.
Blank, H. and Rake, G. *Viral and Rickettsial Diseases of the Skin, Eye and Mucous Membranes of Man.* Boston, Little, Brown, 1955.
Buerk, M. and Blank, H. Disseminated herpes simplex (Kaposi's varicelliform eruption) and the failure of penicillin and aureomycin to influence its course. *N. Eng. J. Med.*, 244:670, 1951.
Hazen, P. and Eppes, R. Eczema herpeticum caused by herpesvirus type 2. *Arch. Dermatol.*, 113:1085, 1977.
Loeffel, E. and Meyer, J. Eczema vaccinatum in Darier's disease. *Arch. Dermatol.*, 102:451, 1970.

Lynch, F. Kaposi's varicelliform eruption: Extensive herpes simplex as a complication of eczema. *Arch. Dermatol. Syph.*, 51:129, 1945.
Otsuka, F. et al. Generalized herpes simplex complicating Hailey-Hailey's disease. *J. Dermatol.* (Tokyo), 8:63, 1981.
Reynolds, A. and Joos, H. Eczema vaccinatum. *Pediatrics*, 22:259, 1958.
Segal, R. and Watson, W. Kaposi's varicelliform eruption in mycosis fungoides. *Arch. Dermatol.*, 114:1067, 1978.
Sussman, S. and Grossman, M. Complications of smallpox vaccination: Effects of vaccinia immune globulin therapy. *J. Pediatr.*, 67:1168, 1965.
Taulbee, K. and Johnson, S. Disseminated cutaneous herpes simplex infection in cutaneous T-cell lymphoma. *Arch. Dermatol.*, 117:114, 1981.
Verbov, J., Munro, D. and Miller, A. Recurrent eczema herpeticum associated with ichthyosis vulgaris. *Br. J. Dermatol.*, 86:638, 1972.

Poxviruses

GENERAL REFERENCES

Joklik, W. The poxviruses. *Ann. Rev. Microbiol.*, 22:359, 1968.
Joklik, W. The poxviruses. *Bacteriol. Rev.*, 30:33, 1966.
Lennette, E. and Schmidt, N. *Diagnostic Procedures for Viral and Rickettsial Infections.* 4th Ed., New York, American Public Health Association, 1969, p. 281.

MILKERS' NODULE

Bowman, K. et al. Cutaneous form of bovine papular stomatitis in man. *JAMA*, 246:2813, 1981.
Davis, C. and Musil, G. Milker's nodule. *Arch. Dermatol.*, 101:305, 1968.
Evins, S., Leavell, U., Jr. and Phillips, J. Intranuclear inclusions in milker's nodules. *Arch. Dermatol.*, 103:91, 1971.
Friedman-Kien, A., Rowe, W. and Banfield, W. Milker's nodules: Isolation of a poxvirus from a human case. *Science*, 140:1335, 1963.
Katzenellenbogen, I. Studies on milkers' nodules. *Dermatologica*, 105:69, 1952.
Nomland, R. and McKee, A. Milkers' nodules: Report of ten cases. *Arch. Dermatol. Syph.*, 65:663, 1952.
Schuler, G. et al. The syndrome of milker's nodules in burn injury: Evidence for indirect transmission. *J. Am. Acad. Dermatol.*, 6:334, 1982.
Thomas, V. Biochemical and electron microscopic studies of the replication and composition of milker's nodule virus. *J. Virol.*, 34:244, 1980.

ORF

Cutler, T. Orf: Report of a case. *Clin. Exp. Dermatol.*, 6:205, 1981.
Guss, S. Contagious ecthyma (sore mouth, orf). *Mod. Vet. Pract.*, 61:335, 1980.
Joklik, W. The poxviruses. *Bacteriol. Rev.*, 30:33, 1966.
Kingery, L. and Dahl, J. Ecthyma contagiosum in man: Data concerning its incidence in several Western states. *Arch. Dermatol. Syph.*, 51:359, 1945.
Leavell, U., Jr. Orf. In: *Dermatology in General Practice.* 2nd Ed., Fitzpatrick, T. et al., eds., New York, McGraw-Hill, 1979, p. 1623.
Leavell, U., Jr., McNamara, M. and Muelling, R. Ecthyma contagiosum (orf). *South. Med. J.*, 58:239, 1965.
——. Orf. *JAMA*, 204:657, 1968.
Lennette, E. and Schmidt, N. *Diagnostic Procedures for Viral and Rickettsial Infections.* 4th Ed., New York, American Public Health Association, 1969, p. 281.
Tarnick, M. et al. Vorkommen von Ekthyma contagiosum (orf) beim Menschen. *Dermatol. Wochenschr.*, 162:402, 1976.
Wheeler, C., Cawley, E. and Johnson, J. Ecthyma contagiosum (orf). *Arch. Dermatol. Syph.*, 71:481, 1955.
Yeh, H. and Soltani, K. Ultrastructural studies in human orf. *Arch. Dermatol.*, 109:390, 1974.

SMALLPOX

Bremen, J. and Arita, I. The confirmation and maintenance of smallpox eradication. *N. Eng. J. Med.*, 303:1263, 1980.
Councilman, W., Magrath, G. and Brinckerhoff, W. The pathological anatomy and histology of variola. *J. Med. Res.*, 11:12, 1904.
Dixon, C. *Smallpox*. London, Churchill, 1962.
Fenner, F. Global eradication of smallpox. *Rev. Infect. Dis.*, 4:916, 1982.
Michelson, H. and Ikeda, K. Microscopic changes in variola. *Arch. Dermatol. Syph.*, 15:138, 1927.
Rao, A., Prahlad, I. and Swaminathan, M. A study of 1000 cases of smallpox. *J. Indian Med. Assoc.*, 35:296, 1960.
Wesselhoeft, C. The differential diagnosis of chicken pox and smallpox. *N. Eng. J. Med.*, 230:15, 1944.

MOLLUSCUM CONTAGIOSUM

Aloi, F. and Pippione, M. Molluscum contagiosum occurring in an epidermal cyst. *J. Cutan. Pathol.*, 12:163, 1985.
Fellner, M. and Osowsky, M. Molluscum contagiosum in an epidermal inclusion cyst. *Internat. J. Dermatol.*, 18:160, 1979.
Henao, M. and Freeman, R. Inflammatory molluscum contagiosum: Clinicopathological study of seven cases. *Arch. Dermatol.*, 90:479, 1964.
Lutzner, M. Molluscum contagiosum, verruca and zoster viruses. *Arch. Dermatol.*, 87:436, 1963.
Mescon, H., Gray, M. and Moretti, G. Molluscum contagiosum: A histochemical study. *J. Invest. Dermatol.*, 23:293, 1954.
Middelkamp, J. and Munger, B. The ultrastructure and histogenesis of molluscum contagiosum. *J. Pediatr.*, 64:888, 1964.
Rake, G. and Blank, H. The relationship of host and virus in molluscum contagiosum. *J. Invest. Dermatol.*, 15:81, 1950.
Steffen, C. and Markman, J. Spontaneous disappearance of molluscum contagiosum. *Arch. Dermatol.*, 116:923, 1980.
Sutton, J. and Burnett, J. Ultrastructural changes in dermal and epidermal cells of skin infected with molluscum contagiosum virus. *J. Ultrastruct. Res.*, 26:177, 1969.

Cat-Scratch Disease

Daniels, W. and MacMurray, F. Cat-scratch disease. *Arch. Int. Med.*, 88:736, 1951.
Emmons, R. et al. Continuing search for the etiology of cat-scratch disease. *J. Clin. Microbiol.*, 4:112, 1976.
Johnson, W. and Helwig, E. Cat-scratch disease: Histopathologic changes in the skin. *Arch. Dermatol.*, 100:148, 1969.
Margileth, A. Cat-scratch disease; Nonbacterial regional lymphadenitis: The study of 145 patients and review of the literature. *Pediatrics*, 42:803, 1968.
Pickerill, R. and Milder, J. Transverse myelitis associated with cat-scratch disease in an adult. *JAMA*, 24:2840, 1981.
Spaulding, W. and Hennessy, J. Cat-scratch disease: A study of eighty-three cases. *Am. J. Med.*, 28:504, 1960.
Warwick, W. and Good, R. Cat-scratch disease in Minnesota. I. Evidence for its epidemic occurrence. *Am. J. Dis. Child.*, 100:228, 1960.
—— Cat-scratch disease in Minnesota. II. The family epidemics. *Am. J. Dis. Child.*, 100:236, 1960.
—— Cat-scratch disease in Minnesota. III. Evaluation of the intradermal skin test to cat-scratch disease antigen. *Am. J. Dis. Child.*, 100:241, 1960.
Wear, D. et al. Cat-scratch disease: A bacterial infection. *Science*, 221:1403, 1983.
Zitelli, B. Neck masses in children: Adenopathy and malignant disease. *Pediatr. Clin. North. Am.*, 4:813, 1981.

Lymphogranuloma Venereum

Becker, L. Lymphogranuloma venereum. *Internat. J. Dermatol.*, 15:26, 1976.

Geller, S. et al. Rectal biopsy in early lymphogranuloma venereum proctitis. *Am. J. Gastroenterol.*, 74:433, 1980.

Kornblith, B. Observations on lymphogranuloma venereum: Clinical pathological study of sixty cases, with observations on the histopathology of the Frei test. *Surg. Gynecol. Obstet.*, 63:99, 1936.

Koteen, H. Lymphogranuloma venereum. *Medicine*, 24:1, 1945.

Olansky, S. and Prentz, D. Lymphogranuloma venereum. In: *Communicable and Infectious Diseases.* 7th Ed., Top, F. and Wehrle, P., eds., St. Louis, Mosby, 1972, p. 378.

Philip, R., Hill, D. and Greaves, A. Study of *Chlamydiae* in patients with lymphogranuloma venereum and urethritis attending a venereal disease clinic. *Br. J. Venereol. Dis.*, 47:114, 1971.

Schachter, J. Chlamydial infections. *N. Eng. J. Med.*, 298:428, 490, 1978.

—— Confirmatory serodiagnosis of lymphogranuloma venereum proctitis may yield false-positive results due to other chlamydial infections of the rectum. *Sex. Transm. Dis.*, 8:26, 1981.

Schachter, J. and Dawson, C. Lymphogranuloma venereum. *JAMA*, 236:915, 1976.

Sheldon, W. and Heyman, A. Lymphogranuloma venereum: A histologic study of the primary lesion, bubonulus and lymph nodes in cases proved by isolation of the virus. *Am. J. Pathol.*, 23:653, 1947.

Sonck, C. Lymphogranuloma inguinale. Klinische, epidemiologische und immunologische Aspekte. *Hautarzt*, 23:280, 1972.

Terho, P. *Chlamydia trachomatis* and clinical genital infections: A general review. *Infection*, 10 (1, suppl.):S5, 1982.

Thorsteinsson, S. et al. Lymphogranuloma venereum: A cause of cervical lymphadenopathy. *JAMA*, 235:1882, 1976.

Diseases Caused by Protozoa

LEISHMANIASIS

Leishmaniasis is a disease produced by infection with parasites of the Leishmania genus. The vector is the sandfly of the genus Phlebotomus.

There are three types:

1. Cutaneous leishmaniasis (Oriental leishmaniasis). This is caused by *Leishmania tropica* and is prevalent in the Middle East and India. Acute lesions begin as papules which evolve into ulcers (Fig. A). There are acute and chronic forms, as well as leishmaniasis recidivans and a disseminated anergic type.
2. Mucocutaneous leishmaniasis (American leishmaniasis). This is caused by *Leishmania brasiliensis* and is prevalent in South America. Cutaneous lesions (Fig. C) are similar to those of Oriental sore. Mucous membrane lesions either form by extension of cutaneous lesions or independently. There is also a disseminated anergic form.
3. Visceral leishmaniasis (kala-azar). This is caused by *Leishmania donovani* and occurs in both the Old and New Worlds. It is a systemic disease involving the reticuloendothelial system.

Microscopic features (Oriental leishmaniasis)

1. There is an infiltrate composed principally of large histiocytes (averaging 30 microns in diameter) which contain Leishmania organisms (Fig. B).
   Lymphoid cells and a few plasma cells are present.
2. The organisms can be demonstrated with H&E (Fig. D) or Giemsa stain and appear as round or oval structures averaging 3 microns in diameter. Most organisms are intracellular, but some are present in the intercellular spaces. The organism does not have a capsule, and is composed of a round nucleus and a smaller, rod-like paranucleus tangential to the nucleus. The paranucleus stains red with Giemsa stain.
3. After ulceration, many neutrophils are present in the infiltrate.
4. Older lesions show a decrease in histiocytes and organisms and the development of a tuberculoid infiltrate. The picture may resemble lupus vulgaris, but lacks caseation necrosis.
5. The disseminated anergic type of leishmaniasis resembles the acute type. Leishmaniasis recidivans shows a picture in between the acute and chronic type.

LEISHMANIASIS

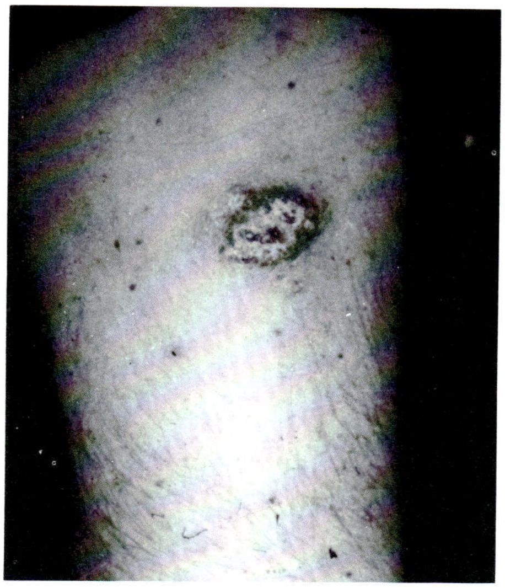

A

Courtesy Dr. Nur Or

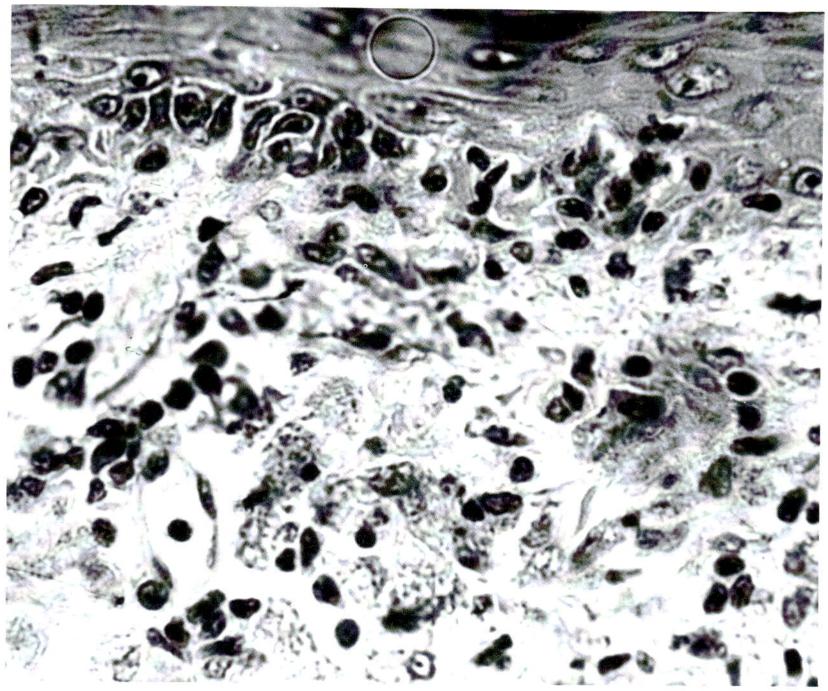

B X780

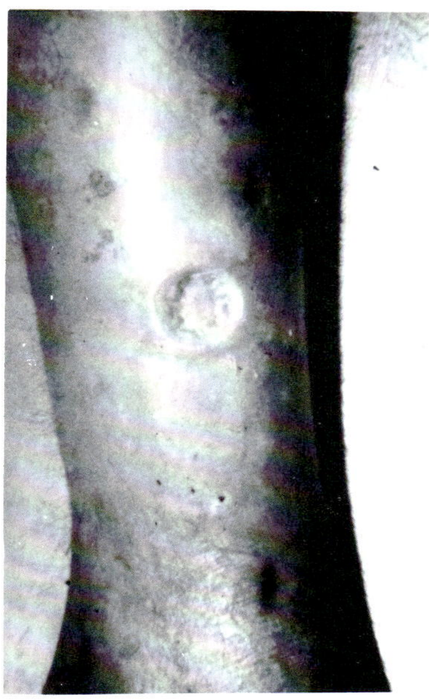

C

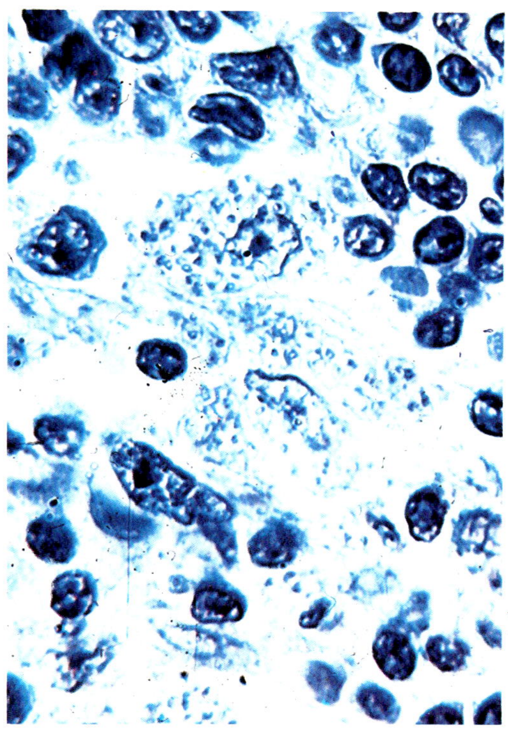

D X1400

LEISHMANIASIS continued

LEISHMANIASIS

Comment

1. Lesions of mucocutaneous leishmaniasis have a histologic picture similar to that of Oriental leishmaniasis, but generally contain fewer organisms (except in the disseminated anergic form of mucocutaneous leishmaniasis).
2. Kala-azar does not generally have cutaneous lesions; however, cutaneous lesions may occasionally develop after recovery from the systemic illness (post-kala-azar dermal leishmaniasis). Cutaneous lesions include hypopigmented and erythematous macules, as well as nodules. The macules show nonspecific inflammation. The nodules show a granulomatous component. Organisms are few in all types of cutaneous lesions of kala-azar.

Diseases Caused by Arthropods

SCABIES

Scabies is caused by the mite *Acarus scabiei* and is characterized by cutaneous lesions called *burrows*. These are thread-like, superficial lesions, often associated with vesicles and pustules (Figs. A,B), which represent a channel within the horny layer, produced by the female mite. Burrows are most common in the interdigital skin, palms, flexor surfaces of the wrists, umbilical area, anterior axillary folds, nipples of women, and genitals of men. Because of the pruritus, excoriations rapidly follow the initial lesions (Fig. C). A papular, pruritic eruption may be present. A rare variant called *Norwegian scabies* generally occurs in mentally defective and debilitated individuals and is characterized by extensive infestation, with resultant severe inflammation, hyperkeratosis, and crusting (Fig. D). Severe scabies can have nodular lesions. Nodular lesions are common in infants. After successful treatment, pruritic papular and nodular lesions may persist.

SCABIES

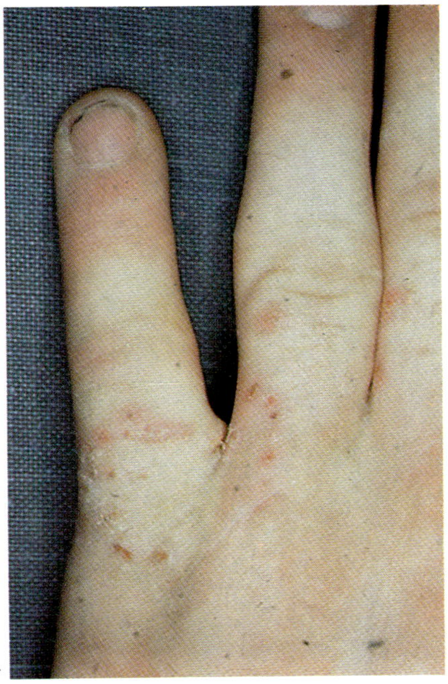
A

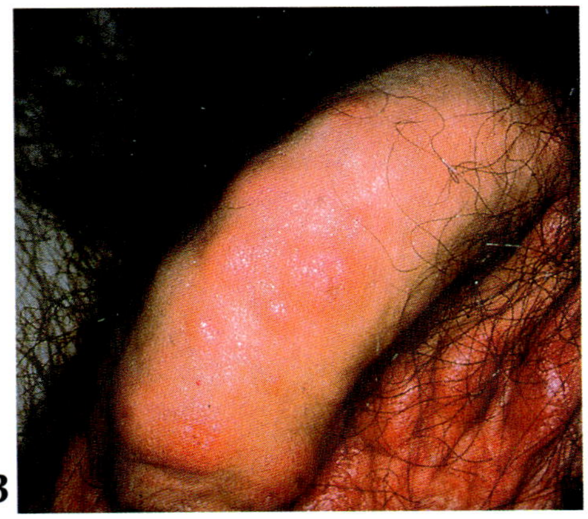
B

Courtesy Dr. Nicholas Fiumara

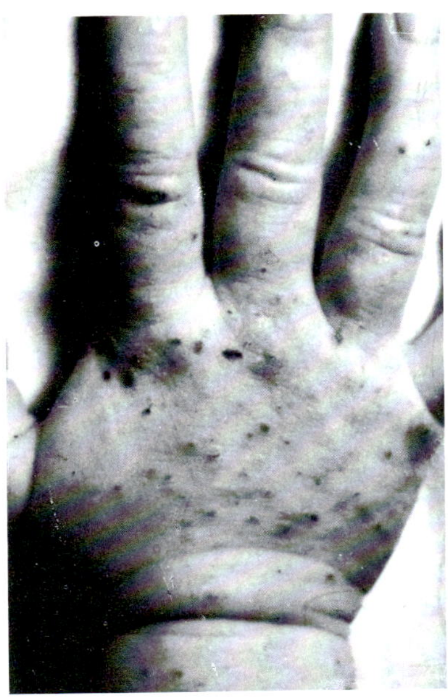
C

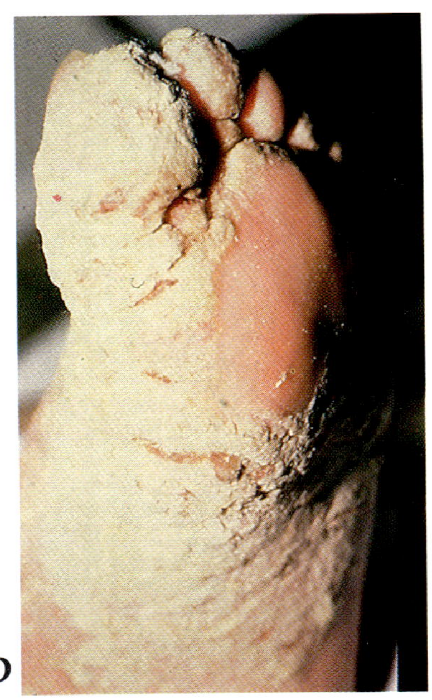
D

SCABIES continued

SCABIES

Microscopic features

1. The burrow is present in the horny layer, with the female mite and eggs at its end (Figs. A,B). At the blind end, the burrow may extend slightly into the malpighian layer. The epidermis beneath the mite may show intracellular and extracellular edema with or without vesicle formation.
2. The dermis shows a nonspecific chronic inflammatory infiltrate (Fig. B). This can be very dense in nodular lesions, resulting in a resemblance to lymphoma. Atypical mononuclear cells can be present. Usually, there are many eosinophils.
3. *Norwegian scabies* shows large numbers of burrows (Fig. B), in addition to hyperkeratosis and crusting.
4. Scrapings of the burrow, placed in potassium hydroxide solution (KOH), mineral oil, or immersion oil may reveal mites and eggs when examined directly under the microscope (Fig. C).

DEMODEX FOLLICULORUM

Demodex folliculorum is a mite which lives in follicular openings and sebaceous ducts, particularly those of the face (Fig. D). It also may be present in the collecting ducts of the nipple. The organism is almost universally present after the age of five. Its role in producing disease in humans is the subject of controversy. It has been proposed that it may play a role in the pathogenesis of rosacea and rosacea blepharitis.

An additional species, *Demodex brevis*, has been described.

SCABIES AND DEMODEX FOLLICULORUM

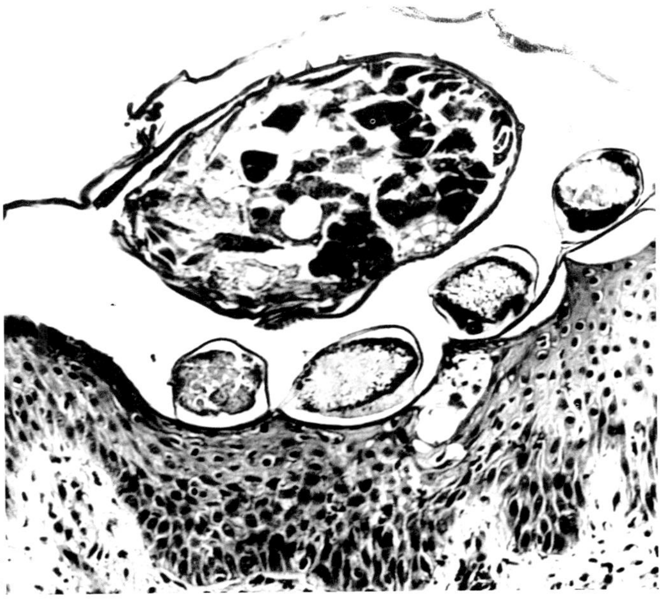

A
X180

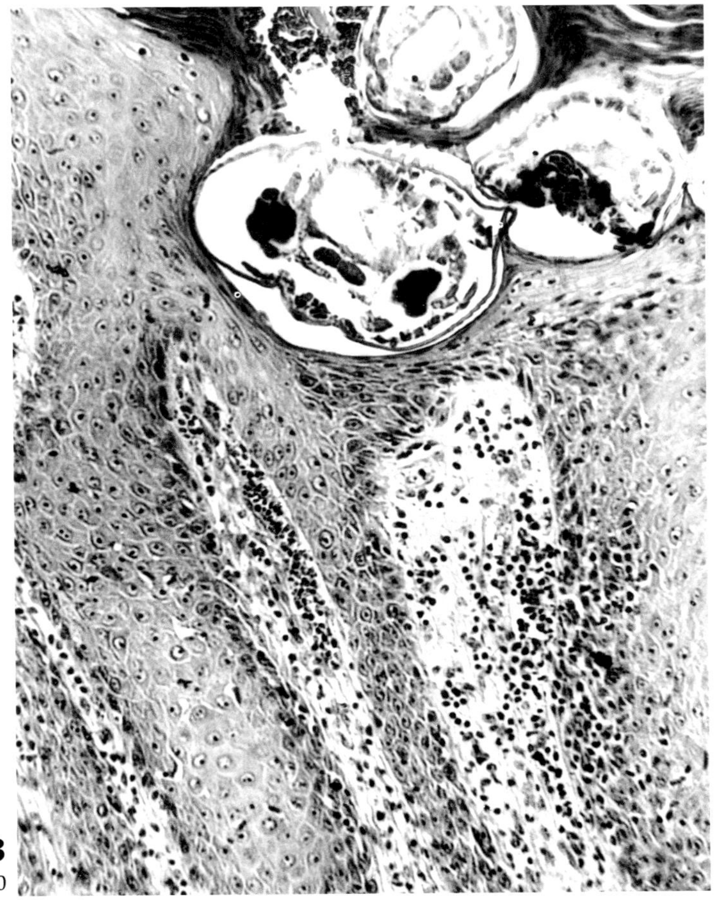

B
X210

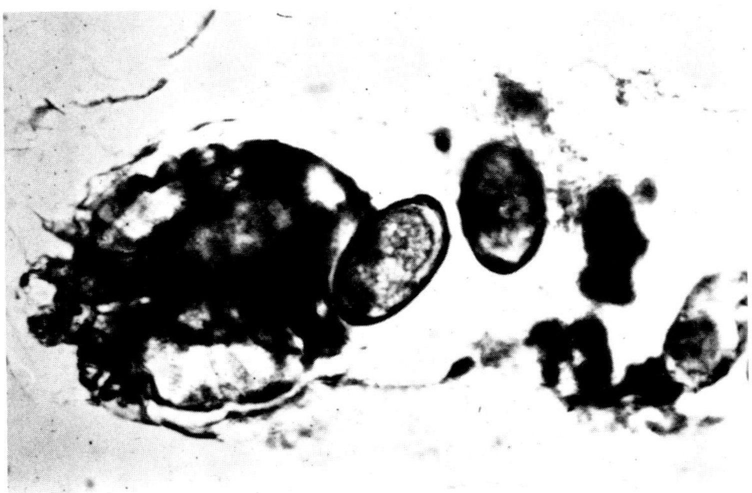

C
X180

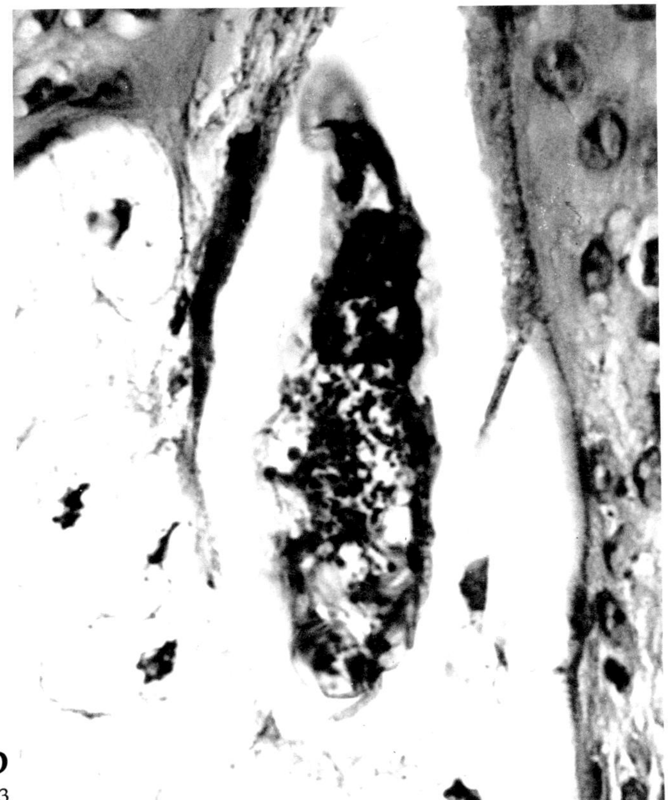

D
X923

PEDICULOSIS (LOUSE INFESTATION)

Lice are flattened, wingless insects. Three types commonly cause human disease: *Pediculus humanus var. capitis* (head louse), *Pediculus humanus var. corporis* (body louse), and *Phthirus pubis* (pubic louse). Pubic lice can also infest other apocrine areas, such as eyelashes and axillae. Lice can transmit infectious diseases, such as typhus, relapsing fever, and trench fever.

The incidence of head lice is highest in children. The diagnosis is made by the demonstration of eggs glued to hairs (nits). Fig. A shows a nit observed directly under the microscope.

The eggs of the body louse are laid in clothing in contact with the skin. The infestation is usually transmitted by clothing or bedclothing, but sometimes the lice can travel directly to a new host. Body lice produce intense itching, with excoriations, papules, and wheals. Hyperpigmentation can develop. Fig. B is a magnified view of a body louse.

Pubic lice (crab lice) are usually transmitted by sexual contact, but there can be transmission by bedclothing. The genital region and adjacent abdomen are typically involved; other apocrine areas, such as the axillae and eyelashes can be affected, as mentioned. Itching is usually intense. Bluish macules may develop on the sides of the trunk and inner thighs. Diagnosis is confirmed by demonstrating lice or eggs. Fig. C shows a magnified view of a pubic louse.

Comment

The stings of Hymenoptera (bees, wasps, and hornets) may produce acute necrotic reactions or subacute to chronic inflammatory reactions. Tick bites may produce nodular lesions that can be diagnostically perplexing. Fleas, mosquitoes, and bedbugs may produce bites that result in a papular or papulovesicular hypersensitivity reaction called *papular urticaria*. (See p. 115 for further discussion of arthropod bites.)

PEDICULOSIS

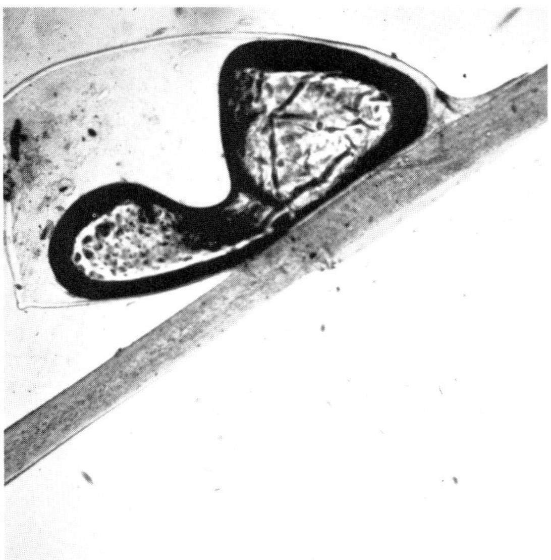

A
X100

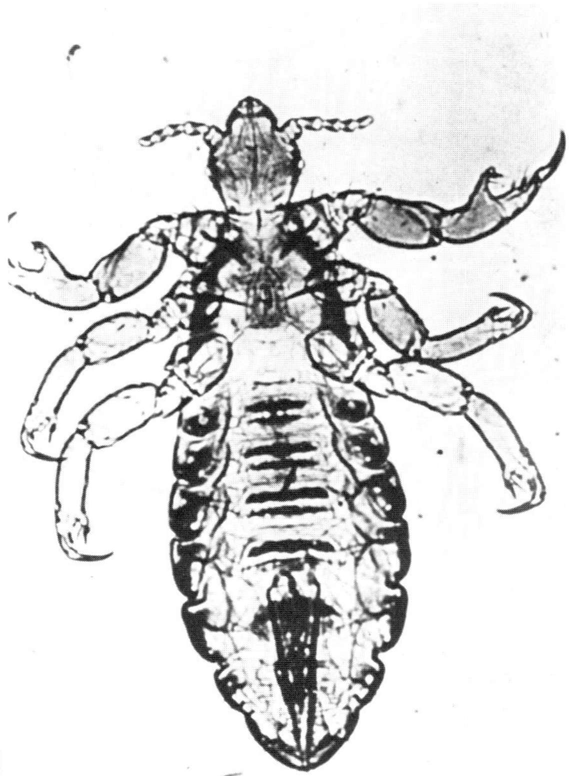

B
X30

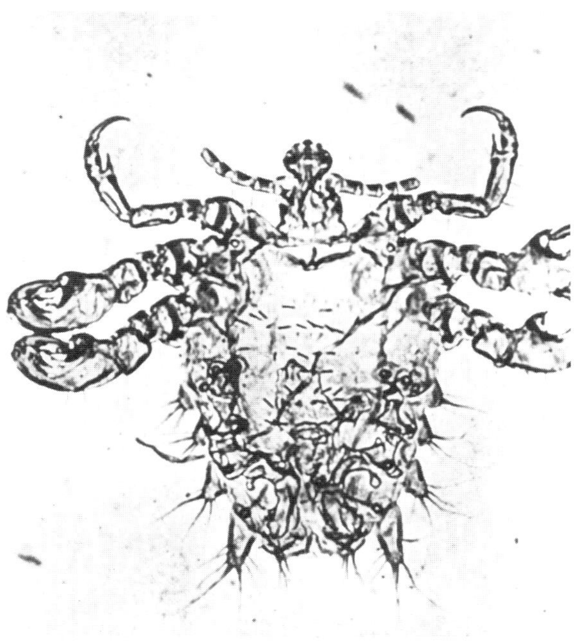

C
X30

Figs. B,C courtesy Dr. Nicholas Fiumara

Suggested Reading

Infectious Diseases: Parasitic

General References

Alfred, D. *Medical Arthropodology: A Laboratory Guide.* Minneapolis, Burgess, 1960.
Brown, H. *Basic Clinical Parasitology.* 3rd Ed., New York, Appleton-Century-Crofts, 1969.
Burrows, R. *Microscopic Diagnosis of the Parasites of Man.* New Haven, Yale Univ. Press, 1965.
Chatterjee, K. *Parasitology in Relation to Clinical Medicine.* 9th Ed., Calcutta, Sree Saraswaty Press, 1973.
Cheng, T. *General Parasitology.* New York, Academic Press, 1973.
Garnham, P. *Immunity to Protozoa.* Oxford, Blackwell, 1963.
Horsfall, W. *Medical Entomology: Arthropods and Human Disease.* New York, Ronald Press, 1962.
Hunter, G. III, Frye, W. and Swartzwelder, J. *A Manual of Tropical Medicine.* 4th Ed., Philadelphia, W. B. Saunders, 1969.
Jeffrey, H. and Leach, R. *Atlas of Medical Helminthology and Protozoology.* Edinburgh, Livingstone, 1966.
Kenney, M. *Scope Monograph on Pathoparasitology: A Color Atlas of Parasites in Tissue Sections.* Kalamazoo, Upjohn Co., 1973.
Levine, M. *Protozoan Parasites of Domestic Animals and Man.* Minneapolis, Burgess, 1961.
McFarlane, L. *A Short Synopsis of Human Protozoology and Helminthology.* Baltimore, Williams & Wilkins, 1969.
Taylor, A. *The Pathology of Parasitic Diseases.* Oxford, Blackwell, 1966.

Leishmaniasis

Adler, S. Immunology of Leishmaniasis. *Israel J. Med. Sci.*, 1:9, 1965.
Barsky, S. et al. Cutaneous leishmaniasis. *Arch. Dermatol.*, 114:1354, 1978.
Bryceson, A. Cutaneous leishmaniasis. *Br. J. Dermatol.*, 94:223, 1976.
Chance, M. The identification of leishmania. *Parasitology*, 17:55, 1979.
Conrad, A., Jr., Manson, R. and Peterkin, G. Cutaneous leishmaniasis: Report of cases occurring in Great Britain and the United States. *Arch. Dermatol. Syph.*, 62:502, 1950.
Convit, J. and Kerdel-Vegas, F. Disseminated cutaneous leishmaniasis: Inoculation of laboratory animals, electron microscopy and fluorescent antibody studies. *Arch. Dermatol.*, 91:439, 1965.
Convit, J., Kerdel-Vegas, F. and Gordon, B. Disseminated anergic cutaneous leishmaniasis. *Br. J. Dermatol.*, 74:132, 1962.
Convit, J., Reyes, O. and Kerdel-Vegas, F. Disseminated anergic American leishmaniasis: Report of three cases of a type clinically resembling lepromatous leprosy. *Arch. Dermatol.*, 76:213, 1957.
Farah, F. and Malak, J. Cutaneous leishmaniasis. *Arch. Dermatol.*, 103:467, 1971.
Girgla, H. et al. Postkala-azar dermal leishmaniasis. *Br. J. Dermatol.*, 97:307, 1977.
Hart, M. et al. Late cutaneous leishmaniasis. *Arch. Dermatol.*, 99:455, 1969.
Kern, F. and Pederson, J. Leishmaniasis in the United States: Report of 10 cases in military personnel. *JAMA*, 226:872, 1973.
Kurban, A. et al. Histopathology of cutaneous leishmaniasis. *Arch. Dermatol.*, 93:396, 1966.
Lagerholm, B., Gip, L. and Lodin, A. The histopathological and cytological diagnosis of cutaneous leishmaniasis in two cases of Leishmania tropica. *Acta Derm. Venereol.*, 48:60, 1968.
Langsjoen, P. Cutaneous leishmaniasis: A report of 10 cases. *Ann. Int. Med.*, 45:623, 1956.
Majumdar, T. Post-kala-azar dermal leishmaniasis. *Dermatol. Internat.* 6:74, 1967.
Manson-Bahr, P. Variations in the clinical manifestations of leishmaniasis caused by *L. tropica. J. Trop. Med. Hyg.*, 67:85, 1964.
Most, H. and Lavietes, P. Kala-azar in American military personnel. *Medicine*, 26:221, 1947.
Nicobis, G. et al. A clinical and histological study of cutaneous leishmaniasis. *Acta Derm. Venereol.* (Stockh.), 58:521, 1978.

Pettit, J. Chronic (lupoid) leishmaniasis. *Br. J. Dermatol.*, 74:127, 1962.
Pham, T. et al. The ultrastructure of Leishmania tropica in the oriental sore. *Ann. Trop. Med. Parasitol.*, 64:1, 1970.
Rau, R., Dubin, H. and Taylor, W. *Leishmania tropica* infections in travellers. *Arch. Dermatol.*, 112:197, 1976.
Sandbank, M. Cutaneous leishmaniasis. Ultrastructural study of three cases. *Arch. Dermatol. Res.*, 257:195, 1976.
Sen Gupta, P. and Bhattacharjee, B. Histopathology of post-kala-azar dermal leishmaniasis. *J. Trop. Med. Hyg.*, 56:110, 1953.
Short, H. Diagnosis of kala-azar. *Trop. Dis. Bull.*, 44:145, 1947.
Simpson, M., Mullins, J. and Stone, O. Disseminated anergic cutaneous leishmaniasis. *Arch. Dermatol.*, 97:301, 1968.
Snow, J., Satulsky, E. and Kean, B. American cutaneous leishmaniasis: Report of twelve cases from the Canal Zone. *Arch. Dermatol. Syph.*, 57:90, 1948.
Walton, B. et al. American cutaneous leishmaniasis. *JAMA*, 228:1256, 1974.
Williams, P. and Coehho, M. de V. Taxonomy and transmission of leishmania. *Adv. Parasitol.*, 16:1, 1979.

Scabies

Berge, T. and Krook, G. Persistent nodules in scabies. *Acta Derm. Venereol.*, 47:20, 1967.
Burkhart, C. Scabies: An epidemiologic reassessment. *Ann. Int. Med.*, 98:498, 1983.
Burks, J., Jr., Jung, R. and George, W. Norwegian scabies. *Arch. Dermatol.*, 74:131, 1956.
Charlesworth, E. and Johnson, J. Epidemic of canine scabies in man. *Arch. Dermatol.*, 110:572, 1974.
Dick, G., Burgdorf, W. and Gentry, W., Jr. Norwegian scabies in Bloom's syndrome. *Arch. Dermatol.*, 115:212, 1979.
Falk, E. and Bolle, R. *In vivo* demonstration of specific immunological hypersensitivity to scabies mite. *Br. J. Dermatol.*, 103:367, 1980.
Falk, E. and Eide, T. Histologic and clinical findings in human scabies. *Internat. J. Dermatol.*, 20:600, 1981.
Fernandez, N., Torres, A. and Ackerman, A. Pathological findings in human scabies. *Arch. Dermatol.*, 113:320, 1977.
Freidman, R. *The Story of Scabies.* New York, Froben Press, 1947.
George, W. Norwegian scabies. *Arch. Dermatol.*, 78:320, 1958.
Haydon, J., Jr. and Caplan, R. Epidemic scabies. *Arch. Dermatol.*, 103:168, 1971.
Hoefling, K. and Schroeter, A. Dermatoimmunopathology of scabies. *J. Am. Acad. Dermatol.*, 3:237, 1980.
Konstantinov, D. and Stanoeva, L. Persistent scabious nodules. *Dermatologica*, 147:321, 1973.
Logan, J., Grant, P. and Keczkes, K. Norwegian scabies and lymphatic leukaemia. *Br. J. Dermatol.*, 79:303, 1967.
Martin, W. and Wheeler, C., Jr. Diagnosis of human scabies by epidermal shave biopsy. *J. Am. Acad. Dermatol.*, 1:335, 1979.
Mellanby, K. The development of symptoms, parasitic infection and immunity in human scabies. *Parasitol.*, 35:197, 1944.
—— *Scabies.* London, Oxford Univ. Press, 1973.
Orkin, M. Resurgence of scabies. *JAMA*, 217:593, 1971.
Orkin, M. and Maibach, H. This scabies pandemic. *N. Eng. J. Med.*, 298:496, 1978.
Orkin, M. et al., eds. *Scabies and Pediculosis.* Philadelphia, JB Lippincott, 1977.
Suzumiya, J. et al. Crusted (Norwegian) scabies with adult T-cell leukemia *Arch. Dermatol.*, 121:903, 1985.
Sweitzer, S. and Winer, L. Norwegian scabies. *Arch. Dermatol. Syph.*, 43:678, 1941.
Thomson, J. et al. Histology simulating reticulosis in persistent nodular scabies. *Br. J. Dermatol.*, 90:421, 1974.

Demodex Folliculorum

Ayres, S., Jr. and Ayres, S., III. Demodectic eruptions (demodicidosis) in the human: 30 years experience with two commonly unrecognized entities: Pityriasis folliculorum (demodex) and acne rosacea (demodex type). *Arch. Dermatol.*, 83:816, 1961.

Ayres, S., Jr. and Mihan, R. Rosacea-like demodicidosis involving the eyelids: A case report. *Arch. Dermatol.*, 95:63, 1967.
Breckenridge, R. Infestation of the skin with *Demodex folliculorum*. *Am. J. Clin. Pathol.*, 23:348, 1953.
Ecker, R. and Winkelmann, R. Demodex Granuloma. *Arch. Dermatol.*, 115:343, 1979.
Grosshans, E., Kremer, M. and Maleville, J. Demodex folliculorum and histogenesis of granulomatous rosacea. *Hautarzt*, 25:166, 1974.
Nutting, W. Hair follicle mites (*Acari demodicidae*) of man. *Internat. J. Dermatol.*, 15:79, 1976.
Riechers, R. and Kopf, A. Cutaneous infestation with *Demodex folliculorum* in man. *J. Invest. Dermatol.*, 52:103, 1969.
Rufli, T. and Murncunagli, Y. The hair follicle mites *Demodex folliculorum* and *Demodex brevis* biology and medical importance. *Dermatologica*, 162:1, 1981.
Spickett, S. Studies on *Demodex folliculorum*. *Parasitol.*, 51:181, 1961.

Pediculosis

Orkin, M. et al., eds., *Scabies and Pediculosis.* Philadelphia, JB Lippincott, 1977.

Chapter 6
Noninfectious Granulomas

In this section some important noninfectious granulomas are discussed. There is no intent to include a comprehensive presentation of noninfectious granulomas in this section.

Certain noninfectious granulomas are presented elsewhere, since they relate to other diseases or categories (e.g., granulomatous folliculitis in acne vulgaris and rosacea, granulomatous panniculitis in erythema nodosum and erythema induratum, and granulomatous reaction to ruptured epidermal cyst).

Noninfectious Granulomas

SARCOIDOSIS

Sarcoidosis is a systemic granulomatous disease of unknown origin which tends to have a benign course. An important feature of sarcoidosis is depressed cellular immunity.

Sarcoidosis has a high incidence in certain ethnic groups, such as American Blacks and Scandinavians.

There is an infrequent transient type and a common chronic type. Features of the subacute transient type of sarcoidosis include fever, hilar adenopathy, erythema nodosum, and iritis. The disease usually ends in a few months. The transient type is usually seen in young persons; the chronic type is usually in persons over 40.

Tissues frequently involved in sarcoidosis include the skin, phalangeal bones, lymph nodes, liver, spleen, kidneys, parotid glands, and eyes.

Cutaneous lesions are varied and include maculopapular lesions, papules (Fig. A), nodules, and plaques (Figs. B,C). The lesions often have a reddish-brown ("apple-jelly") appearance (Figs. A,C). *Lupus pernio* is a cutaneous manifestation characterized by violaceous, boggy plaques, occurring most frequently on the cheeks, ear lobes, and tip of the nose (Fig. D). Annular granulomatous lesions are common. Lesions of sarcoidosis frequently heal by scarring and new lesions may appear in old scars. Rarely, cutaneous lesions of sarcoidosis are atrophic and show ulcerations.

SARCOIDOSIS

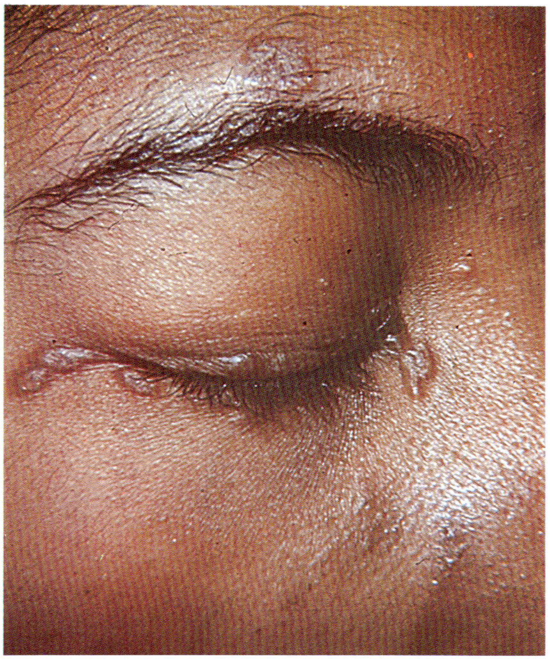

A

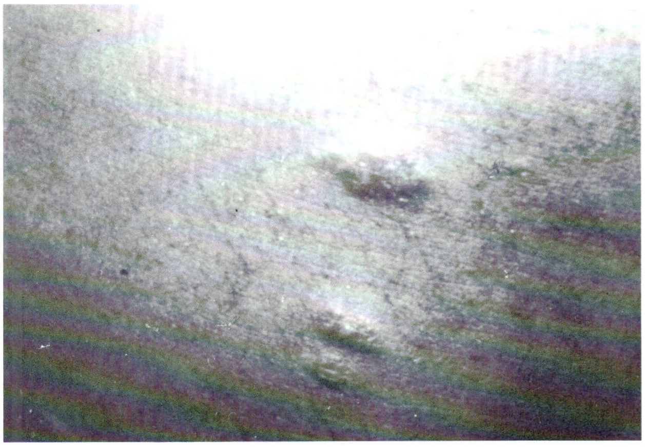

B

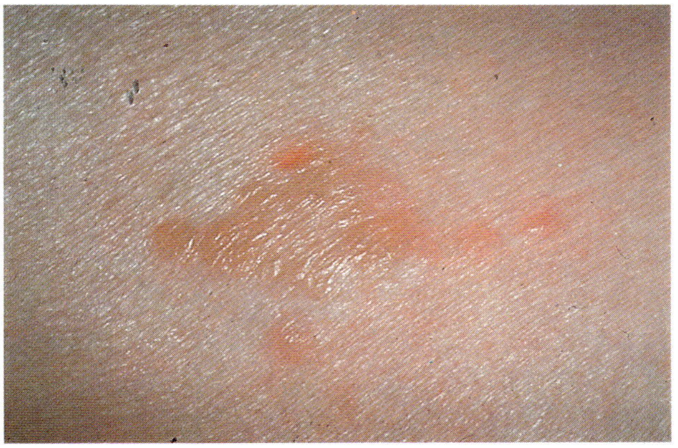

C

Courtesy Dr. Dalal Assaad

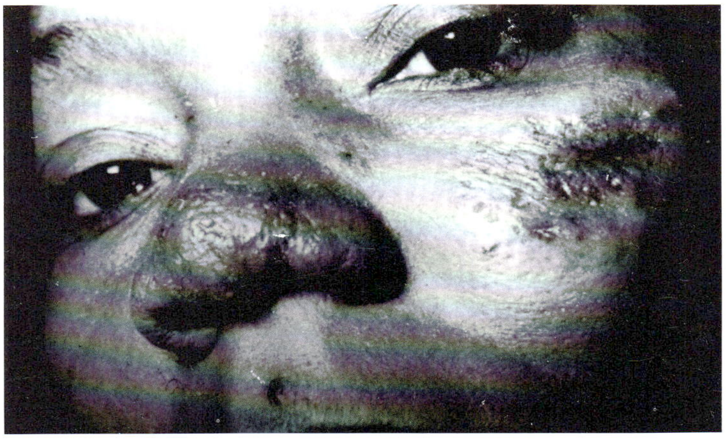

D

SARCOIDOSIS continued ⇨

SARCOIDOSIS

Microscopic features

1. There are many epithelioid tubercles (Figs. A,B) which often occupy the entire dermis and sometimes extend into the subcutaneous fat.
2. The tubercles are called "naked tubercles" since the mononuclear cell infiltrate at the periphery is usually minimal (Figs. A,B,C).
3. In older lesions, irregular, multinucleated giant cells (foreign-body giant cells) are often present (Fig. D). Langhans giant cells are few in number.

SARCOIDOSIS

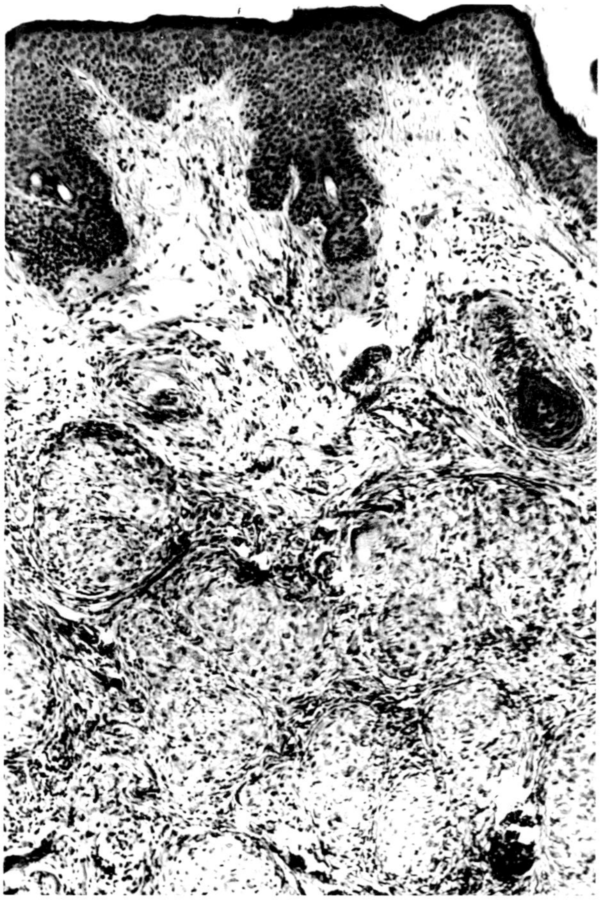

A
X75

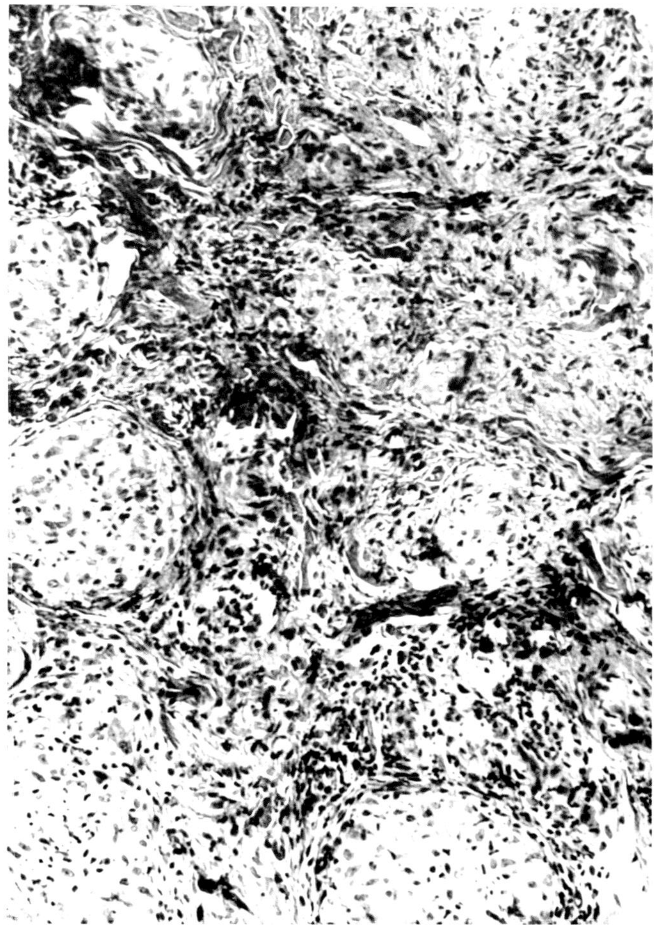

B
X180

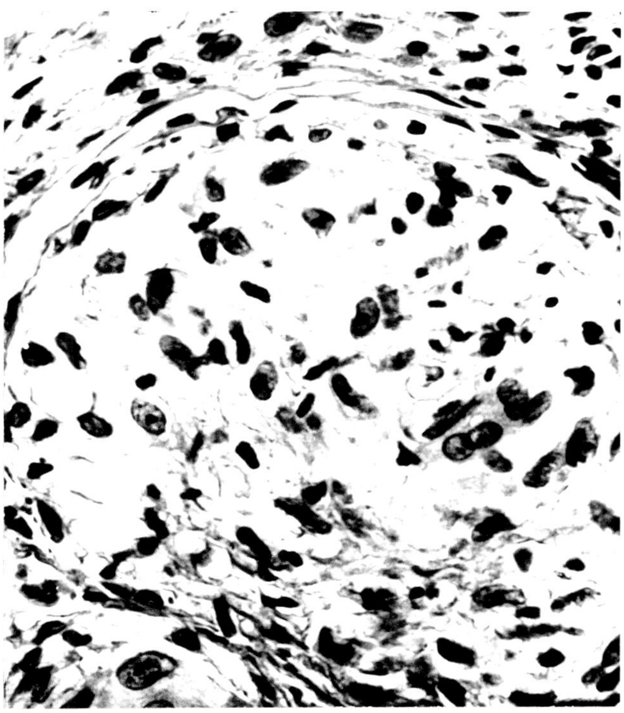

C X530

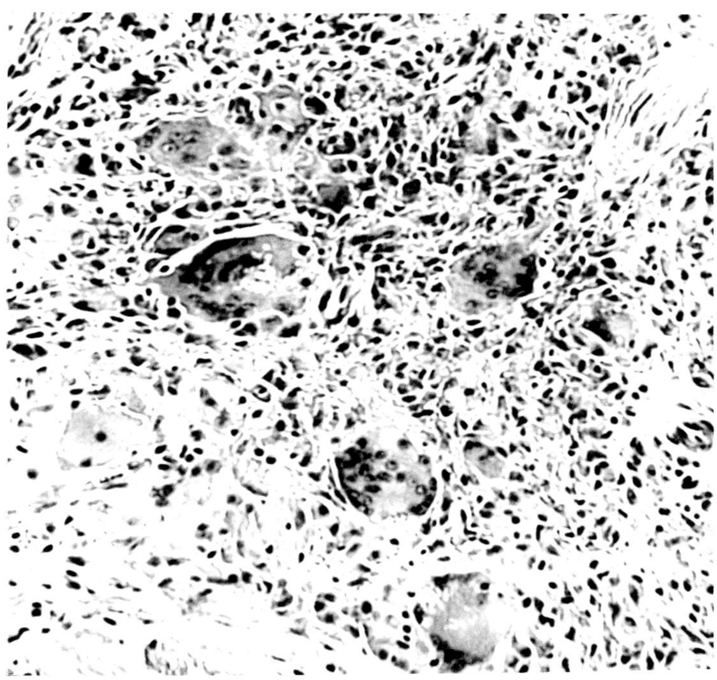

D X250

SARCOIDOSIS continued

SARCOIDOSIS

Microscopic features

4. The giant cells often contain inclusions called *asteroid bodies* (Figs. A,B) and occasionally contain laminated, partially calcified structures called *Schaumann bodies*. (These cellular inclusions are not specific for sarcoidosis.)
5. Occasionally, the mononuclear cell infiltrate around the tubercles can be dense (Fig. C).
6. Caseation necrosis is usually absent, but rarely it is present at the centers of the tubercles (Fig. D).
7. A fine network of reticulum fibers is present around the tubercles.

Microscopic differential diagnosis

1. The histologic pattern of sarcoidosis is not specific. Numerous other conditions can produce a similar histologic picture. "Sarcoidal granuloma" is a generic term used to describe granulomas with naked tubercles and an absence of caseation necrosis. The microscopic picture of sarcoidosis is very similar to that of tuberculoid leprosy, differing principally by the nerve involvement of the latter. Allergic foreign body granulomas (see p. 428) produce a histologic picture similar to that of sarcoidosis, as do anal fissures of Crohn's disease and lesions of cheilitis granulomatosa. Some allergic granulomas can be distinguished histologically from sarcoidosis by the presence of particles that are birefringent with polarized light (e.g., silica granuloma, talc granuloma). Tattoo granulomas can be distinguished by the presence of tattoo pigment.
2. Differentiation from other infectious granulomas is generally dependent on demonstration of the organism and/or immunological studies. Sarcoidosis usually can be distinguished from lupus vulgaris by the following: a) lupus vulgaris usually involves the upper dermis, whereas sarcoidosis usually involves the entire dermis; b) lupus vulgaris, unlike sarcoidosis, usually shows caseation necrosis; c) lupus vulgaris usually has a heavier lymphocytic infiltrate; d) in lupus vulgaris, Langhans giant cells usually predominate.

SARCOIDOSIS

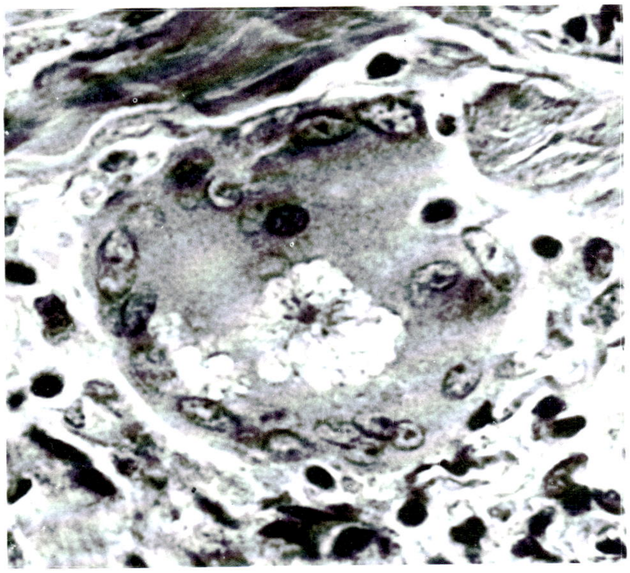

A X810

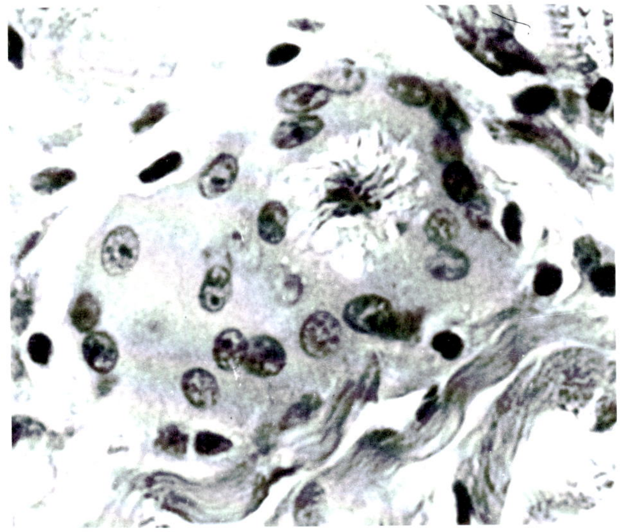

B X810

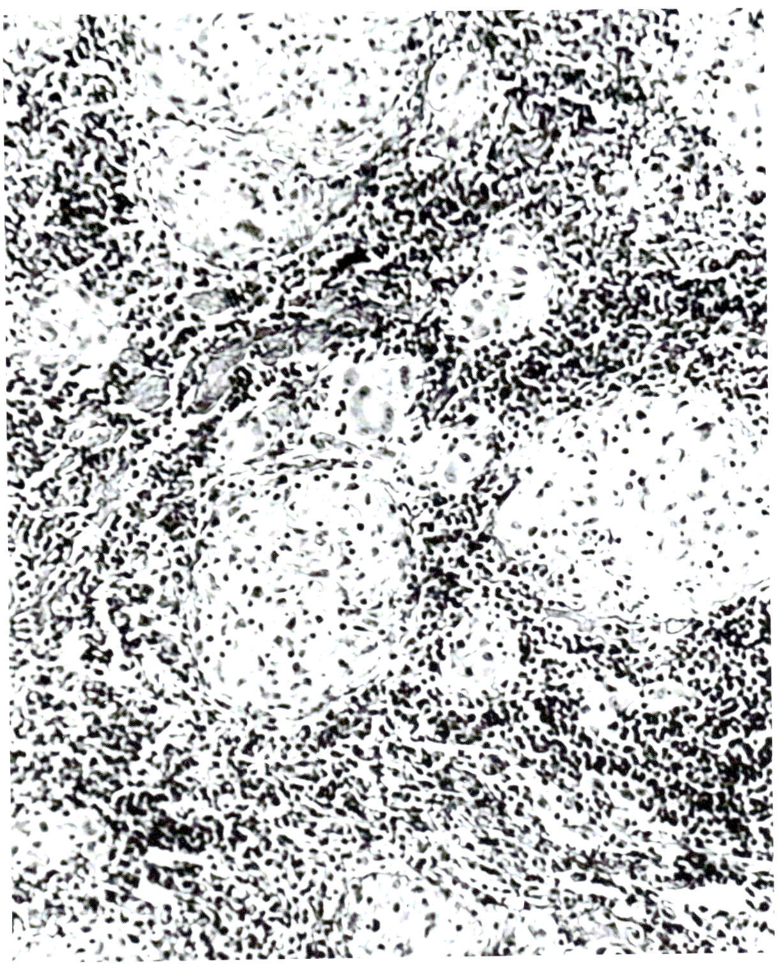

C X210

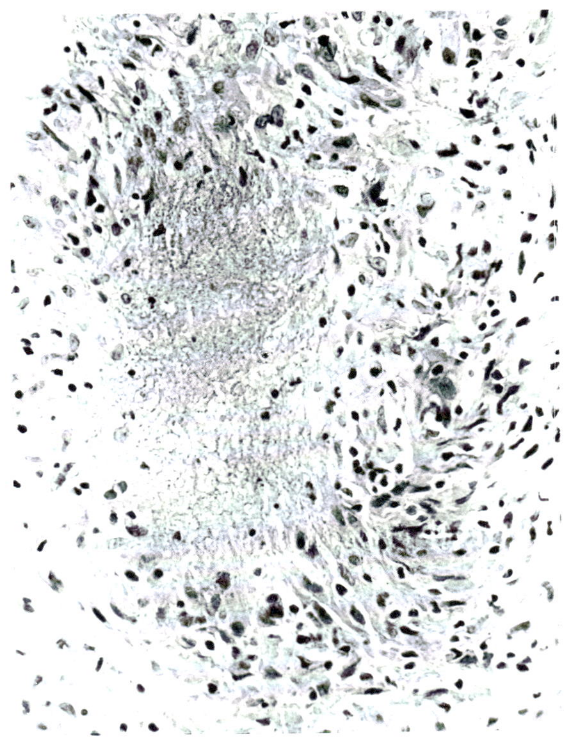

D X200

SARCOIDOSIS continued

SARCOIDOSIS

Comment

1. The Siltzbach-Kveim test consists of an intradermal injection of a preparation of sarcoidal spleen or lymph nodes. A positive reaction is represented by the development in 6 to 8 weeks of a sarcoidal granuloma at the site of the injection. It is positive in 80–90% of the cases.
2. The serum angiotensin converting enzyme reflects enzymatic secretion of epithelioid cells in sarcoidal granulomas and is a helpful test in establishing the diagnosis of sarcoidosis.
3. Asteroid bodies are composed of collagen; Schaumann bodies are residual lysosomal bodies.
4. *Cheilitis granulomatosa* (Miescher-Melkersson-Rosenthal) is characterized by chronic swelling of one or both lips, facial paresis, and occasional swelling of the tongue (scrotal tongue), cheek, eyelids, and forehead. Microscopically, a sarcoidal granuloma is usually present, although the disorder is no longer considered to be a variant of sarcoidosis.
5. Anal fissures are often the presenting feature of Crohn's disease (regional enteritis). Microscopically, subepidermal edema with underlying sarcoidal granulomas are present.

425

NONINFECTIOUS GRANULOMAS continued

LICHEN NITIDUS

Lichen nitidus is a disorder of unknown cause characterized by asymptomatic, small, flat polygonal papules (Fig. A). Lesions vary greatly in number and sometimes are confluent. The penis and flexor surfaces of the forearms are frequently involved.

Microscopic features

1. A focal infiltrate is present just beneath the epidermis in a greatly broadened dermal papilla bordered by elongated rete ridges (Fig. B).
2. The infiltrate is composed of a mixture of lymphocytes, histiocytes, and epithelioid cells (Figs. B,C), with an occasional Langhans giant cell.
3. The overlying epidermis is generally thin (Fig. B), but is sometimes hyperkeratotic or parakeratotic. Hydropic degeneration of basal cells is present and may lead to cleft formation (Fig. B). The thinned epidermis may erode, with possible transepidermal perforation and migration of the infiltrate through the thinned epidermis.

Comment

Older views that lichen nitidus is a tuberculid are no longer held. Some believe that lichen nitidus may represent a variant of lichen planus.

LICHEN NITIDUS

A

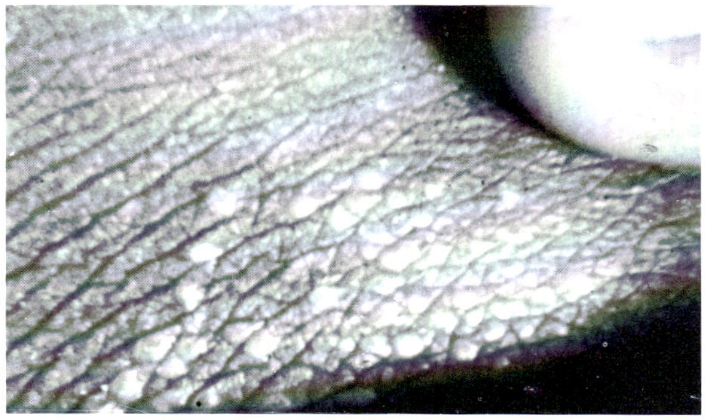

B
X210

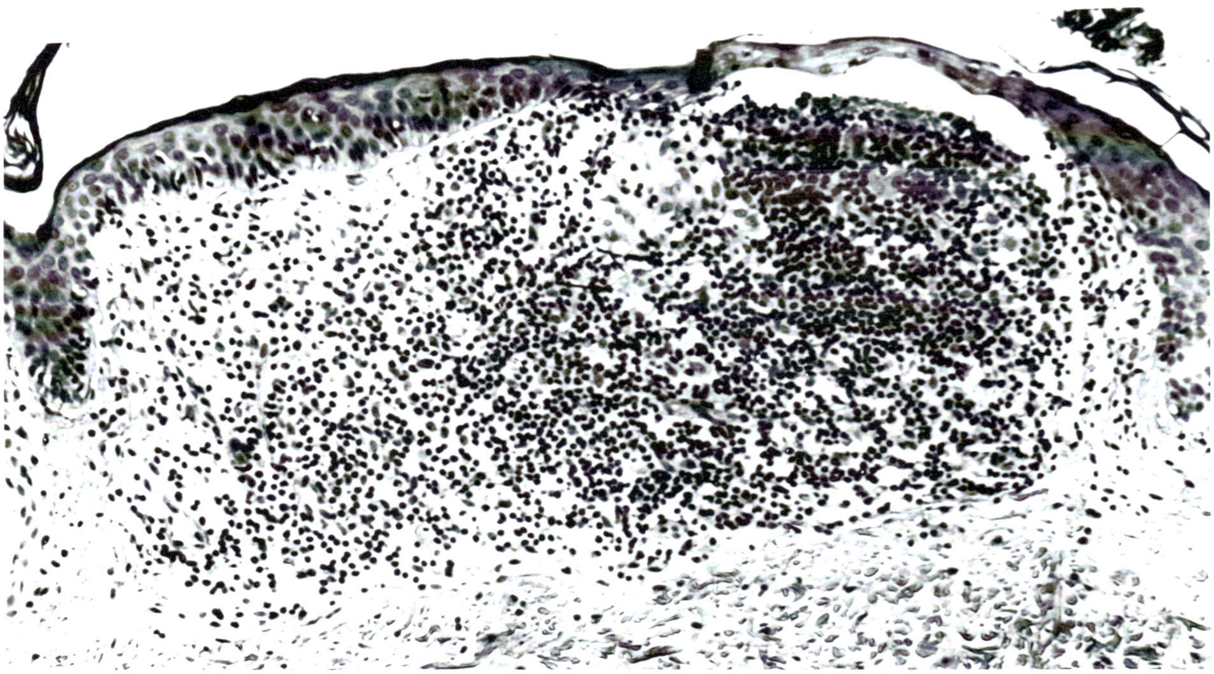

C
X520

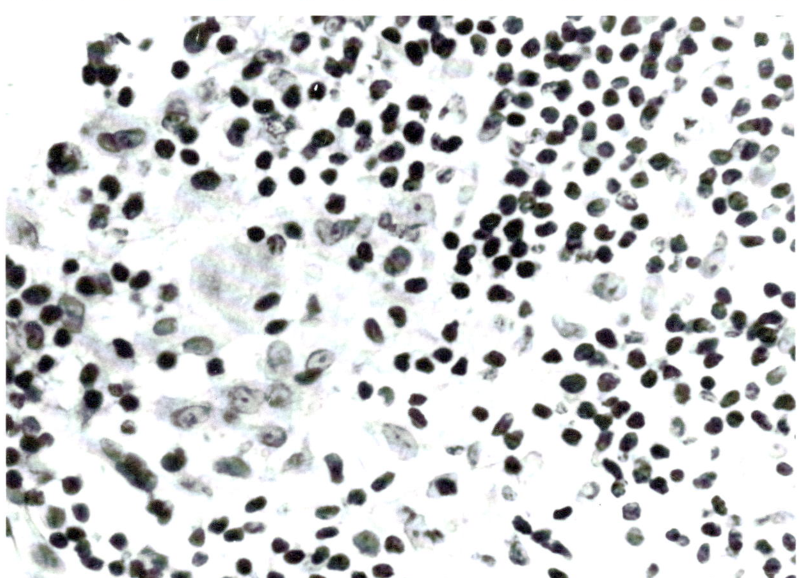

FOREIGN BODY GRANULOMAS

Foreign body granulomas are dermal reactions to exogenous substances. These substances are usually particulate. Materials exogenous to the dermis include those produced within the body (e.g., keratin in folliculitis and ruptured epidermal cyst [See pp. 856]) and those produced outside the body (e.g., sand, wood, talc, insect parts, tattoo pigment, sutures, zirconium, beryllium).

Foreign body granulomas can be allergic or nonallergic. Nonallergic foreign body granulomas generally show a random mixture of inflammatory cells, including foreign body giant cells and sometimes epithelioid cells. Allergic granulomas are characterized by epithelioid tubercles (with or without foreign body giant cells) and varying degrees of caseation necrosis. Allergic foreign body granulomas may be of the sarcoidal type.

Allergic granulomas

Silica (from soil or sand) produces sarcoidal granulomas showing birefringent particles with polariscopic examination. Fig. A (arrow) and Fig. D show respectively a clinical photograph of a silica granuloma and a photomicrograph of a silica granuloma examined with polarized light. Barium from golf balls can produce allergic granulomas with particles that are birefringent with polarized light.

Beryllium (from old type fluorescent light bulbs) and zirconium (in proprietary topical preparations) can produce a sarcoidal granuloma without particles visible with brightfield or polariscopic microscopy. Beryllium granulomas from direct implantation of the substance in the skin can show a significant degree of caseation necrosis; hematogenously disseminated beryllium usually produces no significant caseation necrosis in skin lesions. Figs. B,C show clinical and microscopic photographs of a zirconium granuloma. Tattoos may show epithelioid tubercles with or without caseation necrosis; the coarse pigment granules, visible with brightfield microscopy, usually allow the diagnosis to be made easily. Tattoos may produce an allergic dermatitis; this can be sufficiently intense to result in a patchy infiltrate resembling lymphoma (see p. 1296). Tattoos ordinarily show no inflammatory reaction. The coarse pigment granules are free in the dermis and in macrophages (Fig. E).

ALLERGIC FOREIGN BODY GRANULOMAS

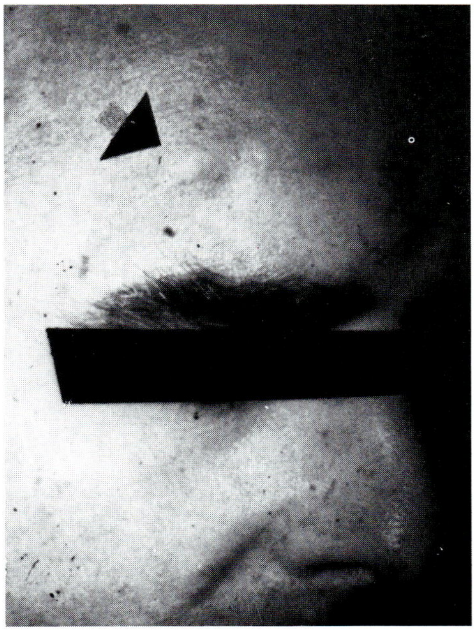
A

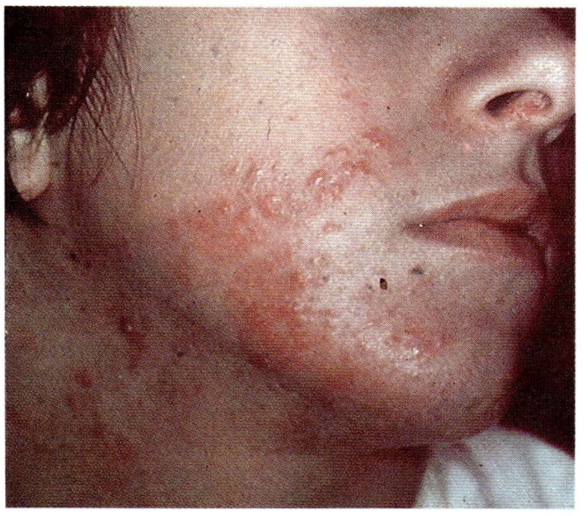
B

Courtesy Dr. Robert Baler

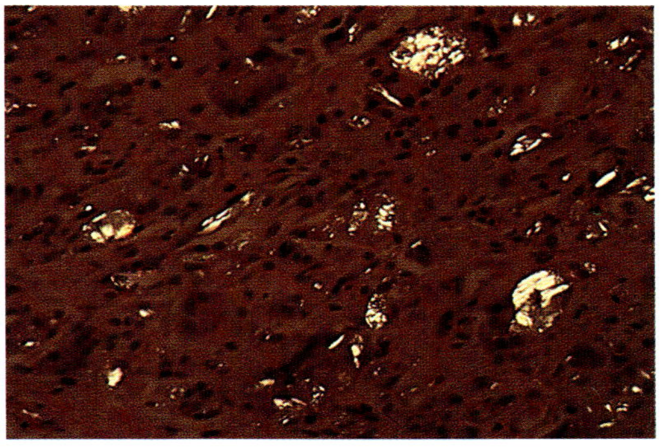
D
X100

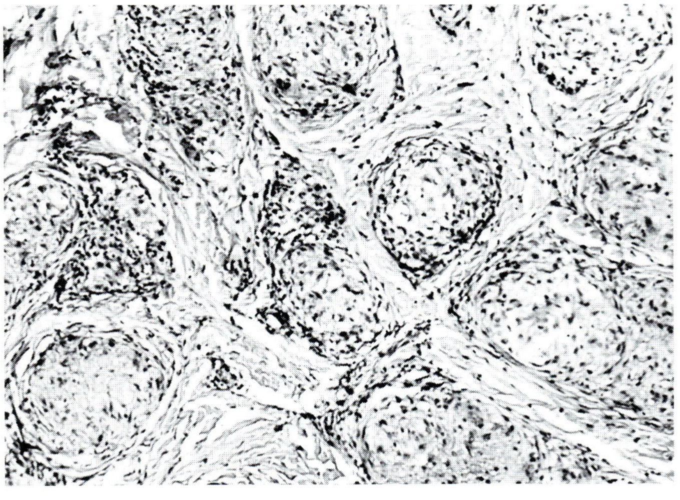
C
X125

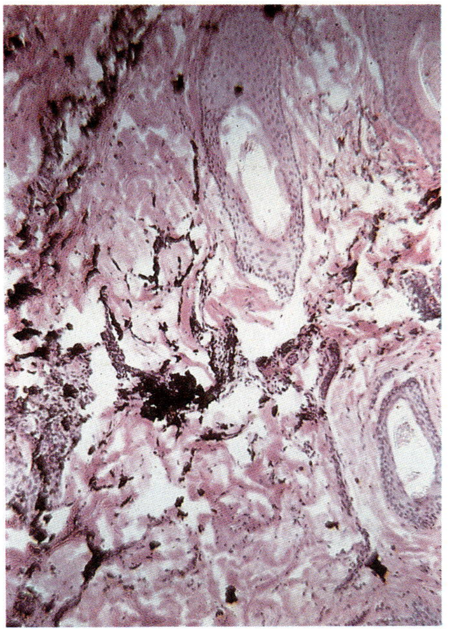
E
X100

FOREIGN BODY GRANULOMAS continued

FOREIGN BODY GRANULOMAS

Nonallergic granulomas

They show a mixture of inflammatory cells, including macrophages and sometimes epithelioid cells, in random arrangement.

Talc granuloma, starch granuloma, and suture granuloma show foreign material that is birefringent with polarized light. The material is largely within macrophages and giant cells. Figs. A, B, and C show photomicrographs of a suture granuloma, seen with brightfield and polariscopic examination. In starch granuloma the ovoid basophilic starch granules show birefringence with polarized light and stain with PAS and methenamine silver stains.

In wood granuloma (e.g., splinter) abscesses surrounded by a granulomatous infiltrate and fibrosis may be present (Fig. D). The wood can be identified by the regular lattice of cellulose cell walls (Figs. D,E). Wood is birefringent with polarized light (Fig. F).

The generic term *paraffinoma* refers to nonallergic granulomas due to oily substances, such as mineral oil, vegetable oils, and silicone gel (which contain vegetable oil and fatty acids, in addition to silicone). The histologic picture in routine sections is characterized by numerous vacuoles, representing spaces formerly occupied by the oily substance (Fig. G). There is a surrounding cellular infiltrate containing many histiocytes and foam cells; fibrosis may be present. The oily substance stains with physicochemical fat stains (e.g., Sudan red) in frozen sections. If the fat is of organic origin, it will also stain with osmic acid or bromide silver stain.

Cholesterol crystals are often seen in granulomas caused by ruptured cysts. In routine sections the crystals are represented by needle-like spaces (Fig. H).

Comment

Interdigital pilonidal sinus results from implantation of hair into the interdigital webs. It has been observed in barbers and dog groomers. There are small tender openings in the webs. Microscopically, the sinus resembles the upper part of a hair follicle and contains hairs. At the deep end of the tract there may be rupture with foreign body granuloma.

NONALLERGIC FOREIGN BODY GRANULOMAS

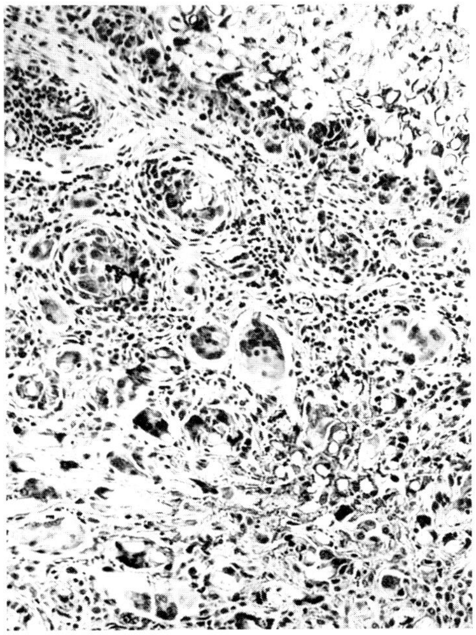

A X120

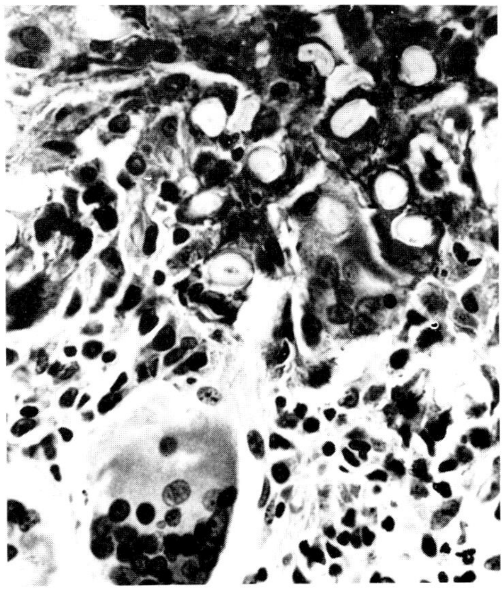

B X340

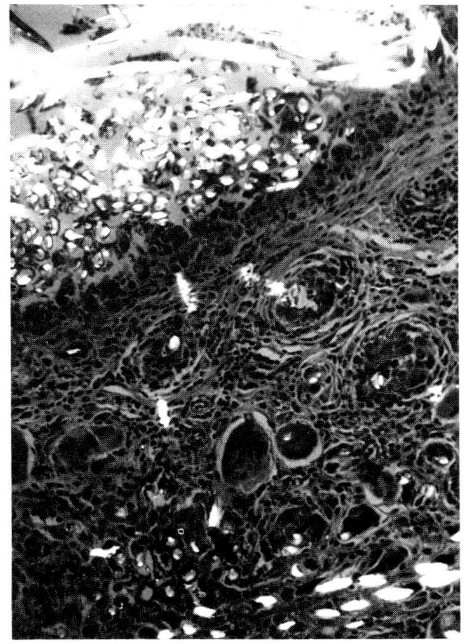

C X120

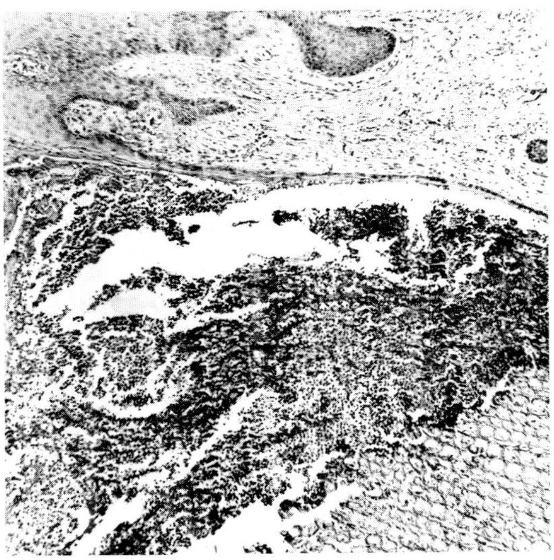

D X80

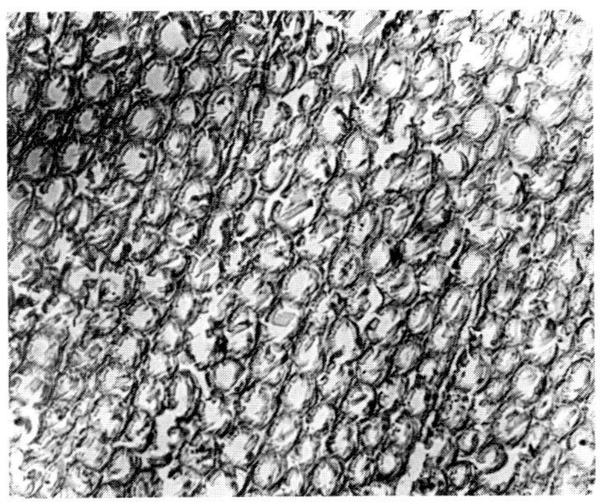

E
X160

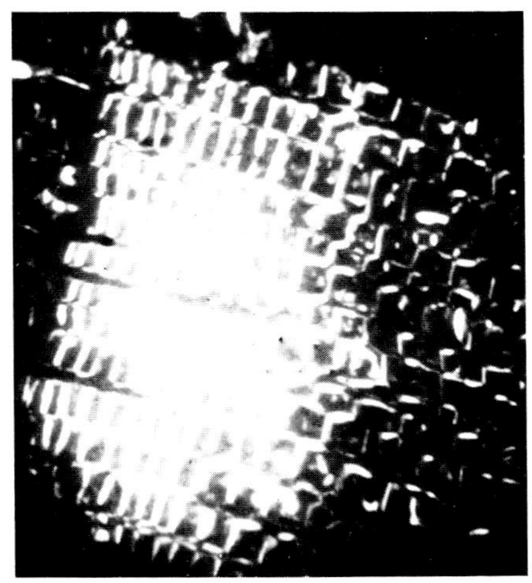

F X160

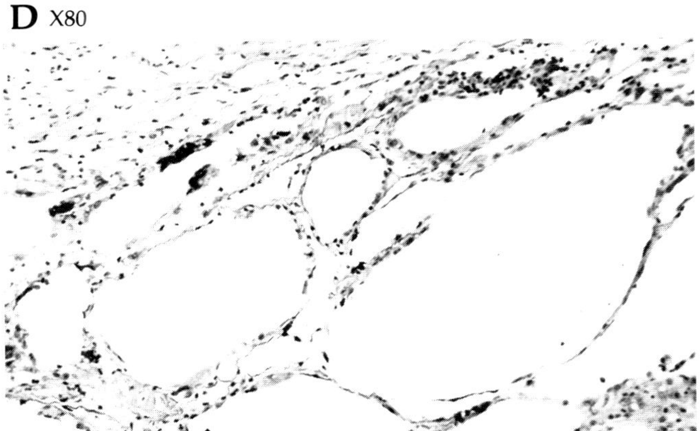

G
X125

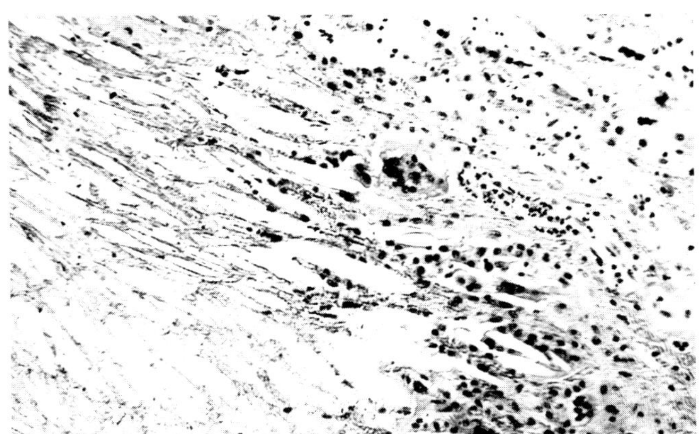

H X110

Suggested Reading

Noninfectious Granulomas

Sarcoidosis

Atwood, W. and Nelson, C. Sarcoidosis. *Med. Clin. N. Am.*, 49:783, 1965.

Azar, H. and Lunardelli, C. Collagen nature of asteroid bodies of giant cells in sarcoidosis. *Am. J. Pathol.*, 57:81, 1969.

Barrie, H. and Bogoch, A. The natural history of the sarcoid granuloma. *Am. J. Pathol.*, 29:451, 1953.

Bjerke, J., Krogh, H. and Matre, R. *In situ* identification of mononuclear cells in cutaneous infiltrates in discoid lupus erythematosus, sarcoidosis and secondary syphilis. *Acta Derm. Venereol.* (Stockh.), 61:371, 1981.

Borda, J. Sarcoidosis. *Arch. Argent. Dermatol.*, 9:261, 1959.

Bornstein, J., Frank, M. and Radner, D. Conjunctival biopsy in the diagnosis of sarcoidosis. *N. Eng. J. Med.*, 267:60, 1962.

Chevrant-Breton, J. et al. Sarcoidose à manifestations cutanées extensives ulcéreuses et atrophiantes. *Ann. Dermatol. Venereol.*, 104:805, 1977.

Clayton, R. et al. Hypopigmented sarcoidosis in the Negro. *Br. J. Dermatol.*, 96:119, 1977.

Crystal, R. et al. Pulmonary sarcoidosis: A disease characterised and perpetuated by activated lung T-lymphocytes. *Ann. Int. Med.*, 94:73, 1981.

Drury, R. Problems in histological interpretation in sarcoidosis. *Postgrad. Med. J.*, 46:478, 1970.

Elgart, M. Skin manifestations of sarcoidosis. *Cutis*, 1:283, 1965.

Gross, M. et al. Nodular subcutaneous sarcoidosis. *Arch. Dermatol.*, 113:1442, 1977.

Hanno, R. et al. Cutaneous sarcoidal granulomas and the development of systemic sarcoidosis. *Arch. Dermatol.*, 117:203, 1981.

Hruza, G. and Kerdel, F. Generalized atrophic sarcoidosis with ulcerations. *Arch. Dermatol.*, 122:320, 1986.

Irgang, S. Sarcoidosis in the Negro. *Cutis*, 5:823, 1969.

Israel, H. The diagnosis of sarcoidosis. *Ann. Int. Med.*, 68:1323, 1968.

Israel, H. and Ostrow, A. Sarcoidosis and aspergillosis. *Am. J. Med.*, 47:243, 1967.

Israel, H. and Sones, M. Selection of biopsy procedures for diagnosis of sarcoidosis. *Arch. Int. Med.*, 113:255, 1964.

Jacques, W. Relationship of asteroid bodies to lipids. *Arch. Pathol.*, 56:68, 1953.

James, D. Dermatological aspects of sarcoidosis. *Quart. J. Med.*, 28:109, 1959.

James, D. and Jones, W. Immunology of sarcoidosis. *Am. J. Med.*, 72:5, 1982.

——. *Sarcoidosis and Other Granulomatous Disorders*. Philadelphia, W. B. Saunders, 1985.

Jasper, P. and Denny, F. Sarcoidosis in Children. *J. Pediatr.*, 73:499, 1968.

Kantor, F., Dwyer, J. and Mangi, R. Sarcoid. *J. Invest. Dermatol.*, 67:470, 1976.

Kauh, Y., Goody, H. and Luscombe, H. Ichthyosiform sarcoidosis. *Arch. Dermatol.*, 114:100, 1978.

Kelly, A. Ichthyosiform sarcoid. *Arch. Dermatol.*, 114:1551, 1978.

Lever, W. and Freiman, D. Sarcoidosis: A Report of an atypical case with erythrodermic lesions, subcutaneous nodes and asteroid inclusion bodies in giant cells. *Arch. Dermatol. Syph.*, 57:639, 1948.

Longcope, W. and Freiman, D. A study of sarcoidosis: Based on a combined investigation of 160 cases including 30 autopsies from the Johns Hopkins Hospital and Massachusetts General Hospital. *Medicine*, 31:1, 1952.

McCoy, R. and Fisher, C. Glomerulonephritis associated with sarcoidosis. *Am. J. Pathol.*, 68:339, 1972.

Mandel, W. *Bibliography on Sarcoidosis (1878–1963)*, Washington, D.C., Pub. #1213, U.S.P.H.S., 1964.

Mankiewicz, E. On the etiology of sarcoidosis. *Canad. Med. Assoc. J.*, 88:593, 1963.

Marten, R. and Warner, J. Subcutaneous nodular sarcoid. *Trans. St. John's Hosp. Dermatol. Soc.*, 53:160, 1967.

Mayock, R. et al. Manifestations of sarcoidosis: Analysis of 145 patients, with a review of nine series selected from the literature. *Am. J. Med.*, 35:67, 1963.

Michelson, H. Uveoparotitis: A sarcoid reaction. *Arch. Dermatol. Syph.*, 39:329, 1939.
Morrison, J. Sarcoidosis in a child, presenting as an erythroderma with keratotic spines and palmar pits. *Br. J. Dermatol.*, 95:93, 1976.
Nozaki, T. Sarcoidosis with lichenoid type eruption. *Jpn. J. Dermatol.*, 82:47, 1972.
Ramasoota, T., Johnson, W. and Graham, J. Cutaneous sarcoidosis and tuberculoid leprosy: A comparative hisopathologic and histochemical study. *Arch. Dermatol.*, 96:259, 1967.
Roberts, W., McAllister, H., Jr., and Ferrans, V. Sarcoidosis of the heart. *Am. J. Med.*, 63:86, 1977.
Ronchese, F. Sarcoid and tuberculosis: Report of a case with autopsy. *Arch. Dermatol. Syph.*, 46:860, 1942.
Scadding, J. *Sarcoidosis*. London, Eyre & Spottiswoode, 1967.
Schaumann, J. On the nature of certain peculiar corpuscles present in the tissue of lymphogranulomatosis benigna. *Acta Med. Scand.*, 106:239, 1941.
Semanzato, G. and Pezzutto, A. Insights into the immunopathogenesis of sarcoidosis. *Immunol. Clin. Sper.*, 1:35, 1982.
Sharma, O. *Sarcoidosis: A Clinical Approach*. Springfield, IL, Thomas, 1975.
Siltzbach, L., ed. Seventh International Conference on Sarcoidosis and Other Granulomatous Diseases. *Ann. N.Y. Acad. Sci.*, 278:1, 1976.
Terzakis, J., Shustak, S. and Stock, E. Talc granuloma identified by x-ray microanalysis. *JAMA*, 239:2371, 1978.
Umbert, P. and Winkelmann, R. Granuloma annulare and sarcoidosis. *Br. J. Dermatol.*, 97:481, 1977.
Vainsencher, D. and Winkelmann, R. Subcutaneous sarcoidosis. *Arch. Dermatol.*, 120:1028, 1984.

Lichen Nitidus

Barber, H. Lichen nitidus. *Br. J. Dermatol.*, 38:143, 1926.
Bardach, H. Perforating lichen nitidus. *J. Cutan. Pathol.*, 8:111, 1981.
Ellis, F. and Hill, W. Is lichen nitidus a variety of lichen planus? *Arch. Dermatol. Syph.*, 38:569, 1938.
Krook, G. Purpura in lichen nitidus generalisatus: Report of a case. *Arch. Derm. Venereol.*, 39:238, 1959.
Lapins, N. et al. Lichen nitidus: A study of forty-three cases. *Cutis*, 21:633, 1978.
Pinkus, H. and Shair, H. Koebner phenomenon in lichen nitidus: Report of two cases. *Arch. Dermatol. Syph.*, 65:82, 1952.
Schuhmachers, R. Lichen nitidus of unusual location. *Hautarzt*, 13:521, 1962.
Tappeiner, S. Zur Stellung des Lichen nitidus im System der Hautkrankheiten. *Dermatologica*, 107:1, 1953.
Trimble, W. and Maloney, E. Lichen nitidus: With a report of two cases. *Arch. Dermatol. Syph.*, 7:452, 1923.
Weiss, R. and Cohen, A. Lichen nitidus of the palms and soles. *Arch. Dermatol.*, 104:538, 1971.
Wilson, H. and Bett, D. Miliary lesions in lichen planus. *Arch. Dermatol.*, 83:920, 1961.

Foreign Body and Other Noninfectious Granulomas

Adams, D. The biology of the granuloma. In: *Pathology of Granulomas*. Ioachim, H., ed., New York, Raven Press, 1983, p. 1.
Arzt, L. Foreign body granulomas and Boeck's sarcoid. *J. Invest. Dermatol.*, 24:155, 1955.
Baler, G. Granulomas from topical zirconium in poison ivy dermatitis. *Arch. Dermatol.*, 91:145, 1965.
Best, W. et al. Sclerosing lipogranuloma of the male genitalia produced by mineral oil. *Proc. Mayo Clin.*, 28:623, 1953.
Björnberg, A. Allergic reaction to cobalt in light blue tattoo markings. *Acta Derm. Venereol.*, 41:259, 1961.
Boros, D. Granulomatous inflammations. *Prog. Allergy*, 24:184, 1978.
Conrad, A., Conrad, A., Jr. and Weiss, R. Sesame oil tumors. *JAMA*, 121:237, 1943.
Danbolt, N. Kveim's reaction and its significance in sarcoidosis research. *Acta Derm. Venereol.*, 42:354, 1962.

Dettinger, G. and Bowers, W. Tissue response to orlon and dacron sutures: A comparison with nylon, cotton, and silk. *Surgery*, 42:325, 1957.
Dickinson, J. Sarcoidal reactions in tattoos. *Arch. Dermatol.*, 100:315, 1969.
Dutra, F. Beryllium granulomas of the skin. *Arch. Dermatol. Syph.*, 60:1140, 1949.
Epstein, E. Silica granuloma of the skin. *Arch. Dermatol.*, 71:24, 1955.
Epstein, W. Foreign body granulomas. In: *Basic and Clinical Aspects of Granulomatous Diseases*. Boros, D. and Yoshida, T., eds., New York, Elsevier, 1980, p. 181.
——. Granuloma formation in man. *Pathobiol. Ann.*, 7:1, 1977.
——. Granulomatous inflammation in skin. In: *Pathology of Granulomas*. Ioachim, H., ed., New York, Raven Press, 1983, p. 21.
Epstein, W. and Allen, J. Granulomatous hypersensitivity after use of zirconium-containing poison oak lotions. *JAMA*, 190:940, 1964.
Epstein, W., Skahen, J. and Krasnobrod, H. Granulomatous hypersensitivity to zirconium: Localization of allergen in tissue and its role in formation of epithelioid cells. *J. Invest. Dermatol.*, 38:223, 1962.
——. The organized epithelioid cell granuloma: Differentiation of allergic (zirconium) from colloidal (silica) types. *Am. J. Pathol.*, 43:391, 1963.
Goldstein, N., ed. Special Issue on Tattoos. *J. Dermatol. Surg. Oncol.*, 5:848, 1979.
Grier, R., Nash, P. and Freiman, D. Skin lesions in persons exposed to beryllium compounds. *J. Ind. Hyg. Toxicol.*, 30:228, 1948.
Harrison, J., Swanson, O. and Lincoln, A. A comparison of the tissue reactions to plastic materials. *Arch. Surg.*, 74:139, 1957.
Ishii, Y. et al. Barium granuloma. *J. Dermatol.*, (Tokyo), 9:153, 1982.
Karkinen-Jaaskelainen, M. et al. Pulmonary berylliosis: Report on a fatal case. *Br. J. Dis. Chest*, 76:290, 1982.
Kasdom, E., Jones, G. and Schlossman, S. Experimental intradermal granuloma formation. *J. Invest. Dermatol.*, 63:411, 1974.
Klaus, S. and Brunsting, L. Melkersson's syndrome (persistent swelling of the face, recurrent facial paralysis and lingua plicata): Report of a case. *Proc. Mayo Clin.*, 34:365, 1959.
Kraissl, C., Kesten, B. and Cimiotti, J. The relation of catgut sensitivity to wound healing. *Surg. Gynecol. and Obst.*, 66:628, 1938.
Krutchkoff, D. and James, R. Cheilitis granulomatosa. *Arch. Dermatol.*, 114:1203, 1978.
Kuchemann, K. and Holm, R. Unusual silica granulomas of the skin with massive involvement of axillary lymph nodes. *Pathol. Res. Pract.*, 164:198, 1979.
Laymon, C. Cheilitis granulomatosa and Melkersson-Rosenthal syndrome. *Arch. Dermatol.*, 83:112, 1963.
Leonard, D. Starch granulomas. *Arch. Dermatol.*, 107:101, 1973.
Loewenthal, L. Reactions in green tattoos: The significance of the valence state of chromium. *Arch. Dermatol.*, 82:237, 1960.
LoPresti, P. and Hambrick, G., Jr. Zirconium granuloma following treatment of Rhus dermatitis. *Arch. Dermatol.*, 92:188, 1965.
McAdams, G. Granulomata caused by absorbable starch glove powder. *Surgery*, 39:329, 1956.
McCallum, D. and Kinmount, P. Dermatological manifestations of Crohn's disease. *Br. J. Dermatol.*, 80:1, 1968.
Madden, J. Reactions to tattoos. *Arch. Dermatol. Syph.*, 40:256, 1939.
Mason, J. and Apisarnthanarax. Migratory silicone granuloma. *Arch. Dermatol.*, 117:366, 1981.
Miescher, G. Essential granulomatous cheilitis. *Dermatologica*, 91:57, 1945.
Neave, H., Frank, S. and Tolmach, J. Cutaneous granuloma following laceration by fluorescent light bulbs. *Arch. Dermatol. Syph.*, 61:401, 1950.
Newcomer, V. et al. Sclerosing lipogranuloma resulting from exogenous lipids. *Arch. Dermatol.*, 73:361, 1956.
Oertel, V. and Johnson, F. Sclerosing lipogranuloma of male genitalia. *Arch. Pathol.*, 101:321, 1977.
Paslin, D., Heaton, C. and Wood, M. Scar biopsy in sarcoidosis. *Dermatologica*, 146:315, 1973.
Postlethwait, R. et al. Wound healing. II. An evaluation of surgical suture material. *Surg. Gynecol. Obst.*, 107:481, 1959.
Radke, H., Nyhus, L. and Bell, J. Starch granuloma: The problems of surgical glove powder. *N.W. Med.*, 60:283, 1961.
Rees, H. Sclerosing lipogranuloma. *Arch. Dermatol.*, 89:277, 1964.
Rhodes, E. and Stirling, G. Granulomatous cheilitis. *Arch. Dermatol.*, 92:40, 1965.
Rostenberg, A., Jr., Brown, R. and Caro, M. Discussion of tattoo reactions with report of a case showing a reaction to a green color. *Arch. Dermatol. Syph.*, 62:540, 1950.

Rubin, L. et al. Granulomas of the axillas caused by deodorants. *JAMA*, 162:953, 1956.
Rupec, M., Treeck, W. and Braun-Falco, O. Zum Paraffingranulom: Eine klinische, histologische und histochemische Studie. *Dermatol. Wochenschr.*, 151:129, 1965.
Shelley, W. and Hurley, H. The allergic origin of zirconium deodorant granulomas. *Br. J. Dermatol.*, 70:75, 1958.
——. The pathogenesis of silica granulomas in man: A non-allergic colloidal phenomenon. *J. Invest. Dermatol.*, 34:107, 1960.
Siltzbach, L. The Kveim test in sarcoidosis: A study of 750 patients. *JAMA*, 178:476, 1961.
Sneddon, I. Berylliosis: A case report. *Br. Med. J.*, 1:1448, 1955.
Sommerville, J. and Milne, J. Pseudo-tuberculoma silicoticum: A form of cutaneous "sarcoid." *Br. J. Dermatol.*, 62:105, 1950.
Steigleder, G., Silva, A., Jr. and Nelson, C. Histopathology of the Kveim test. *Arch. Dermatol.*, 84:828, 1961.
Uber, C. and McReynolds, R. Immunotoxicity of silica. *CRC Crit. Rev. Toxicol.*, 10:303, 1982.
Urbach, F. et al. Generalized paraffinoma (sclerosing lipogranuloma). *Arch. Dermatol.*, 103:277, 1971.
Westermark, P. and Henriksson, T. Granulomatous inflammation of the vulva and penis: A genital counterpart to cheilitis granulomatosa. *Dermatologica*, 158:269, 1979.
White, I., Souteryrand, P. and MacDonald, D. Granulomatous cheilitis. (Miescher). *Clin. Exp. Dermatol.*, 6:391, 1981.
Williams, R. and Skipworth, G. Zirconium granulomas of the glabrous skin following treatment of Rhus dermatitis: Report of two cases. *Arch. Dermatol.*, 80:273, 1959.
Winer, L. et al. Tissue reactions to injected silicone liquids: A report of three cases. *Arch. Dermatol.*, 90:588, 1964.
Winkelmann, R. and Harris, R. Lichenoid delayed hypersensitivity reactions in tattoos. *J. Cutan. Pathol.*, 6:59, 1979.

Chapter 7
Idiopathic Papulosquamous Diseases:

Lichen Planus, Psoriasis, and Pityriasis Rubra Pilaris

These are disorders characterized by scaling papules. Other conditions, including secondary syphilis (p. 298), pityriasis rosea (p. 92), tinea corporis (p. 338), and some drug reactions also may have lesions of this type. In this chapter, idiopathic papulosquamous disorders with more or less distinctive histologic features are discussed.

LICHEN PLANUS

Lichen planus is a disorder of unknown cause. An immune mechanism has been postulated. It is characterized by flat, polygonal papules, with violaceous color, fine scale, and surface striations (Wickham's striae) (Figs. A,B). Lesions often have a linear arrangement (Koebner phenomenon) (Figs. A,B). Pruritus is generally intense. Flexor surfaces of the extremities, particularly the wrists, are frequently involved (Fig. B). Lichen planus may involve hair follicles and mucous membranes. There may be involvement of the nails, with distortion of the nail plate. Involvement of the pharynx, esophagus, gastric mucosa, or anus has been reported. Variants include hypertrophic lichen planus, annular lichen planus, bullous lichen planus, and ulcerative lichen planus.

Microscopic features

1. With the scanning lens, hyperkeratosis and irregular ("saw-tooth") acanthosis are evident, as is the band-like infiltrate impinging on the epidermis (Fig. C).
2. In some cases the band-like infiltrate is separated from the epidermis by a rather edematous zone containing scattered inflammatory cells (Fig. D).

LICHEN PLANUS

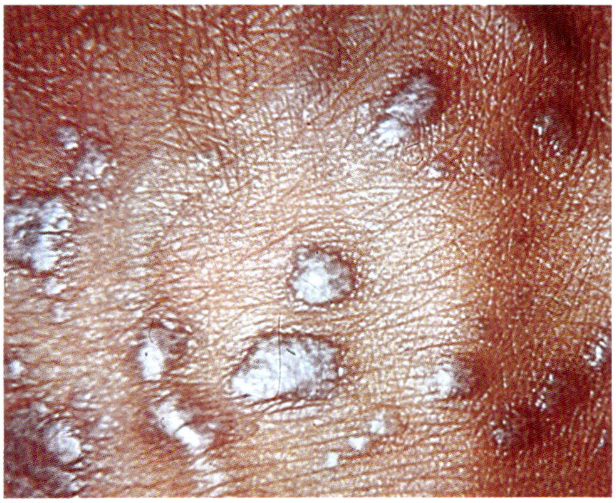

A

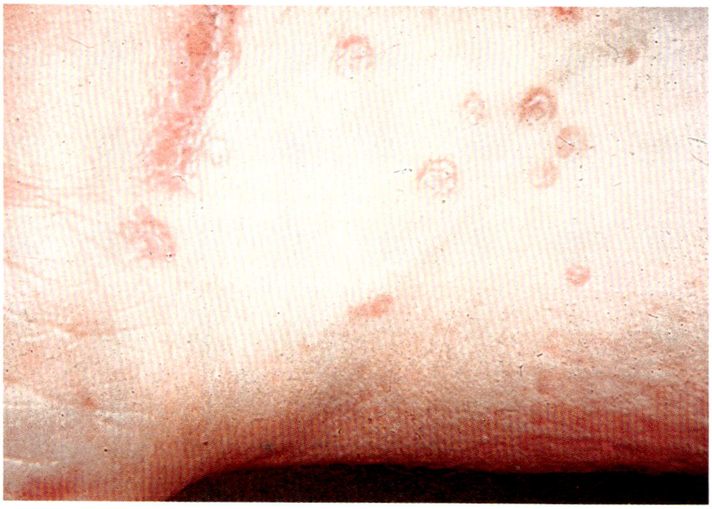

B

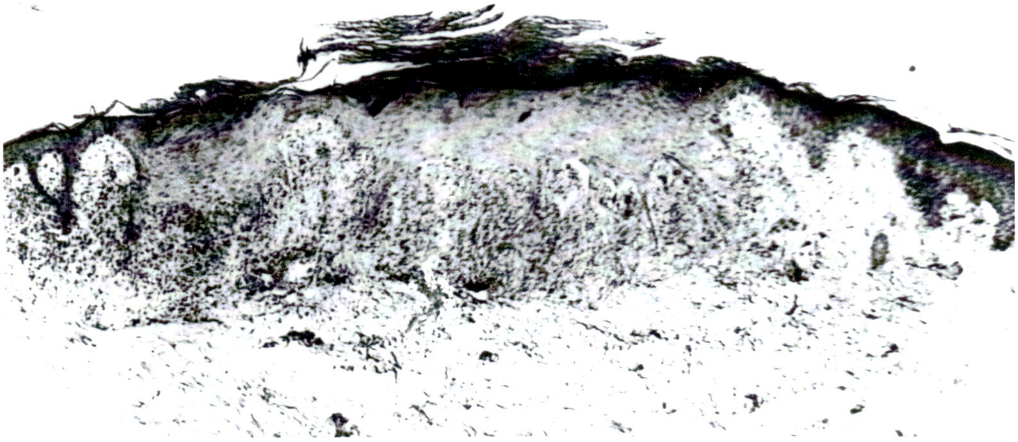

C
X50

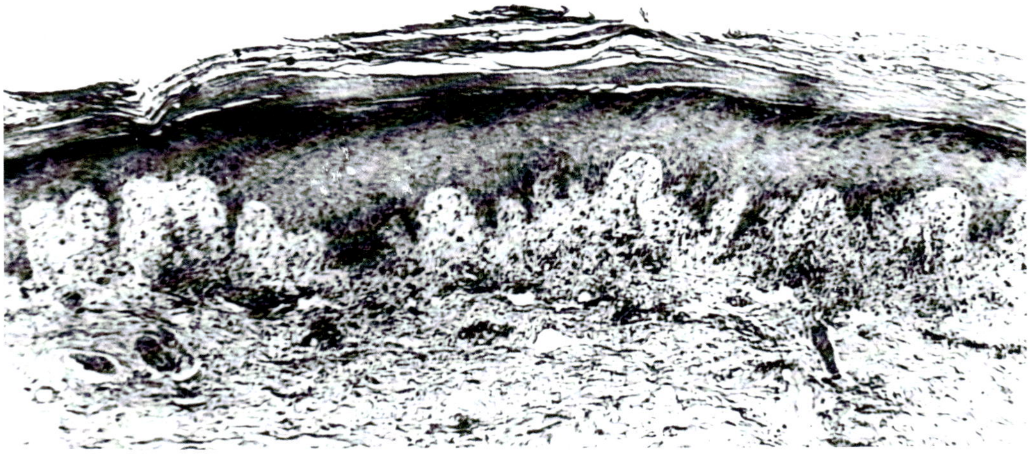

D
X50

LICHEN PLANUS continued

LICHEN PLANUS

Microscopic features

3. Hyperkeratosis, hypergranulosis, and irregular ("saw-tooth") acanthosis are present (Fig. A). Hypergranulosis may be intermittent; keratohyaline granules may be coarser than normal.
4. The basal layer of the epidermis shows hydropic degeneration which may lead to destruction of the basal cells (Fig. B).

   Destruction of the basal cells may result in clefts between the epidermis and dermis (Max Josef spaces) (Figs. C,D).
5. Homogeneous, eosinophilic bodies resembling Russell bodies are generally present in the lower epidermis or upper zone of the dermal infiltrate. These are called *colloid bodies* or *Civatte bodies* (Fig. C, arrow). They represent degenerated keratinocytes.
6. There is a band-like infiltrate in the papillary dermis, impinging on the epidermis (Figs. A,C). It is composed almost entirely of lymphocytes; some histiocytes, and in early lesions, neutrophils may be present. Eosinophils are generally absent. "Melanophages" are often observed in the infiltrate (Fig. E). Histiocytes increase in number in longstanding lesions.
7. The use of antikeratin immune sera has resulted in intense staining of colloid bodies (Fig. F). The staining of colloid bodies demonstrated with immunofluorescence technique (Fig. F) is not considered to have an immunologic basis, but to be due to absorption of immunoglobulins, complement, and fibrin.

LICHEN PLANUS continued

HYPERTROPHIC LICHEN PLANUS

Hypertrophic lichen planus is a variant with clustered, hypertrophic, and hyperkeratotic papules (Fig. A); occasionally lesions have a verrucous appearance (Fig. B). The anterior tibial area is the usual site.

Microscopic features

1. There is extensive irregular acanthosis, hyperkeratosis, and hypergranulosis (Fig. C). Papillomatosis may be present.
2. There is an infiltrate in the upper dermis, but it may not be in a distinct band-like arrangement, and it may not impinge directly on the epidermis, as in the common variety of lichen planus (Fig. C).
3. Hydropic degeneration of the basal layer of the epidermis may or may not (Fig. C) be present.
4. The dermal infiltrate is similar to that of the common variety of lichen planus.

BULLOUS LICHEN PLANUS

In addition to lesions of the common variety of lichen planus, bullae are present (Fig. D).

Microscropic features

1. The bulla is subepidermal and results from extensive destruction of the basal layer (Fig. E).
2. The usual epidermal changes of lichen planus and band-like dermal infiltrate are usually still discernible (Fig. E).

HYPERTROPHIC LICHEN PLANUS

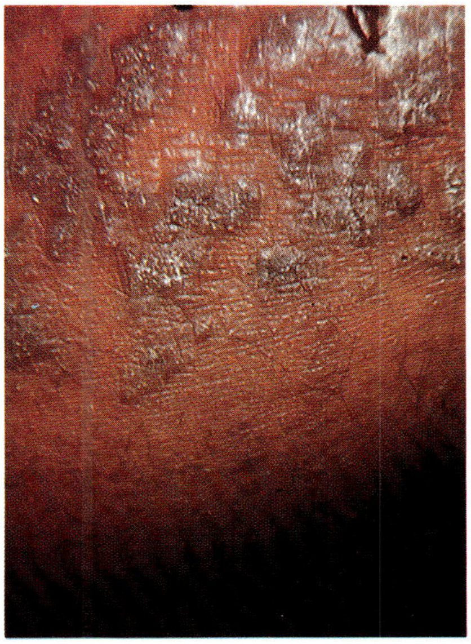
A

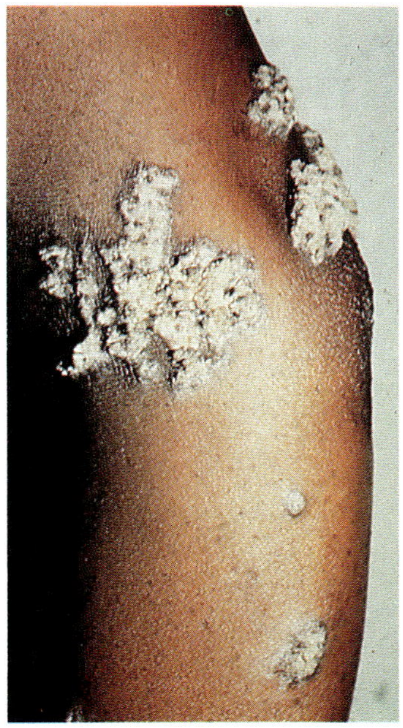
B

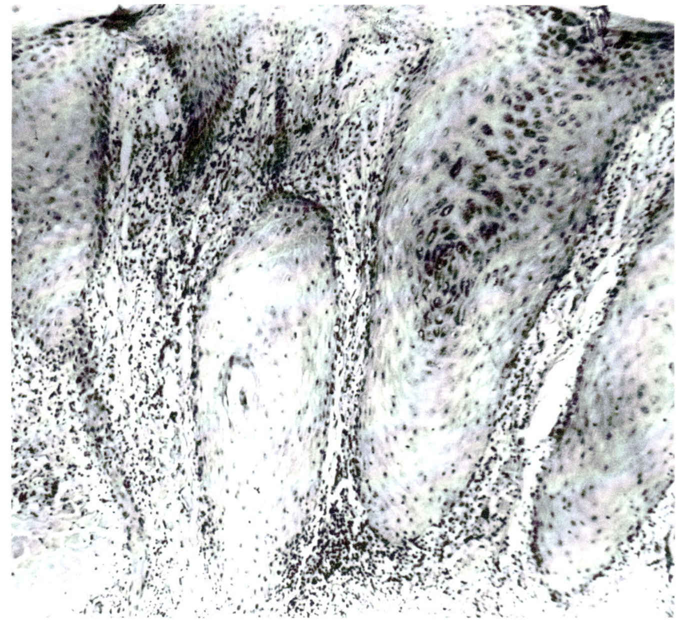
C
X80

BULLOUS LICHEN PLANUS

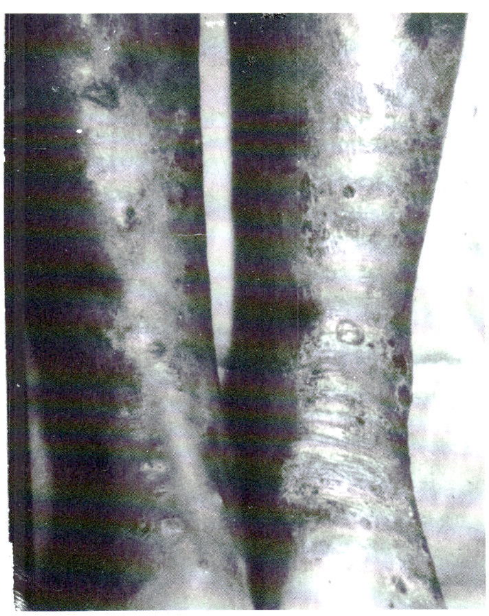
D

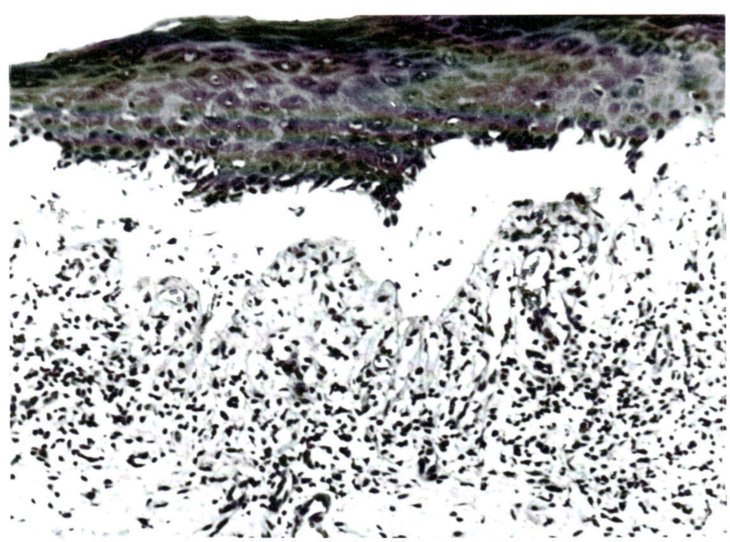
E
X190

LICHEN PLANUS continued ⇨

ANNULAR LICHEN PLANUS

Lesions of annular lichen planus have a resemblance to granuloma annulare (Fig. A), but show surface changes, including scaling.

Microscopic features

The central portions of these lesions may show an atrophic epidermis, but hydropic degeneration of the basal layer and a band-like infiltrate in the papillary dermis are still present (Fig. B).

ANNULAR LICHEN PLANUS

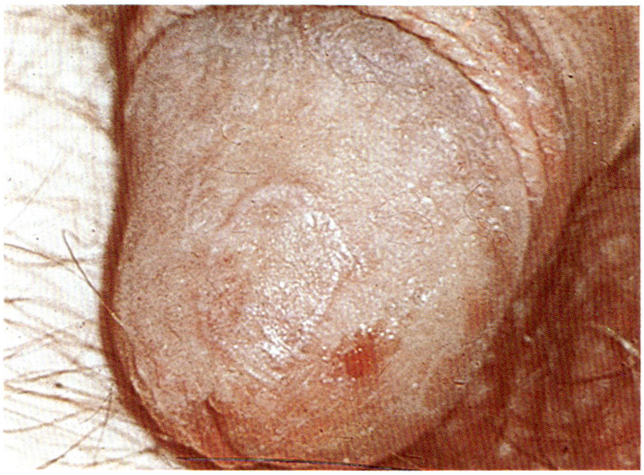

A

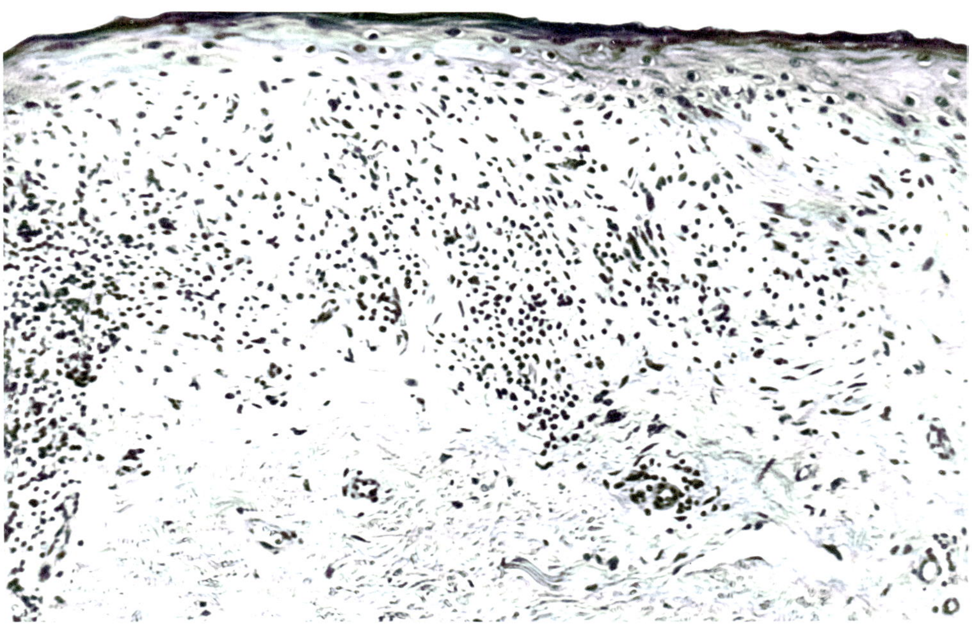

B
X170

LICHEN PLANUS continued

LICHEN PLANUS OF THE MUCOUS MEMBRANES

The oral cavity is the usual site. Lesions have a whitish, lace-like appearance (Figs. A,B). Squamous cell carcinoma is a rare sequel. There may be vesicles or erosions.

Microscopic features

Mucous membrane lesions of lichen planus have a histologic appearance similar to lesions of the glabrous skin. The usual parakeratosis of stratified squamous mucous membrane may be transformed to orthokeratosis and unlike normal stratified squamous mucous membrane, a granular layer is generally visible (Fig. C, arrow).

Distinction from premalignant leukoplakia may be difficult. The key distinguishing feature is the presence of atypia in keratinocytes of premalignant leukoplakia.

LICHEN PLANOPILARIS

Lichen planopilaris refers to lichen planus localized to hair follicles. Initially, there are follicular papules and erythema. Lichen planopilaris of the scalp may progress to a stage of cicatricial alopecia (Fig. D). *Lichen spinulosus et folliculitis decalvans (Graham-Little)* refers to lichen planopilaris with involvement of the glabrous skin and hairy areas, resulting in partial cicatricial alopecia of the scalp and non-cicatricial alopecia of the axillary and pubic areas.

Microscopic features

1. The dense band-like infiltrate impinges on the hair follicle (Figs. E,F).
2. There is hydropic degeneration and destruction of the basal layer of the outer root sheath (Fig. F).
3. Involvement of the hair papilla leads to destruction of the hair follicle, which leaves only a dilated and hyperkeratotic infundibular area.
4. Late lesions show a resemblance to pseudopelade of Brocq (see p. 226). The epidermis is atrophic and there is scattered inflammation and fibrosis in the dermis, with a pronounced loss of pilosebaceous units.

LICHEN PLANUS ERYTHEMATOSUS

This refers to a variant characterized by bright red, soft papules. The histologic picture is the same as that of ordinary lichen planus.

Comment

Graft-versus-host disease is due to transplants of immunocompetent lymphocytes, in most cases via bone marrow transplantation. There is a rare congenital form in which maternal lymphocytes establish themselves in the fetus. The acute phase has cutaneous parallels clinically and microscopically to erythema multiforme; the early lichenoid stage of the chronic phase has clinical and microscopic cutaneous parallels to lichen planus; the late sclerotic stage of the chronic phase has clinical and microscopic cutaneous parallels to scleroderma.

LICHEN PLANUS OF MUCOUS MEMBRANES; LICHEN PLANOPILARIS

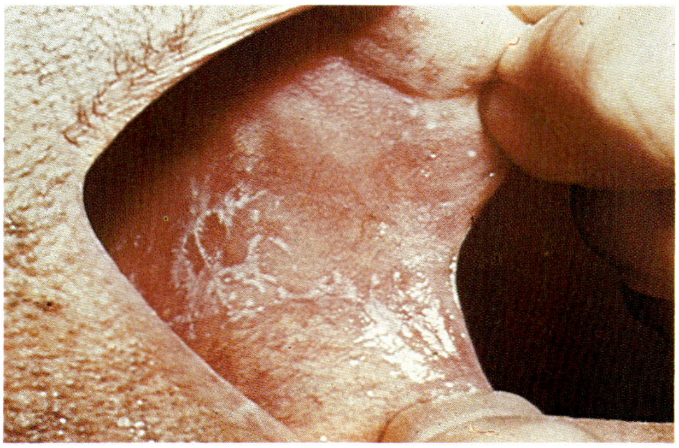

A

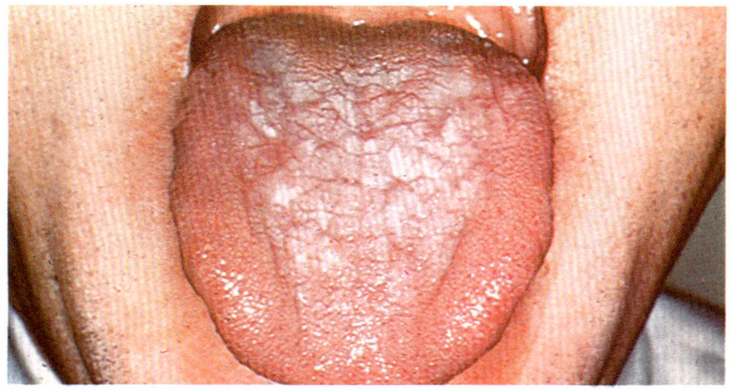

B

Figs. A,B courtesy Dr. Harvey Ansell

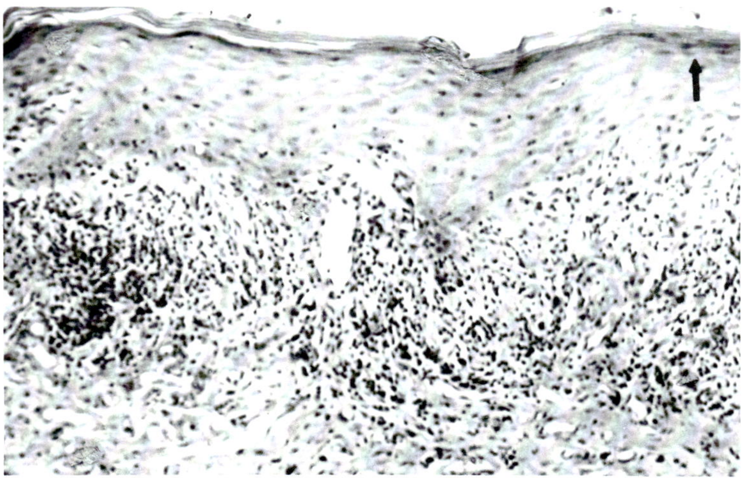

C X120

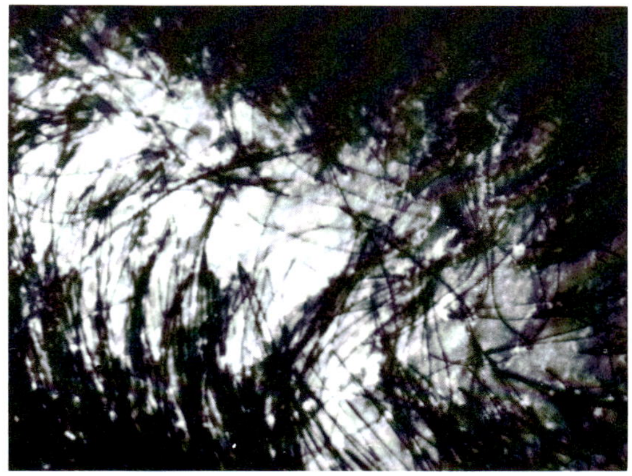

D

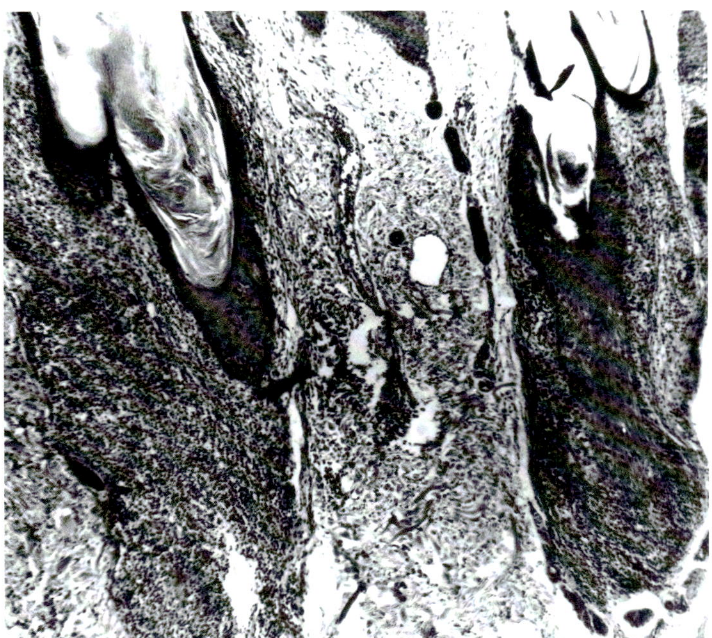

E X80

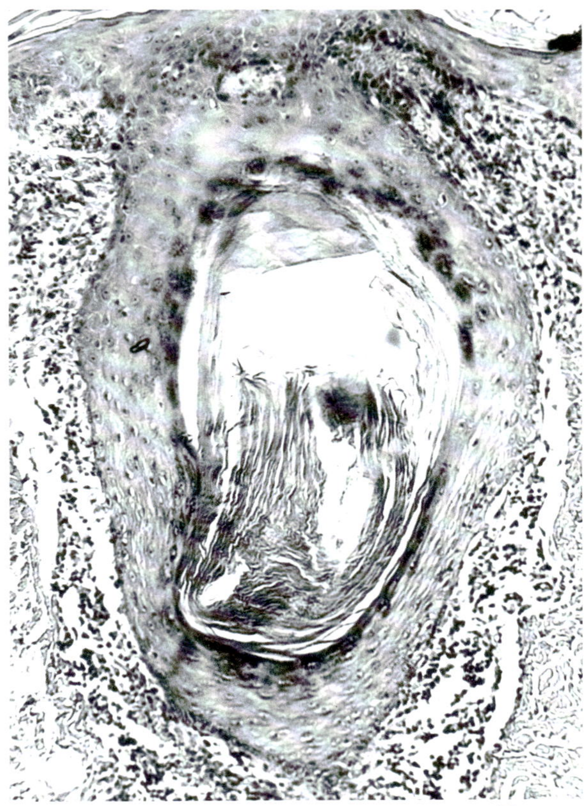

F X120

PSORIASIS

Psoriasis is a chronic disease with a greatly increased rate of epidermal cell replication. The cause in unknown. Heredity appears to play a role. Autoimmune factors have been suggested. Cutaneous lesions are papules and plaques with a silvery scale (Figs. A,B,C,E). The scalp, extensor surfaces of the extremities, and sacral area are sites of predilection. Nail dystrophy, including pitting or gross distortions of the nail plate, are common (Figs. G,H). In Fig. H, the skin adjacent to the nail shows evidence of psoriasis. A form of polyarthritis having some clinical and radiologic similarity to rheumatoid arthritis may be associated with psoriasis.

It has been shown that there is an increased rate of replication of synovial cells in psoriatic arthritis.

Mucous membrane involvement is rare in psoriasis.

Guttate psoriasis is an acute, eruptive variant with numerous small lesions (Fig. C). Psoriatic lesions may show linear arrangement (Fig. C) as a result of trauma (isomorphic or Koebner phenomenon).

Exfoliative erythroderma may develop in psoriasis (Fig. F).

Transitional forms resembling seborrheic dermatitis are common (Fig. D). In such transitional forms, the lesions do not have the usually sharp margination, and they have a greasy scale rather than a silvery scale.

There are a variety of pustular forms of psoriasis (see p. 454). Lithium carbonate can exacerbate psoriasis and induce transformation to the pustular type.

PSORIASIS

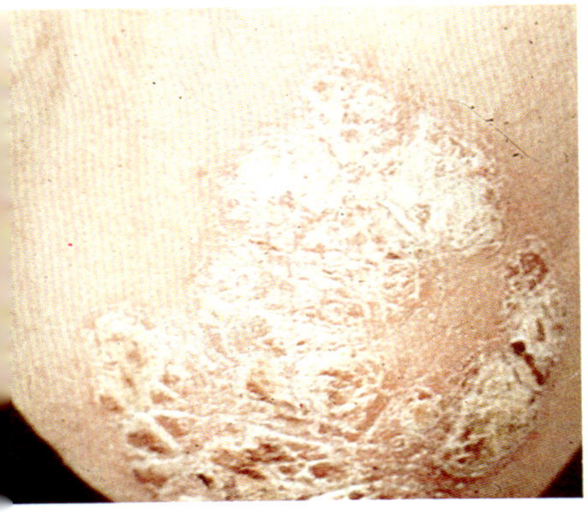

A

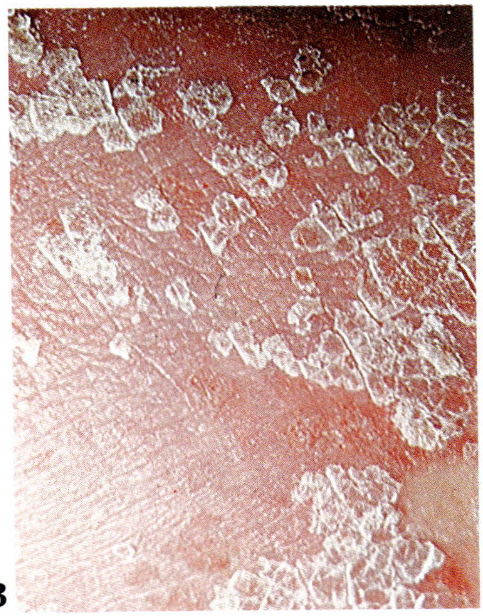

B

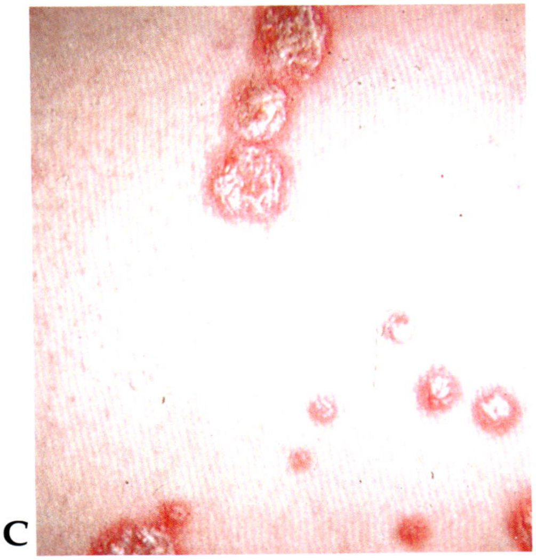

C

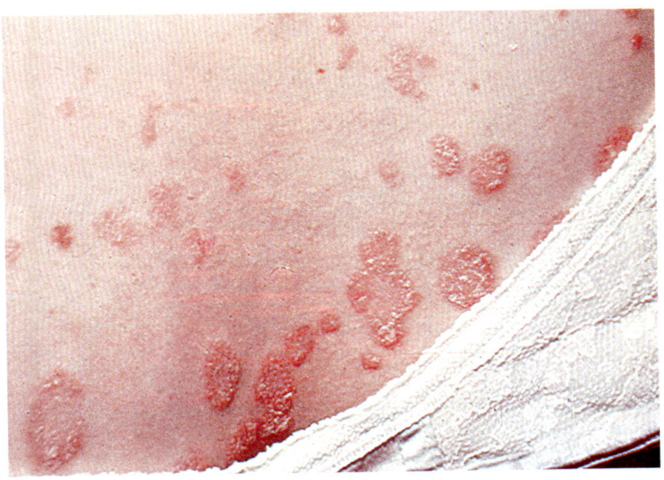

D

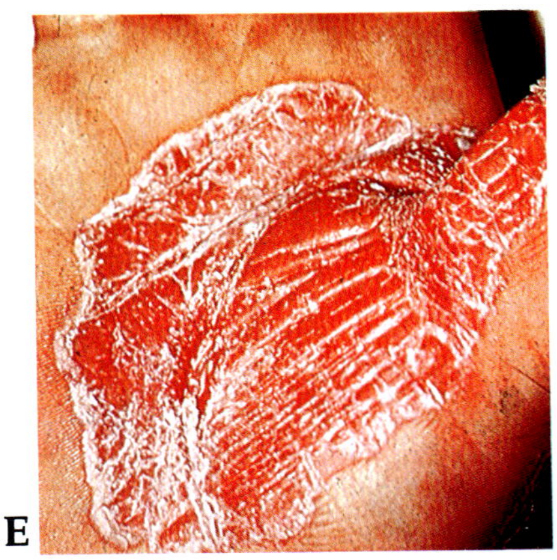

E

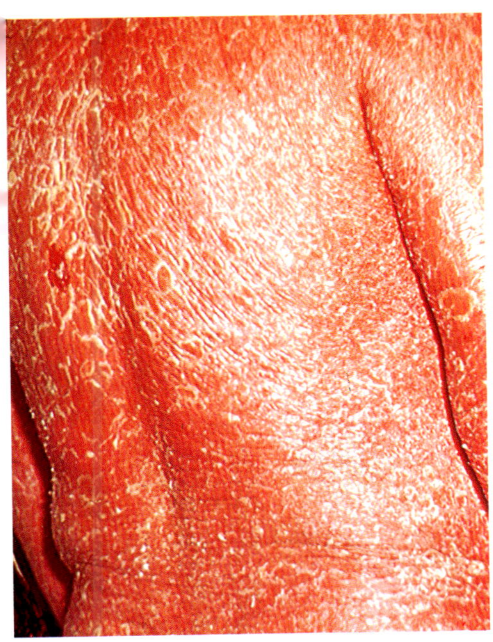

F

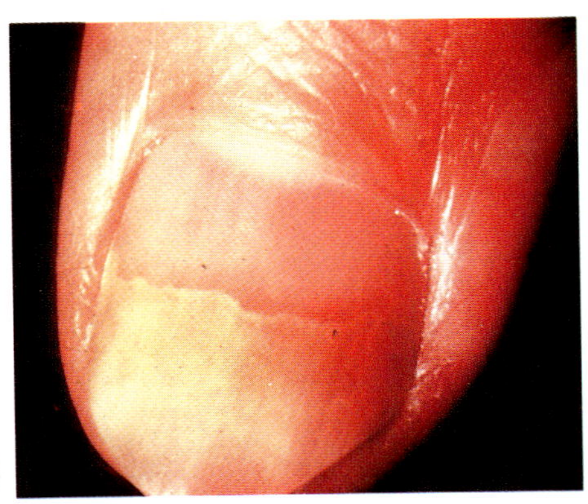

G

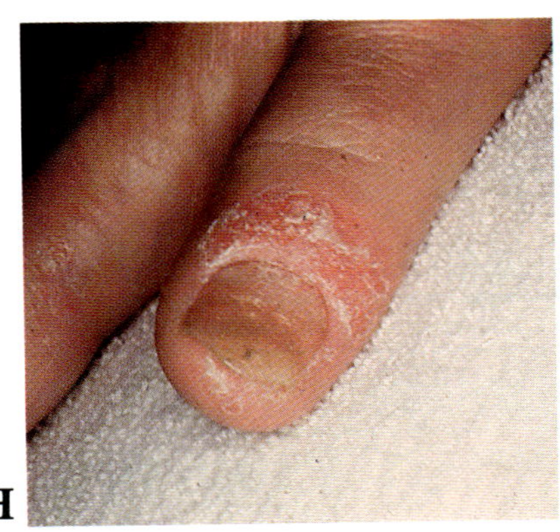

H

PSORIASIS continued ⇨

PSORIASIS

Microscopic features

1. The rete ridges are club-shaped and show regular elongation. Bases of the rete ridges commonly coalesce (Figs. A,B,D,E). Epidermal edema is generally absent. Mitotic figures are frequently observed (Fig. F). There is an increase in nuclear:cytoplasmic ratio in the epidermal cells.
   The granular layer is absent in histologically characteristic lesions of psoriasis.
2. Parakeratosis is present (Figs. B,C). Accumulations of neutrophils are often present in the lower part of the horny layer (Munro microabscesses) (Figs. A,B,C). Some neutrophils may also be present in vacuoles within keratinocytes in the upper malpighian layer (Fig. D). Progression of this change results in the spongiform pustules of pustular psoriasis (see p. 456).
3. Dermal papillae are elongated and edematous; the epidermis overlying the papillae is thin (Figs. A,B,D,E). Capillaries in the papillae are dilated and tortuous.
4. The upper dermis shows a moderate perivascular lymphocytic and histiocytic infiltrate (Figs. B,D,E). In early lesions, accumulations of neutrophils may be present at the tips of the papillae.
5. Lesions of psoriasis do not always show the characteristic histologic features; the pattern may be that of a nonspecific dermatitis. Early scaling papules and the margins of advancing plaques may be sites that are most likely to have a diagnostic histologic pattern.

PSORIASIS

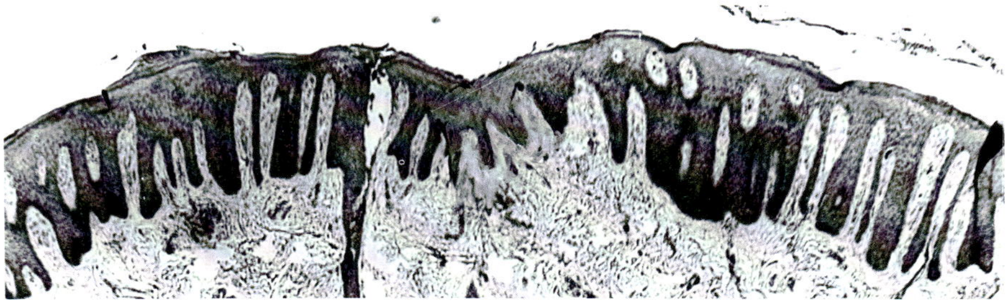

A X40

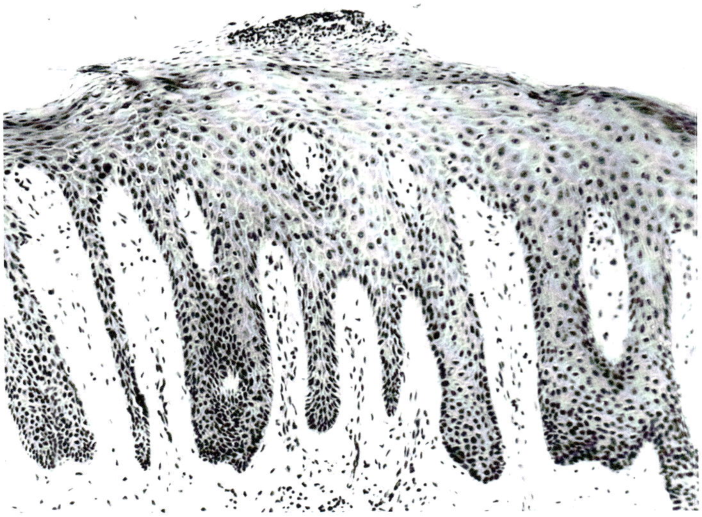

B X120

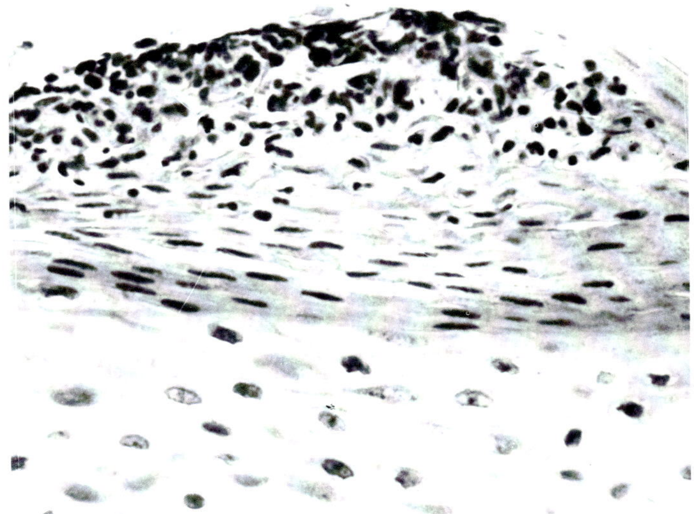

C X580

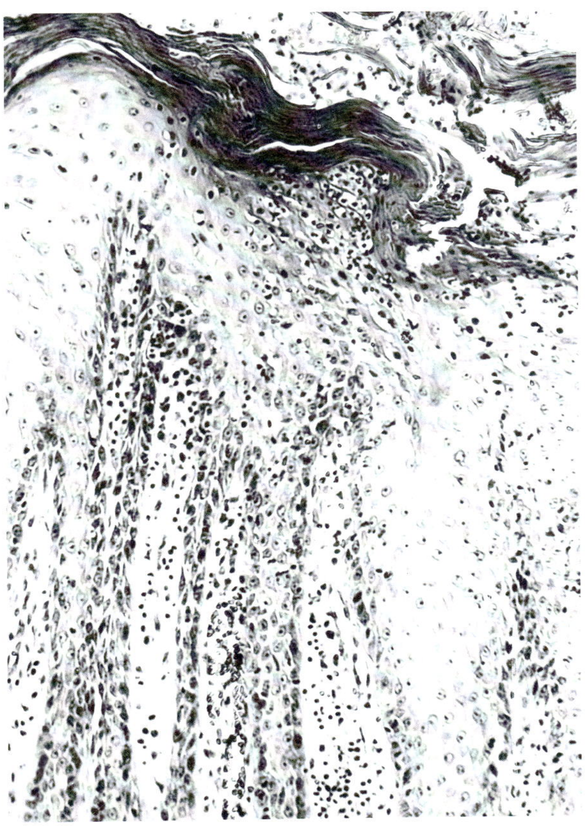

D X160

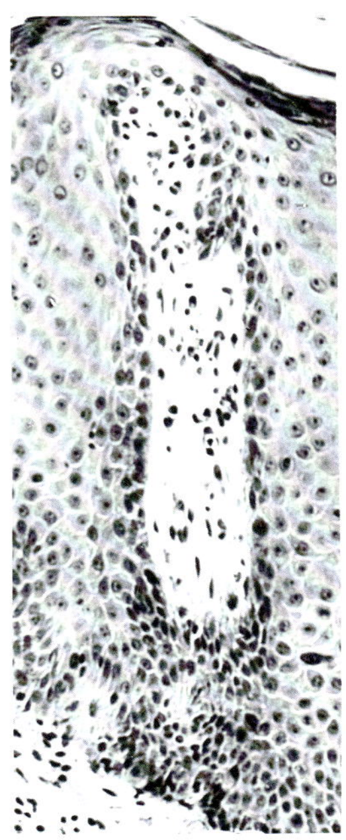

E X210

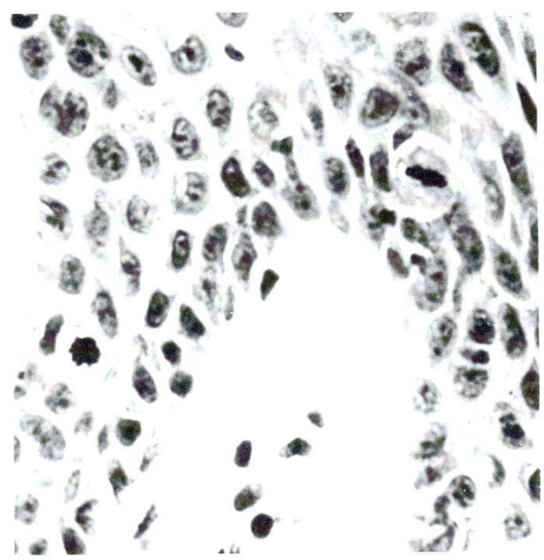

F X580

PSORIASIS continued ⇨

PSORIASIS: PUSTULAR FORMS

1. *Generalized pustular psoriasis of von Zumbusch* is an acute pustular eruption (Fig. A) of skin and mucous membranes accompanied by fever and granulocytosis. It usually develops in patients with pre-existing stable psoriasis, but may occur *de novo*. Generalized pustular psoriasis is often associated with psoriatic arthritis. *Impetigo herpetiformis* is a similar condition and is considered by some authors to be synonymous with generalized pustular psoriasis of von Zumbusch. Impetigo herpetiformis may have an association with pregnancy or parathyroid deficiency.
2. Psoriasiform pustular and hyperkeratotic eruptions of the hands and feet.
   a. *Pustulosis palmaris et plantaris* is a localized form of pustular psoriasis characterized by crops of deep-seated pustules on the palms and soles (Fig. B).
   b. *Acrodermatitis continua of Hallopeau (acropustulosis; dermatitis repens)* refers to a variant of psoriasis with erythematous, crusted, scaling lesions containing multiple pustules which have a predilection for the distal portions of the fingers and toes (Figs. C,D). Secondary nail dystrophy or loss is common (Figs. C,D). Trauma may be an initiating factor. Acrodermatitis continua may be associated with generalized pustular psoriasis.
   c. *Reiter's disease* is characterized by urethritis, arthritis, and conjunctivitis. Stomatitis, with geographic tongue may be present. A significant number of patients develop erosive or psoriasiform cutaneous lesions, generally involving the palms, soles, and glans penis; occasionally there are mucous membrane lesions. Pustules (Figs. E,F) are common and may evolve into conical, hyperkeratotic, scaling lesions (Fig. G) (*keratosis blennorrhagica*). The view that keratosis blennorrhagica is associated with gonococcal urethritis is no longer held.

Comment

Generalized pustular psoriasis may show oral pustules, particularly of the tongue.

PSORIASIS: PUSTULAR FORMS

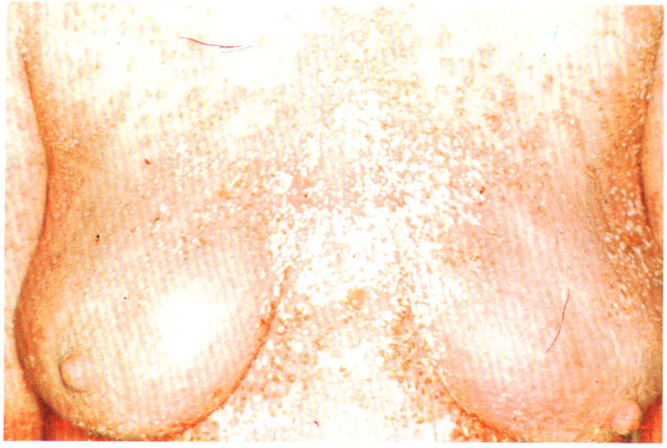

A

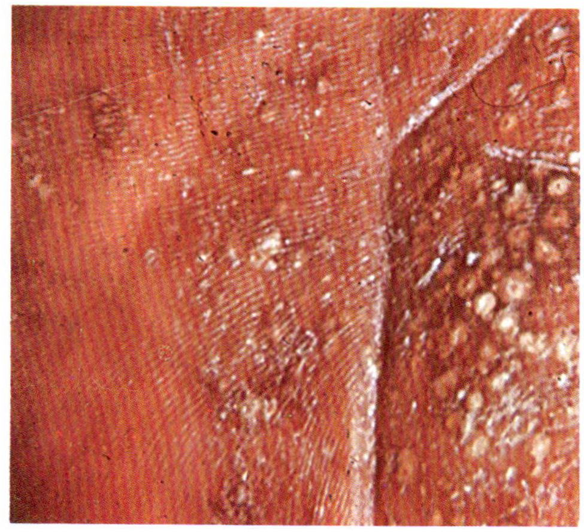

B

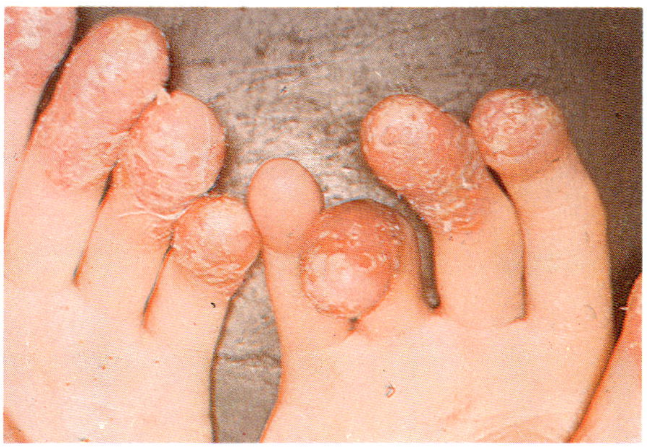

C

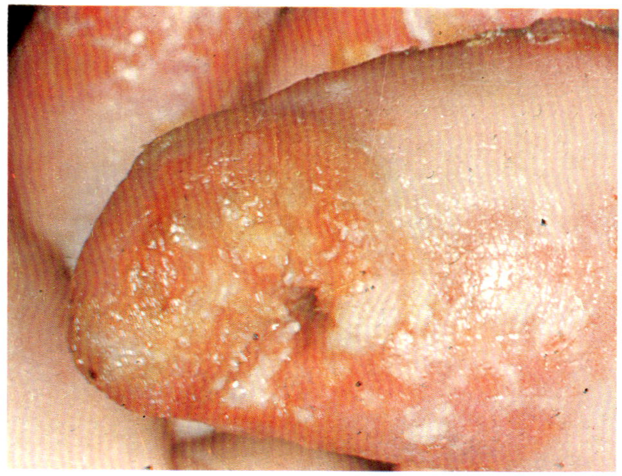

D

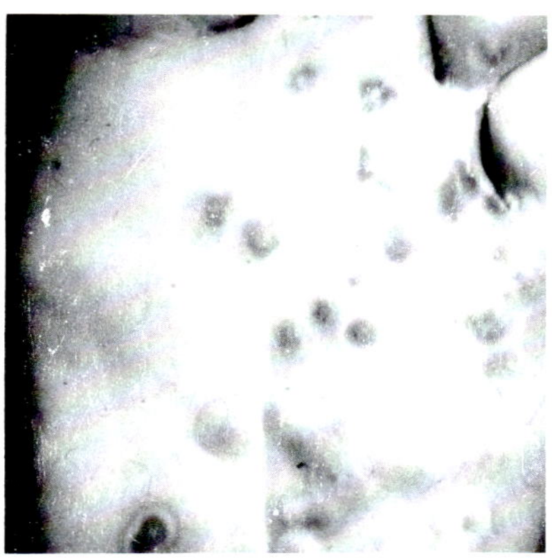

E

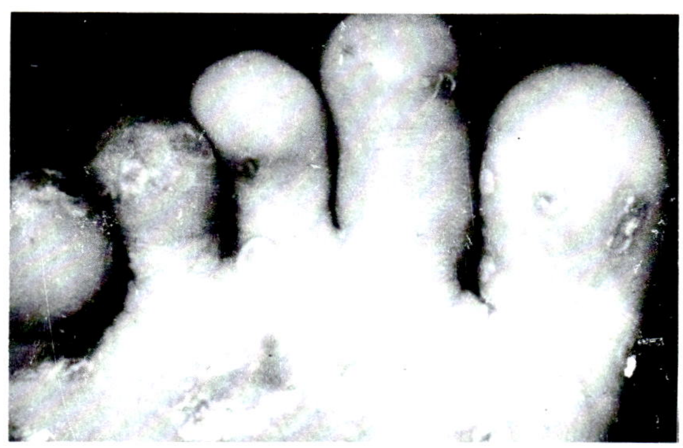

F

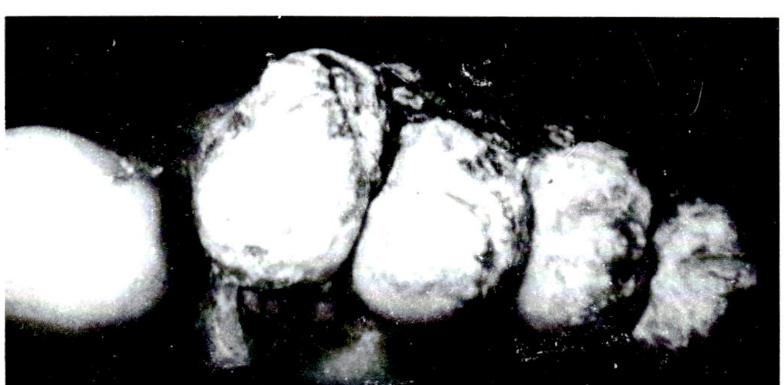

G

Figs. E,F,G courtesy
Dr. Robert Gorlin

PSORIASIS continued ⇨

PSORIASIS: PUSTULAR FORMS

Microscopic features

1. Lesions are characterized by spongiform pustules (Kogoj pustules) which are usually associated with the other histologic features of psoriasis (see p. 452). Spongiform pustules consist of accumulations of neutrophils within vacuolated keratinocytes (Figs. A,B). In well-developed spongiform pustules, neutrophils are present in a meshwork of residual cell walls of keratinocytes (Fig. B, upper part of field).
2. Pustules of pustulosis palmaris et plantaris and pustular bacterid of Andrews are typically mid-epidermal and unilocular (Fig. C). However, spongiform pustules and transitional forms may be present in these disorders. With high magnification (Fig. D) the pustule illustrated in Fig. C shows spongiform elements at its periphery (top of field).
3. Spongiform pustules are not entirely specific for pustular forms of psoriasis and can occasionally be observed in other disorders, such as candidiasis and geographic tongue (migratory glossitis).

PSORIASIS: PUSTULAR FORMS

A X150

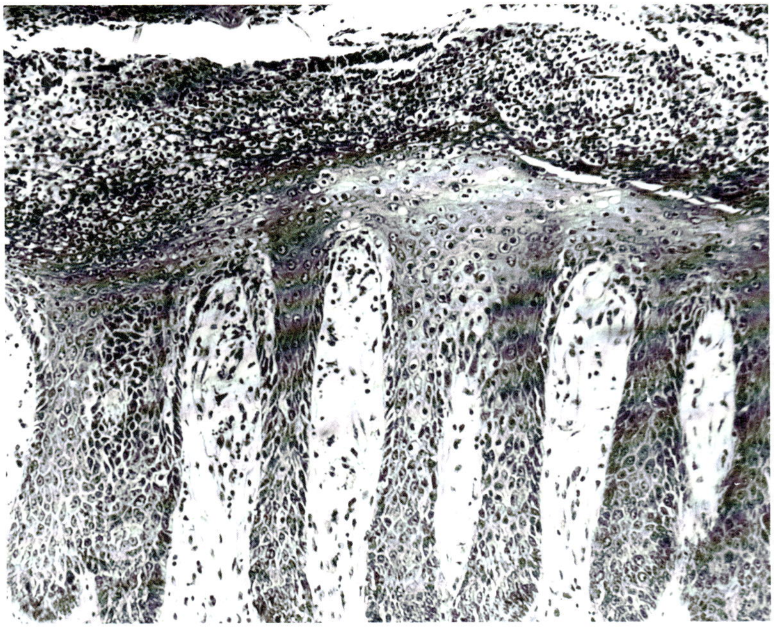

B X730

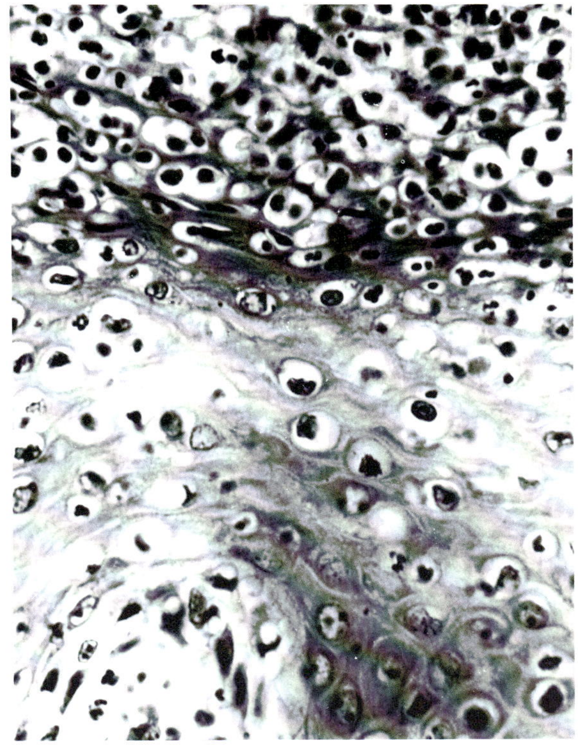

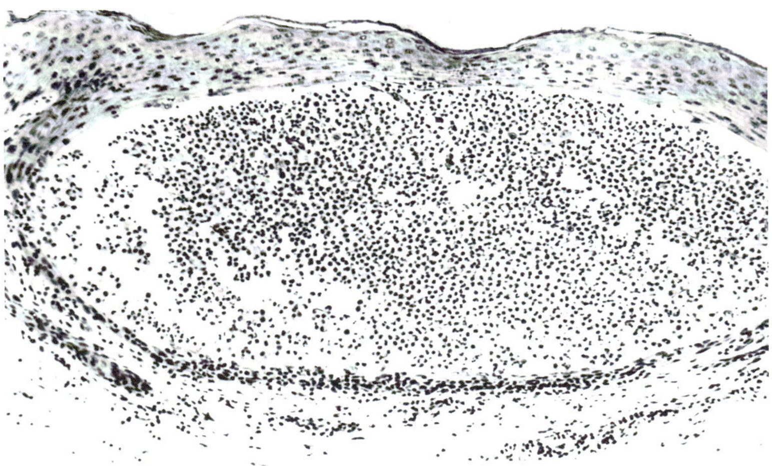

C X140

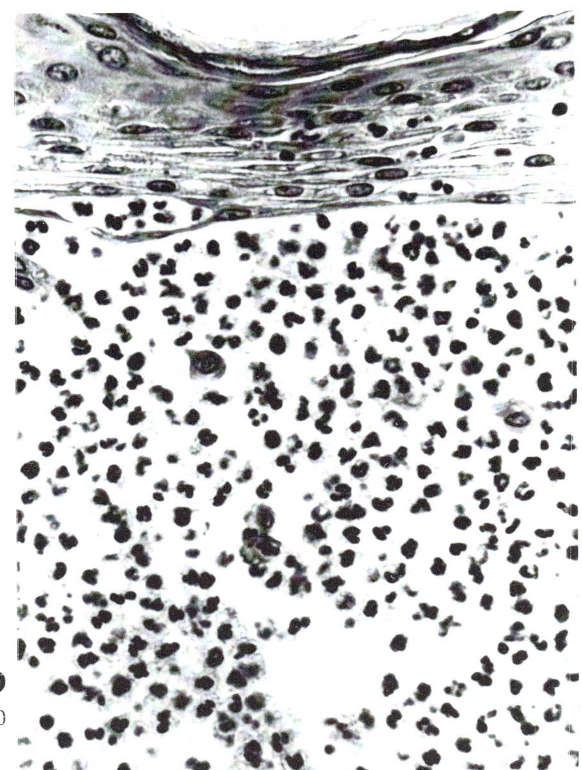

D X630

PSORIASIS continued

PSORIASIS

Microscopic differential diagnosis

1. Seborrheic dermatitis (p. 108) may show histologic features similar to those of psoriasis. However, in seborrheic dermatitis, spongiosis and more extensive inflammatory changes are usually present.
2. Mycosis fungoides may show a psoriasiform epidermal pattern. Differentiation is made on the basis of the Pautrier microabscesses in mycosis fungoides and atypical T lymphocytes in the dermal infiltrate (see p. 1332).

PITYRIASIS RUBRA PILARIS

Pityriasis rubra pilaris is a rare, scaling disease. Primary lesions are follicular and nonfollicular papules. The knuckles and dorsal surfaces of the fingers are common sites of the hyperkeratotic follicular papules (Fig. A). Coalescence of the nonfollicular papules results in scaling, erythematous plaques resembling psoriasis. Salmon-colored areas of the palms and soles (Fig. B) are common. Generalized, scaling erythroderma may be present, often with spared areas; these may show scaling. Nail changes resembling psoriasis may be present. Adult onset pityriasis rubra pilaris, in particular, may resemble psoriasis.

Microscopic features

1. The follicular papules show follicular hyperkeratosis and a mild lymphocytic perifollicular infiltrate (Fig. C). The shoulders of the follicle may show parakeratosis.
2. Histologic changes of chronic dermatitis are seen in nonfollicular lesions. There may be hyperkeratosis with focal parakeratosis.
3. The histologic changes are not specific. Follicular changes similar to those of pityriasis rubra pilaris can be observed in phyrnoderma (vitamin A deficiency) and keratosis pilaris.

Comment

1. It has been proposed by some that there is a relationship between pityriasis rubra pilaris and psoriasis. This is generally not accepted, since pityriasis rubra pilaris does not show classic histologic features of psoriasis.
2. There is an inherited form of pityriasis rubra pilaris which is transmitted as an autosomal dominant trait.
3. A deficiency of vitamin A or abnormal metabolism of vitamin A has been proposed as an etiologic mechanism.

PITYRIASIS RUBRA PILARIS

A 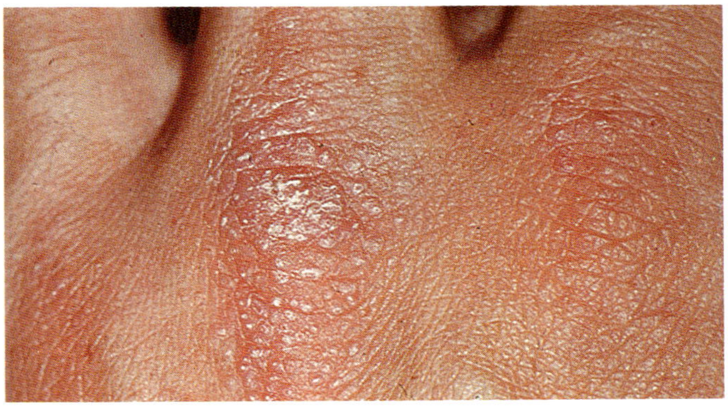

B 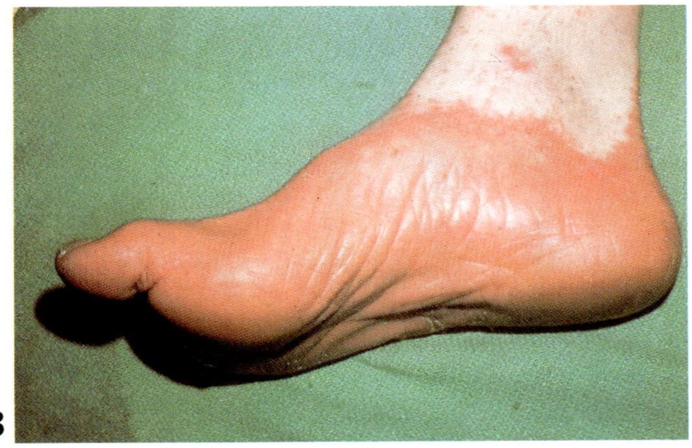

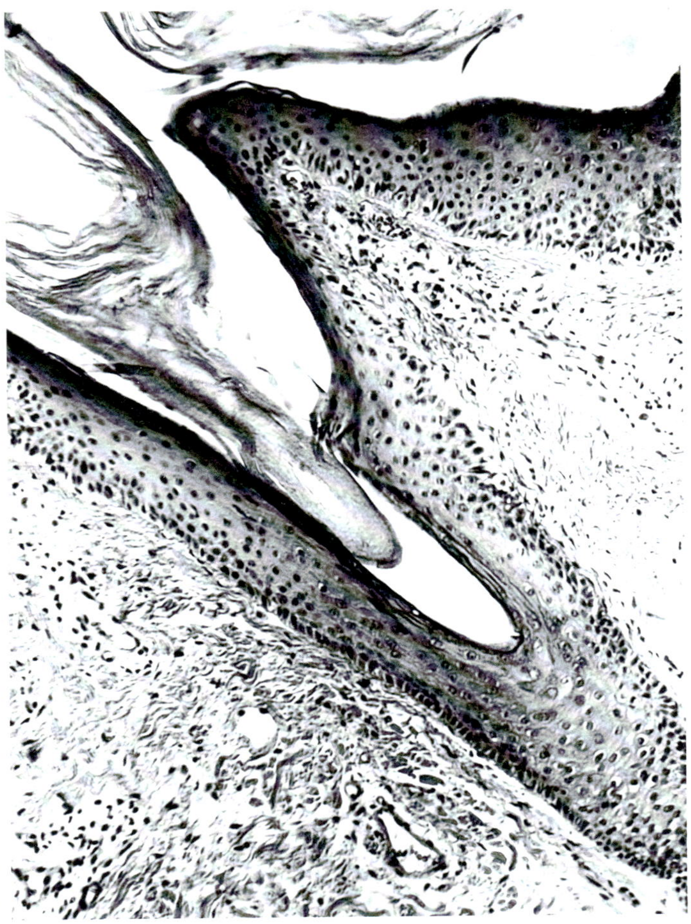

C
X210

Suggested Reading

Papulosquamous Diseases

Lichen planus

Abell, E. et al. The diagnostic significance of immunoglobulin and fibrin deposition in lichen planus. *Br. J. Dermatol.*, 93:17, 1975.

Ahmed, A. et al. Coexistence of lichen planus and systemic lupus erythematosus. *J. Am. Acad. Dermatol.*, 7:478, 1982.

Al-Abdulla, H. Lichen planus actinicus. Thesis submitted to the University of Cairo, 1985.

Alano, A. et al. Lichen planus: Study with antihuman T lymphocytes antigen serum on frozen tissue sections. *Br. J. Dermatol.*, 98:601, 1978.

Altman, J. and Perry, H. The variations and course of lichen planus. *Arch. Dermatol.*, 84:179, 1961.

Andreasen, J. Oral lichen planus. I. A clinical evaluation of 115 cases. *Oral Surg.*, 25:31, 1968.

——. Oral lichen planus. II. A histologic evaluation of ninety-seven cases. *Oral Surg.*, 25:158, 1968.

Arnold, H., Jr. Lichen planus erythematosus: Review, and report of two cases. *Arch. Dermatol.*, 84:741, 1961.

Baart de la Faille-Kuyper, E. and Baart de la Faille, H. An immunofluorescence study of lichen planus. *Br. J. Dermatol.*, 90:365, 1974.

Bhan, A. et al. T cell subsets and Langerhans cells in lichen planus: *In situ* characterization using monoclonal antibodies. *Br. J. Dermatol.*, 105:617, 1981.

Bjorke, J. and Krogh, H. Identification of mononuclear cells *in situ* in skin lesions of lichen planus. *Br. J. Dermatol.*, 98:605, 1978.

Black, M. What is going on in lichen planus? *Clin. Exp. Dermatol.*, 2:303, 1977.

Black, M. and Wilson-Jones, E. The role of the epidermis in the histopathogenesis of lichen planus. *Arch. Dermatol.*, 105:81, 1972.

Braun-Falco, O. et al. Trachyonychie: 20 Nägel-Dystrophie. *Hautarzt*, 32:17, 1981.

Brody, I. The ultrastructure of the epidermis in lichen ruber planus as revealed by electron microscopy. I. Dermoepidermal junction, stratum basale, and lower stratum spinosum. *J. Ultrastruct. Res.*, 28:161, 1969.

——. The ultrastructure of the epidermis in lichen ruber planus as revealed by electron microscopy. II. Cytoplasm and nucleus in certain basal and spinous cells. *J. Ultrastruct. Res.*, 28:178, 1969.

Camisa, C. et al. Bullous lichen planus: Diagnosis by indirect immunofluorescence and treatment with dapsone. *J. Am. Acad. Dermatol.*, 14:464, 1986.

Cooke, B. The oral manifestations of lichen planus: 50 cases. *Br. Dent. J.*, 96:1, 1954.

Cram, D., Kierland, R. and Winkelmann, R. Ulcerative lichen planus of the feet: Bullous variant with hair and nail lesions. *Arch. Dermatol.*, 93:692, 1966.

Cram, D. and Muller, S. Unusual variations of lichen planus. *Mayo Clin. Proc.*, 41:677, 1966.

Davies, M. et al. Is there a relationship between lupus erythematosus and lichen planus? *Br. J. Dermatol.*, 96:145, 1977.

Dilaimy, M. Lichen planus subtropicus. *Arch. Dermatol.*, 112:1251, 1976.

Dostrovsky, A. and Sagher, F. Lichen planus in subtropical countries: Study of an annular type with inverse localization (uncovered surfaces of the skin). *Arch. Dermatol. Syph.*, 59:308, 1949.

Ebner, H. and Gebhart, W. Epidermal changes in lichen planus. *J. Cutan. Pathol.*, 3:167, 1976.

——. Light and electron microscopic studies on colloid and other cytoid bodies. *Clin. Exp. Dermatol.*, 2:311, 1977.

Ebner, H. et al. The epidermal cell proliferation in lichen planus. *Acta Derm. Venereol.* (Stockh.), 57:133, 1977.

El-Labban, N. and Kramer, R. Civatte bodies and the actively dividing epithelial cells in oral lichen planus. *Br. J. Dermatol.*, 90:13, 1974.

Ellis, F. Histopathology of lichen planus based on analysis of one hundred biopsy specimens. *J. Invest. Dermatol.*, 48:143, 1967.

Fordyce, J. and MacKee, G. Clinical types of lichen planus. *J. Cutan. Dis.*, 37:320, 1919.

Gomes, M., Staquet, M. and Thivolet, J. Staining of colloid bodies by keratin antisera in lichen planus. *Am. J. Dermatopathol.*, 3:341, 1981.
Hashimoto, K. Apoptosis in lichen planus and several other dermatoses. *Acta Derm. Venereol.* (Stockh.), 56:187, 1976.
Hintner, H. et al. Lichen planus and bullous pemphigoid. *Acta Derm. Venereol.* (Stockh.), 59 (85, suppl.):71, 1979.
Holmstrup, P. and Pindborg, J. Erythroplakic lesions in relation to oral lichen planus. *Acta Derm. Venereol.* (Stockh.), 59 (85, suppl.):77, 1979.
Horn, R. et al. Immunofluorescent findings and clinical overlap in two cases of follicular lichen planus. *J. Am. Acad. Dermatol.*, 7:203, 1982.
Jamison, T., Cooper, N. and Epstein, W. Lichen planus and discoid lupus erythematosus. Overlap syndrome. *Arch. Dermatol.*, 114:1039, 1978.
Johnson, F. and Fry, L. Ultrastructural observations on lichen planus. *Arch. Dermatol.*, 95:596, 1967.
Kerr, J., Wyllie, A. and Currie, A. Apoptosis: A basic biological phenomenon with wide-ranging implications in tissue kinetics. *Br. J. Cancer*, 26:239, 1972.
Konrad, K. et al. Ultrastructural localization of immunoglobulin and fibrin in lichen planus. *J. Am. Acad. Dermatol.*, 1:233, 1979.
Kronenberg, K., Fretzin, D. and Potter, B. Malignant degeneration of lichen plaus. *Arch. Dermatol.*, 104:304, 1971.
Laur, W., Posey, R. and Waller, J. Lichen planus-like keratosis. *J. Am. Acad. Dermatol.*, 4:329, 1981.
Lin, A. Srolovitz, H. and Billick, R. Familial lichen planus. *Cutis*, 37:135, 1986.
Little, E. Lichen planus. *J. Cutan. Dis.*, 37:639, 1919.
Lumpkin, L. and Helwig, E. Solitary lichen planus. *Arch. Dermatol.*, 93:54, 1966.
Marks, R., Black, M. and Wilson-Jones, E. Epidermal cell kinetics in lichen planus. *Br. J. Dermatol.*, 88:37, 1973.
Morel, P. et al. Lichen plan avec dépôts linéaires d'IgG et de C3 à la jonction dermo-épidermique. *Dermatologica*, 163:117, 1981.
Olson, R. and Everett, M. Epidermal apoptosis: Cell deletion by phagocytosis. *J. Cutan. Pathol.*, 2:53, 1975.
Piepkom, M. Langerhans cells in lichen planus. *Br. J. Dermatol.*, 108:736, 1983.
Presbury, D. and Marks, R. The epidermal disorder in lichen planus: An *in vitro* study. *Br. J. Dermatol.*, 90:373, 1974.
Prieto, J. Pseudopelade of Brocq: Its relationship to some forms of cicatricial alopecias and to lichen planus. *J. Invest. Dermatol.*, 24:323, 1955.
Pullon, P. Ultrastructure of oral lichen planus. *Oral Surg.*, 28:365, 1969.
Ragaz, A. and Ackerman, A. Evolution, maturation, and regression of lesions of lichen planus. *Am. J. Dermatopathol.*, 3:5, 1981.
Sarkany, I., Caron, G. and Jones, H. Lichen planus pemphigoides. *Trans. St. John's Hosp. Dermatol. Soc.*, 50:50, 1964.
Samman, P. Lichen planus: A dermatological centenary. *Br. J. Dermatol.*, 81:306, 1969.
——. Lichen planus: An analysis of 200 cases. *Trans. St. John's Hosp. Dermatol. Soc.*, 46:36, 1961.
Saurat, J. et al. Coexistence d'un lichen plan et d'un pemphigoide bulleuse. *Ann. Dermatol. Venereol.*, 104:368, 1977.
Schmidt, H. Frequency, duration and localization of lichen planus: A study based on 181 patients. *Acta Derm. Venereol.*, 41:164, 1961.
Scott, M., Jr. and Scott, M., Sr. Ungual lichen planus. Lichen planus of the nail. *Arch. Dermatol.*, 115:1197, 1979.
Shapiro, L. and Ackerman, A. Solitary lichen planus-like keratosis. *Dermatologica*, 132:386, 1966.
Sheehan-Dare, R. et al. Oesophageal lichen planus. *Br. J. Dermatol.*, 115:729, 1986.
Shklar, G. Erosive and bullous oral lesions of lichen planus. *Arch. Dermatol.*, 97:411, 1968.
Silver, H., Chargin, L. and Sachs, P. Follicular lichen planus (lichen planopilaris). *Arch. Dermatol. Syph.*, 67:346, 1953.
Summerly, R. and Wilson-Jones, E. The microarchitecture of Wickham's striae. *Trans. St. John's Hosp. Dermatol. Soc.*, 50:157, 1964.
Tan, R., Hayes, J. and Byrom, N. Identification of lymphoid cells in the cutaneous infiltrate of skin reticulosis and lichen planus. *Br. J. Dermatol.*, 93 (11, suppl.):16, 1975.
Tschen, J., Tschen, E. and McGavran, M. Erythema dyschromicum perstans, *J. Am. Acad. Dermatol.*, 2:295, 1980.

Varelzidis, A. et al. Immunohistochemistry in lichen planus. *Dermatologica*, 159:137, 1979.
Warin, R. Epithelioma following lichen planus of the mouth. *Br. J. Dermatol.*, 72:288, 1960.
Weedon, D. Civatte bodies and apoptosis. *Br. J. Dermatol.*, 91:357, 1974.
——. The lichenoid tissue reaction. *J. Cutan. Pathol.*, 12:279, 1985.
White, C. Lichen planus: A critical analysis of sixty-four cases. *J. Cutan. Dis.*, 37:671, 1919.
Wilson, E. On lichen planus. *J. Cutan. Med.*, 3:117, 1869.
Winer, L. and Levitt, H. Lichen planus in the Negro. *Arch. Dermatol. Syph.*, 56:437, 1947.
Zaias, N. The nail in lichen planus. *Arch. Dermatol.*, 101:264, 1970.

Psoriasis

Adachi, K. et al. Prostaglandins and cyclic AMP in epidermis: Evidence for the independent action of prostaglandins and adrenaline on the adenyl cyclase system of pig and human epidermis, normal and psoriatic. *Br. J. Dermatol.*, 92:381, 1975.
Adler, D., Rower, J. and Hashimoto, K. Annular pustular psoriasis. *Arch. Dermatol.*, 117:313, 1981.
Albert, J. and Crone, R. Keratosis blennorrhagica (Reiter's disease?) and its treatment. *Arch. Dermatol.*, 79:581, 1959.
Andrews, G. and Machacek, G. Pustular bacterids of the hands and feet. *Arch. Dermatol. Syph.*, 32:837, 1935.
Ashurst, P. Relapsing pustular eruptions of the hands and feet. *Br. J. Dermatol.*, 76:169, 1964.
Bajaj, A. et al. Impetigo herpetiformis. *Dermatologica*, 155:292, 1977.
Baker, H. Golding, D. and Thompson, M. Psoriasis and arthritis. *Ann. Int. Med.*, 58:909, 1963.
Baker, H. and Ryan, T. Generalized pustular psoriasis: A clinical and epidemiological study of 104 cases. *Br. J. Dermatol.*, 80:771, 1968.
Baumann, R. and Jilson, O. Hyperuricemia and psoriasis. *J. Invest. Dermatol.*, 36:105, 1961.
Beutner, E., ed. *Autoimmunity in Psoriasis*. Boca Raton, FL, CRC Press, 1982, p. 313.
Bollet, A. and Turner, R. Psoriatic arthritis. *Ann. N.Y. Acad. Sci.*, 73:1013, 1958.
Brandrup, F. et al. Psoriasis in monozygotic twins: Variations in expression as individuals with identical genetic constitution. *Acta Derm. Venereol.* (Stockh.), 62:229, 1982.
Braun-Falco, O. The initial psoriatic lesion. In: *Psoriasis, Proceedings of the Second International Symposium of Stanford University*. Farber, E. and Cox, A. eds., New York, Yorke Medical Books, 1976.
Braverman, J., Cohen, I. and O'Keefe, E. Metabolic and ultrastructural studies in a patient with pustular psoriasis (von Zumbusch). *Arch. Dermatol.*, 105:189, 1972.
Brenner, W. and Gschnait, F. Serum uric acid levels in untreated and PUVA-treated patients with psoriasis. *Dermatologica*, 157:91, 1978.
Buchner, A. and Begleiter, A. Oral lesions in psoriatic patients. *Oral Surg.*, 41:327, 1976.
Bullough, W. The epidermal chalone mechanism. *Natl. Cancer Inst. Monograph*, 38:99, 1973.
Burks, J. and Montgomery, H. Histopathologic study of psoriasis. *Arch. Dermatol. Syph.*, 48:479, 1943.
Chopra, D., Cherkas, L. and Flaxman, B. Identification and partial purification of chalone from human epidermis. *Br. J. Dermatol.*, 90:37, 1974.
Chopra, D. and Flaxman, B. Inhibition of mitosis of epidermal cells from psoriasis lesions *in vitro* by extracts from normal human skin. *J. Natl. Cancer Inst.*, 50:281, 1973.
Christophers, E. and Braun-Falco, O. Mechanism of parakeratosis. *Br. J. Dermatol.*, 82:268, 1970.
Colomb, B. and LaBatie, J-P. La pustule spongiforme de Kogoj. Apports de le microscope electronique. *Ann. Dermatol. Venereol.*, 104:707, 1977.
Cox, A. and Watson, W. Histologic variations in lesions of psoriasis. *Arch. Dermatol.*, 106:503, 1972.
Csonka, G. Multiple cases in Reiter's syndrome. *Br. J. Venereol. Dis.*, 45:157, 1969.
Dobson, R. The inheritance of psoriasis. *Arch. Dermatol.*, 116:657, 1980.
Doyle, J. et al. Immunofluorescence in psoriasis. *J. Am. Acad. Dermatol.*, 5:655, 1981.
Eisen, A. and Seegmiller, J. Uric acid metabolism in psoriasis. *J. Clin. Invest.*, 40:1486, 1961.
Elgjo, K. Epidermal chalone and cyclic AMP: An *in vivo* study. *J. Invest. Dermatol.*, 64:14, 1975.
Everall, J. Intractable pustular eruptions of the hands and feet. *Br. J. Dermatol.*, 69:269, 1957.
Farber, E. and Carlsen, R. Psoriasis in childhood. *Calif. Med.*, 105:415, 1966.
Farber, E. and McClintock, R., Jr. A current review of psoriasis. *Calif. Med.*, 108:440, 1968.

Farber, E., Nall, L. and Strefling, A. Psoriasis: A disease of the total skin. *J. Am. Acad. Dermatol.*, 12:150, 1985.

Farber, E., Nall, L. and Watson, W. Natural history of psoriasis in 5,600 patients. *Dermatologica*, 148:1, 1974.

——. Natural history of psoriasis in 61 twin pairs. *Arch. Dermatol.*, 109:207, 1974.

Farber, E., Nall, L. and Watson, W. Natural history of psoriasis in 5,600 patients. *Dermatologica*, 148:1, 1974.

Fry, L. The nature of psoriasis. *Br. J. Dermatol.*, 80:833, 1968.

Gordon, M. and Johnson, W. Histopathology and histochemistry of psoriasis. *Arch. Dermatol.*, 95:402, 1967.

Green, F. Distal interphalangeal joint disease and nail abnormalities. *Ann. Rheum. Dis.*, 27:55, 1968.

Grove, G. Epidermal cell kinetics in psoriasis. *Internat. J. Dermatol.*, 18:111, 1979.

Hancock, J. Surface manifestations of Reiter's disease in the male. *Br. J. Venereol. Dis.*, 36:36, 1960.

Harrist, T. and Mihm, M., Jr. Cutaneous immunopathology. *Hum. Pathol.*, 10:625, 1979.

Hellgren, L. Psoriasis: A statistical, clinical and laboratory investigation of 255 psoriatics and matched healthy controls. *Acta Derm. Venereol.* , 44:191, 1964.

Jablonska, S. et al. Autoimmunity in psoriasis: Relation of disease activity and forms of psoriasis to immunofluorescence findings. *Arch. Dermatol. Res.*, 261:135, 1978.

Jablonska, S. et al. History of psoriasis: The role of polymorphonuclear neutrophils. In: *Autoimmunity in Psoriasis*. Beutner, E., ed., Boca Raton, FL, CRC Press, 1982, p. 22.

Jablonska, S. et al. Immunopathology of psoriasis. *Arch. Dermatol. Res.*, 264:65, 1979.

Khan, M. and Hall, W. Progression of Reiter's syndrome to psoriatic arthritis. *Arch. Int. Med.*, 116:911, 1965.

Khan, S., Peterkin, G. and Mitchell, P. Juvenile generalized pustular psoriasis: A report of five cases and a review of the literature. *Arch. Dermatol.*, 105:67, 1972.

Kimura, S. and Nishikawa, T. An immunohistochemical analysis of the deposited immunoglobulins or fibrinogen in parakeratotic psoriatic horny layer and pemphigus skin lesions. *Arch. Dermatol. Res.*, 261:55, 1978.

Kingery, F., Chinn, H. and Saunders, T. Generalized pustular psoriasis. *Arch. Dermatol.*, 84:912, 1961.

Komura, J., Takigawa, M. and Ofuji, S. Epidermal cell-leukocyte interactions in spongiform pustules of Kogoj. *Arch. Dermatol. Forsch.*, 249:321, 1974.

Krueger, G. Psoriasis: Current concepts of its etiology and pathogenesis. In: *1981 Year Book of Dermatology*. Dobson, R. and Thiers, B., eds., Chicago, Year Book Medical Publishers, 1981, p. 13.

Krueger, G. and Eyre, R. Trigger factors in psoriasis. In: *Dermatology Clinics*. 2nd Ed., Weinstein, G. and Voorhees, J., eds., Philadelphia, W. B. Saunders, 1984, p. 373.

Kulka, J. The lesions ofeReiter's syndrome. *Arthritis Rheum.*, 5:195, 1962.

Lerner, M. and Lerner, A. Congenital psoriasis. *Arch. Dermatol.*, 105:598, 1972.

Lever, W. and Crawford, G. Keratosis blennorrhagica without gonorrhea (Reiter's disease?) *Arch. Dermatol. Syph.*, 49:389, 1944.

Lowe, N. and Ridgway, H. Generalized pustular psoriasis precipitated by lithium carbonate. *Arch. Dermatol.*, 114:1788, 1978.

McFadyen, T. and Lyell, A. Successful treatment of generalized pustular psoriasis (von Zumbusch) by systemic antibiotics controlled by blood culture. *Br. J. Dermatol.*, 85:274, 1971.

Marcelo, C. et al. Cyclic nucleotide levels in psoriatic and normal keratomed epidermis. *J. Invest. Dermatol.*, 72:20, 1979.

Matta, M. Blood and pustule culture in pustular psoriasis. *Br. J. Dermatol.*, 90:309, 1974.

Moll, J. The clinical spectrum of psoriatic arthritis. *Clin. Orthop.*, 143:66, 1979.

Montgomery, M. et al. The mucocutaneous lesions of Reiter's syndrome. *Ann. Int. Med.*, 51:99, 1959.

Muller, S. and Kitzmiller, K. Generalized pustular psoriasis: Report of two cases. *Acta Derm. Venereol.*, 42:504, 1962.

Murphy, F. and Stolman, L. Generalized pustular psoriasis. *Arch. Dermatol.*, 115:1215, 1979.

Neumann, E. and Hard, S. The significance of the epidermal sweat duct unit in the genesis of pustular psoriasis (von Zumbusch) and the microabscess of Munro-Sabouraud. *Acta Derm. Venereol.*, 54:141, 1974.

Norins, A. and Yaffee, H. Psoriasis of the hard palate: Report of a case. *Arch. Dermatol.*, 76:357, 1957.

Orfanos, C. et al. Alterations of cell surfaces as a pathogenetic factor in psoriasis. *Arch. Dermatol.*, 107:38, 1973.

Osterling, R. et al. Impetigo herpetiformis or generalized pustular psoriasis. *Arch. Dermatol.*, 114:1527, 1978.

Ozawa, A. et al. Some recent advances in HLA and skin diseases. *Am. Acad. Dermatol.*, 4:205, 1981.

Pascher, F. and Wood, W. Erythrodermic psoriasis in children: A report of two cases. *Arch. Dermatol.*, 74:173, 1956.

Penneys, N. et al. Pathogenesis of Woronoff ring in psoriasis. *Arch. Dermatol.*, 112:955, 1976.

Perry, H. and Mayne, J. Psoriasis and Reiter's syndrome. *Arch. Dermatol.*, 92:129, 1965.

Pindborg, J., Gorlin, R. and Asboe-Hansen, G. Reiter's syndrome: Review of the literature and report of a case. *Oral Surg.*, 16:551, 1963.

Pinkus, H. and Mehregan, A. The primary histologic lesion of seborrheic dermatitis and psoriasis. *J. Invest. Dermatol.*, 46:109, 1966.

Ragaz, A. and Ackerman, A. Evolution, maturation, and regression of lesions of psoriasis. *Am. J. Dermatopathol.*, 1:199, 1979.

Ross, J. The psoriatic capillary: Its nature and value in the identification of the unaffected psoriatic. *Br. J. Dermatol.*, 76:511, 1964.

Rowe, L., Dixon, W. and Forsythe, A. Mitoses in normal and psoriatic epidermis. *Br. J. Dermatol.*, 98:293, 1978.

Russell, T., Schultes, L. and Kuban, D. Histocompatibility (HL-A) antigens associated with psoriasis. *N. Eng. J. Med.*, 287:738, 1972.

Ryan, T. Microcirculation in psoriasis: Blood vessels, lymphatics and tissue fluid. *Pharmacol. Ther.*, 10:27, 1980.

——. A study of the epidermal capillary unit in psoriasis. *Dermatologica*, 138:459, 1969.

Samitz, M. and Albom, J. Palmar psoriasis. *Arch. Dermatol. Syph.*, 64:199, 1951.

Sanchez, N. et al. Subcorneal pustular dermatosis and pustular psoriasis: A clinicopathologic correlation. *Arch. Dermatol.*, 119:715, 1983.

Sauer, G. and Geha, B. Impetigo herpetiformis: Report of a case treated with corticosteroids. *Arch. Dermatol.*, 83:119, 1961.

Schachter, J. et al. Isolation of Bedsoniae from the joints of patients with Reiter's syndrome. *Proc. Soc. Exp. Biol. Med.*, 122:283, 1966.

Shatin, H., Canizares, O. and Ladany, E. Reiter's syndrome and keratosis blennorrhagica. *Arch. Dermatol.*, 81:551, 1960.

Shelley, W. and Kirschbaum, J. Generalized pustular psoriasis. *Arch. Dermatol.*, 84:73, 1961.

Shuster, S., Watson, A. and Marks, J. Small intestine in psoriasis. *Br. Med. J.*, 3:458, 1967.

Sidi, E., Zagula-Mally, Z. and Hincky, M. *Psoriasis*. Springfield, IL, Thomas, 1968.

Skog, E. Familial acrodermatitis continua (Hallopeau)—psoriasis. *Acta Derm. Venereol.*, 38:345, 1958.

Staricco, R. Altered capillary response to tape stripping in psoriasis and some other dermatoses: Petechial threshold test. *Dermatologica*, 160:315, 1980.

Van Scott, E. and Ekel, T. Kinetics of hyperplasia in psoriasis. *Arch. Dermatol.*, 88:373, 1963.

Voorhees, J. Role of cyclic AMP in the control of epidermal cell growth and differentiation. *Natl. Cancer Inst. Monograph*, 38:47, 1973.

Voorhees, J., Marcelo, C. and Duell, E. Cyclic AMP, cyclic GMP and glucocorticoids as potential metabolic regulators of epidermal proliferation and differentiation. *J. Invest. Dermatol.*, 65:179, 1975.

Voorhees, J. and Mier, P. The epidermis and cyclic AMP. *Br. J. Dermatol.*, 90:223, 1974.

Voorhees, J. et al. Decreased cyclic AMP in the epidermis of lesions of psoriasis. *Arch. Dermatol.*, 105:695, 1972.

Voorhees, J. et al. Increased cyclic GMP and decreased cyclic AMP levels in the hyperplastic abnormally differentiated epidermis of psoriasis. *Life Sciences*, 13:639, 1973.

Voorhees, J. et al. Increased cyclic GMP and decreased cyclic AMP levels in the rapidly proliferating epithelium of psoriasis. In: *The Role of Cyclic Nucleotides in Carcinogenesis*, Vol. 6, Schultz, J. and Gratzner, H. eds., New York, Academic Press, 1973, p. 325.

Wagner, G., Luckasen, J. and Goltz, R. Mucous membrane involvement in generalized pustular psoriasis. *Arch. Dermatol.*, 112:1010, 1976.

Weddell, G. et al. Psoriatic skin. *Arch. Dermatol.*, 91:252, 1965.

Weinberger, H. et al. Reiter's syndrome, clinical and pathologic observations: A long term study of 16 cases. *Medicine*, 41:35, 1962.

Weinstein, G. and Frost, P. Abnormal cell proliferation in psoriasis. *J. Invest. Dermatol.*, 50:254, 1968.

Weinstein, G. and Van Scott, E. Autoradiographic analysis of turnover times of normal and psoriatic epidermis. *J. Invest. Dermatol.*, 45:257, 1965.

White, S. et al. Disturbance of HL-A antigen frequency in psoriasis. *N. Eng. J. Med.*, 287:740, 1972.

Wright, V. Psoriatic arthritis: A comparative radiographic study of rheumatoid arthritis and arthritis associated with psoriasis. *Ann. Rheum. Dis.*, 20:123, 1961.

——. Rheumatism and psoriasis: A re-evaluation. *Am. J. Med.*, 27:424, 1959.

Wright, V. and Reed, W. The link between Reiter's syndrome and psoriatic arthritis. *Ann. Rheum. Dis.*, 23:12, 1964.

Zachariae, H. Pathological findings in internal organs of patients with severe psoriasis. *Acta Derm. Venereol.* (Stockh.), (87, suppl.):87, 1979.

Zaias, N. Psoriasis of the nail. *Arch. Dermatol.*, 99:567, 1969.

Pityriasis Rubra Pilaris

Aguilar, A. et al. Pityriasis rubra pilaris with joint and muscle involvement. *Dermatologica*, 146:361, 1973.

Brunsting, L. and Sheard, C. Dark adaptation in pityriasis rubra pilaris. *Arch. Dermatol. Syph.*, 43:42, 1941.

Davidson, C., Jr., Winkelmann, R. and Kierland, R. Pityriasis rubra pilaris: A follow-up study of 57 patients. *Arch. Dermatol.*, 100:175, 1969.

Griffiths, W. Pityriasis rubra pilaris. *Clin. Exp. Dermatol.*, 5:105, 1980.

Gross, D., Landau, J. and Newcomer, V. Pityriasis rubra pilaris: Report of a case and analysis of the literature. *Arch. Dermatol.*, 99:710, 1969.

Huntley, C. Pityriasis rubra pilaris. *Am. J. Dis. Child.*, 122:22, 1971.

Marshall, J. Case of pityriasis rubra pilaris with lesions of buccal mucosa. *Arch. Dermatol. Syph.*, 66:626, 1952.

Niemi, K. et al. Pityriasis rubra pilaris. *Dermatologica*, 152:109, 1976.

Stanoeva, L., Konstantinov, D. and Ristov, R. Clinical aspect of pityriasis rubra pilaris in childhood. *Dermatologica*, 142:1, 1971.

Chapter 8
Drug Reactions

Mechanisms of drug eruptions vary, but the majority are allergic.

In most instances the histologic changes in drug reactions are nonspecific. In a smaller number of cases, the histologic pattern of a drug reaction will simulate that of an idiopathic histologic entity. Only rarely can a specific drug be suspected on the basis of microscopic cutaneous changes.

Nonspecific reaction patterns produced by drugs include dermatitis, perivasculitis, inflammatory purpura, vasculitis (lymphocytic and leukocytoclastic), noninflammatory purpura, panniculitis (particularly erythema nodosum), and folliculitis.

Histologic changes produced by drugs which simulate more specific histologic entities include erythema multiforme-like eruptions (including erythema multiforme bullosum), lupus erythematosus-like eruptions, lichenoid drug eruptions, and arsenical keratoses.

Fixed drug eruption may be regarded as a variant of erythema multiforme-like drug eruption. It may be localized or generalized and has a tendency to recur in the same sites when the eliciting drug is administered. Clinical manifestations include the morphologic range typical of erythema multiforme. An important feature of fixed drug eruption is the tendency to develop post-inflammatory hyperpigmentation, resulting in a slate blue color. Histologically, this hyperpigmentation is represented by "melanophages" in the dermis as well as by an increase in epidermal melanin (a pattern observed in other types of post-inflammatory hyperpigmentation).

Drug-induced coma and carbon monoxide poisoning may result in intraepidermal or subepidermal bullae and sweat gland necrosis. Eccrine glands become deeply eosinophilic; their nuclei become pyknotic and ultimately disappear.

Lichenoid drug eruptions are often due to antimalarials, phenothiazines, and gold, but can be due to a variety of drugs. The histologic picture may be identical to that of idiopathic lichen planus, but sometimes differs by showing more parakeratosis, spongiosis, and the presence of eosinophils.

Lupus erythematosus-like drug eruptions are often due to hydralazine (apresoline) but can be caused by other drugs (procaine amide, reserpine, hydantoin derivatives, griseofulvin, penicillin, sulfonamides, and methadone). These eruptions parallel spontaneous lupus erythematosus in most respects. However, unlike spontaneous lupus erythematosus, the direct immunofluorescence test does not commonly show antibodies at the epidermal-dermal junction in normal-appearing skin.

Keratoses produced by prolonged ingestion of inorganic trivalent arsenicals can have a histologic pattern resembling that of Bowen's disease (see p. 794).

Penicillamine can induce changes in the skin similar to anetoderma, elastosis perforans serpiginosa, or pemphigus. Anovulatory drugs can produce changes similar to scleroderma.

DRUG REACTIONS continued

FIXED DRUG ERUPTION

Fixed drug eruption may be regarded as a variant of erythema multiforme-like drug eruption. It may be localized or generalized and has a tendency to recur in the same sites when the eliciting drug is administered. Clinical manifestations include the morphologic range of erythema multiforme. Early lesions often have a violaceous color (Figs. A,B); bullae may occur. Late lesions usually show post-inflammatory hyperpigmentation and have a brownish or slate-blue color (Fig. C). Phenolphthalein and the barbiturates are frequent causes.

Microscopic features

1. Early lesions show histologic features of erythema multiforme. There may be hydropic degeneration of the basal layer or extensive epidermal necrosis (Fig. D) such as is observed in toxic epidermal necrolysis. Bullae may form subepidermally, as in erythema multiforme.
2. Late lesions show nonspecific post-inflammatory hyperpigmentation with many "melanophages" in the dermis (Fig. E).

FIXED DRUG ERUPTION

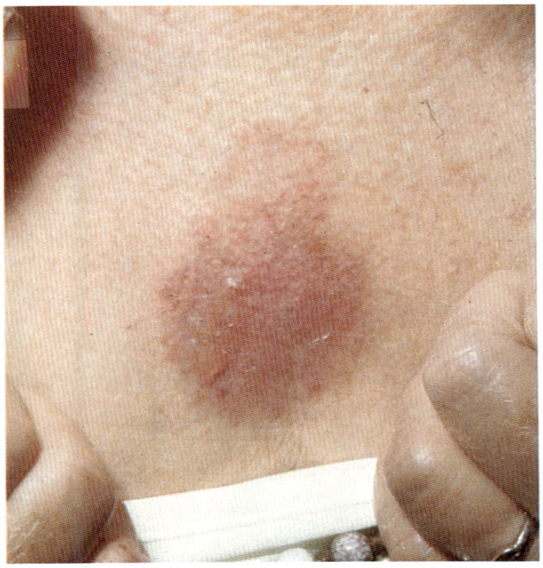

A

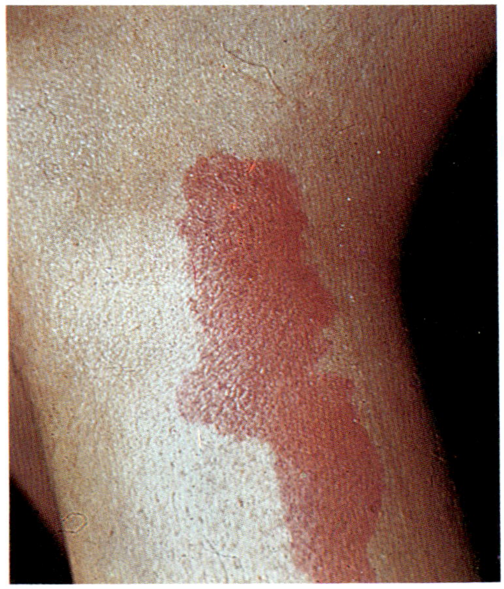

B

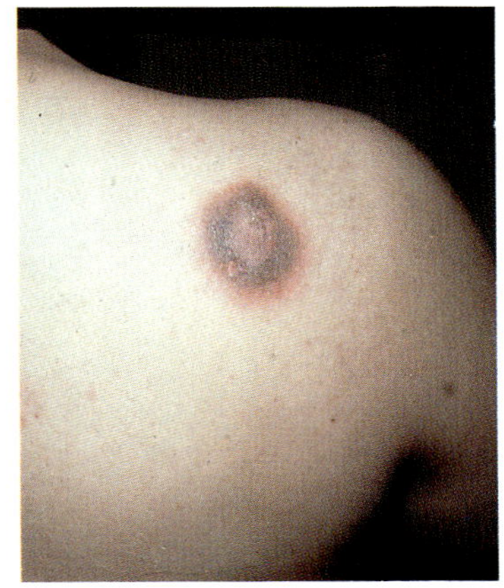

C

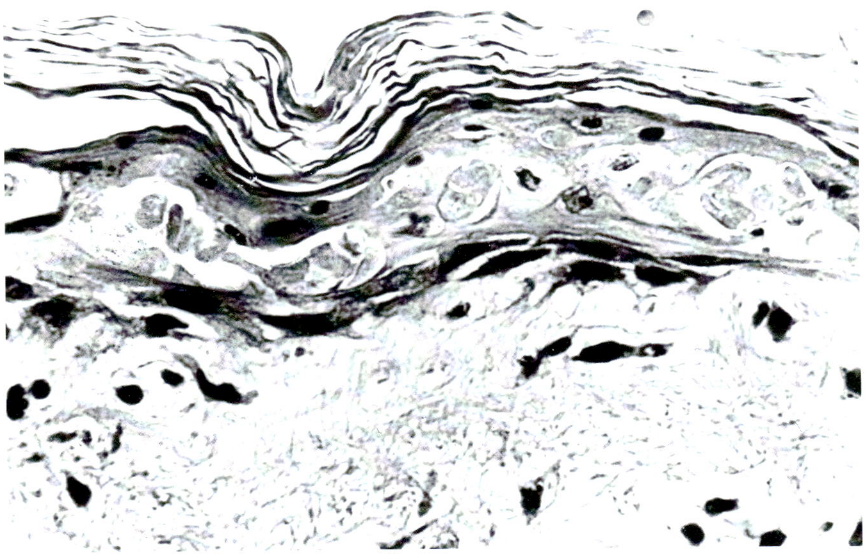

D
X680

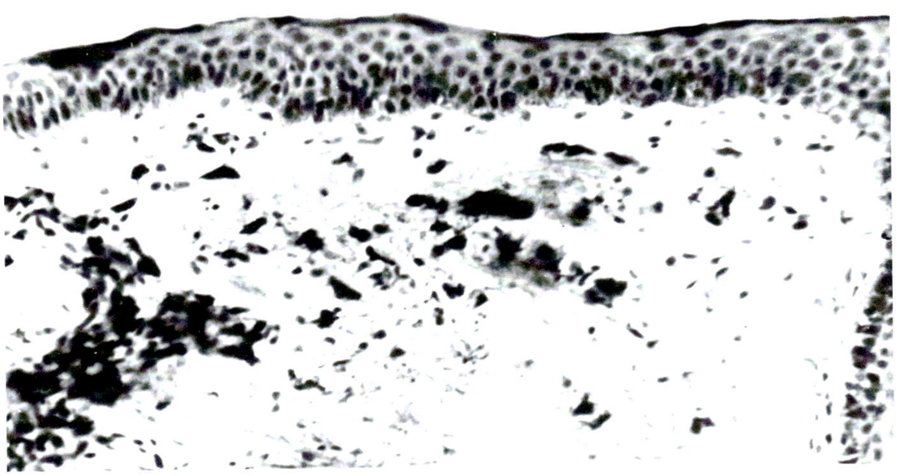

E
X260

Courtesy Dr. John Knox

DRUG REACTIONS continued ⇨

Drug Reactions with Special Histologic Features

BROMODERMA AND IODODERMA

Intake of iodides or bromides may result in verrucous, vegetating lesions (Figs. A,B) (halide granulomas) or acneiform eruptions (Fig. C). Such halide reactions may be a manifestation of delayed hypersensitivity. Acneiform eruptions are more common in iododerma.

Microscopic features

1. The epidermis shows pseudoepitheliomatous hyperplasia. Intraepidermal abscesses containing neutrophils, eosinophils, and histiocytes (Figs. D,E) are present.
2. A dermal infiltrate is present, composed of a mixture of inflammatory cells (Figs. D,E). Abscesses may develop in the dermis.
3. Extensive capillary proliferation is present (Figs. D,E), and is often accompanied by hemorrhage and necrosis.
4. Iododerma generally shows less epithelial proliferation than bromoderma and a greater tendency towards ulceration. Histiocytes in the dermal infiltrate in iododerma may show mitotic activity and nuclear hyperchromasia, which results in a resemblance to mycosis cells of mycosis fungoides (see p. 1332).

Microscopic differential diagnosis

1. Bromoderma and iododerma are differentiated from blastomycosis and other deep mycoses by the absence of organisms and giant cells (see p. 358).
2. Pemphigus vegetans (see p. 538) can usually be differentiated from halide granuloma by the presence of acantholysis.

Comment

Fluoride from fluoride gel applied to gums may produce a papular or nodular eruption of the posterior auricular area and neck. This application is used to prevent caries during irradiation therapy. The inflammation is mild. There are neutrophils and eosinophils with microabscesses in the epidermis.

BROMODERMA AND IODODERMA

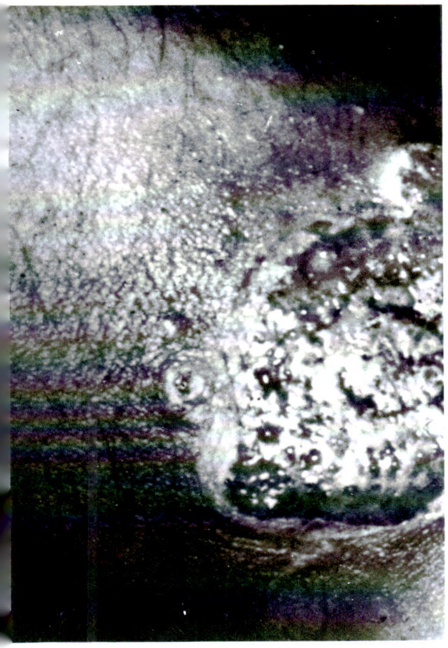
A

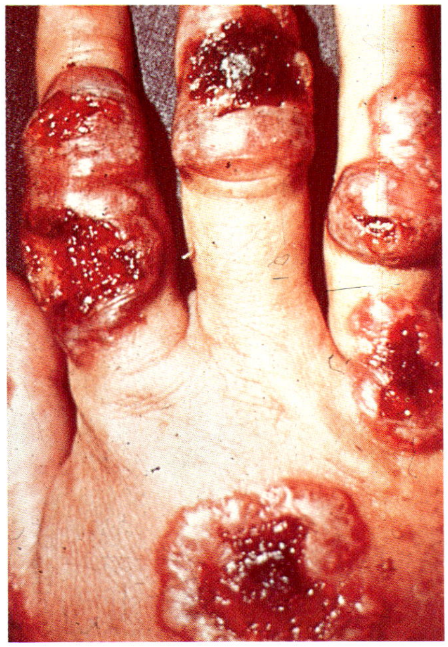
B Courtesy Dr. Harvey Ansell

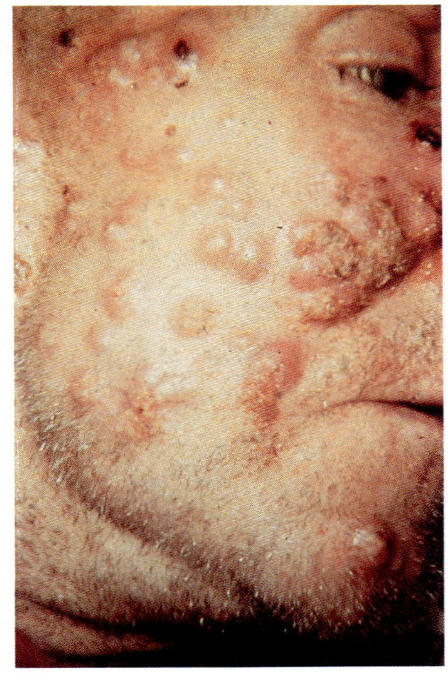
C

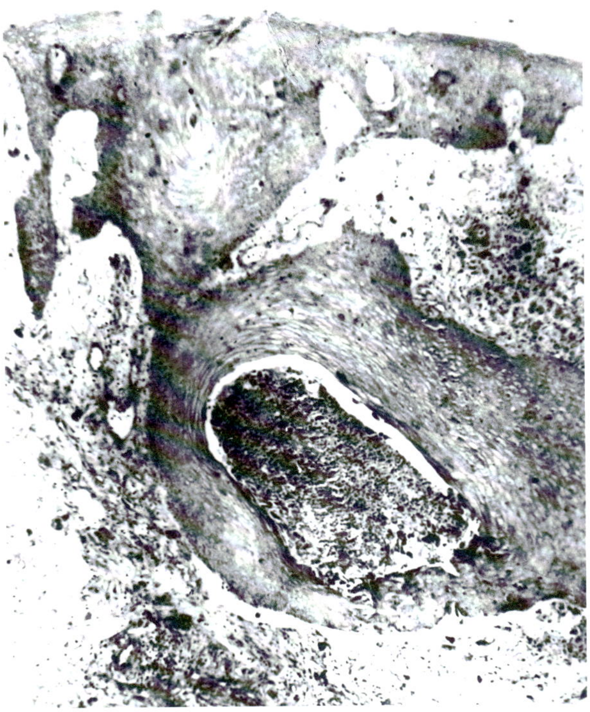
D
X120

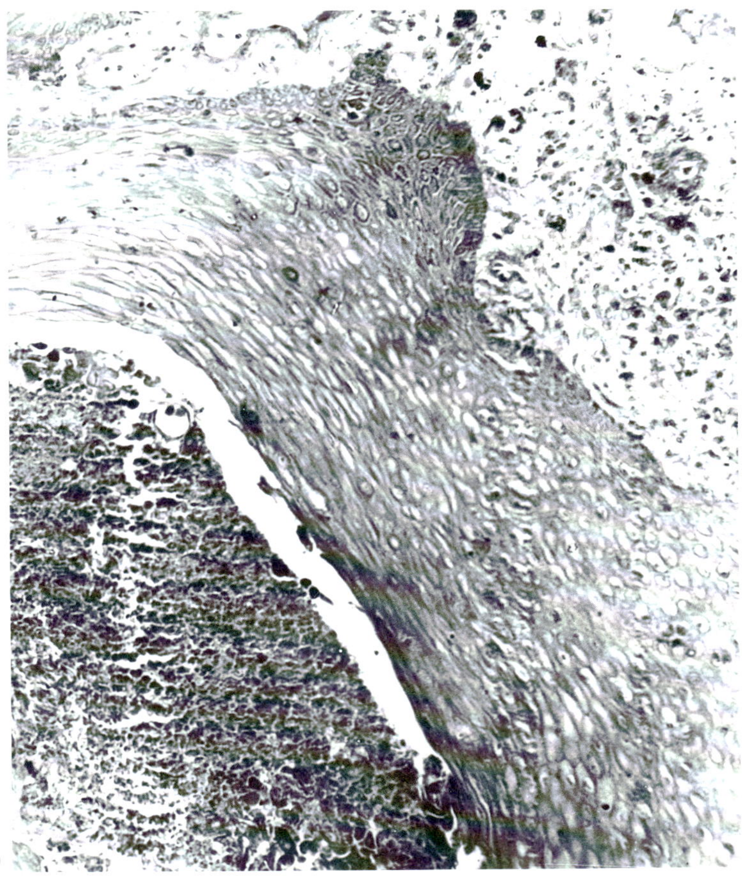
E
X440

DRUG REACTIONS continued

Drug Reactions with Special Histologic Features

ARGYRIA, CHRYSIASIS, AND LOCALIZED MERCURIALISM

Systemic administration of silver or gold salts may result in a diffuse slate-gray pigmentation on the exposed areas of the body (Fig. B); prolonged topical application of silver salts may result in similar changes of the sclerae (Fig. A). With silver salts, but not with gold salts, there may be pigmentation of the oral mucosa. Prolonged topical application of mercury salts may also result in slate-gray discoloration of the skin.

Microscopic features

1. With brightfield microscopy, gold or silver particles appear as brownish granules about 1 micron or less in diameter; they are refractile with darkfield microscopy.
2. Silver granules are absent in the epidermis. They are deposited in the tissue spaces of the dermis (Fig. C), in the membrana propria of sweat glands (Fig. D), in the connective tissue sheaths around hair follicles and sebaceous glands, in dermal phagocytes (Fig. C), in arrectores pilorum, and in the elastic fibers. There is an associated increase in melanin in both the basal epidermis and in dermal "melanophages." The clinical manifestations of argyria are due principally to this increased melanization. The increased melanization is limited to the exposed parts of the body.
3. Gold particles are present in the epidermis and endothelial cells as well as in phagocytes of the dermis. They are sometimes present in the tissue spaces, but are absent in membrana propria of sweat glands.

   As in argyria, melanin is increased both in the epidermis and dermis, and this is the cause of the bluish-gray discoloration of the skin.
4. Localized mercurialism shows a picture similar to that of argyria.

Comment

Antimalarials can produce a grayish pigmentation of the pretibial skin and of the oral mucosa, mainly the hard palate.

ARGYRIA

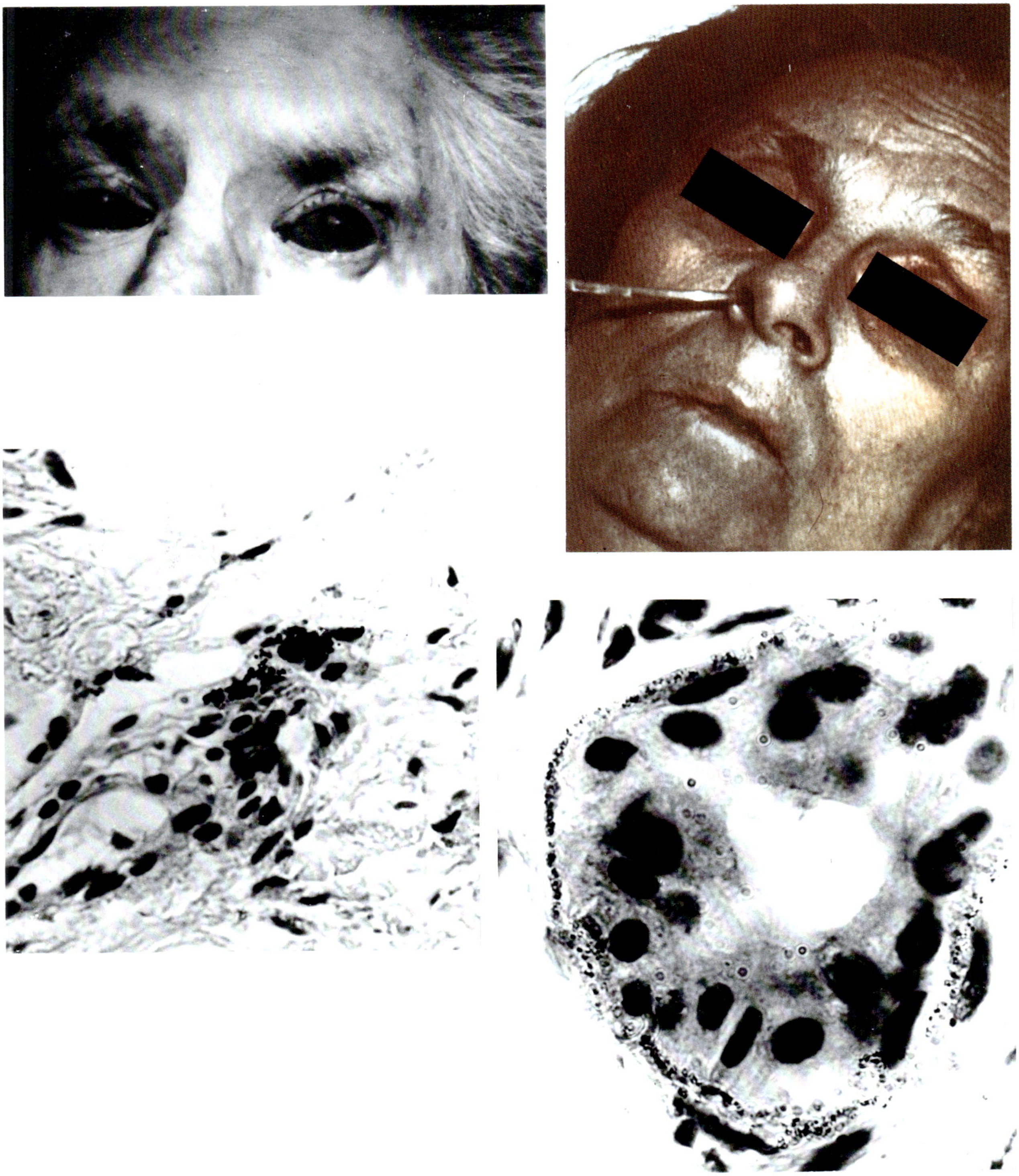

A

B

C
X820

D
X1300

Suggested Reading

Drug Reactions

General References

Alexander, H. *Reactions with Drug Therapy*. Philadelphia, W. B. Saunders, 1955.

Arndt, K. and Jick, H. Rates of cutaneous reactions to drugs. *JAMA*, 235:918, 1976.

Brown, E. Problems of drug allergy, *JAMA*, 1577:814, 1955.

Cohen, S. and Feldman-Armstrong, M. *Drug Interactions*. Baltimore, Williams & Wilkins, 1974.

Dash, C. and Jones, H. *Mechanisms in Drug Allergy*. Baltimore, Williams & Wilkins, 1972.

Davidson, B. et al. Cimetidine-associated exacerbation of cutaneous lupus erythematosus. *Arch. Int. Med.*, 142:101, 1982.

de Weck, A. Drug reactions. In: *Immunological Diseases*. 2nd Ed., Sampter, M. ed., Boston, Little, Brown, 1971, p. 415.

Emmett, E. Phototoxicity from exogenous agents. *Photochem. Photobiol.*, 30:429, 1979.

Fellner, M. and Baer, R. Cutaneous reaction to drugs. *Med. Clin. N. Amer.*, 49:709, 1965.

Friedlander, M., Chisari, F. and Baer, H. Role of inflammatory response of skin and lymph nodes in induction of sensitization to simple chemicals. *J. Immunol.*, 111:164, 1973.

Girard, J. et al. Immunological mechanisms and diagnostic tests in allergic drug reactions. *Ann. Clin. Res.*, 3:74, 1976.

Leroy, J. et al. Deux cas de pigmentation cutanée au cours de traitements par la minocycline. *Ann. Dermatol. Venereol.*, 108:871, 1981.

Levantine, A. and Almeyda, J. Cutaneous reactions to food and drug additives. *Br. J. Dermatol.*, 91:359, 1974.

——. Drug reactions. XXIV: Cutaneous reactions to cytostatic agents. *Br. J. Dermatol.*, 90:239, 1974.

McGrae, J., Jr. and Zelickson, A. Skin pigmentation secondary to minocycline therapy. *Arch. Dermatol.*, 116:1262, 1980.

Mullick, F. et al. Drug related vasculitis. *Hum. Pathol.*, 10:313, 1979.

Neumann, H. and van Joost, T. Adverse reactions of the skin to metroprolol and beta-adrenergic-blocking agents. *Dermatologica*, 162:330, 1981.

Rosenheim, M. and Moulton, R. *Sensitivity Reactions to Drugs*. Oxford, Blackwell, 1958.

Samter, M. and Parker, C. *Hypersensitivity to Drugs*. New York, Pergamon Press, 1972.

Saurat, J. et al. Cell-mediated hypersensitivity in skin reactions to drugs. *Clin. Allerg.*, 3:427, 1973.

Stewart, G. and McGovern, J. *Penicillin Allergy: Clinical and Immunological Aspects*. Springfield, IL, Thomas, 1970.

Swidler, G. *Handbook of Drug Interactions*. New York, Wiley-Interscience, 1971.

Warrington, R. et al. Drug hypersensitivities with special reference to penicillin. In: *Immediate Hypersensitivity, Modern Concepts and Developments*. Bach, M., ed., New York/Basel, Dekker, 1978, p. 749.

Lichenoid Drug Reactions

Bereston, E. Lichenoid dermatitis: Observation of two hundred cases from the Dermatology Section, Medical Branch, DeWitt General Hospital, Auburn, California. *J. Invest. Dermatol.*, 7:69, 1946.

Buckley, W. Lichenoid eruptions following contact dermatitis. *Arch. Dermatol.*, 78:454, 1958.

Dinsdale, R., Ormerod, T. and Walker, A. Lichenoid eruption due to chlorpropamide. *Br. Med. J.*, 1:100, 1968.

Feder, A. Clinical observations on atypical lichen planus and related dermatoses presumably due to atabrine toxicity. *Ann. Int. Med.*, 31:1078, 1949.

Fry, L. Skin disease from colour developers. *Br. J. Dermatol.*, 77:456, 1965.

Groth, O. Lichenoid dermatitis resulting from treatment with the phenothiazine derivatives metopromazine and laevomepromazine. *Acta Derm. Venereol.*, 41:168, 1961.

Holt, P. and Navaratnum, A. Lichenoid eruption due to methyldopa. *Br. Med. J.*, 3:234, 1974.

Reinhardt, L. et al. Lichenoid eruption produced by captopril. *Cutis,* 31:98, 1983.
Sarkany, I. Lichen planus following quinidine therapy. *Br. J. Dermatol.,* 79:123, 1967.
Wilson, D. Eczematous and pigmentary lichenoid dermatitis: Atypical lichen planus: Preliminary report. *Arch. Dermatol. Syph.,* 54:377, 1946.
Winer, L. and Leeb, A. Lichenoid eruptions: A histopathological study. *Arch. Dermatol. Syph.,* 70:274, 1954.

Lupus Erythematosus-like Drug Reactions

Alarcon-Segovia, D. et al. Clinical and experimental studies on the hydralazine syndrome and its relationship to systemic lupus erythematosus. *Medicine,* 46:1, 1967.
Blomgren, S., Condemi, J. and Vaughan, J. Procainamide-induced lupus erythermatosus: Clinical and laboratory observations. *Am. J. Med.,* 52:338, 1972.
Blumenkrantz, N. and Asboe-Hansen, G. Connective-tissue effects of drugs causing lupoid syndrome. *Acta Derm. Venereol.,* 54:35, 1974.
Condemi, J. et al. Antinuclear antibodies following hydralazine toxicity. *N. Eng. J. Med.,* 276:486, 1967.
Dubois, E. Procainamide induction of a systemic lupus erythematosus-like syndrome. *Medicine,* 48:217, 1969.
Dubois, E., Tallman, E. and Wonka, R. Chlorpromazine-induced systemic lupus erythematosus: Case report and review of the literature. *JAMA,* 221:595, 1972.
Gaultier, C. et al. Lupus induit par l'isoniazide. *Ann. Pediat.* (Paris), 19:459, 1972.
Hahn, B. et al. Immune responses to hydralazine and nuclear antigens in hydralazine-induced lupus erythematosus. *Ann. Int. Med.,* 76:365, 1972.
Lee, S., Rivero, I. and Siegel, M. Activation of systemic lupus erythematosus by drugs. *Arch. Int. Med.,* 117:620, 1966.
Leigh, I. Mepacrine (quinacrine) pigmentation in systemic lupus erythematosus: New data from an ultrastructural, biochemical and analytical electron microscopy investigation. *Br. J. Dermatol.,* 101:147, 1979.
Sheldon, P. and Williams, W. Procainamide-induced systemic lupus erythematosus. *Ann. Rheum. Dis.,* 29:236, 1970.
Ullman, S. et al. Drug-induced lupus erythematosus syndrome: Immunopathologic, electron microscopic and serologic studies. *Acta Derm. Venereol.,* 54:387, 1974.
Weiss, R. and Swift, S. The significance of a positive lupus erythematosus phenomenon. *Arch. Dermatol.,* 72:103, 1955.
Whittle, T., Jr. and Ainsworth, S. Procainamide-induced systemic lupus erythematosus. *Arch. Pathol.,* 100:469, 1976.

Drug-induced Coma Associated with Sweat Gland Necrosis and Bullae

Brehmer-Anderson, E. and Pederson, N. Sweat gland necrosis and bullous changes in acute drug intoxication. *Acta Derm. Venereol.,* 49:157, 1969.
Herschthal, D. and Robinson, M. Blisters of the skin in coma induced by amitriptyline and clorazepate dipotassium. *Arch. Dermatol.,* 115:499, 1979.
Leavell, U., Farley, C. and McIntire, J. Cutaneous changes in a patient with carbon monoxide poisoning. *Arch. Dermatol.,* 99:429, 1969.
Mandy, S. and Ackerman, A. Characteristic traumatic skin lesions in drug-induced coma. *JAMA,* 213:253, 1970.
Varma, A., Fisher, B. and Sarin, M. Diazepam induced coma with bullae and eccrine sweat gland necrosis. *Arch. Int. Med.,* 137:1207, 1977.

Penicillamine-Induced Dermatoses

Bardach, H. and Gebhart, W. Penicillamininduzierte dermolytische Dermatose bei einer Patientin mit Morbus Wilson. *Dermatologica,* 162:473, 1981.
Bardach, H., Gebhart, W. and Niebauer, G. "Lumpy-bumpy" elastic fibers in the skin and lungs of a patient with penicillamine-induced elastosis perforans serpiginosa. *J. Cutan. Pathol.,* 6:243, 1979.

Charles, R. In discussion of Davis, W.: Wilson's disease and penicillamine-induced anetoderma. *Arch. Dermatol.*, 113:976, 1977.
Davis, W. Wilson's disease and penicillamine-induced anetoderma. *Arch. Dermatol.*, 113:976, 1977.
Degos, R. et al. Pemphigus chez un malade traité par pénicillamine pour maladie de Wilson. *Bull. Soc. Fr. Dermatol. Syph.*, 76:751, 1969.
From, E. and Frederiksen, P. Pemphigus vulgaris following D-penicillamine. *Dermatologica*, 152:358, 1976.
Greer, K., Askew, F. and Richardson, D. Skin lesions induced by penicillamine. *Arch. Dermatol.*, 112:1267, 1976.
Guilaine, J., Benhamon, J. and Molas, G. Élastome perforant verruciforme chez un malade traité par pénicillamine pour maladie de Wilson. *Bull. Soc. Fr. Dermatol. Syph.*, 79:450, 1972.
Hashimoto, K., McEvoy, B. and Belcher, R. Ultrastructure of penicillamine-induced skin lesions. *J. Am. Acad. Dermatol.*, 4:300, 1981.
Katz, R. Penicillamine-induced skin lesions. *Arch. Dermatol.*, 95:196, 1967.
Kirsch, N. and Hukill, P. Elastosis perforans serpiginosa induced by penicillamine. *Arch. Dermatol.*, 113:630, 1977.
Kristensen, J. and Wadskov, S. Penicillamine-induced pemphigus foliaceus. *Acta Derm. Venereol.* (Stockh.), 57:69, 1977.
Marsden, R. et al. Pemphigus foliaceus induced by penicillamine. *Br. Med. J.*, 2:1423, 1976.
Pass, F. et al. Elastosis perforans serpiginosa during penicillamine therapy for Wilson disease. *Arch. Dermatol.*, 108:713, 1973.
Sparrow, G. Penicillamine pemphigus and the nephrotic syndrome occurring simultaneously. *Br. J. Dermatol.*, 98:103, 1978.

Fixed Drug Eruption

Chargin, L. and Leifer, W. Fixed eruptions due to the arsphenamines. *J. Invest. Dermatol.*, 3:443, 1940.
De Dobbeleer, G. and Achten, G. Fixed drug eruption, ultrastructural study of dyskeratotic cells. *Br. J. Dermatol.*, 96:239, 1977.
Klevansky, H. and Kingsley, H. Fixed drug eruptions caused by dyes. *S. Afr. Med. J.*, 38:216, 1964.
Savin, J. Current cases of fixed drug eruptions. *Br. J. Dermatol.*, 83:546, 1970.
Shelley, W., Schlappner, O. and Heiss, H. Demonstration of intercellular immunofluorescence and epidermal hysteresis in bullous fixed drug eruption due to phenolphthalein. *Br. J. Dermatol.*, 86:118, 1972.
Stritzler, C. and Kopf, A. Fixed drug eruption caused by 8-chlortheophylline in dramamine with clinical and histologic studies. *J. Invest. Dermatol.*, 34:319, 1960.
Tarnowski, W. Fixed drug eruption due to tetracyclines. *Acta Derm. Venereol.*, 50:117, 1970.
Welsh, A. *The Fixed Eruption: A Possible Hazard of Modern Drug Therapy.* Springfield, IL, Thomas, 1961.
Welsh, A. and Ede, M. The fixed eruption: A possible hazard of modern drug therapy. *Arch. Dermatol.*, 84:1004, 1961.
Wyatt, E., Greaves, M. and Søndergaard, J. Fixed drug eruption (phenolphthalein): Evidence for a blood-borne mediator. *Arch. Dermatol.*, 106:671, 1972.

Halide Eruptions

Aquilina, J. and Bissell, G. Fungating iododerma treated with hydrocortisone. *JAMA*, 158:727, 1955.
Blasik, L. and Spencer, S. Fluoroderma. *Arch. Dermatol.*, 115:1334, 1979.
Heydenreich, G. and Larsen, P. Iododerma after high dose urography in an oliguric patient. *Br. J. Dermatol.*, 97:567, 1977.
Hollander, L. and Fetterman, G. Fatal iododerma: The eleventh case reported in the literature. *Arch. Dermatol. Syph.*, 34:228, 1936.
Jones, L., Pariser, H. and Murray, P. Recurrent iododerma. *Arch. Dermatol.*, 78:353, 1958.
Leibl, K. Bromoderma tuberosum. *Derm. Wschr.*, 137:681, 1958.
Perroud, H. and Delacrétaz, J. Iodides végétantes. *Ann. Dermatol. Venereol.*, 104:154, 1977.

Rosenberg, F. et al. Vegetating iododerma: An immunologic mechanism. *Arch. Dermatol.*, 105:900, 1972.
Teller, H. Bromoderma und Iododerma tuberosum. *Derm. Wschr.*, 143:273, 1961.

Argyria

Burge, K. and Winkelmann, R. Mercury pigmentation: An electron microscopic study. *Arch. Dermatol.*, 102:51, 1960.
Harker, J. and Hunter, D. Occupational argyria. *Br. J. Dermatol.*, 47:441, 1935.
Hill, W. and Montgomery, H. Argyria: With special reference to the cutaneous histopathology. *Arch. Dermatol. Syph.*, 44:588, 1941.
Hill, W. and Pillsbury, D. *Argyria: The Pharmacology of Silver*. Baltimore, Williams & Wilkins, 1939.
Johannson, E. et al. Generalized argyria. *Clin. Exp. Dermatol.*, 7:169, 1982.
Lamar, L. and Bliss, B. Localized pigmentation of the skin due to topical mercury. *Arch. Dermatol.*, 93:450, 1966.
Mehta, A., Dawson-Butterworth, K. and Woodhouse, M. Argyria: Electron microscopic study of a case. *Br. J. Dermatol.*, 78:175, 1966.
Prose, P. An electron microscopic study of human generalized argyria. *Am. J. Pathol.*, 42:293, 1963.
Reymond, J., Stoebner, P. and Amblard, P. Argyrie cutanée. *Ann. Dermatol. Venereol.*, 107:251, 1980.

Chrysiasis

Driver, J. and Weller, J. Untoward results from the use of gold compounds: Report of a fatal case. *Arch. Dermatol. Syph.*, 23:87, 1931.
Penneys, N., Ackerman, A. and Gottlieb, N. Gold dermatitis: Clinical and histologic study. *Arch. Dermatol.*, 109:372, 1974.
Roenigk, H. and Handel, D. Gold vasculitis. *Arch. Dermatol.*, 109:253, 1974.
Schamberg, J. Chrysoderma: A permanent gold staining of the skin. *Arch. Dermatol. Syph.*, 18:862, 1928.
Schmidt, O. Chrysiasis. *Arch. Dermatol. Syph.*, 44:446, 1941.
Wigley, J. Some observations on the deposition of gold in the skin. *Br. J. Dermatol.*, 44:69, 1932.

Chapter 9
Connective Tissue Diseases

The designation "connective tissue diseases" includes a diverse group of disorders having important morphologic and immunologic features in common. The old designation was "collagen diseases," and a more recent designation was "connective tissue immunopathies." Although autoimmunity is a key feature in this group of disorders, all of the observed phenomena cannot be explained on this basis.

Connective tissue and vascular changes are important in this group of disorders.

Lupus erythematosus, dermatomyositis, scleroderma, rheumatic fever, and rheumatoid arthritis are among disorders considered to be in this category. Discussion of rheumatoid nodule is in the chapter on degenerative dermatoses since the histologic features are similar to those of granuloma annulare and necrobiosis lipoidica.

Connective tissue diseases

LUPUS ERYTHEMATOSUS

It is now generally agreed that lupus erythematosus encompasses a spectrum of clinical and laboratory manifestations. At one end of the spectrum is discoid lupus erythematosus (DLE), with localized skin (and/or mucous membrane) lesions; at the other end of the spectrum is systemic lupus erythematosus (SLE), which is associated with systemic lesions. An older view that DLE and SLE are separate diseases has been generally rejected; however, conversion of well-established cases of DLE into SLE is uncommon.

Intermediate types include disseminated DLE, with widespread cutaneous lesions and mild systemic involvement, and subacute cutaneous lupus erythematosus, which shows widespread nonscarring cutaneous lesions (often annular and polycyclic), severe photosensitivity, and mild systemic illness.

Photosensitivity plays an important role in the development of skin lesions of both DLE and SLE.

Immunologic changes are most pronounced in SLE and least pronounced in DLE. The antinuclear antibody test (ANA) is positive in significant titers in only a minority of patients with DLE but is positive in a high percentage of patients with SLE. The lupus band test indicates the presence of immune complex at the epidermal-dermal junction and is positive in involved skin in 90% of cases of DLE and SLE. In uninvolved skin, the lupus band test is almost always negative in DLE. It is positive in 50% of patients with SLE. The LE cell test is negative in DLE and frequently positive in SLE. The LE cell test and anti-native DNA test are regarded as having a high specificity for SLE. There is a subset of SLE, with a negative ANA test, anticytoplasmic antibodies, photosensitivity eruption, and a low incidence of renal disease.

Diagnosis of SLE is made on considering a spectrum of clinical and laboratory data. The American Rheumatism Association (ARA) has delineated a series of clinical and laboratory findings from which they recommend a diagnosis of SLE if four are present simultaneously.

Systemic manifestations of SLE include arthralgia, nephritis, serositis, seizures, psychoses, Raynaud's phenomenon, fever, and malaise.

Cutaneous lesions are present in all cases of DLE, but not in all cases of SLE. Cutaneous lesions in DLE tend to be more specific than those of SLE, both clinically and histologically. When specific histologic changes of LE are present, histologic findings cannot make a definite distinction between DLE and SLE. Hyperkeratosis and inflammation tend to be more pronounced in DLE than in SLE. Nonspecific histologic patterns in SLE include perivasculitis, vasculitis, and edema. Occasionally, lesions are present which resemble malignant atrophic papulosis. Livedo reticularis or thrombophlebitis may occur.

COMPARISON OF CLINICAL AND LABORATORY FEATURES OF DLE AND SLE

	DLE	SLE
1. Prognosis	good	variable; may be poor
2. Cutaneous lesions	always present	present in 80% of cases
3. Symptoms of systemic illness	absent	may be present; include fever and malaise
4. Systemic lesions	absent	present: include polyserositis, endocarditis, glomerulitis, CNS disease, peripheral neuropathy, and hemolytic anemia
5. Laboratory findings		
thrombocytopenia	absent	frequently present
leukopenia	absent	frequently present
anemia	absent	frequently present
sedimentation rate	normal	usually elevated
LE cell test	negative	frequently positive
ANA test	4% to 33% positive	usually positive in a significant titer
Biologic false positive STS	absent	common
Demonstration of antibody at basement zone of epidermis (direct immunoflourescent test [lupus "band" test])	positive in lesions only	positive in lesions and may be positive in uninvolved skin; "cytoid" bodies may be present

The LE cell test is based on observation of LE bodies in phagocytes. The LE body is a nucleus that has interacted with ANA with subsequent extrusion from the cell. LE bodies may be found in systemic lesions of LE and are called *hematoxylin bodies* there.

LUPUS ERYTHEMATOSUS continued ⇨

Cutaneous lesions of lupus erythematosus

Discoid lupus erythematosus

The central areas of the face (Figs. A,B,C,D,E,F), forehead, scalp (Fig. H), and ears are most frequently involved, but lesions may appear in any area of the skin, as well as the lips and oral mucosa (Fig. G). Lesions may be solitary, few in number, or (in the disseminated type) numerous and generalized. Early lesions are well-defined, infiltrated erythematous areas. With progression, focal hyperkeratotic areas appear ("carpet tack" or "grains of sand" pattern) (Figs. B,C,D). The hyperkeratotic areas correspond to "follicular plugs" observed microscopically. Verrucous hyperkeratotic areas may be present. Atrophy (Figs. E,F), telangiectasia, hyperpigmentation and hypopigmentation (Figs. E,F), and scarring alopecia are common sequelae of longstanding lesions of DLE. Ulceration and, rarely, squamous cell carcinoma, may develop in longstanding lesions.

A rare variant of DLE is *lupus profundus*, a nodular panniculitis.

LUPUS ERYTHEMATOSUS

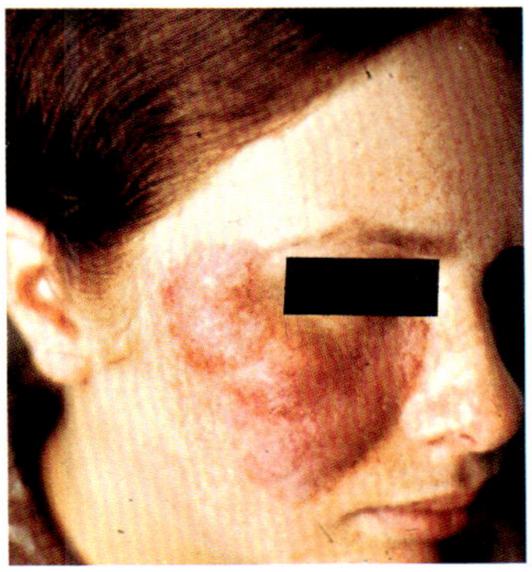

A

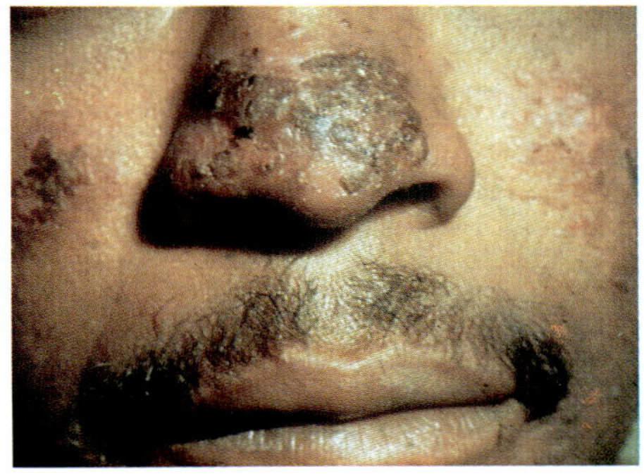

B

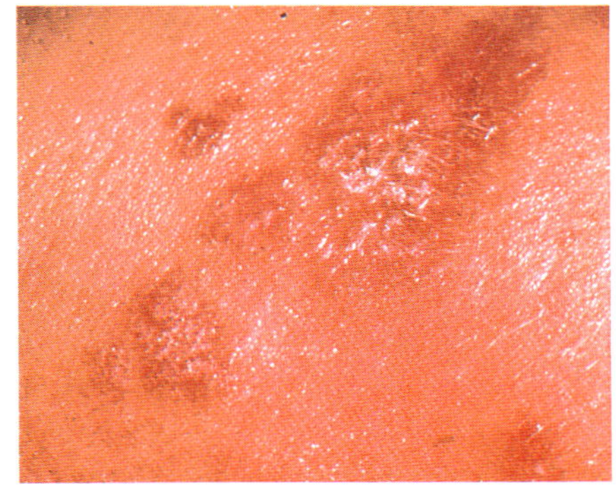

C

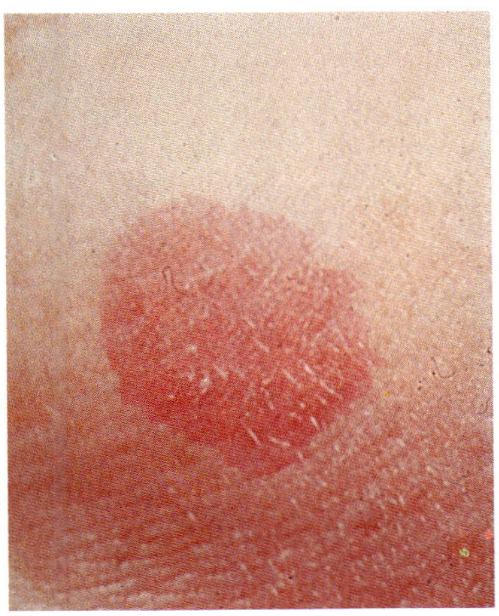

D

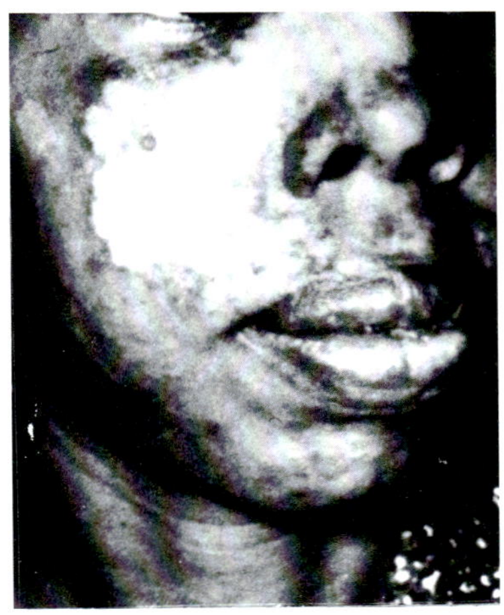

E

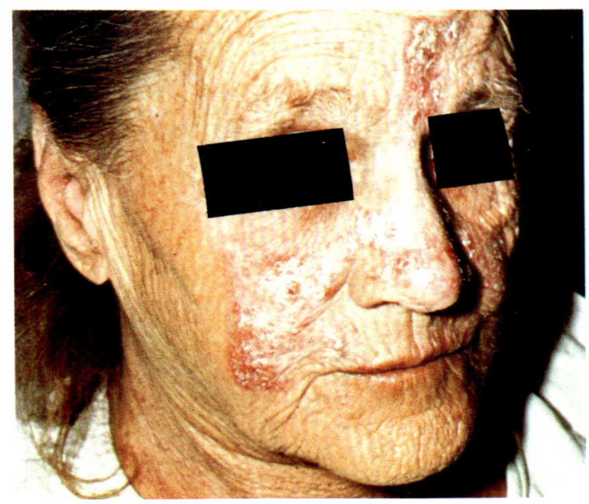

F

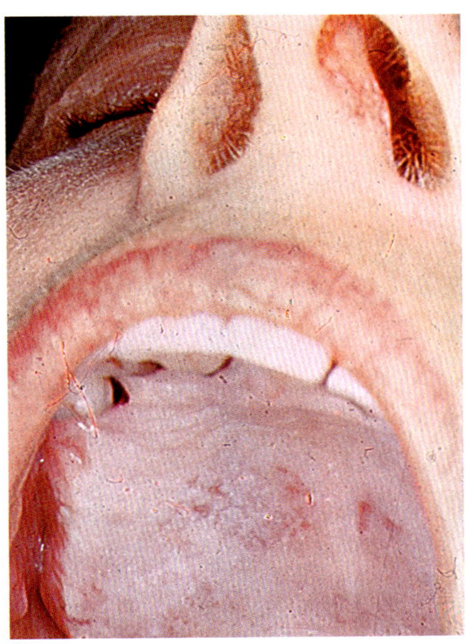

G

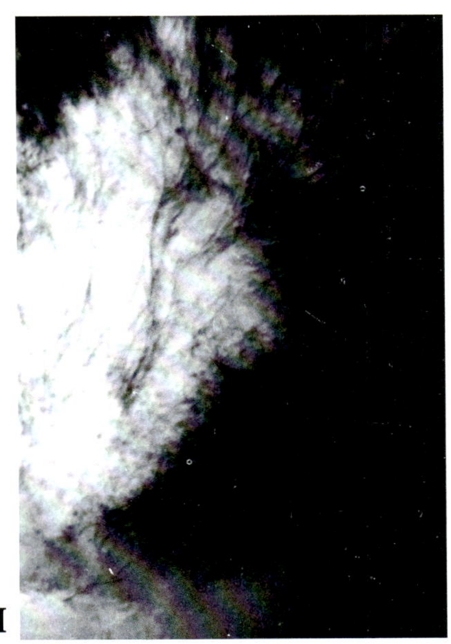

H

LUPUS ERYTHEMATOSUS continued ⇨

Cutaneous lesions of lupus erythematosus

Systemic lupus erythematosus

Cutaneous lesions of systemic lupus erythematosus are quite varied, but generally appear as erythematous areas in the central portions of the face ("butterfly" rash) (Fig. A). Vesicles occasionally develop. Hyperkeratosis, atrophy, and pigmentary changes are generally not as evident as in DLE, but sometimes the cutaneous lesions may be identical to those of DLE.

Diffuse maculopapular, erythematous, and scaling lesions are common. Other cutaneous manifestations of SLE include inflammatory purpura, bullae (Fig. B), and ulcerations. Poikiloderma may be present (Fig. C). Note relationship to sun exposure in the illustration. Areas of reticulate telangiectatic erythema may appear on the extremities, particularly in the periungual skin.

Lupus profundus (Fig. D) is more common in SLE than in DLE; there are subcutaneous nodules. Subcutaneous nodules resembling rheumatoid nodules may also occur in SLE.

Lesions of urticarial vasculitis may be present (showing leukocytoclastic vasculitis microscopically). Lesions clinically and histologically identical to those of Degos disease may be seen.

LUPUS ERYTHEMATOSUS

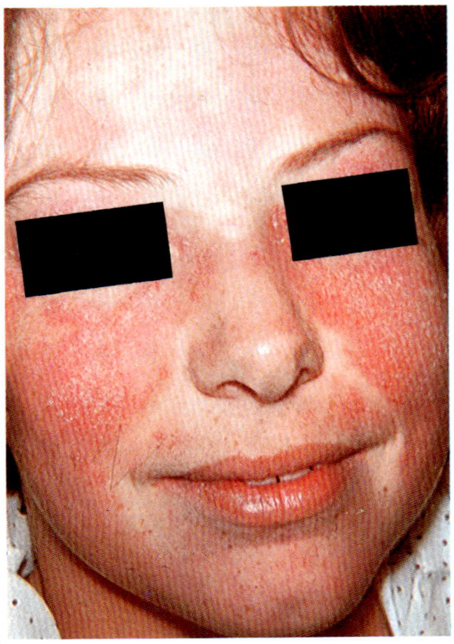

A

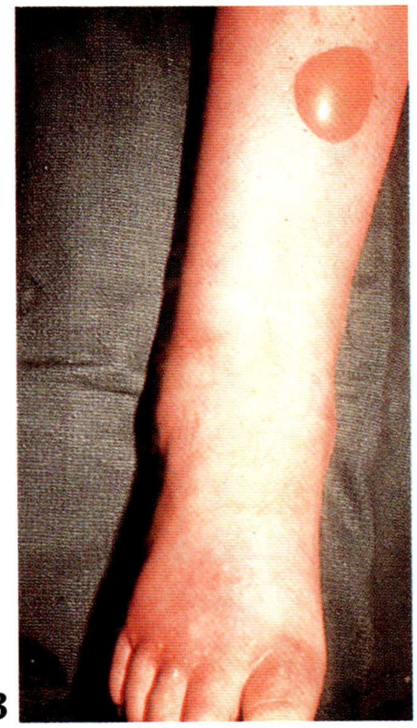

B

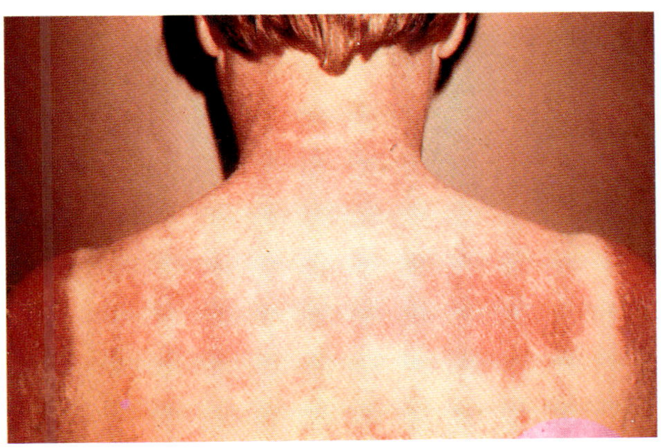

C

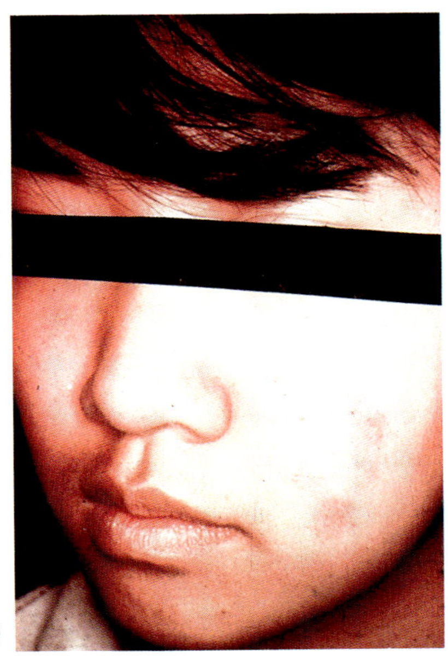

D

LUPUS ERYTHEMATOSUS continued

LUPUS ERYTHEMATOSUS

Microscopic features

Histologic changes of DLE and SLE tend to differ only in degree, and unequivocal differentiation cannot be made histologically. Some lesions of SLE are entirely nonspecific histologically.

1. There is hyperkeratosis with hyperkeratotic invaginations of the epidermis (Figs. A,B). These invaginations are called "follicular plugs," although they do not always correspond to follicular openings. "Keratotic plugging" is a better designation.
2. The epidermis is usually atrophic (Fig. B), although in rare cases it may be hypertrophic and verrucous.
3. There is liquefaction (hydropic) degeneration of the basal cells of the epidermis (Figs. B,C) and outer root sheath; in some fields this change may be minimal or absent (Fig. A).
4. The upper dermis often shows edema (Fig. B), hemorrhage, capillary dilatation (Fig. C), and "melanophages" (Fig. C).
5. There is a dense, patchy infiltrate composed principally of lymphoid cells; this has a tendency to surround cutaneous appendages, particularly pilosebaceous units (Figs. A,B).
6. The subcutaneous fat is often involved in SLE, and less often in DLE. There is nonspecific panniculitis; mucoid degeneration of fat and thickening of trabeculae separating fat lobules may be present. In lupus profundus the changes in the fat are more pronounced; in this form of LE, lymphoid follicles may be observed, as well as calcification.
7. There may be an increase in dermal ground substance (hyaluronic acid). This is usually more evident in SLE than in DLE.

LUPUS ERYTHEMATOSUS

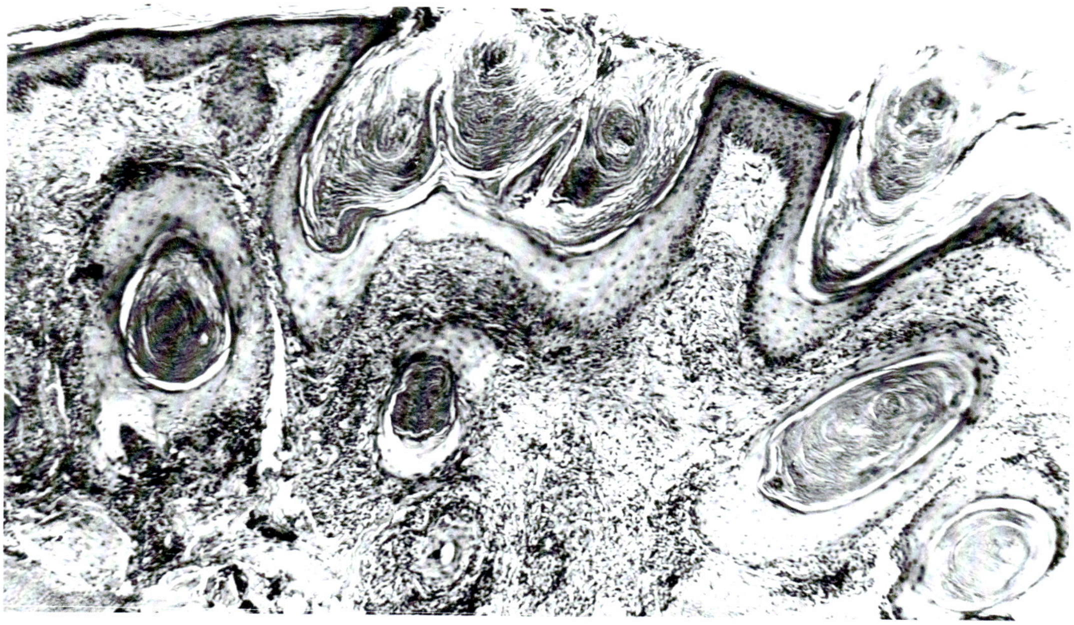

A
X60

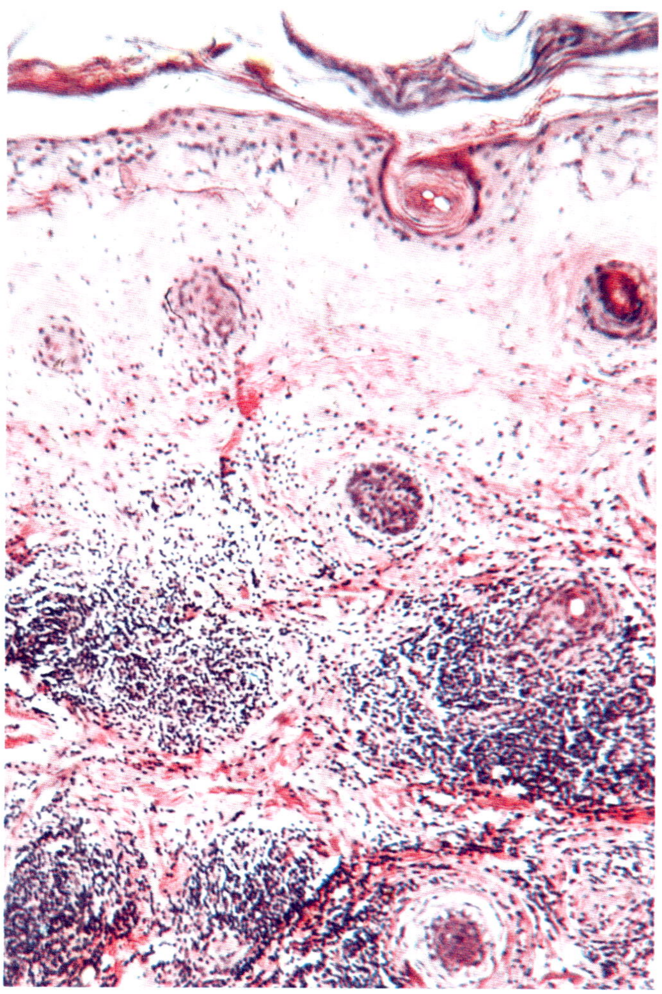

B X80

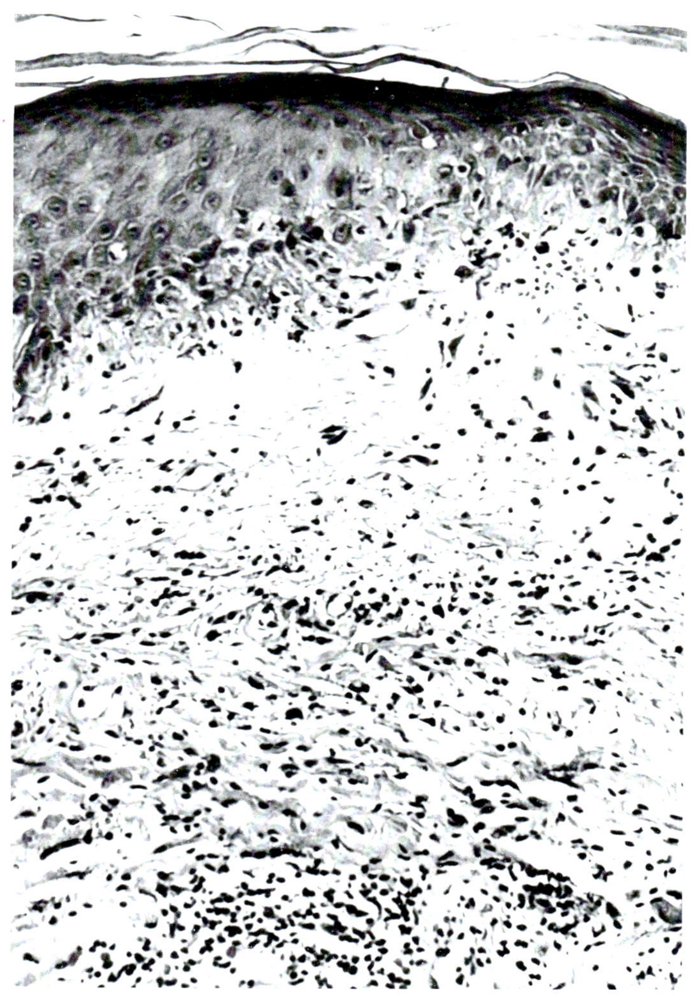

C X220

LUPUS ERYTHEMATOSUS continued

LUPUS ERYTHEMATOSUS

Microscopic features
(high magnification of the epidermal-dermal junction)

1. There is hydropic degeneration of the basal layer (Figs. A,B,C,D).
2. Thickening of the basement zone due to deposition of PAS-positive immune complex and complement and/or PTAH-positive fibrin is present (Fig. B). In SLE, PAS-positive, diastase-resistant fibrinoid material is also deposited around capillaries and between collagen bundles. This occurs more often in SLE than in DLE.
3. Severe hydropic degeneration of the basal layer may lead to epidermal-dermal separation (Fig. B). Well-formed subepidermal bullae may also be present.
4. Colloid bodies similar to those observed in lichen planus (see p. 440) may be present (Fig. C, arrow).
5. Edema of the papillary dermis is generally evident (Figs. A,B,C,D).
6. "Melanophages" and extravasated red blood cells are often observed in the papillary dermis (Fig. D).

LUPUS ERYTHEMATOSUS

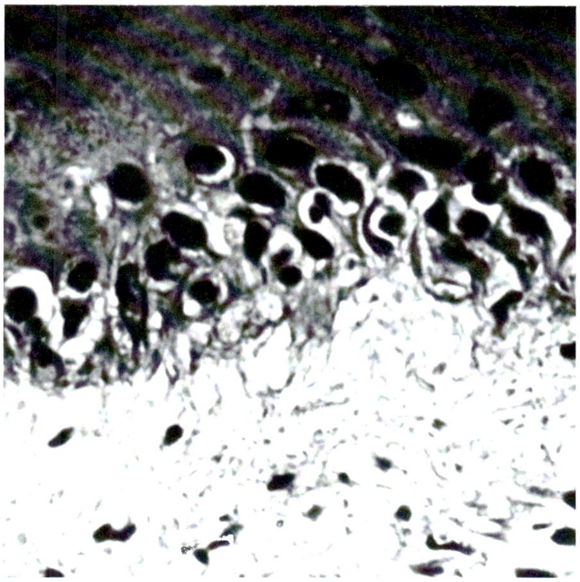

A X600

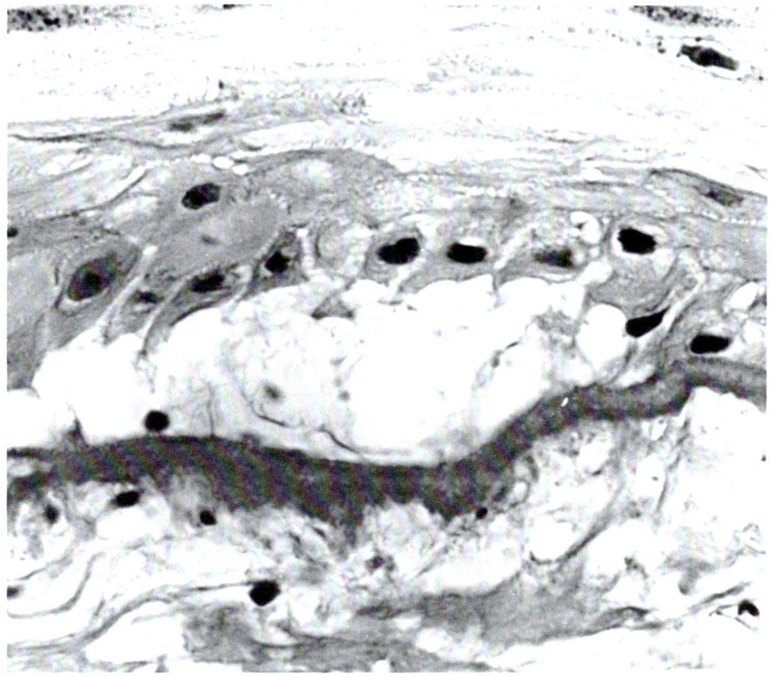

B X600

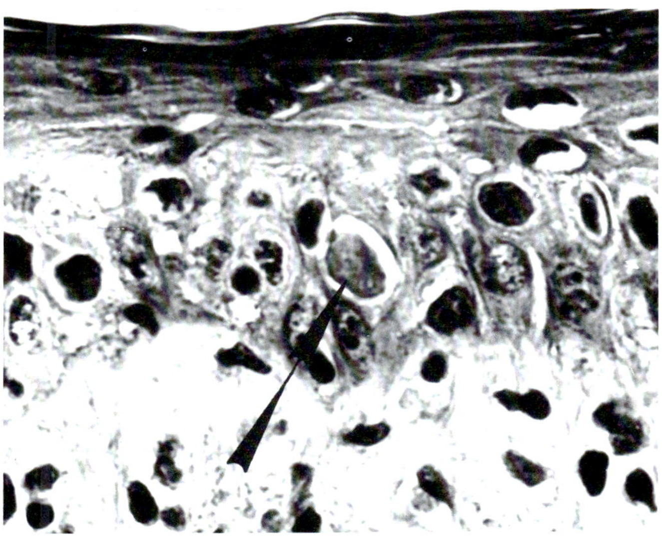

C X600

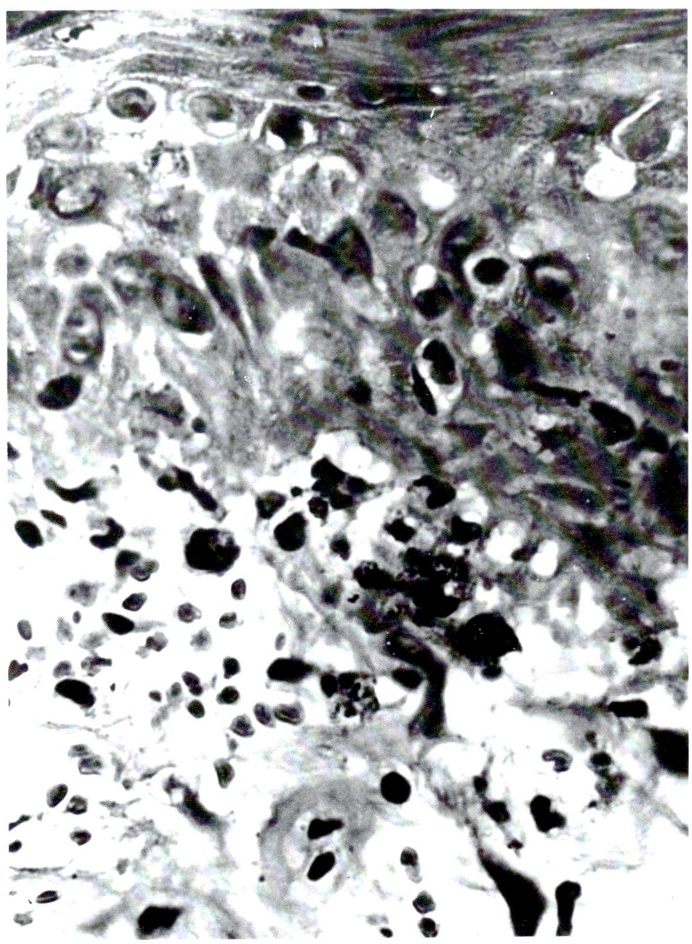

D X640

LUPUS ERYTHEMATOSUS continued

LUPUS ERYTHEMATOSUS

Microscopic variations

1. In late lesions, telangiectasia may be pronounced (Fig. A). The histologic picture may be identical to that of idiopathic poikiloderma (see p. 616), with epidermal atrophy, hydropic degeneration of the basal layer, a band-like infiltrate in the upper dermis, and "pigmentary incontinence" characterized by "melanophages."
2. Progression of epidermal-dermal separation may lead to bulla formation (Fig. B). This is more common in SLE than in DLE.
3. Hydropic damage may be observed in the basal layer of the outer root sheath of hair follicles (Figs. C,D). This change, together with the surrounding infiltrate, produces a resemblance to lichen planopilaris (see p. 448).

Microscopic differential diagnosis

1. Lichen sclerosus et atrophicus (see p. 656) also shows hyperkeratosis with follicular plugging, epidermal atrophy, hydropic degeneration of the basal layer, and edema of the upper dermis. However, lichen sclerosus et atrophicus can usually be identified by the extreme degree of the edema of the upper dermis as well as by its "ground-glass" quality. Also, lichen sclerosus et atrophicus generally shows sclerosis of the deeper dermis, which is absent in lupus erythematosus.
2. There is a resemblance between atrophic solar keratosis (see p. 782) and lupus erythematosus. Distinction can generally be made on the basis of nuclear atypia in epidermal cells of solar keratosis. However, in some instances differentiation can be very difficult, particularly since lesions of lupus erythematosus are often present in sun-exposed areas, which show solar damage of collagen.
3. Lupus erythematosus must also be differentiated from other conditions showing a patchy dermal infiltrate, such as lymphoma and secondary syphilis. In such cases, differentiation can generally be made on the basis of the epidermal changes of lupus erythematosus, as well as on the basis of the specific histologic features associated with other conditions.
4. Dermatomyositis may show cutaneous changes identical to those of lupus erythematosus (see p. 502).
5. Polymorphous light eruption of the plaque type and some forms of lymphocytic infiltration of the skin of Jessner-Kanof may be variants of lupus erythematosus, differing by the degree of epidermal change (see p. 500).
6. Erythema dyschromicum perstans shows hydropic damage of the basal layer of the epidermis, but lacks hyperkeratotic plugging, epidermal atrophy, and a patchy periappendageal infiltrate.
7. Bullous lupus erythematosus may be difficult to distinguish from other subepidermal bullous dermatoses.

LUPUS ERYTHEMATOSUS

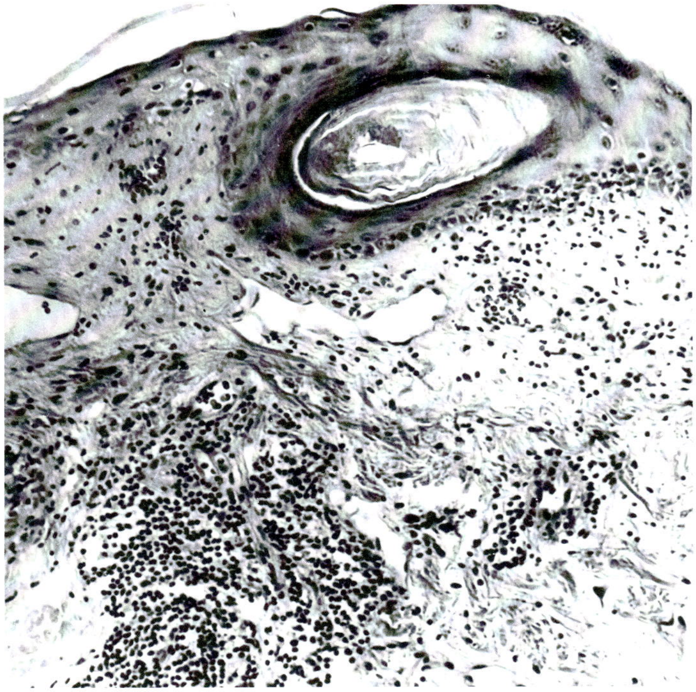

A
X160

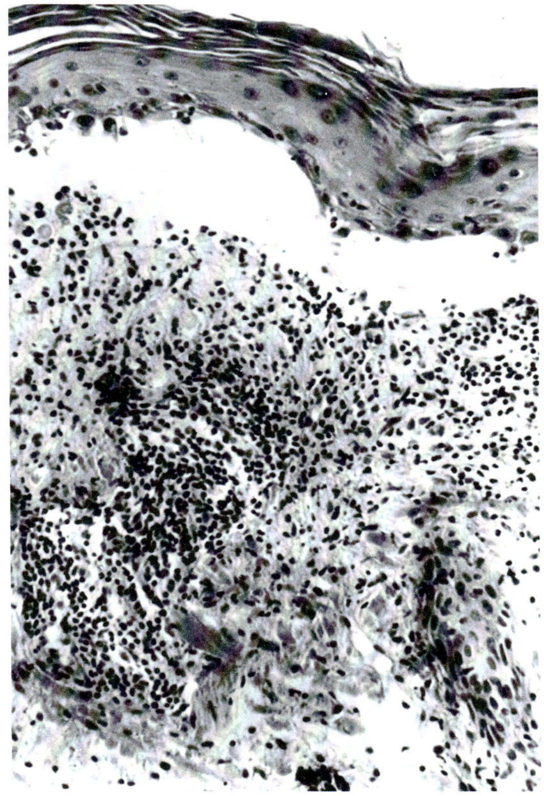

B
X157

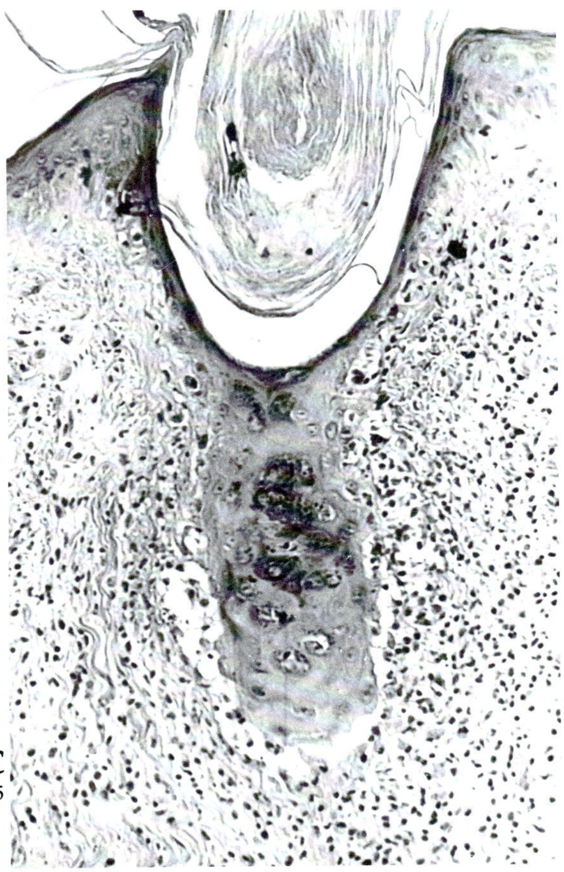

C
X195

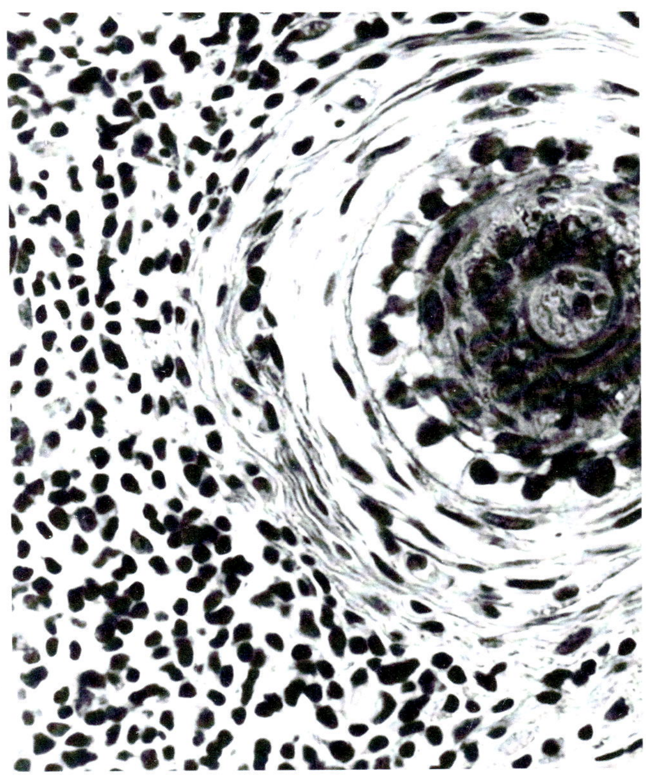

D X530

LUPUS ERYTHEMATOSUS continued ⇨

HISTOLOGIC COMPARISON OF DLE AND SLE

1. Hyperkeratosis and hyperkeratotic plugging are more pronounced in DLE.
2. Atrophy of the malpighian layer of the epidermis is usually more pronounced in SLE.
3. Liquefaction degeneration of the basal layer is usually more pronounced in SLE.
4. Edema, vasodilatation and hemorrhage in the upper dermis are more pronounced in SLE.
5. Bullous lesions are more common in SLE.
6. The dermal infiltrate is usually more pronounced in DLE.
7. Atrophy and disappearance of the pilosebaceous units are more common in DLE.
8. Deposition of PAS-positive fibrinoid material around capillaries and between collagen bundles which is observed in SLE, is not as frequently observed in DLE, although PAS-positive thickening of the basement zone is not uncommon in DLE. Mucinous changes may be observed in the dermis in SLE.
9. Scarring is more common in DLE.
10. Late development of squamous cell carcinoma is more common in lesions of DLE.

SYSTEMIC LESIONS OF SLE

Systemic lesions of SLE often show a necrotizing vasculitis involving small arteries and arterioles, with deposition of fibrinoid material in the vessel walls. Fibrous thickening of vessel walls is common. The spectrum of kidney changes includes mesangial lupus nephritis, focal proliferative glomerular lesions, diffuse proliferative glomerulonephritis, and membranous glomerulonephritis.

Comment

1. *Lichen planus/lupus erythematosus overlap syndrome* shows features of both diseases. Most reported cases have had features of discoid lupus erythematosus (DLE), but a few have had features of systemic lupus erythematosus (SLE). Chronic bluish-red patches with tendency towards atrophy have been described in the overlap syndrome.
2. SLE is frequently associated with systemic scleroderma or dermatomyositis. This has been called overlap syndrome. Overlap syndrome is different from mixed connective tissue disease (MCTD) which is considered to be a distinct entity, which features scleroderma, SLE, rheumatoid arthritis, and myositis. Patients with MCTD have antibodies to an extractable nuclear antigen (ENA).

LUPUS ERYTHEMATOSUS continued ⌜

IMMUNOFLUORESCENCE TESTS FOR LE

1. The lupus band test is a direct immunofluorescence test for the presence of immunoglobulins and complement at the basement zone. 3 mm or 4 mm specimens of unfixed skin are submitted either frozen, wrapped in saline-impregnated gauze, or immersed in phosphate-buffered saline. Specimens are snap-frozen in liquid nitrogen and stored at −70°C. Cryostat sections are stained with fluorescein-conjugated antisera to IgA, IgG, IgM, and C3. A positive test is characterized by a granular band along the epidermal-dermal junction (Figs. A,B).

   When involved skin is tested for diagnosis, over 90% of specimens of DLE and SLE are positive.

   When uninvolved, sun-exposed skin is taken for diagnostic purposes, over 80% of patients with untreated SLE are positive, whereas the lupus band test is almost always negative in DLE. The specimen is usually taken from the dorsal surface of the forearm.

   When uninvolved, sun-protected skin (usually from the buttock or volar aspect of the forearm) is taken for prognostic purposes, there is a correlation between incidence of positivity of the LE band test and the severity of renal disease in SLE.
2. The ANA test is an indirect immunofluorescence test which uses mouse liver sections as substrate. With a serum dilution of 1:20 there is a positive test in over 90% of patients with untreated SLE. At this titer approximately 20% of patients with DLE, most patients with systemic scleroderma, and up to 5% of normal individuals show positivity. A titer of 1:160 or above with a peripheral nuclear staining pattern is considered to be virtually diagnostic of SLE. SLE tends to have homogeneous (Fig. C) or peripheral (Fig. D) patterns, whereas scleroderma tends to produce speckled or nucleolar patterns.

POLYMORPHOUS LIGHT ERUPTION OF THE PLAQUE TYPE; LYMPHOCYTIC INFILTRATION OF THE SKIN OF JESSNER; HYDROA VACCINIFORME; ACTINIC RETICULOID

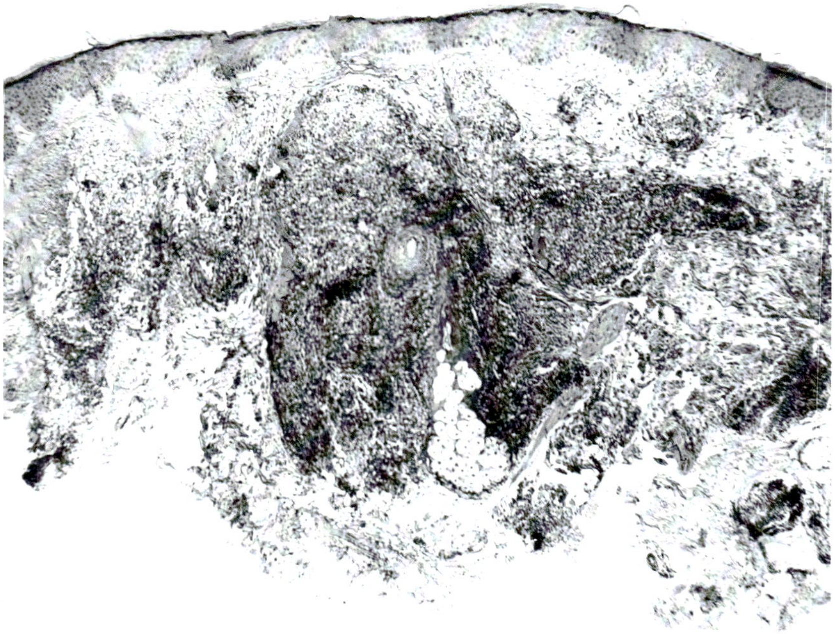

A
X55

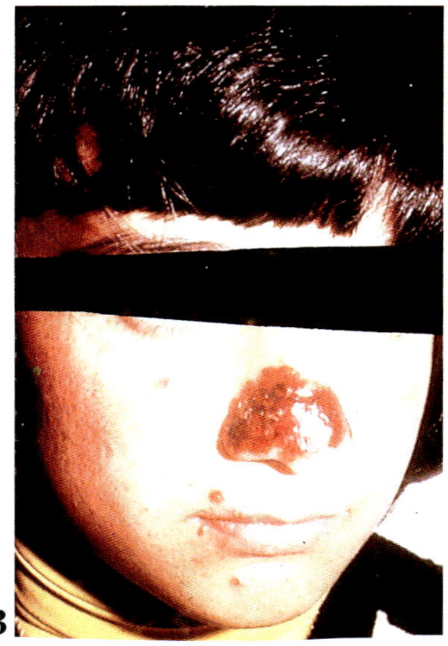

B

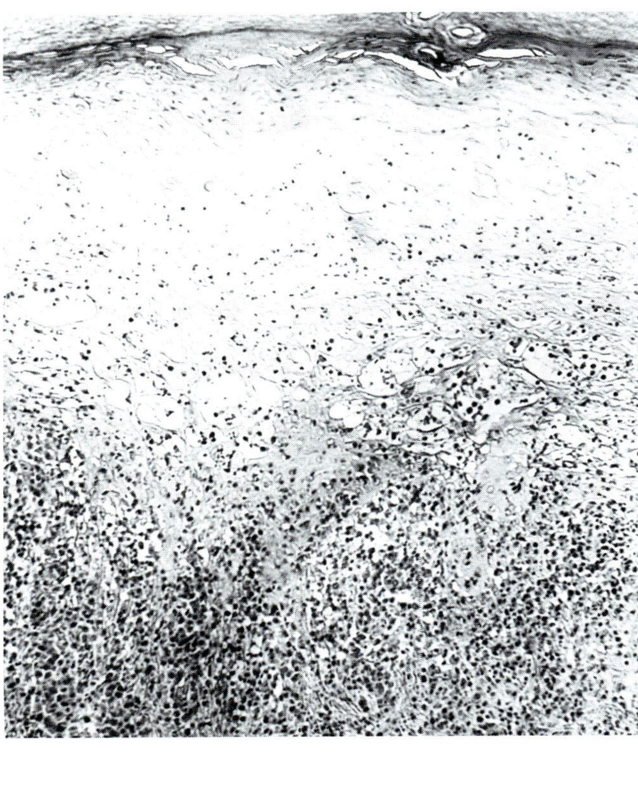

C
X120

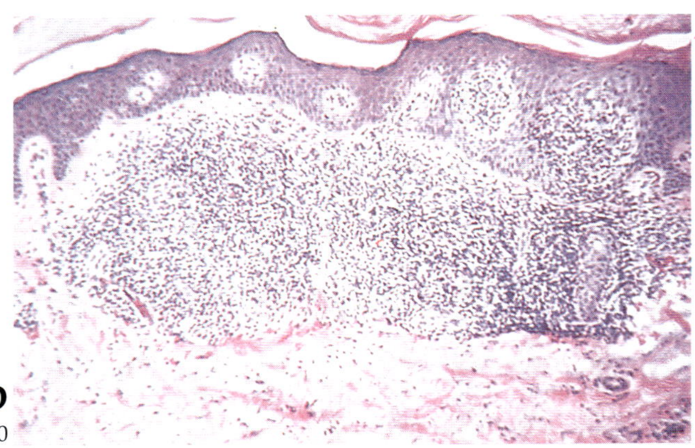

D
X100

DERMATOMYOSITIS

Dermatomyositis affects skin and skeletal muscle. Changes in other organs are rare. Polyarthritis, dysphagia, and vasculitis of the gastrointestinal tract and peripheral nerves are seen in the juvenile form. In cases where cutaneous involvement is absent, the term *polymyositis* is used. Females are affected more often than males; peaks of incidence occur before the age of ten and between the ages of forty and sixty.

There is a possible association between dermatomyositis and internal malignancy in adults. When the tumor is removed, symptoms of dermatomyositis may subside.

Cutaneous Lesions

A wide variety of cutaneous lesions may be observed; some have a general similarity to lesions of systemic lupus erythematosus, and others to lesions of scleroderma. Periungual erythema and telangiectasia are common.

Heliotrope erythema, a violaceous discoloration of the eyelids associated with edema (Fig. A) is fairly characteristic of dermatomyositis. Erythematous or violaceous plaques may develop elsewhere.

Lesions of dermatomyositis may progress to a stage of poikiloderma (Fig. B). Sclerodermatous changes and calcification are common.

Slightly erythematous, shiny plaques may occur over the joints of the hand (Gottron's sign) (Fig. C). Periungual telangiectasia, erythema, or mucous membrane lesions may occur.

Raynaud's phenomenon is common in adults with dermatomyositis.

Skeletal Muscle Involvement

Symptoms include tenderness and weakness. Flexor muscles of the neck and proximal musculature of the extremities are most frequently involved. Ocular, pharyngeal, and esophageal muscles may also be affected. Rarely, there is involvement of cardiac muscle.

Muscle atrophy is a late change.

Microscopic features (skin)

1. In most cutaneous lesions, the histologic picture is that of a nonspecific perivasculitis (see p. 120).

   There may be focal accumulations of mucin (acid mucopolysaccharides) in the dermis. A panniculitis with focal areas of mucinous degeneration may be present.
2. In some instances, the histologic picture parallels that of systemic lupus erythematosus (Figs. D,E; E = bullous lesion) (see p. 490).

DERMATOMYOSITIS: SKIN CHANGES

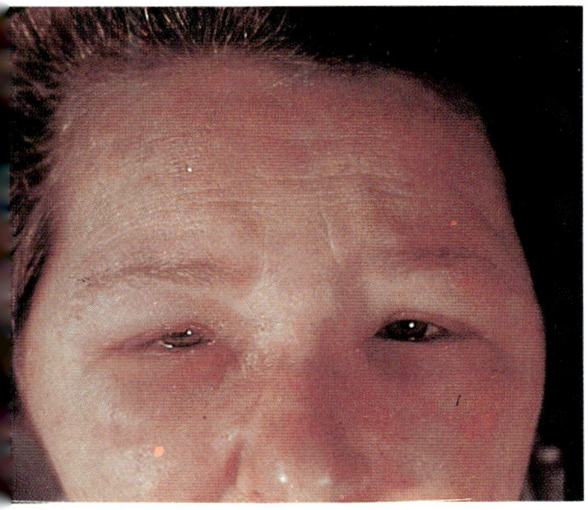

A

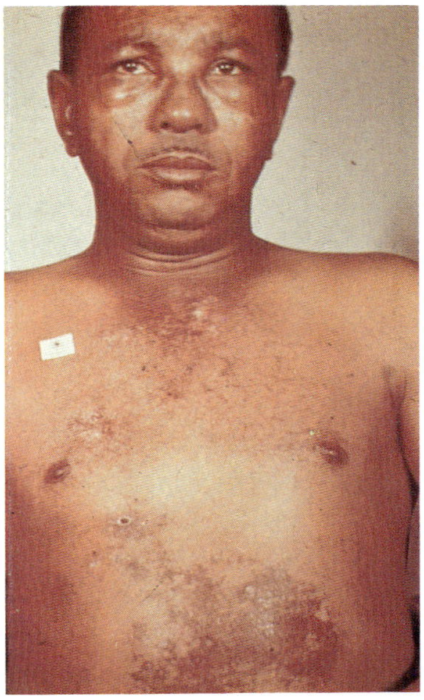

B

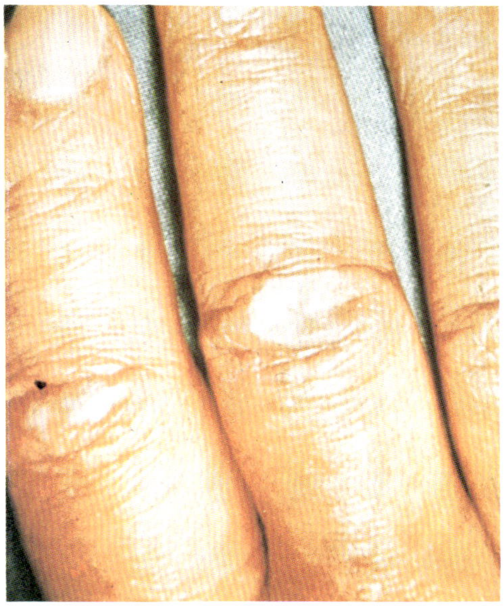

C

Figs. B,C courtesy Dr. John Knox

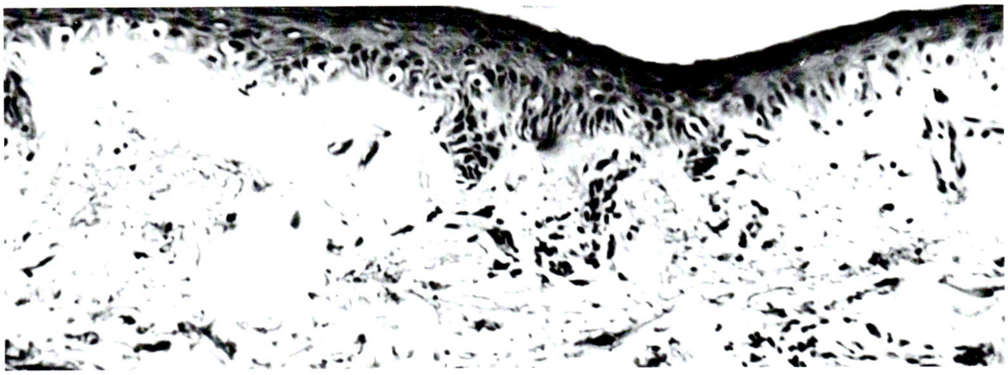

D
X190

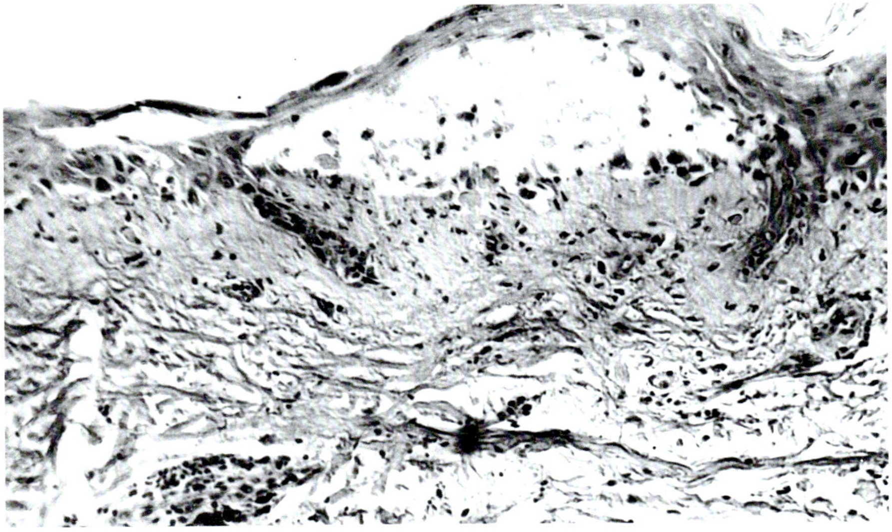

E
X150

DERMATOMYOSITIS continued

DERMATOMYOSITIS

Microscopic features (muscle)

1. Alterations in skeletal muscle have a focal distribution which may be related to small vessel infarcts.
2. Muscle changes include loss of transverse striations (Figs. C,D), hyalinization (Figs. C,D), vacuolization (Fig. D), fragmentation (Figs. C,D), and basophilia.
3. An infiltrate composed of lymphocytes, plasma cells, and histiocytes is present (Figs. A,B,C). Phagocytosis of fragmented muscle fibers may be observed.
4. Late lesions show proliferation of sarcolemmal nuclei and progressive fibrosis.

Comment

1. *Immunofluorescence tests in differential diagnosis of dermatomyositis.* The lupus band test is the most important test in distinguishing LE from dermatomyositis. This is negative in dermatomyositis. The ANA test is usually negative in dermatomyositis. The test for antibodies to ribonucleoprotein is also usually negative. This test, in conjunction with a negative test for ribonuclease-sensitive extractable nuclear antigen excludes mixed connective tissue disease (MCTD).
2. Paramyxovirus-like bodies have been found with electron microscopy in lesions of dermatomyositis and systemic lupus erythematosus. The etiologic significance of this finding is uncertain.

DERMATOMYOSITIS: MUSCLE CHANGES

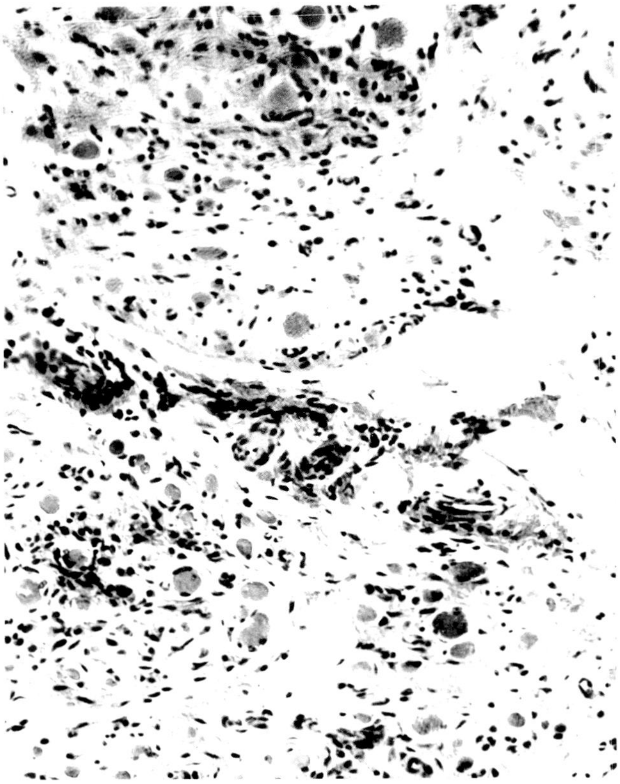

A X150

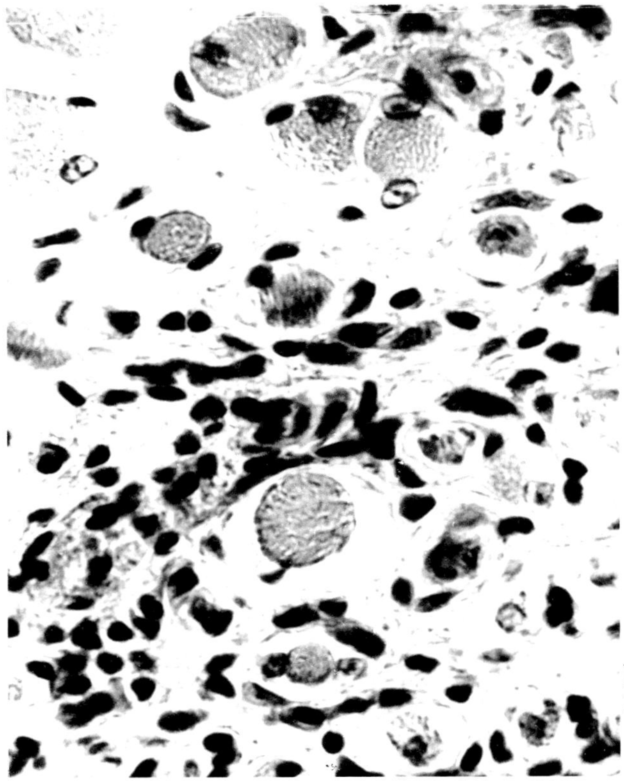

B X670

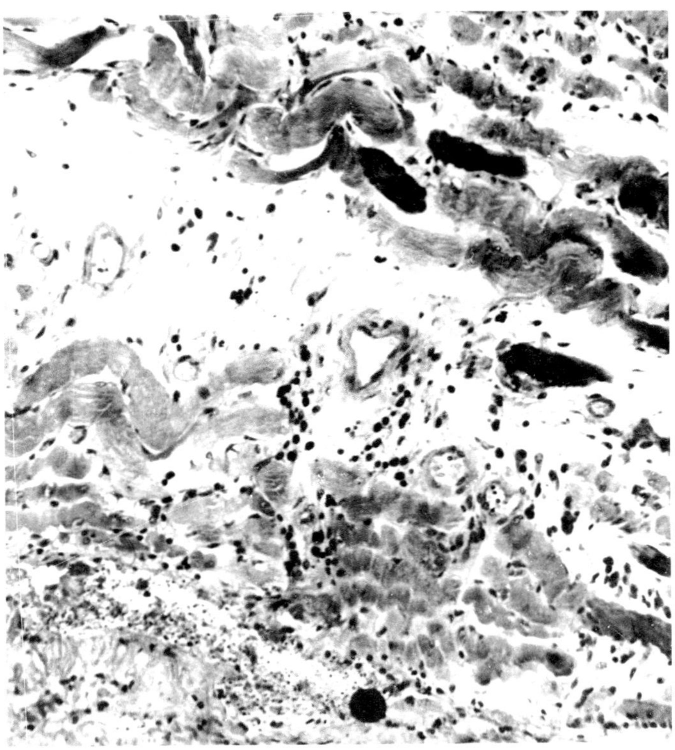

C X250

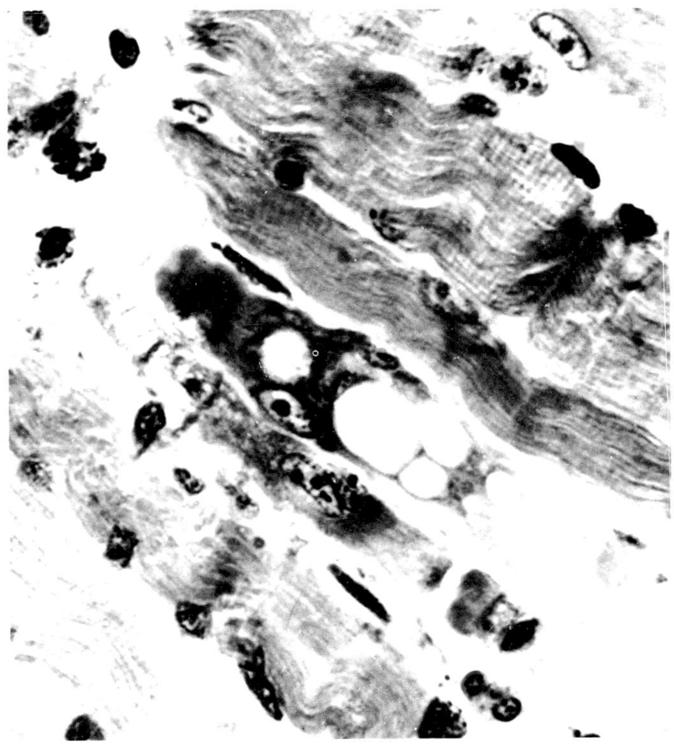

D X810

SCLERODERMA

Scleroderma is characterized by thickening of connective tissue. There are two principal types: *circumscribed scleroderma (morphea)*, and *systemic scleroderma (progressive systemic sclerosis)*. Transformation of circumscribed scleroderma into systemic scleroderma is rare. Women are more often affected than men.

CIRCUMSCRIBED SCLERODERMA (MORPHEA)

Three types are recognized: guttate, plaque, and linear. The plaque type is most common. Early lesions usually are violaceous (Fig. A), sometimes with an enlarging yellowish-white sclerotic center (Fig. B). As lesions progress, the inflammatory halo tends to disappear (Fig. C), leaving an ivory-white, indurated area. Guttate scleroderma is almost always associated with lesions of the plaque type, differing by their smaller size and more superficial involvement. Guttate lesions resemble lichen sclerosus et atrophicus (see p. 654), but they lack the keratotic plugs. Morphea and lichen sclerosus et atrophicus (LSA) may coexist; whether or not they are variants of the same disease has been controversial. Lesions of linear scleroderma may have a unilateral distribution and may lead to hemiatrophy of the face or extremities. Linear scleroderma involving the frontoparietal region is called *coup de sabre*. Hemiatrophy may be associated with atrophy of underlying muscles and bone. Spinal deformities, especially spina bifida, may be associated with linear scleroderma. In generalized morphea, lesions are widely disseminated; a mixture of all three types may be present. Bullous lesions may occur in generalized morphea.

CIRCUMSCRIBED SCLERODERMA

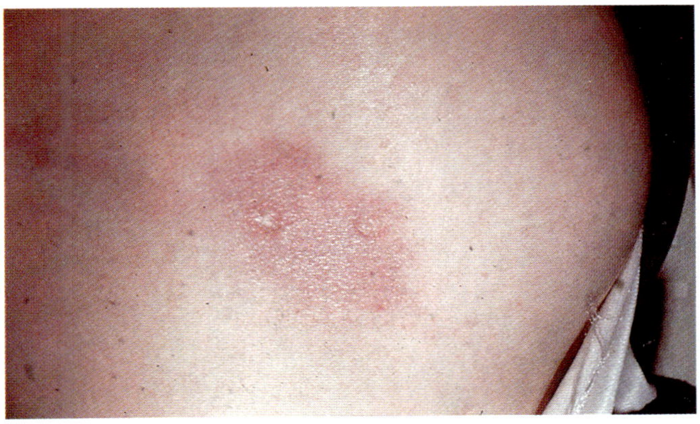
A

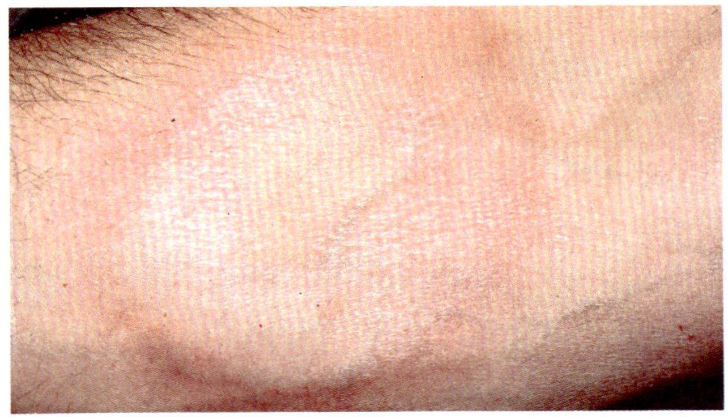
B

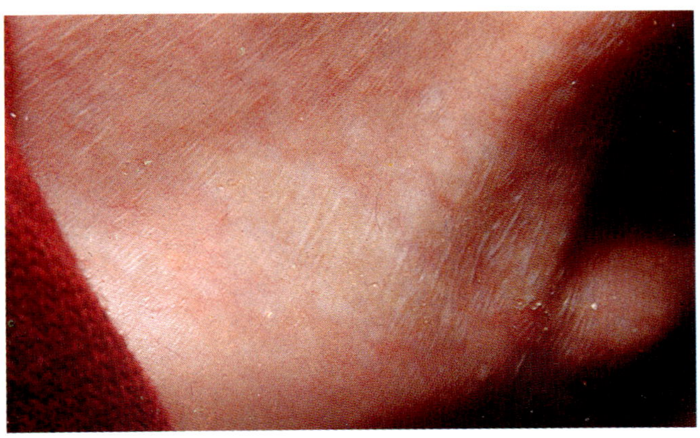
C

SCLERODERMA continued

CIRCUMSCRIBED SCLERODERMA

Microscopic features (circumscribed scleroderma)

1. Initially, there is a lymphocytic perivasculitis (Fig. C) with considerable edema of the walls of the involved vessels. There is also a lymphocytic infiltrate between collagen bundles (Fig. B) which may extend into subcutaneous fat, and which may surround sweat glands (Fig. D).
2. As lesions progress, the inflammatory infiltrate decreases. The dermis becomes thickened and the collagen fibers become hypertrophic, densely aggregated, and often hyalinized. Fibroblast nuclei are decreased in number (Fig. A).
3. The late sclerotic stage shows changes identical to those of systemic scleroderma. The collagen fibers are uniformly thickened and hyalinized. Pilosebaceous units are decreased in number or absent, and the eccrine glands are surrounded by sclerotic collagen fibers ("bound down" appearance). The subcutaneous fat becomes extensively collagenized.
4. The epidermis remains normal in appearance, but the papillary dermis often appears dense and homogeneous.
5. In linear scleroderma, the fascia may show fibrosis and sclerosis; striated muscles may show vacuolization, and there may be edema and inflammation between muscle fibers.
6. There may be epidermal atrophy in morphea.
7. Subepidermal bullae may be present in morphea profunda.

Comment

Since the dermis from the back normally is deep and has rather coarse collagen fibers in the reticular dermis, it is desirable to obtain an adjacent control biopsy of clinically normal skin, when assessing lesions for scleroderma in this area.

CIRCUMSCRIBED SCLERODERMA

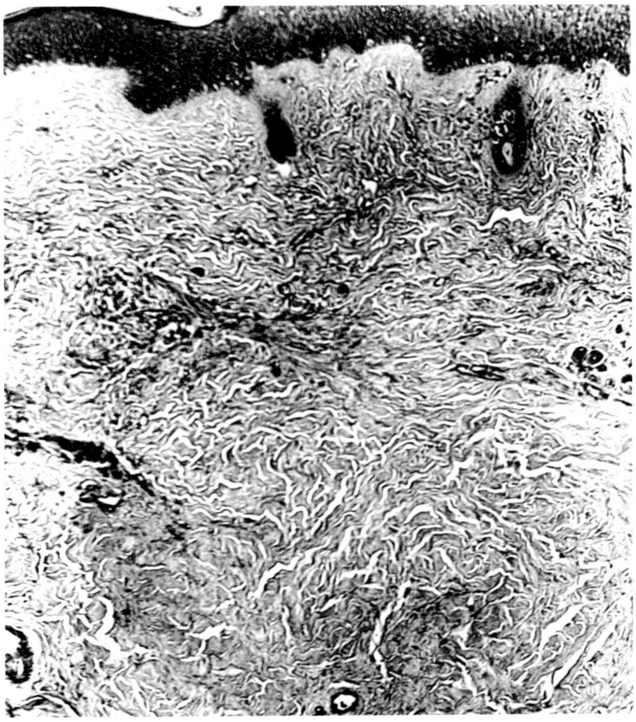

A
X100

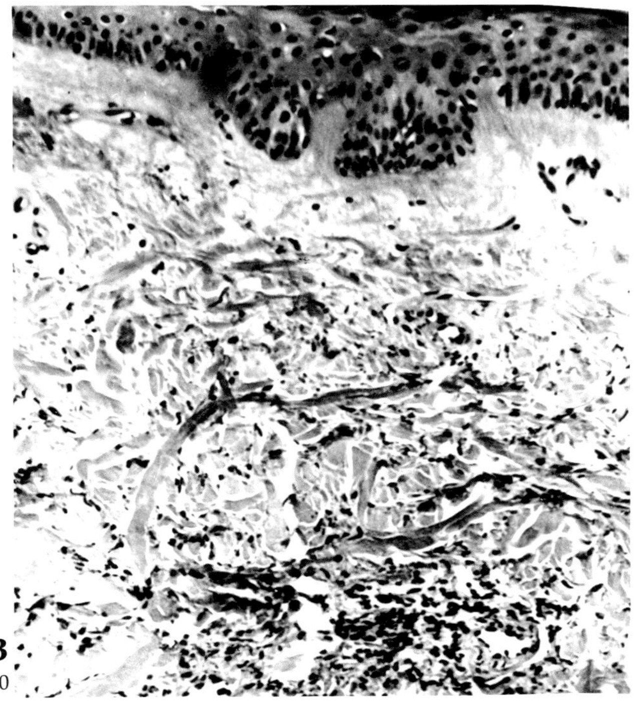

B
X250

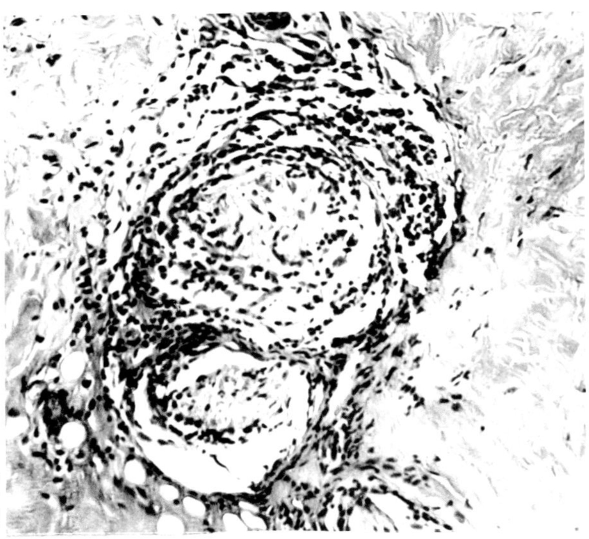

C
X185

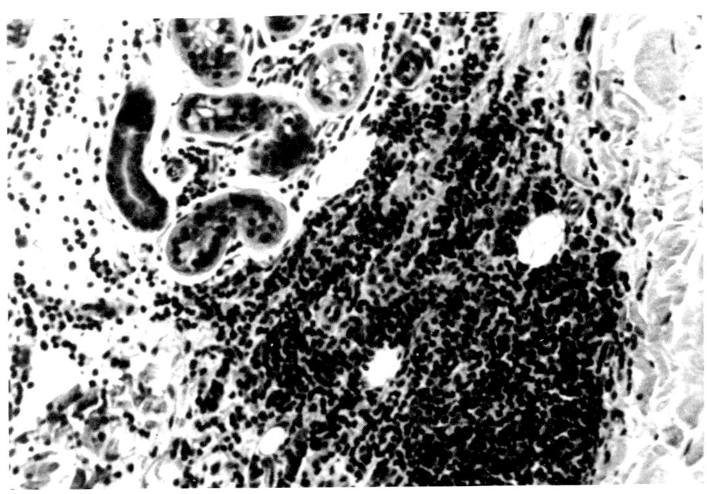

D
X220

SCLERODERMA continued

SYSTEMIC SCLERODERMA

In addition to skin, systemic scleroderma involves viscera. Common visceral sites include the gastrointestinal tract, especially the esophagus, lungs, heart, and kidneys. Cutaneous lesions often begin in acral areas (face and distal parts of the extremities), with progression proximally. This type of systemic scleroderma is called *acrosclerosis*. Acrosclerosis is associated with Raynaud's phenomenon, which may precede other manifestations of scleroderma. Much less commonly, lesions begin on the trunk (diffuse systemic scleroderma). In such cases, there is no association with Raynaud's phenomenon. Cutaneous lesions of systemic scleroderma are usually diffuse, but sometimes circumscribed morphea-like lesions may be present. There is induration of the skin. Acrosclerosis may show macular telangiectasias of the face and hands, ulceration of the fingertips and knuckles, and calcinosis cutis on the extremities. Diffuse hyperpigmentation may be present in diffuse systemic scleroderma. There may be claw-like deformities in acrosclerosis (Fig. A). Fig. B shows scleroderma of the hands, with characterisitic shiny, smooth, indurated skin. The face in acrosclerosis may become drawn and taut (Fig. C), with difficulty in opening the mouth completely. Involvement of skeletal muscle occurs in systemic scleroderma, a parallel to dermatomyositis that may produce difficulty in differential diagnosis. Weakness, atrophy, contractures of muscles and tendons, as well as ankyloses of the joints, may be present. CRST syndrome (Fig. D) is a type of acrosclerosis which tends to have a relatively favorable prognosis. It is characterized by calcinosis, Raynaud's phenomenon, sclerodactyly, and telangiectasia. It is also known as the CREST syndrome because of the frequency of esophageal involvement and dysphagia.

SYSTEMIC SCLERODERMA

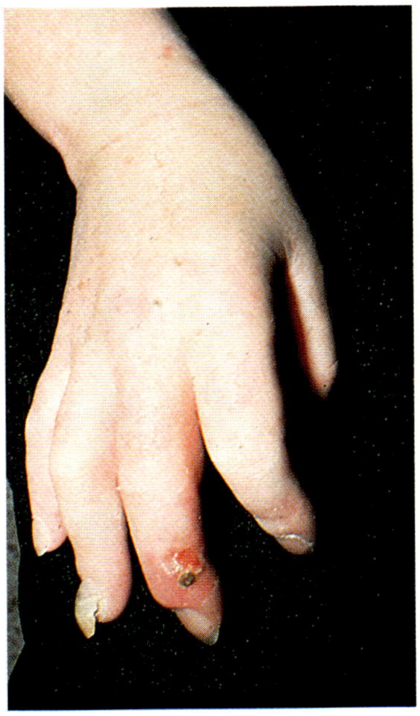

A

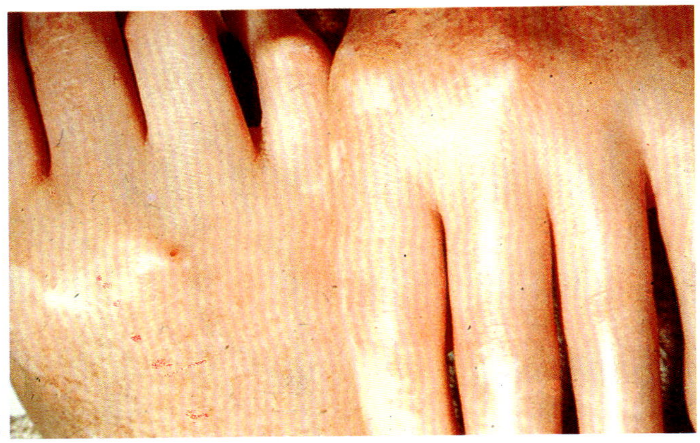

B

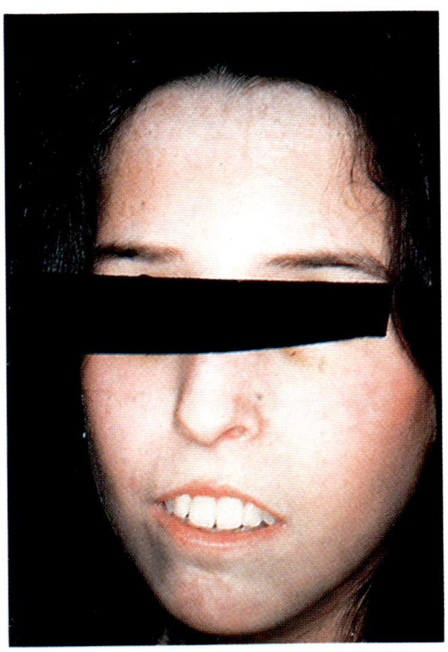

C

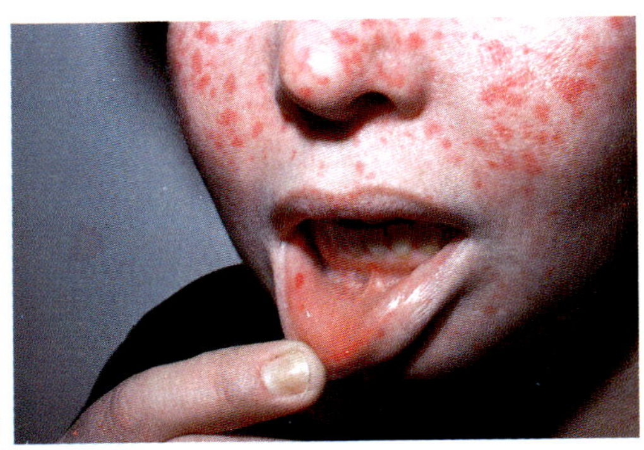

D

SCLERODERMA continued

SYSTEMIC SCLERODERMA

Microscopic features

1. Systemic scleroderma shows histologic changes similar to those of circumscribed scleroderma (see p. 506). The pronounced inflammatory infiltrate associated with early lesions of circumscribed scleroderma is not observed, but early lesions may show some inflammation.
2. Early changes include deposition of fibrinoid material in the dermis and thickening of the walls of cutaneous vessels.
3. Late lesions show typical thickening and hyalinization of collagen fibers (Figs. A,B). Foci of calcification may be present, especially in the subcutaneous tissue.
4. Pilosebaceous units disappear, and eccrine glands become "bound down" by thickened collagen (Figs. B,C).
5. The epidermis is generally normal, but may become atrophic in late stages.
6. Muscle changes parallel those of dermatomyositis (see p. 504).
7. Visceral lesions are characterized by sclerosis and thickening of vessels.

Comment

Since the dermis from the back normally is deep and has rather coarse collagen fibers in the reticular dermis, it is desirable to obtain an adjacent control biopsy of clinically normal skin when assessing lesions for scleroderma in this area.

SYSTEMIC SCLERODERMA

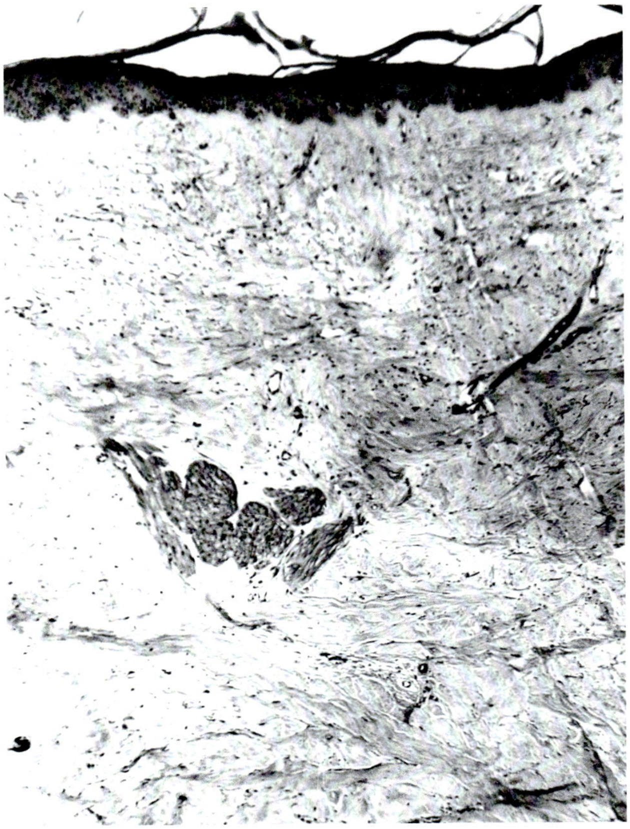

A
X50

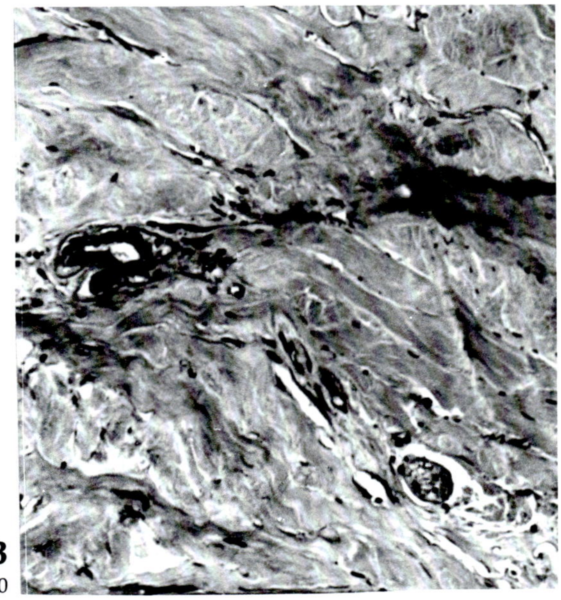

B
X220

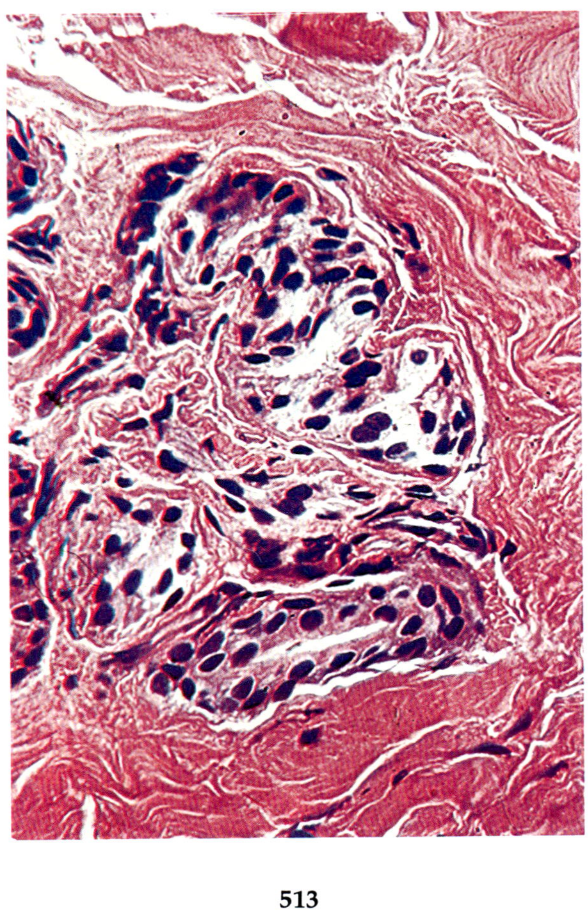

C
X820

SCLERODERMA continued

SCLERODERMA

Comment: conditions with parallels to scleroderma

1. *Atrophoderma of Pasini and Pierini* is characterized by large, sharply circumscribed depressed areas on the trunk with a bluish color; the subcutaneous fat is severely damaged and may be absent. The histologic changes are essentially those of scleroderma. Some authors regard atrophoderma of Pasini and Pierini as a variant of morphea.
2. *Progeria of adults (Werner's syndrome)* is a rare disorder transmitted as an autosomal recessive trait. It is characterized by premature aging of the skin and other organs. The skin of the extremities is indurated, and ulcerations are common. Underlying fat and skeletal muscles become atrophic. The histologic picture may closely resemble the late stage of scleroderma.
3. *In pachydermoperiostosis,* clubbing of the digits is associated with periosteal new bone formation, thickening of skin of the face, cutis verticis gyrata, and ptosis.

   The primary form is a hereditary disorder transmitted as an autosomal dominant gene with variable penetrance. Secondary pachydermoperiostosis is usually secondary to pulmonary disease, such as carcinoma of the bronchus, pleural mesothelioma, or lung abscess.

   Cutaneous lesions have a microscopic resemblance to scleroderma. There is an increase in hyaluronic acid in the ground substance.
4. *Eosinophilic fasciitis (Shulman's syndrome)* is now widely regarded as a variant of morphea. There is typically an acute onset with diffuse swelling and induration of affected areas—usually the limbs. Tenderness is usually present, along with dimpling or ridging. Moderate blood eosinophilia and hypergammaglobulinemia are commonly observed. The microscopic picture is characterized by sclerosis of the fascia accompanied by a chronic inflammatory infiltrate which may contain an admixture of eosinophils.

   Scleroderma-like changes may occur in the lower dermis and subcutaneous fat. There may be arthralgia and myositis.

SCLERODERMA

Comment: conditions with parallels to scleroderma

5. *Graft-versus-host disease* is due to transplants of immunocompetent lymphocytes, in most cases via bone marrow transplantation. There is a rare congenital form in which maternal lymphocytes establish themselves in the fetus. The acute phase has cutaneous parallels clinically and microscopically to erythema multiforme; the early lichenoid stage of the chronic phase has clinical and microscopic parallels to lichen planus; the late sclerotic stage of the chronic phase has clinical and microscopic cutaneous parallels to scleroderma.
6. *Scleredema adultorum* (Buschke) is characterized by generalized brawny edema. It may follow infections, and persistent cases may be associated with diabetes mellitus. There is thickening of the dermis and a diffuse deposition of hyaluronic acid, which gives the collagen fibers a fenestrated appearance. Late stages resemble scleroderma. The process begins in the face and then extends to the neck and upper trunk. Sometimes the term *scleredema* is used alone since the condition can occur in children.
7. *Acro-osteolysis* refers to lytic changes in the distal phalanges. There are familial, idiopathic (nonfamilial), and occupational types. The idiopathic and occupational types may be associated with cutaneous lesions similar to those of scleroderma.
8. *Melorheostosis* refers to linear hyperostosis of an extremity. The overyling skin may show thickening similar to that observed in scleroderma.

Immunofluorescence tests in scleroderma

The presence of antinuclear antibodies in the sera of about two thirds of patients with systemic scleroderma, with titers that often reach levels seen in SLE, is evidence of the role of autoimmunity. The ANA pattern is typically speckled or nucleolar. Antinucleolar antibodies can be observed in epidermal cells of clinically normal skin in systemic scleroderma. Anticentromere antibodies have been reported in CRST syndrome.

Suggested Reading

Connective Tissue Diseases

General References

Beutner, E. et al. *Immunopathology of the Skin: Labeled Antibody Studies*. Stroudsburg, Penn., Dowden, Hutchinson and Ross, 1973.

Duthie, J. and Alexander, W. *Rheumatic Diseases*. Edinburgh, Universities Press, 1968.

Gardner, D. *Pathology of the Connective Tissue Diseases*. London, Arnold, 1965.

Good, R. and Fisher, D. *Immunobiology*. Stamford, Conn., Sinauer Associates, 1971.

Samter, M. *Immunological Diseases*. 2nd Ed., Boston, Little, Brown, 1971.

Sell, S. *Immunology, Immunopathology, and Immunity*. New York, Harper & Row, 1972.

Sinkovics, J. Working hypothesis: Viral etiology of autoimmune diseases. *N. Eng. J. Med.*, 280:903, 1969.

Tuffanelli, D. and LaPerriere, R. Connective tissue diseases. *Pediatr. Clin. N. Am.*, 18:925, 1971.

Lupus Erythematosus

Abell, E., Black, M. and Marks, R. Immunoglobulin and complement deposits in the skin in inflammatory dermatoses: An immunofluorescence study. *Br. J. Dermatol.*, 91:281, 1974.

Appel, G. et al. Renal involvement in systemic lupus erythematosus (SLE): A study of 56 patients emphasizing histologic classification. *Medicine* (Baltimore), 57:371, 1978.

Baer, R. and Harber, L. Photobiology of lupus erythematosus. *Arch. Dermatol.*, 92:124, 1965.

Baldwin, D. et al. Lupus nephritis: Clinical course as related to morphologic forms and their transitions. *Am. J. Med.*, 62:12, 1977.

Bangert, J. et al. Subacute cutaneous lupus erythematosus and discoid lupus erythematosus: Comparative histopathologic findings. *Arch. Dermatol.*, 120:332, 1984.

Bardawil, W. et al. Disseminated lupus erythematosus, scleroderma, and dermatomyositis as manifestations of sensitization to DNA-protein. *Am. J. Pathol.*, 34:607, 1958.

Beck, J. and Rowell, N. Discoid lupus erythematosus: A study of the clinical features and biochemical and serological abnormalities in 120 patients with observations on the relationship of this disease to systemic lupus erythematosus. *Quart. J. Med.*, 35:119, 1966.

Berk, S. and Blank, H. Ultraviolet light and cytoplasmic tubules in lupus erythematosus. *Arch. Dermatol.*, 109:364, 1963.

Biesecker, G. et al. Cutaneous localization of the membrane attack complex in discoid and systemic lupus erythematosus. *N. Eng. J. Med.*, 306:264, 1982.

Black, M. and Hudson, P. Atrophie blanche lesions closely resembling malignant atrophic papulosis (Degos disease) in systemic lupus erythematosus. *Br. J. Dermatol.*, 95:649, 1976.

Burch, P. and Rowell, N. Lupus erythematosus: Analysis of the sex- and age-distribution of the discoid and systemic forms of the disease in different countries. *Acta Derm. Venereol.*, 50:293, 1970.

Burnham, T. Antinuclear antibodies. *Arch. Dermatol.*, 114:1343, 1978.

Burnham, T. and Fine, G. The immunofluorescent "band" test for lupus erythematosus. *Arch. Dermatol.*, 103:24, 1971.

——. The immunofluorescent "band" test for lupus erythematosus. *Br. J. Dermatol.*, 84:176, 1971.

——. The immunofluorescent "band" test for lupus erythematosus. I. Morphologic variations of the band of localized immunoglobulins at the dermal-epidermal junction in lupus erythematosus. *Arch. Dermatol.*, 99:413, 1969.

Burnham, T. et al. The immunofluorescent tumor imprint technique. *Arch. Dermatol.*, 99:611, 1969.

Callen, J. Chronic cutaneous lupus erythematosus. *Arch. Dermatol.*, 118:412, 1982.

Chorzelski, T., Jablonska, S. and Blaszczyk, M. Immunopathologic investigations in lupus erythematosus. *J. Invest. Dermatol.*, 52:333, 1969.

Chubick, A. and Gilliam, J. A review of mixed connective tissue disease. *Internat. J. Dermatol.*, 17:123, 1978.

Codman, G., Deitch, A. and Klemperer, P. The composition of the LE and hematoxylin bodies of systemic lupus erythematosus. *Am. J. Pathol.*, 34:1, 1958.

Cruickshank, B. The basic pattern of tissue damage and pathology of systemic lupus erythematosus. In: *Lupus Erythematosus: A Review of the Current Status of Discoid and Systemic Lupus Erythematosus and their Variants.* Dubois, E., ed., New York, Blakiston, 1966, p. 10.

Davies, M. and Marks, R. Evolution of the lesion of discoid lupus erythematosus: A comparison with lichen planus. *Br. J. Dermatol.*, 97:313, 1977.

Decker, J. et al. Systemic lupus erythematosus: Evolving concepts. *Ann. Int. Med.*, 91:587, 1979.

Dimant, J. et al. The clinical significance of Raynaud's phenomenon in systemic lupus erythematosus. *Arthritis Rheum.*, 22:815, 1979.

Dubois, E. *Lupus Erythematosus.* New York, McGraw-Hill, 1966.

Dubois, E. and Tuffanelli, D. Clinical manifestations of systemic lupus erythematosus: Computer analysis of 520 cases. *JAMA*, 190:104, 1964.

Ellis, F. and Bundick, W. Histology of lupus erythematosus. *Arch. Dermatol.*, 70:311, 1954.

Epstein, J., Tuffanelli, D. and Dubois, E. Light sensitivity and lupus erythematosus. *Arch. Dermatol.*, 91:483, 1965.

Fisher, D. et al. Polymorphous light eruption and lupus erythematosus. *Arch. Dermatol.*, 101:458, 1970.

——. Polymorphous light eruption and lupus erythematosus: Differential diagnosis by fluorescent microscopy. *Arch. Dermatol.*, 101:458, 1970.

Fries, J. The clinical aspects of systemic lupus erythematosus. *Med. Clin. North. Am.*, 61:229, 1977.

Gilliam, J. and Sontheimer, R. Distinctive cutaneous subsets in the spectrum of lupus erythematosus. *J. Am. Acad. Dermatol.*, 4:471, 1981.

Gilliam, J. et al. Immunoglobulin in clinically uninvolved skin in systemic lupus erythematosus: Association with renal disease. *J. Clin. Invest.*, 53:1434, 1974.

Golitz, L. Collagen diseases. *J. Cutan. Pathol.*, 12:358, 1985.

Grund, J. Chronic lupus erythematosus: Report of an unusual case with concomitant subcutaneous edematous nodes and swellings: Historical review. *Arch. Dermatol. Syph.*, 61:20, 1950.

Györkey, F. et al. A morphologic study on the occurrence and distribution of structures resembling viral nucleocapsids in collagen diseases. *Am. J. Med.*, 53:148, 1972.

Györkey, F. et al. Systemic lupus erythematosus and myxovirus. *N. Eng. J. Med.*, 280:333, 1069.

Hahn, B., Yardley, J. and Stevens, M. "Rheumatoid" nodules in systemic lupus erythematosus. *Ann. Int. Med.*, 72:49, 1970.

Haim, S. and Shafrir, A. The nature of discoid lupus erythematosus. *Acta Derm. Venereol.*, 50:86, 1970.

Hall, R. et al. Bullous eruption of lupus erythematosus. *Ann. Int. Med.*, 97:165, 1982.

Hargraves, M., Richmond, H. and Morton, R. Presentation of two bone marrow elements: The "tart" cell and the "L.E." cell. *Proc. Mayo Clin.*, 23:25, 1948.

Harrist, T. and Mihm, M., Jr. Cutaneous immunopathology: The diagnostic use of direct and indirect immunofluorescence techniques in dermatologic diseases. (Review). *Hum. Pathol.*, 10:625, 1979.

Harvey, A. et al. Systemic lupus erythematosus: A review of the literature and clinical analysis of 138 cases. *Medicine*, 33:291, 1954.

Haserick, J. and Kellum, R. *Primer for Patients with Lupus Erythematosus.* 2nd Ed., Southern Pines, NC, Pilot Press, 1973.

Hashimoto, K. Paramyxovirus-like inclusion in so-called collagen and autoimmune diseases. *Progr. Dermatol.*, 5:1, 1070.

Hashimoto, K. and Thompson, D. Discoid lupus erythematosus: Electron microscopic studies of paramyxovirus-like structures. *Arch. Dermatol.*, 101:565, 1970.

Hughs, G. Diagnosis of systemic lupus erythematosus. *Br. J. Haematol.*, 25:409, 1973.

Irgang, S. Lupus erythematosus in the Negro. *N. Y. J. Med.*, 66:727, 1966.

Jager, B. Disseminated lupus erythematosus: Report of two cases with unusual clinical manifestations. *Arch. Dermatol. Syph.*, 46:362, 1942.

Kennedy, C. and Gold, S. Subacute cutaneous lupus erythematosus. *Clin. Exp. Dermatol.*, 6:673, 1981.
Klemperer, P., Pollack, A. and Baehr, G. Pathology of disseminated lupus erythematosus. *Arch. Pathol.*, 32:569, 1941.
Kobayasi, T. and Asboe-Hansen, G. Ultrastructure of systemic lupus erythematosus skin: Dermo-epidermal junction. *Acta Derm. Venereol.*, 53:417, 1973.
Lang, P., Smith, G., Jr. and Green, W., Jr. Vacuolar myopathy in lupus erythematosus. *JAMA*, 191:49, 1965.
Levy, S. et al. Immunofluorescent and electron-microscopic findings in the uninvolved skin of patients with systemic lupus erythematosus. *Acta Derm. Venereol.* (Stockh.), 59:427, 1979.
McCreight, W. and Montgomery, H. Cutaneous changes in lupus erythematosus: Histopathologic aspects, with special reference to vascular changes. *Arch. Dermatol. Syph.*, 61:1, 1950.
Maciejewski, W. Annular erythema as an unusual manifestation of chronic disseminated lupus erythematosus. *Arch. Dermatol.*, 116:450, 1980.
Maddison, P., Provost, T. and Reichlin, M. Serological findings in patients with "ANA-negative" systemic lupus erythematosus. *Medicine* (Baltimore), 60:87, 1981.
Marten, R. and Blackburn, E. Lupus erythematosus: Clinical and histopathological studies in seventy-seven cases. *Arch. Dermatol.*, 73:1, 1956.
Millard, L. and Rowell, N. Abnormal laboratory test results and their relationship to prognosis in discoid lupus erythematosus. *Arch. Dermatol.*, 115:1055, 1979.
Ogawa, K. Ultrastructure of cutaneous lesions in lupus erythematosus. *J. Dermatol.* (Tokyo), 8:175, 1981.
Olansky, A. et al. Bullous systemic lupus erythematosus. *J. Am. Acad. Dermatol.*, 7:511, 1982.
O'Loughlin, S., Schroeter, A. and Jordan, R. Chronic urticaria-like lesions in systemic lupus erythematosus. *Arch. Dermatol.*, 114:879, 1978.
——. A study of lupus erythematosus with particular reference to generalized discoid lupus. *Br. J. Dermatol.*, 99:1, 1978.
Ores, R. and Mandel, E. LE cells in biopsies of positive deoxyribonucleic acid skin tests. *Br. J. Dermatol.*, 84:217, 1971.
Panet-Raymond, G. and Johnson, W. Lupus erythematosus and polymorphous light eruption: Differentiation by histochemical procedures. *Arch. Dermatol.*, 108:785, 1973.
Pascher, F., Sims, C. and Pensky, N. Lupus erythematosus profundus: Report of a case including a comparative study of the histopathology with that of chronic discoid lupus erythematosus. *J. Invest. Dermatol.*, 25:347, 1955.
Pehamberger, H., Konrad, K. and Holubar, K. Immunoelectron microscopy of skin in lupus erythematosus. *J. Cutan. Pathol.*, 5:319, 1978.
Percy, J. and Smyth, C. The immunofluorescent skin test in systemic lupus erythamatosus. *JAMA*, 208:485, 1969.
Peterson, W., Jr. and Gokcen, M. Antinuclear factors in chronic discoid lupus erythematosus. *Arch. Dermatol.*, 86:783, 1962.
Pohle, E. and Tuffanelli, D. Study of cutaneous lupus erythematosus. *Arch. Dermatol.*, 97:520, 1968.
Pollak, V. Antinuclear antibodies in families of patients with systemic lupus erythematosus. *N. Eng. J. Med.*, 271:165, 1964.
Provost, T. The relationship between discoid lupus erythematosus and systemic lupus erythematosus. *Am. J. Dermatol.*, 1:181, 1979.
——. Subsets in systemic lupus erythematosus. *J. Invest. Dermatol.*, 72:110, 1979.
Provost, T. et al. Lupus band test in untreated SLE patients. *J. Invest. Dermatol.*, 74:407, 1980.
Prunieras, M. and Montgomery, H. Histopathology of cutaneous lesions in systemic lupus erythematosus. *Arch. Dermatol.*, 74:177, 1956.
Prystowsky, S. and Gilliam J. Discoid lupus erythematosus as part of a larger disease spectrum. *Arch. Dermatol.*, 111:1448, 1975.
Prystowsky, S. et al. Chronic cutaneous lupus erythematosus (DLE): A clinical and laboratory investigation of 80 patients. *Medicine* (Baltimore), 55:1983, 1976.
Quismorio, F., Dubois, E. and Chandor, S. Soft-tissue calcification in systemic lupus erythematosus. *Arch. Dermatol.*, 111:352, 1975.
Reed, W. et al. Hereditary inflammatory vasculitis with persistent nodules: A genetically-determined new entity probably related to lupus erythematosus. *Br. J. Dermatol.*, 87:299, 1972.
Romero, R. et al. Unusual variant of lupus erythematosus on lichen planus. Clinical, histopathologic and immunofluorescent studies. *Arch. Dermatol.*, 113:741, 1977.

Ropes, M. Observations on the natural course of disseminated lupus erythematosus. *Medicine*, 43:387, 1964.

Rowell, N. Laboratory abnormalities in the diagnosis and management of lupus erythematosus. *Br. J. Dermatol.*, 84:210, 1971.

Sánchez, N., Peters, M. and Winkelmann, R. The histopathology of lupus erythematosus panniculitis. *J. Am. Acad. Dermatol.*, 5:673, 1981.

Scott, A. and Rees, E. The relationship of systemic lupus erythematosus and discoid lupus erythematosus: A clinical and hematological study. *Arch. Dermatol.*, 79:422, 1959.

Sharp, G. and Anderson, P. Current concepts in the classification of connective tissue diseases: Overlap syndromes and mixed connective tissue disease (MCTD). *J. Am. Acad. Dermatol.*, 2:269, 1980.

Sharp, G., Irwin, W. and Tan, E. Mixed connective tissue disease: An apparently distinct rheumatic disease syndrome associated with a specific antibody to an extractable nuclear antigen (ENA). *Am. J. Med.*, 52:148, 1972.

Shrank, A. and Doniach, D. Discoid lupus erythematosus: Correlation of clinical features with serum auto-antibody pattern. *Arch. Dermatol.*, 87:677, 1963.

Sontheimer, R., Thomas, J. and Gilliam, J. Subacute cutaneous lupus erythematosus: A cutaneous marker for a distinct lupus erythematosus subset. *Arch. Dermatol.*, 115:1409, 1979.

Tan, E. et al. Deoxyribonucleic acid (DNA) and antibodies to DNA in the serum of patients with systemic lupus erythematosus. *J. Clin. Invest.*, 45:1732, 1966.

Tuffanelli, D. Lupus erythematosus panniculitis (profundus): Clinical and immunologic studies. *Arch. Dermatol.*, 103:231, 1971.

Tuffanelli, D. and Dubois, E. Cutaneous manifestations of systemic lupus erythematosus. *Arch. Dermatol.*, 90:377, 1964.

Tuffanelli, D., Kay, D. and Fukuyama, K. Dermal-epidermal junction in lupus erythematosus. *Arch. Dermatol.*, 99:652, 1969.

——. Dermal-epidermal junction in lupus erythematosus. *Arch. Dermatol.*, 99:652, 1969.

Ueki, H., Wolff, H. and Braun-Falco, O. Cutaneous localization of human gammaglobulins in lupus erythematosus. *Arch. Derm. Forsch.*, 248:297, 1974.

Uitto, J. et al. Verrucous lesions in patients with discoid lupus erythematosus. *Br. J. Dermatol.*, 98:507, 1978.

Verbov, J. *Systemic Lupus Erythematosus: Clinical and Theoretical Aspects.* New York, MSS Information Corp., 1973.

Wechsler, H. and Stavrides, A. Systemic lupus erythematosus with anti-Ro antibodies. *J. Am. Acad. Dermatol.*, 6:73, 1982.

Weigand, D., Burgdorf, W. and Gregg, L. Dermal mucinosis in discoid lupus erythematosus. *Arch. Dermatol.*, 117:735, 1981.

Winkelmann, R. Spectrum of lupus erythematosus. *J. Cutan. Pathol.*, 6:457, 1979.

Worthingon, J., Jr., Baggenstoss, A. and Hargraves, M. Significance of hematoxylin bodies in the necropsy diagnosis of systemic lupus erythematosus. *Am. J. Pathol.*, 35:955, 1959.

Zweiman, B., Tomar, R. and Gross, P. Lupus erythematosus profundus following thrombocytopenic purpura. *Arch. Dermatol.*, 111:347, 1975.

Mixed Connective Tissue Disease

Gilliam, J. and Prystowky, S. Mixed connective tissue disease syndrome. *Arch. Dermatol.*, 113:583, 1977.

Prystowky, S. and Tuffanelli, D. Speckled (particulate) epidermal nuclear IgG deposition in normal skin. *Arch. Dermatol.*, 114:705, 1978.

Sharp, G. and Anderson, P. Current concepts in the classification of connective tissue diseases. *J. Am. Acad. Dermatol.*, 2:269, 1980.

Sharp, G. et al. Mixed connective tissue disease: An apparently distinct rheumatic disease syndrome associated with a specific antibody to an extractable nuclear antigen (ENA). *Am. J. Med.*, 52:148, 1972.

Polymorphous Light Eruption—Lymphocytic Infiltration of the Skin (Jessner-Kanof)—Actinic Reticuloid—Hydroa Vacciniforme

Barthelmes, H. and Sonnichsen, M. Differential diagnosis of chronic discoid lupus erythematosus and lymphocytic infiltration of Jessner and Kanof by immunofluorescent histology. *Arch. Klin. Exp. Dermatol.*, 232:384, 1968.

Bickers, D. et al. Hydroa vacciniforme. *Arch. Dermatol.*, 114:1193, 1978.

Birt, A. and Davis, R. Hereditary polymorphic light eruption of American Indians. *Internat. J. Dermatol.*, 14:105, 1975.

Brody, R. and Bergfeld, W. Actinic reticuloid. *Internat. J. Dermatol.*, 20:374, 1981.

Calnan, C. Lymphocytic infiltration of the skin (Jessner). *Br. J. Dermatol.*, 69:169, 1957.

Calnan, C. and Meara, R. Actinic prurigo (Hutchinson's summer prurigo). *Clin. Exp. Dermatol.*, 2:365, 1977.

Degos, R. et al. Actino-réticulose: Photo-allergie avec infiltrat hématodermique. *Ann. Dermatol. Syph.*, 97:121, 1970.

Epstein, J. Polymorphous light eruption. *J. Am. Acad. Dermatol.*, 3:329, 1980.

Fisher, D. et al. Polymorphous light eruption and lupus erythematosus. *Arch. Dermatol.*, 101:458, 1970.

Frain-Bell, W., Hetherington, A. and Johnson, B. Contact allergic sensitivity to chrysanthemum and the photosensitivity dermatitis and actinic reticuloid syndrome. *Br. J. Dermatol.*, 101:491, 1979.

Frain-Bell, W. and Johnson, B. Contact allergic sensitivity to plants and the photosensitivity dermatitis and actinic reticuloid syndrome. *Br. J. Dermatol.*, 101:503, 1979.

Frain-Bell, W., MacKenzie, L. and Witham, E. Chronic polymorphous light eruption. *Br. J. Dermatol.*, 81:885, 1969.

Frain-Bell, W. et al. The syndrome of chronic photosensitivity dermatitis and actinic reticuloid. *Br. J. Dermatol.*, 91:617, 1974.

Gottlieb, B. and Winkelmann, R. Lymphocytic infiltration of the skin. *Arch. Dermatol.*, 86:626, 1962.

Guardiola, A. and Sánchez, J. Actinic reticuloid. *Internat. J. Dermatol.*, 19:154, 1980.

Holzle, E. et al. Polymorphous light eruption: Experimental reproduction of skin lesions. *J. Am. Acad. Dermatol.*, 7:111, 1982.

Ive, F. et al. "Actinic reticuloid": A chronic dermatosis associated with severe photosensitivity and histologic resemblance of lymphoma. *Br. J. Dermatol.*, 81:469, 1969.

Jaschke, E., Reinken, L. and Frisch, A. Hydroa vacciniforme Bazin. *Hautarzt*, 26:11, 1975.

Jensen, N. and Sneddon, I. Actinic reticuloid with lymphoma. *Br. J. Dermatol.*, 82:287, 1970.

Jessner, M. and Kanof, N. Lymphocytic infiltration of the skin. *Arch. Dermatol.*, 68:447, 1953.

Johnson, S., Cripps, D. and Norback, D. Actinic reticuloid: A clinical, pathologic, and action spectrum study. *Arch. Dermatol.*, 115:1078, 1979.

Kaidbey, K. and Messenger, J. The clinical spectrum of persistent light reactor. *Arch. Dermatol.*, 120:1441, 1984.

Krieger, B. Lymphocytic infiltration of the skin (Jessner). *Arch. Dermatol.*, 100:247, 1969.

Lester, R. et al. Immunologic concepts of light reactions in lupus erythematosus and polymorphous light eruptions. *Arch. Dermatol.*, 96:1, 1967.

McGrae, J. and Perry, H. Hydroa vacciniforme. *Arch. Dermatol.*, 87:618, 1963.

Morison, W. and Stern, R. Polymorphous light eruption: A common reaction uncommonly recognized. *Acta Derm. Venereol.* (Stockh.), 62:237, 1982.

Neild, V. et al. Actinic reticuloid with Sézary cells. *Clin. Exp. Dermatol.*, 7:143, 1982.

Panet-Raymond, G. and Johnson, W. Lupus erythematosus and polymorphous light eruption: Differentiation by histochemical procedures. *Arch. Dermatol.*, 108:785, 1973.

Perrot, H. et al. Sarcome ganglionnaire généralisé au cours de l'évolution d'une actino-réticulose. *Ann. Dermatol. Venereol.*, 105:33, 1978.

Ralfkiaer, E. et al. Photosensitive dermatitis with actinic reticuloid syndrome: An immunohistological study of the cutaneous infiltrate. *Br. J. Dermatol.*, 114:47, 1986.

Scheen, S., III, Connolly, S. and Dicken, C. Actinic prurigo. *J. Am. Acad. Dermatol.*, 5:183, 1981.

Thomsen, K. The development of Hodgkin's disease in a patient with actinic reticuloid. *Clin. Exp. Dermatol.*, 2:109, 1977.

Dermatomyositis

Arundell, F., Wilkinson, R. and Haserick, J. Dermatomyositis and malignant neoplasms in adults: A survey of twenty years' experience. *Arch. Dermatol.*, 82:772, 1960.

Banker, B. and Victor, M. Dermatomyositis (systemic angiopathy) of childhood. *Medicine*, 45:261, 1966.

Barnes, B. Dermatomyositis and malignancy: A review of the literature. *Ann. Int. Med.*, 84:68, 1976.

Bohan, A. et al. A computer-assisted analysis of 153 patients with polymyositis and dermatomyositis. *Medicine* (Baltimore), 56:255, 1977.

Boylan, R. and Sokoloff, L. Vascular lesions in dermatomyositis. *Arthritis Rheum.*, 3:379, 1960.

Braverman, I. *Skin Signs of Systemic Diseases*. 2nd Ed. Philadelphia, W. B. Saunders, 1981, p. 302.

Callen, J. Dermatomyositis. (Review). *Internat. J. Dermatol.*, 18:423, 1979.

Callen, J. et al. The relationship of dermatomyositis and polymyositis to internal malignancy. *Arch. Dermatol.*, 116:295, 1980.

Carpenter, S. and Karpati, G. The major inflammatory myopathies of unknown cause. *Ann. Pathol.*, 16:205, 1981.

Christianson, H., Brunsting, L. and Perry, H. Dermatomyositis: Unusual features, complications, and treatment. *Arch. Dermatol.*, 74:581, 1956.

Crowe, W. et al. Clinical and pathogenetic implications of histopathology in childhood polydermatomyositis. *Arthritis Rheum.*, 25:126, 1982.

Curtis, A., Heckaman, J. and Wheeler, A. Study of the autoimmune reaction in dermatomyositis. *JAMA*, 178:571, 1961.

Degos, R. et al. The prognosis of adult dermatomyositis. *Trans. St. John's Hosp. Dermatol. Soc.*, 57:98, 1971.

Dowling, G. and Freudenthal, W. Dermatomyositis and poikiloderma atrophicans vasculare: A clinical and histological comparison. *Br. J. Dermatol.*, 50:519, 1938.

Everett, M. and Curtis, A. Dermatomyositis: A review of nineteen cases in adolescents and children. *Arch. Int. Med.*, 100:70, 1957.

Gonzalez-Angulo, A., Fraga, A. and Mintz, G. Submicroscopic alterations in capillaries of skeletal muscles in polymyositis. *Am. J. Med.*, 45:873, 1968.

Guy, W., Grauer, R. and Jacob, F. Poikilodermatomyositis. *Arch. Dermatol. Syph.*, 40:867, 1939.

Györkey, F. et al. A morphologic study on the occurrence and distribution of structures resembling viral nucleocapsids in collagen diseases. *Am. J. Med.*, 53:148, 1972.

Hashimoto, K. et al. Dermatomyositis: Electron microscopic, immunologic, and tissue culture studies of paramyxovirus-like inclusions. *Arch. Dermatol.*, 103:120, 1971.

Haupt, H. and Hutchins, G. The heart and cardiac conduction system in polymyositis-dermatomyositis: A clinicopathologic study of 16 autopsied patients. *Am. J. Cardiol.*, 50:998, 1982.

Herd, J. and Vaughan, J. Calcinosis universalis complicating dermatomyositis—Its treatment with Na_2EDTA: Report of two cases in children. *Arthritis Rheum.*, 7:259, 1964.

Horn, R. Poikilodermatomyositis: Report of a case with complete postmortem examination. *Arch. Dermatol. Syph.*, 44:1086, 1941.

Janis, J. and Winkelmann, R. Histopathology of the skin in dermatomyositis: A histopathologic study of 55 cases. *Arch. Dermatol.*, 97:640, 1968.

Kehoe, R. et al. Cardiac conduction defects in polymyositis. *Ann. Int. Med.*, 94:41, 1981.

Kinney, T. and Maher, M. Dermatomyositis: A study of five cases. *Am. J. Pathol.*, 16:561, 1940.

Medsger, T., Jr., Robinson, H. and Masi, A. Factors affecting survivorship in polymyositis: A life-table study of 124 patients. *Arthritis Rheum.*, 14:249, 1971.

Muller, S., Winkelmann, R. and Brunsting, L. Calcinosis in dermatomyositis: Observations on course of disease in children and adults. *Arch. Dermatol.*, 79:669, 1959.

Norton, W., Velayos, E. and Robinson, L. Endothelial inclusions in dermatomyositis. *Ann. Rheum. Dis.*, 29:67, 1970.

O'Leary, P. and Waisman, M. Dermatomyositis: A study of forty cases. *Arch. Dermatol. Syph.*, 41:1001, 1940.

Oxhandler, R. et al. Pathology of skeletal muscle in mixed connective tissue disease. *Arthritis Rheum.*, 20:985, 1977.

Pachman, L. and Cooke, N. Juvenile dermatomyositis: A clinical and immunologic study. *J. Pediatr.*, 96:226, 1980.

Pollock, J. Toxoplasmosis appearing to be dermatomyositis. *Arch. Dermatol.*, 115:736, 1979.
Ringel, S. et al. Sjögren's syndrome and polymyositis or dermatomyositis. *Arch. Neurol.*, 39:157, 1982.
Sewell, R. et al. Calcinosis in juvenile dermatomyositis. *Skeletal Radiol.*, 3:137, 1978.
Shafiq, S., Milhorat, A. and Gorycki, M. Electron microscopic study of muscular degeneration and vascular changes in polymyositis. *J. Pathol.*, 94:139, 1967.
Sullivan, D. et al. Prognosis in childhood dermatomyositis. *J. Pediatr.*, 80 (Pt. 1):555, 1972.
Swartz, M. Myositis. In: *Principles and Practice of Infectious Diseases*. Mandel, G. et al., eds., New York, John Wiley & Sons, 1979, p. 818.
Wainger, C. and Lever, W. Dermatomyositis: A report of three cases with postmortem observations. *Arch. Dermatol. Syph.*, 59:196, 1949.
Walton, J. and Adams, R. *Polymyositis*. Edinburgh, Livingstone, 1958.
Weston, W. and Throne, E. Profound T lymphopenia in dermatomyositis with cancer. *N. Eng. J. Med.*, 291:208, 1974.
Whitaker, J. and Engel, W. Vascular deposits of immunoglobulin and complement in idiopathic inflammatory myopathy. *N. Eng. J. Med.*, 286:333, 1972.
Williams, R., Jr. Dermatomyositis and malignancy: A review of the literature. *Ann. Int. Med.*, 50:1174, 1959.
Wolfe, J. et al. Antinuclear antibody with distinct specificity for polymyositis. *J. Clin. Invest.*, 59:176, 1977.

Scleroderma

Alpert, L. and Warner, R. Systemic sclerosis. *Am. J. Med.*, 45:568, 1968.
Barnett, A. *Scleroderma (Progressive and Systemic)*. Springfield, IL, Thomas, 1974.
Basler, R. and Kohnen, P. Localized hemosiderosis as a sequela of acne. *Arch. Dermatol.*, 114:1695, 1978.
Bauer, E. and Uitto, J. Collagen in cutaneous diseases. *Internat. J. Dermatol.*, 18:251, 1979.
Bennett, R. et al. Survival in scleroderma. *Ann. Rheumat. Dis.*, 30:581, 1971.
Burnham, T. Antinuclear antibodies. *Arch. Dermatol.*, 114:1343, 1978.
Carr, R., Heisel, E. and Stevenson, T. CRST syndrome: A benign variant of scleroderma. *Arch. Dermatol.*, 92:519, 1965.
Chazen, E., Cook, C. and Cohen, J. Morphea. *J. Pediatr.*, 60:385, 1962.
Christianson, H. et al. Localized scleroderma: A clinical study of two hundred thirty-five cases. *Arch. Dermatol.*, 74:629, 1956.
Cooper, S. et al. Increase in fibronectin in the deep dermis of involved skin in progressive systemic sclerosis. *Arthrit. Rheum.*, 22:983, 1979.
Curtis, A. and Jansen, T. The prognosis of localized scleroderma. *Arch. Dermatol.*, 78:749, 1958.
D'Angelo, W. et al. Pathologic observations in systemic sclerosis (scleroderma). *Am. J. Med.*, 46:428, 1969.
Diaz-Perez, J., Connolly, S. and Winkelmann, R. Disabling pansclerotic morphea of children. *Arch. Dermatol.*, 116:169, 1980.
Dilley, J. and Perry, H. Bilateral linear scleroderma *en coup de sabre*. *Arch. Dermatol.*, 97:688, 1968.
Douvar, A. Identification of a nuclear protein (Scl-70) as a unique target of human antinuclear antibodies in scleroderma. *J. Biol. Chem.*, 254:10514, 1979.
Farmer, E. and Hood, A. Graft-versus-host disease. In: *Update: Dermatology in General Medicine*. Fitzpatrick, T. et al., eds., New York, McGraw-Hill, 1983, p. 28.
Farmer, R., Gifford, R., Jr. and Hines, E., Jr. Prognostic significance of Raynaud's phenomenon and other clinical characteristics of systemic scleroderma: A study of 271 cases. *Circulation*, 21:1088, 1960.
Fennell, R., Jr., Reddy, C. and Vazquez, J. Progressive systemic sclerosis and malignant hypertension: Immunohistochemical study of renal lesions. *Arch. Pathol.*, 72:209, 1961.
Finch, W. et al. Bleomycin-induced scleroderma. *J. Rheumatol.*, 7:651, 1980.
Fisher, E. and Rodnan, G. Pathologic observations concerning the cutaneous lesion of progressive systemic sclerosis: An electron microscopic histochemical and immunohistochemical study. *Arthrit. Rheum.*, 3:536, 1960.
——. Pathologic observations concerning the kidney in progressive systemic sclerosis. *Arch. Pathol.*, 65:29, 1958.
Fleischmajer, R. Relationship between morphea and lichen sclerosus et atrophicus. Am. J. Dermatopathol., 2:283, 1980.

Fleischmajer, R., Damiano, V. and Nedwich, A. Alteration of subcutaneous tissue in systemic scleroderma. *Arch. Dermatol.*, 105:59, 1972.

Fleischmajer, R. and Nedwich, A. Generalized morphea. I. Histology of the dermis and subcutaneous tissue. *Arch. Dermatol.*, 106:509, 1972.

Fleischmajer, R., Perlish, J. and Duncan, M. Scleroderma: A model for fibrosis. *Arch. Dermatol.*, 119:957, 1983.

Fleischmajer, R. et al. Skin capillary changes in early systemic scleroderma. *Arch. Dermatol.*, 112:1553, 1976.

Fritzler, M. et al. The CREST syndrome: A distinct serologic entity with anticentromere antibodies. *Am. J. Med.*, 69:520, 1980.

Gay, R. et al. Collagen types synthesized in dermal fibroblast cultures from patients with early progressive systemic sclerosis. *Arthrit. Rheum.*, 23:190, 1980.

Haggani, M. and Holti, G. Systemic sclerosis with pulmonary fibrosis and oat cell carcinoma. *Acta Derm. Venereol.*, 53:369, 1973.

Hayes, R. and Rodnan, G. The ultrastructure of skin in progressive sclerosis (scleroderma). *Am. J. Pathol.*, 63:433, 1971.

Hickman, J. and Sheils, W. Progressive facial hemiatrophy: Report of a case with marked homolateral involvement. *Arch. Int. Med.*, 113:716, 1964.

Hoskins, L. et al. Functional and morphologic alterations of the gastrointestinal tract in progressive systemic sclerosis (scleroderma). *Am. J. Med.*, 33:459, 1962.

Hulsmans, R. et al. Hereditary deficiency of C2 in association with linear scleroderma "en coup de sabre." *Arch. Dermatol.*, 122:76, 1986.

Ikai, K. et al. Morphea-like cutaneous changes in a patient with systemic scleroderma. *Dermatologica*, 158:438, 1979.

Ingram, J. Morphoea and systemic sclerosis. *Br. J. Dermatol.*, 76:238, 1964.

Jablonska, S. Relationship between morphea and lichen sclerosus et atrophicus. *Am. J. Dermatopathol.*, 2:285, 1980.

Jablonska, S., Askansas, Z. and Leszczynski, S. *Scleroderma and Pseudoscleroderma: Systemic Scleroderma, Morphea and Allied Conditions*. Warsaw, Polish Medical Pub., 1965.

Kass, H., Hanson, V. and Patrick, J. Scleroderma in childhood. *J. Pediatr.*, 68:243, 1966.

Keiser, H., Stein, H. and Sjoerdsma, A. Increased protocollagen proline hydroxylase activity in sclerodermatous skin. *Arch. Dermatol.*, 104:57, 1971.

Kobayasi, T. and Asboe-Hansen, G. Ultrastructure of generalized scleroderma. *Acta Derm. Venereol.*, 52:81, 1972.

Lapenas, D., Rodnan, G. and Cavallo, T. Immunopathology of the renal vascular lesion of progressive systemic sclerosis (scleroderma). *Am. J. Pathol.*, 91:243, 1978.

Leroy, E. Connective tissue synthesis by scleroderma skin fibroblasts in cell culture. *J. Exp. Med.*, 135:1351, 1972.

Mackel, A. et al. Antibodies to collagen in scleroderma. *Arthrit. Rheum.*, 25:522, 1982.

Medsger, T. et al. Survival with systemic sclerosis (scleroderma): A life-table analysis of clinical and dermographic factors in 309 patients. *Ann. Int. Med.*, 75:369, 1971.

Minkin, W. and Rabhan, N. Office nail fold capillary microscopy using ophthalmoscope. *J. Am. Acad. Dermatol.*, 7:190, 1982.

Miyashi, Y. et al. Linear melorheostotic scleroderma with hypertrichosis. *Arch. Dermatol.*, 115:1233, 1979.

Moroi, Y. et al. Antibody to centromere (kinetocore) in scleroderma sera. *Proc. Natl. Acad. Sci. USA*, 77:1627, 1980.

Muller, S., Brunsting, L. and Winkelmann, R. Calcinosis cutis: Its relationship to scleroderma. *Arch. Dermatol.*, 80:15, 1959.

Nielsen, A., Brun, B. and Secher, L. Calcinosis in generalized scleroderma. *Acta Derm. Venereol.* (Stockh.), 60:301, 1980.

O'Leary, P., Montgomery, H. and Ragsdale, W., Jr. Dermatohistopathology of various types of scleroderma. *Arch. Dermatol.*, 75:78, 1957.

Piper, W. and Helwig, E. Progressive systemic sclerosis: Visceral manifestations in generalized scleroderma. *Arch. Dermatol.*, 72:535, 1955.

Rodnan, G., Myerowitz, R. and Justh, G. Morphologic changes in the digital arteries of patients with progressive systemic sclerosis (scleroderma) and Raynaud phenomenon. *Medicine* (Baltimore), 59:393, 1980.

Rodnan, G. et al. Skin thickness and collagen content in progressive systemic sclerosis and localized scleroderma. *Arthrit. Rheum.*, 22:130, 1979.

Rowell, N. The prognosis of systemic sclerosis. *Br. J. Dermatol.*, 95:57, 1976.

Rubin, L. Linear scleroderma: Association with abnormalities of the spine and nervous system. *Arch. Dermatol. Syph.*, 58:1, 1948.

Sackner, M. *Scleroderma*. New York, Grune & Stratton, 1966.

Serup, J. Assessment of epidermal atrophy in localized scleroderma (morphea). *Dermatologica*, 172:205, 1986.

Stuart, J. et al. Evidence for cell-mediated immunity to collagen in progressive systemic sclerosis. *J. Lab. Clin. Med.*, 88:601, 1976.

Su, D. and Person, J. Morphea profunda: A new concept and a histopathologic study of 23 cases. *Am. J. Dermatopathol.*, 3:251, 1981.

Su, W. and Greene, S. Bullous morphea profunda. *Am. J. Dermatopathol.*, 8:144, 1986.

Synkowski, D., Lobitz, W., Jr. and Provost, T. Bullous scleroderma. *Arch. Dermatol.*, 117:135, 1981.

Talbott, J. et al. Dermatomyositis with scleroderma, calcinosis and renal endarteritis associated with focal cortical necrosis: Report of a case in which the condition simulated Addison's disease, with comment on metabolic and pathologic studies. *Arch. Int. Med.*, 63:476, 1939.

Templeton, H. Localized scleroderma with bullae. *Arch. Dermatol. Syph.*, 43:361, 1941.

Tuffanelli, D. and Winkelmann, R. Systemic scleroderma: A clinical study of 727 cases. *Arch. Dermatol.*, 84:359, 1961.

Uitto, J. et al. Connective tissue in scleroderma. *Acta Derm. Venereol.*, 51:401, 1968.

Uitto, J. et al. Scleroderma: Increased biosynthesis of triplehelical type I and type III procollagens associated with unaltered expression of collagenase by skin fibroblasts in culture. *J. Clin. Invest.*, 64:921, 1979.

Velayos, E. et al. The "CREST" syndrome: Comparison with SS (scleroderma). *Arch. Int. Med.*, 139:1240, 1979.

Viraben, R. and Dupre, A. Eosinophilic fasciitis (Shulman syndrome) in association with morphea, immunologic disturbance and profuse achromia. *Dermatologica*, 174:93, 1987.

Wagers, L., Young, A., Jr. and Ryan, S. Linear melorheostotic scleroderma. *Br. J. Dermatol.*, 86:297, 1972.

Wuthrich, R., Roenigk, H., Jr. and Steck, W. Localized scleroderma. *Arch. Dermatol.*, 111:98, 1975.

Atrophoderma of Pasini and Pierini

Canizares, O. et al. Idiopathic atrophoderma of Pasini and Pierini. *Arch. Dermatol.*, 77:42, 1958.

Jablonska, S. and Szczepanski, A. Atrophoderma Pasini-Pierini: Is it an entity? *Dermatologica*, 125:226, 1962.

Kee, C., Brothers, W. and New, W. Idiopathic atrophoderma of Pasini and Pierini with coexistent morphea: A case report. *Arch. Dermatol.*, 82:100, 1960.

Miller, R. Idiopathic atrophoderma: Report of a case and nosologic study. *Arch. Dermatol.*, 92:653, 1965.

Progeria of Adults (Werner's Syndrome)

Boatwright, H., Wheeler, C. and Cawley, E. Werner's syndrome. *Arch. Int. Med.*, 90:243, 1952.

DeBusk, F. The Hutchinson-Gilford progeria syndrome. *J. Pediatr.*, 80:697, 1972.

Feingold, M. and Kidd, R. Progeria and scleroderma in infancy. *Am. J. Dis. Child.*, 122:61, 1971.

Östenjö, B. Werner's syndrome: Progeria genito-dystrophicum. *Acta Derm. Venereol.* , 33:497, 1953.

Reed, R., Seville, R. and Tattersall, R. Werner's syndrome. *Br. J. Dermatol.*, 65:165, 1953.

Tao, L., Stecker E. and Gardner, H. Werner's syndrome and acute myeloid leukemia. *Can. Med. Assoc. J.*, 105:951, 1971.

Pachydermoperiostosis

Curth, H., Firschein, I. and Alpert, M. Familial clubbed fingers. *Arch. Dermatol.*, 83:828, 1961.

Fischer, D., Singer, D. and Feldman, S. Clubbing: A review, with emphasis on hereditary acropachy. *Medicine*, 43:459, 1964.

Hambrick, G., Jr. and Carter, D. Pachydermoperiostosis: Touraine-Solente-Gole syndrome. *Arch. Dermatol.*, 94:594, 1966.

Rimoin, D. Pachydermoperiostosis (idiopathic clubbing and periostosis): Genetic and physiologic considerations. *N. Eng. J. Med.*, 272:923, 1965.

Vogl, A. and Goldfischer, S. Pachydermoperiostosis: Primary or idiopathic hypertrophic osteoarthropathy. *Am. J. Med.*, 33:166, 1962.

Eosinophilic Fasciitis

Barnes, L. et al. Eosinophilic fasciitis. *Am. J. Pathol.*, 96:493, 1979.

Barrière, H. et al. Syndrome de Shulman. *Ann. Dermatol. Venereol.*, 107:643, 1980.

Chevrant-Breton, J. et al. Le syndrome de Shulman: Fasciite avec éosinophilie; pseudosclérodermie à éosinophiles: A propos de deux cas. *Ann. Dermatol. Venereol.*, 104:616, 1977.

Coyle, H. and Chapman, R. Eosinophilic fasciitis (Shulman syndrome) in association with morphoea and systemic sclerosis. *Acta Derm. Venereol.*, 60:181, 1980.

Fleischmajer, R. et al. Scleroderma, eosinophilia, and diffuse fasciitis. *Arch. Dermatol.*, 114:1320, 1978.

Golitz, L. Fasciitis with eosinophilia: The Shulman syndrome. *Internat. J. Dermatol.*, 19:552, 1980.

Hintner, H. et al. Fasziitis mit Eosinophilie. Das Shulman Syndrom. *Hautarzt*, 32:75, 1981.

King, D. et al. Generalized morphea with peripheral eosinophilia, fasciitis and myositis. *Internat. J. Dermatol.*, 19:149, 1980.

Krauser, R. and Tuthill, R. Eosinophilic fasciitis. *Arch. Dermatol.*, 113:1092, 1977.

Lupton, G. and Goette, D. Localized eosinophilic fasciitis. *Arch. Dermatol.*, 115:85, 1979.

Michet, C., Jr., Doyle, J. and Ginsburg, W. Eosinophilic fasciitis: Report of 15 cases. *Mayo Clin. Proc.*, 56:27, 1981.

Moore, T. and Zuckner, J. Eosinophilic fasciitis. *Semin. Arthrit. Rheum.*, 9:228, 1980.

Moutsopoulos, H. et al. Diffuse fasciitis and eosinophilia: A cliniopathologic study. *Am. J. Med.*, 68:701, 1980.

Rodnan, G. et al. Eosinophilic fasciitis: Report of seven cases of a newly recognized scleroderma-like syndrome. *Arthrit. Rheum.*, 18:422, 1975.

Seibold, J. et al. Circulating immune complexes in eosinophilic fasciitis. *Arthrit. Rheum.*, 25:1180, 1982.

Shewmake, S., Lopez, P. and McGlamory, J. The Shulman syndrome. *Arch. Dermatol.*, 114:556, 1978.

Shulman, L. Diffuse fasciitis with hypergammaglobulinemia and eosinophilia: A new syndrome? (abstr.). *J. Rheumatol.*, 1 (1, suppl.):46, 1974.

Solomon, G. et al. Eosinophilic fasciitis responsive to cimetidine. *Ann. Int. Med.*, 97:547, 1982.

Su, W. and Person, J. Morphea profunda. *Am. J. Dermatopathol.*, 3:251, 1981.

Torres, V. and George, W. Diffuse eosinophilic fasciitis. *Arch. Dermatol.*, 113:1591, 1977.

Weinstein, D. and Schwartz, R. Eosinophilic fasciitis. *Arch. Dermatol.*, 114:1047, 1978.

Graft-versus-Host Disease

De Dobbeleer, G., Ledoux-Corbusier, M. and Achtern, G. Graft-versus-host reaction: An ultrastructural study. *Arch. Dermatol.*, 111:1597, 1975.

Farmer, E. and Hood, A. Graft-versus-host disease. In: *Update: Dermatology in General Medicine*. Fitzpatrick, T. et al., eds., New York, McGraw-Hill, 1983, p. 28.

Gluckman, E. et al. Graft-versus-host disease in recipients of syngeneic bone marrow. *Lancet*, 1:253, 1980.

Glucksberg, H. et al. Clinical manifestations of graft-versus-host disease in human recipients of marrow from HL-A-matched sibling donors. *Transplantation*, 18:295, 1975.

Graham-Brown, R. and Sarkany, I. Scleroderma-like changes due to chronic graft-versus-host disease. *Clin. Exp. Dermatol.*, 8:531, 1983.

Grogan, T., Odom, R. and Burgess, J. Graft-versus-host reaction. *Arch. Dermatol.*, 113:806, 1977.

Hood, A. et al. Graft-versus-host reaction. *Arch. Dermatol.*, 113:1087, 1977.

Janin-Mercier, A. et al. The lichen planus-like and sclerotic phases of the graft-versus-host disease in man. *Acta Derm. Venereol.* (Stockh.), 61:187, 1981.

Mascaro, J. et al. Acute and chronic graft-versus-host reaction in skin: Report of two cases. *Br. J. Dermatol.*, 102:461, 1980.

Morhenn, V. and Maibach, H. Graft-versus-host reaction in a newborn. *Acta Derm. Venereol.* (Stockh.), 54:133, 1974.

Parkman, R., Rappeport, J. and Rosen, F. Human graft-versus-host disease. *J. Invest. Dermatol.*, 74:276, 1980.

Peck, G., Herzig, G. and Elias, P. Toxic epidermal necrolysis in a patient with graft-versus-host reaction. *Arch. Dermatol.*, 105:561, 1972.

Rappeport, J. et al. Acute graft-versus-host disease in recipients of bone marrow transplants from identical twin donors. *Lancet*, 2:717, 1979.

Rodu, B. and Gockerman, J. Oral manifestations of the chronic graft-versus-host reaction. *JAMA*, 249:504, 1983.

Rosen, R. et al. Acute leukemia and granulocyte transfusion: Fatal graft-versus-host reaction following transfusion of cells obtained from normal donors. *J. Pediatr.*, 93:268, 1978.

Saurat, J. et al. The lichen planus-like eruption after bone marrow transplantation. *Br. J. Dermatol.*, 93:675, 1975.

Schmitt, D. and Thivolet, J. Lymphocyte-epidermis interactions in malignant epidermotrophic lymphomas. *Acta Derm. Venereol.* (Stockh.), 60:1, 1980.

Shulman, H. et al. Chronic cutaneous graft-versus-host disease in man. *Am. J. Pathol.*, 91:545, 1978.

Spielvogel, R., Goltz, R. and Kersey, J. Scleroderma-like changes in chronic graft-versus-host disease. *Arch. Dermatol.*, 113:1424, 1977.

Storb, R. et al. Marrow transplantation in thirty "untransfused" patients with severe aplastic anemia. *Ann. Int. Med.*, 92:30, 1980.

Tsoi, M. et al. Deposition of IgM and C at the dermoepidermal junction in acute and chronic cutaneous graft-versus-host disease in man. *J. Immunol.*, 120:1485, 1978.

Ullman, S. Immunoglobulins and complement in skin in graft-versus-host disease. *Ann. Int. Med.*, 85:205, 1976.

Scleredema Adultorum

Carrington, P. et al. Scleredema adultorum. *Internat. J. Dermatol.*, 23:514, 1984.

Cohn, B., Wheeler, C., Jr. and Briggaman, R. Scleredema adultorum of Buschke and diabetes mellitus. *Arch. Dermatol.*, 101:27, 1970.

Curtis, A. and Shulak, B. Scleredema adultorum. *Arch. Dermatol.*, 92:526, 1965.

Fleischmajer, R., Faludi, G. and Krol, S. Scleredema and diabetes mellitus. *Arch. Dermatol.*, 101:21, 1970.

Fleischmajer, R. and Perlish, J. Glycosaminoglycans in scleroderma and scleredema. *J. Invest. Dermatol.*, 58:129, 1972.

Greenberg, L. et al. Scleredema "adultorum" in children. *Pediatrics*, 32:1044, 1963.

Kövary, P. et al. Monoclonal gammopathy in scleredema. *Arch. Dermatol.*, 117:536, 1981.

Krakowski, A., Covo, J. and Berlin, C. Diabetic scleredema. *Dermatologica*, 146:193, 1973.

Leinwand, I. Generalized scleredema: Report with autopsy findings. *Ann. Int. Med.*, 34:226, 1951.

McNaughton, F. and Keczkes, K. Scleredema adultorum and diabetes mellitus (scleredema diutinum). *Clin. Exp. Dermatol.*, 8:41, 1983.

Vallee, B. Scleredema: A systemic disease. *N. Eng. J. Med.*, 235:207, 1946.

Acro-osteolysis

Fine, R. Acro-osteolysis: Vinyl chloride induced "scleroderma." *Internat. J. Dermatol.*, 15:676, 1976.

Markowitz, S. et al. Occupational acro-osteolysis. *Arch. Dermatol.*, 106:219, 1972.

Meyerson, L. and Meier, G. Cutaneous lesions in acro-osteolysis. *Arch. Dermatol.*, 106:224, 1972.

Veltmann, G., Lange, C. and Stein, G. Die Vinylkrankheit. *Hautarzt*, 29:177, 1978.

Chapter 10
Bullous Dermatoses

Bullae are classified by the mechanism and site of their formation. The difference between vesicles and bullae is only a matter of size. Here we are using the term *bullae* in its generic sense, encompassing all blistering lesions.

CLASSIFICATION OF BLISTERS

Site of Formation	*Mode of Formation*	*Disease*
subcorneal	Detachment of horny layer	Impetigo; subcorneal pustular dermatosis; erythema toxicum neonatorum; miliaria crystallina
Intraepidermal	Intercellular edema (spongiosis) and intracellular edema	Dermatitis (eczema); incontinentia pigmenti; miliaria rubra
	Degeneration of keratinocytes	Epidermolytic hyperkeratosis; friction blister; epidermal type of erythema multiforme
	Acantholysis (separation of keratinocytes due to loss of intercellular cement substance and/or loss of desmosomes)	Pemphigus (vulgaris and foliaceus); Hailey-Hailey disease; Darier's disease; Grover's disease; warty dyskeratoma; acantholytic solar keratosis and squamous cell carcinoma; viral blisters (herpes simplex; varicella; herpes zoster; variola; hand-foot-and-mouth disease)
Subepidermal	Degeneration of basal cells	Lichen planus; lupus erythematosus; lichen sclerosus et atrophicus; epidermolysis bullosa, epidermal type
	Degeneration of basement membrane zone	Bullous pemphigoid; cicatricial pemphigoid; dermatitis herpetiformis; herpes gestationis; erythema multiforme, dermal type; epidermolysis bullosa, junctional and dystrophic types; urticaria pigmentosa; porphyria cutanea tarda

In this chapter we will restrict discussion to entities in which blister formation is the key identifying characteristic; other entities with blisters are discussed elsewhere.

Acantholytic Bullous Dermatoses

Pemphigus

Pemphigus is a group of acantholytic bullous disorders characterized by loss of intercellular cement substance and loss of desmosomes.

It is probably of autoimmune etiology, with pathogenesis based on autoantibodies to intercellular cement substance.

There are two types of pemphigus, each with a variant:

- Pemphigus vulgaris
  - variant: Pemphigus vegetans
- Pemphigus foliaceus
  - variant: Pemphigus erythematosus

Whether or not pemphigus vulgaris and pemphigus foliaceus should be considered expressions of the same disease is controversial. Cases are on record of patients with coexisting lesions of both types or with evolution of lesions from one type to another.

PEMPHIGUS VULGARIS

Pemphigus vulgaris is generally fatal when untreated. The era of corticosteroid therapy has changed the prior outlook of almost inevitable fatality.

Onset is usually in middle age; there is a predilection for Jews and other Mediterranean groups.

Penicillamine can induce pemphigus vulgaris or pemphigus foliaceus; pemphigus vulgaris is induced less frequently than pemphigus foliaceus.

Lesions of pemphigus vulgaris start as flaccid bullae, which rapidly rupture to form large, denuded areas (Figs. A, B).

Mucous membranes, particularly the oral mucosa, are often involved. Frequently, initial lesions involve the oral mucosa.

Microscopic features

1. The earliest change is intercellular edema (spongiosis) in the lower epidermis; this may be accompanied by a migration of eosinophils into the epidermis. This has been called eosinophilic spongiosis (Fig. C).
2. The stage of spongiosis is followed by suprabasal acantholysis leading to suprabasal clefts (Fig. D) and bullae.
3. In fully formed blisters, the dermis is lined by a single row of basal cells, many of which have been separated from each other by a loss of intercellular bridges; the bulla cavity often contains detached acantholytic epidermal cells (Fig. F).
4. In older (denuded) lesions (Fig. E), the dome of the blister is lost, leaving only the row of basal cells at the base. The inflammatory reaction may destroy the row of basal cells in the center of the lesion.
5. In older blisters, regeneration of epithelium may result in multiple layers of epithelial cells at the base (Fig. G, right side of field).
6. Early lesions show only a slight mixed dermal inflammatory infiltrate, but later lesions may have a dense infiltrate, including many eosinophils and plasma cells.
7. Papillomatous projections lined by epithelial cells are called *villi* (Fig. E).

PEMPHIGUS VULGARIS

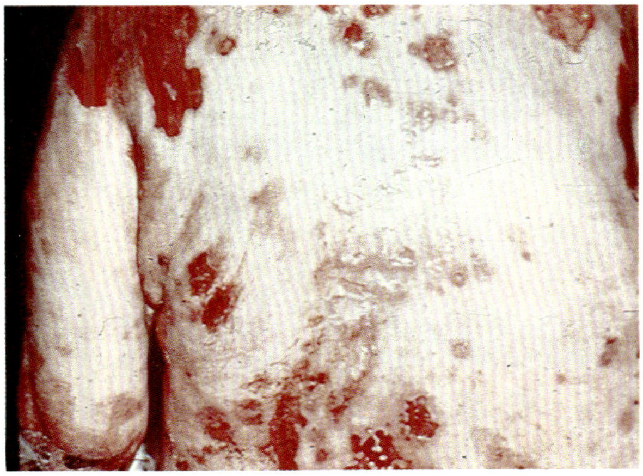

A

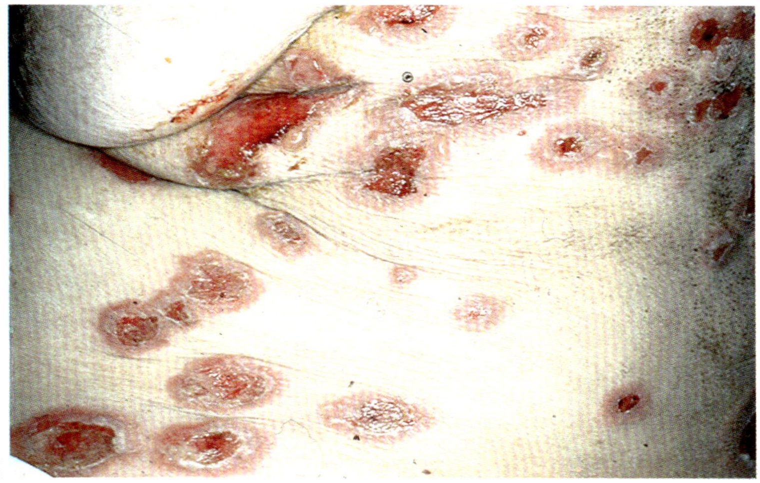

B

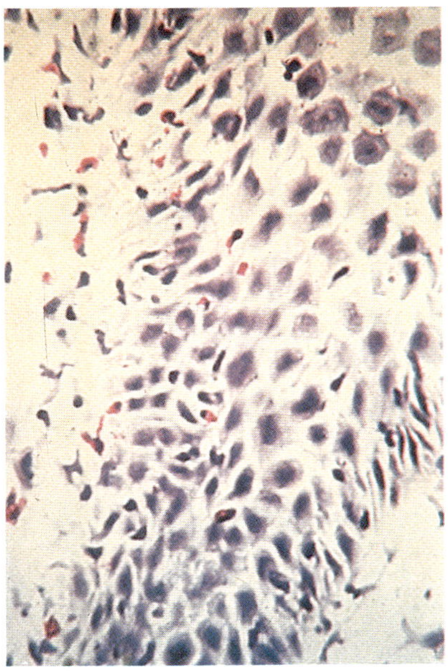

C
X400

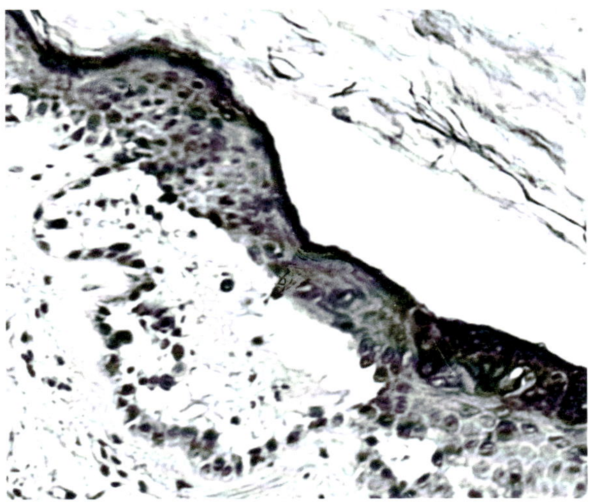

D
X260

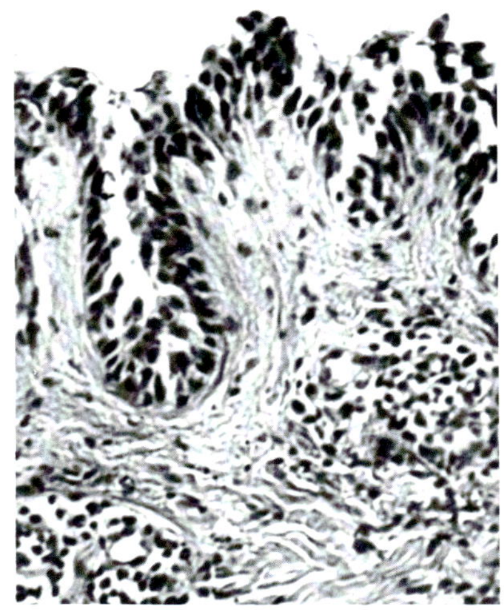

E
X180

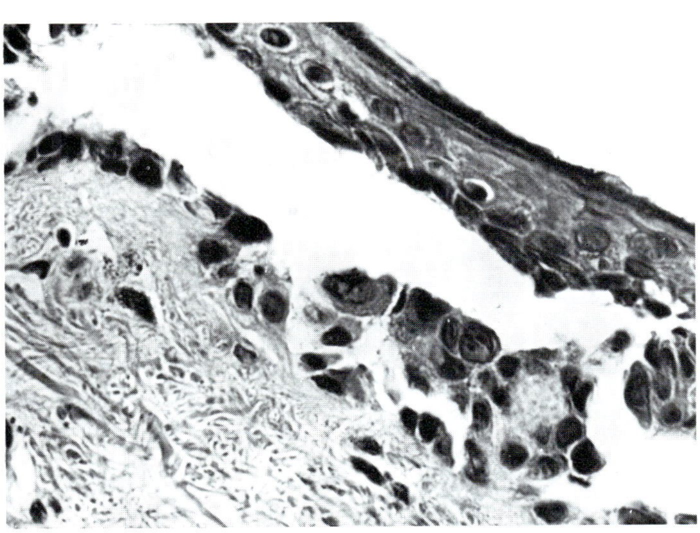

F
X540

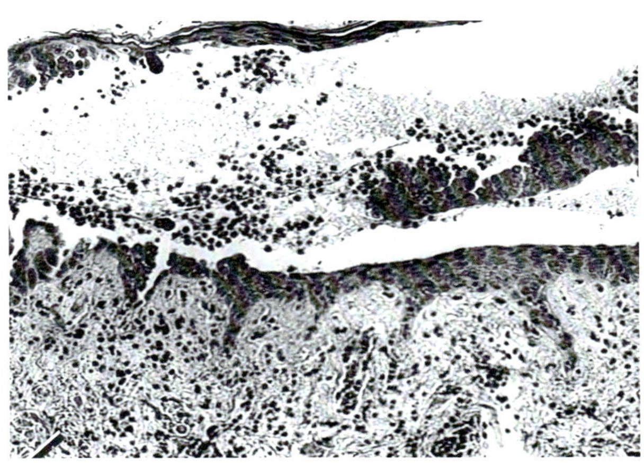

G
X130

PEMPHIGUS continued

PEMPHIGUS VULGARIS

Microscopic features

8. Suprabasal acantholysis often involves the outer root sheath (Figs. A,B).
9. Dyskeratosis is not a typical feature of pemphigus vulgaris, but it can occasionally be seen. There is an element of dyskeratosis in the fields shown on the opposite page.

Comment

It is desirable to obtain an early lesion for histologic diagnosis of pemphigus vulgaris, since old lesions may not show diagnostic changes. Ideally, a lesion small enough to be removed *in toto* with a biopsy punch should be obtained.

PEMPHIGUS VULGARIS

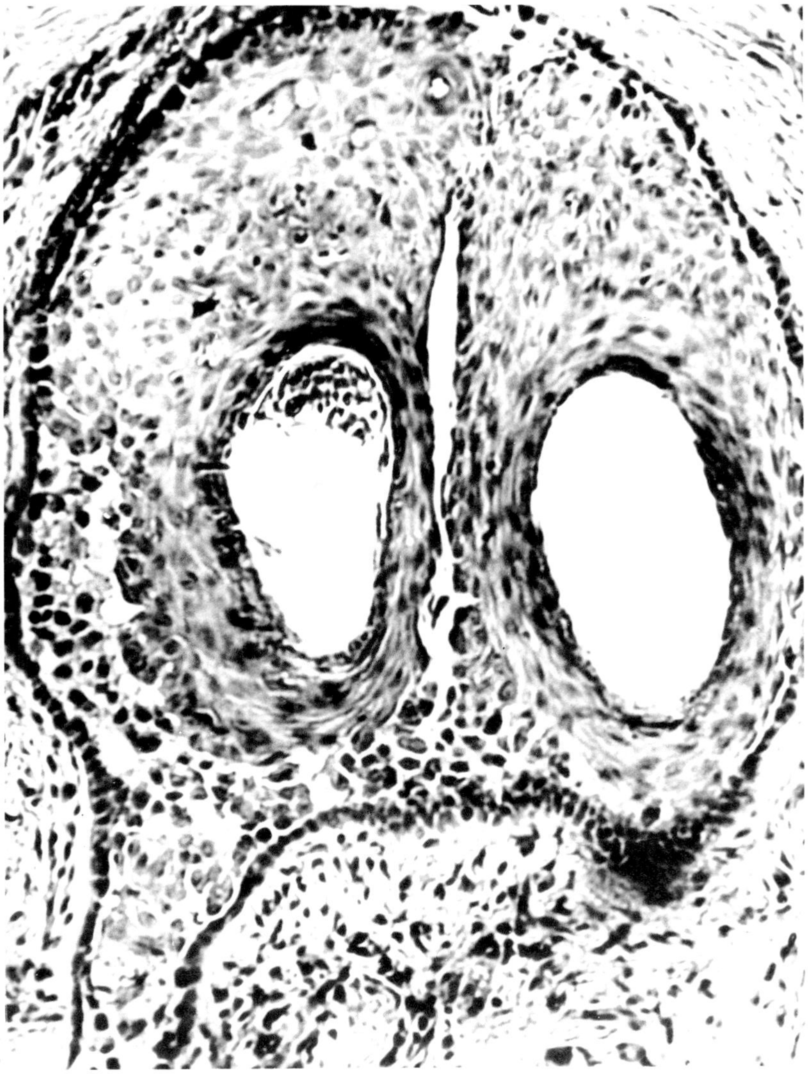

A
X260

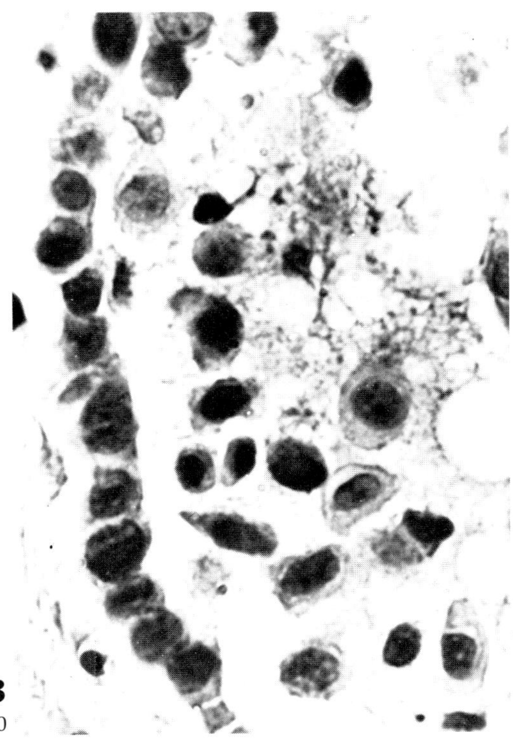

B
X720

PEMPHIGUS continued ⇨

PEMPHIGUS VULGARIS OF THE MUCOUS MEMBRANES

The oral mucosa and vermilion border of the lips are frequently involved. Bullae rupture easily, resulting in denuded, crusting areas (Fig. A). Only fresh lesions are observed intact (Fig. B).

Microscopic features

1. Histologic features parallel those of the skin. Suprabasal acantholysis leads to cleft and bulla formation (Fig. C).
2. A dense dermal infiltrate may be present (Fig. C).

Microscopic differential diagnosis of pemphigus vulgaris (see chart, p. 554)

1. Acantholytic solar keratoses show suprabasal acantholysis but can usually be distinguished from pemphigus vulgaris by the presence of nuclear atypia of keratinocytes.
2. Grover's disease (transient acantholytic dermatosis or TAD) can show acantholytic changes indistinguishable from those in pemphigus vulgaris, although the acantholytic areas tend to be smaller than those in pemphigus vulgaris. Distinction can be made by immunofluorescence testing. Pemphigus vulgaris shows intercellular epidermal antibodies; Grover's disease does not.

PEMPHIGUS VULGARIS: MUCOUS MEMBRANES

A

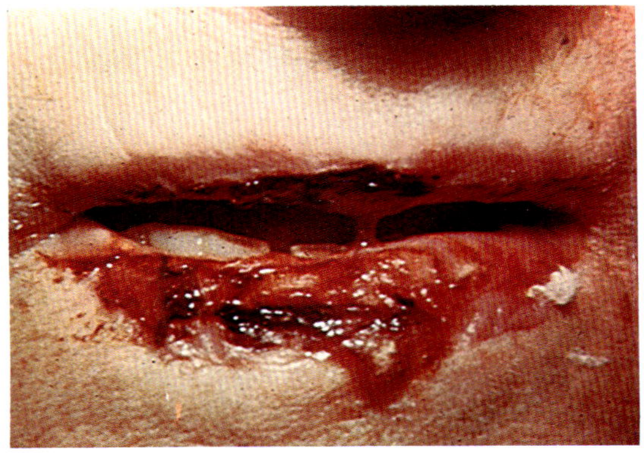

B

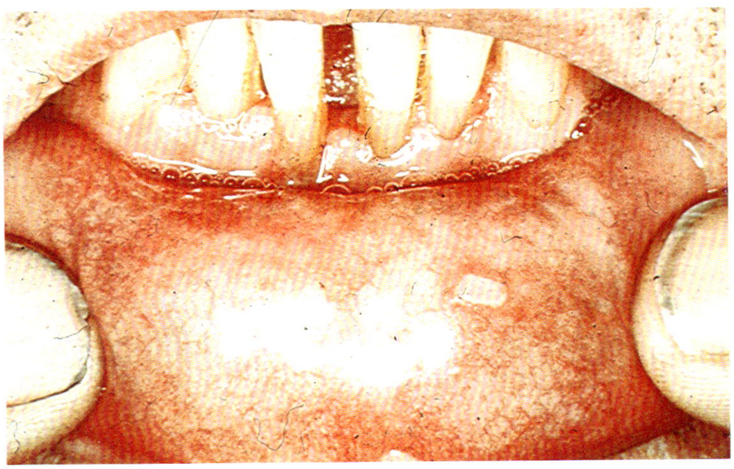

C
X200

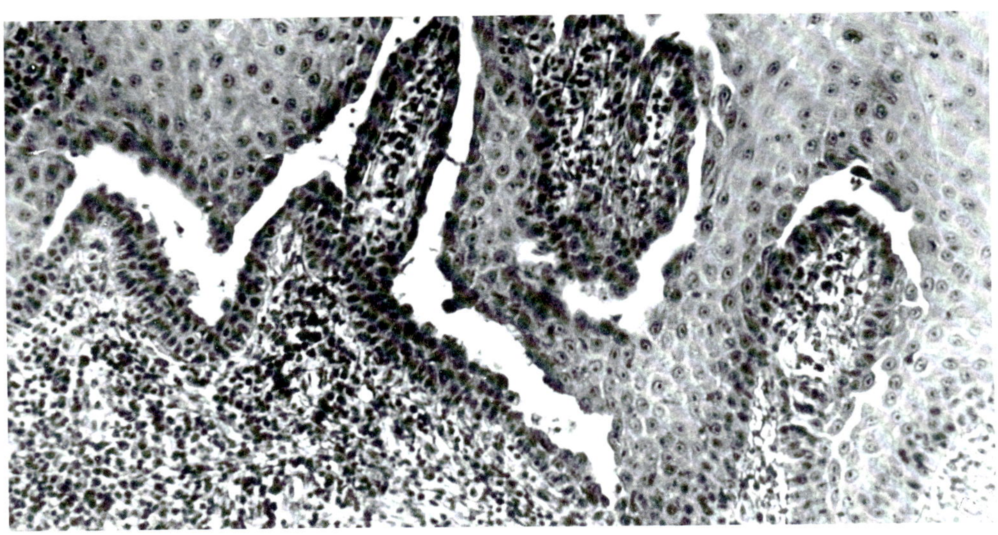

PEMPHIGUS continued ⇨

PEMPHIGUS VULGARIS

Immunofluorescence testing in pemphigus

Direct immunofluorescence testing. Unfixed, frozen sections of perilesional or normal skin are used. Fluorescein-labeled antihuman immunoglobulins and C3 are applied. A positive test is indicated by fluorescence of the intercellular spaces (Fig. A). IgG is almost always present. In many patients, IgA, IgM, or C3 may also be present.

Indirect immunofluorescence testing. Substrate consists of unfixed, frozen sections of monkey or guinea pig esophagus. First the patient's serum at various dilutions is applied and then fluorescein-labeled antihuman IgG. A positive test is indicated by fluorescence of the intercellular spaces (Fig. B).

In general, the antibody titer is proportional to the severity of disease, but exceptions are not uncommon. In early localized pemphigus vulgaris the indirect fluorescent antibody test may be negative. Direct immunofluorescence testing is more sensitive.

Comment

Mixed bullous disease refers to the coexistence of various combinations of acantholytic and subepidermal bullous dermatoses, including pemphigus vulgaris, pemphigus foliaceus, dermatitis herpetiformis, and bullous pemphigoid.

PEMPHIGUS VEGETANS

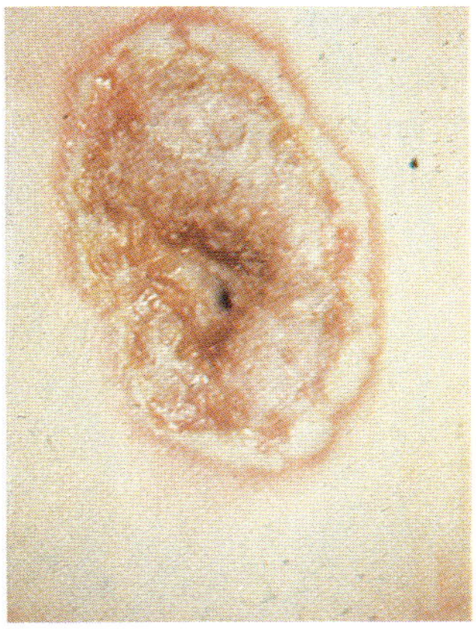
A

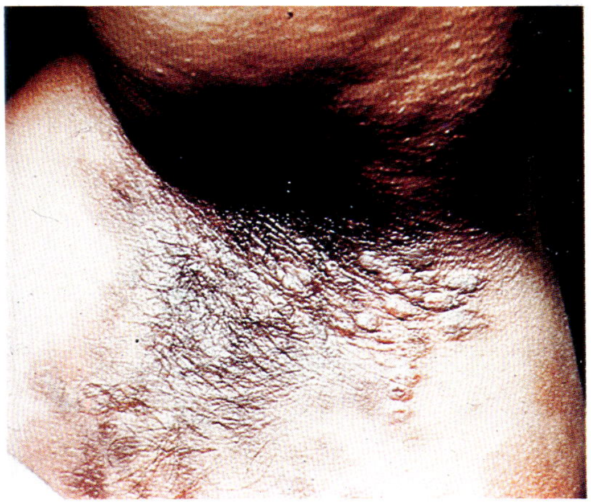
B

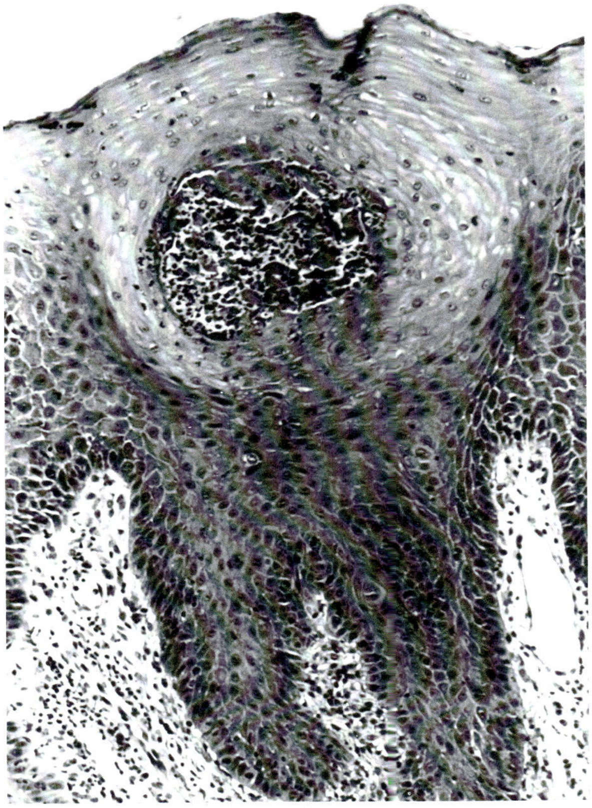
C
X175

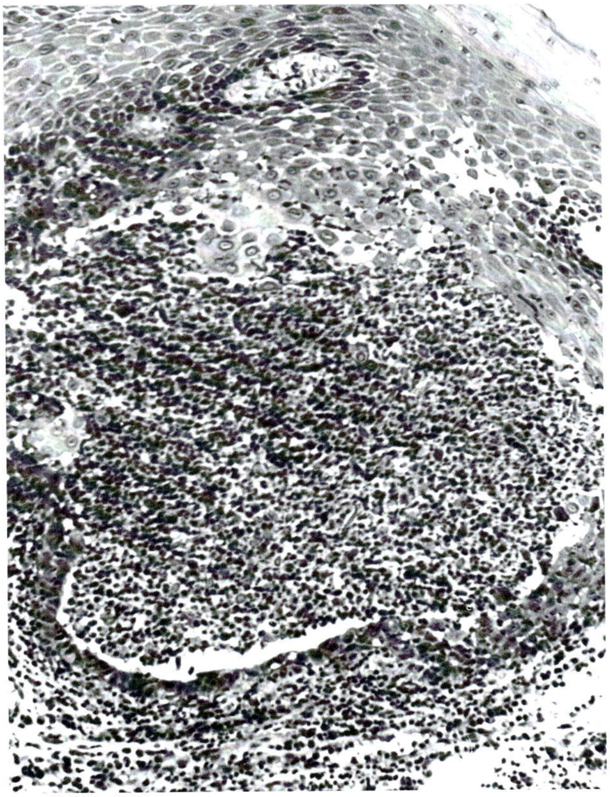
D
X160

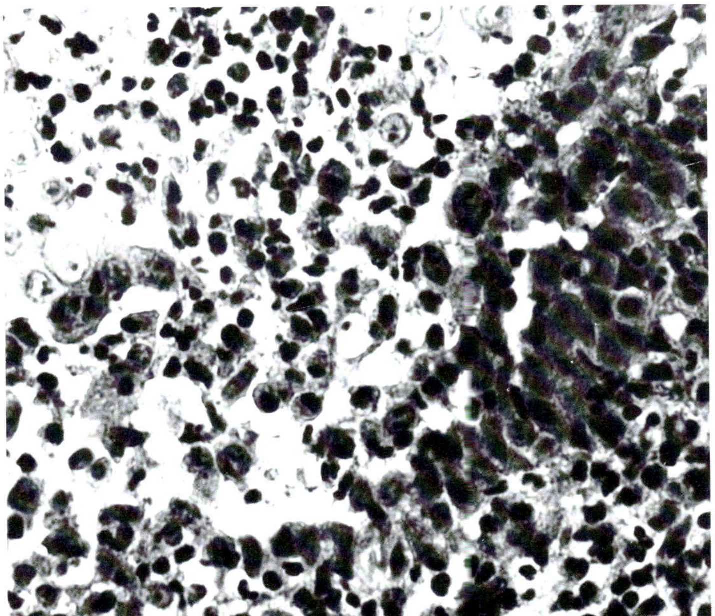
E
X520

PEMPHIGUS continued

PEMPHIGUS FOLIACEUS

Pemphigus foliaceus is less severe than pemphigus vulgaris; however, fatal cases occur in the older age groups. The age of onset is more variable than in pemphigus vulgaris, and there does not seem to be an ethnic predisposition.

Early lesions are shallow, flaccid blisters which rapidly evolve into areas of superficial denudation, scaling, and crusting (Figs. A,B). The initial site is often the central area of the face. Eventually, wide areas of the skin may be involved and generalized exfoliation may occur. Advancing lesions are often sharply marginated and serpiginous.

Oral lesions are uncommon.

Early stages of pemphigus foliaceus may have lesions resembling dermatitis herpetiformis—grouped papules, vesicles, or bullae.

Pemphigus erythematosus (Senear-Usher) is a variant of pemphigus foliaceus in which lesions tend to remain localized in the central area of the face, scalp, chest, and upper back. Lesions resemble seborrheic dermatitis or lupus erythematosus.

Microscopic features

1. The key feature is acantholysis high in the epidermis, usually in the granular layer or adjacent to it (Figs. C,D). This results in a bulla with superficial location, with acantholysis at the dome and base (Figs. C,D).
2. There may be an early stage of eosinophilic spongiosis, as in pemphigus vulgaris.
3. Occasionally, acantholytic separations occur at lower levels of the epidermis (Fig. E), and rarely these are present in a suprabasal location, making differentiation from pemphigus vulgaris difficult.

PEMPHIGUS FOLIACEUS

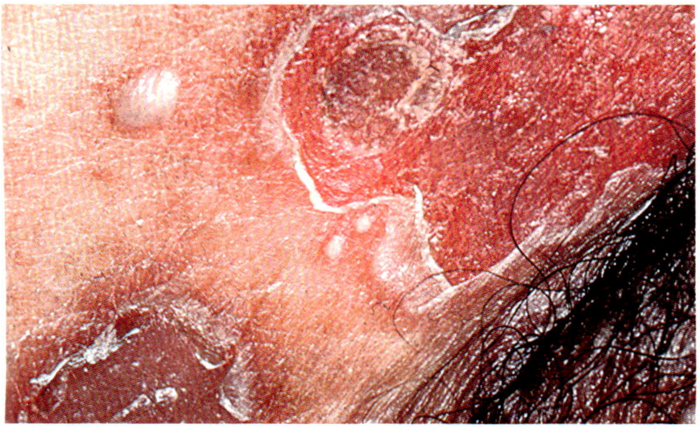

A

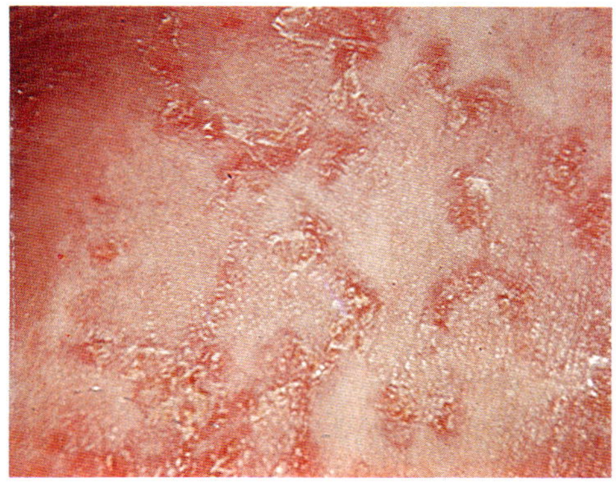

B

C X180

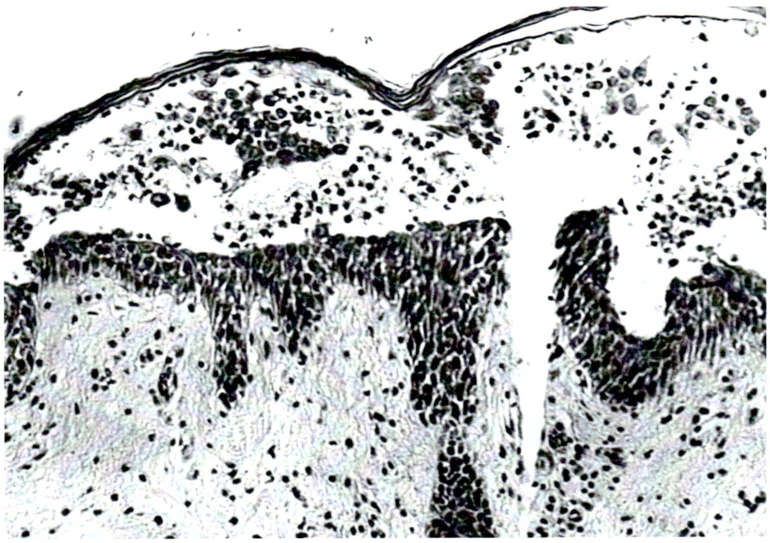

D X520

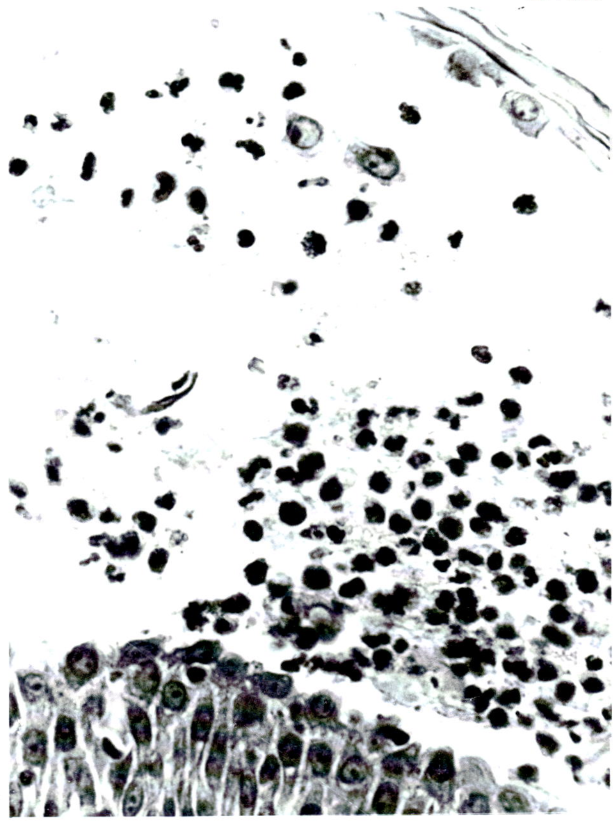

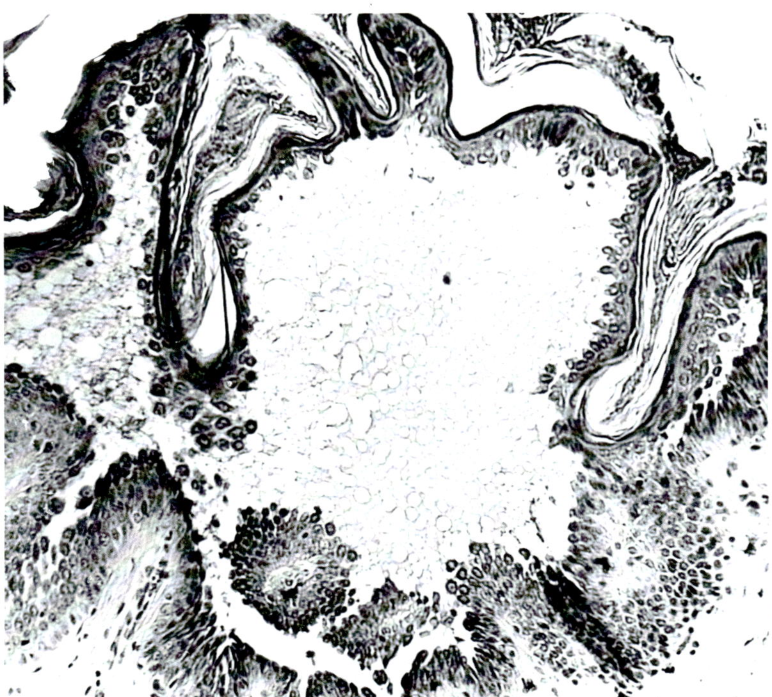

E X160

PEMPHIGUS continued ⇨

PEMPHIGUS FOLIACEUS

Microscopic features

4. In some lesions, intact bullae are not present, but acantholysis is evident in the upper epidermis (Fig. A).
5. Grains (ellipsoid dyskeratotic, acantholytic cells) are present in the upper epidermis (Figs. A,B).
6. Older lesions show acanthosis and papillomatosis (Fig. A). Hyperkeratosis, parakeratosis, and hyperkeratotic follicular plugs may be observed.
7. The dermis contains an inflammatory infiltrate of varying intensity; eosinophils are often present.

PEMPHIGUS FOLIACEUS

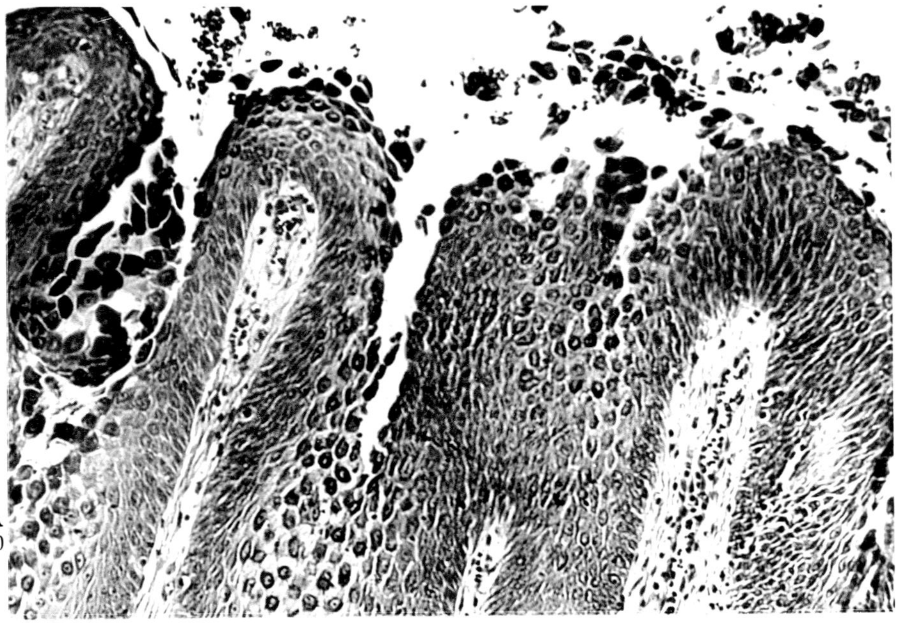

A
X180

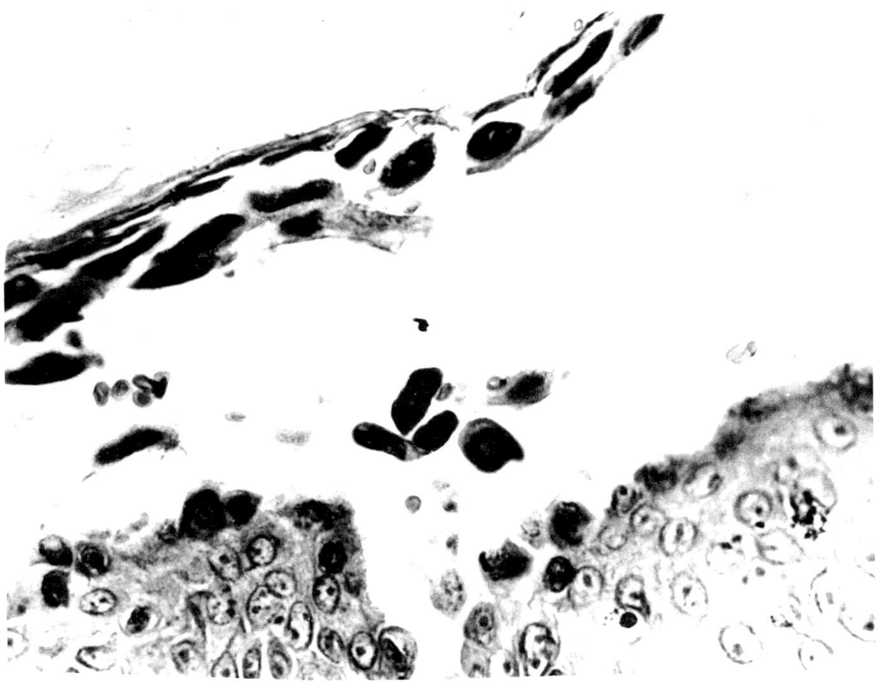

B
X530

PEMPHIGUS continued ⇨

PEMPHIGUS FOLIACEUS

Microscopic differential diagnosis (see p. 554)

1. There is a resemblance to impetigo or subcorneal pustular dermatosis (Fig. A); however, pemphigus foliaceus can usually be distinguished by the presence of significant acantholysis (Figs. A,B) and dyskeratosis (grains).

Comment

1. Intercellular antibodies can be demonstrated in pemphigus foliaceus by immunofluorescence testing, as in pemphigus vulgaris.
2. *Fogo selvagem* is a form of pemphigus foliaceus endemic to Brazil.

PEMPHIGUS FOLIACEUS

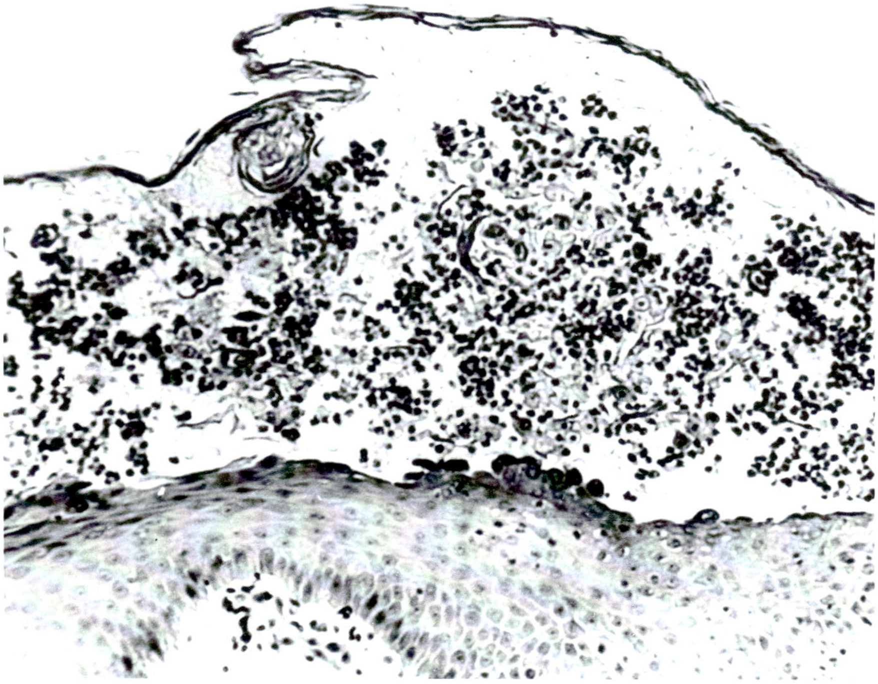

A X75

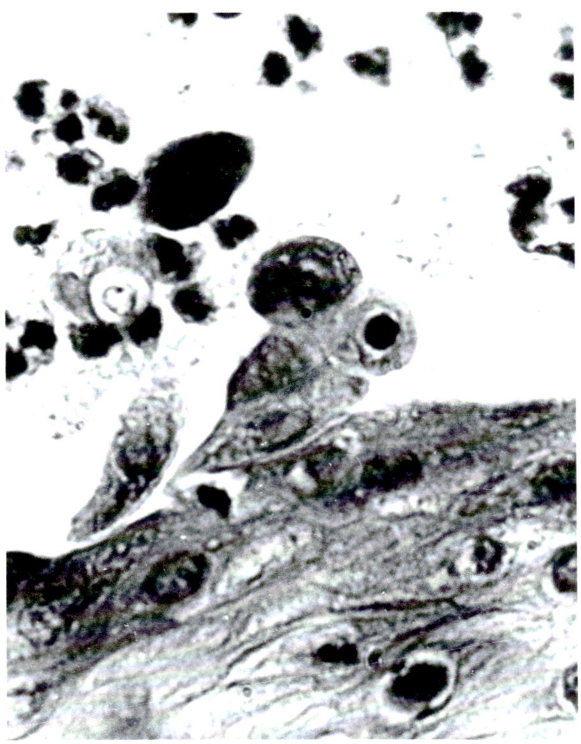

B X660

FAMILIAL BENIGN CHRONIC PEMPHIGUS (HAILEY-HAILEY)

Familial benign chronic pemphigus has a probable dominant mode of inheritance with incomplete penetrance. Onset is usually during the second or third decade of life. Lesions are elicited by trauma or infection.

Initial lesions are vesicles on an erythematous base, which evolve into denuded areas with crusting and vegetations (Fig. A). A sharply marginated border may be present, resulting in a resemblance to lesions of pemphigus foliaceus. Healing occurs without scarring, but occasionally with hyperpigmentation. Sites of predilection are the intertriginous areas and the sides (Fig. A) and nape of the neck. Mucosal lesions are infrequent. Haily-Hailey disease is believed to be based on a defect in cellular cohesion, either via a defect in cement substance or desmosomes. The theory that the disorder represents a bullous variant of Darier's disease is not widely accepted.

Microscopic features

1. Lesions are characterized by suprabasal acantholysis resulting in clefts and bullae (Figs. B,C,D,E).
2. Acantholytic separation of epidermal cells is also extensive at higher levels of the epidermis, producing a "tumbling brick wall" appearance (Figs. B,C,D,E). The stratum corneum may be involved (Figs. D,E).
3. Papillomatosis with villus formation may be observed (Fig. E); strands of proliferating epidermal cells may extend downward into the dermis.
4. Moderate dyskeratosis may be present, with cells resembling grains and *corps ronds* of Darier's disease (Figs. D,E).

Microscopic differential diagnosis (see p. 554)

Comment

Intercellular antibody has not been demonstrated with the indirect immunofluorescence test. This can help in the differentiation from pemphigus vulgaris.

HAILEY-HAILEY DISEASE

B
X250

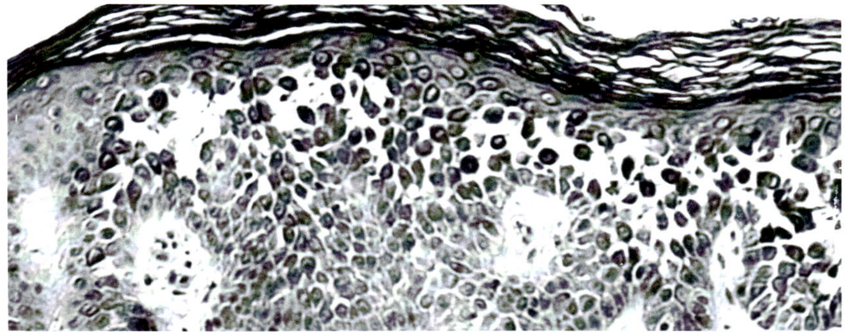

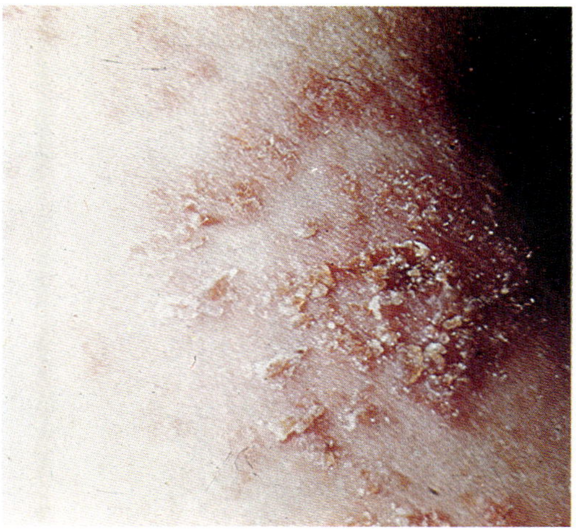

A

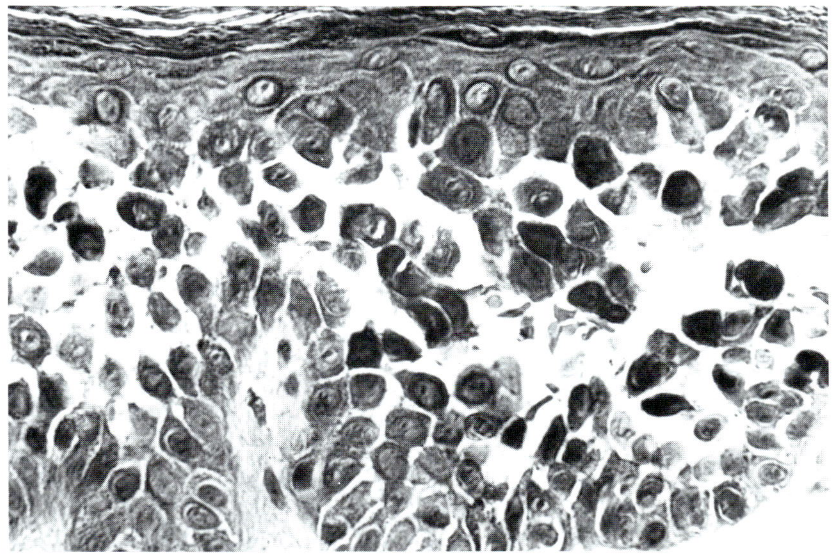

C
X750

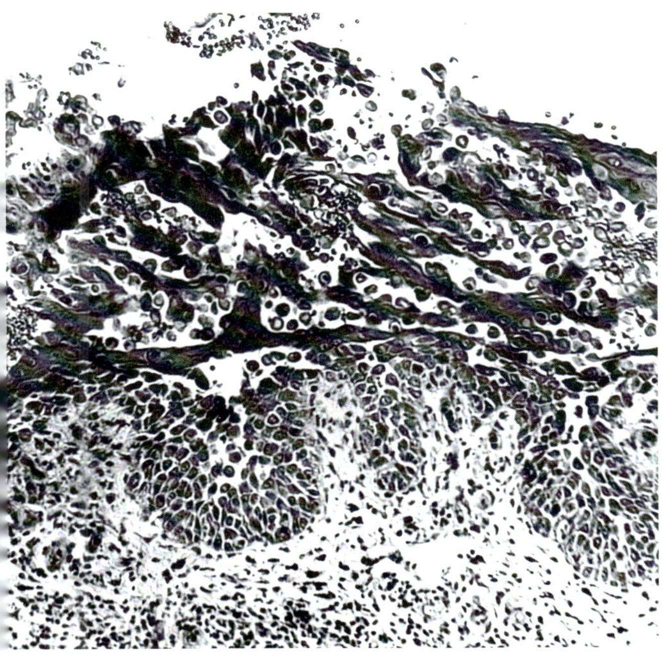

D
X150

E
X150

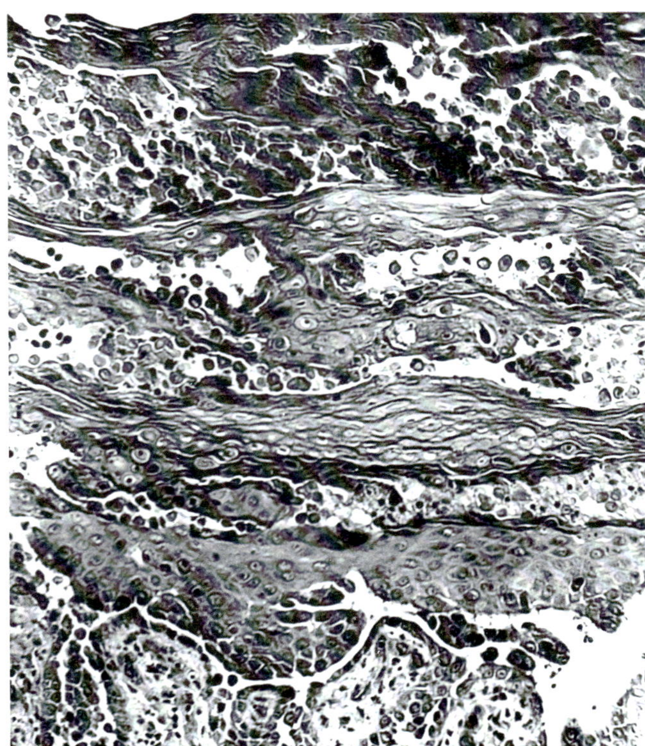

DARIER'S DISEASE (KERATOSIS FOLLICULARIS)

Darier's disease is an inherited disorder transmitted as an autosomal dominant trait (sometimes with incomplete penetrance). Onset is usually during childhood, but can occur later. Lesions are small keratotic papules which tend to coalesce and form a brownish greasy scale (Figs, A,B). Predisposed sites are the face, chest, back, and extremities.

Lesions are not limited to the follicular openings. Lesions may occur on the palms and soles. Small papules are often present on the hands and feet, resembling acrokeratosis verruciformis of Hopf.

Lesions of Darier's disease are believed to form via abnormalities in desmosomes.

Papules may occur on the oral mucosa. Nail involvement includes subungual keratosis and longitudinal ridging of the nail plate.

Microscopic features

1. Microscopic intraepidermal separations form by suprabasal acantholysis (Figs. C,D). Early clefts are called *lacunae* (Fig. D, arrow).
2. Papillomatosis results in villus formation (Figs. C, D). Strands of epidermis may extend downward into the dermis (Fig. D), at times resulting in pseudoepitheliomatous hyperplasia.
3. Hyperkeratosis is usually extensive (Fig. C); hyperkeratotic plugs are present both within follicular orifices and outside of follicular orifices.
4. Dyskeratotic, acantholytic cells called grains and *corps ronds* are present (see next page).

DARIER'S DISEASE

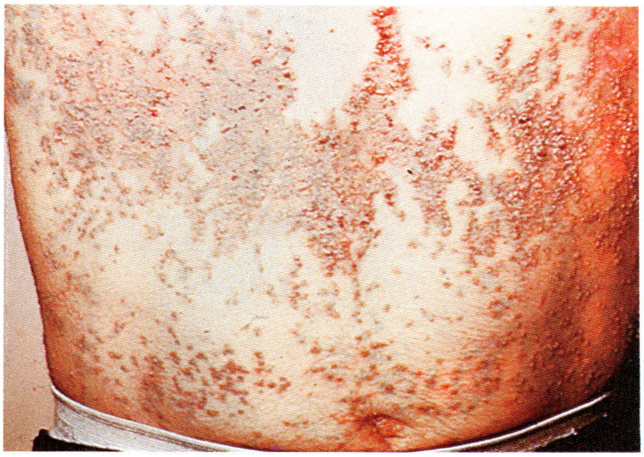

A

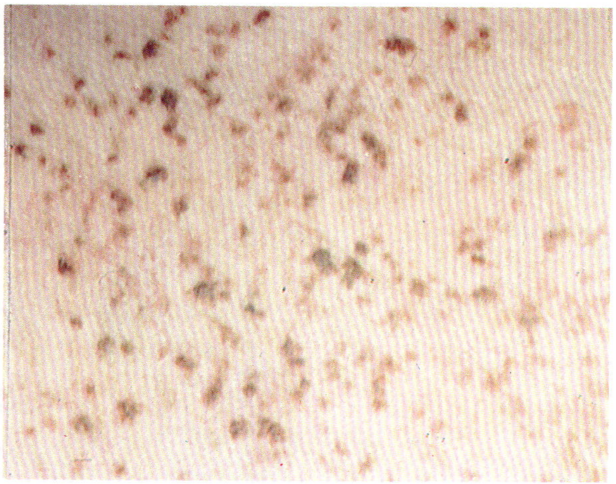

B

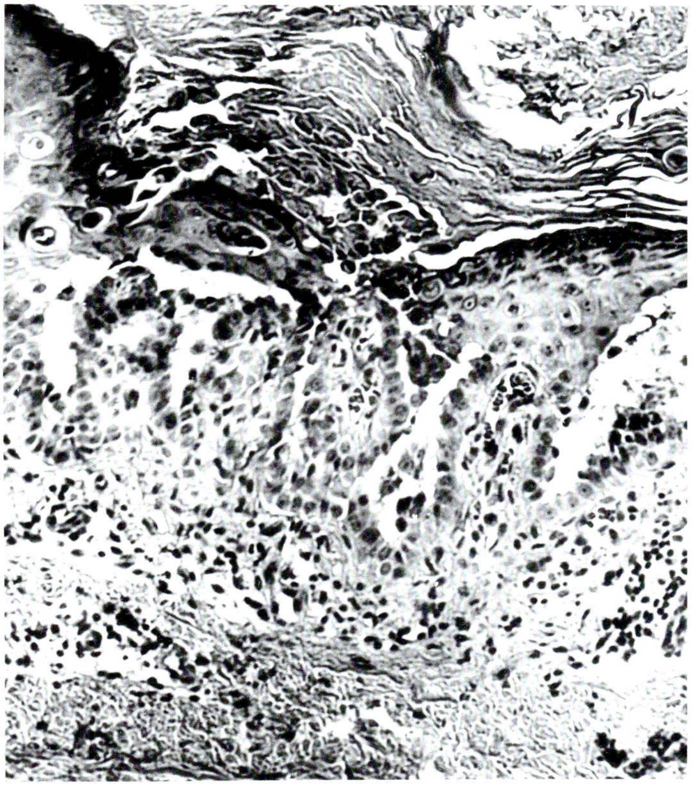

C X200

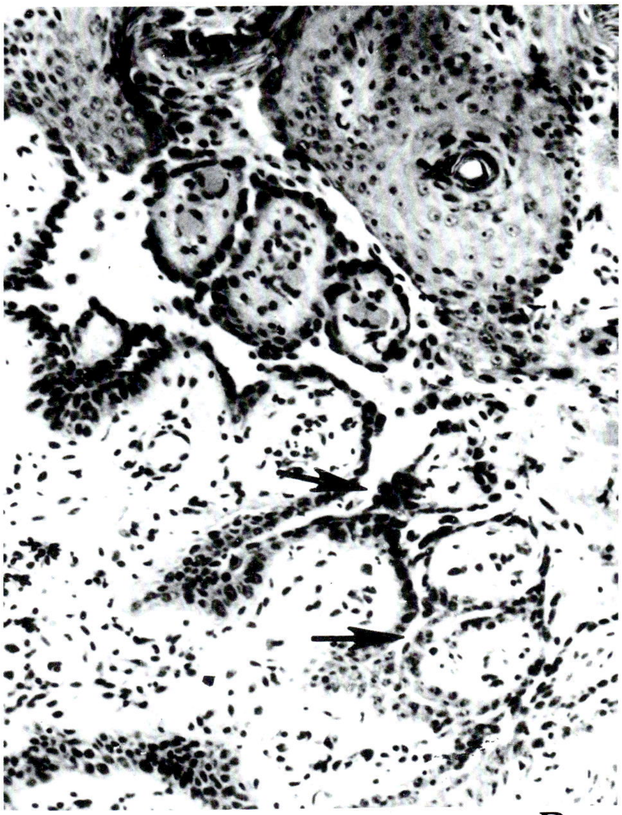

D X190

DARIER'S DISEASE continued

DARIER'S DISEASE

Microscopic features

5. Dyskeratotic, acantholytic cells called *grains* and *corps ronds* are shown in more detail. Grains (G-Fig. B) are ellipsoid dyskeratotic cells in the stratum corneum which resemble parakeratotic cells. They are larger than parakeratotic cells and have a more eosinophilic cytoplasm. In addition, they typically show acantholytic separation. *Corps ronds* (Fig. A; C-Fig. B) are round dyskeratotic cells with a central pyknotic nucleus, surrounded by a halo and an outer ring of homogeneous, eosinophilic cytoplasm.
6. Early suprabasal acantholytic clefts (lacunae) are shown in more detail in Figs. A,B.

Microscopic differential diagnosis (see chart p. 554)

The histologic pattern of Darier's disease is not specific. Warty dyskeratoma shows a similar histologic picture, but differs by having a crateriform architecture. Grover's disease (TAD) may show a histologic picture identical to that of Darier's disease. In addition, similar changes can be seen as a coincidental finding in a variety of dermatoses, including benign papillomas. The histopathologic pattern observed in Darier's disease has been given a generic designation—*acantholytic dyskeratosis.*

DARIER'S DISEASE

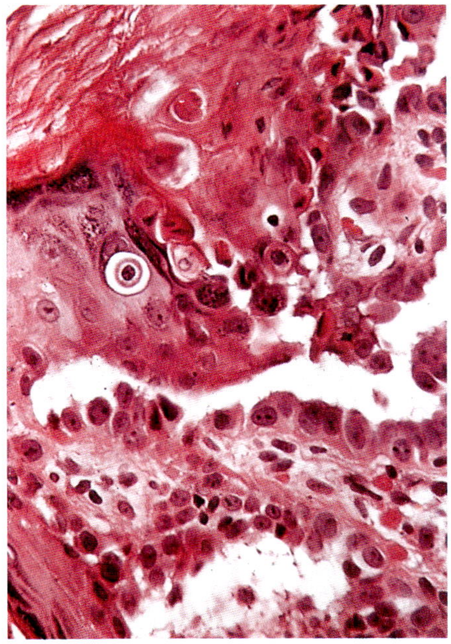

A
X400

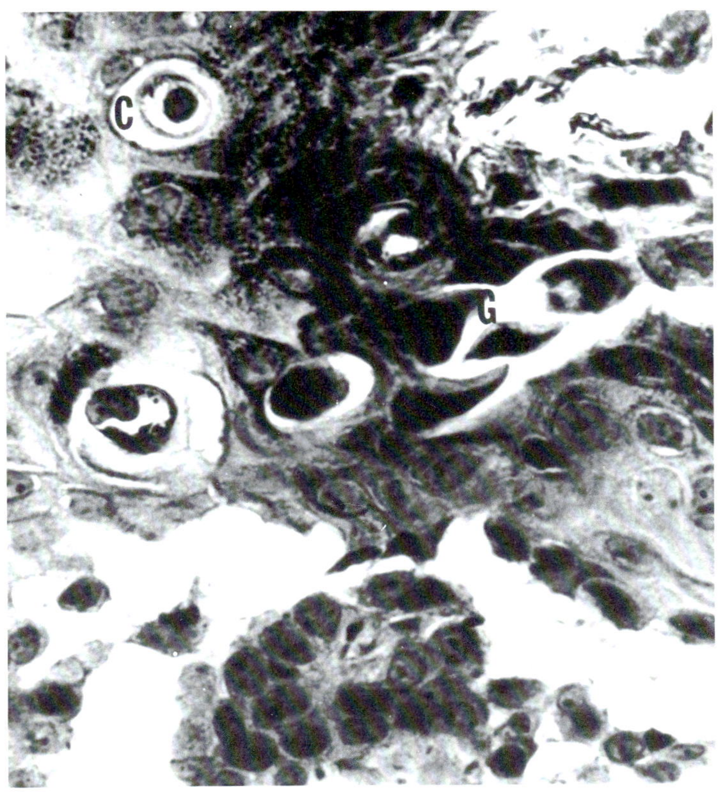

B
X550

GROVER'S DISEASE (TRANSIENT ACANTHOLYTIC DERMATOSIS)

Grover's disease is characterized by scattered, pruritic erythematous papules or papulovesicles, usually on the trunk (Fig. A). Bullous and erythematous plaque variants have been reported. Grover's disease may be precipitated by sun exposure and exacerbated by heat. There is a predilection for middle-aged or elderly males. Spontaneous resolution within two weeks to three months is the rule, but persistence for several years has been reported.

Microscopic features

A variety of acantholytic patterns may occur, including patterns seen in pemphigus vulgaris, pemphigus foliaceus, Hailey-Hailey disease, and Darier's disease. Sometimes acantholytic cells are observed in areas of spongiosis.

Microscopic differential diagnosis (see p. 554)

A specific microscopic diagnosis is not possible. The small size of the acantholytic areas and the presence of a mixture of acantholytic patterns are histologic features that can be suggestive of Grover's disease. Negative tests for intercellular antibodies help make the distinction from pemphigus. Clinical data are essential.

GROVER'S DISEASE

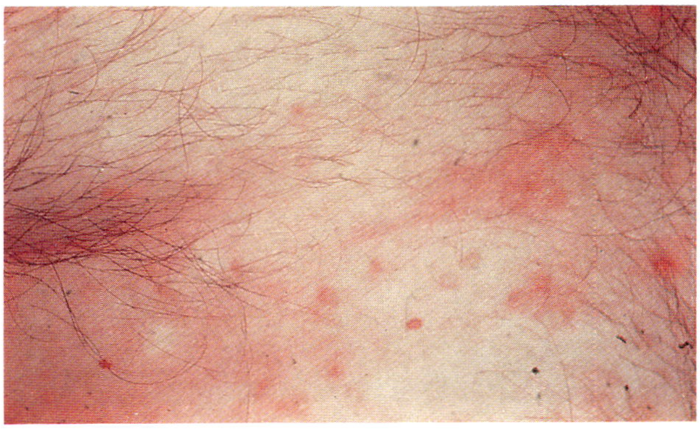

A

KEY DIFFERENTIAL DIAGNOSTIC FEATURES OF ACANTHOLYTIC BULLAE

1. Pemphigus vulgaris: suprabasal acantholysis, which may involve hair follicles.
2. Pemphigus vegetans: suprabasal acantholysis and intraepidermal abscesses composed of eosinophils.
3. Pemphigus foliaceus and pemphigus erythematosus: acantholysis high in the epidermis; grains in the stratum corneum and stratum granulosum.
4. Darier's disease: suprabasal acantholysis with grains and *corps ronds* in the stratum corneum and stratum granulosum.
5. Hailey-Hailey disease: extensive acantholysis involving all layers of the epidermis; some dyskeratosis may be present.
6. Grover's disease (TAD): the acantholytic foci tend to be small. The histologic pattern can simulate that seen in pemphigus vulgaris, pemphigus foliaceus, Hailey-Hailey disease, or Darier's disease. Immunofluorescence tests can distinguish pemphigus vulgaris or foliaceus from Grover's disease. In Grover's disease, intercellular antibodies are not found.
7. Solar keratosis: suprabasal acantholysis with nuclear atypia of the basal cells.
8. Viral vesicles: widespread acantholysis with balloon cells and inclusion bodies.

Subepidermal Bullous Dermatoses

Determining cleavage site of subepidermal bullous dermatoses

Cleavage site of subepidermal bullous dermatoses can be determined by electron microscopy (see p. 586) or by modified indirect immunofluorescence techniques delineating 3 components of the basement zone:

1. Bullous pemphigoid antibodies delineating the lamina lucida.
2. Anti-type IV collagen antibodies, delineating a component of the basal lamina.
3. Antilaminin antibodies delineating a noncollagenous protein found throughout the basal lamina.

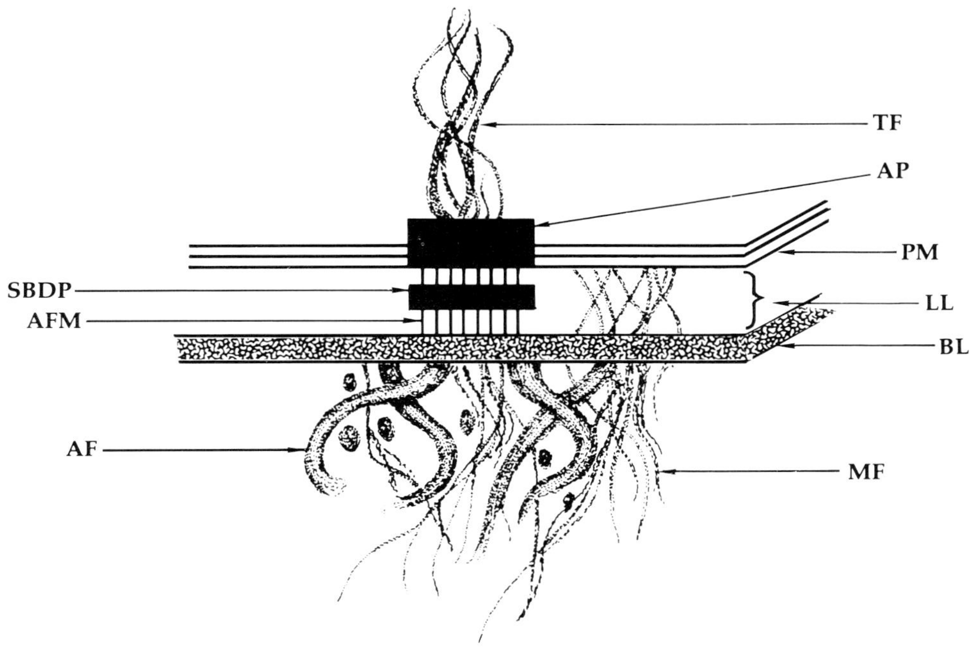

Schematic View of Epidermal-Dermal Junction

TF = Tonofilaments
AP = Attachment plaque of half-desmosome
PM = Trilaminar plasma membrane of basal cell
LL = Lamina lucida
BL = Basal lamina
MF = Microfilament
AF = Anchoring fibril
AFM = Anchoring filament
SBDP = Sub-basal cell dense plaque

Subepidermal Bullous Dermatoses

DERMATITIS HERPETIFORMIS (DUHRING'S DISEASE)

Dermatitis herpetiformis is a chronic disorder of possible autoimmune etiology. Males are affected more often than females. Lesions are grouped papules or vesicles (Fig. B); some degree of erythema or urticaria may be present. Pruritus is generally intense, and often excoriations are the dominant presenting feature (Fig. A).

Lesions often have a symmetrical, bilateral distribution. Predisposed sites include the scalp, extensor surfaces of the extremities, scapular areas, and buttocks. Oral lesions are uncommon.

Dermatitis herpetiformis may be associated with gluten enteropathy.

Therapy with sulfapyridine and the sulfones is effective. Some consider the therapeutic response as essential in confirming the diagnosis.

Microscopic features

1. Characteristic changes of dermatitis herpetiformis are best seen in biopsies taken from erythematous areas in the vicinity of early blisters.
2. Early lesions show accumulations of neutrophils and nuclear fragments at the tips of the dermal papillae (Fig. D), accompanied by degeneration of collagen.
3. Later, neutrophils and some eosinophils fill the papillae and result in papillary microabscess formation (Fig. C).

DERMATITIS HERPETIFORMIS

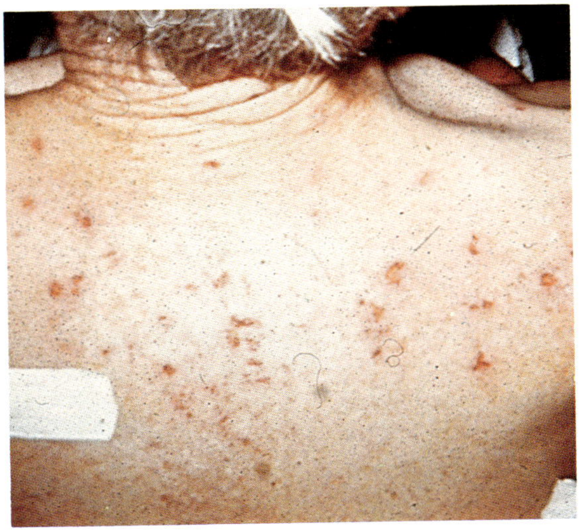

A Courtesy Dr. John Knox

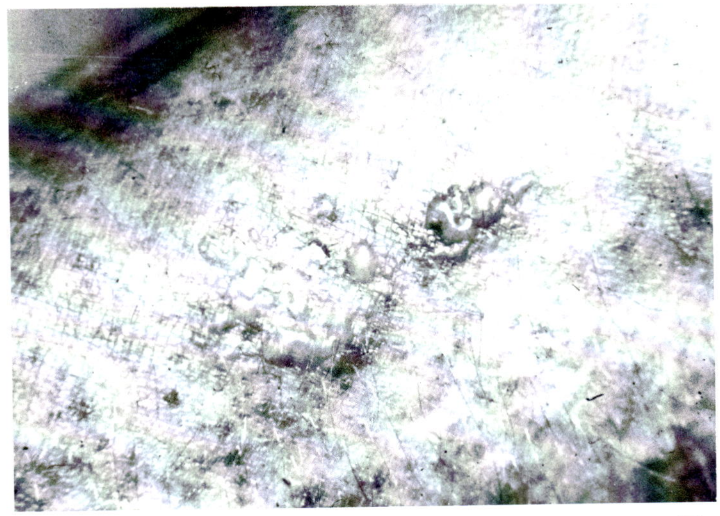

B

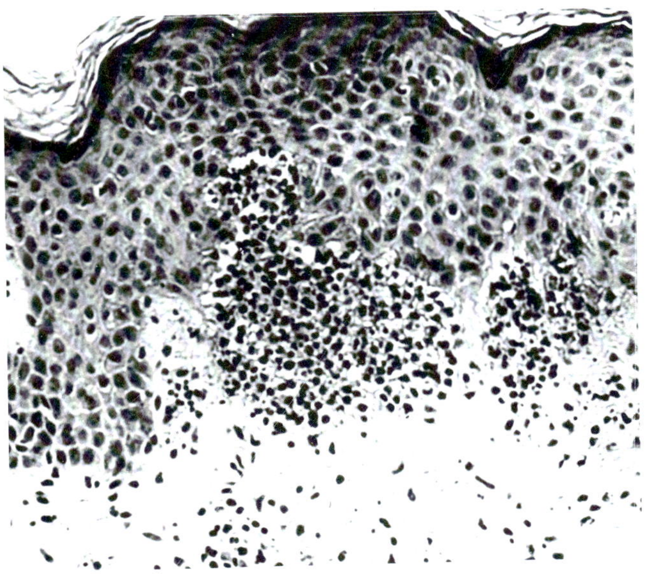

C X220

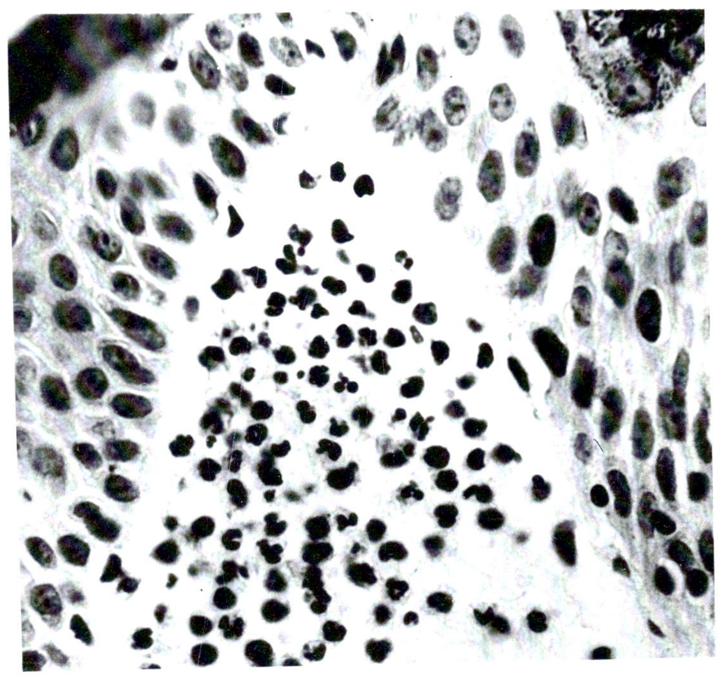

D X150

DERMATITIS HERPETIFORMIS continued

DERMATITIS HERPETIFORMIS

Microscopic features

4. Papillary abscesses evolve into subepidermal clefts (Fig. A) and then into small subepidermal bullae (Fig. B), which may fuse, resulting in large subepidermal bullae (Fig. D).
5. The dermis shows a variable inflammatory infiltrate and at times a leukocytoclastic vasculitis (Fig. C).

Microscopic differential diagnosis (see p. 586)

The main problem in histologic differential diagnosis of dermatitis herpetiformis is distinction from bullous pemphigoid. Both diseases show papillary microabscesses in early lesions, with neutrophils predominating in dermatitis herpetiformis and eosinophils predominating in bullous pemphigoid. However, differentiation on the basis of neutrophil:eosinophil ratio is not always reliable; clinical and immunofluorescence data are important in making an accurate diagnosis. Because of differences in therapy, the distinction of dermatitis herpetiformis from bullous pemphigoid has practical significance.

Comment

Dermatitis herpetiformis shows deposits of IgA at the epidermal-dermal junction at the tips of dermal papillae (see p. 560). In "classic" dermatitis herpetiformis these deposits are granular. Some authors consider cases with linear, rather than granular IgA deposits, as a separate entity, possibly identical with linear IgA dermatosis of childhood. Described differentiation from "classic" dermatitis herpetiformis includes absence of gluten-sensitive enteropathy and a tendency to have predominantly bullous rather than papulovesicular lesions. Circulating anti-basement membrane zone antibodies of the IgA class are rare in "classic" dermatitis herpetiformis but are said to be present in about a third of patients with linear IgA dermatosis.

Classic dermatitis herpetiformis is rare in children, but bullous pemphigoid and linear IgA dermatosis occur more often, usually in preschool age children. Annular and serpiginous erythematous patches with bullae at their periphery have been described in linear IgA dermatosis of childhood.

DERMATITIS HERPETIFORMIS

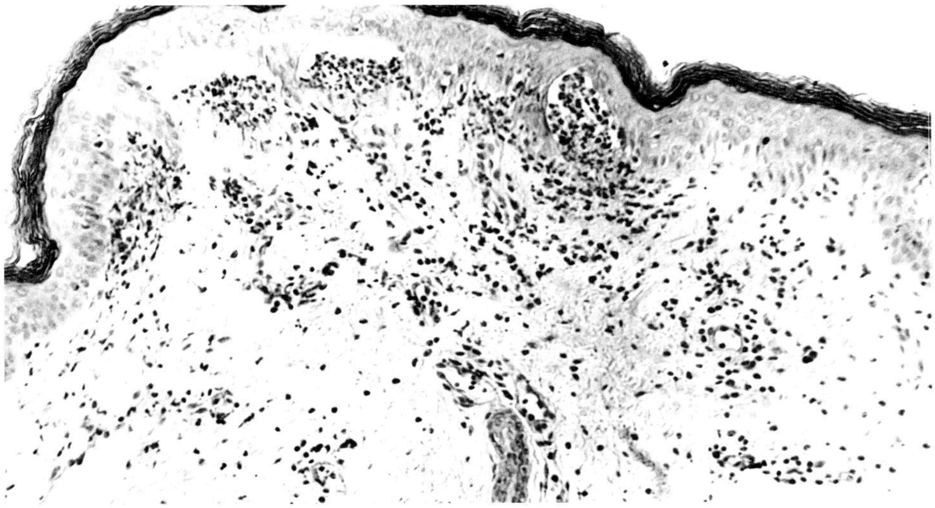

A
X180

B X200

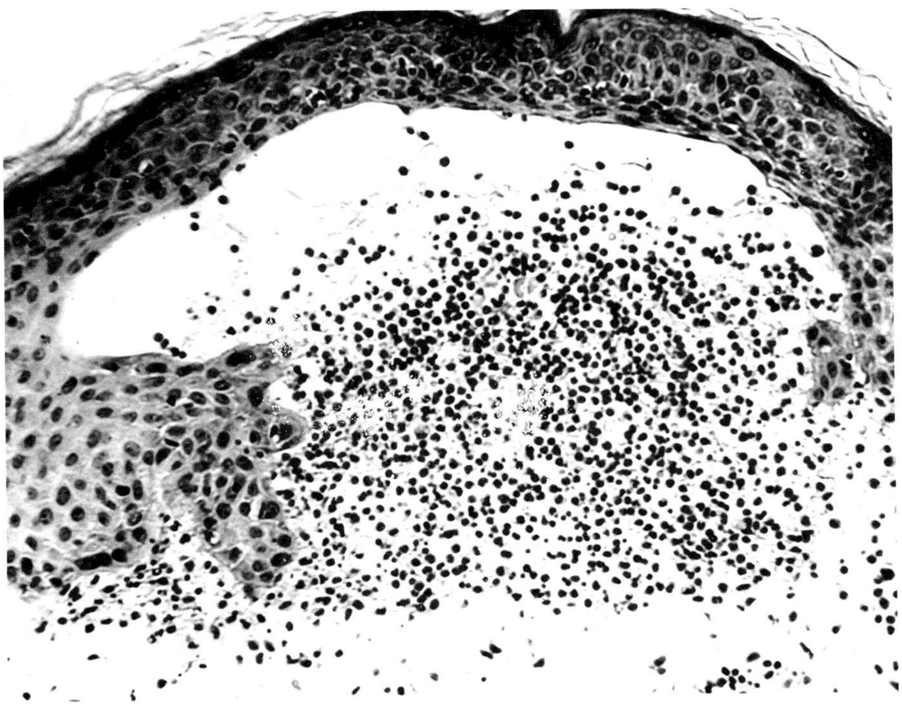

C X660

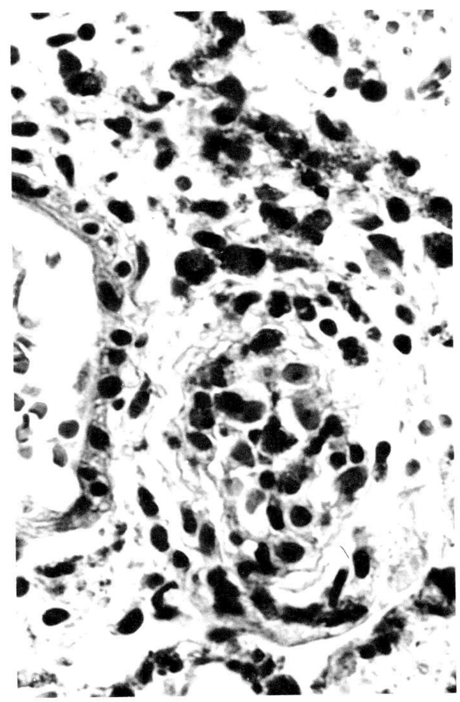

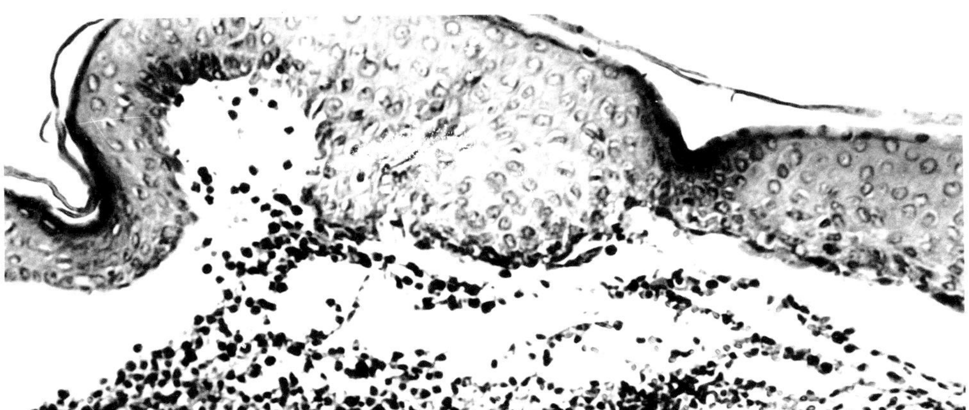

D
X260

DERMATITIS HERPETIFORMIS continued ⇨

DERMATITIS HERPETIFORMIS

Immunofluorescence testing

In "classic" dermatitis herpetiformis, granular deposits of IgA can be demonstrated at the basement membrane zone at the tips of dermal papillae by the direct immunofluorescence method (Fig. A). In linear IgA dermatosis, the IgA has a linear, rather then granular, distribution. Specimens for immunofluorescence testing should be taken at sites away from lesions. Other immunoglobulins or C3 may also be present.

Circulating anti-basement zone IgA is only rarely observed in "classic" dermatitis herpetiformis, but is present more often in patients with linear IgA dermatosis.

DERMATITIS HERPETIFORMIS: IMMUNOFLUORESCENCE

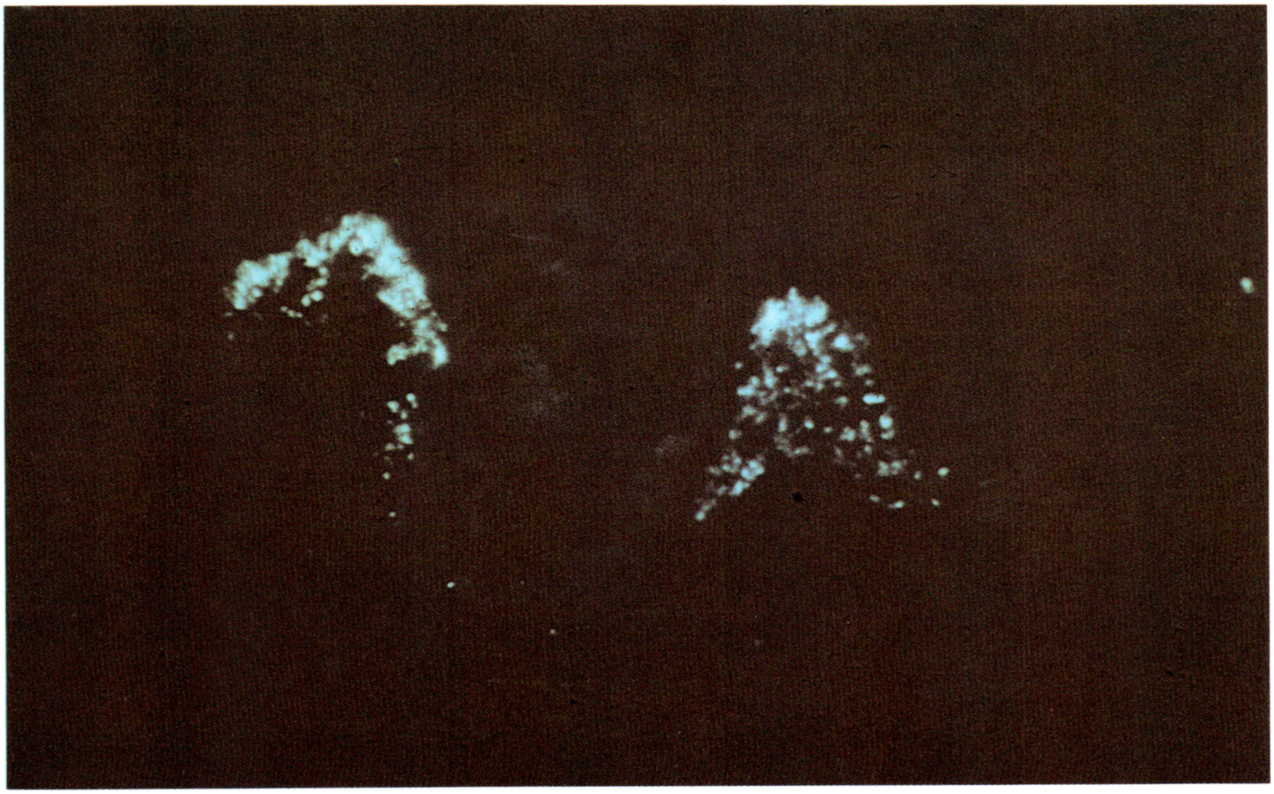

A
X220

Courtesy Dr. Soyu Shu, Dr. Ernst Beutner

BULLOUS PEMPHIGOID

Bullous pemphigoid is a disorder with a possible autoimmune etiology which usually affects the elderly, but which can occur in young adults or children. Unlike pemphigus vulgaris, there is no racial predilection, and the prognosis tends to be good. Typical lesions are large, tense blisters (Fig. A), which are sometimes hemorrhagic or surrounded by erythema. Zones of erythema or edema without blisters can be present (Fig. B). Flexural areas are often involved. Sometimes there are vesicular lesions, which may be grouped, producing a resemblance to dermatitis herpetiformis. Vegetating lesions may occur, especially in the axillae and groin. Localized lesions may occur, most commonly on the lower extremities. The oral mucosa is often involved. Bullous pemphigoid and linear IgA bullous disease may be associated with immune nephritis.

Microscopic features

1. Bullae form subepidermally (Fig. D).
2. Microvacuoles may be observed beneath the basal layer before frank subepidermal bulla formation develops (Fig. C).
3. Epidermal regeneration occurs rapidly at the base of bullae, producing bullae with an intraepidermal location (Fig. E). This picture could represent any of the subepidermal bullous dermatoses.
4. The degree of inflammation in the bulla and beneath it varies. There is usually a mixture of inflammatory cells; eosinophils are generally abundant. Occasionally leukocytoclastic vasculitis may be present.
5. At the tips of dermal papillae adjacent to bullae, accumulations of eosinophils and neutrophils are sometimes present (Fig. F). The proportion of eosinophils in these papillary abscesses is usually greater than in the papillary microabscesses of dermatitis herpetiformis.

Microscopic differential diagnosis (see p. 586)

The main problem in histologic differential diagnosis of bullous pemphigoid is distinction from dermatitis herpetiformis. Both diseases show papillary microabscesses in early lesions, with neutrophils predominating in dermatitis herpetiformis and eosinophils predominating in bullous pemphigoid. However, differentiation on the basis of neutrophil:eosinophil ratio is not always reliable; clinical and immunofluorescence data are important in making an accurate diagnosis. Because of differences in therapy, the distinction of dermatitis herpetiformis from bullous pemphigoid has practical significance.

BULLOUS PEMPHIGOID

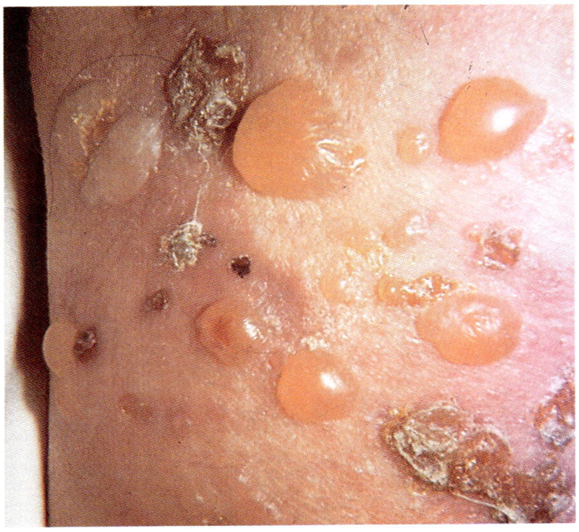

A

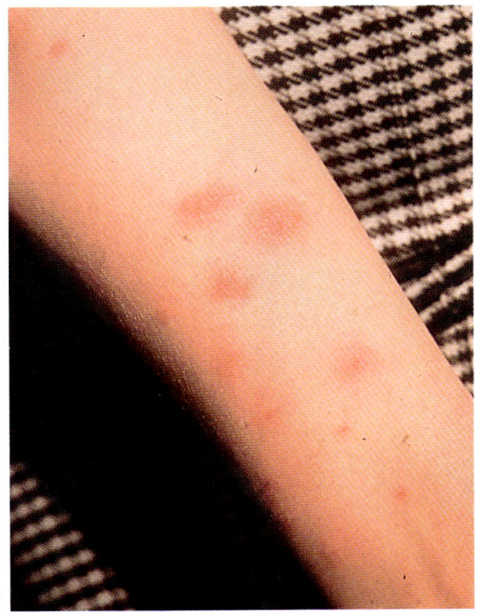

B

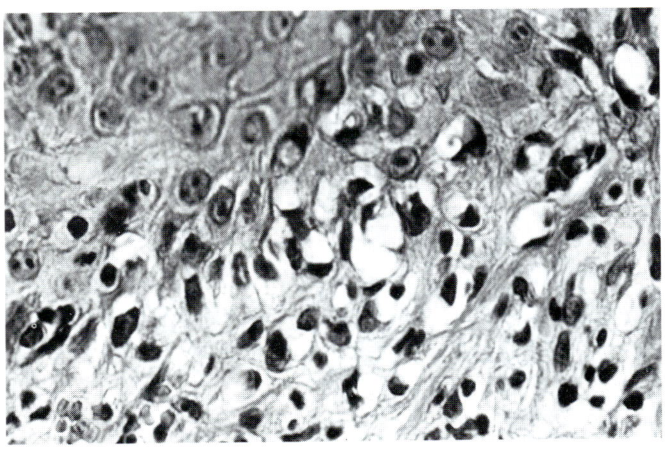

C X630

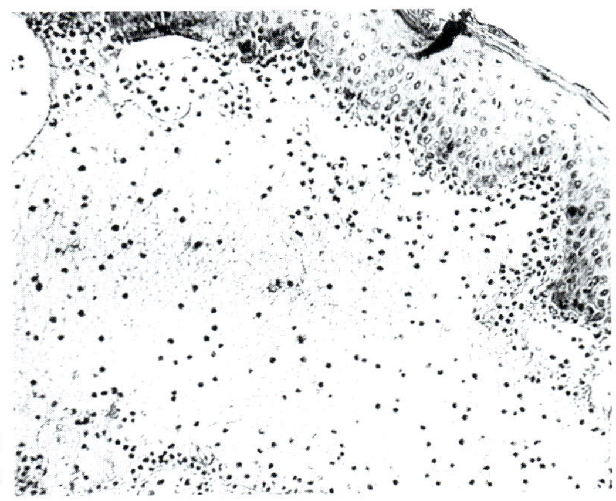

D X125

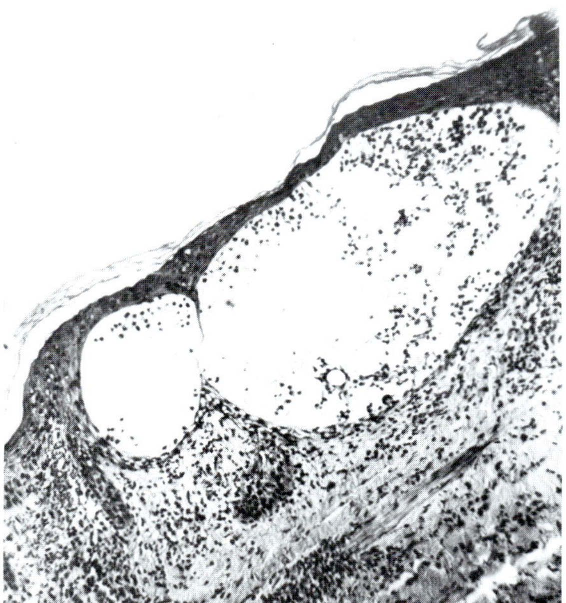

E X60

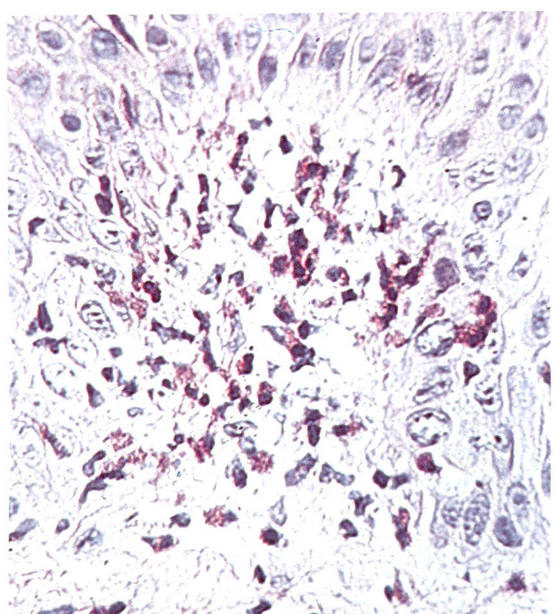

F X520

BULLOUS PEMPHIGOID cont

BULLOUS PEMPHIGOID

Immunofluorescence testing

Direct immunofluorescence testing. Perilesional skin is used. A positive immunofluorescence test is indicated by the presence of linear immunofluorescence along the basement zone (Fig. A). Positivity is noted in virtually all patients with bullous pemphigoid. Typically the immunoglobulin is IgG. C3, IgM, or IgA may be present.

Indirect immunofluorescence testing. Circulating antibodies are found in about 7.0% of patients and can be demonstrated, using guinea pig or monkey esophagus as substrate (Fig. B). The antibodies are IgG. There is no correlation between intensity of the disease and titer.

BENIGN MUCOUS MEMBRANE PEMPHIGOID

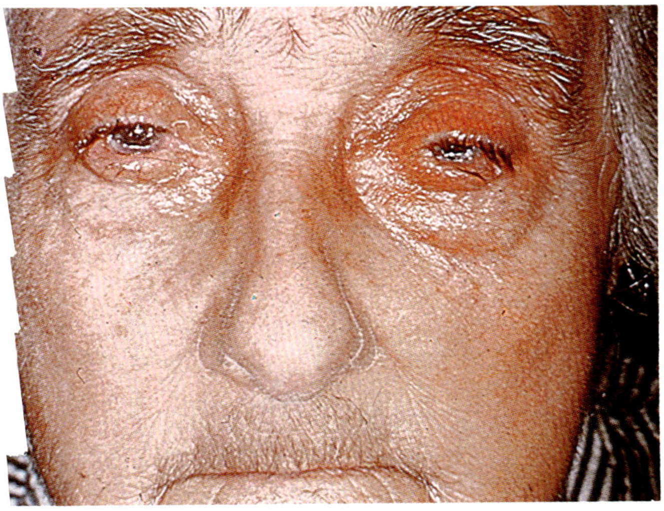

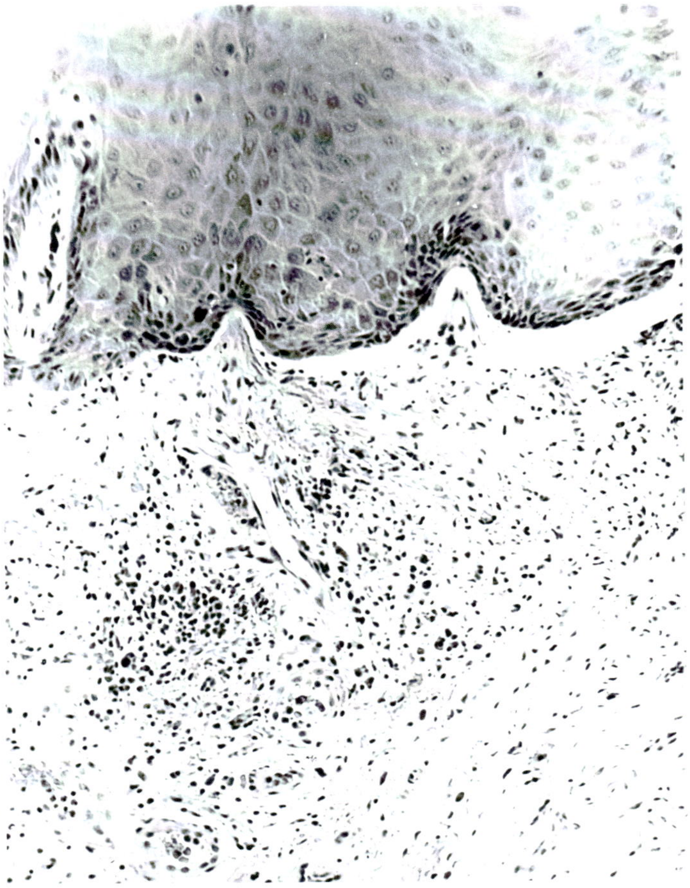

B
X200

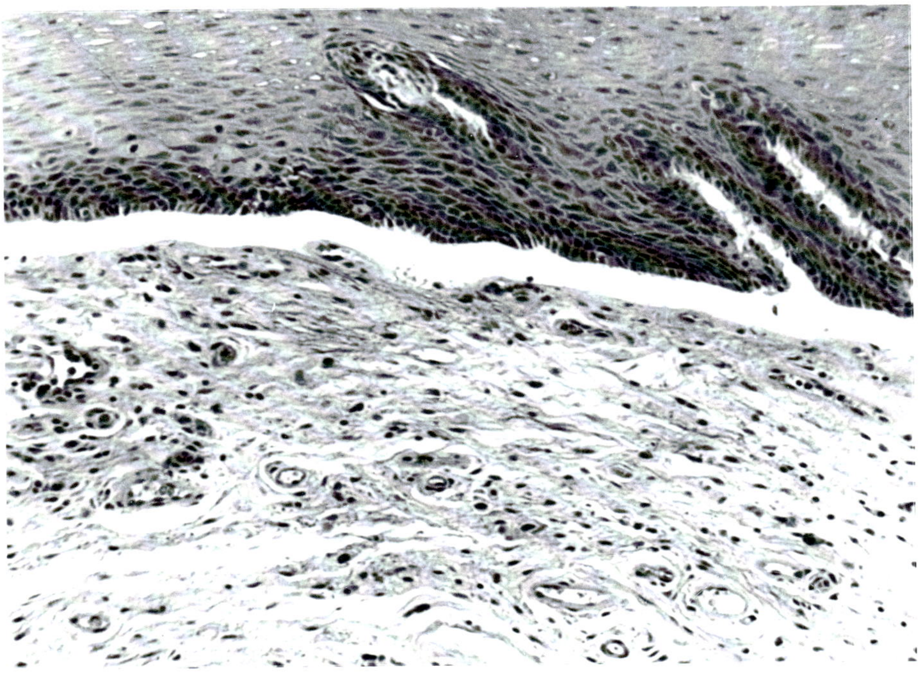

C
X200

HERPES GESTATIONIS

Herpes gestationis is a rare eruption occurring during pregnancy and the postpartum period. It is associated with increased fetal mortality. There are areas of erythema and edema, as well as vesicles and bullae; pruritus is typically intense. Oral lesions are not usually present. Herpes gestationis has a clinical resemblance to bullous pemphigoid. The abdomen (Fig. A) is often the first area involved. An increased fetal mortality rate has been reported, as well as some instances of a vesiculobullous eruption in the newborn.

Microscopic features

1. Microscopic features are not specific.
2. Both subacute dermatitis and subepidermal bullae may be observed.
3. Necrosis of the basal epidermis with formation of colloid bodies has been reported.
4. An inflammatory infiltrate containing a high percentage of eosinophils is usually present. The eosinophils may show fragmentation of their nuclei ("nuclear dust").

Microscopic differential diagnosis

There is a resemblance to dermatitis or subepidermal bullous dermatoses, depending on the stage of the lesion observed. The many eosinophils, some with nuclear fragments, can produce a resemblance to bullous pemphigoid. Bullous pemphigoid does not usually show a necrotic element. The histologic picture parallels the spectrum of erythema multiforme.

Immunofluorescence testing

Direct immunofluorescence testing of perilesional skin typically shows C3 along the basement zone. Other complement factors or immunoglobulins may be present. Circulating anti-basement membrane IgG is rarely present. Most patients have a thermostable serum IgG (HG factor) capable of fixing C3 at the basement membrane zone of normal human skin *in vitro*.

HERPES GESTATIONIS

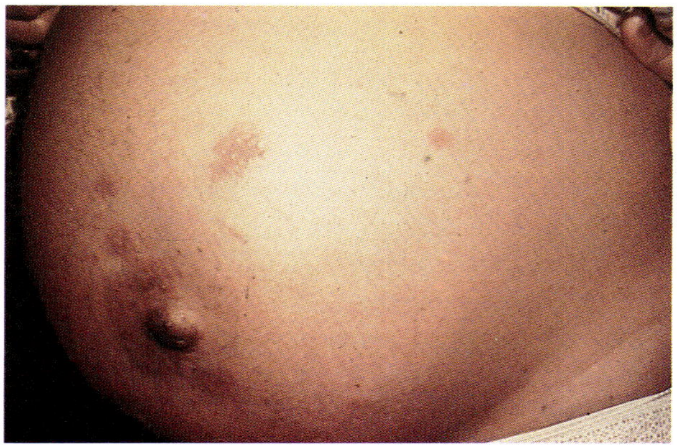

A

ERYTHEMA MULTIFORME

Erythema multiforme is an acute syndrome which may be idiopathic or which may represent a hypersensitization reaction to a variety of antigens, including antigens associated with infections (e.g., herpes simplex), drugs, and possibly neoplasms. Fixed drug eruption (see p. 472) is generally considered to be a localized variant of erythema multiforme.

Cutaneous lesions are varied; they include erythema, macules, papules, vesicles, and bullae. Vesiculobullous lesions are frequently surrounded by an erythematous ring (iris or target lesions) (Figs. A,B). Hemorrhagic lesions are common.

Microscopic features

1. There is a range of histologic patterns corresponding in a general way with the range of clinical lesions. Patterns include dermatitis, perivasculitis, lymphocytic vasculitis, and both spongiotic (intraepidermal) and subepidermal bullae (Figs. D,E). Whether or not leukocytoclastic vasculitis is observed in erythema multiforme has been controversial. In the authors' experience leukocytoclastic vasculitis can occur.
2. Epidermal necrosis (Fig. C) often occurs in erythema multiforme with or without bullae; there may be individual cells showing eosinophilic necrosis, as well as hydropic degeneration of the basal epidermis.
3. The dermal infiltrate consists of a mixture of inflammatory cells, mostly lymphoid cells, with a frequent component of eosinophils.
4. The classification of erythema multiforme into epidermal, mixed epidermal-dermal, and dermal types is somewhat misleading, since these patterns appear as part of a spectrum rather than as clearly defined entities.
5. When subepidermal bullae form (Fig. D), they may be preceded by a stage of edema of the papillary dermis (Fig. E).
6. A definite diagnosis of erythema multiforme on purely histologic grounds is not possible, although the presence of significant epidermal necrosis is a suggestive feature.

ERYTHEMA MULTIFORME

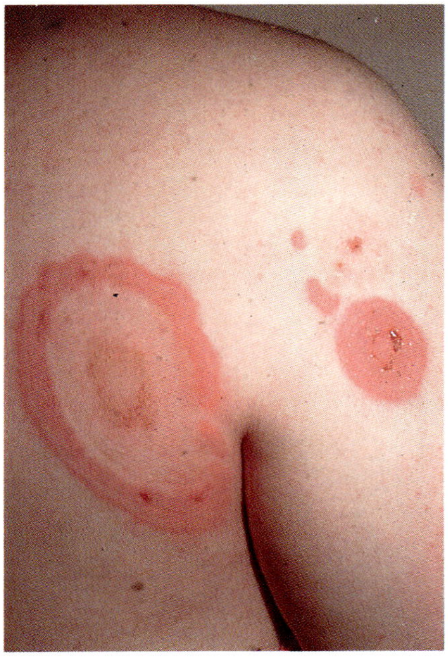
A

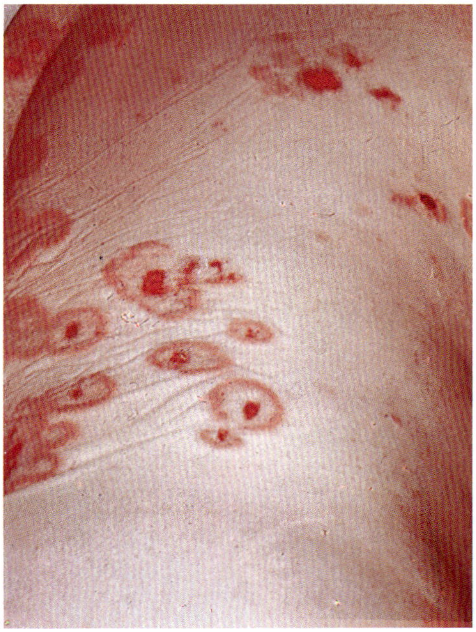
B

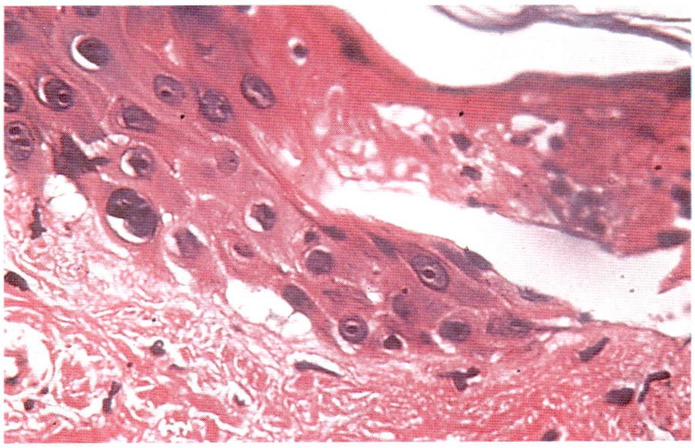
C
X500

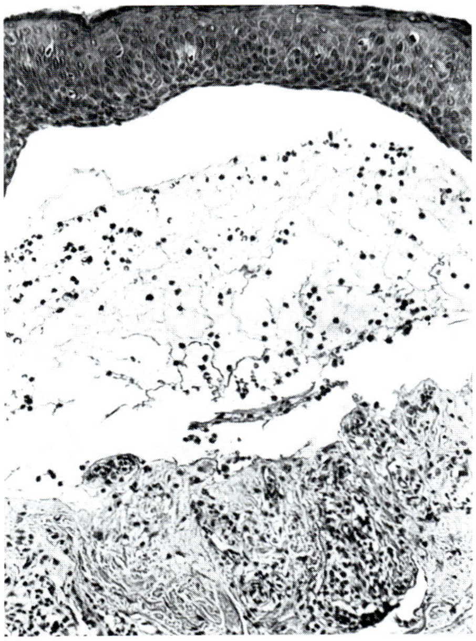
D
X140

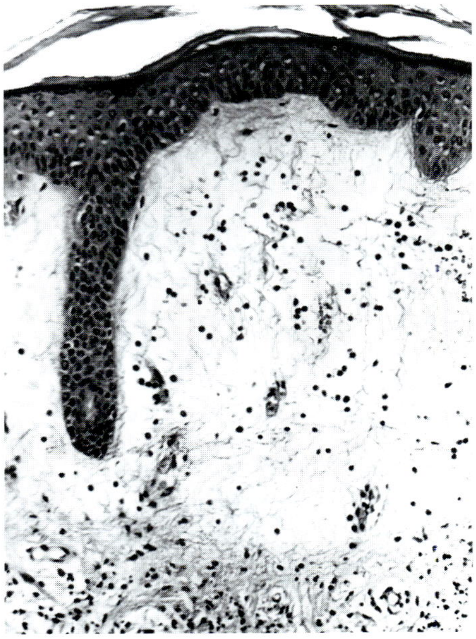
E
X140

ERYTHEMA MULTIFORME continued

ERYTHEMA MULTIFORME

Microscopic features

7. Regeneration occurs rapidly at the base of subepidermal bullae (Figs. A,B), resulting in bullae with an intraepidermal location. Regenerating epithelial cells are often elongated, with their long axes parallel to the base of the bulla (Figs. A,B).
8. The domes of bullae often show necrosis (Fig. A).
9. Necrotic, eosinophilic epithelial cells may be present in the epidermis adjacent to bullae.
10. A leukocytoclastic (Fig. C) or lymphocytic vasculitis may be present, and this may extend into the subcutaneous fat (Fig. D).

Microscopic differential diagnosis (see p. 586)

Subepidermal bullae of erythema multiforme are nonspecific and can be indistinguishable from mature lesions of bullous pemphigoid or dermatitis herpetiformis, as well as lesions of other subepidermal bullous dermatoses.

Comment

1. Basement zone antibody is not demonstrable with the indirect immunofluorescent technique, in contrast to bullous pemphigoid.
2. Subepidermal bullae and sweat gland necrosis have been reported in drug-induced coma and carbon monoxide poisoning. This pattern may represent a variant of erythema multiforme.
3. *Graft-versus-host disease* is due to transplants of immunocompetent lymphocytes, in most cases via bone marrow transplantation. There is a rare congenital form in which maternal lymphocytes establish themselves in the fetus. The acute phase has cutaneous parallels clinically and microscopically to erythema multiforme; the early lichenoid stage of the chronic phase has clinical and microscopic parallels to lichen planus; the late sclerotic stage of the chronic phase has clinical and microscopic cutaneous parallels to scleroderma.

ERYTHEMA MULTIFORME

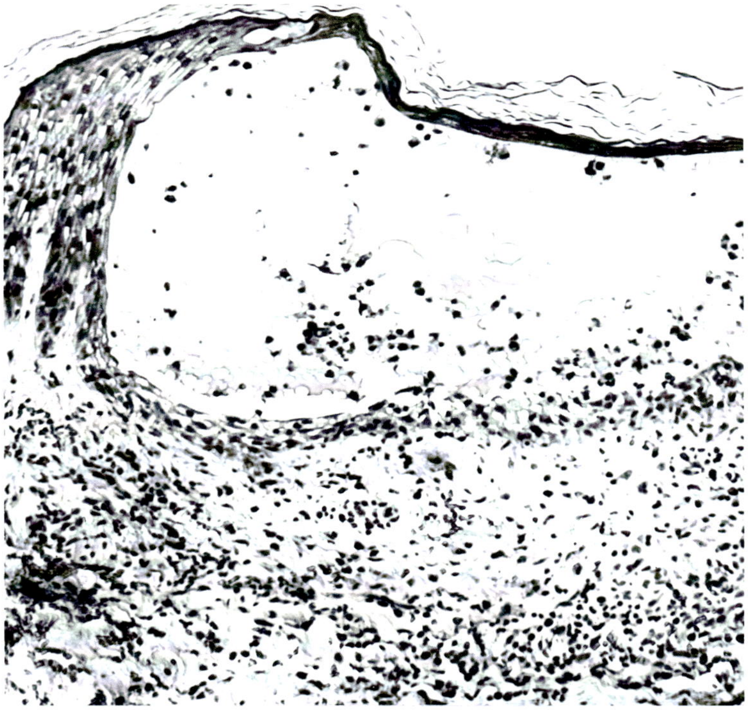

A X180

B X520

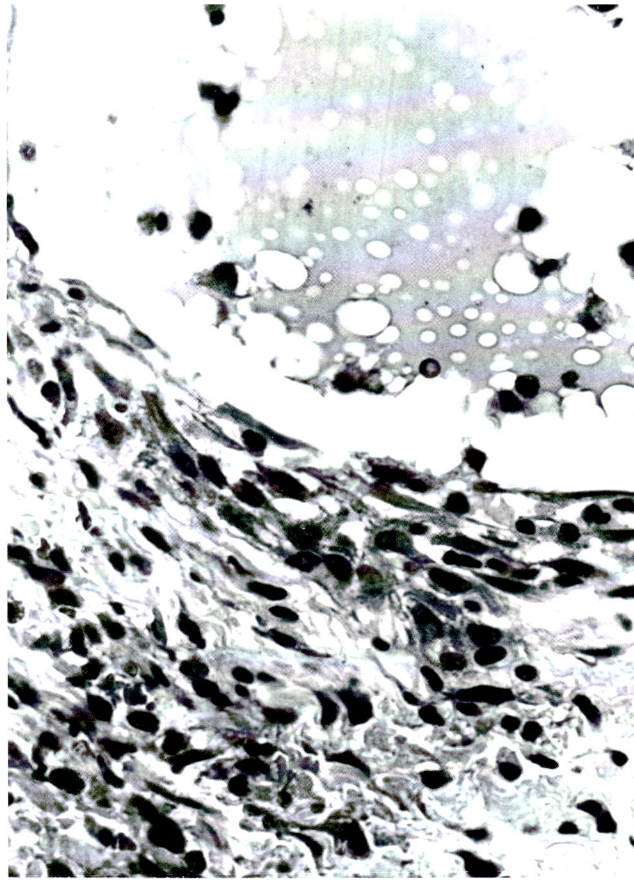

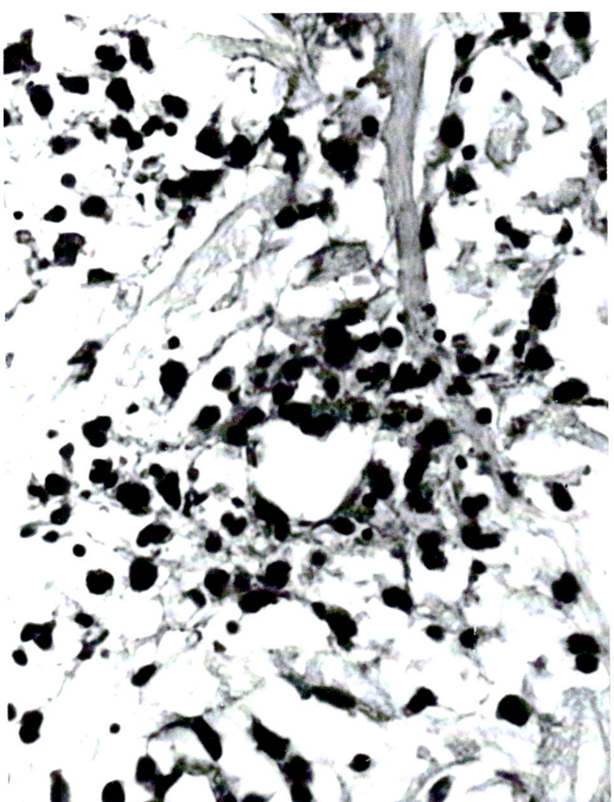

C X650

D X170

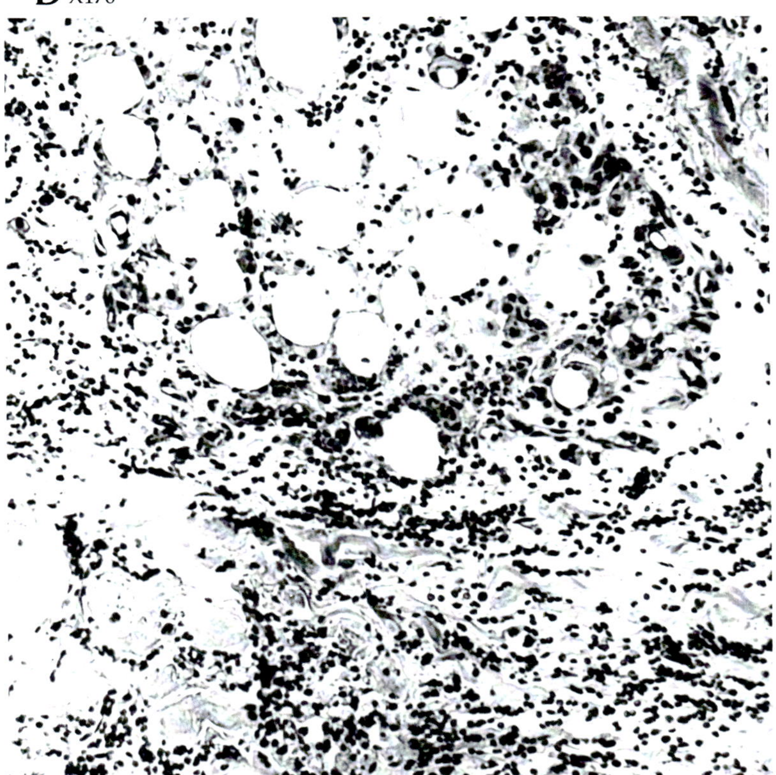

ERYTHEMA MULTIFORME continued ⇨

ERYTHEMA MULTIFORME: STEVENS-JOHNSON SYNDROME

Stevens-Johnson syndrome is a severe bullous variant of erythema multiforme involving skin and mucous membranes. High fever and malaise are generally present.

The bullous lesions are necrotic and hemorrhagic (Fig. A).

Microscopic features

1. The basic histologic picture is the same as that of erythema multiforme bullosum (Fig. B) (see p. 570).
2. The dermal infiltrate is generally very dense, and hemorrhage is extensive (Fig. B). Epidermal necrosis is often present.

ERYTHEMA MULTIFORME: TOXIC EPIDERMAL NECROLYSIS (LYELL'S SYNDROME; SCALDED SKIN SYNDROME)

The term *toxic epidermal necrolysis* has also been applied to a form of staphylococcal bullous impetigo (Ritter's disease) (see p. 284). As used here, the term applies to another severe variant of erythema multiforme bullosum, with high fever, malaise, and necrotic bullae. Necrotic domes of bullae detach in large sheets, leaving denuded areas resembling second degree burns (Fig. C).

Microscopic features

1. The basic histologic picture is that of erythema multiforme bullosum (see p. 570).
2. The domes of the bullae show severe necrosis (Fig. D).

Comment

Necrolytic migratory erythema (glucagonoma syndrome) has clinical and microscopic parallels to the more necrotizing forms of erythema multiforme. This syndrome is believed to be related to deficiency of amino acids, which are consumed in large amounts in the synthesis of glucagon. Glucagonoma syndrome is usually associated with glucagon-secreting alpha cell tumors of the pancreas, but can be associated with glucagonemia related to hepatic cirrhosis. The syndrome can also be due to lowered amino acid levels from malabsorption. Skin lesions consist of erosions, erythema, and fragile vesicles and pustules. Peripheral spreading and central clearing can result in circinate lesions. The microscopic picture corresponds to variants of erythema multiforme with epidermal necrosis. Sometimes there are subepidermal bullae. Other manifestations of glucagonoma syndrome include weight loss, anemia, mild adult-onset diabetes, and high elevation of serum glucagon.

ERYTHEMA MULTIFORME: STEVENS-JOHNSON SYNDROME

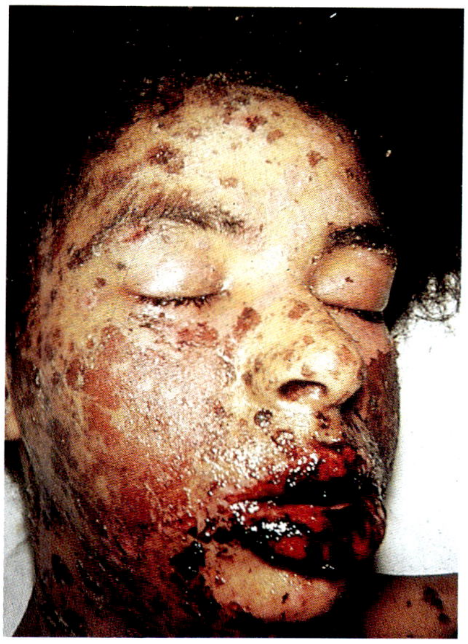

A

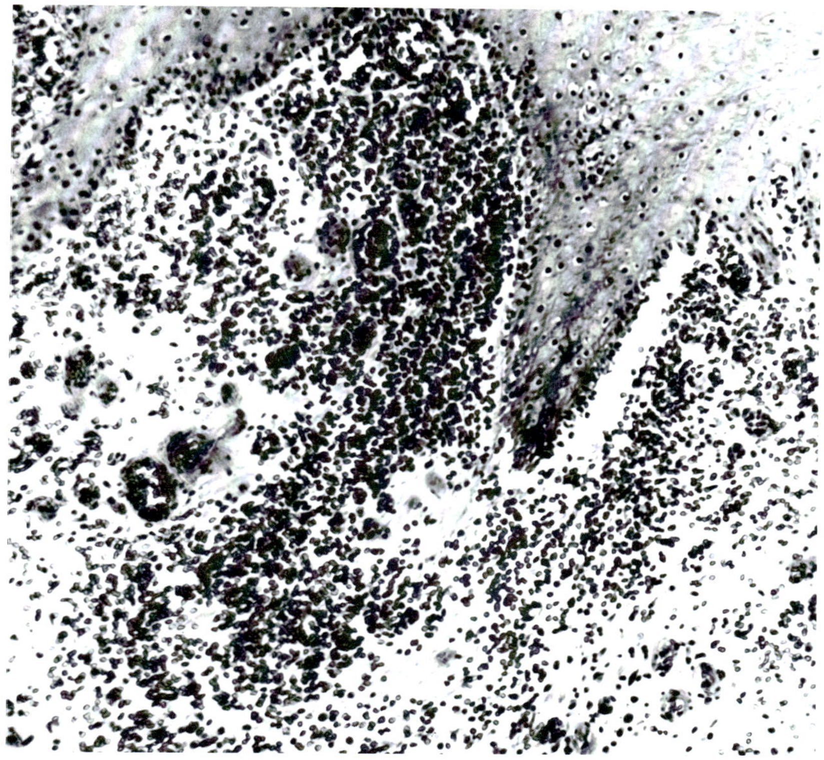

B
X200

ERYTHEMA MULTIFORME: TOXIC EPIDERMAL NECROLYSIS

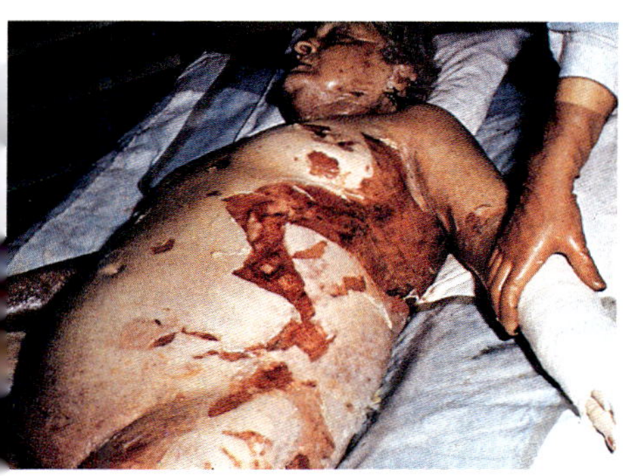

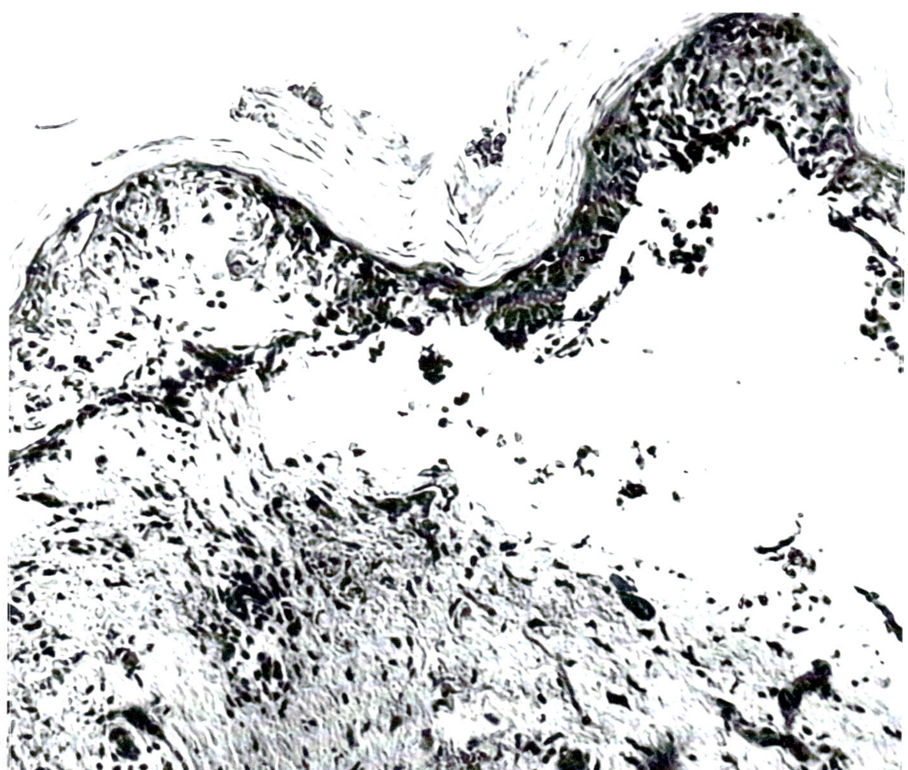

D
X260

PORPHYRIA

Porphyrins are pigments which are intermediates in the biosynthetic pathway of heme. Porphyria encompasses a group of disorders characterized by enzymatic defects in this pathway. Most of the types of porphyria are hereditary, and most have cutaneous manifestations based on the photosensitizing properties of porphyrins. The clinical and microscopic features of skin lesions of the various types of porphyria are, for the most part, similar.

The table on the opposite page summarizes features of various types of porphyria.

In this section, we will consider porphyria cutanea tarda and erythropoietic protoporphyria.

CLASSIFICATION OF THE PORPHYRIAS

	Type; Heredity; Onset	Cutaneous Manifestations	Extracutaneous Manifestations	Urine	Feces	Erythrocytes	Enzymatic Defect
Erythropoietic Porphyria	Ery; Rec; Infancy	Blisters; Severe scarring	Red teeth; Hemolytic anemia	Uro I	Copro I	Uro I; Stable fluorescence	Uroporphyrinogen III cosynthetase
Erythropoietic Protoporphyria	Ery; Dom; Childhood	Burning; Edema; Thickening; Rarely, blisters	Rarely, fatal liver disease	Negative	Protoporphyrin continuously	Protoporphyrin; Transient fluorescence	Ferrochelatase; (Heme synthetase)
Hepatoerythrocytic Porphyria	Ery and Hep; Rec; Childhood	Blisters; Severe scarring; Thickening	Decreased liver function	Uro I; Uro III	Copro I; Copro III	Protoporphyrin	?Ferrochelatase and uroporphyrinogen decarboxylase
Acute Intermittent Porphyria (AIP)	Hep; Dom; Young adulthood	Negative	Abdominal pain; Neuropathy; Psychoses	ALA, PBG continuously	Negative	Negative	Uroporphyrinogen I synthetase
Porphyria Variegata	Hep; Dom; Young adulthood	Same as PCT	Same as AIP	ALA, PBG during attacks	Protoporphyrin continuously	Negative	Protoporphyrinogen oxidase
Porphyria Cutanea Tarda (PCT)	Hep; Dom; Middle age	Blisters; Scarring; Thickening	Decreased liver function; Siderosis	Uro III; Continuous fluorescence		Negative	Uroporphyrinogen III decarboxylase
Hereditary Coproporphyria	Hep; Dom; Young adulthood	Same as PCT	Same as AIP	Copro, ALA, PBG during attacks	Copro continuously	Negative	Coproporphyrinogen oxidase

AIP = acute intermittent porphyria
Ery = erythropoietic
Hep = hepatic
Dom = autosomal dominant
Rec = autosomal recessive
Uro = uroporphyrin
Copro = coproporphyrin
ALA = delta-aminolevulinic acid
PBG = porphobilinogen
PCT = porphyria cutanea tarda

From *Histopathology of the Skin*, 6th edition, by Walter F. Lever and Gundula Schaumburg-Lever, Lippincott, Philadelphia, 1983.

PORPHYRIA CUTANEA TARDA

Porphyria cutanea tarda is the most common type of porphyria. Increased uroporphyrin levels are associated with hepatic damage; there is often a background of alcoholism. Most cases are acquired, but occasionally porphyria cutanea tarda is transmitted as an autosomal dominant trait. Onset is usually in middle age.

Cutaneous lesions are varied and generally occur on the exposed areas, due to the photosensitizing effects of the porphyrins. Skin changes include erosions and bullae (Figs. B,C), milia, hyperpigmentation (Fig. A), hypertrichosis, and diffuse sclerosis. Scarring alopecia is common.

Microscopic features

1. Bullae form subepidermally (Fig. D) above the PAS-positive basement zone.
2. Papillae at the base of the bullae are well preserved, but slightly edematous (Fig. D). This "festooning" is rather characteristic.
3. Inflammatory changes in the dermis are minimal (Figs. D,E).
4. Collagen fibers show varying degrees of thickening and hyalinization (Fig. E).
5. PAS-positive, diastase-resistant hyaline deposits are present in the perivascular areas of the upper dermis, and in severe cases, in the perivascular areas of the deep dermis. Acid mucopolysaccharides may also be present.

Microscopic differential diagnosis (see p. 586)

Comment

1. *Pseudoporphyria* is a condition that mimics porphyria cutanea tarda clinically and histologically, but usually has no abnormality of porphyrin excretion. It has been associated with treatment with Furosemide, nalidixic acid, tetracycline hydrochloride, sulfonamides, and naproxen.
2. In erythropoietic protoporphyria, lesions elicited by exposure to light include edema, followed by induration and sometimes vesicles. Lesions of erythropoietic protoporphyria may resemble those of hydroa vacciniforme. PAS-positive, diastase-resistant perivascular hyaline deposits are typically present. The hyaline material may contain lipid and acid mucopolysaccharides.

PORPHYRIA CUTANEA TARDA

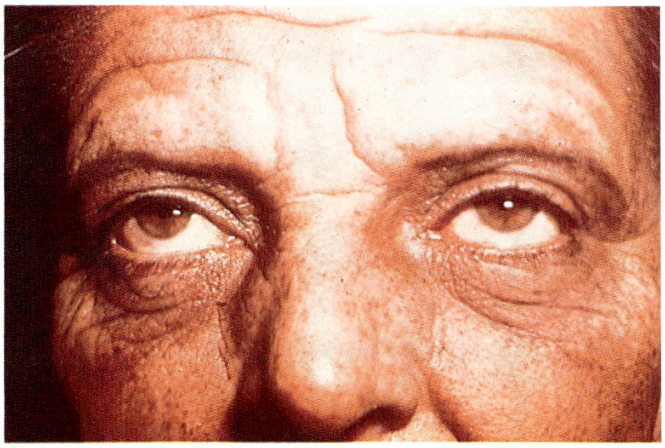

A

Figs. A,B,C courtesy Dr. Harvey Ansell

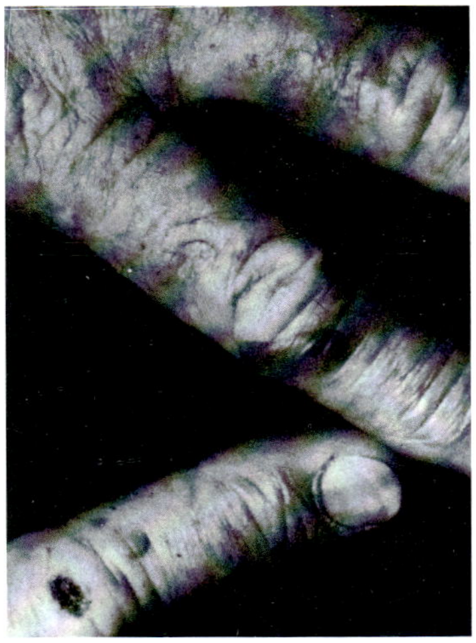

B

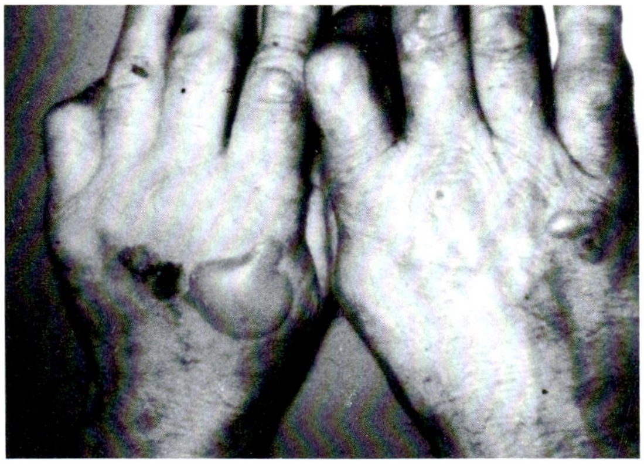

C

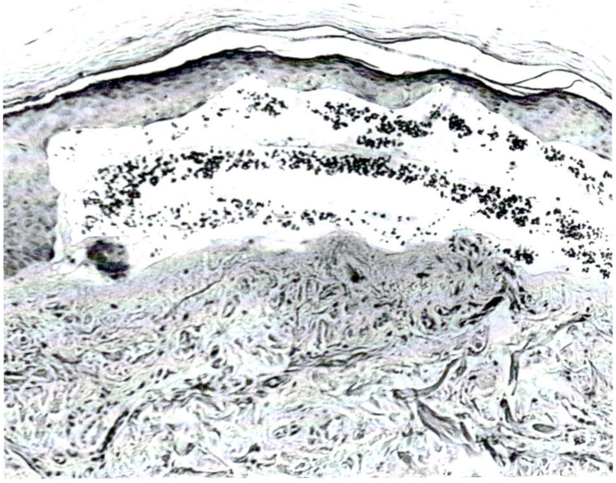

D
X190

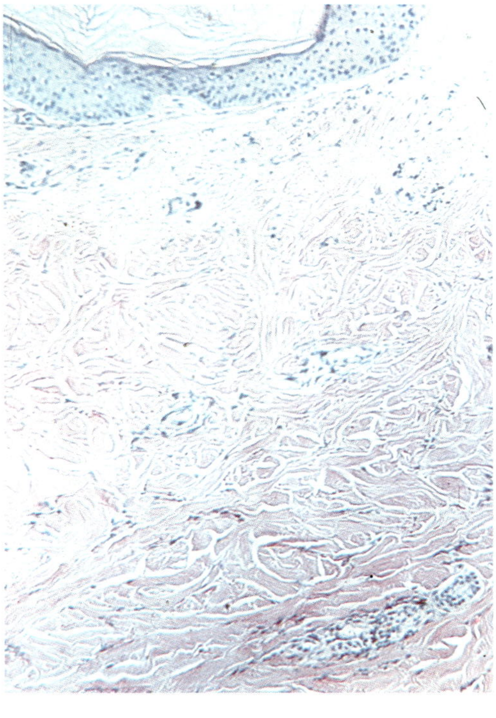

E
X190

EPIDERMOLYSIS BULLOSA

Epidermolysis bullosa (EB) encompasses a group of disorders, mostly hereditary, in which blisters form in response to trauma; these disorders are sometimes called *mechanobullous disorders*. Clinical features of the types of epidermolysis bullosa overlap, and the microscopic pattern in all of them is characterized by subepidermal bulla formation. Electron microscopic analysis is a key procedure in the current scheme of classification.

The mildest forms of EB show blisters without scarring. Milia are common in all forms. The more severe forms show varying degrees of dystrophic scarring, varying tendency towards mucosal involvement, and varying dystrophic changes in hair and nails. The severe cases may be fatal.

In EB simplex and EB of Cockayne, blisters heal without scarring; in the latter form, blisters are limited to the hands and feet. In these disorders, the blisters form in the lower portion of the basal cells of the epidermis, although in EB of Cockayne there is rapid regeneration and the cleavage may appear to be within the spinous layer in biopsies. Both show dominant genetic transmission. There is a severe form of epidermolysis bullosa simplex with extensive blistering that improves with age.

In EB letalis (Fig. A), blisters have little tendency to heal; scarring is not observed. Oral lesions and nail changes occur. The blister forms in the lamina lucida. There is recessive genetic transmission.

In generalized benign atrophic EB, lesions heal with superficial atrophic scars. Oral lesions, alopecia, and nail changes are observed. The blister forms in the lamina lucida. There is recessive genetic transmission.

Both recessive and dominant forms of EB dystrophica show scarring; mucosal and nail changes can be observed. Changes are more severe in the recessive form, with ulcers and dystrophic scars (Fig. B) which can result in fibrous binding of the digits. Squamous cell carcinoma can be a sequel. Esophageal stenosis may occur in the recessive form. In both forms of EB dystrophica, the blisters form in the uppermost dermis, in the region of the anchoring fibrils.

EB acquisita arises in adult life. Blisters induced by trauma lead to atrophic scars; the nails and oral mucosa may be affected. This disorder is not hereditary. Blisters form in the uppermost dermis. Linear deposits of immunoglobulins and complement at the basement zone suggest an autoimmune pathogenesis. There have been suggestions that EB acquisita is a manifestation of cicatricial pemphigoid. However, in cicatricial pemphigoid, the immunoglobulins and complement are found above the basal lamina, not below it, as in EB acquisita.

EPIDERMOLYSIS BULLOSA

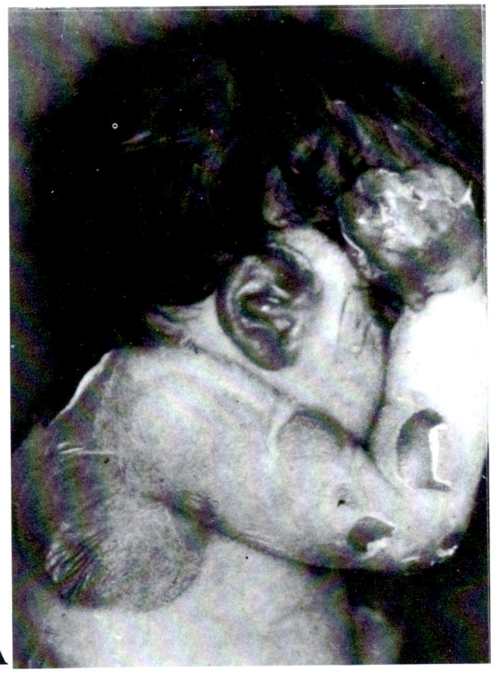

A

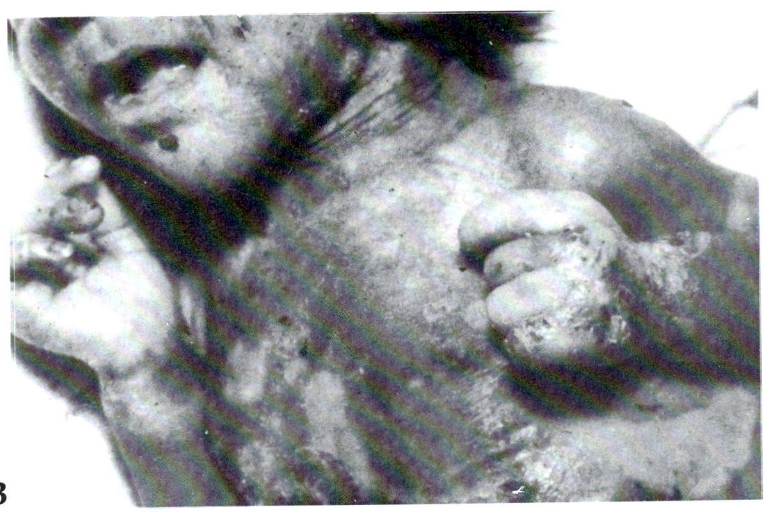

B

Courtesy Dr. Robert Gorlin

EPIDERMOLYSIS BULLOSA continued

EPIDERMOLYSIS BULLOSA

Microscopic features

1. Bullae are observed subepidermally (Fig. A).
2. In epidermolysis bullosa simplex and epidermolysis bullosa of Cockayne, bullae form subepidermally, but due to rapid regeneration, bullae may be intra-epidermal when observed histologically, with similar appearance to friction blisters (see below).
3. There may be inflammation beneath the blisters (Fig. A).
4. In the scarring forms of EB, fibrosis is observed beneath the blisters.

Microscopic differential diagnosis (see p. 586)

Comment

Friction blisters typically occur on the palms and soles of normal individuals as a result of repetitive or prolonged trauma. There is cleavage of the epidermis due to degeneration of keratinocytes. The clefts are usually observed beneath the stratum granulosum (Fig. B). Degenerated keratinocytes may be seen at the margins of the cleft.

EPIDERMOLYSIS BULLOSA

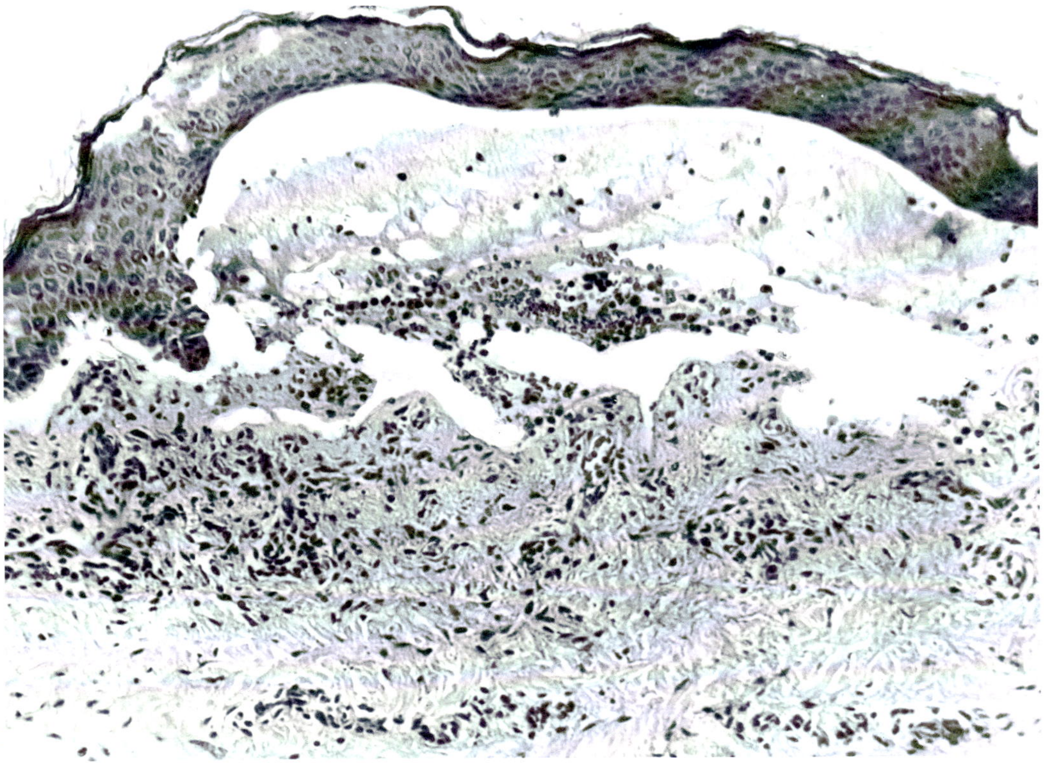

A
X165

FRICTION BLISTER

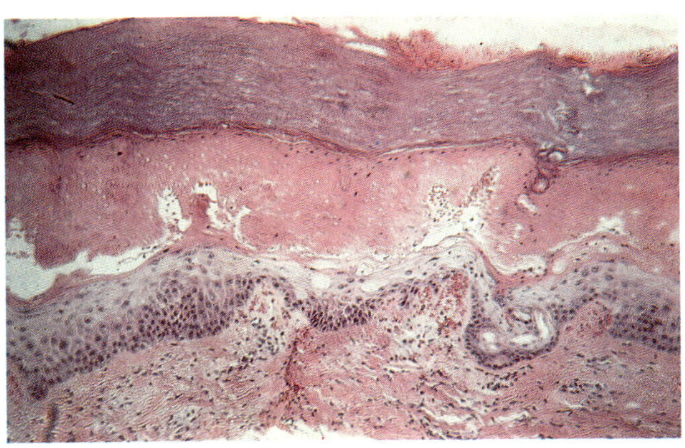

B
X100

BURNS

Burns are necrotic lesions of the skin induced by a variety of stimuli, including heat and cold (thermal burns), electricity, chemicals, and ultraviolet light.

The degree and depth of the necrosis vary with the intensity of the stimulus. In first degree burns, the necrosis is limited to the upper epidermis. In second degree burns, there is necrosis of the epidermis and upper dermis. In addition, second degree burns are characterized by separation of the epidermis and dermis. Third degree burns show necrosis of the entire thickness of the skin, with possible involvement of subcutaneous tissue and muscle.

Electrical burns are of special interest in dermatopathology, since electrosurgery is used to treat or remove some skin lesions, and specimens submitted for histologic examination may show electrical burns.

A common type of burn is sunburn. Fig. A shows a second degree sunburn with numerous blisters.

Microscopic features

1. Burns show varying degrees of coagulation necrosis of tissue, with vacuolization and pyknosis of nuclei. In the epidermis, perinuclear halos may be present. There is an alteration of normal staining characteristics of tissue components. Illustrated is a second degree thermal burn, showing extensive coagulation necrosis and subepidermal bulla (Fig. B).
2. Electrical burns show, in addition to subepidermal bulla formation, a special feature—pronounced elongation of basal cells of the epidermis, resulting in a fringe lining the domes of the bullae (Figs. C,D). The dermis at the base of the blisters shows coagulation necrosis (Figs. C,D).
3. Inflammation occurs as a late feature, at the periphery of necrotic areas.

SECOND DEGREE BURN

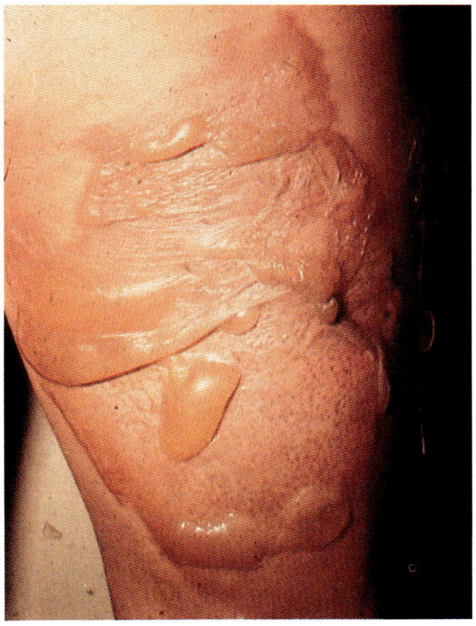

A

Courtesy Dr. Hein Ter Poorten

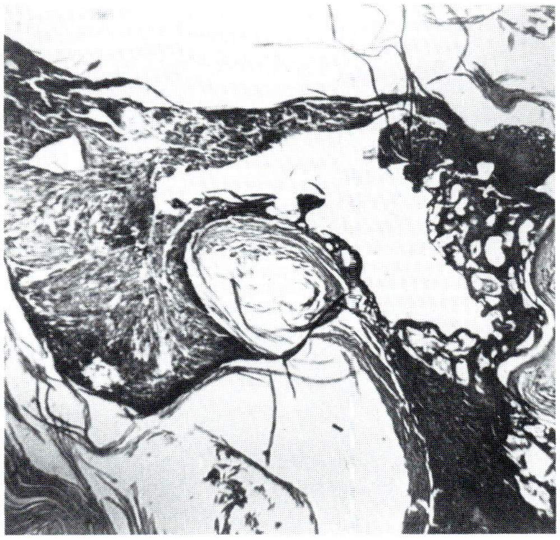

B
X120

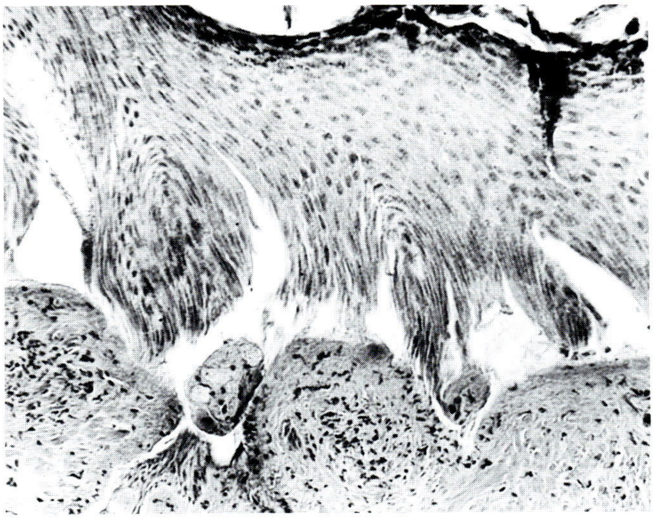

C
X125

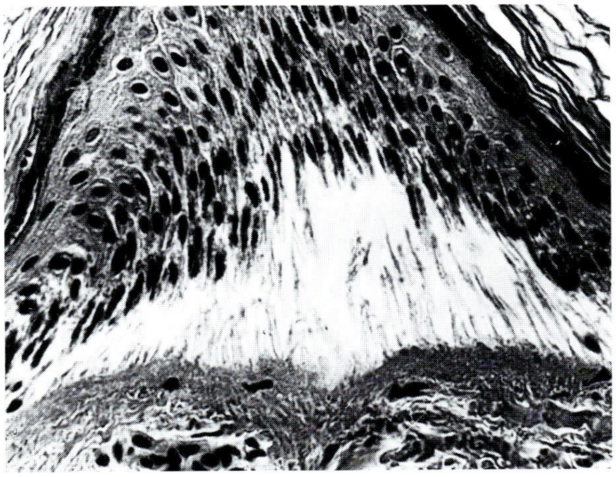

D
X340

In general, the microscopic differential diagnosis of subepidermal bullae is not as clear-cut as that of intraepidermal bullae; differences cited in the chart are not always present, but are helpful when correlated with the clinical features.

KEY DIFFERENTIAL DIAGNOSTIC FEATURES OF SUBEPIDERMAL BULLAE

Bullous pemphigoid	Papillary dermal abscesses are present, composed primarily of eosinophils.
Dermatitis herpetiformis	Papillary dermal abscesses are present, composed primarily of neutrophils.
Erythema multiforme bullosum	Necrosis and dyskeratosis may be observed in the epidermal dome of the bulla and adjacent epidermis.
Cicatricial pemphigoid	Dermal fibrosis is pronounced.
Porphyria cutanea tarda	Well-formed papillae generally remain at the base of the bulla. Dermal inflammation is typically minimal or absent. The collagen shows scleroderma-like changes. Papillae contain hyaline material similar to that of lipoid proteinosis.
Epidermolysis bullosa	Well-formed papillae generally remain at the base of the bulla. Dermal inflammation is typically minimal or absent. There may be fibrosis.
Second degree burn (electrical)	A fringe of elongated basal cells ("goat's whiskers") is present.
Second degree burn (thermal)	Coagulation necrosis of dome and base of bulla is present.

Ultrastructural Cleavage Plane of Subepidermal Bullous Dermatoses

Dermatitis Herpetiformis: Discontinuities in basal lamina
Bullous pemphigoid
- Noninflammatory lesions: In lamina lucida
- Inflammatory lesions: Discontinuities in basal lamina

Herpes gestationis: Above basal lamina
Cicatricial pemphigoid: Cleavage plane similar to that of bullous pemphigoid
Erythema Multiforme
- Dermal type: Beneath basal lamina
- Mixed type or
- Epidermal type: In some cases basal lamina destroyed; in other cases cleavage above basal lamina

Porphyria cutanea tarda: Above basal lamina
Epidermolysis bullosa
- EB simplex } In lower part of basal cells
- EB of hands and feet } In lower part of basal cells
- EB letalis } In lamina lucida
- Generalized atrophic benign EB } In lamina lucida
- EB dystrophica (dominant and recessive) } In regions of anchoring fibrils
- EB acquisita } In regions of anchoring fibrils

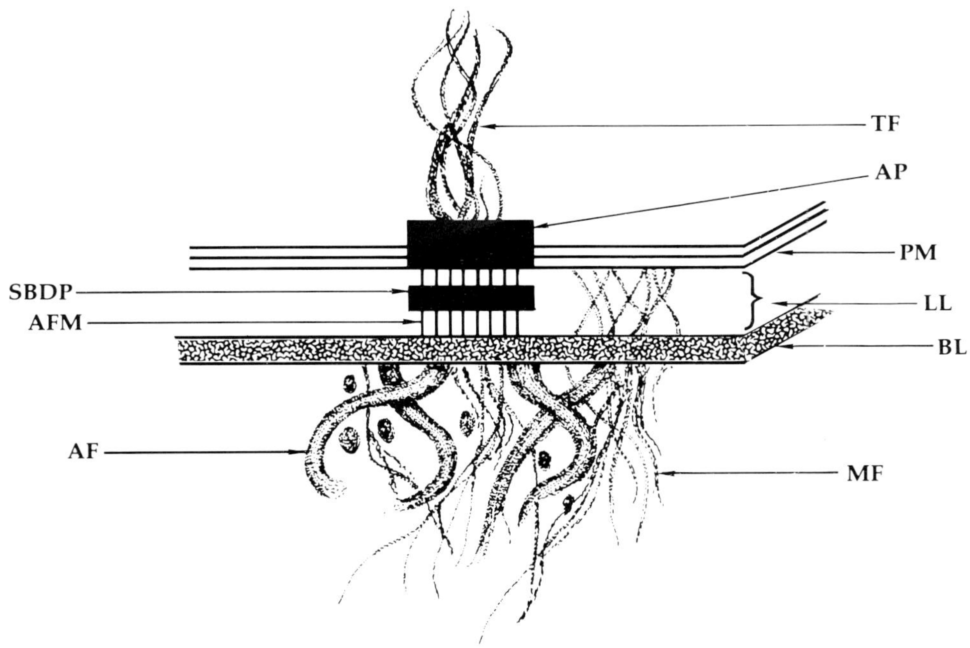

Schematic View of Epidermal-Dermal Junction

TF = Tonofilaments
AP = Attachment plaque of half-desmosome
PM = Trilaminar plasma membrane of basal cell
LL = Lamina lucida
BL = Basal lamina
MF = Microfilament
AF = Anchoring fibril
AFM = Anchoring filament
SBDP = Sub-basal cell dense plaque

BULLOUS DERMATOSES continued

Subcorneal Bullous Dermatoses

SUBCORNEAL PUSTULAR DERMATOSIS (SNEDDON-WILKINSON)

This chronic disorder is of unknown cause. It is characterized by recurrent crops of vesiculopustules (Fig. A) which are sometimes surrounded by a zone of erythema. Lesions often have an annular arrangement (Fig. B), and have a predilection for the flexor surfaces of the extremities and abdomen. Middle-aged women are commonly affected.

A variety of conditions have been reported with Sneddon-Wilkinson disease. These include IgA paraproteinemia, leukocytoclastic vasculitis, erythema multiforme, pyoderma gangrenosum, systemic lupus erythematosus, bullous pemphigoid, and polyarthritis.

Microscopic features

1. Vesicles and pustules have a subcorneal location (Fig. C), and contain many neutrophils and a few eosinophils. A few acantholytic cells are sometimes present.
2. The underlying epidermis and dermis show features of subacute dermatitis (see p. 98).

Microscopic differential diagnosis

1. Subcorneal pustular dermatosis cannot be distinguished from impetigo histologically. Gram stain is not a reliable method for making the distinction, but bacterial culture of pustule contents may be of value.
2. Acute mucocutaneous candidiasis may show a histologic picture identical to that of subcorneal pustular dermatosis or impetigo, but PAS stain typically shows spores and hyphae in candidiasis. An additional feature that may be present in candidiasis is spongiform pustulation as seen in pustular psoriasis (see p. 350).
3. Spongiform pustulation is not typically present in subcorneal pustular dermatosis, but some authors have suggested that subcorneal pustular dermatosis is a form of pustular psoriasis and have described cases of subcorneal pustular dermatosis evolving into pustular psoriasis.

Comment

1. Subcorneal pustular dermatosis may respond to sulfapyridine, or sulfone therapy.
2. *Acropustulosis of infancy* is a disorder in which recurrent crops of small vesiculopustules develop in the acral areas. Spontaneous resolution occurs in about two years. Histologically, subcorneal pustules are observed, which are identical to those of subcorneal pustular dermatosis or impetigo.

SUBCORNEAL PUSTULAR DERMATOSIS

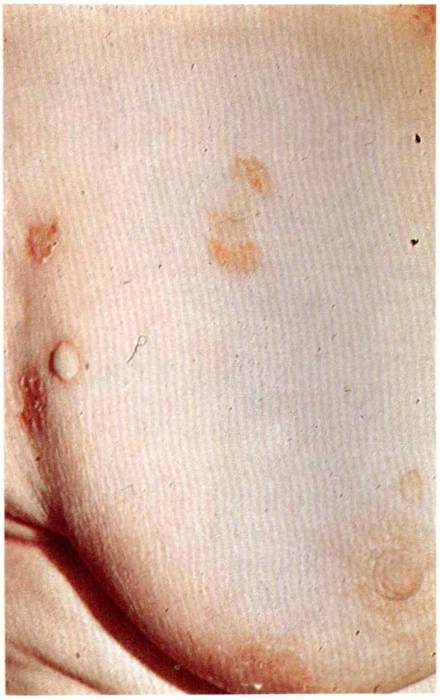

A

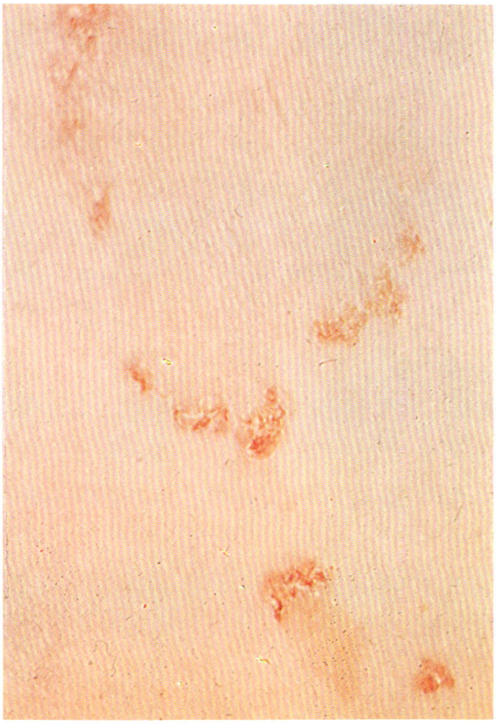

B

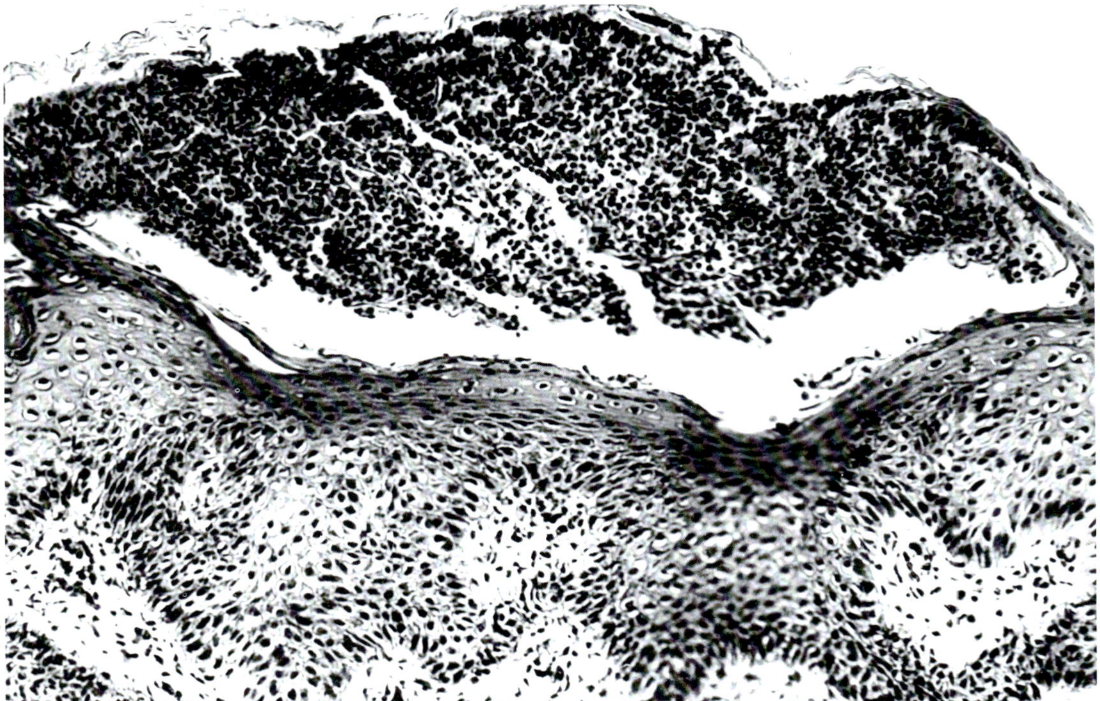

C
X180

Suggested Reading

Bullous Dermatoses: Acantholytic

Pemphigus

GENERAL REFERENCES

Ahmed, A. et al. Pemphigus: Current concepts. *Ann. Int. Med.*, 92:396, 1980.

Asboe-Hansen, G. Blister-spread induced by finger pressure: A diagnostic sign of pemphigus. *J. Invest. Dermatol.*, 34:5, 1960.

Beutner, E., Chorzelski, T. and Jordon, R. *Autosensitization in Pemphigus and Bullous Pemphigoid.* Springfield, IL, Thomas, 1970.

Beutner, E. et al. *Immunopathology of the Skin Labeled Antibody Studies.* Stroudsburg, PA, Dowden, Hutchinson and Ross, 1973.

Creswell, S. et al. Correlation of circulating intercellular antibody titers in pemphigus with disease activity. *Clin. Exp. Dermatol.*, 6:477, 1981.

Hashimoto, J. et al. Anti-cell surface pemphigus autoantibody stimulates plasminogen activator activity of human epidermal cells. A mechanism for the loss of epidermal cohesion and blister formation. *J. Exp. Med.*, 157:259, 1983.

Judd, K. and Lever, W. Correlation of antibodies in skin and serum with disease severity in pemphigus. *Arch. Dermatol.*, 115:428, 1979.

Judd, K. and Mescon, H. Comparison of different epithelial substrates useful for indirect immunofluorescent testing of sera from patients with active pemphigus. *J. Invest. Dermatol.*, 72:314, 1979.

Kennedy, C., Hodge, L. and Sanderson, K. Skin changes caused by D-penicillamine treatment of arthritis: Report of three cases with immunological findings. *Clin. Exp. Dermatol.*, 3:107, 1978.

Knight, A., Black, M. and Delaney, J. Eosinophilic spongiosis: Clinical, histologic and immunofluorescent correlation. *Clin. Exp. Dermatol.*, 1:141, 1976.

Krain, L. Pemphigus: Epidemiologic and survival characteristics of 59 patients, 1955–73. *Arch. Dermatol.*, 110:862, 1974.

Lagerholm, B., Frithz, A. and Borglund, E. Light and electron microscopic aspects of pemphigus herpetiformis (eosinophilic spongiosis) in comparison with other acantholytic disorders. *Acta Derm. Venereol.* (Stockh.), 59:305, 1979.

Lever, W. Pemphigus. *Medicine*, 32:1, 1953.

——. *Pemphigus and Pemphigoid*, Springfield, IL, Thomas, 1965.

Lever, W. and Hashimoto, K. The etiology and treatment of pemphigus and pemphigoid. *J. Invest. Dermatol.*, 53:373, 1969.

Miescher, P. and Muller-Eberhard, H. *Textbook of Immunopathology.* Vol. 2, New York, Grune & Stratton, 1968.

Pearson, R. Advances in the diagnosis and treatment of blistering diseases: A selective review. *Year Book of Dermatology.* Chicago, Year Book, 1977.

Santa Cruz, D. et al. Pemphigus-like lesions induced by D-penicillamine: Analysis of clinical, histopathological and immunofluorescence features in 34 cases. *Am. J. Dermatopathol.*, 3:85, 1981.

Stanley, J. et al. Pemphighus antibodies identify a cell surface glycoprotein synthesized by human and mouse keratinocytes. *J. Clin. Invest.*, 70:281, 1982.

Troy, J. et al. Penicillamine-associated pemphigus: Is it really pemphigus? *J. Am. Acad. Dermatol.*, 4:547, 1981.

Pemphigus Vulgaris

Arundell, F. Pemphigus biopsies. *Arch. Dermatol.*, 98:28, 1968.

Beutner, E., Jordon, R. and Chorzelski, T. The immunopathology of pemphigus and bullous pemphigoid. *J. Invest. Dermatol.*, 51:63, 1968.

Beutner, E. et al. Autoantibodies in pemphigus vulgaris: Response to an intercellular substance of epidermis. *JAMA*, 192:682, 1965.

Blank, H. and Burgoon, C. Abnormal cytology of epithelial cells in pemphigus vulgaris: A diagnostic aid. *J. Invest. Dermatol.*, 18:213, 1952.
Chorzelski, T., von Weiss, J. and Lever, W. Clinical significance of autoantibodies in pemphigus. *Arch. Dermatol.*, 93:570, 1966.
Civatte, A. Diagnostic histopathologique de la dermatite polymorphe douloureuse ou maladie de Duhring-Brocq. *Ann. Derm. Syph.* (Ser. 8), 3:1, 1943.
Director, W. Pemphigus vegetans: A clinicopathologic correlation. *Arch. Dermatol. Syph.*, 66:343, 1952.
——. Pemphigus vulgaris: A clinicopathologic study. *Arch. Dermatol. Syph.*, 65;155, 1952.
Emmerson, R. and Wilson-Jones, E. Eosinophilic spongiosis in pemphigus. *Arch. Dermatol.*, 97:252, 1968.
Forman, L. Pemphigus vegetans of Hallopeau. *Arch. Dermatol.*, 114:627, 1978.
Fukuyama, K. et al. Immuno-histochemical method of localization of antibodies in cutaneous disease. *Am. J. Clin. Pathol.*, 54:410, 1970.
Hashimoto, K. and Lever, W. An ultrastructural study of cell junctions in pemphigus vulgaris. *Arch. Dermatol.*, 101:287, 1970.
Jablonska, S. and Chorzelski, T. Utilization of immunofluorescence in the diagnosis of bullous diseases, lupus erythematosus and certain other dermatoses. *Internat. J. Dermatol.*, 14:83, 1975.
Jordon, R., Ihrig, J. and Perry, H. Childhood pemphigus vulgaris. *Arch. Dermatol.*, 100:176, 1969.
Jordon, R. et al. Classic and alternate pathway activation of complement in pemphigus vulgaris lesions. *J. Invest. Dermatol.*, 63:256, 1974.
Jordon, R. et al. Negative complement immunofluorescence in pemphigus. *J. Invest. Dermatol.*, 57:407, 1971.
Knight, A., Delaney, T. and Black, M. Eosinophilic spongiosis, a clinical, histological and immunofluorescent correlation. *Br. J. Dermatol.*, 93:13, 1975.
Krain, L. and Bierman, S. Pemphigus vulgaris and internal malignancy. *Cancer*, 33:1091, 1974.
LeRoy, D. et al. Pemphigus végétant à type clinique de dermatite pustuleuse chronique de Hallopeau. *Ann. Dermatol. Venereol.*, 109:549, 1982.
Murphy, P. and Harrell, E. Pemphigus vulgaris in childhood. *Am. J. Dis. Child.*, 123:70, 1972.
Nelson, C. Pemphigus vegetans of Hallopeau. *Arch. Dermatol.*, 114:627, 1978.
Nelson, C. et al. Pemphigus vegetans of Hallopeau. *Arch. Dermatol.*, 113:942, 1977.
Neumann, H. and Faber, W. Pyodermite végétante of Hallopeau. *Arch. Dermatol.*, 116:1169, 1980.
Pearson, R., O'Donoghue, M. and Kaplan, S. Pemphigus vegetans: Its relationship to eosinophilic spongiosis and favorable response to dapsone. *Arch. Dermatol.*, 116:65, 1980.
Rook, A. and Whimster, I. The histological diagnosis of pemphigus. *Br. J. Dermatol.*, 62:443, 1950.
Ruzicka, T. and Goetz, G. Beobachtungen bei der Pyodermite végétante Hallopeau. *Z. Haut.*, 54:24, 1979.
Sams, W. and Jordon, R. Pemphigus antibodies: Their role in disease. *J. Invest. Dermatol.*, 56:474, 1971.
Sams, W., Jr. and Jordon, R. Correlation of pemphigus and pemphigoid antibody titers with activity of disease. *Br. J. Dermatol.*, 84:7, 1971.
Wolff, K. and Schreiner, E. Ultrastructural localization of pemphigus autoantibodies within the epidermis. *Nature*, 229:59, 1971.

Mixed Bullous Disease

Barranco, V. Mixed bullous disease. *Arch. Dermatol.*, 110:221, 1974.
Chorzelski, T. et al. Coexistence of pemphigus and bullous pemphigoid. *Arch. Dermatol.*, 109:849, 1974.
DeMento, F. and Grover, R. Acantholytic herpetiform dermatitis. *Arch. Dermatol.*, 107:883, 1973.
Eng, A. and Moncada, B. Bullous pemphigoid and dermatitis herpetiformis Histopathologic differentiation of bullous pemphigoid and dermatitis herpetiformis. *Arch. Dermatol.*, 110:51, 1974.
Floden, C. and Gentele, H. A case of clinically typical dermatitis herpetiformis (Duhring) presenting acantholysis. *Acta Derm. Venereol.*, 35:128, 1955.

Honeyman, J. et al. The enigma of bullous pemphigoid and dermatitis herpetiformis. *Arch. Dermatol.*, 106:22, 1972.
Meer, J. van der. Granular deposits of immunoglobulins in the skin of patients with dermatitis herpetiformis: An immunofluorescent study. *Br. J. Dermatol.*, 81:493, 1969.
Winkelmann, R. and Roth, H. Dermatitis herpetiformis with acantholysis or pemphigus with response to sulfonamides. *Arch. Dermatol.*, 82:385, 1960.

Pemphigus Foliaceus

Bean, S. and Lynch, F. Senear-Usher syndrome (pemphigus erythematosus). *Arch. Dermatol.*, 101:642, 1970.
Bystryn, J., Abel, E. and DeFeo, C. Pemphigus foliaceus: Subcorneal intercellular antibodies of unique specificity. *Arch. Dermatol.*, 110:857, 1974.
Chorzelski, T., Jablonska, S. and Blaszczyk, M. Immunopathological investigation in the Senear-Usher syndrome (coexistence of pemphigus and lupus erythematosus). *Br. J. Dermatol.*, 80:211, 1968.
Furtado, T. Histopathology of pemphigus foliaceus. *Arch. Dermatol.*, 80:66, 1959.
Giannetti, A. Immunofluorescence studies in Senear-Usher syndrome. *Arch. Dermatol. Forsch.*, 248:287, 1974.
Guimaraes Proenca, N. and Rivitti, E. Antiepithelial antibodies in Brazilian pemphigus foliaceus. *Internat. J. Dermatol.*, 16:799, 1977.
Jablonska, S. et al. Pathogenesis of pemphigus erythematosus. *Arch. Dermatol. Res.*, 258:135, 1977.
Lagerholm, B. and Frithz, A. Submicroscopic aspect of the keratinization, dyskeratinization and acantholysis of fogo selvagem. *Acta Derm. Venereol.* (Stockh.), 58:37, 1978.
Perry, H. Pemphigus foliaceus. *Arch. Dermatol.*, 83:52, 1961.
Perry, H. and Brunsting, L. Pemphigus foliaceus: Further observations. *Arch. Dermatol.*, 91:10, 1965.
Schroeter, A., Sams, W., Jr. and Jordon, R. Immunofluorescent studies of pemphigus foliaceus in a child. *Arch. Dermatol.*, 100:736, 1969.
Siakia, N. and MacConnell, L. Senear-Usher syndrome and internal malignancy. *Br. J. Dermatol.*, 87:1, 1972.
Wilgram, G., Caulfield, J. and Madgic, E. An electron microscopic study of acantholysis and dyskeratosis in pemphigus foliaceus. *J. Invest. Dermatol.*, 43:287, 1964.

Familial Benign Chronic Pemphigus (Hailey-Hailey)

Berger, R. and Lynch, P. Familial benign chronic pemphigus: Surgical treatment and pathogenesis. *Arch. Dermatol.*, 104:380, 1971.
Botvinick, I. Familial benign pemphigus with oral mucous membrane lesions. *Cutis*, 12:371, 1973.
Chorzelski, T. Experimentally induced acantholysis in Hailey's benign pemphigus. *Dermatologica*, 124:21, 1962.
De Dobbeleer, G. and Achten, G. Disrupted desmosomes in induced lesions of familial benign chronic pemphigus. *J. Cutan. Pathol.*, 6:418, 1979.
Ellis, F. Vesicular Darier's disease (so-called benign familial pemphigus: A variant of Darier's disease). *Arch. Dermatol. Syph.*, 61:715, 1950.
Finnerud, C. and Szymanski, F. Chronic benign familial pemphigus: A possible vesicular variant of keratosis follicularis. *Arch. Dermatol. Syph.*, 61:737, 1950.
Ganor, S. and Sagher, F. Keratosis follicularis (Darier) and familial benign chronic pemphigus (Hailey-Hailey) in the same patient. *Br. J. Dermatol.*, 77:24, 1965.
Gottlieb, S. and Lutzner, M. Hailey-Hailey disease: An electron microscopic study. *J. Invest. Dermatol.*, 54:368, 1970.
Hailey, H. and Hailey, H. Familial benign chronic pemphigus. *Arch. Dermatol. Syph.*, 39:679, 1939.
Heinze, R. Pemphigus chronicus benignus familiaris (Gougerot-Hailey-Hailey) mit Schleimhautbeteiligung bei einer Diabetikerin. *Dermatol. Monatsschr.*, 165:862, 1979.
Herzberg, J. Pemphigus Gougerot/ Hailey-Hailey. *Arch. Klin. Exp. Dermatol.*, 202:21, 1955.
Izumi, A., Shmunes, E. and Wood, M. Familial benign chronic pemphigus: The role of trauma including contact sensitivity. *Arch. Dermatol.*, 104:177, 1971.

Kahn, D. and Hutchinson, E. Esophageal involvement in familial benign chronic pemphigus. *Arch. Dermatol.*, 109:718, 1974.
Marsch, W. and Stüttgen, G. Generalized Hailey-Hailey disease. *Br. J. Dermatol.*, 99:553, 1978.
Nicolis, G. et al. Keratosis follicularis and familial benign chronic pemphigus in the same patient. *Dermatologica*, 159:346, 1979.
Palmer, D. and Perry, H. Benign familial chronic pemphigus. *Arch. Dermatol.*, 86:493, 1962.
Pinkus, H. and Epstein, S. Familial benign chronic pemphigus: Report of a case. *Arch. Dermatol. Syph.*, 53:119, 1946.
Václavínková, Y. and Neumann, E. Vaginal involvement in familial benign chronic pemphigus (morbus Hailey-Hailey). *Acta Derm. Venereol.* (Stockh.), 62:80, 1982.
Wilgram, G. and Caulfield, J. and Lever, W. An electron microscopic study of acantholysis and dyskeratosis in Hailey and Hailey disease. *J. Invest. Dermatol.*, 39:373, 1962.
Wilkin, J. Chronic benign familial pemphigus. *Arch. Dermatol.*, 114:136, 1978.
Winer, L. and Leeb, A. Benign familial pemphigus: Cytology and nosology. *Arch. Dermatol. Syph.*, 67:77, 1953.
Witkowski, J. and Parish, L. Familial benign chronic pemphigus: Papular variant. *Arch. Dermatol.*, 108:842, 1973.

Darier's Disease (Keratosis Follicularis)

Ackerman, A. Focal acantholytic dyskeratosis. *Arch. Dermatol.*, 106:702, 1972.
Binnick, S. and Fleischmajer, R. Unilateral keratosis follicularis. *Arch. Dermatol.*, 113:1459, 1977.
Carapeto, F. and Armijo, M. Maladie de Darier à minimes lésions ou variété Darier-like de la maladie de Grover. *Ann. Dermatol. Venereol.*, 106:279, 1979.
Caulfield, J. and Wilgram, G. An electron-microscope study of dyskeratosis and acantholysis in Darier's disease. *J. Invest. Dermatol.*, 41:57, 1963.
Delacrétaz, J. and Christeler, A. Dyskératose acantholytique régionale. *Dermatologica*, 163:113, 1981.
Ellis, F. Keratosis follicularis is not primarily a follicular disease. *Arch. Dermatol. Syph.*, 50:27, 1944.
Getzler, N. and Flint, A. Keratosis follicularis: A study of one family. *Arch. Dermatol.*, 93:545, 1966.
Gisslén, H. and Mobacken, H. Acute adult-onset Darier-like dermatosis. *Br. J. Dermatol.*, 98:217, 1978.
Gorlin, R. and Chaudhry, A. The oral manifestation of keratosis follicularis. *Oral Surg.*, 12:1468, 1959.
Gottlieb, S. and Lutzner, M. Darier's disease. *Arch. Dermatol.*, 107:225, 1973.
Graham, J. and Helwig, E. Isolated dyskeratosis follicularis. *Arch. Dermatol.*, 77:377, 1958.
Jones, W., Nix, T., Jr. and Clark, W., Jr. Hemorrhagic Darier's disease. *Arch. Dermatol.*, 89:523, 1964.
Klein, A., Burns, L. and Leyden, J. Rectal mucosa involvement in keratosis follicularis. *Arch. Dermatol.*, 109:560, 1974.
Leeming, J. Acquired linear naevus showing histological features of keratosis follicularis. *Br. J. Dermatol.*, 81:128, 1969.
Mann, P. and Haye, K. An electron microscope study on the acantholytic and dyskeratotic process in Darier's disease. *Br. J. Dermatol.*, 82:561, 1970.
Panja, R. Acrokeratosis verruciformis (Hopf): A clinical entity? *Br. J. Dermatol.*, 96:643, 1977.
Peck, G. et al. Cornifying Darier disease: A unique variant. *Arch. Dermatol.*, 112:495, 1976.
Sato, A., Anton-Lamprecht, J. and Schnyder, U. Ultrastructure of dyskeratosis in morbus Darier. *J. Cutan. Pathol.*, 4:173, 1977.
Starink, T. and Woerdeman, M. Unilateral systematized keratosis follicularis: A variant of Darier's disease or an epidermal nevus (acantholytic dyskeratotic epidermal nevus)? *Br. J. Dermatol.*, 105:207, 1981.
Weathers, D., Olansky, S. and Sharpe, L. Darier's disease with mucous membrane involvement: A case report. *Arch. Dermatol.*, 100:50, 1969.
White, J. A case of keratosis (ichthyosis) follicularis. *J. Cutan. Genito-Urin. Dis.*, 7:201, 1889.

Incidental Acantholytic Dyskeratosis and Epidermolytic Hyperkeratosis

Ackerman, A. Focal acantholytic dyskeratosis. *Arch. Dermatol.*, 106:702, 1972.

——. Histopathologic concept of epidermolytic hyperkeratosis. *Arch. Dermatol.*, 102:253, 1970.

Ackerman, A. and Reed, R. Epidermolytic variant of solar keratosis. *Arch. Dermatol.*, 107:104, 1973.

Botet, M. and Sánchez, J. Vesiculation of focal acantholytic dyskeratosis in acral lentiginous malignant melanoma. *J. Dermatol. Surg. Oncol.*, 5:798, 1979.

Gebhart, W. and Kidd, R. Das solitäre epidermolytische Akanthom. *Z. Haut.*, 47:1, 1972.

Hirone, T. and Fukushiro, R. Disseminated epidermolytic acanthoma. *Acta Derm. Venereol.* (Stockh.), 53:393, 1973.

Mehregan, A. Epidermolytic hyperkeratosis. *J. Cutan. Pathol.*, 5:76, 1978.

Miyamoto, Y. et al. Disseminated epidermolytic acanthoma. *J. Cutan. Pathol.*, 6:272, 1979.

Nagashima, M. and Matsuoka, S. So-called granular degeneration as incidental histopathological finding. *Jpn. J. Dermatol.*, (Series B), 81:494, 1971.

Niizuma, K. Isolated epidermolytic acanthoma. *Dermatologica*, 159:30, 1979.

Shapiro, L. and Baraf, C. Isolated epidermolytic acanthoma. *Arch. Dermatol.*, 101:220, 1970.

Stern, J., Wolf, J., Jr. and Rosen, T. Focal acantholytic dyskeratosis in pityriasis rosea. *Arch. Dermatol.*, 115:497, 1979.

Grover's Disease (Transient Acantholytic Dermatosis)

Bystryn, J. Immunofluorescence studies in transient acantholytic dermatosis (Grover's disease). *Am. J. Dermatopathol.*, 1:325, 1979.

Chalet, M., Grover, R. and Ackerman, A. Transient acantholytic dermatosis. *Arch. Dermatol.*, 113:431, 1977.

Fawcett, H. and Miller, J. Persistent acantholytic dermatosis related to actinic damage. *Br. J. Dermatol.*, 109:349, 1983.

Fishman, H. Acute eruptive Darier disease. *Arch. Dermatol.*, 111:221, 1975.

Gisslén, H. and Mobacken, H. Acute adult-onset Darier-like dermatosis. *Br. J. Dermatol.*, 98:217, 1978.

Grover, R. Transient acantholytic dermatosis. *Arch. Dermatol.*, 101:426, 1970.

——. Transient acantholytic dermatosis: Electron microscope study. *Arch. Dermatol.*, 104:26, 1971.

Grover, R. and Duffy, J. Transient acantholytic dermatosis: Electron microscope study of the Darier type. *J. Cutan. Pathol.*, 2:111, 1975.

Heenan, P. and Quirk, C. Transient acantholytic dermatosis. *Br. J. Dermatol.*, 102:515, 1980.

Horiuchi, Y., Umezawa, A. and Kamimura, K. Erythematous plaque variant of transient acantholytic dermatosis. *Cutis*, 38:48, 1986.

Kanzaki, T. and Hashimoto, K. Transient acantholytic dermatosis with involvement of oral mucosa. *J. Cutan. Pathol.*, 5:23, 1978.

Millns, J. et al. Positive cutaneous immunofluorescence in Grover's disease. *Arch. Dermatol.*, 116:515, 1980.

Pehamberger, H. et al. Transient acantholytic dermatosis Grover. *Z. Haut.*, 52:841, 1977.

Sanchez, N. and Ackerman, A. Subcorneal pustular dermatosis: A variant of pustular psoriasis. *Acta Derm. Venereol.* (Stockh.), 59 (85, suppl.):147, 1979.

Sanchez, N., Perry, H. and Muller, S. On the relationship between subcorneal pustular dermatosis and pustular psoriasis. *Am. J. Dermatopathol.*, 3:385, 1981.

Simon, R. et al. Persistent acantholytic dermatosis: A variant of transient acantholytic dermatosis (Grover's disease). *Arch. Dermatol.*, 112:1429, 1976.

Waisman, M. et al. Bullous transient acantholytic dermatosis. *Arch. Dermatol.*, 112:1440, 1976.

Wolff, H., Chalet, M. and Ackerman, A. Transitorische akantholytische Dermatose (Grover). *Hautarzt*, 28:78, 1977.

Wolff, K. Transient acantholytic dermatosis (Grover). *Derm. Monatsschr.*, 158:533, 1972.

Bullous Dermatoses: Subepidermal

Dermatitis Herpetiformis; Chronic Dermatosis of Childhood

Ackerman, A. and Tolman, M. Papular dermatitis herpetiformis in childhood. *Arch. Dermatol.*, 100:286, 1969.

Bean, S. et al. Chronic non-hereditary blistering disease in children. *Am. J. Dis. Child.*, 122:137, 1971.

Brow, J. et al. The small intestinal mucosa in dermatitis herpetiformis. I. Severity and distribution of the small intestinal lesion and associated malabsorption. *Gastroenterology*, 60:355, 1971.

Chorzelski, T. and Jablonska, S. IgA linear dermatosis of childhood (chronic bullous disease of childhood). *Br. J. Dermatol.*, 101:535, 1979.

——. IgA-lineäre Dermatose. *Hautarzt*, 32:546, 1981.

Chorzelski, T. et al. Linear IgA bullous dermatosis: In: *Immunopathology of the Skin*. Beutner, E. et al., eds., New York, John Wiley & Sons, 1979, p. 316.

Connor, B., Marks, R. and Wilson Jones, E. Dermatitis herpetiformis. *Trans. St. John's Hosp. Dermatol. Soc.*, 58:191, 1972.

Dabrowski, J. et al. Immunoelectron microscopic studies in IgA linear dermatosis. *Arch. Dermatol. Res.*, 265:289, 1979.

Eng, A. and Moncada, B. Bullous pemphigoid and dermatitis herpetiformis. *Arch. Dermatol.*, 110:51, 1974.

Esterly, N. et al. Chronic bullous dermatosis of childhood. *Arch. Dermatol.*, 113:42, 1977.

Evans, C. and Fraser, I. The natural history of dermatitis herpetiformis. *Trans. St. John's Hosp. Dermatol. Soc.*, 49:108, 1963.

Fraser, N. et al. Serum complement (C3) and immunoglobulin levels in dermatitis herpetiformis. *Br. J. Dermatol.*, 85:314, 1971.

Fry, L. and Johnson, F. Electron microscopic study of dermatitis herpetiformis. *Br. J. Dermatol.*, 81:44, 1969.

Fry, L. and Seah, P. Dermatitis herpetiformis : An evaluation of diagnostic criteria. *Br. J. Dermatol.*, 90:137, 1974.

Jablonska, S. and Chorzelski, T. Dermatose à IgA linéaire. *Ann. Dermatol. Venereol.*, 106:651, 1979.

——. When and how to use sulfones in bullous diseases. *Internat. J. Dermatol.*, 20:103, 1981.

Jablonska, S. et al. Dermatitis herpetiformis and bullous pemphigoid: Intermediate and mixed forms. *Arch. Dermatol.*, 112:45, 1976.

Jordon, R. et al. Childhood bullous dermatitis herpetiformis. *Arch. Dermatol.*, 101:629, 1970.

Katz, S. and Strober, W. The pathogenesis of dermatitis herpetiformis. (Review) *J. Invest. Dermatol.*, 70:63, 1978.

Katz, S. et al. Dermatitis herpetiformis: The skin and the gut. *Ann. Int. Med.*, 93:857, 1980.

Katz, S. et al. HL-A8: A genetic link between dermatitis herpetiformis and gluten-sensitive enteropathy. *J. Clin. Invest.*, 51:2977, 1972.

Kint, A., Geerts, M. and De Brauwere, D. Diagnostic criteria in dermatitis herpetiformis. *Dermatologica*, 153:266, 1976.

Lancaster-Smith, M. et al. Antireticulin antibodies in dermatitis herpetiformis and adult coeliac disease: Their relationship to a gluten free diet and jejunal histology. *Br. J. Dermatol.*, 92:37, 1975.

Lawley, T. et al. Small intestinal biopsies and HLA types in dermatitis herpetiformis patients with granular and linear IgA skin deposits. *J. Invest. Dermatol.*, 74:9, 1980.

Leonard, J. et al. Linear IgA disease in adults *Br. J. Dermatol.*, 107:301, 1982.

Ljunghall, K. et al. Circulating reticulin autoantibodies of IgA class in dermatitis herpetiformis. *Br. J. Dermatol.*, 100:173, 1979.

Lyell, A. Dermatitis herpetiformis enteropathy. *Br. J. Dermatol.*, 81:228, 1969.

Marks, J. Dogma and dermatitis herpetiformis. *Clin. Exp. Dermatol.*, 2:189, 1977.

Marsden, R. et al. A study of benign chronic bullous dermatosis of childhood. *Clin. Exp. Dermatol.*, 5:159, 1980.

Pehamberger, H., Konrad, K. and Holubar, K. Circulating IgA antibasement membrane antibodies in linear dermatitis herpetiformis (Duhring): Immunofluorescence and immunoelectron-microscopic studies. *J. Invest. Dermatol.*, 69:490, 1977.

——. Juvenile dermatitis herpetiformis: An immunoelectron-microscopic study. *Br. J. Dermatol.*, 101:271, 1979.

Reunala, T. et al. Herpes gestationis. *Br. J. Dermatol.*, 96:563, 1977.

Schaumburg-Lever, G. et al. Herpes gestationis: Histology and ultrastructure. *J. Invest. Dermatol.*, 107:888, 1973.

Seah, P. and Fry, L. Immunoglobulins in the skin in dermatitis herpetiformis and their relevance in diagnosis. *Br. J. Dermatol.*, 92:157, 1975.

Seah, P. et al. Immunoglobulins in the skin in dermatitis herpetiformis and coeliac disease. *Lancet*, 1:611, 1972.

Seah, P. et al. Tissue antibodies in dermatitis herpetiformis and adult coeliac disease. *Lancet*, 1:834, 1971.

Shuster, S., Watson, A. and Marks, J. Coeliac syndrome in dermatitis herpetiformis. *Lancet*, 1:1101, 1968.

Smith, S. et al. Linear IgA bullous dermatosis V dermatitis herpetiformis: Quantitative measurements of dermoepidermal alterations. *Arch. Dermatol.*, 120:324, 1984.

Thune, P. et al. Immunological and gastrointestinal abnormalities in dermatitis herpetiformis. *Internat. J. Dermatol.*, 18:136, 1979.

Tolman, M., Moschella, S. and Schneidermann, R. Dermatitis herpetiformis: Specific entity or clinical complex? *J. Invest. Dermatol.*, 32:557, 1959.

Van Der Meer, J. et al. IgA antibasement membrane antibodies in a boy with pemphigoid. *Arch. Dermatol.*, 113:1462, 1977.

Yaoita, H. Identification of IgA binding structures in skin of patients with dermatitis herpetiformis. *J. Invest. Dermatol.*, 71:213, 1978.

Yaoita, H., Gullino, M. and Katz, S. Herpes gestationis: Ultrastructure and ultrastructural localization on *in-vivo*-bound complement. *J. Invest. Dermatol.*, 66:383, 1976.

Yaoita, H. and Katz, S. Circulating IgA anti-basement membrane zone antibodies in dermatitis herpetiformis, *J. Invest. Dermatol.*, 69:558, 1977.

——. Immunoelectron-microscopic localization of IgA in skin of patients with dermatitis herpetiformis. *J. Invest. Dermatol.*, 67:502, 1976.

Zone, J. et al. Circulating immune complexes of IgA type in dermatitis herpetiformis. *J. Invest. Dermatol.*, 75:152, 1980.

Bullous Pemphigoid

Ahmed, A., Chu, T. and Provost, T. Bullous pemphigoid: Clinical and serologic evaluation for associated malignant neoplasms. *Arch. Dermatol.*, 113:969, 1977.

Ahmed, A., Maize, J. and Provost, T. Bullous pemphigoid: Clinical and immunologic follow-up after successful therapy. *Arch. Dermatol.*, 113:1043, 1977.

Bean, S. et al. Vesicular pemphigoid. *Arch. Dermatol.*, 112:1402, 1976.

Charles, A. Electronmicroscopic observation on pemphigoid. *Br. J. Dermatol.*, 72:439, 1960.

Chorzelski, T. and Cormane, R. The presence of complement "bound" *in vivo* in the skin of patients with pemphigoid. *Dermatologica*, 137:134, 1968.

Chorzelski, T. et al. Coexistence of pemphigus and bullous pemphigoid. *Arch. Dermatol.*, 109:849, 1974.

Chorzelski, T. et al. Immunofluorescence studies in the diagnosis of dermatitis herpetiformis and its differentiation from bullous pemphigoid. *J. Invest. Dermatol.*, 56:373, 1971.

Cormane, R. and Szabo, E. Immuno-histopathology of the skin in pemphigoid. *Br. J. Dermatol.*, 83:435, 1970.

Dubertret, L. et al. Cellular events leading to blister formation in bullous pemphigoid. *Br. J. Dermatol.*, 103:615, 1980.

Dvorak, A. et al. Bullous pemphigoid: An ultrastructural study of the inflammatory response. *J. Invest. Dermatol.*, 78:91, 1982.

Eng, A. and Moncada, B. Bullous pemphigoid and dermatitis herpetiformis. *Arch. Dermatol.*, 110:51, 1974.

Hodge, L. et al. Bullous pemphigoid: The frequency of mucosal involvement and concurrent malignancy related to indirect immunofluorescence findings. *Br. J. Dermatol.*, 105:65, 1981.

Honeyman, J. et al. The enigma of bullous pemphigoid and dermatitis herpetiformis. *Arch. Dermatol.*, 106:22, 1972.

Jablonska, S. et al. Dermatitis herpetiformis and bullous pemphigoid: Intermediate and mixed forms. *Arch. Dermatol.*, 112:45, 1976.

Jablonska, S. et al. Juvenile dermatitis herpetiformis in the light of immunofluorescence studies. *Br. J. Dermatol.*, 85:307, 1971.

Jordan, R., Triftshauser, C. and Schroeter, A. Direct immunofluorescent studies of pemphigus and bullous pemphigoid. *Arch. Dermatol.*, 103:486, 1971.
Kumar, V. et al. Coexistence of bullous pemphigoid and systemic lupus erythematosus. *Arch. Dermatol.*, 114:1187, 1978.
Kuokkanen, K. and Helin, H. Pemphigoid vegetans. *Arch. Dermatol.*, 117:56, 1981.
Lever, W. *Pemphigus and Pemphigoid*. Springfield, IL, Thomas, 1965.
——. Pemphigus and pemphigoid: A review of the advances made since 1964. *J. Am. Acad. Dermatol.*, 1:2, 1979.
Naito, K., Morioka, S. and Ogawa, H. The pathogenic mechanisms of bullous pemphigoid in blister formation. (abstr.) *J. Invest. Dermatol.*, 76:420, 1981.
Person, J. and Rogers, R., III. Bullous pemphigoid responding to sulfapyridine and the sulfones. *Arch. Dermatol.*, 113:610, 1977.
——. Bullous and cicatricial pemphigoid: Clinical, histopathogenic, and immunopathologic correlations. *Mayo Clin. Proc.*, 52:54, 1977.
Person, J. Rogers, R., III and Perry, H. Localized pemphigoid. *Br. J. Dermatol.*, 95:531, 1976.
Prakken, J. and Woerdeman, M. "Pemphigoid" (para-pemphigus): Its relationship to other bullous dermatoses. *Br. J. Dermatol.*, 67:92, 1955.
Provost, T. et al. Unusual subepidermal bullous diseases with immunologic features of bullous pemphigoid. *Arch. Dermatol.*, 115;156, 1979.
Sams, W., Jr. and Jordon, R. Correlation of pemphigoid and pemphigus antibody titres with activity of disease. *Br. J. Dermatol.*, 84:7, 1971.
Schaumburg-Lever, G., Orfanos, G. and Lever, W. Electron microscopic study of bullous pemphigoid. *Arch. Dermatol.*, 113:622, 1972.
Schmidt, B. et al. Ultrastructural localization of *in vivo*-bound complement in bullous pemphigoid. *J. Invest. Dermatol.*, 65:217, 1975.
Simon, C. and Winkelmann, R. Bullous pemphigoid and glomerulonephritis. *J. Am. Acad. Dermatol.*, 14:456, 1986.
Sneddon, I. and Church, R. Diagnosis and treatment of pemphigoid: Report on 22 cases. *Br. Med. J.*, 2:1360, 1955.
van Joost, T. et al. Subepidermal bullous autoimmune disease associated with immune nephritis. *J. Am. Acad. Dermatol.*, 14:214, 1986.
Weber, L. et al. Immunofluorescent localization of type IV collagen and laminin in human skin and its application in junctional zone pathology. *Br. J. Dermatol.*, 106:267, 1982.
Winkelmann, R. and Su, W. Pemphigoid vegetans. *Arch. Dermatol.*, 115:446, 1979.

Benign Mucous Membrane Pemphigoid (Cicatricial Pemphigoid)

Bean, S. Cicatricial pemphigoid. *Arch. Dermatol.*, 110:552, 1974.
Bean, S. et al. Cicatricial pemphigoid: Immunofluorescent studies. *Arch. Dermatol.*, 106:195, 1972.
Behlen, C., II, and Mackey, D. Benign mucous membrane pemphigus with a generalized eruption. *Arch. Dermatol.*, 92:566, 1965.
Brauner, G. and Jimbow, K. Benign mucous membrane pemphigoid: An unusual case with electron microscopic findings. *Arch. Dermatol.*, 106:535, 1972.
Braun-Falco, O., Wolff, H. and Ponce, E. Disseminiertes vernarbendes Pemphigoid. *Hautarzt*, 32:233, 1981.
Brunsting, L. and Perry, H. Benign pemphigoid? A report of seven cases with chronic, scarring, herpetiform plaques about the head and neck. *Arch. Dermatol.*, 75:489, 1957.
Caputo, R., Bellone, A. and Crosti, C. Pathogenesis of the blister in cicatricial pemphigoid and in bullous pemphigoid. *Arch. Dermatol. Forsch.*, 247:181, 1973.
Carroll, J. and Kuwabara, T. Ocular pemphigus: An electron microscopic study of the conjunctival and corneal epithelium. *Arch. Ophthalmol.*, 80:683, 1968.
Carruthers, J., Black, M. and Ramnarain, N. Immunopathological studies in herpes gestationis. *Br. J. Dermatol.*, 96:35, 1977.
Chorzelski, T. et al. Herpes gestationis with identical lesions in the newborn. *Arch. Dermatol.*, 112:1129, 1976.
Church, R. and Sneddon, I. Ocular pemphigus with generalized bullous eruption. *Br. J. Dermatol.*, 68:128, 1956.
Cram, D., Griffith, M. and Fukuyama, K. Pemphigus-like antibodies in cicatricial pemphigoid. *Arch. Dermatol.*, 109:235, 1974.
Dabelsteen, E. et al. Demonstration of basement membrane autoantibodies in patients with benign mucous membrane pemphigoid. *Acta Derm. Venereol.*, 54:189, 1974.

Griffith, M. et al. Immunofluorescent studies in mucous membrane pemphigoid. *Arch. Dermatol.*, 109:195, 1974.

Hanno, R., Foster, D. and Bean, S. Brunsting-Perry cicatricial pemphigoid associated with bullous pemphigoid. *J. Am. Acad. Dermatol.*, 3:470, 1980.

Hertz, K. et al. Herpes gestationis: A clinicopathological study. *Arch. Dermatol.*, 112:1543, 1976.

Holubar, K., Honigsmann, H. and Wolff, K. Cicatricial pemphigoid. *Arch. Dermatol.*, 108:50, 1973.

Honigsmann, H. et al. Herpes gestationis: Fine structural pattern of immunoglobulin deposits in the skin *in vivo*. *J. Invest. Dermatol.*, 66:389, 1976.

Jacoby, W., Jr. et al. Cicatricial pemphigoid (Brunsting-Perry type). Case report and immunofluorescence findings. *Arch. Dermatol.*, 114:779, 1978.

Katz, A. et al. Immunopathologic study of herpes gestationis in mother and infant. *Arch. Dermatol.*, 113:1069, 1977.

Kocsis, M. et al. Immunofluorescence studies in herpes gestationis. *Acta Derm. Venereol.* (Stockh.), 55:25, 1975.

Kristensen, E. and Norn, M. Benign mucous membrane pemphigoid. I. Secretion of mucus and tears. *Acta Ophthalmol.*, 52:266, 1974.

Lever, W. Pemphigus. *Medicine*, 32:1, 1953.

——. Pemphigus conjunctivae with scarring of the skin: Report of three additional cases. *Arch. Dermatol. Syph.*, 49:113, 1944.

——. Pemphigus conjunctivae with scarring of the skin: Report of three cases. *Arch. Dermatol. Syph.*,46:875, 1942.

McCarthy, P. and Shklar, G. Benign mucous-membrane pemphigus. *N. Eng. J. Med.*, 258:726, 1958.

Michel, B. et al. Cicatricial pemphigoid of Brunsting-Perry: Immunofluorescent studies. *Arch. Dermatol.*, 113:1403, 1977.

Nieboer, C. et al. Immunoelectron-microscopic findings in cicatricial pemphigoid: Their significance in relation to epidermolysis bullosa acquisita. *Br. J. Dermatol.*, 106:419, 1982.

Provost, T. et al. Unusual subepidermal bullous diseases with immunologic features of bullous pemphigoid. *Arch. Dermatol.*, 115:156, 1979.

Razzaque, A. et al. Localized cicatricial pemphigoid (Brunsting-Perry). A transplantation experiment. *Arch. Dermatol.*, 102:932, 1984.

Rogers, R., III. et al. Immunopathology of cicatricial pemphigoid: Studies of complement deposition. *J. Invest. Dermatol.*, 68:39, 1977.

Schaumburg-Lever, G., Orfanos, C. and Lever, W. Electron microscopic study of bullous pemphigoid. *Arch. Dermatol.*, 106:662, 1972.

Slepyan, A., Burks, J. and Fox, J. Persistent denudation of the scalp in cicatricial pemphigoid: Treatment by skin grafting. *Arch. Dermatol.*, 84:444, 1961.

Sneddon, I. Cicatricial pemphigoid and skin grafts. *Arch. Dermatol.*, 86:226, 1962.

Soudakoff, P. and Whalman, H. Ocular pemphigus: Report of a case with the histologic findings in the cornea. *Am. J. Ophthalmol.*, 36:231, 1953.

Susi, F. and Shklar, G. Histochemistry and fine structure of oral lesions of mucous membrane pemphigoid. *Arch. Dermatol.*, 104:244, 1971.

Tagami, H. and Imamura, S. Benign mucous membrane pemphigoid: Demonstration of circulating and tissue-bound membrane antibodies. *Arch. Dermatol.*, 109:711, 1974.

Herpes Gestationis

Bushkell, L., Jordon, R. and Goltz, R. Herpes gestationis: New immunologic findings. *Arch. Dermatol.*, 110:65, 1974.

Carruthers, J. Herpes gestationis: A reappraisal. *Clin. Exp. Dermatol.*, 3:199, 1978.

Carruthers, J. and Black, M. Immunopathological findings in herpes gestationis. *Br. J. Dermatol.*, 93:17, 1975.

Carruthers, J. et al. Immunopathological studies in herpes gestationis. *Br. J. Dermatol.*, 96:35, 1977.

Harrington, C. and Bleehen, S. Herpes gestationis: Immunopathological and ultrastructural studies. *Br. J. Dermatol.*, 100:389, 1979.

Hentschel, U. Herpes gestationis (Milton), *Dermatol. Monatsschr.*, 159:904, 1973.

Hertz, K. et al. Herpes gestationis: A clinicopathologic study. *Arch. Dermatol.*, 112:1543, 1976.

Holmes, R. Herpes gestationis and bullous pemphigoid: A disease spectrum. *Br. J. Dermatol.*, 103:535, 1980.

Hönigsmann, H. et al. Herpes gestationis: Fine structural pattern of immunoglobulin deposits in the skin *in vivo*. *J. Invest. Dermatol.*, 66:389, 1976.
Jablonska, S. et al. Immunologic phenomena in herpes gestationis. *Arch. Dermatol. Forsch.*, 252:267, 1975.
Jordon, R. et al. The immunopathology of herpes gestationis: Immunofluorescent studies and characterization of "HG factor." *J. Clin. Invest.*, 57:1426, 1976.
Katz, S. et al. Herpes gestationis: Immunopathology and characterization of the HG factor. *J. Clin. Invest.*, 57:1434, 1976.
Lawley, T. et al. Fetal and maternal risk factors in herpes gestationis. *Arch. Dermatol.*, 114:552, 1978.
Piérard, J., Thiery, M. and Kint, A. Histologie et ultrastructure de l'herpes gestationis. *Arch. Belg. Dermatol. Syph.*, 25:321, 1969.
Schaumburg-Lever, G. et al. Herpes gestationis: Histology and ultrastructure. *Arch. Dermatol.*, 107:888, 1973.
Shornick, J. et al. Herpes gestationis: Clinical and histologic features of twenty-eight cases. *J. Am. Acad. Dermatol.*, 8:214, 1983.
Winton, G. and Lewis, C. Dermatoses of pregnancy. *J. Am. Acad. Dermatol.*, 6:977, 1982.

Erythema Multiforme, Stevens-Johnson Syndrome, Toxic Epidermal Necrolysis

Aberer, W. et al. Stevens-Johnson Syndrom und toxische epidermale Nekrolyse nach Sulfonamideinnahme. *Hautarzt*, 33:484, 1982.
Ackerman, A., Penneys, N. and Clark, W., Jr. Erythema multiforme exudativum: Distinctive pathological process. *Br. J. Dermatol.*, 84:554, 1971.
Ashby, D. and Lazar, T. Erythema multiforme exudativum major (Stevens-Johnson syndrome). *Lancet*, 1:1091, 1951.
Bedi, T. and Pinkus, H. Histopathological spectrum of Erythema multiforme. *Br. J. Dermatol.*, 95:243, 1976.
Bianchi, J. Drugs as etiologic factors in Stevens-Johnson syndrome. *Am. J. Med.*, 44:390, 1968.
Bluefarb, S. and Szanto, P. Erythema multiforme associated with acute renal tubular necrosis. *Arch. Dermatol.*, 92:367, 1965.
Bushkell, L., Mackel, S. and Jordon, R. Erythema multiforme: Direct immunofluorescence studies and detection of circulating immune complexes. *J. Invest. Dermatol.*, 74:372, 1980.
Cannell, H., Churcher, G. and Milton-Thompson, G. Stevens-Johnson syndrome associated with Mycoplasma pneumoniae infection. *Br. J. Dermatol.*, 81:196, 1969.
Carroll, O., Bryan, P. and Robinson, R. Stevens-Johnson syndrome associated with long acting sulfonamides. *JAMA*, 195:691, 1966.
Caulfield, J. and Wilgram, G. An electron microscopic study of blister formation in erythema multiforme. *J. Invest. Dermatol.*, 39:307, 1962.
Comaish, J. and Kerr, D. Erythema multiforme and nephritis. *Br. Med. J.*, 2:84, 1961.
Costello, M. Erythema multiforme exudativum (erythema bullosum malignans-pluriorificial type): Personal observations of cases in Willard Parker Hospital for Contagious Diseases (1932–1946). *J. Invest. Dermatol.*, 8:127, 1947.
Coursin, D. Stevens-Johnson syndrome: Nonspecific parasensitivity reaction? *JAMA*, 198:113, 1966.
Finland, M., Jolliffe, L. and Parker, F., Jr. Pneumonia and erythema multiforme exudativum: Report of four cases and three autopsies. *Am. J. Med.*, 4:473, 1948.
Foy, H., Kenny, G. and Koler, J. Mycoplasma pneumoniae in Stevens-Johnson syndrome. *Lancet*, 2:550, 1966.
Henz, M. and Feinberg, M. Localized erythema multiforme due to lymphatic obstruction. *Br. J. Dermatol.*, 106:95, 1982.
Howland, W. et al. Erythema multiforme: Clinical, histopathologic, and immunologic study. *J. Am. Acad. Dermatol.*, 10:438, 1984.
Huff, J. and Weston, W. Clinical and laboratory features of recurrent erythema multiforme. (abstr.) *J. Invest. Dermatol.*, 76:331, 1981.
Huff, J. et al. Mixed cryoglobulinemia, ^{125}I C1q binding and skin immunofluorescence in erythema multiforme. *J. Invest. Dermatol.*, 74:375, 1980.
Hunter, J. and Davison, A. Toxic epidermal necrolysis associated with pentazocine therapy and severe reversible renal failure. *Br. J. Dermatol.*, 88:287, 1980.

Imamura, S. et al. Erythema multiforme: Demonstration of immune complexes in the sera and skin lesions. *Br. J. Dermatol.*, 102:161, 1980.
Kazmierowski, J. and Wuepper, K. Erythema multiforme: Immune complex vasculitis of the superficial cutaneous microvasculature. *J. Invest. Dermatol.*, 71:366, 1978.
Kazmierowski, J. et al. Herpes simplex antigen in immune complexes of patients with erythema multiforme. *JAMA*, 247:2547, 1982.
Kopf, A., Grupper, C. and Baer, R. Eruptive nevocytic nevi after severe bullous disease. *Arch. Dermatol.*, 113:1080, 1977.
Lyell, A. Toxic epidermal necrolysis (the scalded skin syndrome): A reappraisal. *Br. J. Dermatol.*, 100:69, 1979.
Lyell, A. et al. Mycoplasmas and erythema multiforme. *Lancet*, 2:1116, 1967.
Macdonald, A. and Feiwel, M. Isolation of herpes virus from erythema multiforme. *Br. Med. J.*, 2:570, 1972.
MacVicar, D., Graham, J. and Burgoon, C., Jr. Dermatitis herpetiformis, erythema multiforme and bullous pemphigoid: A comparative histopathological and histochemical study. *J. Invest. Dermatol.*, 41:289, 1963.
Orfanos, C., Schaumburg-Lever, G. and Lever, W. Dermal and epidermal types of erythema multiforme. *Arch. Dermatol.*, 109:682, 1974.
Osler, W. On the visceral manifestations of the erythema group of skin diseases. *Am. J. Med. Sci.*, 127:1, 1904.
——. The visceral lesions of the erythema group. *Br. J. Dermatol.*, 12:227, 1900.
Piérard, J. and Whimster, I. The histopathological diagnosis of dermatitis herpetiformis, bullous pemphigoid and erythema multiforme. *Br. J. Dermatol.*, 73:253, 1961.
Prutkin, L. and Fellner, M. Erythema multiforme bullosum. *Acta Derm. Venereol.*, 51:429, 1971.
Safai, B. et al. Erythema multiforme: Report of two cases and speculation on immune mechanisms involved in the pathogenesis. *Clin. Immunol. Immunopathol.*, 7:379, 1977.
Shklar, G. Oral lesions of erythema multiforme: Histologic and histochemical observations. *Arch. Dermatol.*, 92:495, 1965.
Sieber, O., Jr. et al. Stevens-Johnson syndrome associated with Mycoplasma pneumoniae infection. *JAMA*, 200:79, 1967.
Sontheimer, R., Garibaldi, R. and Krueger, G. Stevens-Johnson syndrome associated with *Mycoplasma pneumoniae* infections. *Arch. Dermatol.*, 114:241, 1978.
Stevens, A. and Johnson, F. A new eruptive fever associated with stomatitis and ophthalmia: Report of two cases in children. *Am. J. Dis. Child.*, 24:526, 1922.
Tonneson, M. and Soter, N. Erythema multiforme. *J. Am. Acad. Dermatol.*, 1:357, 1979.
Williamson, D. Erythema multiforme in infectious mononucleosis. *Br. J. Dermatol.*, 91:345, 1974.
Yaffee, H. Erythema multiforme caused by Coxsackie B 5: A possible association with epidemic pustular stomatitis of children. *Arch. Dermatol.*, 82:737, 1960.

Necrolytic Migratory Erythema (Glucagonoma Syndrome)

Barber, S. and Hamer, J. Skin rash in patient receiving glucagon. *Lancet*, 2:1138, 1976.
Becker, S., Kahn, D. and Rothman, S. Cutaneous manifestations of internal malignant tumors. *Arch. Dermatol. Syph.*, 45:1069, 1942.
Binnick, A. et al. Glucagonoma syndrome. *Arch. Dermatol.*, 113:749, 1977.
Doll, D. Necrolytic migratory erythema. *Arch. Dermatol.*, 116:861, 1980.
Domen, R. et al. The glucagonoma syndrome. *Arch. Int. Med.*, 140:262, 1980.
Doyle, J., Schroeter, A. and Rogers, R., III. Hyperglucagonemia and necrolytic migratory erythema in cirrhosis, possible pseudoglucagonoma syndrome. *Br. J. Dermatol.*, 101:581, 1979.
Goodenberger, D. et al. Necrolytic migratory erythema without glucagonoma. *Arch. Dermatol.*, 115:1429, 1979.
Kahan, R., Perez-Figaredo, R. and Neimanis, A. Necrolytic migratory erythema. *Arch. Dermatol.*, 113:792, 1977.
Leichter, S. Clinical and metabolic aspects of glucagonoma. *Medicine* (Baltimore), 59:100, 1980.
Lewis, A. The glucagonoma syndrome. *Internat. J. Dermatol.*, 18:17, 1979.
Mallinson, C. et al. A glucagonoma syndrome. *Lancet*, 2:1, 1974.
Norton, J. et al. Amino acid deficiency and the skin rash associated with glucagonoma. *Ann. Int. Med.*, 91:213, 1979.

Ohyama, K. et al. Ultrastructural studies of necrolytic migratory erythema. *Arch. Dermatol.*, 118:679, 1982.
Pedersen, N., Jonsson, L. and Holst, J. Necrolytic migratory erythema and glucagon cell tumor of the pancreas: The glucagonoma syndrome. *Acta Derm. Venereol.* (Stockh.), 56:391, 1976.
Sweet, R. A dermatosis specifically associated with a tumor of pancreatic alpha cells. *Br. J. Dermatol.*, 90:301, 1974.
Wilkinson, D. Necrolytic migratory erythema with carcinoma of the pancreas. *Trans. St. John's Hosp. Dermatol. Soc.*, 59:244, 1973.

Porphyria

Baer, R. et al. Erythropoietic protoporphyria. *Dermatologica*, 135:5, 1967.
Benedetto, A., Kushner, J. and Taylor, J. Porphyria cutanea tarda in three generations of a single family. *N. Eng. J. Med.*, 298:358, 1978.
Charles, R., Beidler, J. and Johnson, B. Erythropoietic protoporphyria . *Arch. Pathol.*, 97:79, 1974.
Corey, T. et al. Variegate porphyria: Clinical and laboratory features. *J. Am. Acad. Dermatol.*, 2:36, 1980.
Cripps, D. and Goldfarb, S. Erythropoietic protoporphyria: Hepatic cirrhosis. *Br. J. Dermatol.*, 98:349, 1978.
Cruces Prado, M. et al. Two cases of infantile and familial porphyria cutanea tarda. *Dermatologica*, 161:205, 1980.
Czarnecki, D. Hepatoerythropoietic porphyria. *Arch. Dermatol.*, 116:307, 1980.
Dean, G. *The Porphyrias: A Story of Inheritance and Environment*. London, Pitman Medical Pub., 1973.
del C Batelle, A. Prophyrins and porphyrias: Etiopathogenesis, clinics and treatment. *Int. J. Biochem.*, 12:671, 1980.
De Leo, V. et al. Erythropoietic protoporphyria: Ten years' experience. *Am. J. Med.*, 60:8, 1976.
de Verneuil, H. et al. Familial and sporadic porphyria cutanea: Two different diseases. *Hum. Genet.*, 44:145, 1978.
Donaldson, E., McCall, A. and Magnus, I. Erythropoietic protoporphyria: Two deaths from hepatic cirrhosis. *Br. J. Dermatol.*, 84:14, 1971.
Elder, G. Enzymatic defects in porphyria: An overview. *Semin. Liver Dis.*, 2:87, 1982.
Elder, G. et al. Identification of two types of porphyria cutanea tarda by measurement of erythrocyte uroporphyrinogen decarboxylase. *Clin. Sci.*, 58:477, 1980.
Epstein, J., Tuffanelli, D. and Epstein, W. Cutaneous changes in the porphyrias. *Arch. Dermatol.*, 107:689, 1973.
Epstein, J. et al. Porphyria-like cutaneous changes induced by tetracycline hydrochloride photosensitization. *Arch. Dermatol.*, 112:661, 1976.
Feldaker, M., Montgomery, H. and Brunsting, L. Histopathology of porphyria cutanea tarda. *J. Invest. Dermatol.*, 24:131, 1955.
Fromke, V. et al. Porphyria variegata: Study of a large kindred in the United States. *Am. J. Med.*, 65:80, 1978.
Goldstein, B. and Harber, L. Erythropoietic protoporphyria: Lipid peroxidation and red cell membrane damage associated with photohemolysis. *J. Clin. Invest.*, 51:892, 1972.
Goodwin, T. *Porphyrins and Related Compounds*. New York, Academic Press, 1968.
Grossman, M. et al. Porphyria cutanea tarda: Clinical features and laboratory findings in 40 patients. *Am. J. Med.*, 67:277, 1979.
Hanno, R. and Callen, J. Porphyria cutanea tarda as a cause of bullous dermatosis of hemodialysis: A case report and review of the literature. *Cutis*, 28:261, 1981.
Harber, L. and Bickers, D. Porphyria and pseudoporphyria. *J. Invest. Dermatol.*, 82:207, 1984.
——. The porphyrias: Basic science aspects, clinical diagnosis and management. In: *Yearbook of Dermatology—1975*. Malkinson, F. and Pearson, R., eds., Chicago, Yearbook Medical Pub., 1975, p. 9.
Hunter, G. Clinical manifestations of the porphyrias: A review. *Aust. J. Dermatol.*, 20:120, 1979.
Judd, L., Henderson, D. and Hill, D. Naproxen-induced pseudoporphyria: A clinical and ultrastructural study. *Arch. Dermatol.*, 122:451, 1986.
Kappas, A. et al. The porphyrias. In: *The Metabolic Basis of Inherited Disease*, 5th Ed., Stanbury, J. et al., eds., New York, McGraw-Hill, 1983, p. 1301.

Keczkes, K. and Barker, D. Malignant hepatoma associated with acquired cutaneous porphyria. *Arch. Dermatol.*, 112:78, 1976.

Kint, A. A comparative electron microscopic study of the perivascular hyaline from porphyria cutanea tarda and from lipoid proteinosis. *Arch. Klin. Exp. Dermatol.*, 239:203, 1970.

Kushner, J., Barbuto, A. and Lee, G. An inherited enzymatic defect in porphyria cutanea tarda. *J. Clin. Invest.*, 58:1089, 1976.

Kushner, J., Lee, G. and Nacht, S. Role of iron in pathogenesis of porphyria cutanea tarda. *J. Clin. Invest.*, 51:3044, 1972.

Lichtenstein, J., Babb, E. and Felsher, B. Porphyria cutanea tarda (PCT) in a patient with chronic renal failure on hemadialysis. *Br. J. Dermatol.*, 104:575, 1981.

McColl, K. et al. Abnormal haem biosynthesis in chronic alcoholics. *Eur. J. Clin. Invest.*, 11:461, 1981.

McColl, K. et al. Acute ethanol ingestion and haem biosynthesis in healthy subjects. *Eur. J. Clin. Invest.*, 10:107, 1980.

Magnus, I. The cutaneous porphyrias. *Semin. Hematol.*, 5:380, 1968.

——. *Dermatological Photobiology*. London, Blackwell, 1976.

——. Photobiological aspects of porphyria. *Proc. R. Soc. Med.*, 61:196, 1968.

Mann, R. and Harman, R. Porphyria cutanea tarda and sarcoidosis. *Clin. Exp. Dermatol.*, 7:619, 1982.

Marver, H. and Schmid, R. The porphyrias. In: *The Metabolic Basis of Inherited Disease*. 3rd Ed., Stanbury, J., Wyngarrden, J. and Fredrickson, D., eds., New York, McGraw-Hill, 1972, p. 1087.

Mathews-Roth, M. Erythropoietic protoporphyria: Diagnosis and treatment. *N. Eng. J. Med.*, 297:98, 1977.

Mustajoki, P. Variegate porphyria. *Ann. Int. Med.*, 89:238, 1978.

——. Variegate porphyria: Twelve years experience in Finland. *Q. J. Med.*, 49:191, 1980.

Ozasa, S. et al. Erythropoietic protoporphyria. *J. Dermatol.* (Tokyo), 4:85, 1977.

Pathak, M. and West, J. Porphyrias: Office procedures and laboratory tests for diagnosis of prophyrin abnormalities. *Acta Derm. Venereol.* (Stockh.), (100, suppl.):91, 1982.

Perrot, H. et al. Porphyria cutanea tarda-like dermatosis by hemodialysis. *Arch. Dermatol. Res.*, 259, 177, 1977.

Pimstone, N. Porphyria cutanea tarda. *Semin. Liver Dis.*, 2:125, 1982.

Poh-Fitzpatrick, M. Laboratory testing in the porphyrias. *Internat. J. Dermatol.*, 18:453, 1979.

Poh-Fitzpatrick, M., Masullo, A. and Grossman, M. Porphyria cutanea tarda associated with chronic renal failure and hemodialysis. *Arch. Dermatol.*, 116:191, 1980.

Poh-Fitzpatrick, M. et al. Porphyria cutanea tarda in two patients treated with hemodialysis for chronic renal failure. *N. Eng. J. Med.*, 299:292, 1978.

Reed, W. et al. Erythropoietic protoporphyria. *JAMA*, 214:1060, 1970.

Rimington, C. et al. Porphyria and photosensitivity. *Quart. J. Med.*, 36:29, 1967.

Roenigk, H. and Gottlieb, N. Estrogen-induced porphyria cutanea tarda. *Arch. Dermatol.*, 102:260, 1970.

Ryan, E. and Madill, G. Electron microscopy of the skin in erythropoietic protoporphyria. *Br. J. Dermatol.*, 80:561, 1968.

Saltzer, E., Redeker, A. and Wilson, J. Porphyria cutanea tarda. *Arch. Dermatol.*, 98:496, 1968.

Suurmond, D., van Steveninck, J. and Went, L. Some clinical and fundamental aspects of erythropoietic protoporphyria. *Br. J. Dermatol.*, 82:232, 1970.

Tschudy, D. Porphyrin metabolism and the porphyrias. In: *Duncan's Diseases of Metabolism: Genetic and Biochemical Basis of Disease*. 7th Ed., Bondy, P. and Rosenberg, L. eds., Philadelphia, W. B. Saunders, 1974.

Tschudy, D. and Lamon, J. Porphyrin metabolism and the porphyrias. In: *Duncan's Diseases of Metabolism*, 8th Ed., Bondy, P. and Rosenberg, L. eds., Philadelphia, W. B. Saunders, 1980, p. 939.

Weidmann, A. Porphyria cutanea tarda. *Dermatol. Internat.*, 4:201, 1965.

Epidermolysis Bullosa

Anton-Lamprecht, I. Electron microscopy in the early diagnosis of genetic disorders of the skin. *Dermatologica*, 157:65, 1978.

Anton-Lamprecht, I. and Schnyder, U. Epidermolysis bullosa dystrophica dominans—ein Defekt der anchoring fibrils? *Dermatologica*, 147:289, 1973.

——. Zur Ultrastruktur der Epidermolysen mit junktionaler Blasenbildung. *Dermatologica*, 159:377, 1979.

Bauer, E. et al. The role of human skin collagenase in epidermolysis bullosa. *J. Invest. Dermatol.*, 68:119, 1977.

Bergenholtz, A. and Olsson, O. Epidermolysis bullosa hereditaria. I. Epidermolysis bullosa hereditaria letalis. *Acta Derm. Venereol.*, 48:220, 1968.

Briggaman, R. and Wheeler, C., Jr. Epidermolysis bullosa dystrophica—recessive: A possible role of anchoring fibrils in the pathogenesis. *J. Invest. Dermatol.*, 65:203, 1975.

Buchbinder, L. Severe infantile epidermolysis bullosa simplex: Dowling-Meara type. *Arch. Dermatol.*, 122:190, 1986.

Dahl, M. Epidermolysis bullosa acquisita: A sign of cicatricial pemphigoid. *Br. J. Dermatol.*, 101:475, 1979.

Eisen, A. Human skin collagenase: Relationship to the pathogenesis of epidermolysis bullosa dystrophica. *J. Invest. Dermatol.*, 52:449, 1969.

Eisen, A., Bauer, E. and Jeffrey, J. Animal and human collagenases. *J. Invest. Dermatol.*, 55:359, 1970.

Gedde-Dahl, T. Classification of epidermolysis bullosa. In: *Pädiatrische Dermatologie*. Herzberg, J., ed., Stuttgart, Shattauer, 1977.

Gedde-Dahl, T. and Anton-Lamprecht, I. Epidermolysis bullosa. In: *Principles and Practice in Medical Genetics*. Emory, A. and Rimoin, D., eds. New York, Livingstone, 1981.

Haber, R. et al. Hereditary epidermolysis bullosa. *J. Am. Acad. Dermatol.*, 13:252, 1985.

Haneke, E. and Anton-Lamprecht, I. Ultrastructure of blister formation in epidermolysis bullosa hereditaria. V. Epidermolysis bullosa simplex localisata Type Weber-Cockayne. *J. Invest. Dermatol.*, 78:219, 1982.

Hashimoto, I. et al. Ultrastructural studies in epidermolysis bullosa hereditaria: II. Dominant dystrophic types of Cockayne and Touraine. *Arch. Dermatol. Res.*, 255:285, 1976.

——. Ultrastructural studies in epidermolysis bullosa hereditaria. III. Recessive dystrophic types with dermolytic blisters (Hallopeau-Siemens types and inverse type). *Arch. Dermatol. Res.*, 256:137, 1976.

Hashimoto, K. Electron microscopy for diagnosis of selected dermatoses. *Semin. Dermatol.*, 3:36, 1984.

Hintner, H. and Wolff, K. Generalized atrophic benign epidermolysis bullosa. *Arch. Dermatol.*, 118:375, 1982.

Hintner, H. et al. Immunofluorescence mapping of antigen determinants within the dermal-epidermal junction in mechanobullous diseases. *J. Invest. Dermatol.*, 76:113, 1981.

Johnson, S. and Test, A. Epidermolysis bullosa simplex of the hands and the feet: A genetic study of the hereditary type. *Arch. Dermatol. Syph.*, 53:610, 1946.

Kobayashi, T. Dermo-epidermal junction in the recessive type of epidermolysis bullosa. *Acta Derm. Venereol.*, 47:57, 1967.

Lamb, J. and Halpert, B. Epidermolysis bullosa of the newborn. *Arch. Dermatol. Syph.*, 55:369, 1947.

Lazarus, G. Collagenase and connective tissue metabolism in epidermolysis bullosa. *J. Invest. Dermatol.*, 58:242, 1972.

Livden, J. et al. Epidermolysis bullosa acquisita with Crohn's disease. *Acta Derm. Venereol.* (Stockh.), 58:241, 1978.

Lowe, L., Jr. Hereditary epidermolysis bullosa. *Arch. Dermatol.*, 95:587, 1967.

Nieboer, C. et al. Epidermolysis bullosa acquisita. *Br. J. Dermatol.*, 102:383, 1980.

Orlando, R. et al. Epidermolysis bullosa: Gastrointestinal manifestations. *Ann. Int. Med.*, 81:203, 1974.

Paller, A. The generalized atrophic benign form of junctional epidermolysis bullosa: Experience with four patients in the United States. *Arch. Dermatol.*, 122:704, 1986.

Pass, F. and Dobson, R. Epidermolysis bullosa acquisita: A disease of dermal connective tissue. *Arch. Dermatol.*, 91:219, 1965.

Passarge, E. Epidermolysis bullosa hereditaria simplex: Kindred affected in 4 generations. *J. Pediatr.*, 67:819, 1965.

Pearson, R. Studies on the pathogenesis of epidermolysis bullosa. *J. Invest. Dermatol.*, 39:551, 1962.

Pearson, R., Potter, B. and Strauss, F. Epidermolysis bullosa hereditaria letalis. *Arch. Dermatol.*, 109:349, 1974.
Pearson, R. and Spargo, B. Electron microscope studies of dermal-epidermal separation in human skin. *J. Invest. Dermatol.*, 36:213, 1961.
Peltier, F. et al. Epidermolysis bullosa letalis associated with congenital pyloric atresia. *Arch. Dermatol.*, 117:728, 1981.
Reed, W. et al. Epidermolysis bullosa dystrophica with epidermal neoplasms. *Arch. Dermatol.*, 110:894, 1974.
Richter, B. and McNutt, N. The spectrum of epidermolysis bullosa acquisita. *Arch. Dermatol.*, 115:1325, 1979.
Roberts, M. et al. Epidermolysis bullosa letalis: Report of three cases with particular reference to the histopathology of the skin. *Pediatrics*, 25:283, 1960.
Roenigk, H., Jr., Ryan, J. and Bergfeld, W. Epidermolysis bullosa acquisita. *Arch. Dermatol.*, 103:1, 1971.
——. Epidermolysis bullosa acquisita. *Arch. Dermatol.*, 103:1, 1971.
Schachner, L., Lazarus, G. and Dembitzer, H. Epidermolysis bullosa hereditaria letalis. *Br. J. Dermatol.*, 96:51, 1977.
Schäffer, G. Two cases of epidermolysis bullosa hereditaria letalis. *Acta Derm. Venereol.*, 31:704, 1951.
Stricklin, G. et al. Human skin collagenase in recessive dystrophic epidermolysis bullosa. *J. Clin. Invest.*, 69:1373, 1982.
Turner, T. Two cases of junctional epidermolysis bullosa (Herlitz-Pearson). *Br. J. Dermatol.*, 102:97, 1980.
Wechsler, H., Krugh, F. and Domonkos, A. Polydysplastic epidermolysis bullosa and development of epidermal neoplasms. *Arch. Dermatol.*, 102:374, 1970.
Winstock, D. Oral aspects of epidermolysis bullosa. *Br. J. Dermatol.*, 74:431, 1962.
Yaoita, H. et al. Epidermolysis bullosa acquisita: Ultrastructural and immunological studies. *J. Invest. Dermatol.*, 76:288, 1981.

Burns

Ablin, R. and Holder, I. IgG and complement-fixing pseudointercellular antibodies after thermal injury. *Arch. Dermatol.*, 109:887, 1974.
Chorzelski, T. et al. Can pemphigus be provoked by a burn? *Br. J. Dermatol.*, 85:320, 1971.
Foley, F. Pathology of cutaneous burns. *Surg. Clin. North. Am.*, 50:1200, 1970.
Gaughan, L., Bergeron, J. and Mullins, J. Giant basal cell epithelioma developing in acute burn site. *Arch. Dermatol.*, 99:594, 1969.
Moritz, A. Studies of thermal injury. III. The pathology and pathogenesis of cutaneous burns: An experimental study. *Am. J. Pathol.*, 23:915, 1947.
Sevitt, S. Histological changes in burned skin. In: *Burns: Pathology and Therapeutic Applications*. London, Butterworth & Co., 1957, p. 18.
Winer, L. and Levin, G. Changes in the skin as a result of electric current. *Arch. Dermatol.*, 78:386, 1958.

Bullous Dermatoses: Subcorneal

Subcorneal Pustular Dermatosis (Sneddon-Wilkinson)

Barsky, S. and Cornbleet, T. Subcorneal pustular dermatosis: A report of 2 cases. *J. Invest. Dermatol.*, 32:69, 1959.
Burns, R. and Fine, G. Subcorneal pustular dermatosis. *Arch. Dermatol.*, 80:72, 1959.
Chimenti, S. and Ackerman, A. Is subcorneal pustular dermatosis of Sneddon and Wilkinson an entity *sui generis*? *Am. J. Dermatopathol.*, 3:363, 1981.
Ellis, F. Subcorneal pustular dermatosis. *Arch. Dermatol.*, 78:580, 1958.
Feuerman-Pogorzelski, E. Subcorneal pustular dermatosis Sneddon-Wilkinson with face lesions: The first case in Israel. *Acta Derm. Venereol.*, 41:240, 1961.
Lin, R. et al. Subcorneal pustular dermatosis with polyarthritis. *Cutis*, 37:123, 1986.

Marks, J. and Shuster, S. Small-intestinal mucosa in pemphigoid and subcorneal pustular dermatosis. *Arch. Dermatol.*, 100:136, 1969.
Marsden, J. and Millard, L. Pyoderma gangrenosum, subcorneal pustular dermatosis and IgA paraproteinaemia. *Br. J. Dermatol.*, 114:125, 1986.
Ryatt, K. et al. Subcorneal pustular dermatosis and IgA gammopathy. *Acta Derm. Venereol.* (Stockh.), 61:560, 1981.
Schieferstein, G. et al. Subcorneal pustular dermatosis of Sneddon-Wilkinson: A long-term immunologic case study. *Arch. Derm. Res.*, 276:65, 1984.
Sneddon, I. and Wilkinson, D. Subcorneal pustular dermatosis. *Br. J. Dermatol.*, 68:385, 1956.
——. Subcorneal pustular dermatosis. *Br. J. Dermatol.*, 100:61, 1979.

Acropustulosis of Infancy

Jarratt, M. and Ramsdell, W. Infantile acropustulosis. *Arch. Dermatol.*, 115:834, 1979.
Kahn, G. and Rywlin, A. Acropustulosis of infancy. *Arch. Dermatol.*, 115:831, 1979.
Laudren, A., Chevrant-Breton, J. and Lancien, G. Acropustulose infantile: Un cas. *Ann. Dermatol. Venereol.*, 112:251, 1985.
Sturman, S. Infantile acropustulosis. *Semin. Dermatol.*, 3:50, 1984.

Chapter 11
Degenerative Dermatoses

"Degeneration" is an admittedly vague and somewhat outmoded biologic concept. However, there is a large group of skin disorders characterized by processes of change or deterioration that are not well understood. The designation "degenerative dermatoses" is convenient and appropriate for these disorders.

SOLAR DEGENERATION OF THE SKIN (SOLAR ELASTOSIS)

The skin changes usually considered to be due to aging are actually related primarily to the cumulative effects of ultraviolet light. Such changes increase with time only because cumulative ultraviolet exposure increases with time. The UVB component of sunlight is largely responsible for photoaging of the skin. Sun-damaged skin shows changes of poikiloderma: wrinkling, varying degrees of atrophy, mottled hyperpigmentation and hypopigmentation, and telangiectasia. Fig. A shows sun-damaged skin with many solar keratoses. The skin may have a yellowish color. All of the cited changes are not necessarily present. Special variants of solar degeneration of the skin include *cutis rhomboidalis nuchae,* in which the skin of the back of the neck is furrowed and thickened, and *Favre-Racouchot syndrome* (nodular elastosis with cysts and comedones) characterized by yellowish nodules and comedones in the periorbital area (Fig. B). A variant of this syndrome is *actinic comedonal plaque,* a solitary lesion with small nodules and dilated hair follicles, on the arms or face.

Individuals with fair skin, albinism, or xeroderma pigmentosum are particularly susceptible to solar skin damage.

Solar-damaged skin tends to develop certain neoplasms: solar keratoses, squamous cell carcinoma, basal cell carcinoma, lentigo maligna, and lentigo maligna melanoma. With the exception of basal cell carcinoma, which rarely metastasizes whether it is on sun-exposed skin or not, malignant neoplasms related to cumulative solar damage are typically less malignant than their non-sun-related counterparts.

Aging changes in skin not exposed to sunlight include thinning of the skin and loss of subcutaneous fat.

Microscopic features

1. A zone of altered connective tissue is present in the upper third of the dermis; this is usually separated from the epidermis by a narrow band of morphologically normal connective tissue (Figs. C,D,E).
2. With H&E, this altered connective tissue appears as basophilic, granular, amorphous material (Fig. D), or as basophilic, thickened, and curled fibers (Fig. C). With special stains, such as Giemsa stain, an acid mucopolysaccharide component may be demonstrable.
3. The altered connective tissue has an affinity for elastic tissue stains (Fig. E). It is brownish-black with acid orcein Giemsa stain.
4. The pigmentary mottling may not be apparent with H&E stain; with Fontana-Masson stain, the uneven melanization of the basal epidermis may be visible.
5. In Favre-Racouchot syndrome, comedones (Fig. D) and milia are also present.

SOLAR DEGENERATION OF THE SKIN

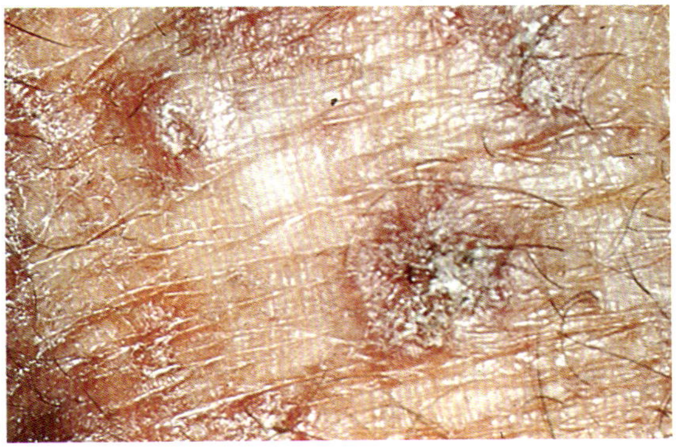

A

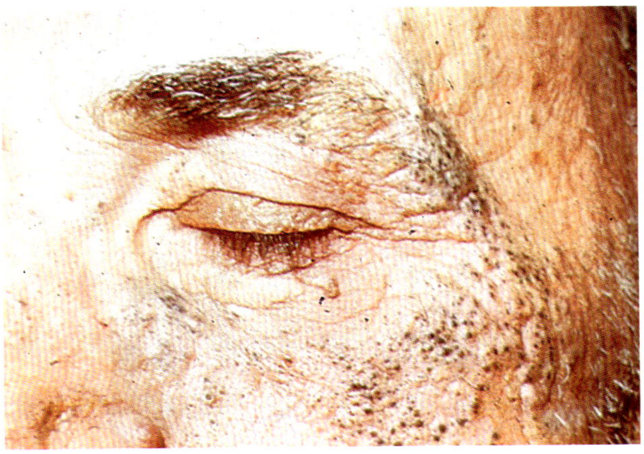

B

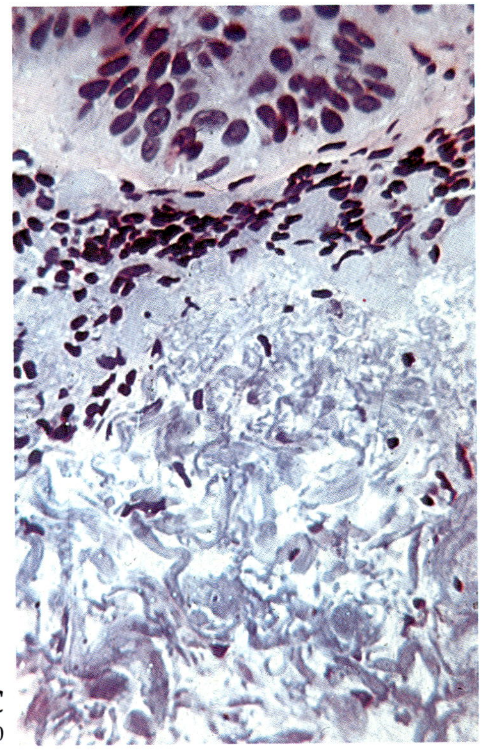

C
X520

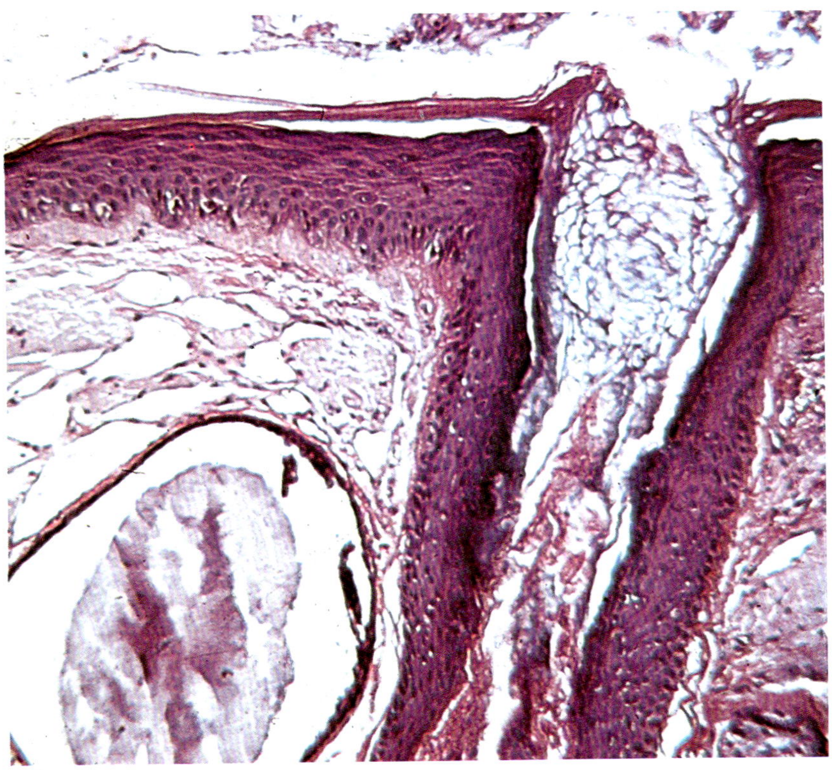

D
X180

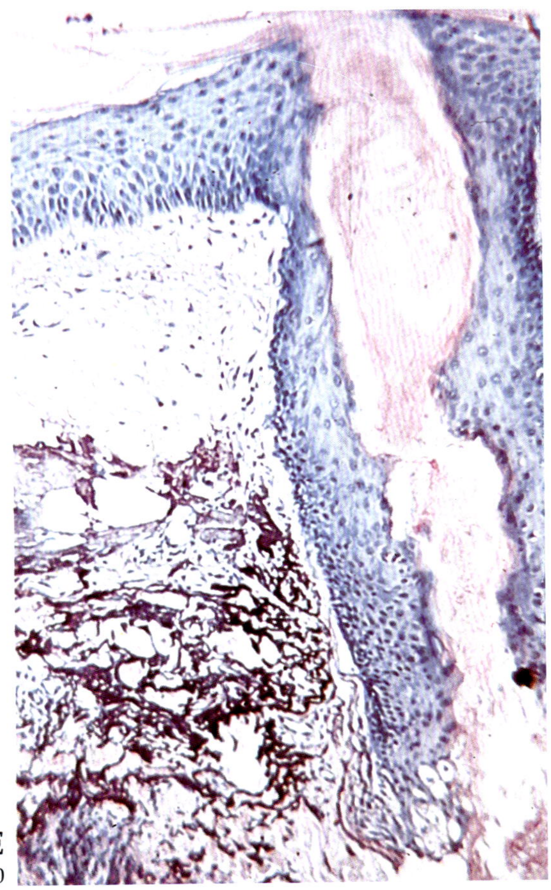

E
X180

ACID ORCEIN GIEMSA STAIN

SOLAR DEGENERATION continued

SOLAR DEGENERATION OF THE SKIN

Comment

1. The nature of the elastotic material has been a controversial subject. The prevailing view is that it derives neither from collagen nor elastin, but represents a new, abnormal material produced by fibroblasts.
2. Sudanophilic substances may be present in solar elastosis.

DEGENERATIVE DERMATOSES continued

RADIODERMATITIS

Acute radiodermatitis follows the administration of a high single dose of ionizing radiation or multiple high doses given over a very short period of time. It is characterized by dusky erythema, followed by blisters, and in severe cases, ulceration. Healing is followed by the development of epidermal atrophy, hyperpigmentation, and telangiectasia.

The histologic changes are analogous to those of a burn.

CHRONIC RADIODERMATITIS

Chronic radiodermatitis develops years after a course of radiotherapy; it may also develop from very small doses of ionizing radiation received over a period of years (as in occupational exposure).

The appearance of the skin in chronic radiodermatitis resembles its appearance in areas of solar degeneration. There is mottled hyperpigmentation and hypopigmentation, atrophy, and telangiectasia (Figs. A,C). Ulceration, premalignant keratoses, and carcinomas (Fig. B) may develop, particularly in instances of prolonged occupational exposure. Squamous cell carcinomas developing at sites of chronic radiodermatitis tend to be more malignant than those related to solar skin damage.

Microscopic features

1. The epidermis is flattened (Figs. D,E), but a few elongated rete ridges may be present, as well as foci of hyperkeratosis. Epithelial cells may show some degeneration, with loss of morphologic detail.
2. The dermis shows extensive edema and homogenization of collagen (Figs. D,E), as well as newly-formed, basophilic collagen fibers.
3. Large fibroblastic nuclei may be present in the upper dermis (Figs. E,F,G).
4. Telangiectatic capillaries are present just below the epidermis (Figs. D,E). Vessels of the deeper dermis generally have thickened, fibrotic walls and occasionally are thrombosed. This may result in ulceration.
5. Epidermal appendages are reduced in number; loss of eccrine glands, however, is usually minimal.
6. Epidermal changes similar to those of solar keratosis gradually develop.
7. Basal cell carcinomas and squamous cell carcinomas may develop in areas of radiation damage. Squamous cell carcinomas are frequently of the spindle cell type.

Microscopic differential diagnosis

1. The connective tissue changes in chronic radiodermatitis tend to be more extensive and deeper than those of solar elastosis, and the altered connective tissue tends to be more eosinophilic and more homogeneous.
2. Chronic radiodermatitis has a resemblance to necrobiosis lipoidica, but the connective tissue changes tend to be more widespread. There is less inflammation and usually no granulomatous element.
3. There is less homogenization of connective tissue in scleroderma.

CHRONIC RADIODERMATITIS

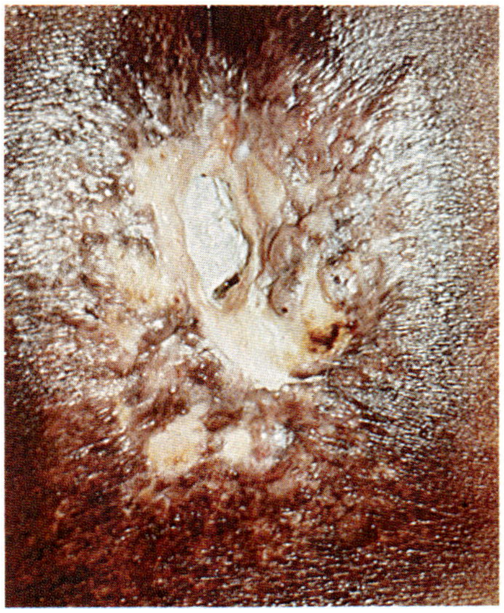

A

B

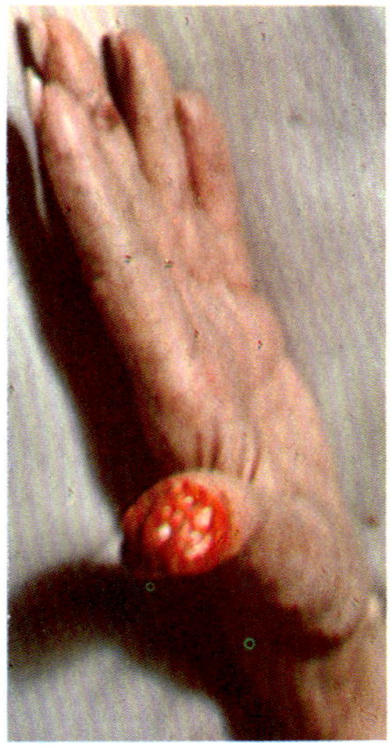

C

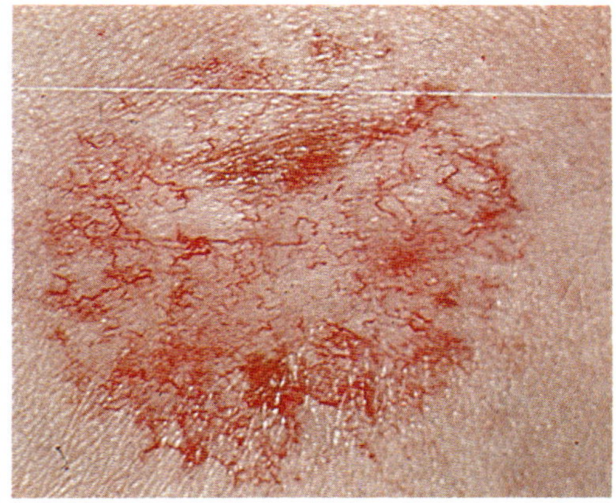

Figs. A,B,C courtesy Dr. M. Legg

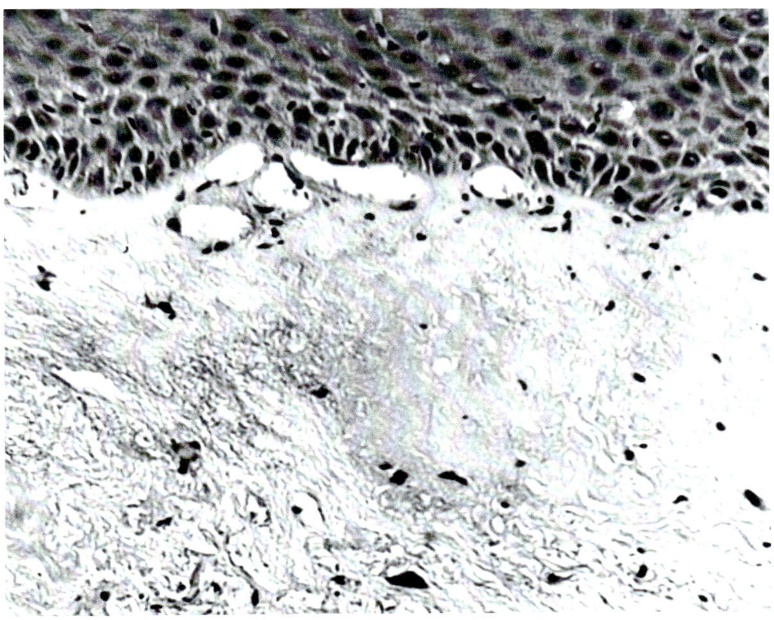

D
X230

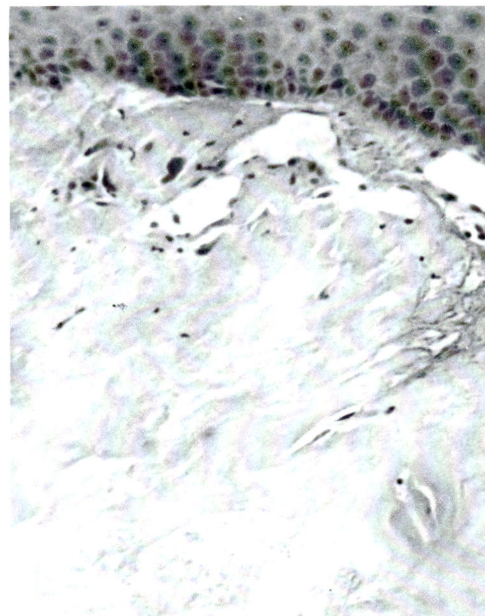

E X200

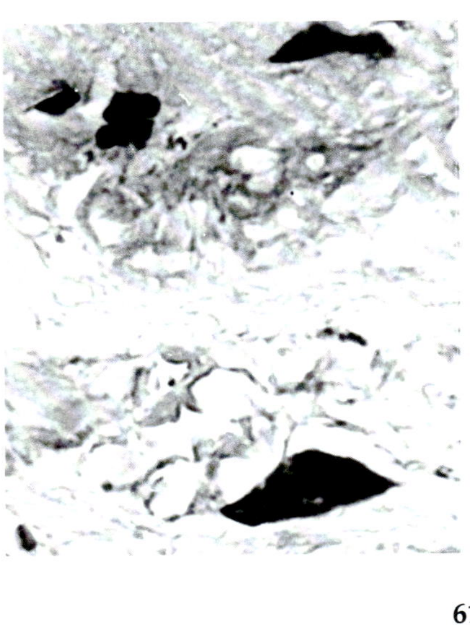

F
X770

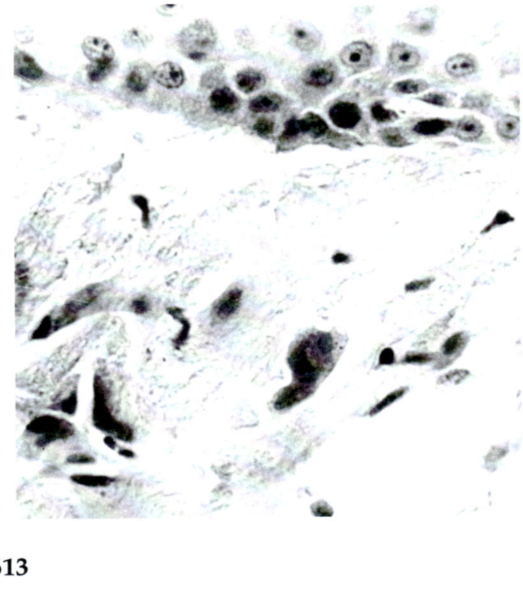

G
X600

POIKILODERMA

Congenital or associated with hereditary disorders

Poikiloderma congenitale (Rothmund-Thomson)

Hartnup disease

Bloom's syndrome

Dyskeratosis congenita

Xeroderma pigmentosum (see p. 244)

Idiopathic acquired

Poikiloderma atrophicans vasculare (see p. 616)

Parapsoriasis variegata (see p. 94)

Poikiloderma of Civatte (see p. 616)

Secondary to other acquired disorders

Solar degeneration (see p. 608)

Chronic radiodermatitis (see p. 612)

Lupus erythematosus (see p. 488)

Dermatomyositis (see p. 502)

Mycosis fungoides (see p. 1330)

POIKILODERMA

Poikiloderma refers to skin showing mottled hyperpigmentation and hypopigmentation, telangiectasia, and atrophy. Poikiloderma occurs in many conditions (see chart, previous page); in addition, there are forms of poikiloderma that are considered entities *sui generis*: a congenital form which is recessively inherited (poikiloderma congenitale of Rothmund-Thomson), and acquired forms (poikiloderma atrophicans vasculare and poikiloderma of Civatte).

Skin changes of poikiloderma congenitale are widespread and resemble those of xeroderma pigmentosum (see p. 244). Associated features include photosensitivity, endocrine disorders, skeletal abnormalities, and cataracts. *Hartnup disease, Bloom's syndrome*, and *dyskeratosis congenita* show similar cutaneous changes.

Poikiloderma atrophicans vasculare (Fig. A) arises in adult life and is characterized by symmetrical, diffuse areas of poikiloderma. Poikiloderma atrophicans vasculare should be considered not associated with other disorders only when proven otherwise. We have already cited the association of poikiloderma with mycosis fungoides, lupus erythematosus, and dermatomyositis. Some authors consider poikiloderma atrophicans vasculare to be synonymous with parapsoriasis variegata. Large plaque parapsoriasis grades into parapsoriasis variegata; both clinical patterns can represent precursor stages of mycosis fungoides. Repeated biopsies, sometimes taken over a span of years, may be required to demonstrate definite histologic evidence of mycosis fungoides (see p. 1330).

Poikiloderma of Civatte (Fig. B) arises in middle-aged women and involves the sides of the face and neck. It may be related to sun exposure.

Microscopic features

1. There is atrophy of the epidermis and hydropic degeneration of the basal cells (Figs. C,D). Colloid bodies may be present.
2. A mixed chronic inflammatory infiltrate composed principally of lymphoid cells is present beneath the epidermis (Figs. C,D).
3. Later lesions develop telangiectasia (Fig. D) in the upper dermis. "Melanophages" appear as the inflammatory infiltrate regresses. In contrast to scleroderma, the thickness of the dermis is decreased.
4. Poikiloderma associated with other disease entities may show histologic features of those entities (e.g., poikiloderma associated with mycosis fungoides may show atypical T lymphocytes in the infiltrate).

POIKILODERMA

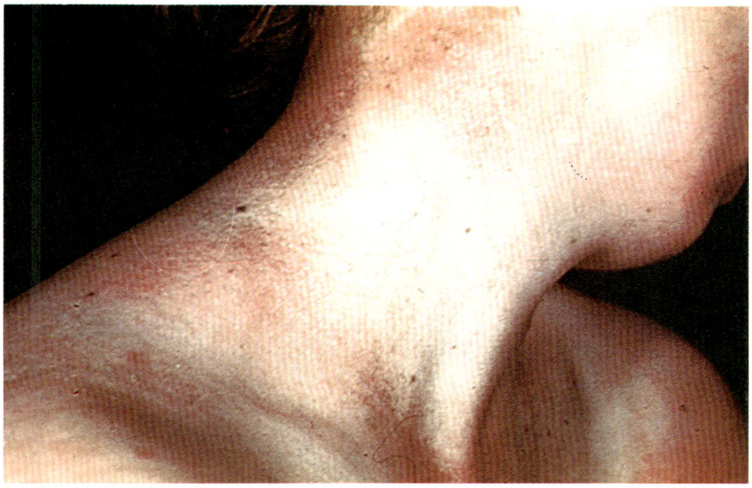

A Courtesy Dr. Ramon Fusaro, Dr. J. Koh

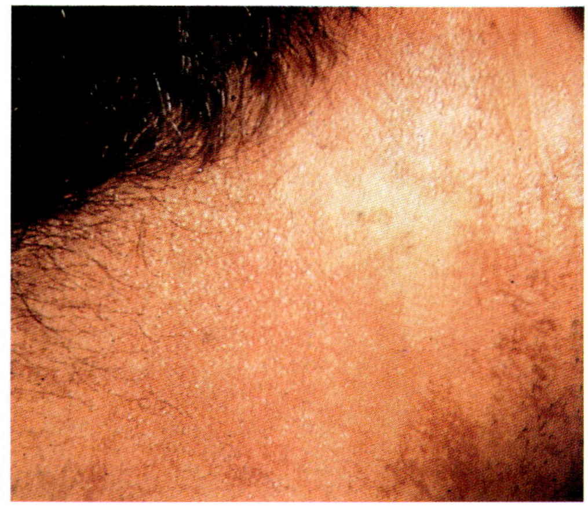

B

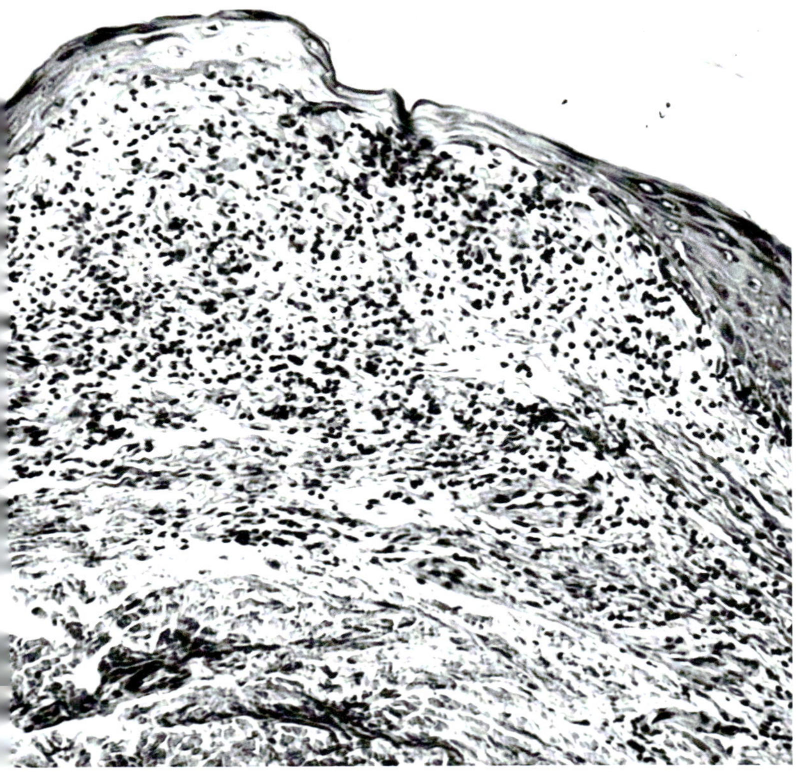

C
X250

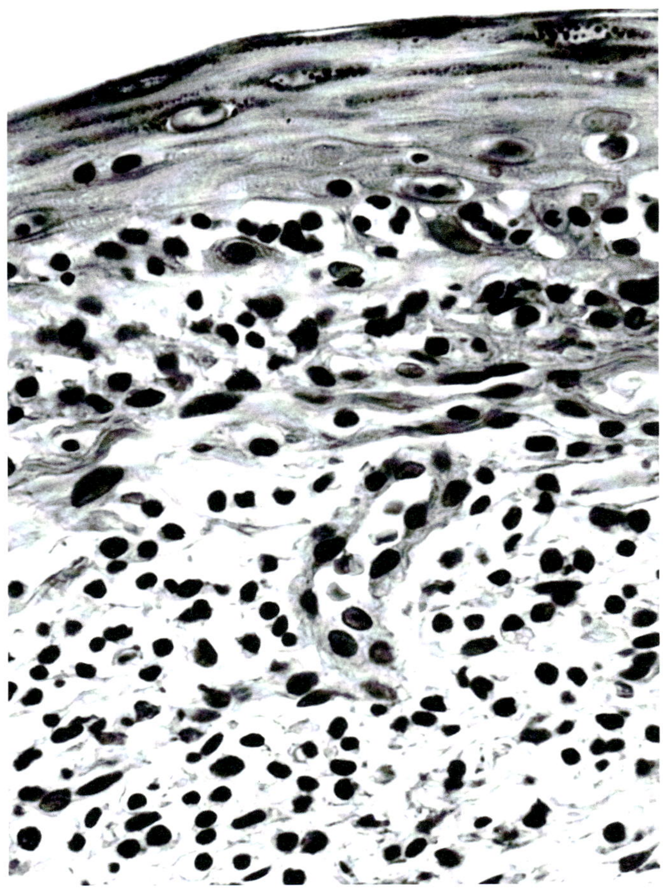

D
X700

ACRODERMATITIS CHRONICA ATROPHICANS

Acrodermatitis chronica atrophicans is a disorder of unknown etiology affecting individuals in the older age groups. Incidence is highest in Europe.

Lesions progress from an early stage of inflammation to a late stage of extreme atrophy of all layers of the skin (Fig. A). Atrophy of the skin and subcutaneous fat may allow the subcutaneous veins to be seen. Occasionally, fibrous thickenings resulting in a resemblance to scleroderma may be observed.

There is a predilection for the extensor surfaces of the extremities.

It has been suggested that acrodermatitis chronica atrophicans may be caused by a group B arbovirus amenable to penicillin therapy and transmitted by a tick. An alternative possibility is that acrodermatitis chronica atrophicans is the end result of Lyme disease, caused by a tick-borne spirochaete.

Microscopic features

1. The epidermis is atrophic (Figs. B,C); sometimes there is mild hyperkeratosis.
2. A band-like infiltrate composed principally of lymphoid cells is present in the upper dermis; this is separated from the epidermis by a narrow zone of connective tissue (Figs. B,C). In addition, there are scattered areas of inflammation in the deeper dermis and fat (Fig. C).
3. The dermis shows edema and atrophy of collagen fibers (Figs. B,C); with progression, the thickness of the dermis is decreased, and there is atrophy of the subcutaneous fat. There is loss of elastic tissue.
4. Sebaceous glands and hairs are often entirely absent (Figs. B,C), but eccrine glands are generally unaffected.
5. There may be moderate vascular dilatation and thickening.
6. Fibrous bands show a picture resembling that of scleroderma.

ACRODERMATITIS CHRONICA ATROPHICANS

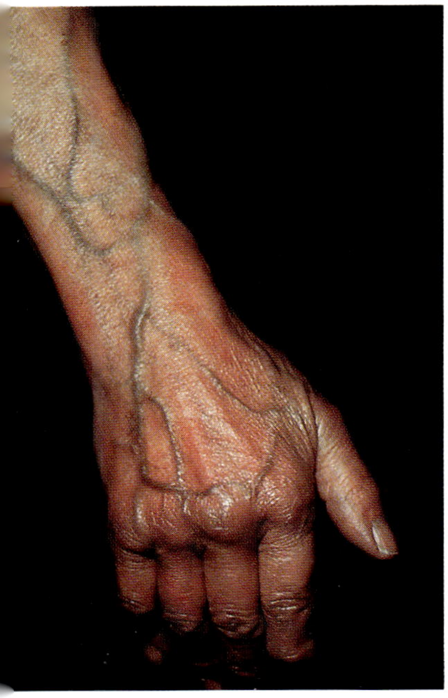

A

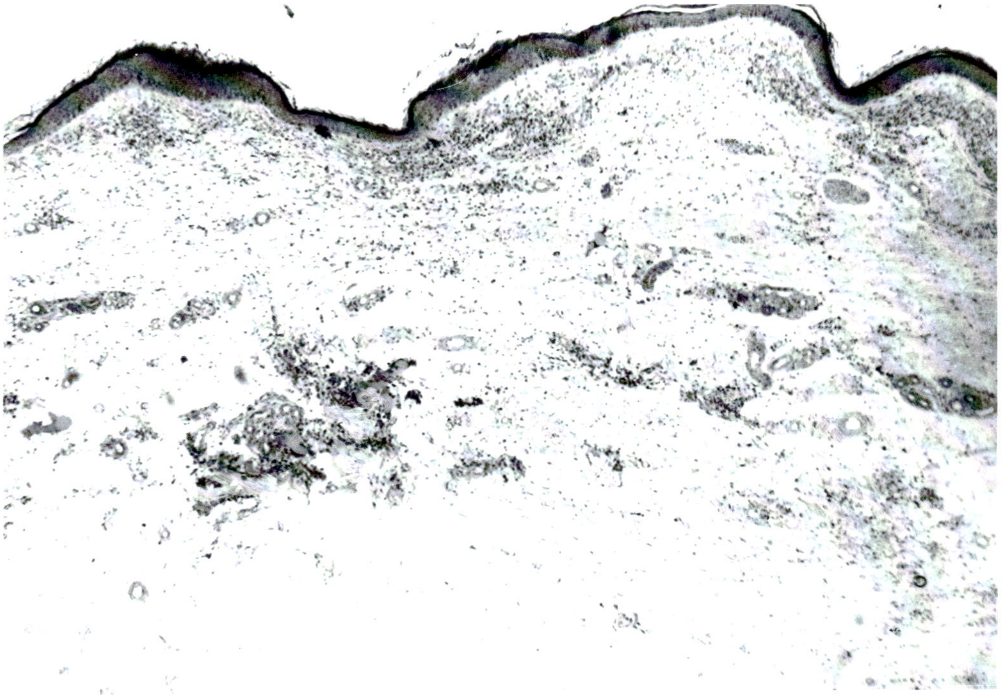

B
X40

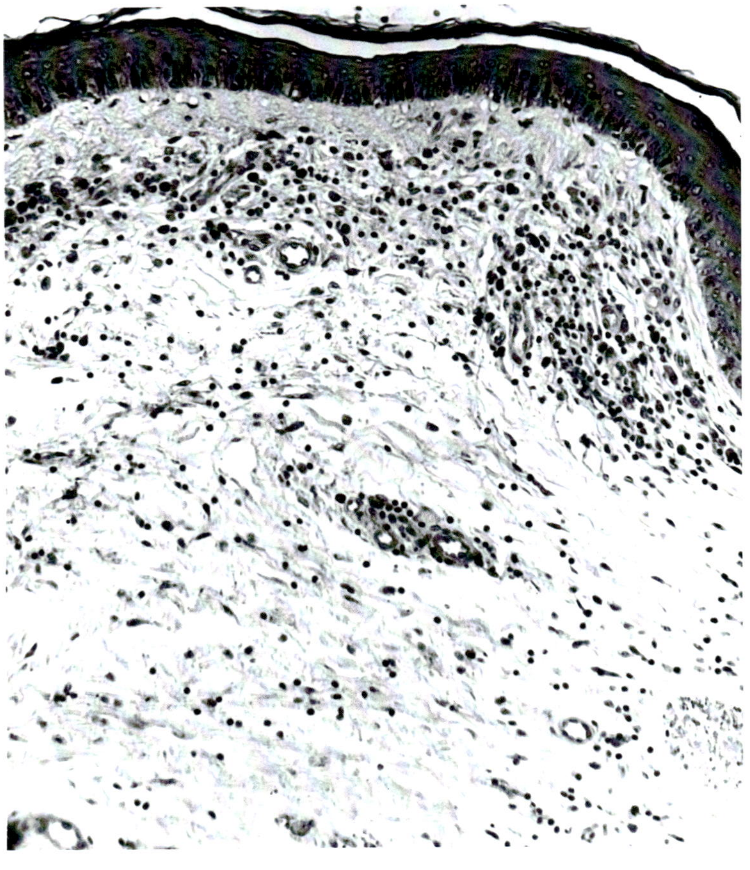

C
X200

ANETODERMA (MACULAR ATROPHY)

Anetoderma is characterized by atrophic, depressed patches, which may show hernia-like bulging of the skin, due to loss of elastic fibers. The usual location is the trunk (Fig. A).

Two types have been described: a noninflammatory type (Schweninger-Buzzi type) and a type with an initial stage of inflammation (Jadassohn type). Clear-cut distinction between the two is not always possible.

The cause is unknown.

The previous suggestion that there is a type of anetoderma secondary to diseases such as syphilis, tuberculosis, and lupus erythematosus is now generally doubted.

Microscopic features

1. In anetoderma of Schweninger-Buzzi, and in the late stage of anetoderma of Jadassohn, elastic tissue stains show a localized area devoid of elastic fibers (Figs. B,C). The surrounding elastic fibers may be coarse and clumped (Figs. B,C). Collagen fibers in the affected area show swelling and fragmentation.
2. In the early stage of the Jadassohn type of anetoderma there is a perivasculitis or leukocytoclastic vasculitis.

Comment

There has been a recent report of anetoderma following prolonged treatment with penicillamine.

ANETODERMA

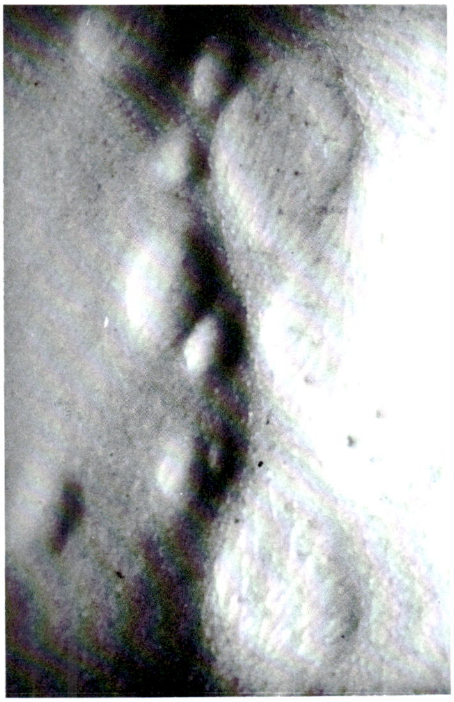

A

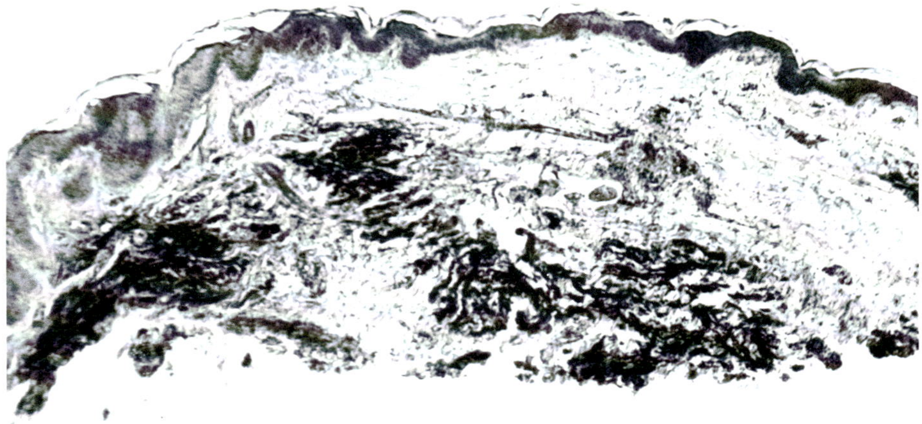

B X50

VERHOEFF-VAN GIESON STAIN

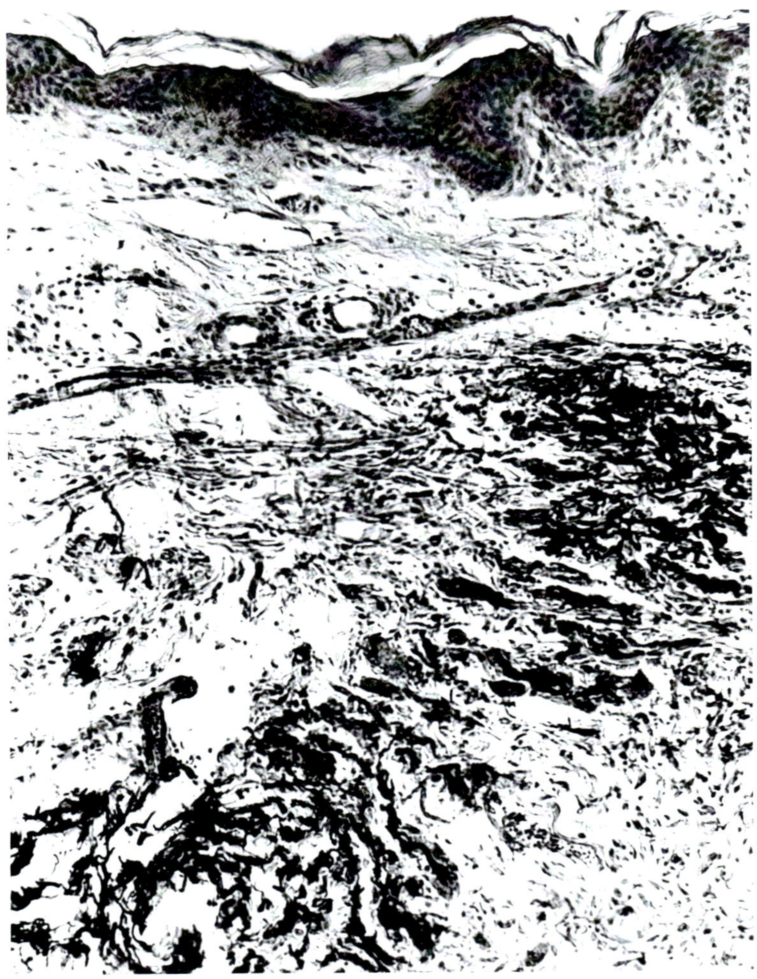

C
X150

VERHOEFF-VAN GIESON STAIN

STRIAE DISTENSAE

Striae distensae are bands of wrinkled, depressed skin (Fig. A). Initial lesions are reddish, but they eventually become white. Both stress damage and increased glucocorticoid levels are factors in their development. Striae distensae can be observed in obesity, pregnancy, Cushing's disease, adolescence, and the therapeutic use of corticosteroids. Breasts, abdomen, thighs, buttocks, and inguinal areas are common sites.

Microscopic features

1. Centers of lesions show absence of elastic fibers.
2. At the periphery of lesions, breakage and retraction of elastic fibers can be demonstrated with elastic stains, such as Verhoeff-Van Gieson stain (Fig. B). The broken ends of elastic fibers are curled.
3. The collagen fibers may appear stretched.
4. The epidermis may be thinned.
5. The dermis may show a decrease in thickness.

Microscopic differential diagnosis

The elastic fiber alterations may have some resemblance to those observed in anetoderma. Clinically, the two conditions are quite dissimilar.

STRIAE DISTENSAE

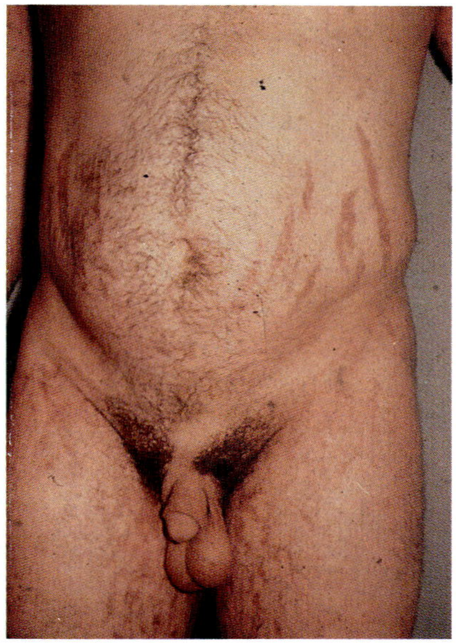

A

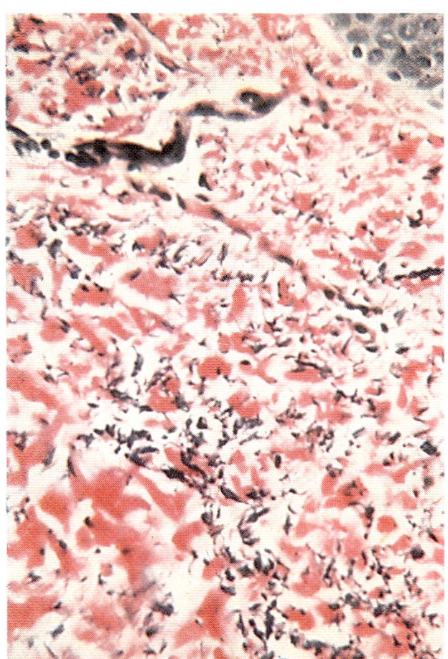

B
X520

VERHOEFF-VAN GIESON STAIN

STEROID ATROPHY

Therapeutic local application of corticosteroids, either by injection or by topical application may produce atrophy of the skin. Atrophy caused by topical application of corticosteroids is more likely to occur if fluorinated corticosteroids are used, if intertriginous areas are involved, and if there is use of plastic film occlusion. Illustrated is an example of atrophy due to corticosteroid injection, showing a pronounced depression (Fig. A). Another example (Fig. B) shows diffuse thinning of the skin, allowing blood vessels to be visualized.

Atrophy of the skin due to local application of corticosteroids sometimes resolves spontaneously.

Microscopic features

1. The key feature is decrease in the depth of the dermis due to loss of collagen fibers (Fig. C).
2. There may be atrophy of the epidermis.

STEROID ATROPHY

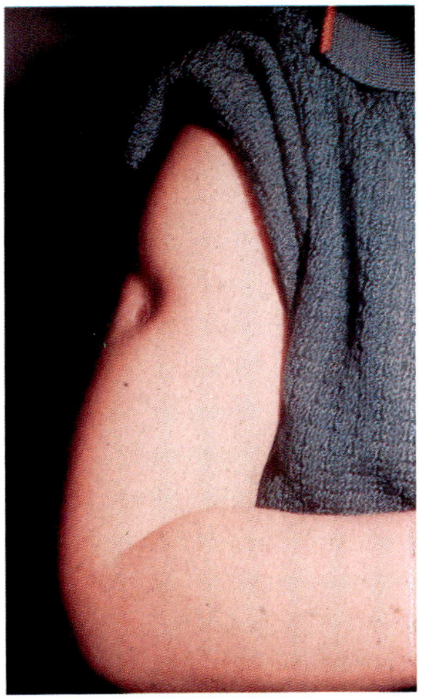

A

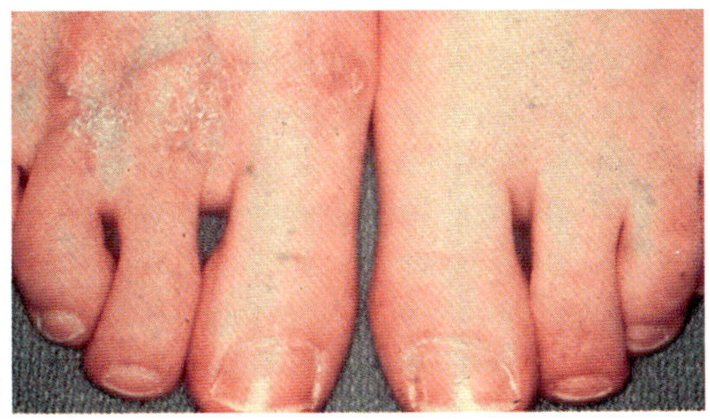

B

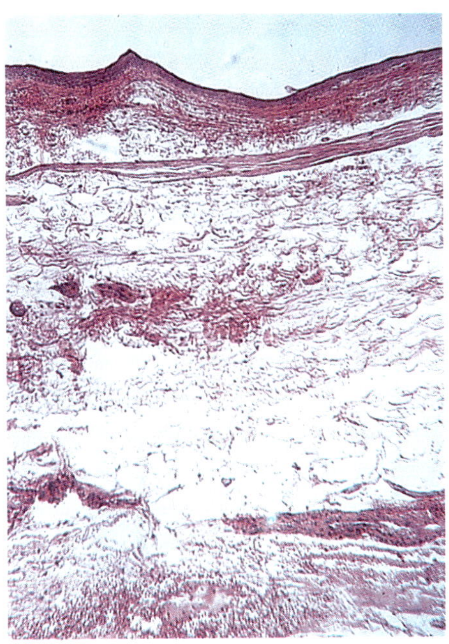

C
X60

Degenerative dermatoses

PERFORATING DERMATOSES

A group of dermatoses has been recognized, having the common feature of a transepidermal canal. In some of these disorders, it is believed that the canal forms as a passageway to eliminate abnormal dermal material.

Disorders with transepidermal canals

Chondrodermatitis nodularis helicis

Elastosis perforans serpiginosa

Calcific elastosis

Kyrle's disease

Perforating folliculitis

Reactive perforating collagenosis

Perforating granuloma annulare

CHONDRODERMATITIS NODULARIS HELICIS

The disorder is characterized by tender nodules on the helix. The nodules are usually solitary and often involve the free margin. Occasionally they are located on the anthelix (Fig. A). Hyperkeratosis and crusting may be present. Incidence is highest in older men. Although the cause is unknown, trauma and exposure to temperature extremes are believed to be predisposing factors.

Microscopic features

1. There is an epidermal invagination (Fig. B) which contains a hyperkeratotic and para-
keratotic plug. In some instances, a crusted ulcer is present (Fig. C).
2. Beneath the invagination or ulcer there is a zone of fibrinoid collagen degeneration (Fig. C, arrow) with loss of connective tissue nuclei. This is surrounded by a zone of granulation tissue (Fig. D). Fig. B also shows the zone of collagen degeneration (D), the zone of granulation tissue (G), and cartilage (C).
3. Changes in the cartilage vary. There may be thickening of the perichondrium as well as loss of nuclei, loss of basophilia and decrease in morphologic detail (Fig. E). Calcification and ossification may occur.

Comment

1. It is no longer widely believed that changes in the cartilage are secondary to the cutaneous changes. Histologic changes in the cartilage are now believed to be due to aging, with no relationship to the focal lesion of chondrodermatitis nodularis helicis.
2. It is now widely believed that the epidermal channel or ulcer forms as a mechanism to eliminate the altered collagen. Therefore, chondrodermatitis nodularis helicis can be considered one of the perforating dermatoses.
3. Some authors have described glomus-like vascular formations in chondrodermatitis nodularis helicis and have explained the pain on this basis.
4. *Relapsing polychondritis* is an intermittent and progressive inflammation of cartilaginous structures throughout the body. Typical features include auricular chondritis, respiratory tract chondritis, polyarthritis, and ocular inflammation. There is a significant mortality rate, primarily because of respiratory tract or cardiac valve involvement. Purpuric or erythema nodosum-like skin lesions may occur. The microscopic picture is characterized by inflammation and degeneration of cartilage. Skin lesions show vasculitis.

CHONDRODERMATITIS NODULARIS HELICIS

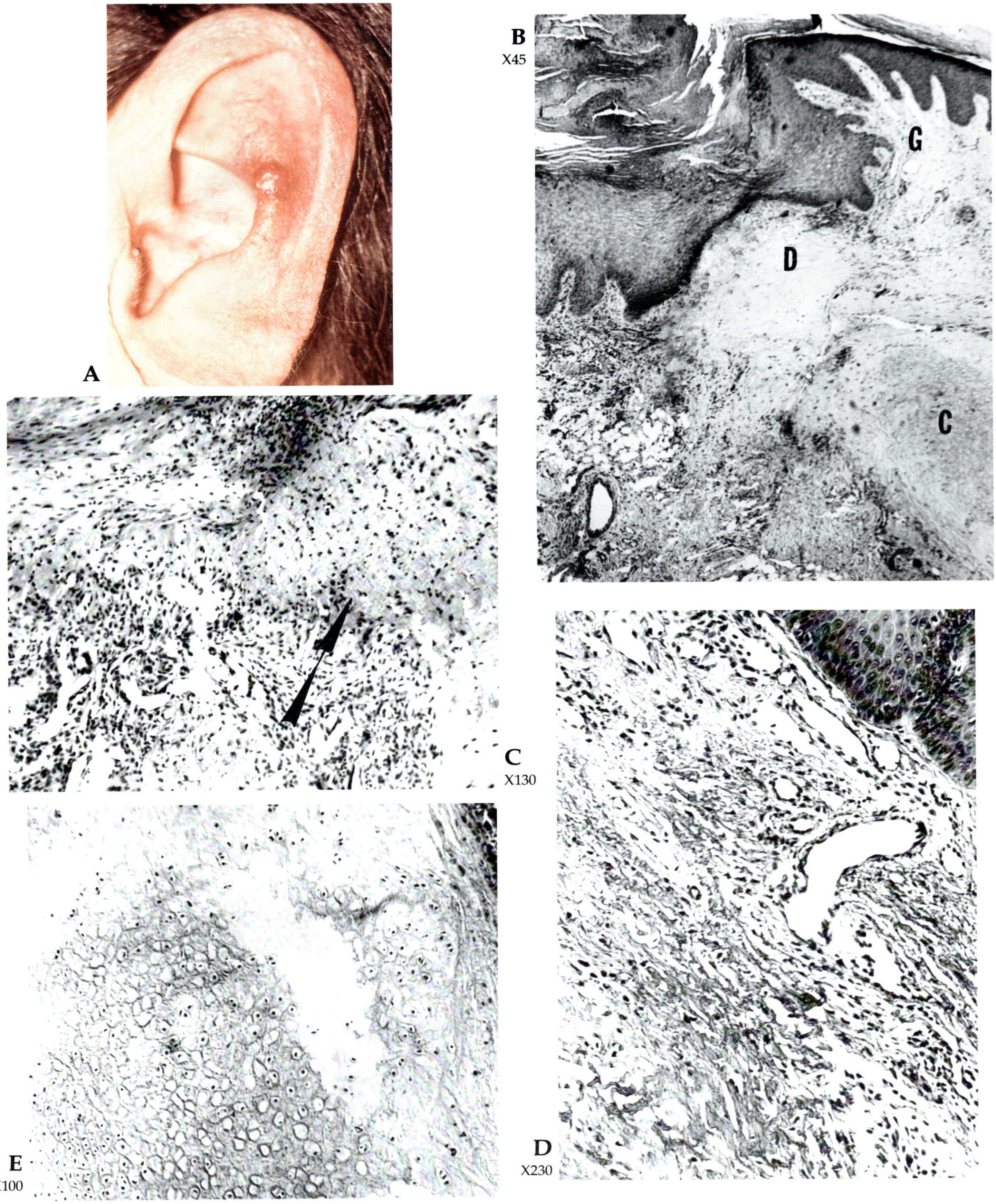

A

B X45

C X130

E X100

D X230

ELASTOSIS PERFORANS SERPIGINOSA

Elastosis perforans serpiginosa is a rare condition characterized by keratotic papules with an annular arrangement (Figs. A,B). The sides and back of the neck are common sites. The cause is unknown. Rarely, lesions are disseminated.

In some instances there is an association with Mongolism, pseudoxanthoma elasticum, Ehlers-Danlos syndrome, or Marfan's syndrome. There has been a recent report of elastosis perforans serpiginosa associated with renal disease.

It has been proposed that the pathogenesis of elastosis perforans serpiginosa may involve an increase in tropoelastin and a decrease in mature elastin.

Microscopic features

1. There is an invagination (Fig. C) filled with a hyperkeratotic and parakeratotic plug. In its lower portion, the plug contains basophilic, necrotic material and eosinophilic refractile fibers. The eosinophilic fibers have been regarded as elastic fibers which no longer take elastic tissue stains.
2. The epidermis adjacent to the plug is acanthotic (Figs. C,D).
3. The upper dermis, adjacent to the acanthotic epidermis, shows an inflammatory infiltrate (Fig. C) which may contain foreign body giant cells.
4. With elastic tissue stains, such as acid orcein Giemsa stain (Figs. C,D), the elastic fibers in the papillary dermis and dermal papillae adjacent to the plug are revealed as coarse and increased in number. Material taking the elastic tissue stain may be present in the plug and in a narrow channel through the epidermis, connecting the plug with the dermis.

Microscopic differential diagnosis (see chart, p. 632)

Comment

1. Penicillamine may induce lesions clinically identical to idiopathic elastosis perforans serpiginosa, but histologically somewhat different. There is less hyperplasia of elastic fibers in the papillary dermis and more hyperplasia in the mid- and deep dermis in the penicillamine induced variant. A unique feature of penicillamine induced elastosis perforans serpiginosa is the presence of budding of the elastic fibers of the mid- and deep dermis.
2. *Calcific elastosis* (perforating calcific elastosis) has been referred to as perforating pseudoxanthoma elasticum, but is not a variant of pseudoxanthoma elasticum. Calcific elastosis is one of the perforating dermatoses. It is observed in multiparous, middle-aged women, and appears as a pigmented periumbilical patch that may contain hyperkeratotic papules, verrucous areas, or a verrucous border. The histologic picture is similar to that of pseudoxanthoma elasticum, except that the altered, calcified elastic fibers are extruded through a transepidermal canal containing a hyperkeratotic plug.

ELASTOSIS PERFORANS SERPIGINOSA

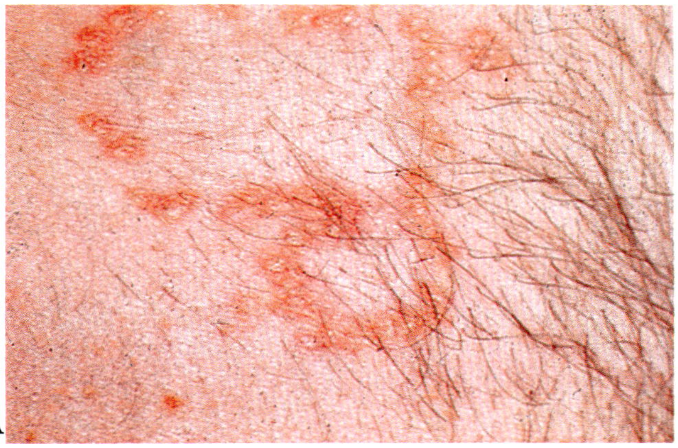

A

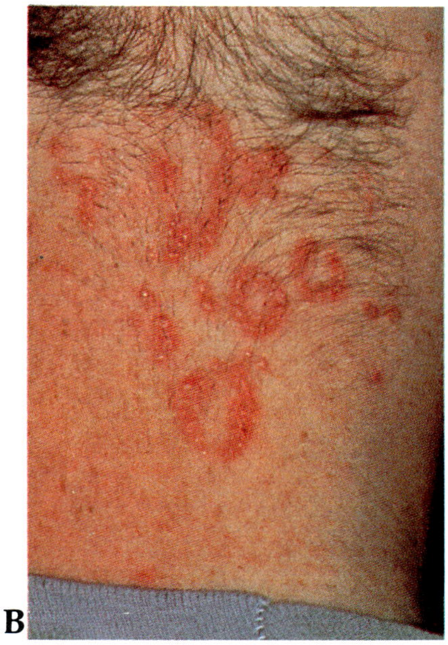

B

Courtesy Dr. Arnold Gellman

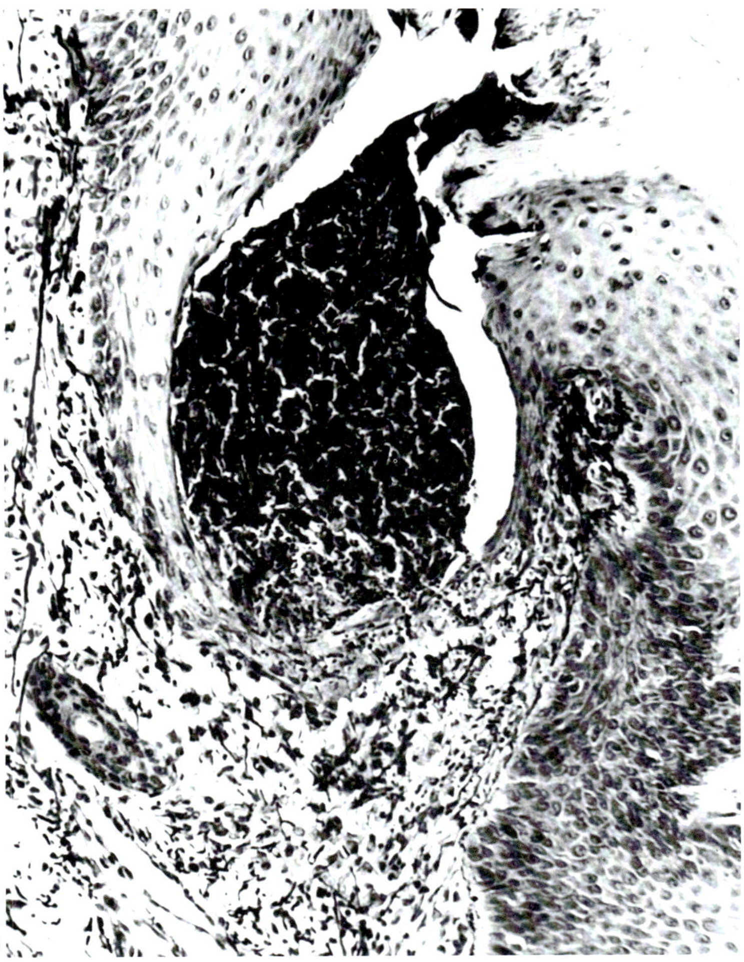

C

X450

ACID ORCEIN GIEMSA STAIN

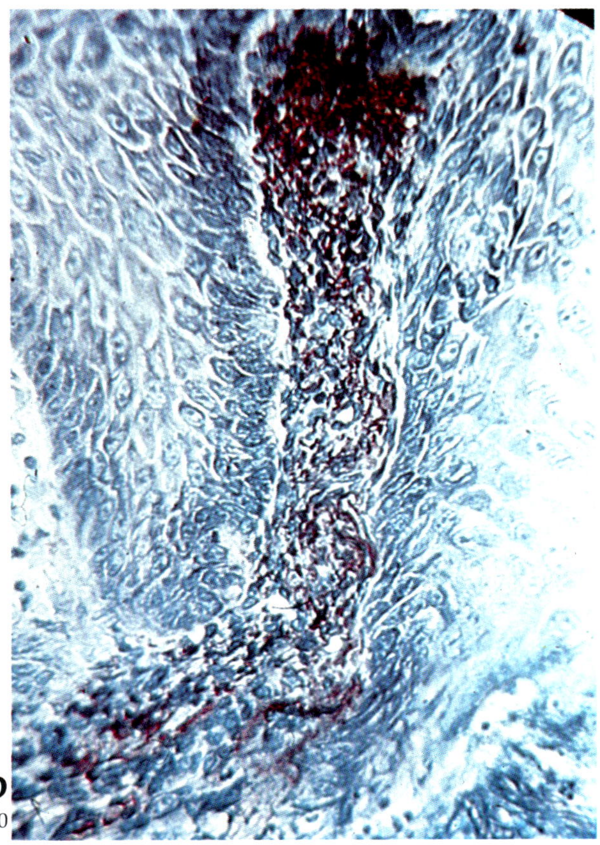

D

X450

ACID ORCEIN GIEMSA STAIN

KYRLE'S DISEASE (HYPERKERATOSIS FOLLICULARIS ET PERIFOLLICULARIS IN CUTEM PENETRANS)

Kyrle's disease is a rare condition characterized by papules with conical keratotic plugs (Figs. A,B); the papules are located at the follicular orifices or near them. Lesions may be widely distributed and tend to be numerous on the extremities. Lesions may coalesce to form verrucous areas. The cause of Kyrle's disease is unknown. There is evidence of an association with diabetes mellitus or the prediabetic state. Kyrle's disease has been reported in patients receiving hemodialysis for chronic renal failure. Many cases have no association with diabetes mellitus or chronic renal disease.

Microscopic features

1. There is a large hyperkeratotic and parakeratotic plug penetrating the epidermis (Fig. C). Parakeratotic, dyskeratotic, and vacuolated cells may extend to the basal layer of the epidermis.
2. The lower part of the plug contains granular necrotic material (Fig. D).
3. At the base of the plug, the epidermis is thinned or absent (Figs. C,D).
4. There is an inflammatory infiltrate (Fig. D), and often a foreign body granuloma is found in the dermis at the site of penetration of the keratotic material. Degenerated granulomatous material may move into the transepidermal canal. The hyperkeratotic and parakeratotic plug does not always penetrate to the dermis.
5. There are no elastic tissue abnormalities.

Microscopic differential diagnosis (see chart, below)

Comment

It has been suggested that Kyrle's disease represents a focal disorder of epidermal keratinization, in which keratinization is more rapid than keratinocyte proliferation, leading to a transepidermal canal.

MICROSCOPIC DIFFERENTIAL DIAGNOSIS OF THE PERFORATING DERMATOSES

	Kyrle's disease	*Perforating folliculitis*	*Elastosis perforans serpiginosa*	*Reactive perforating collagenosis*
Keratotic material within invagination	present	present	present	present
Site of invagination	at or near follicular openings	follicular openings	random	random
Elastic tissue abnormalities	none	none	coarse elastic fibers in papillary dermis	none
Collagen abnormalities	none	none	none	necrobiotic collagen is present in the papillary dermis and in the keratotic plug

KYRLE'S DISEASE

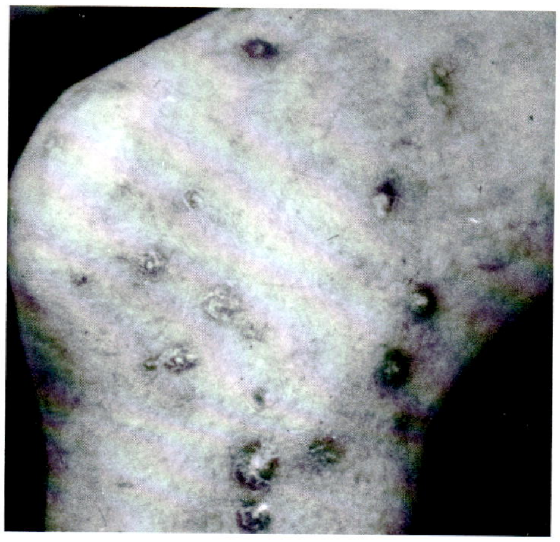
A

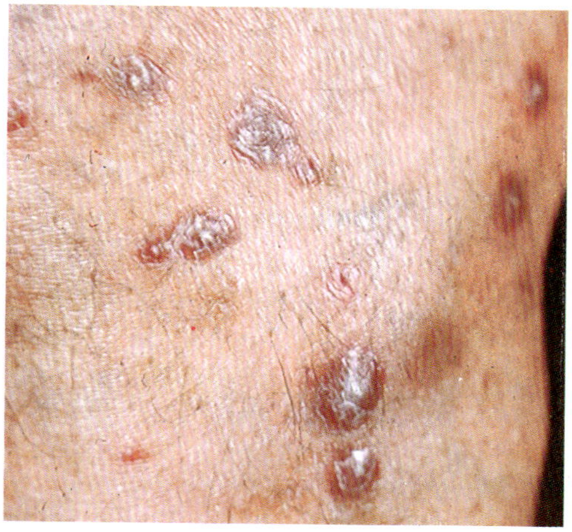
B

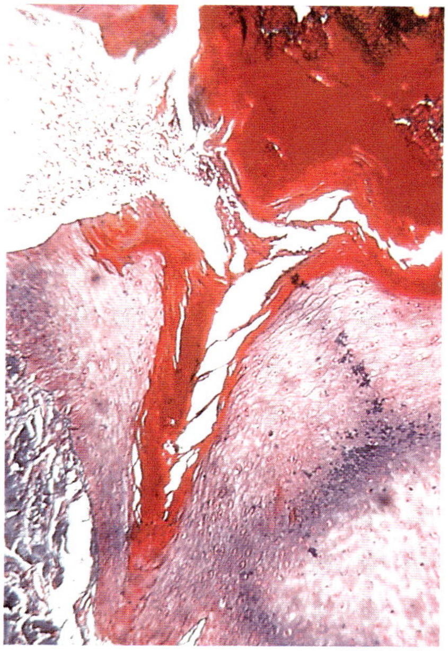
C
X120
TRICHROME STAIN

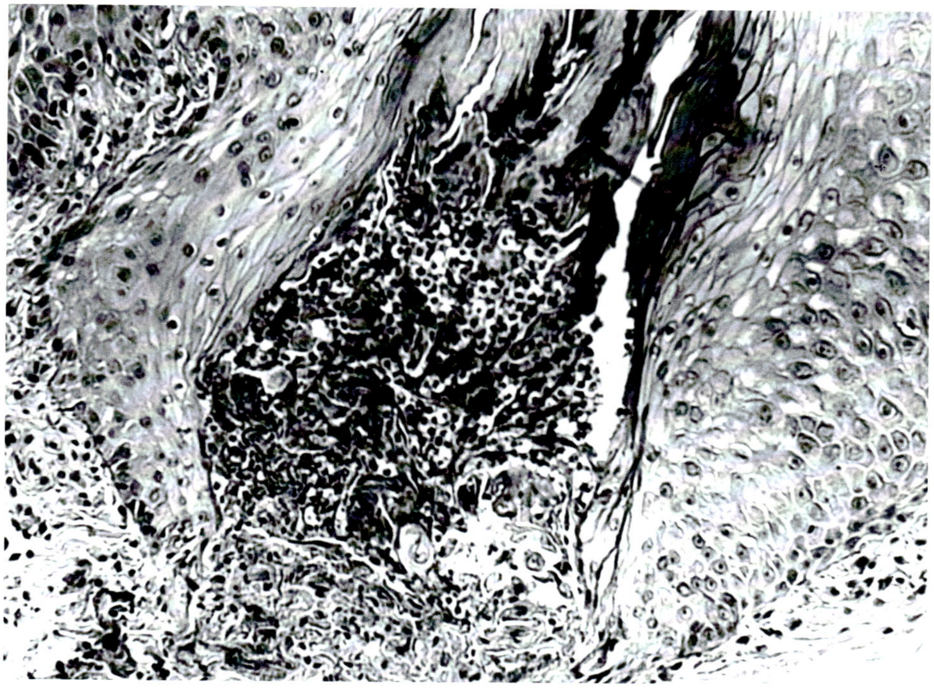
D
X230

PERFORATING FOLLICULITIS

This was a common disorder whose incidence appears to have decreased recently. There is a close clinical resemblance to Kyrle's disease. Unlike Kyrle's disease, lesions do not have a tendency to coalesce, and they are located exclusively in hair follicles. The condition can be associated with diabetes mellitus and renal failure.

Microscopic features

1. The picture parallels that of Kyrle's disease, except that the transepithelial canal is located in the follicular infundibulum (Figs. A,B). Eosinophilic fibers are present in the canal. These are believed to be degenerated elastic fibers that have lost their orceinophilic staining property.
2. There are no elastic tissue abnormalities in the dermis.

Microscopic differential diagnosis (see chart, p. 632)

Comment

It has been suggested that the spring action of rolled-up thin hair is responsible for the initial break in the follicular wall.

PERFORATING FOLLICULITIS

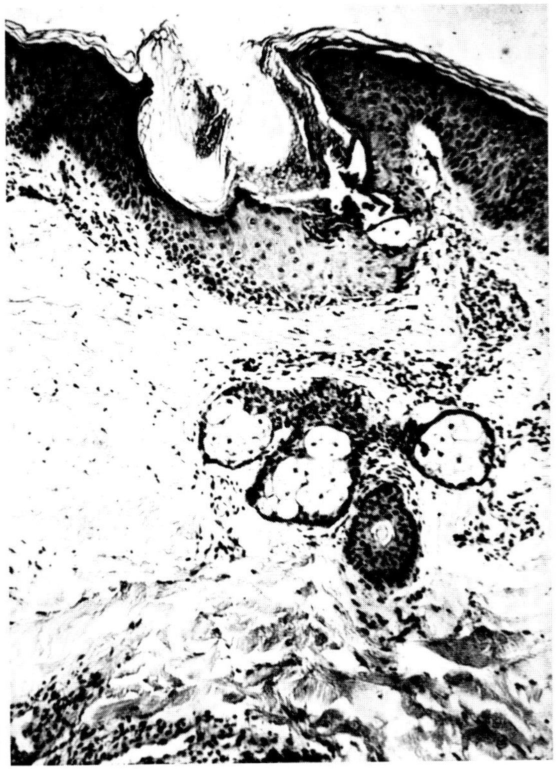

A
X120

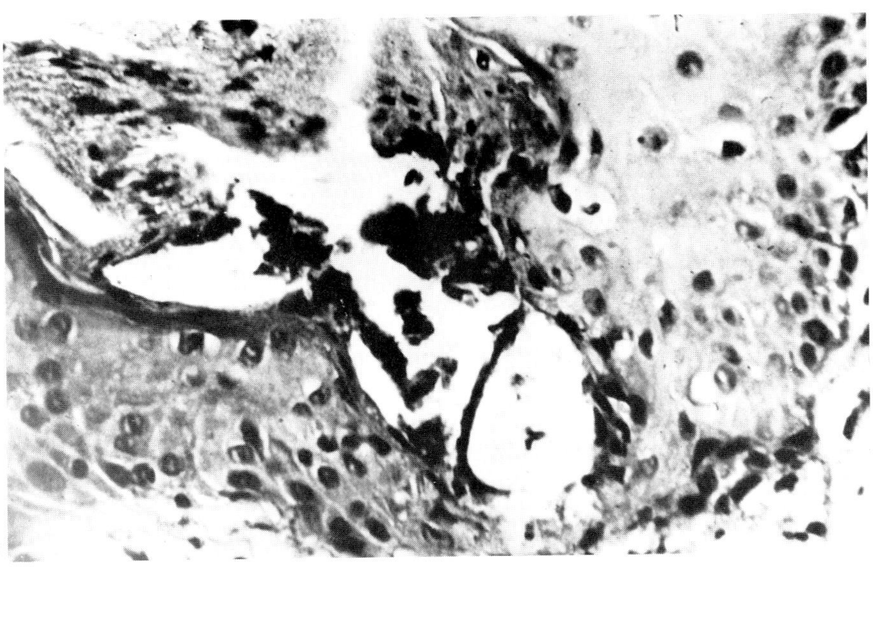

B
X540

REACTIVE PERFORATING COLLAGENOSIS

Reactive perforating collagenosis is a rare disorder in which umbilicated papules develop in response to trauma. There may be autosomal recessive inheritance.

The extensor surfaces of the extremities are common sites (Fig. A).

Onset is usually in infancy or childhood. Some cases start in adult life; these cases may be associated with severe diabetes mellitus with chronic renal insufficiency. Lesions tend to involute in 6 to 10 weeks, and new lesions may continue to appear. Scars may be present in the involved areas.

Microscopic features

1. The initial microscopic change is an accumulation of necrobiotic basophilic collagen in a widened papilla with surrounding inflammatory reaction (Fig. B).
2. A hyperkeratotic and parakeratotic plug subsequently develops in an invagination of dermis overlying the widened papilla (Fig. C). The adjacent epidermis is acanthotic and may show channels of degenerating collagen extending from the epidermal-dermal junction to the plug.
3. There is regeneration of epidermis at the base of the invagination after the degenerated dermal material has been eliminated (Fig. D).
4. There is no increase in elastic fibers in the dermis and no stainable elastic fibers in the plug.

REACTIVE PERFORATING COLLAGENOSIS

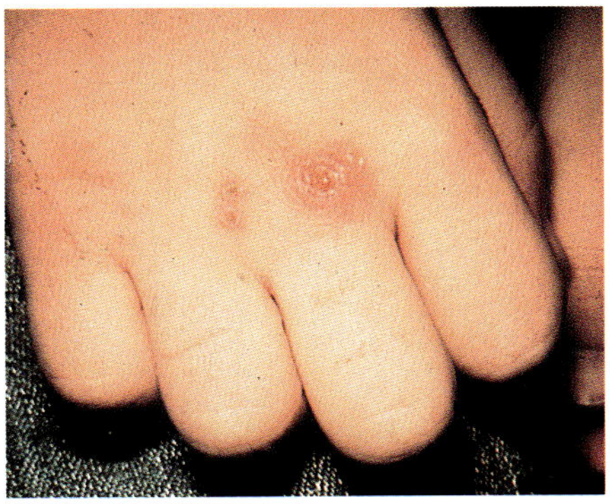

A

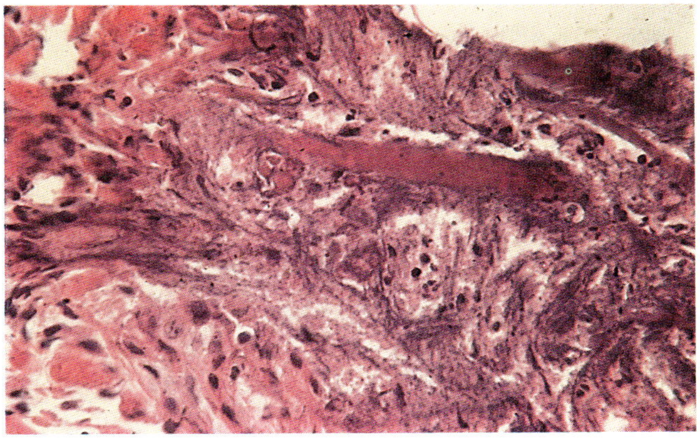

B
X540

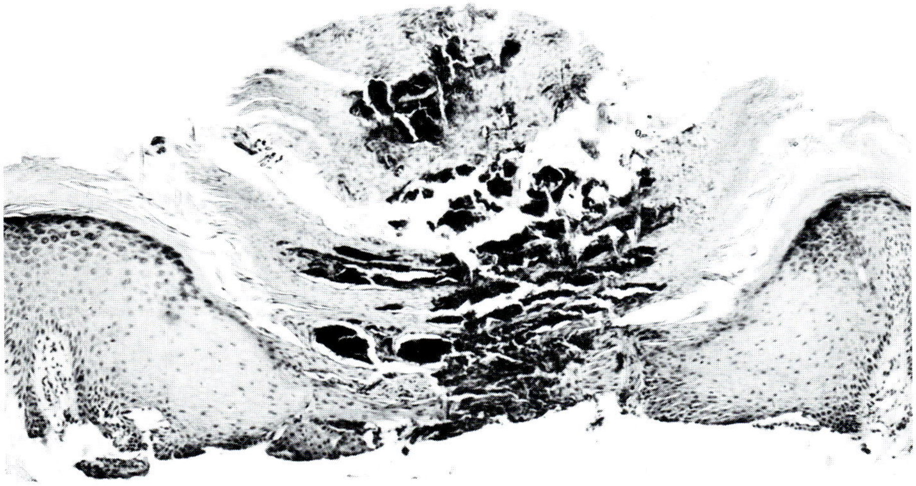

C
X120

Figs. C,D courtesy Dr. Amir Mehregan

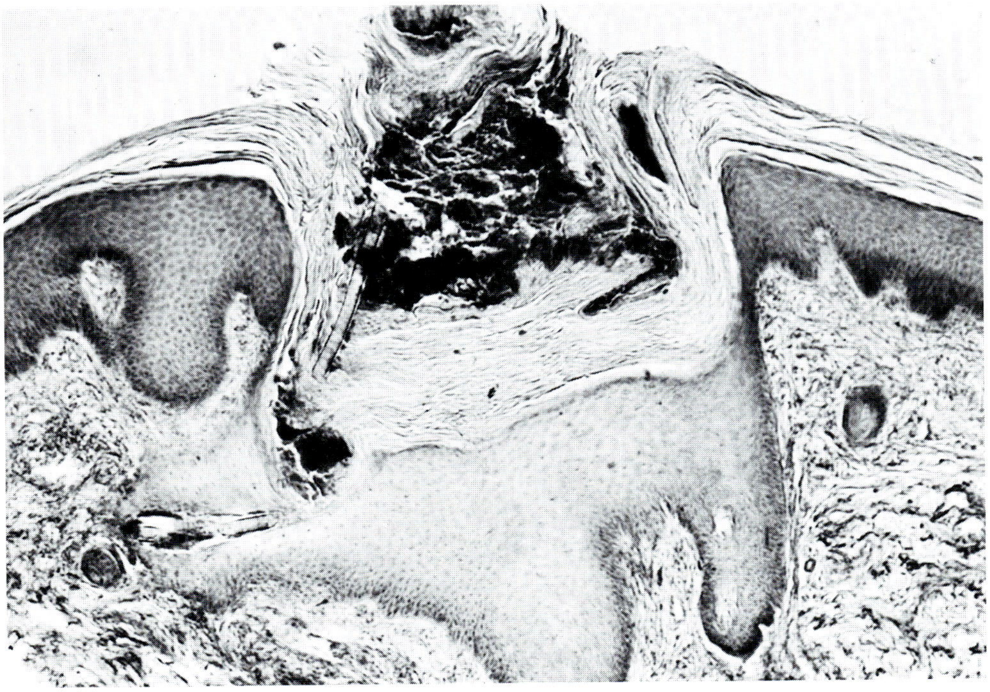

D
X120

Degenerative dermatoses

NECROBIOTIC DISORDERS

Granuloma annulare, necrobiosis lipoidica, and rheumatoid nodule have in common degeneration of connective tissue referred to as necrobiosis.

The term "necrobiosis" is rather archaic and imprecise. The definition "physiologic death of tissue" does not apply here. Partial death of connective tissue may be more applicable to these disorders. We retain the term because it is still being used.

The necrobiotic disorders may show a granulomatous response to the degenerated material, and this granuloma may have a palisading pattern.

There is a perforating variant of granuloma annulare, and this variant is one of the perforating disorders.

A newly described entity with histologic changes similar to those of necrobiotic disorders is the allergic reaction to injected bovine collagen.The histologic pattern resembles granuloma annulare.

GRANULOMA ANNULARE

Granuloma annulare is a fairly common disorder of unknown cause, with a predilection for children and young adults. Lesions are papules or nodules in ring formation (Figs. A,B). When the papules and nodules are closely approximated or fused, the rings appear uninterrupted (Fig. A). The hands and feet are common sites. Rings of granuloma annulare are usually solitary or few in number, but occasionally may be disseminated (Fig. C). Generalized papular granuloma annulare has been reported to have an association with diabetes mellitus or AIDS. Infrequently, granuloma annulare may appear as erythematous patches on which papules develop. Other variants include perforating granuloma annulare, in which the degenerated collagen is eliminated via a transepidermal canal, and subcutaneous granuloma annulare. Subcutaneous granuloma annulare has clinical and microscopic features similar to rheumatoid nodule. Whether to call such lesions granuloma annulare or pseudorheumatoid nodule is moot. Granuloma annulare and necrobiosis lipoidica may coexist.

Microscopic features

1. In the focal histologic type of granuloma annulare there is a circumscribed area of extensive collagen degeneration surrounded by lymphoid cells, histiocytes, and fibroblasts in palisade arrangement (Figs. D,E). The degenerated collagen is usually basophilic due to mucin content.
2. There is a scattered mixed inflammatory infiltrate in the dermis. Occasionally this contains a high percentage of eosinophils.
3. Neutral and acid mucopolysaccharides are generally present in the areas of collagen degeneration. In some instances, lipid droplets can be demonstrated in frozen sections with fat stain.
4. Rarely, giant cells and groups of epithelioid cells may be present.
5. Subcutaneous nodules of granuloma annulare show the histologic changes described above, but the degenerated collagen tends to be eosinophilic, with a resemblance to rheumatoid nodule.

GRANULOMA ANNULARE

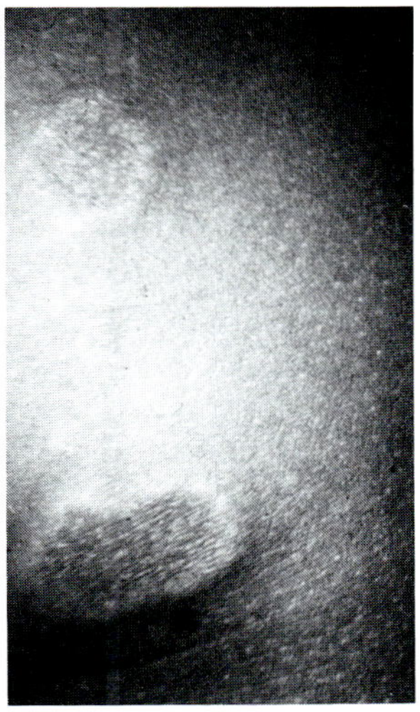

A

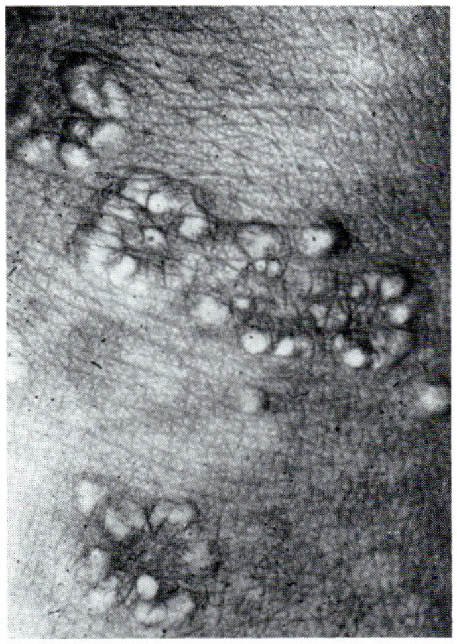

B

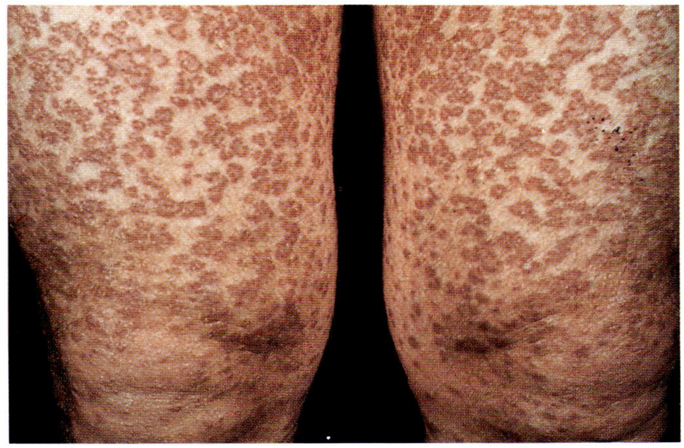

C

Courtesy Dr. Paul Birnbaum

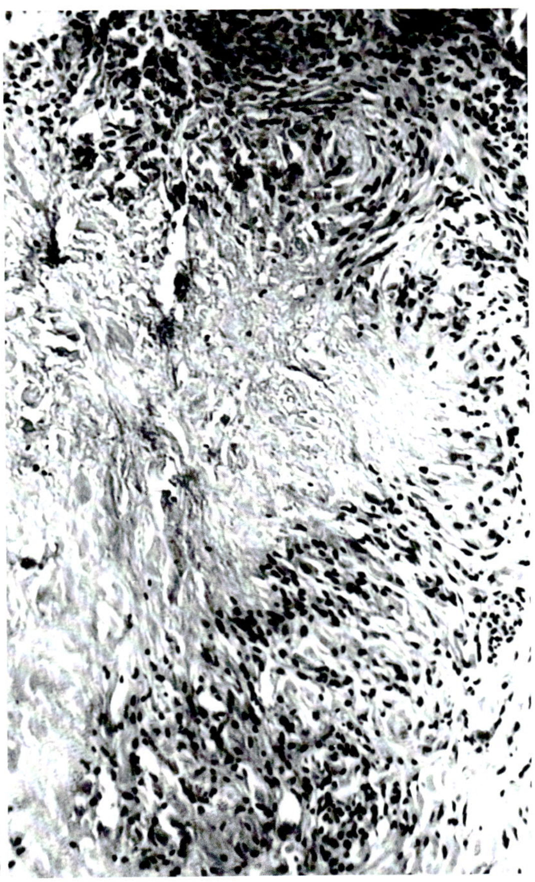

D
X190

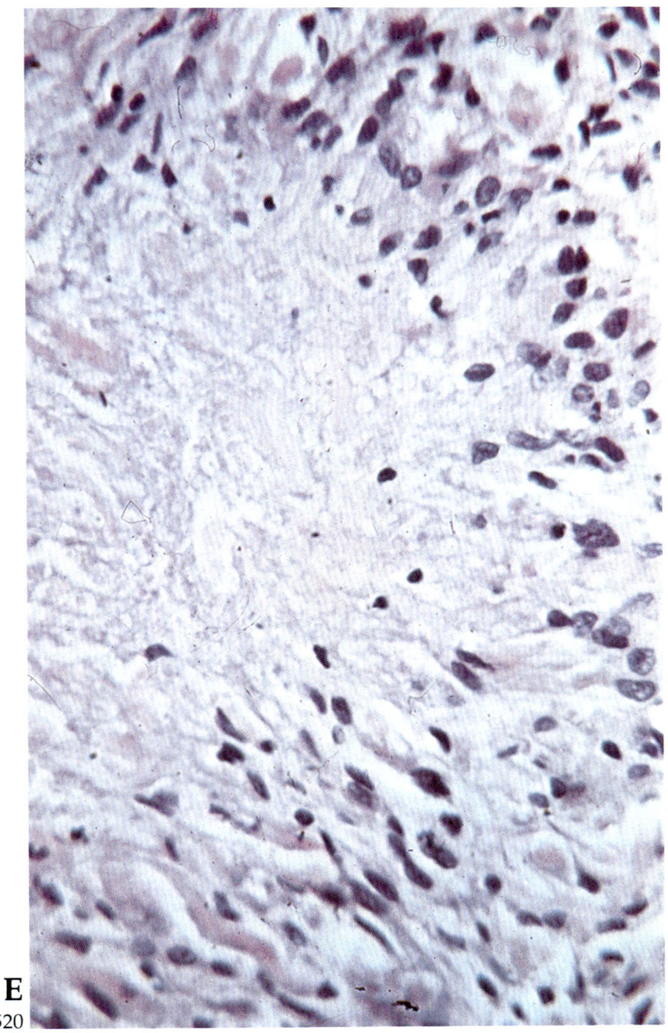

E
X520

GRANULOMA ANNULARE continued

GRANULOMA ANNULARE

Microscopic features

6. In the more common diffuse histologic type of granuloma annulare, there are scattered areas of partial degeneration of collagen (Figs. C,D), intermingled with lymphoid cells, histiocytes, and fibroblasts, often in linear arrangement (Figs. A,B). With low magnification, collagen degeneration may not be readily apparent (Fig. A), but the diagnosis may be suspected by the linear arrangement of the infiltrate.

Microscopic differential diagnosis (see p. 652)

1. The diffuse type of granuloma annulare has a histologic resemblance to dermatofibroma. The proliferating epidermis, usually present in dermatofibroma can help make the distinction.
2. Surprisingly, degenerating foam cells in eruptive xanthoma can resemble degenerated collagen in granuloma annulare. Fat stains of frozen sections may not make the distinction, since extracellular lipid may present in granuloma annulare. Clinical and laboratory data are important.
3. Histologic distinction of granuloma annulare from necrobiosis lipoidica can be difficult. Necrobiosis lipoidica generally shows more extensive areas of collagen degeneration, has a greater tendency towards granuloma formation (with more giant cells), and usually shows more pronounced vascular changes. The collagen degeneration in necrobiosis lipoidica tends to be more eosinophilic than in granuloma annulare. Clinical information may be essential in distinguishing these entities.

GRANULOMA ANNULARE

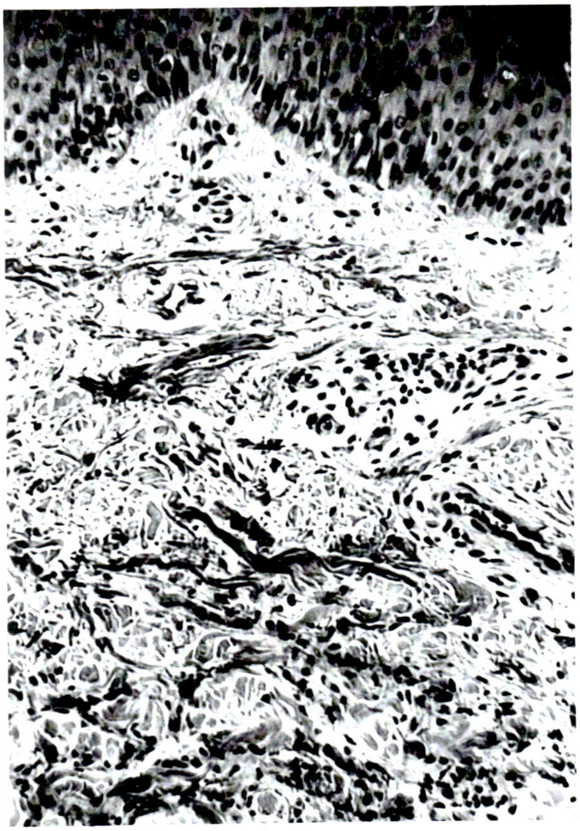

A
X170

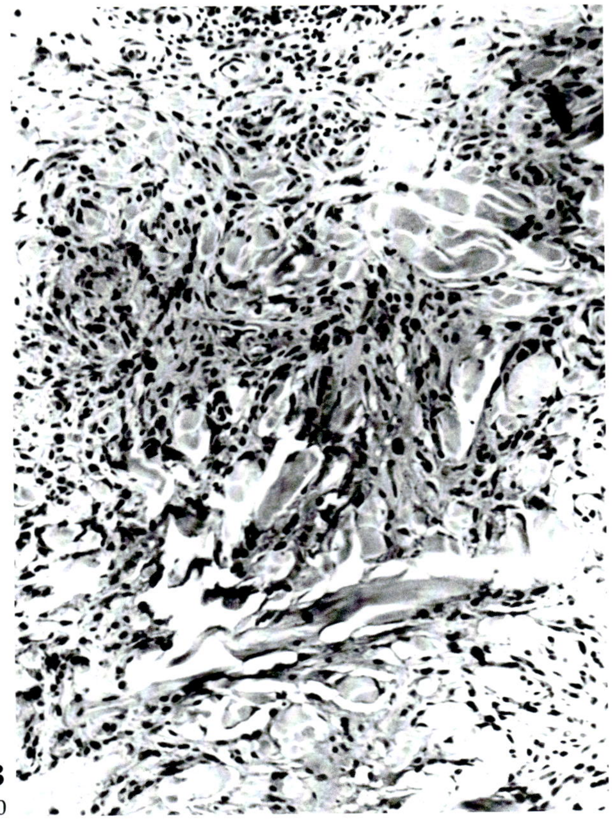

B
X150

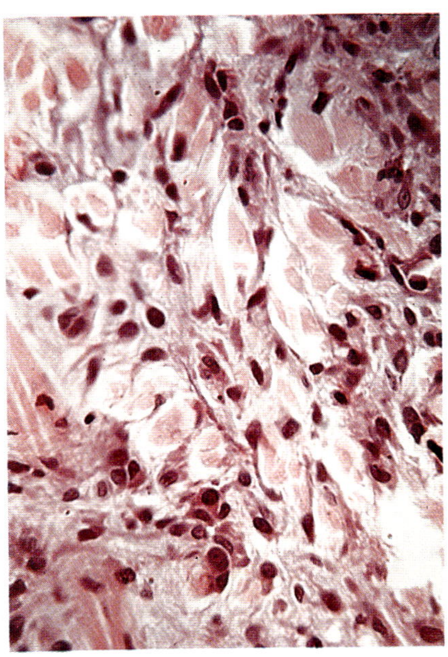

C
X540

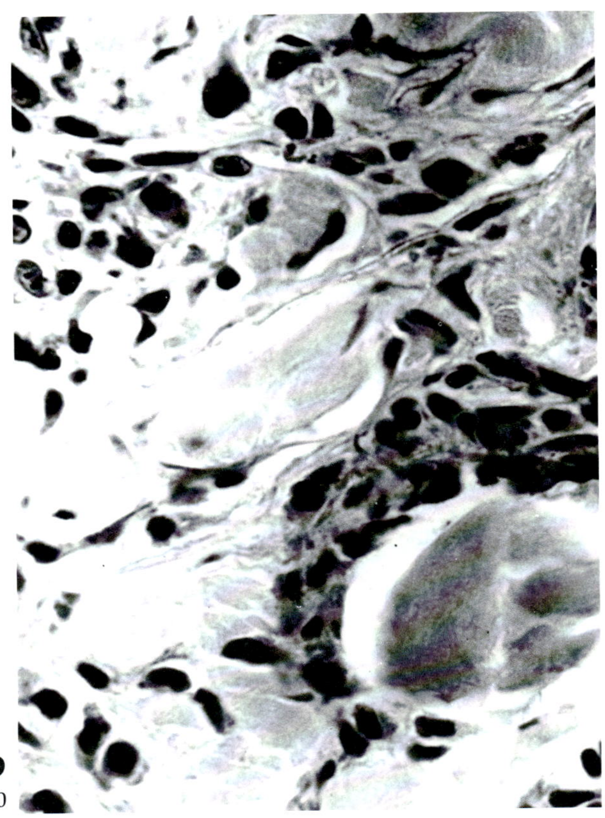

D
X670

GRANULOMA ANNULARE continued ⇨

GRANULOMA ANNULARE

Comment

Annular elastolytic granuloma (actinic granuloma) is an entity that has been the subject of considerable controversy. Lesions are elevated rings with hypopigmented centers—having a clinical resemblance to granuloma annulare. The usual location is the face (Fig. A). Some authors consider this entity to be a variant of granuloma annulare; others consider it a granulomatous response to solar degeneration of connective tissue, as the name *actinic granuloma* indicates. The basic process may be a granulomatous destruction of elastic tissue or a cell-mediated immune response to actinically damaged elastic fibers. Key histologic features are loss of elastic tissue accompanied by giant cells containing phagocytosed fragments of elastic fibers (Fig. B).

It is of interest that intracellular elastin has been observed in generalized granuloma annulare, deep granuloma annulare, granuloma multiforme (an African variant of granuloma annulare), and elastosis perforans serpiginosa. This was not found in necrobiosis lipoidica.

ANNULAR ELASTOLYTIC GRANULOMA

A

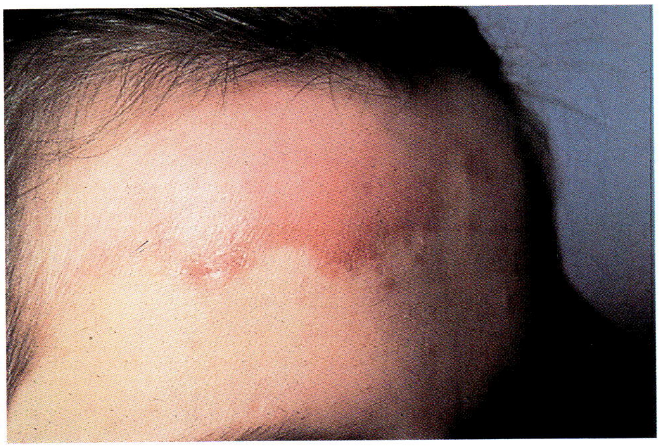

Figs. A,B courtesy Dr. Dalal Assaad

B
X420

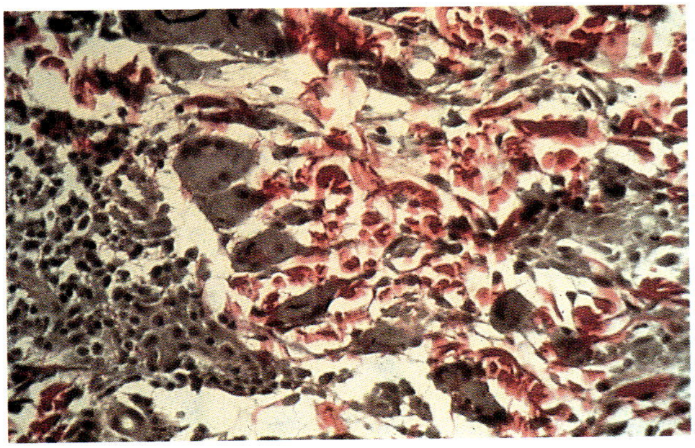

VERHOEFF-VAN GIESON STAIN

GRANULOMA ANNULARE continued ⇨

PERFORATING GRANULOMA ANNULARE

This is a rare form characterized by localized (Figs. A,B) or generalized umbilicated lesions.

Microscopic features

1. The epidermis shows a transepidermal elimination canal or ulceration (Figs. C,D). The dermis shows the usual changes of granuloma annulare (Fig. C).
2. There is a focus of collagen degeneration just below the transepidermal elimination canal or ulceration (Figs. C,D).

PERFORATING GRANULOMA ANNULARE

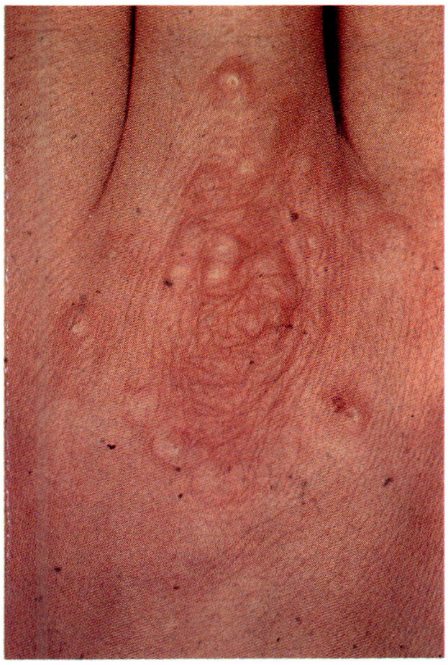

A

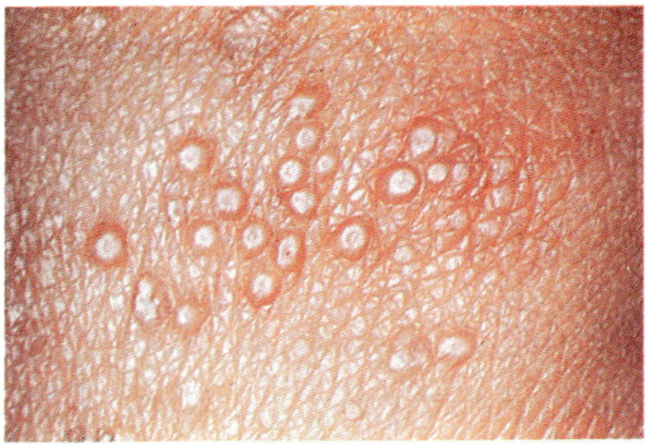

B

Courtesy Dr. John Walter

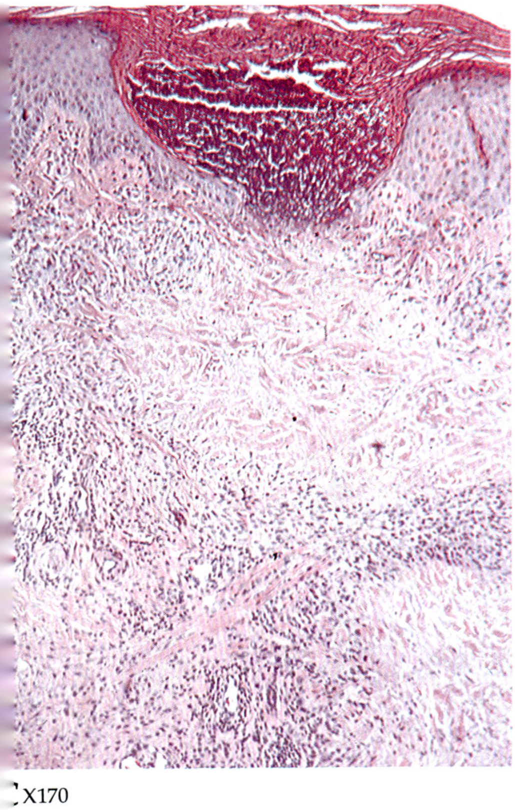

C X170

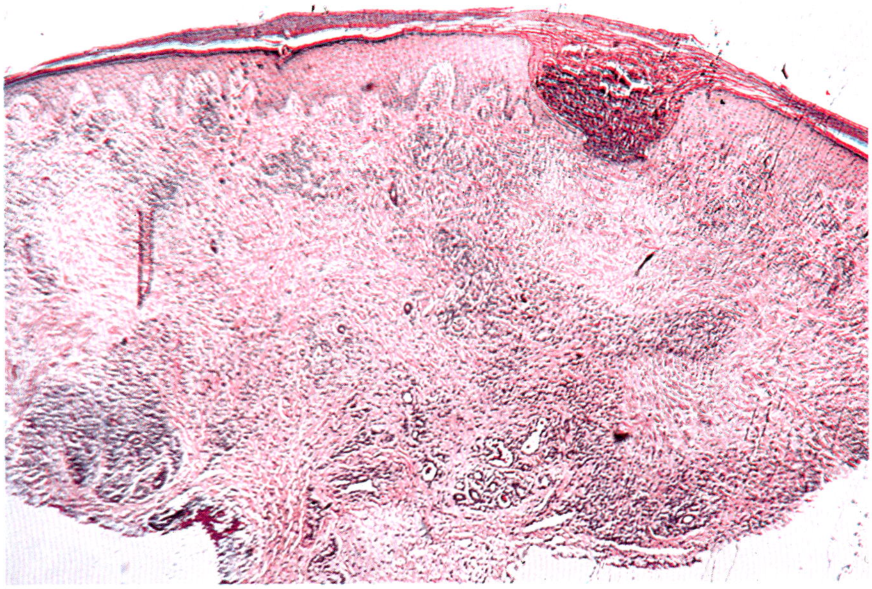

D X40

NECROBIOSIS LIPOIDICA

Necrobiosis lipoidica has a much higher incidence in women than in men, and it is often associated with clinically evident or latent diabetes mellitus.

Lesions may be unilateral or bilateral and occur principally on the anterior and lateral surfaces of the lower legs (Fig. A). Other reported sites include the thighs, hands, forearms, face, and scalp. Early lesions are nodules and plaques with a deeply violaceous color (Fig. A). With progression, a yellowish central area develops. Late lesions have an atrophic, translucent yellowish appearance, with visible superficial vessels (Fig. B). Ulceration may occur. Lesions outside the legs may resemble granuloma annulare. A rare perforating variant of necrobiosis lipoidica has been described, with transfollicular elimination of degenerated material.

Microscopic features

1. Large areas of collagen degeneration are present in the dermis. These are characterized by fragmentation of the fibers, deposits of neutral mucopolysaccharides, and occasionally deposits of acid mucopolysaccharides. Affected collagen fibers show loss of structural detail (Fig. C) and generally are eosinophilic (Figs. C,D).
2. A granulomatous infiltrate is often present (Fig. D).
3. The epidermis may be normal, atrophic, or ulcerated.

NECROBIOSIS LIPOIDICA

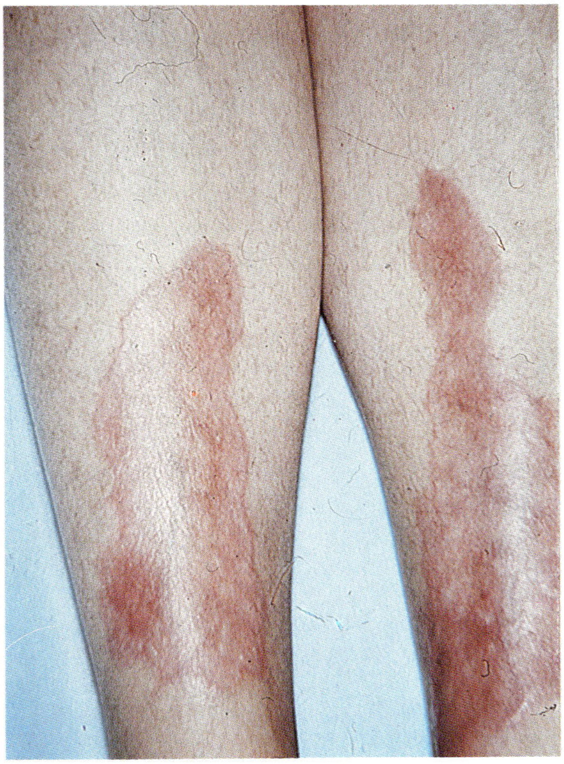
A

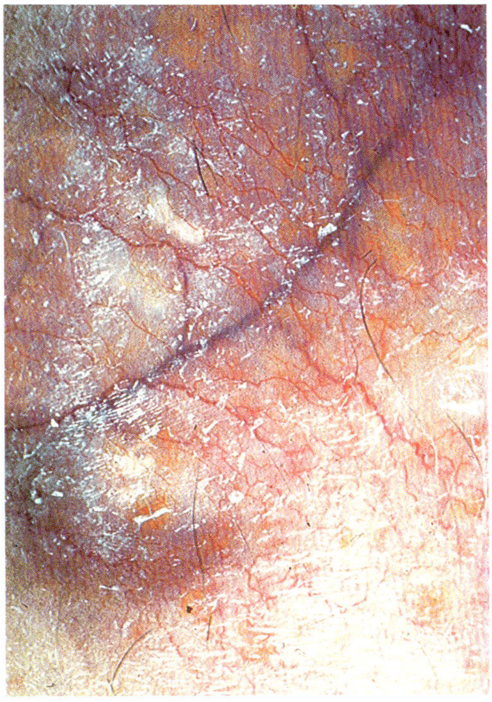
B

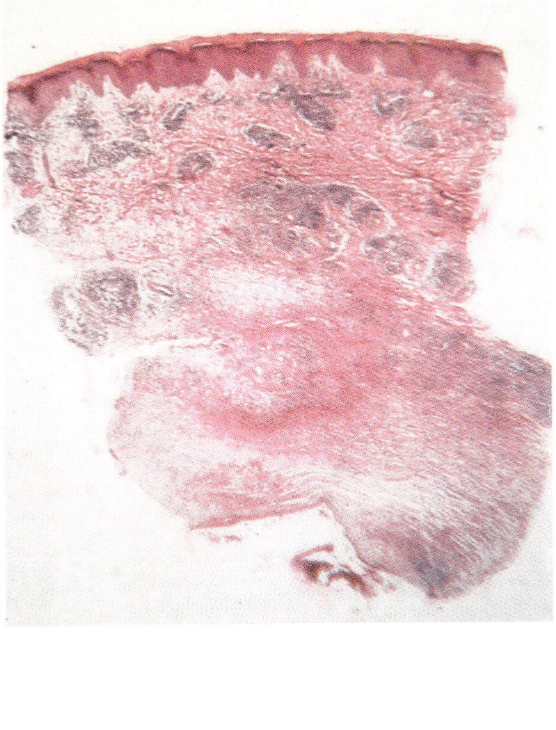
C
X30

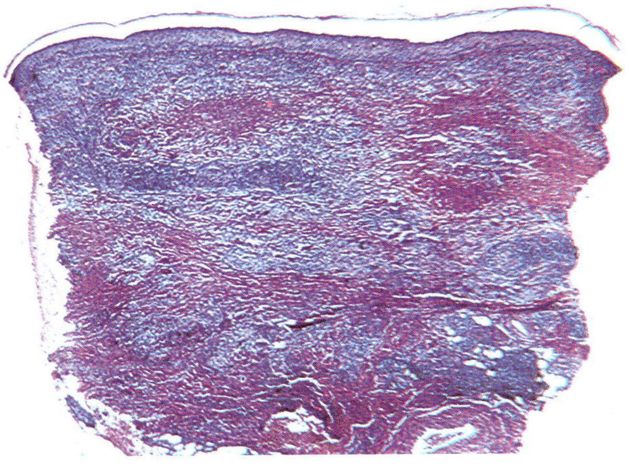
D
X30

NECROBIOSIS LIPOIDICA continued

NECROBIOSIS LIPOIDICA

Microscopic features

4. With higher magnification, loss of structural detail, edema, and thickening of collagen fibers are evident (Fig. D).
5. The granulomatous infiltrate in areas of collagen degeneration (Figs. C,E) may be extensive. The term *granulomatosis disciformis* has been used to describe lesions in which the granulomatous component is prominent. Palisading granulomas may be observed.
6. Foreign body giant cells are common (Fig. A). In the section illustrated, the foreign body giant cell appears to be engulfing degenerated collagen. A lymphoid cell infiltrate (Fig. A) may be present around the area of degenerating collagen.
7. A diffuse inflammatory infiltrate and occasionally a leukocytoclastic vasculitis (Fig. B) may be present.
8. Fat stains (frozen sections) demonstrate extracellular lipid deposits.
9. Blood vessels show thickening of their walls and endothelial proliferation; this is most pronounced in lesions from the lower legs. The vessel changes may be related to the diabetic or prediabetic state. PAS-positive, diastase-resistant material may be present in the vessel walls.

Microscopic differential diagnosis (see p. 652)

Comment

Pretibial pigmented patches (diabetic dermopathy) are atrophic lesions occurring in about 20% of diabetics. Their histologic appearance is nonspecific. There is chronic inflammation, hemosiderin deposition, and thickening of blood vessels (diabetic microangiopathy).

The vessels may have deposits of PAS-positive, diastase-resistant material.

Lesions often develop in response to trauma, and are sometimes associated with subepidermal bullae on the dorsal surfaces of the hands (bullosis diabeticorum).

NECROBIOSIS LIPOIDICA

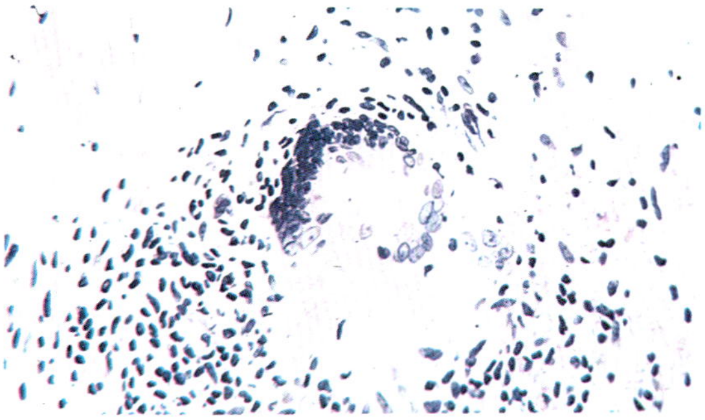

A
X180

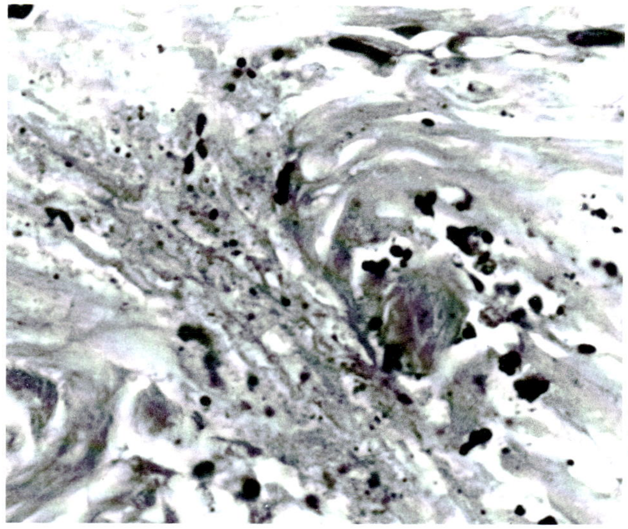

B
X770

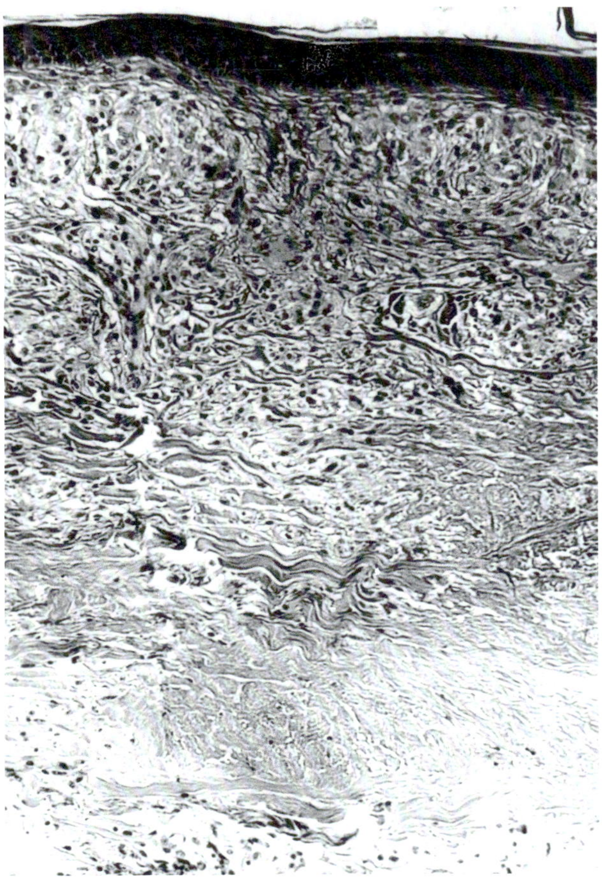

C
X130

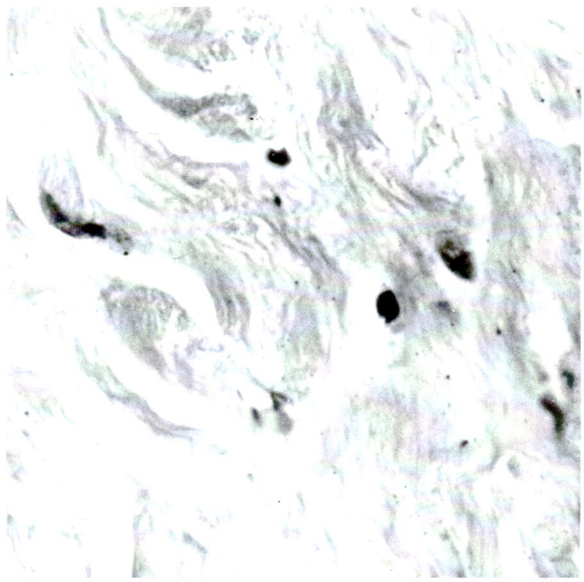

D
X770

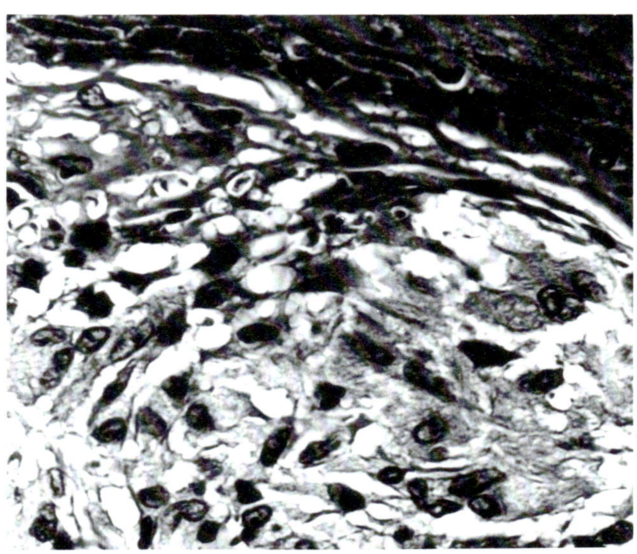

E
X520

RHEUMATOID NODULE

Subcutaneous nodules may develop near joints or bony prominences in rheumatic fever or rheumatoid arthritis (Fig. A).

Rheumatoid nodules rarely occur in lupus erythematosus. They also may be observed in the absence of rheumatic disease or lupus erythematosus.

Microscopic features

1. Early lesions show granulation tissue.
2. Large foci of fibrinoid degeneration of collagen then develop around blood vessels.
3. Fully formed lesions show large areas of eosinophilic fibrinoid degeneration of collagen surrounded by histiocytes and fibroblasts in palisade arrangement (Figs. B,C). The stroma between these foci shows granulation tissue and fibrosis.
4. Lipid may be present in areas of degeneration or in the granulomatous areas.

Microscopic differential diagnosis

Some helpful features in the histologic differential diagnosis of granuloma annulare, necrobiosis lipoidica, and rheumatoid nodule

1. Degenerated collagen in granuloma annulare is usually basophilic, whereas in necrobiosis lipoidica and rheumatoid nodule it is usually eosinophilic.
2. Rheumatoid nodules are subcutaneous, whereas lesions of granuloma annulare and necrobiosis lipoidica are primarily intradermal.
3. Collagen changes are usually more widespread in necrobiosis lipoidica than in granuloma annulare. In addition, giant cells, histiocytes, and epithelioid cells are usually more numerous in necrobiosis lipoidica.

RHEUMATOID NODULE

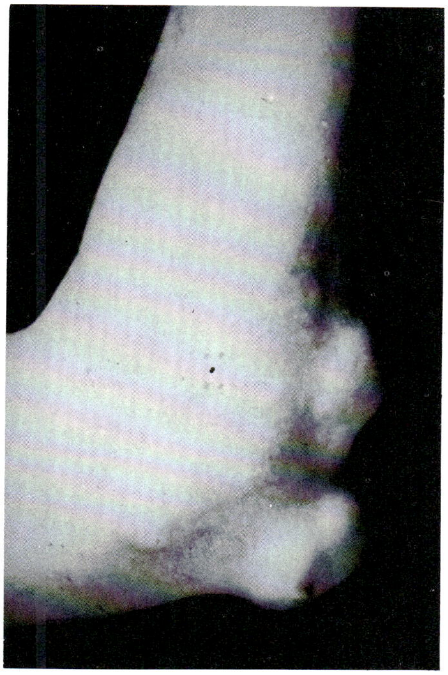

A

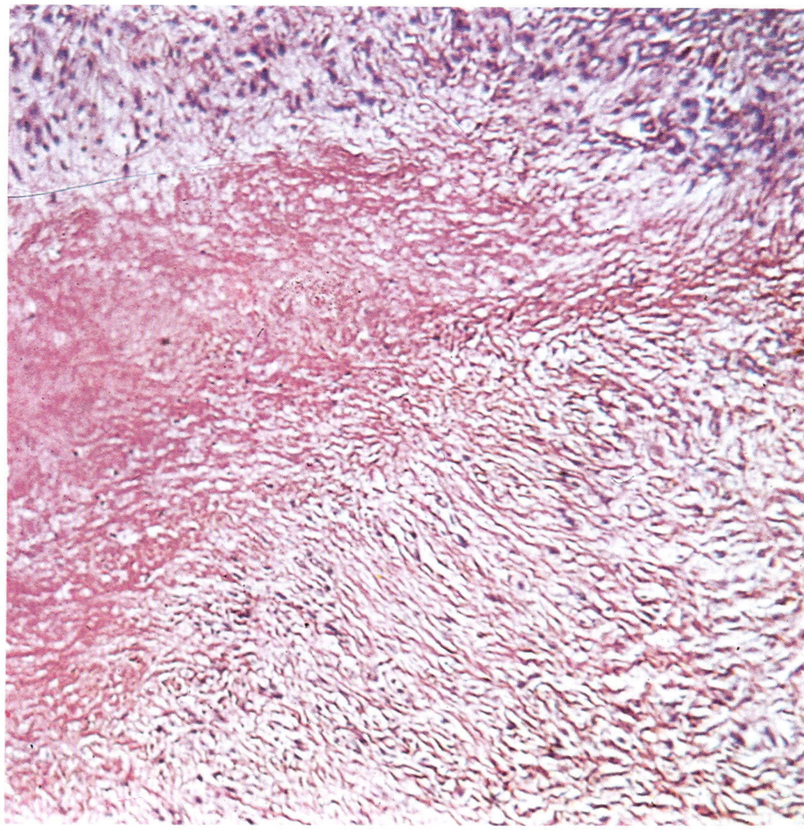

B
X210

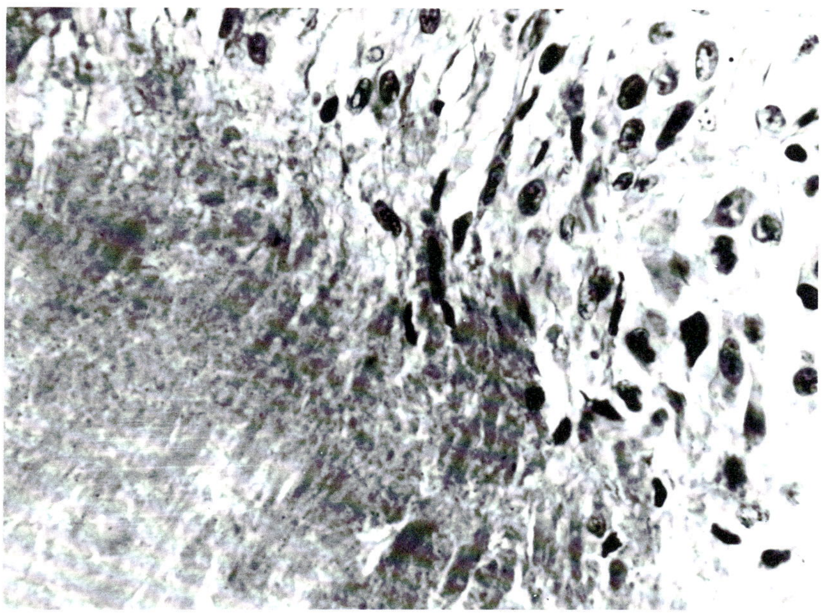

C
X520

LICHEN SCLEROSUS ET ATROPHICUS

Lichen sclerosus et atrophicus has some clinical and microscopic resemblance to localized scleroderma. Most authors consider lichen sclerosus et atrophicus to be completely distinct from scleroderma, but some consider it a variant. Women are affected more often than men. Inherited factors may play a role in the development of lichen sclerosus et atrophicus.

Initial lesions are polygonal, slightly umbilicated whitish papules (Fig. A). These tend to coalesce and evolve into depigmented, atrophic patches (Figs. B,C,D,E,F). Bullous components may be present, which can become hemorrhagic.

The female genitals and adjacent perianal areas are frequently involved (Figs. C,D). This is called *kraurosis vulvae*. Kraurosis vulvae is often confused with leukoplakia. Unlike leukoplakia, however, the lesions are atrophic rather than hypertrophic. Also unlike leukoplakia, kraurosis vulvae only rarely culminates in *squamous cell carcinoma*. The genitals are also commonly involved in males. Involvement of the glans penis (Fig. E) is called *balanitis xerotica obliterans*. Squamous cell carcinoma is a rare sequel of balanitis xerotica obliterans.

LICHEN SCLEROSUS ET ATROPHICUS

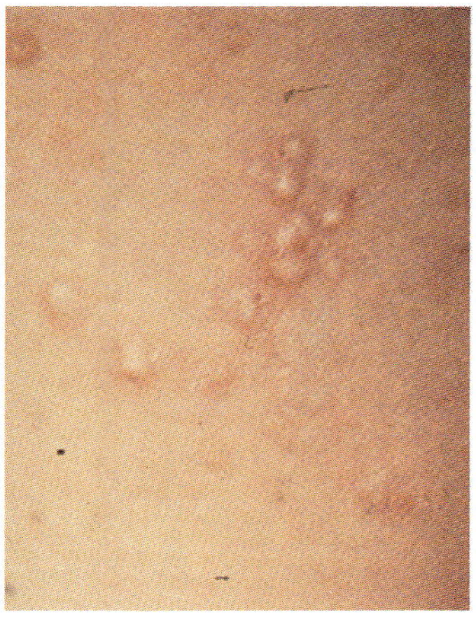

A

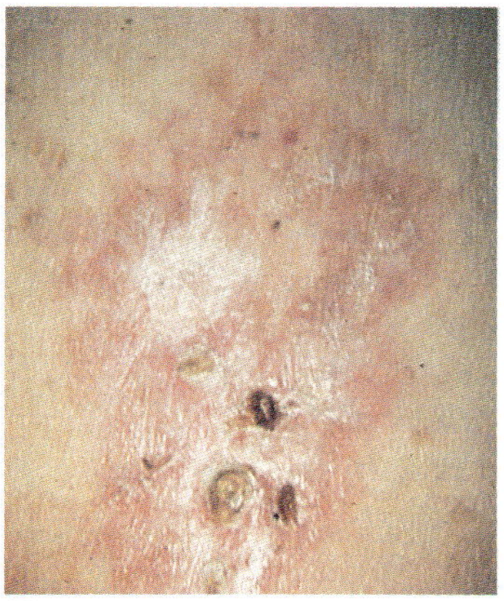

B

Figs. A,B courtesy Dr. Henry Jolly

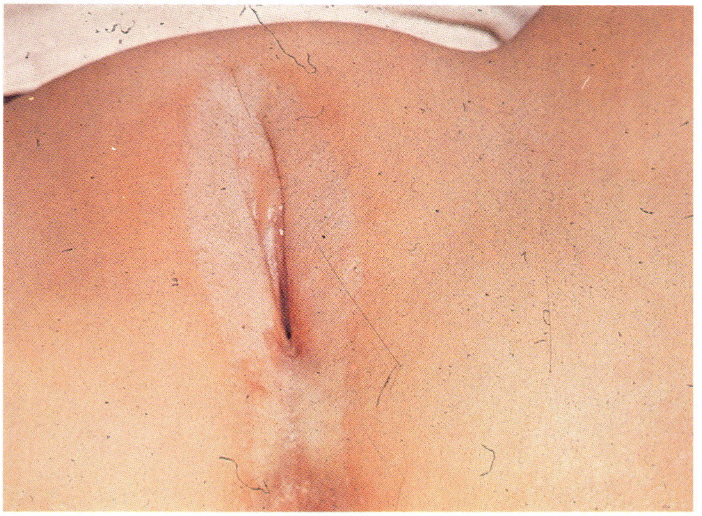

C

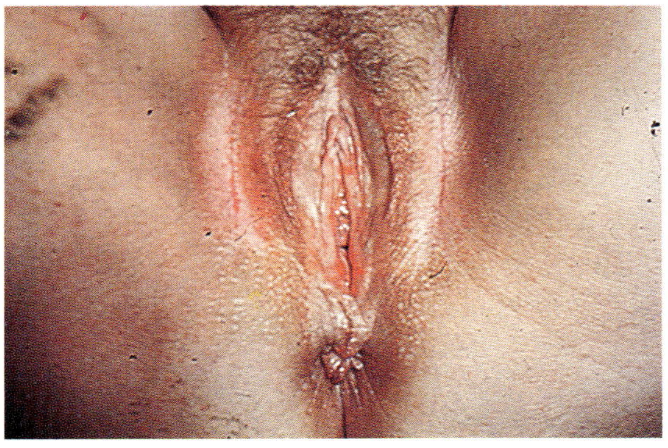

D

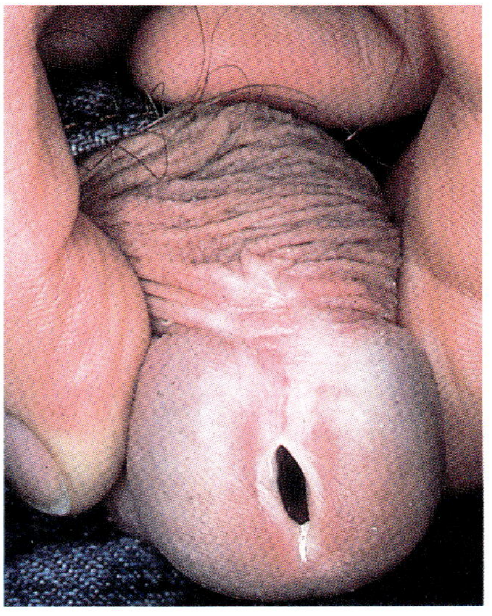

E

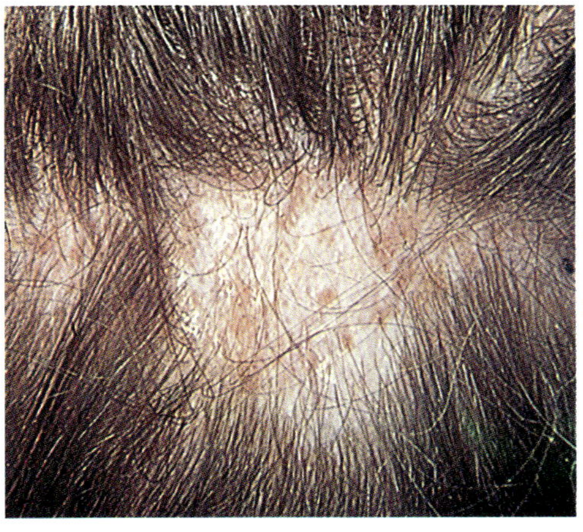

F

LICHEN SCLEROSUS ET ATROPHICUS continued ⇨

Degenerative dermatoses

LICHEN SCLEROSUS ET ATROPHICUS

Microscopic features

1. There is atrophy of the epidermis with hyperkeratosis and keratotic plugging (Figs. A,B). Hydropic damage is present in the basal layer (Figs. B,C,D).
2. A zone of severe edema and homogenization of collagen is present in the upper dermis ("ground glass" edema) (Figs. A,B,C). Elastic fibers are decreased in this zone and hemorrhage may be present.
3. There is an infiltrate composed principally of lymphoid cells (Figs. B,C) in the dermis, just below the zone of edema. In early lesions the infiltrate is located at higher levels of the dermis.

LICHEN SCLEROSUS ET ATROPHICUS

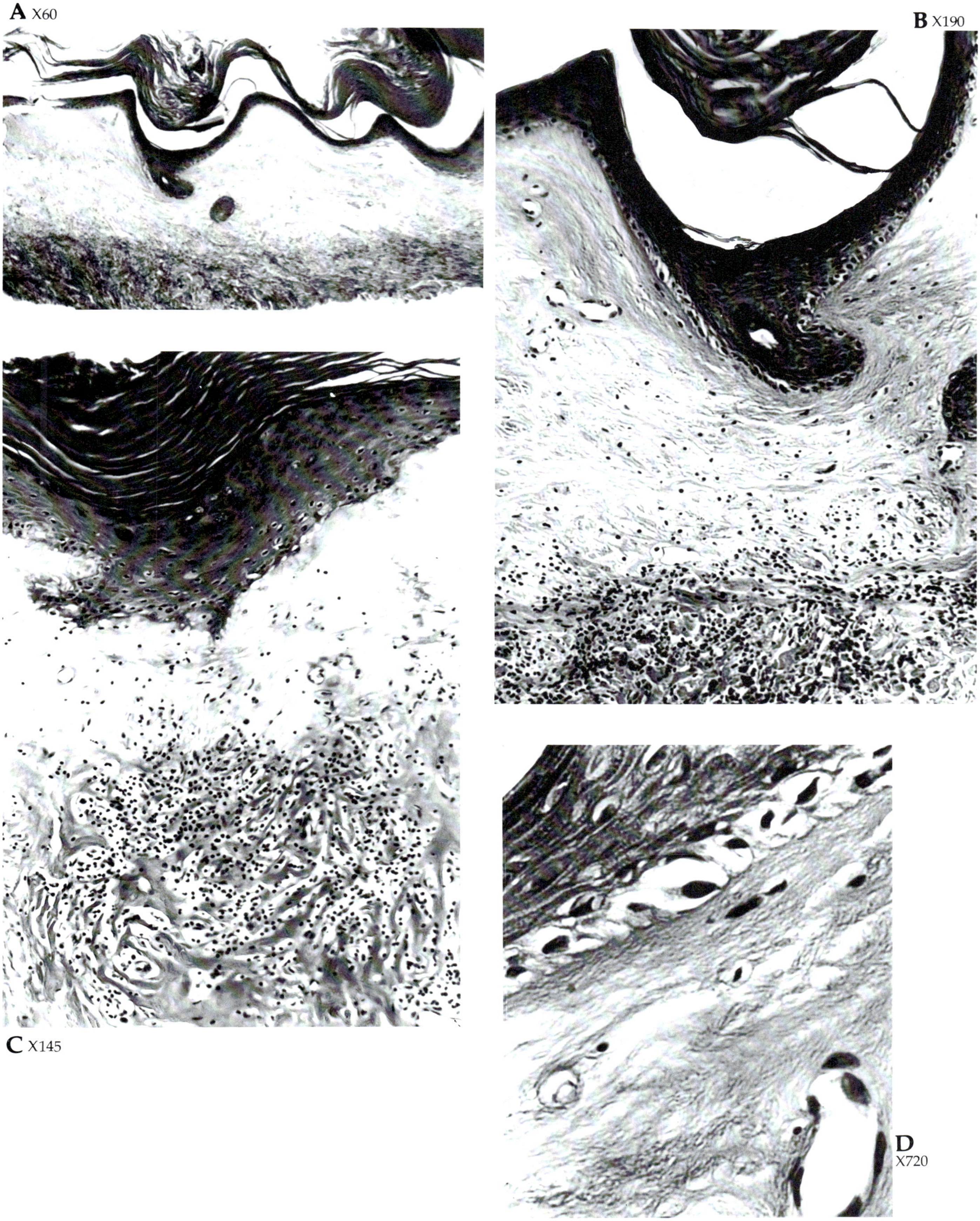

A X60

B X190

C X145

D X720

LICHEN SCLEROSUS ET ATROPHICUS continued ⇨

LICHEN SCLEROSUS ET ATROPHICUS

Microscopic features

4. Hydropic damage of the basal layer of the epidermis and severe edema of the upper dermis may result in subepidermal bullae (Fig. A).
5. In longstanding lesions, the collagen fibers in the lower dermis may show thickening and homogenization (Fig. B).

Microscopic differential diagnosis

1. The sclerotic changes in collagen in the late lesions produce a resemblance to scleroderma. However, differentiation from scleroderma can usually be made on the basis of the changes in the basal layer and edema of the upper dermis in lichen sclerosus et atrophicus.
2. Changes in the epidermis are similar to those of lupus erythematosus. The "ground glass" edema of the upper dermis in lesions of lichen sclerosus et atrophicus facilitates microscopic differentiation, as does the deep sclerosis.

LICHEN SCLEROSUS ET ATROPHICUS

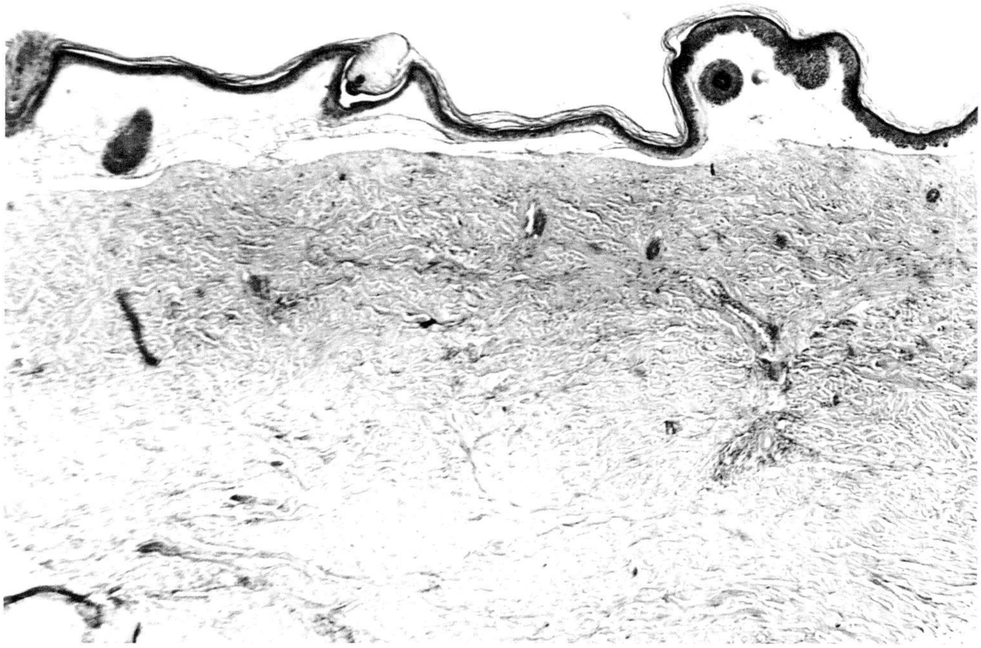

A
X43

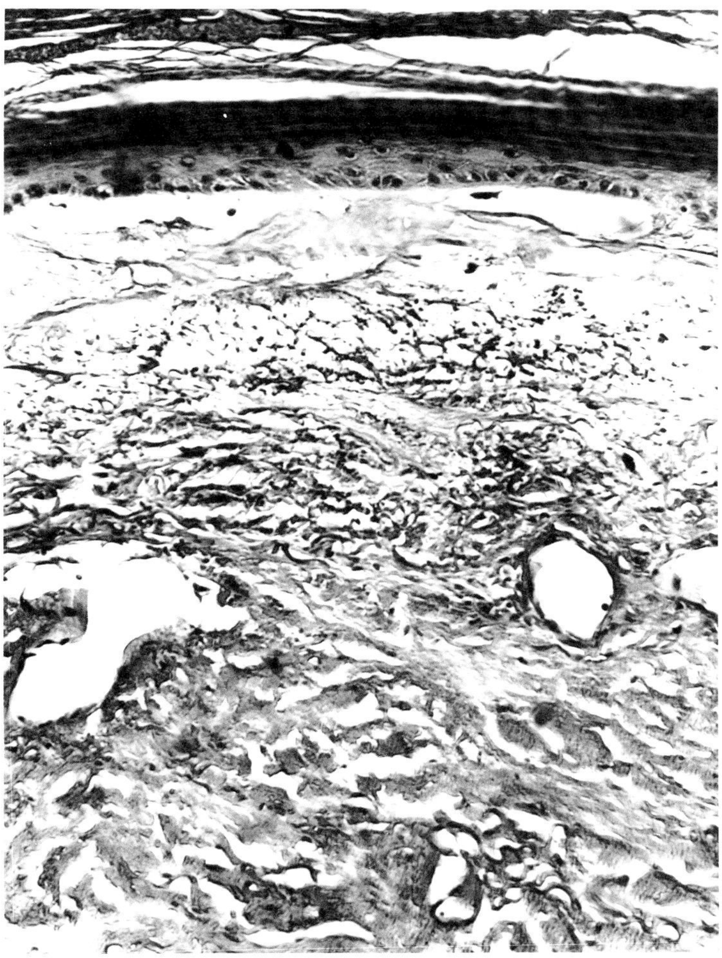

B
X190

Degenerative dermatoses

MUCINOSES

Accumulation of mucin in the skin is observed in a wide variety of conditions. In this section we will discuss some conditions in which accumulation of mucin is a dominant or key feature. There are numerous conditions in which deposition of mucin is a minor or secondary feature.

I. Mucinoses associated with thyroid dysfunction
  - Generalized myxedema
  - Pretibial myxedema

II. Mucinoses associated with abnormal gamma globulin
  - Lichen myxedematosus

III. Other mucinoses
  - Mucous cyst of the oral mucosa
  - Digital mucous cyst
  - Alopecia mucinosa
  - Reticular erythematous mucinosis (REM)
  - Scleredema
  - The genetic mucopolysaccharidoses

The genetic mucopolysaccharidoses are hereditary disorders characterized by the accumulation of mucopolysaccharides in various tissues due to specific lysosomal enzyme deficiencies.

There are marked differences in clinical expression, hereditary transmission, and enzymatic abnormality in the various types of mucopolysaccharidoses. Examples are the Hurler and Hunter syndromes.

Common clinical features seen in this group of disorders include dwarfism, skeletal abnormalities, hepatosplenomegaly, corneal opacity, mental deterioration, and cardiorespiratory disease.

In the skin, metachromatic granules are present within fibroblasts, in eccrine glands, and sometimes in epidermal cells. Circulating lymphocytes show metachromatic granules in smear preparations.

CIRCUMSCRIBED MYXEDEMA (PRETIBIAL MYXEDEMA)

Circumscribed myxedema occurs in Graves' disease, which includes non-nodular goitrous hyperthyroidism and exophthalmos. All three components need not be present. Patients may be euthyroid or hypothyroid. About 50% of the patients have a circulating IgG called LATS (long-acting thyroid stimulator). Lesions may be waxy, indurated plaques with dilated follicular openings (Fig. A) or nodules (Fig. B). The anterior tibial areas are the usual sites, but there may be involvement of the dorsal aspects of the feet. Localized myxedema associated with Graves' disease may occur in unusual locations, such as the shoulders, neck, and pinnae.

Microscopic features

1. Extensive areas of basophilic, stringy mucin deposition are present in the mid-dermis (Fig. C,D).
2. Fibroblasts are not increased in number in the involved areas, but they often have a stellate configuration.
3. The mucin is hyaluronic acid and takes stains for acid mucopolysaccharides (see p. 5).

Comment

1. *Generalized myxedema* occurs in patients with hypothyroidism. The skin is diffusely pale, swollen, and dry. Broadening of the nose, as well as swelling of the eyelids and feet may be present. With routine stains, histologic abnormalities are not generally apparent; there may be slight separation of collagen fibers. With stains for acid mucopolysaccharides, small amounts of mucin can be demonstrated in the vicinity of blood vessels and around hair follicles.
2. *Scleredema adultorum (Buschke)* is characterized by generalized brawny edema. It may follow infections, and persistent cases may be associated with diabetes mellitus. There is thickening of the dermis and a diffuse deposition of hyaluronic acid, which gives collagen fibers a fenestrated appearance. Late stages resemble scleroderma. The process begins on the face and extends to the neck and upper trunk. Sometimes the term scleredema is used alone, since the disorder can occur in children.

CIRCUMSCRIBED MYXEDEMA

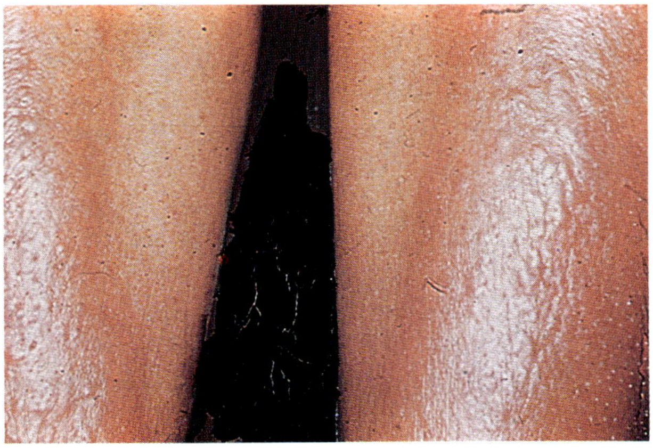

A

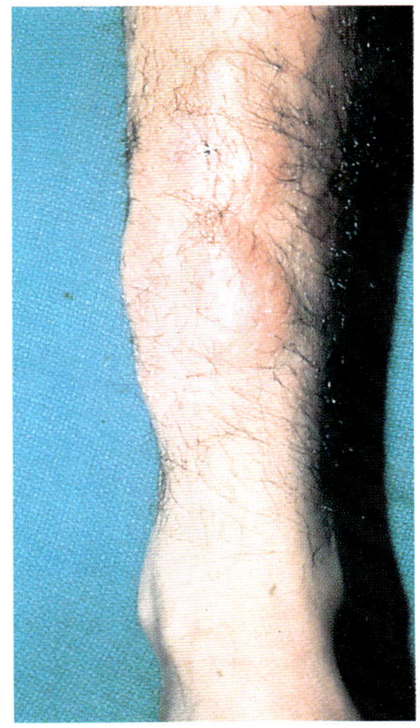

B

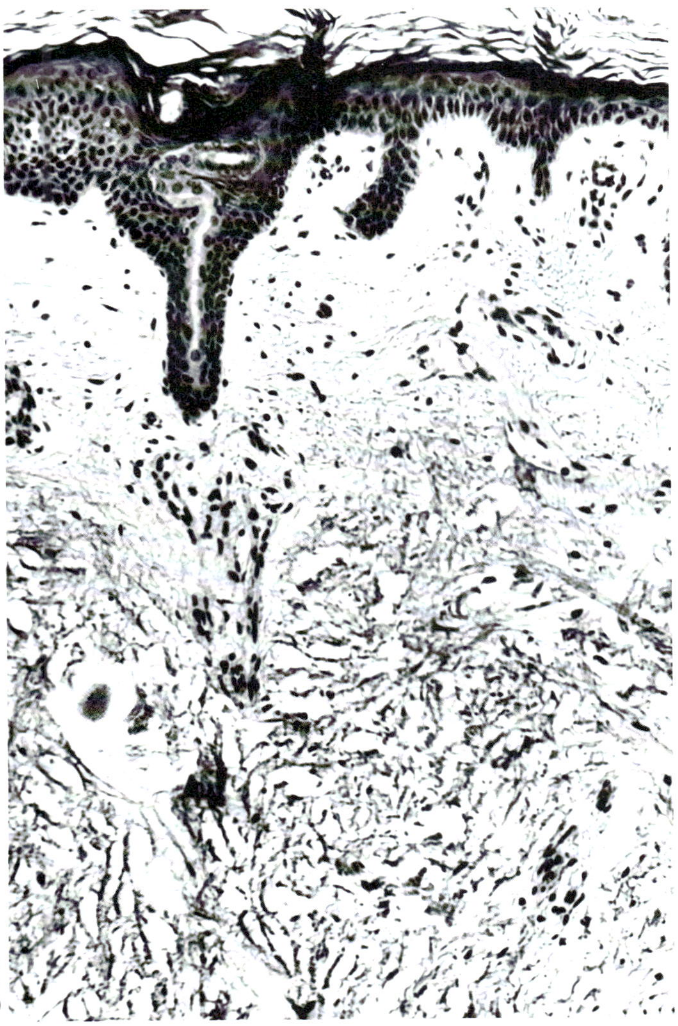

C
210

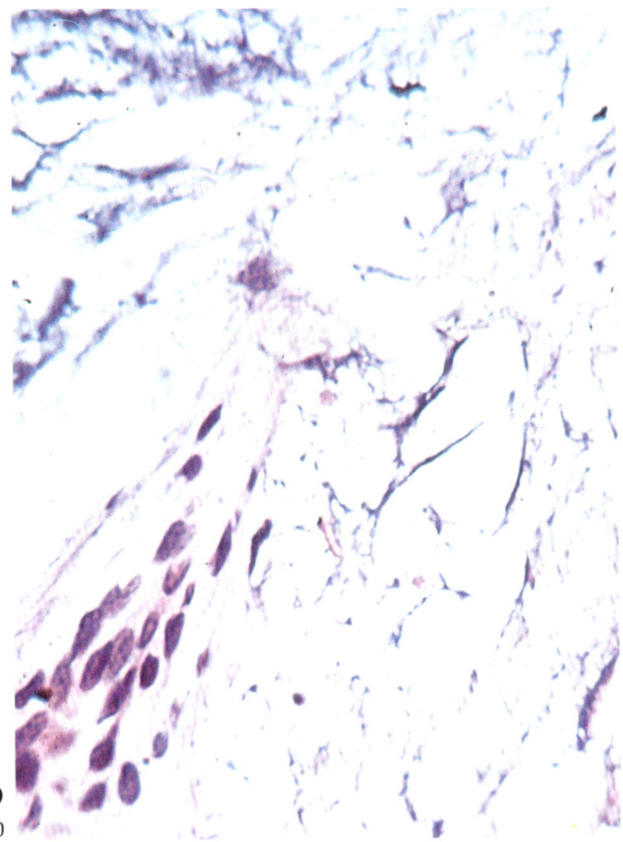

D
X860

LICHEN MYXEDEMATOSUS (PAPULAR MUCINOSIS)

Lichen myxedematosus is characterized by a widespread eruption of soft papules and nodules (Fig. B). In a variant called *scleromyxedema* there is, in addition, diffuse thickening of the skin (Fig. A) and erythema. Accentuation of the skin folds is observed, and is most pronounced on the face (Fig. A). Unlike scleroderma, the thickened skin is freely movable. The face, ears, and arms are sites of predilection.

Lichen myxedematosus is not associated with thyroid dysfunction, but is believed to be associated with deposition of an abnormal gamma globulin (IgG) and hyperplasia of marrow plasma cells. Scleromyxedema has been reported to be associated with bizarre neurologic symptoms, scleroderma involving the kidneys, or multiple myeloma. Definite association with multiple myeloma has not been established.

Microscopic features

1. There is a circumscribed deposition of mucin in the upper dermis (Figs. C,D). This takes stains for acid mucopolysaccharides such as Hale's colloidal iron stain (Fig. E).
2. There is a great increase in fibroblasts in the involved area. Many of them have a stellate configuration (Figs. C,D).
3. In scleromyxedema, changes are more extensive than in papular mucinosis.

Comment

Lichen myxedematosus has been classified into four clinical types:

1. Generalized lichenoid papular type (this has been considered synonymous with scleromyxedema by many authors).
2. Discrete papular type.
3. Lichenoid plaques, localized or generalized.
4. Urticarial plaques and nodular eruption that eventually changes to the generalized lichenoid form.

LICHEN MYXEDEMATOSUS

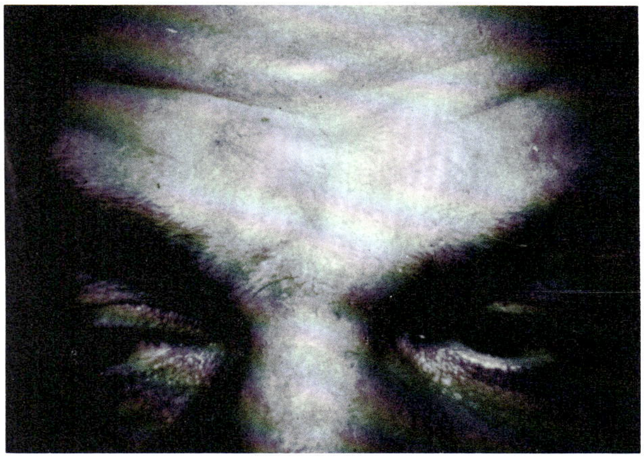

A

Courtesy Dr. Mauray Tye

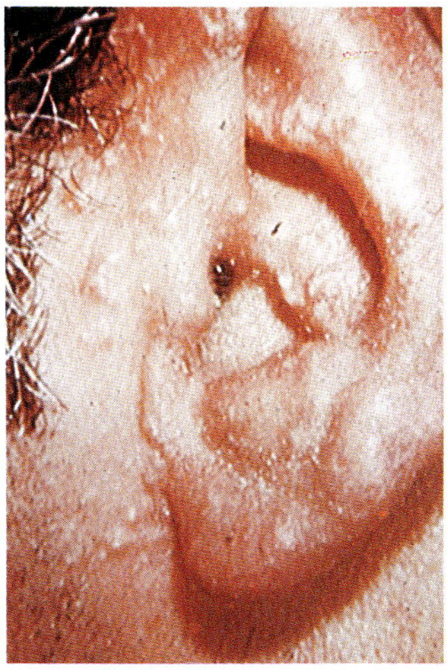

B

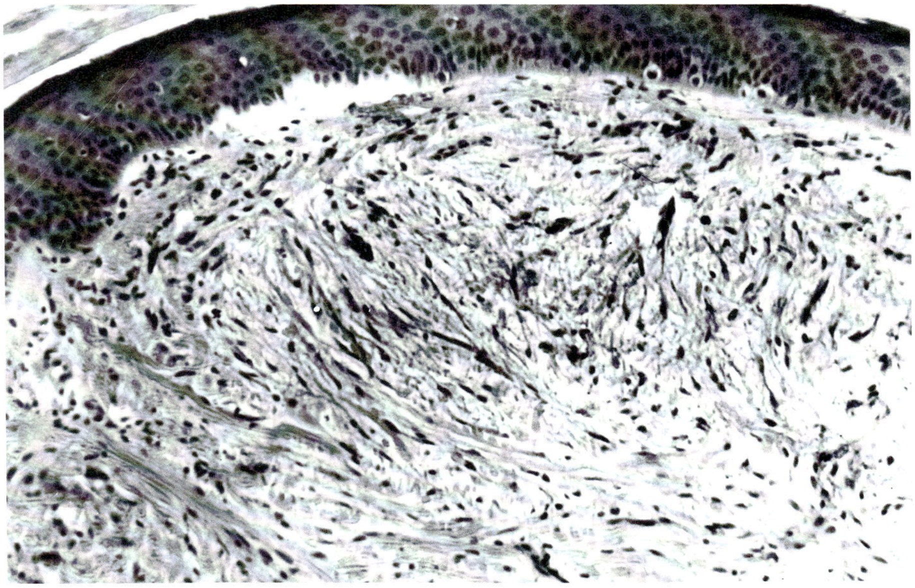

C
X200

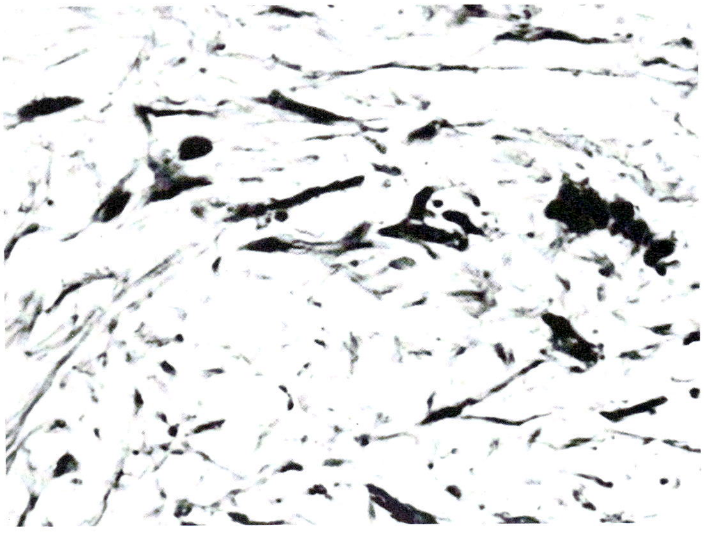

D
X810

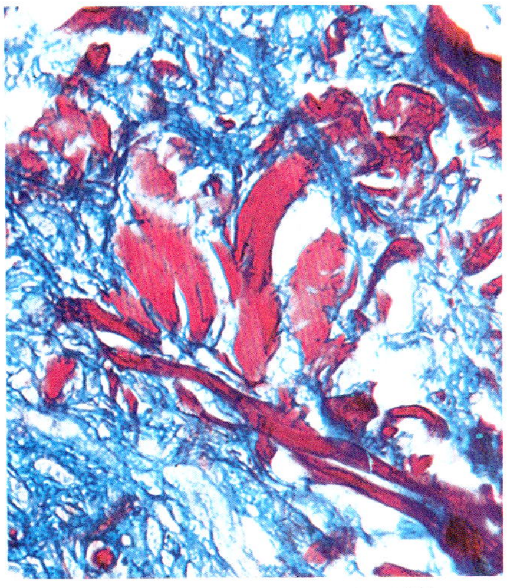

E
X810

HALE'S COLLOIDAL IRON STAIN

Courtesy Dr. William Clendenning and Dr. Thomas Watt

DIGITAL MUCOUS CYST

Digital mucous cysts are translucent, globular lesions, generally located on the dorsal surface of the distal phalanx of the finger (Fig. A). Occasionally, similar lesions may be located on the corresponding area of the toes. When the cyst is located under the posterior nail fold, it may cause a longitudinal groove in the nail plate.

Microscopic features

1. A greatly enlarged dermal papilla shows stringy, basophilic mucin deposition and numerous stellate fibroblasts (Figs. B,C).
2. Adjacent rete ridges are greatly elongated and appear to "wrap around" the area of mucin deposition (Figs B,C).
3. The mucin takes stains for acid mucopolysaccharides (see p. 5).

Comment

The pathogenesis of digital mucous cyst is uncertain. One view holds that lesions are analogous to those of focal mucinosis (cutaneous myxoma) (see p. 984), with localized overproduction of hyaluronic acid by fibroblasts. Another view holds that the mucin (hyaluronic acid) is derived from the joint fluid of the distal interphalangeal joint via a pedicle.

DIGITAL MUCOUS CYST

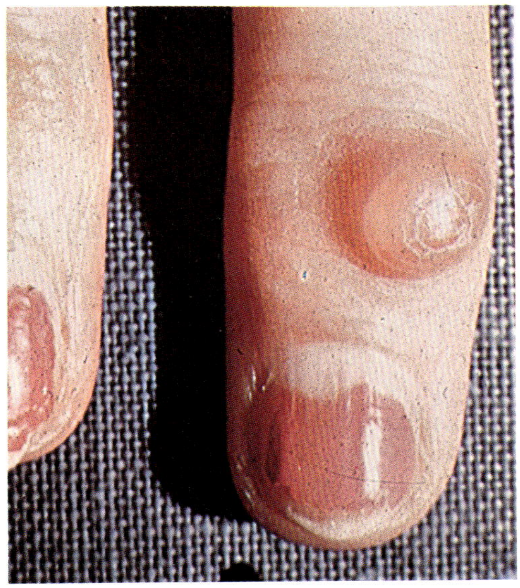

A

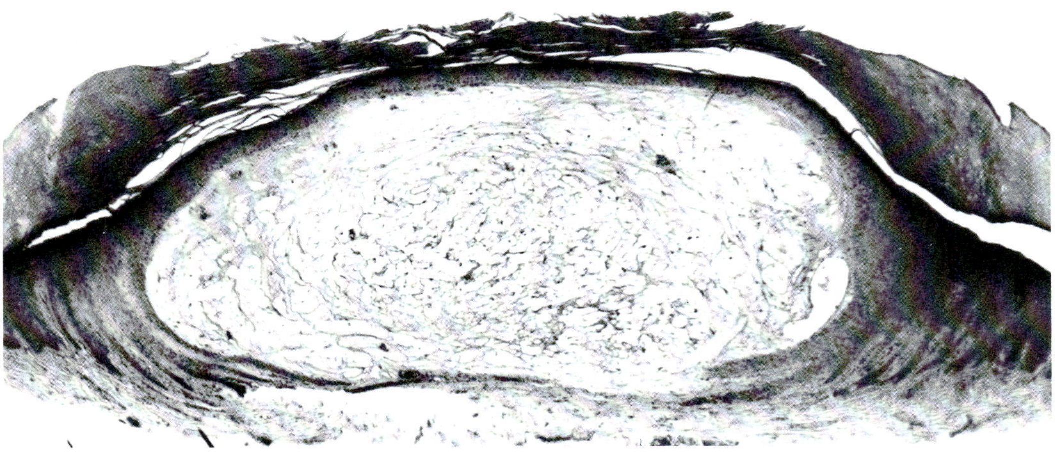

B
X53

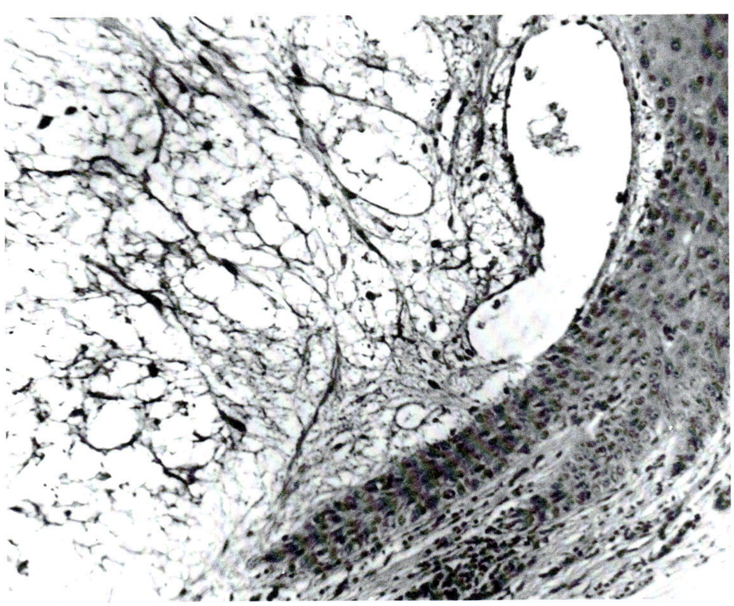

C
X180

MUCOUS CYST OF THE ORAL MUCOSA

The cysts occur on the lower lip (Fig. A) and less frequently on the tongue or other sites in the oral mucosa. They are believed to form as a result of traumatic rupture of salivary ducts. Sometimes the cysts are associated with cheilitis glandularis (see below).

Microscopic features

1. The wall of the cyst is composed of a dense aggregation of histiocytes, fibroblasts, and lymphocytes (Figs. B,C). Macrophages containing mucin are often present at the periphery of the cyst (Fig. C, lower part of field).
   A ruptured salivary duct may empty into the cyst cavity.
2. The mucin in the cyst is sialomucin. It is PAS-positive (Fig. D), but also shows staining reactions for acid mucopolysaccharides.
3. Sometimes there is a projection of squamous epithelium partially encompassing the cyst (Fig. B, left side of field).

Comment

Cheilitis glandularis results in diffuse swelling, usually involving the lower lip. Mucus can be expressed from the affected area. Ectopic salivary glands are present in the lip area, and are often surrounded by chronic inflammation (sialoadenitis). Since the everted lip is exposed to solar radiation, twenty percent of the cases develop squamous cell carcinoma. Mucous cysts are occasionally observed in affected areas.

MUCOUS CYST OF THE ORAL MUCOSA

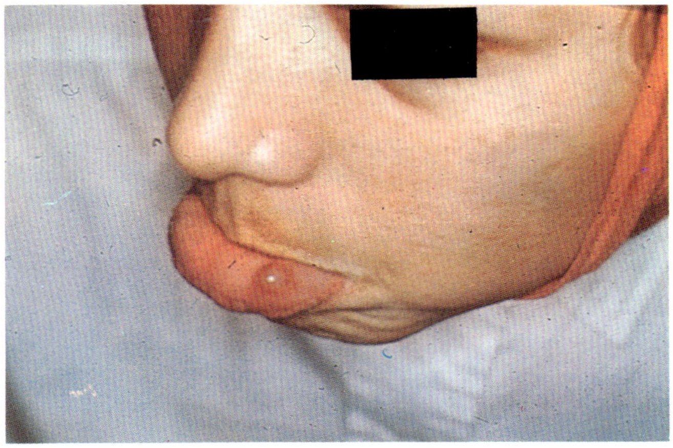

A

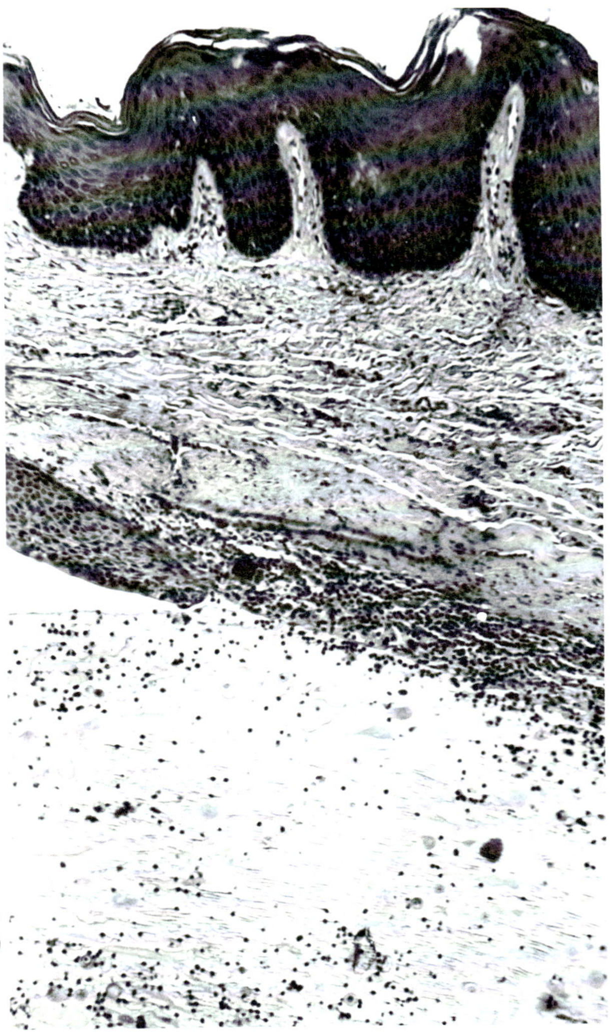

B
X200

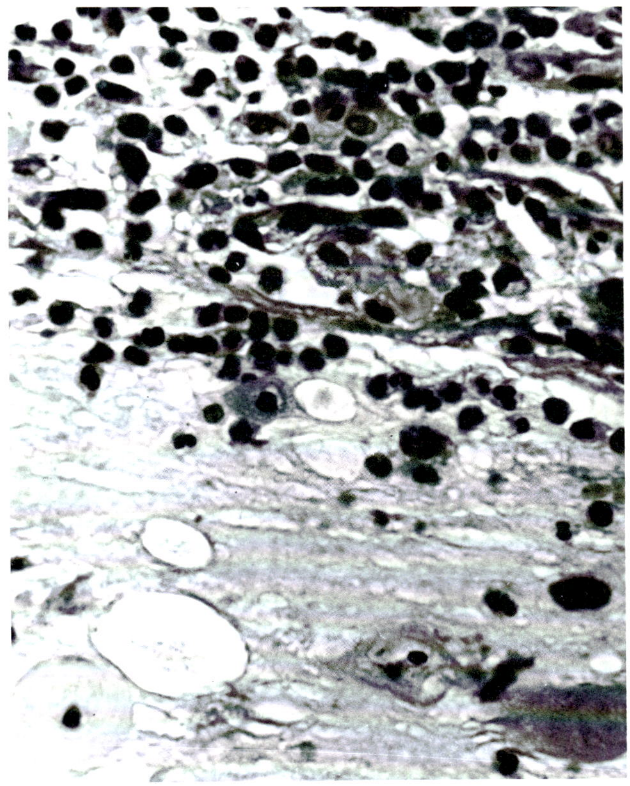

C
X700

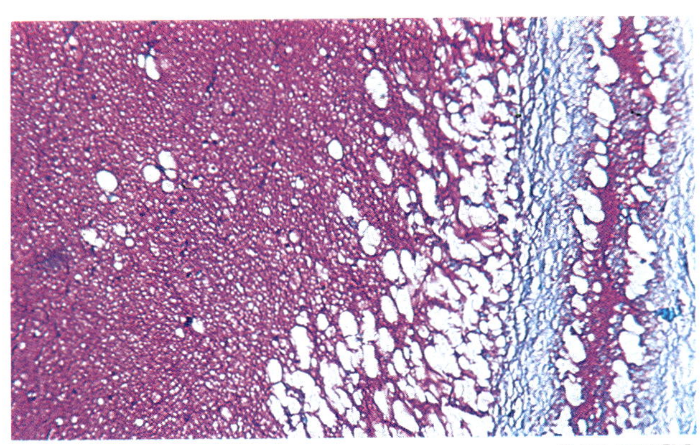

D
X120

PAS STAIN

ALOPECIA MUCINOSA (FOLLICULAR MUCINOSIS)

Alopecia mucinosa is characterized by grouped follicular papules or glistening, erythematous plaques (Figs. A,B). Lesions are associated with clinically evident hair loss, only in hairy areas.

The cause is unknown, but some cases are secondary to cutaneous lymphoma, particularly mycosis fungoides. Some use the term *follicular mucinosis* to differentiate secondary from primary alopecia mucinosa.

Microscopic features

1. The initial change is intercellular and intracellular edema involving the outer root sheath (Fig. C).
2. This is followed by disruption of cells and accumulation of mucin in cystic spaces (Figs. D,E). The mucin takes stains for acid mucopolysaccharides (see p. 5). It is, for the most part, digested with hyaluronidase.

ALOPECIA MUCINOSA

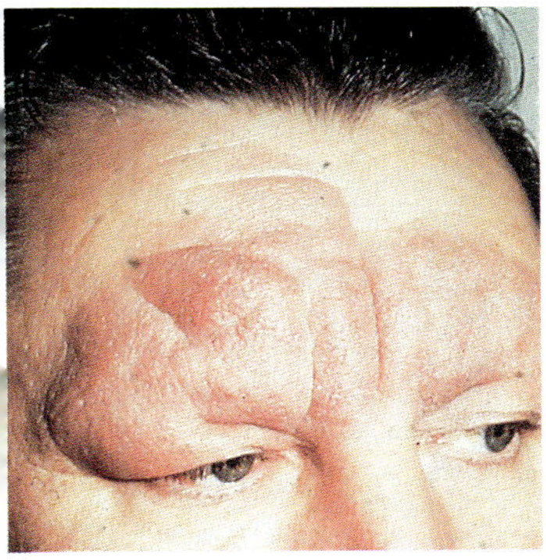

A

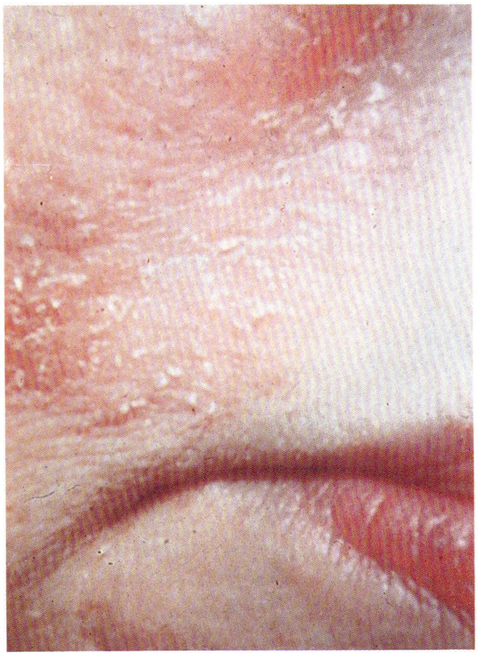

B

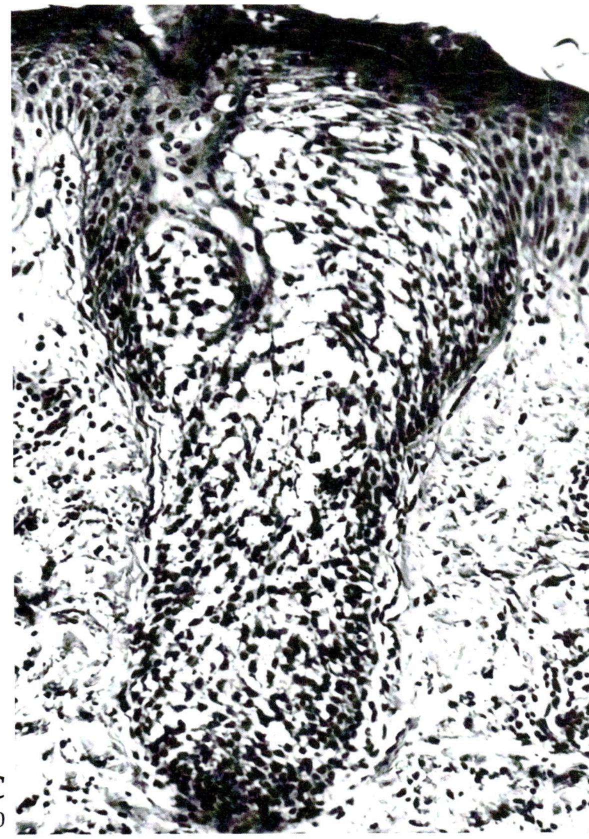

C
X200

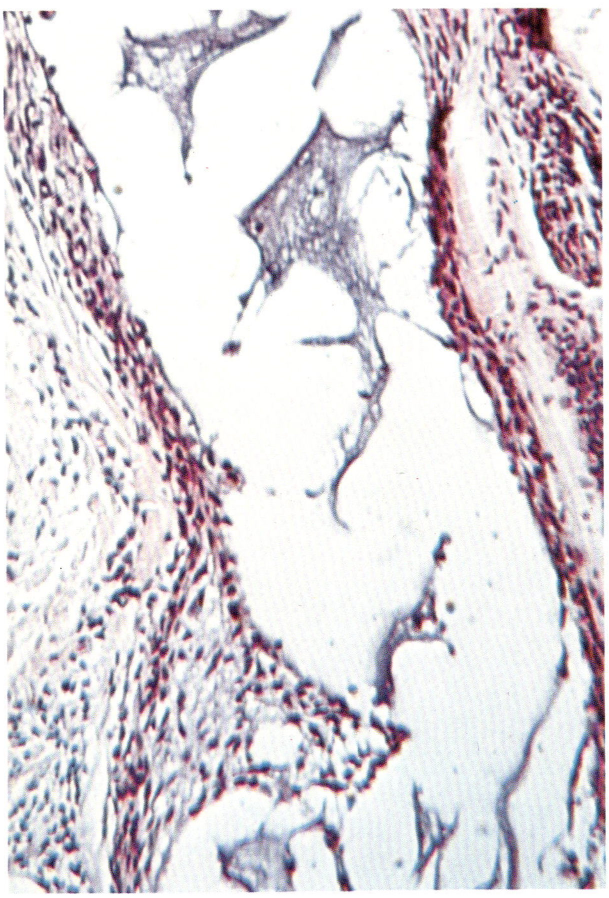

D
X200

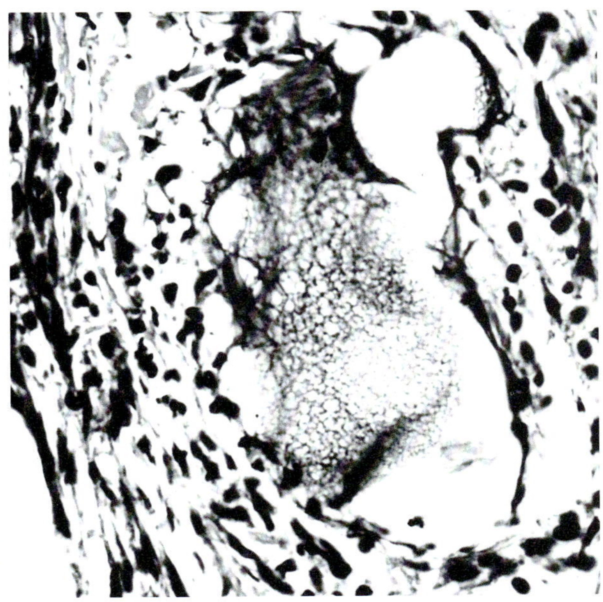

E
X520

ALOPECIA MUCINOSA continued ⇨

ALOPECIA MUCINOSA

Microscopic features

3. Mucinous changes also occur in sebaceous glands (Fig. A).
4. Foci of mucinous degeneration may be present in the dermis (Fig. B). These areas may contain PAS-positive, diastase-resistant material.
5. The dermis shows an inflammatory infiltrate of varying composition (Fig. C). In secondary alopecia mucinosa, the infiltrate contains tumor cells of the underlying lymphoma.
6. Dendritic cells with metachromatic granules may be present in the basal layer of the epidermis and outer root sheath. By electron microscopy these have been shown to be mast cells and cells combining features of mast cells and melanocytes.

Comment

1. Occasionally, no mucin is observed histologically. This may be due to its removal during processing.
2. *Reticular erythematous mucinosis* is characterized by reticulated erythematous patches with irregular margins. It is typically located on the trunk. Macular and papular lesions are present. The histologic picture shows small deposits of mucin, which are most apparent in the papular lesions. There is also nonspecific inflammation which tends to be perivascular and perifollicular. The mucin may not be evident in the macular lesions.
3. It has been postulated that spongiosis is the result of deposition of water-binding acid mucopolysaccharides in intercellular spaces. This has been demonstrated in mycosis fungoides. Follicular mucinosis may represent an extreme example of this phenomenon.

ALOPECIA MUCINOSA

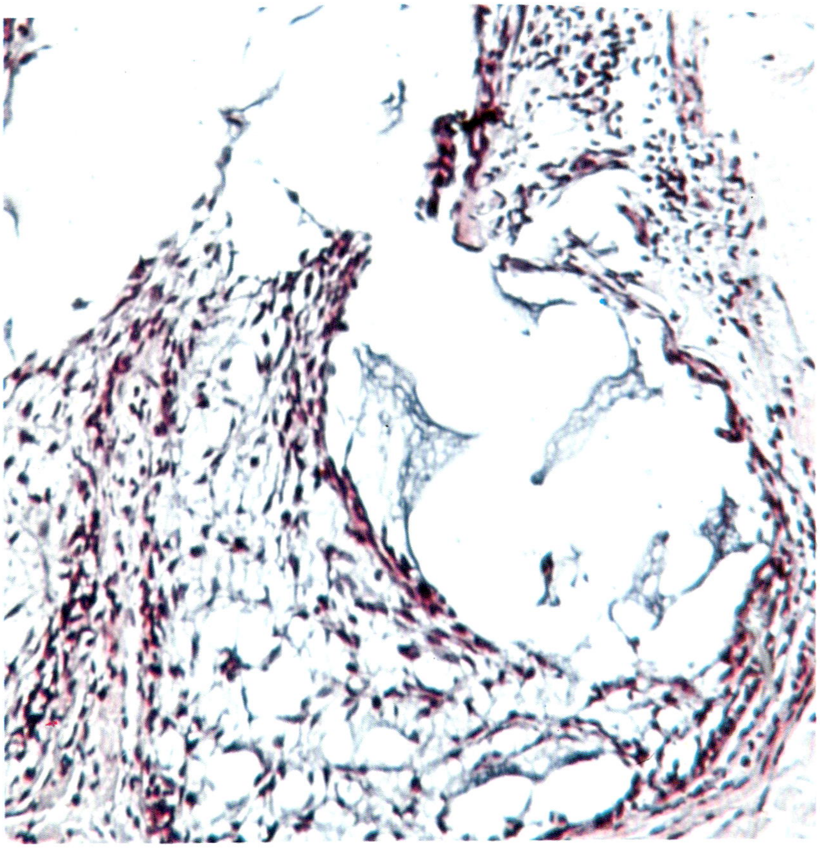

A
X400

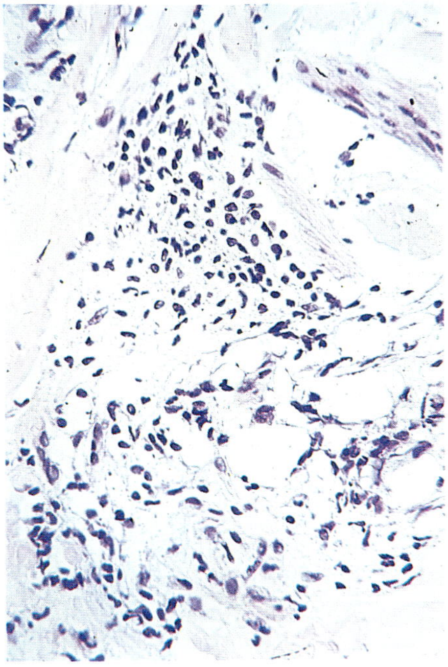

B
X400

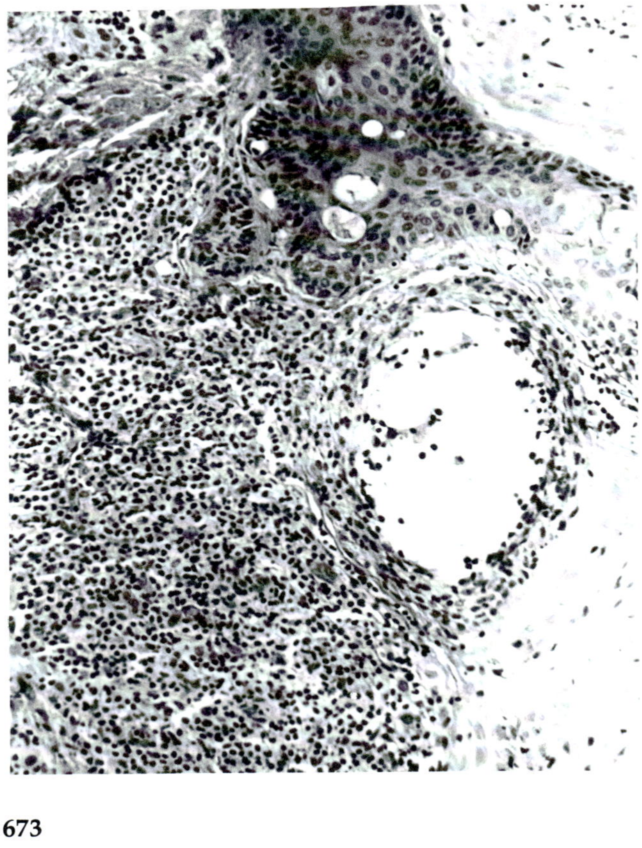

C
X190

CALCIFICATION AND OSSIFICATION

Calcium deposits in the skin (calcinosis cutis) may be the result of metabolic or local factors. *Metabolic (metastatic) calcinosis cutis* is due either to hypercalcemia or hyperphosphatemia (which may be caused by hyperparathyroidism or hypervitaminosis D). Other factors that can cause metastatic calcinosis cutis include excessive intake of milk or alkali, and destructive processes involving bone. Local factors (causing *dystrophic calcinosis cutis*) include trauma, systemic scleroderma, dermatomyositis, pseudoxanthoma elasticum, sclerema neonatorum, and tumors (e.g., calcifying epithelioma of Malherbe, apocrine mixed tumor). Calcinosis cutis may occasionally be idiopathic.

Areas of calcification are indurated papules, nodules, or plaques (Fig. A).

Ossification may develop in pre-existing cutaneous lesions (e.g., calcifying epithelioma of Malherbe, apocrine mixed tumor, inflamed hair follicles, epidermal cysts). Ossification may also occur as a primary hamartoma (osteoma cutis). Such lesions are often multiple. In *Albright's hereditary osteodystrophy*, multiple cutaneous osteomas are present. Osteomas are seen as part of the Gardner syndrome.

Microscopic features

1. With hematoxylin and eosin (Fig. B), calcium appears as deeply basophilic, granular material; calcium stains black with von Kossa's stain.
2. Deposits of calcium are frequently surrounded by a foreign body granuloma and fibrosis.
3. Areas of ossification are more eosinophilic than areas of calcification (Fig. C). At times, osteoblasts and bone marrow elements can be observed in areas of ossification.

CALCIFICATION

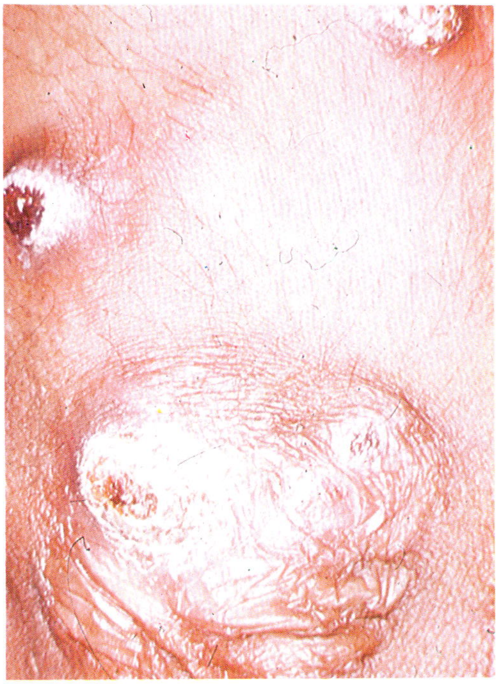

A

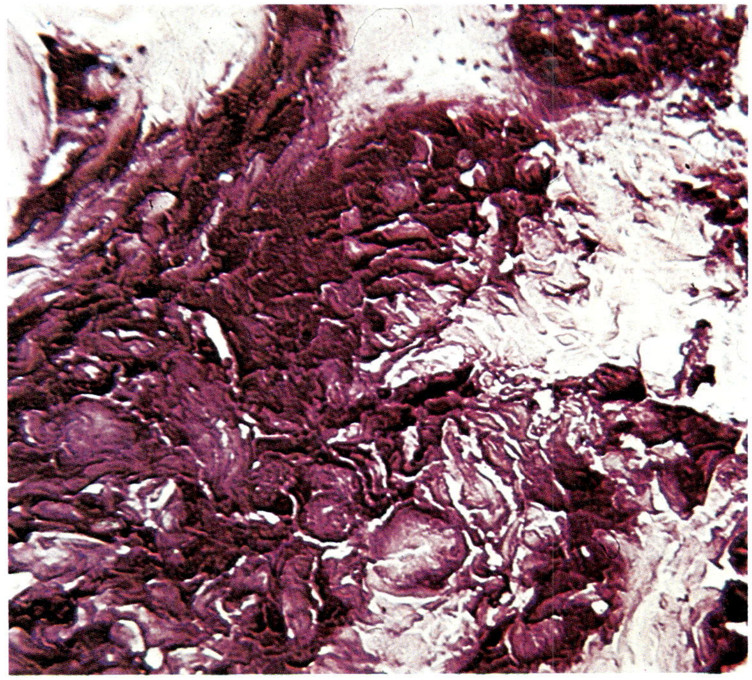

B
X170

OSSIFICATION

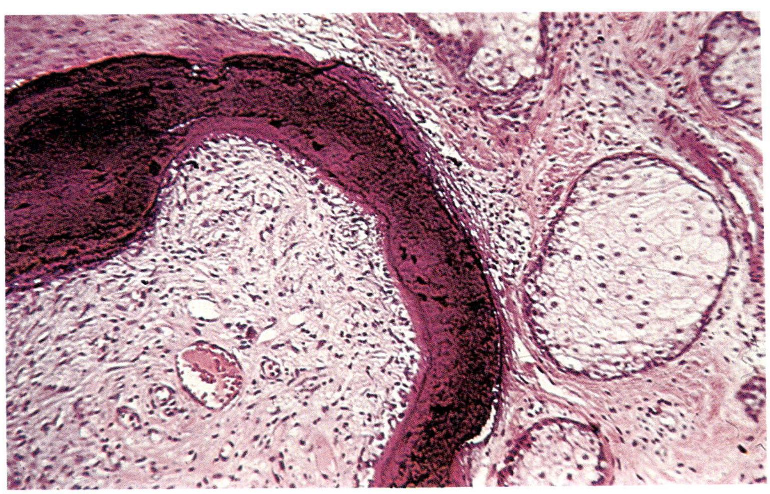

C
X190

CALCIFICATION AND OSSIFICATION

Comment

1. *Subepidermal calcified nodule* is a special form of localized calcification, usually found on the face and extremities. The lesion is usually solitary (Fig. A) and may be verrucous. It may be present at birth or may develop later in life. There is evidence that subepidermal calcified nodule may develop from pre-existing tumors, possibly nevocellular nevi or hamartomas of sweat glands.

   Microscopically, globular calcium deposits are in the upper dermis (Figs. B,C) and occasionally in the deep dermis. Often they are arranged in nests (Fig. C). Some of the globules may contain structures resembling nuclei (arrow – Fig. D). A foreign body granuloma may be present. The epidermis may be hypertrophic with papillomatosis (Fig. B). Transepidermal elimination of calcium has been reported to occur in subepidermal calcified nodule.
2. *Idiopathic calcinosis of the scrotum* consists of multiple asymptomatic nodules of the scrotal skin.

SUBEPIDERMAL CALCIFIED NODULE

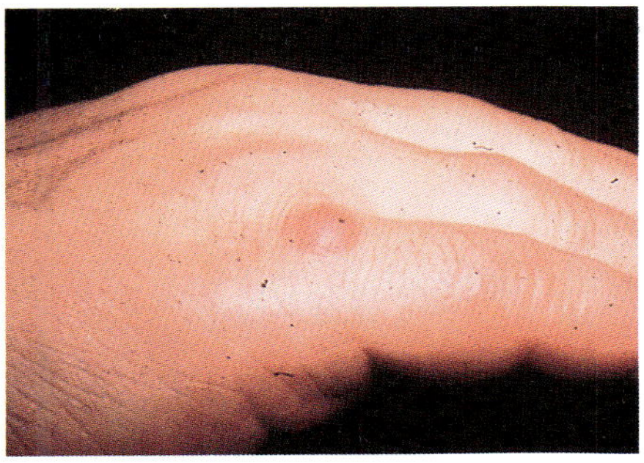

A

Courtesy Dr. Hein Ter Poorten

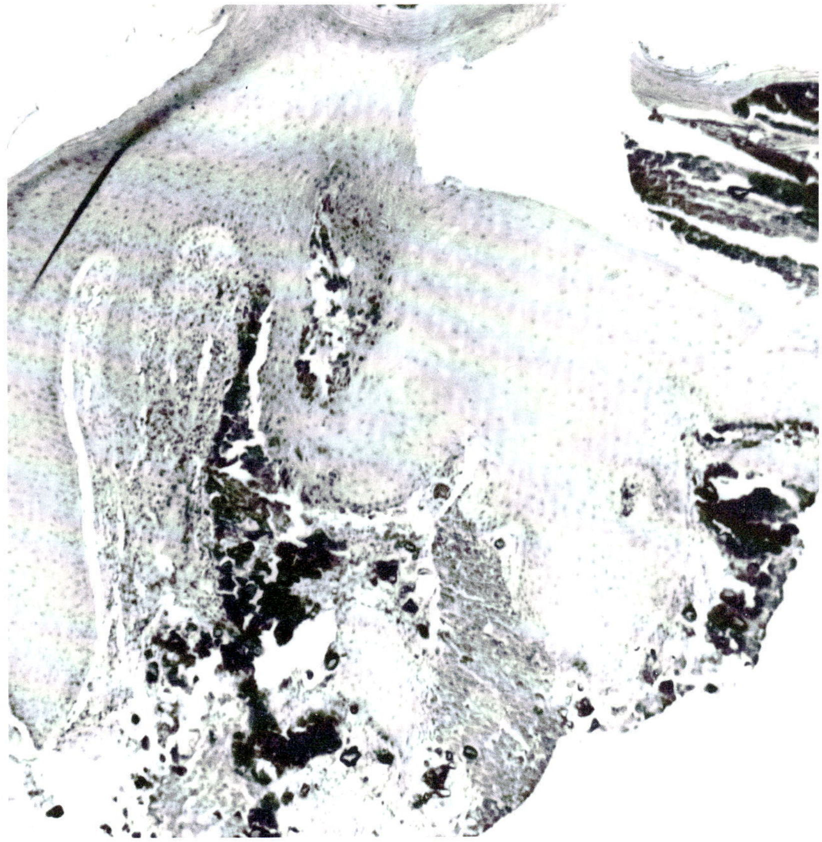

B
X100

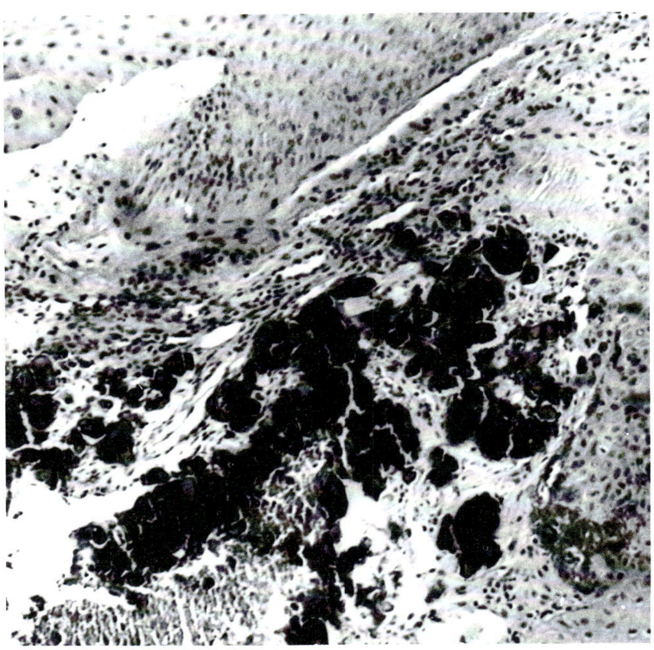

C
X190

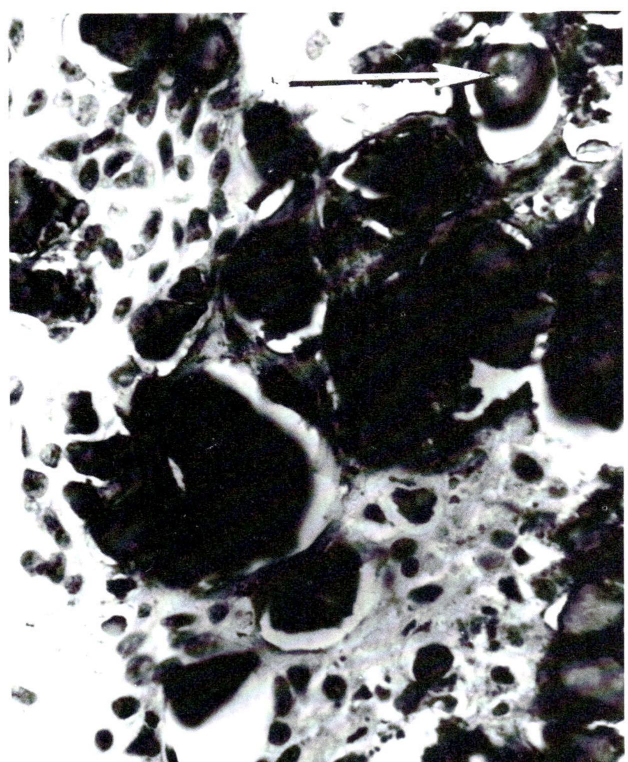

D
X530

VITILIGO

Vitiligo is a common acquired focal loss of cutaneous pigment. Lesions may be localized or widespread. Symmetry is often present (Figs. A,B); periorificial distribution is common. Sometimes hairs in affected areas are white. Loss of pigment in vitiligo ranges from partial to complete. Peripheral to depigmented areas, there may be hyperpigmentation. Ocular disturbances, including fundal pigment disturbances, may occur in vitiligo.

The cause is unknown. There may be a dominantly inherited predisposition to vitiligo. An autoimmune basis has been proposed, in which specific antibodies to melanocytes have been postulated. A clinical association with disorders suspected to be of autoimmune origin, such as Addison's disease, hyperthyroidism, hypothyroidism, pernicious anemia, and rheumatic diseases, has been noted. There is also an association between vitiligo and alopecia areata; vitiligo may be present in the Vogt-Koyanagi syndrome.

Microscopically, there is a loss of epidermal melanocytes, reflected by a decrease or absence of epidermal melanization. In routine sections a definitive diagnosis of vitiligo cannot be made, but loss of melanin is consistent with vitiligo. Fontana-Masson stain can help delineate loss of melanin and melanocytes, especially if there is a control biopsy of adjacent normal skin. Dopa stain can help delineate loss of epidermal melanocytes. At the edge of vitiliginous lesions, melanocytes may appear large and have long dendritic processes filled with melanin granules. There may be a dermal inflammatory infiltrate at the periphery of lesions.

Whether or not there is an increase in Langerhans cells accompanying loss of melanocytes in vitiligo has been the subject of controversy.

Comment

Idiopathic guttate hypomelanosis is characterized by numerous small hypopigmented and achromic macules with irregular borders. There is a predilection for the exposed areas of the extremities. It has been suggested that the condition may be related to the effects of aging and solar exposure.

VITILIGO

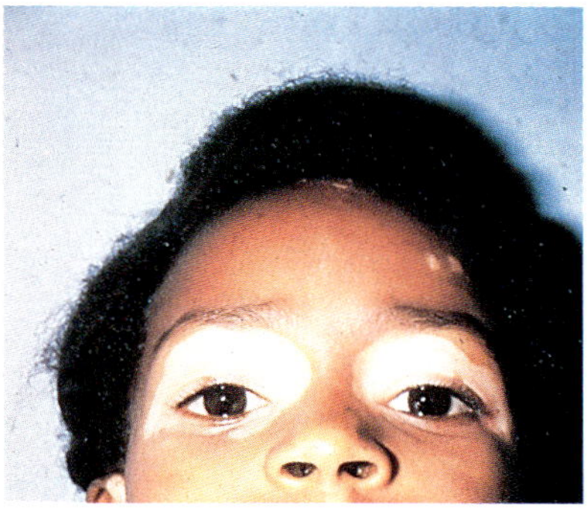

A

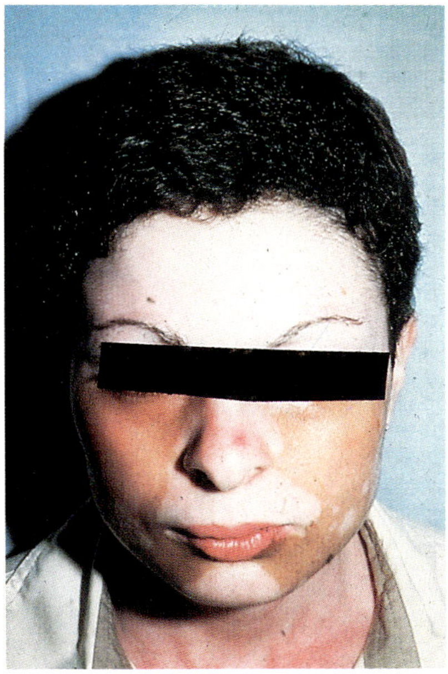

B

Amyloidosis

Amyloid is an eosinophilic, fibrillar substance with a characteristic ultrastructure and x-ray diffraction pattern. A variety of conditions are associated with deposition of amyloid. Its protein composition varies with its origin. A polysaccharide component is present. The following is a widely accepted classification of amyloidosis. Primary amyloidosis is sometimes called "immunocyte-derived amyloidosis," and secondary amyloidosis is sometimes called "reactive systemic amyloidosis."

Classification of amyloidosis

1. Primary amyloidosis
   a. Hereditary types
   b. Idiopathic types
      1. Systemic
      2. Localized
         a. Lichenoid type (lichen amyloidosus)
         b. Macular type
         c. Nodular type
2. Secondary systemic amyloidosis

Cutaneous lesions are observed in the primary idiopathic forms of amyloidosis.

In routine H&E sections, amyloid appears as a moderately eosinophilic, homogeneous material. The most reliable special stain is considered to be alkaline Congo red used with paraffin sections. With this method, amyloid stains orange-red and may show greenish birefringence with polarized light (see p. 684). Although this greenish birefringence is considered important in identifying amyloid, it may not always be present, possibly due to variability of amyloid. Thickness of sections may be a factor in obtaining a positive reaction.

Fluorescence is observed when amyloid is stained with thioflavin T and examined with a fluorescence microscope. The PAS stain is positive. A useful method for distinguishing amyloid from solar elastosis is the acid orcein Giemsa stain. With this method, amyloid is blue and solar elastotic material is brownish-black. Amyloid in unfixed, frozen sections shows metachromasia when stained with crystal violet. None of these methods is specific for amyloid since colloid (see p. 686) shows similar staining reactions.

Comment

The amyloid in lichen amyloidosus and macular amyloidosis is believed to derive from basal cells, transformed by apoptosis.

AMYLOIDOSIS continued ⇨

PRIMARY IDIOPATHIC SYSTEMIC AMYLOIDOSIS

Amyloid is deposited in mesenchymal tissues and in skeletal and smooth muscle. Walls of blood vessels and perivascular areas are frequently involved. Fatal cases are often due to involvement of the heart, kidney, or gastrointestinal tract.

The skin and tongue are frequently affected (Figs. A,B,C). Cutaneous lesions are waxy papules and nodules, frequently with a purpuric component (Fig. A). Lichenoid, macular, or poikiloderma-like lesions may occur in primary idiopathic systemic amyloidosis. Lesions can be widely disseminated but tend to be particularly numerous on the face, particularly on the eyelids (Fig. A). Bullae occur occasionally. In the absence of cutaneous lesions, biopsy from the rectal or oral mucosa, or subcutaneous tissue, can help establish the diagnosis.

Cases of primary idiopathic systemic amyloidosis are associated with some abnormality of marrow plasma cells, including multiple myeloma, nodular lymphoma, immunoblastic lympadenopathy, Waldenström's macroglobulinemia, heavy chain disease, or agammaglobulinemia. Paraproteinemia is often present.

Microscopic features

Amyloid is deposited in the dermis and subcutaneous tissue. Infiltration of amyloid may be present in blood vessels, a feature which explains the hemorrhagic component seen clinically. The membrana propria of sweat glands may be involved. In the subcutaneous fat, amyloid rings around fat cells may be present.

Comment

Secondary systemic amyloidosis typically involves parenchymal organs. The skin is not clinically involved. The disorder may occur as a result of a variety of chronic inflammatory diseases, including rheumatoid arthritis, osteomyelitis, stasis ulcer, hidradenitis suppurativa, and lepromatous leprosy. Key clinical features are hepatosplenomegaly and nephrotic syndrome.

A skin biopsy, despite absence of clinical involvement, may be of value in making a diagnosis of secondary amyloidosis. Amyloid may be present in the fat (amyloid rings), as well as in the deeper dermal vessels and adnexa.

PRIMARY IDIOPATHIC SYSTEMIC AMYLOIDOSIS

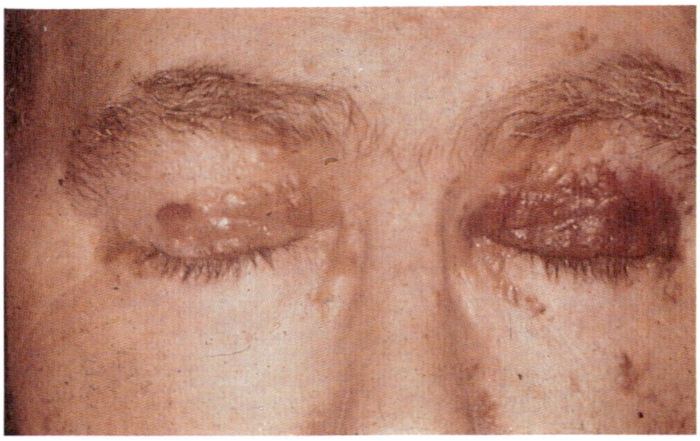

A

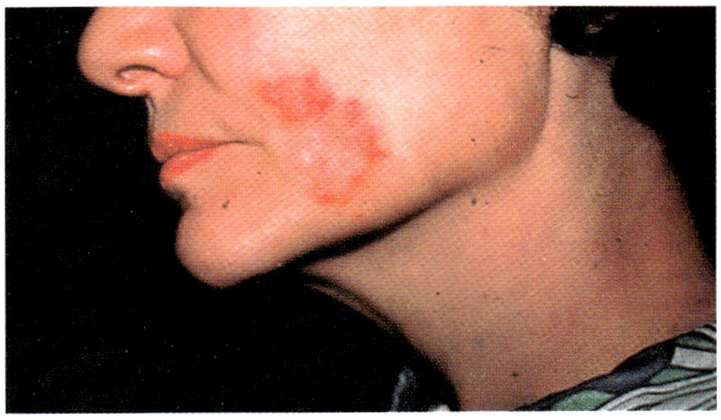

B

Courtesy Dr. Herbert Mescon

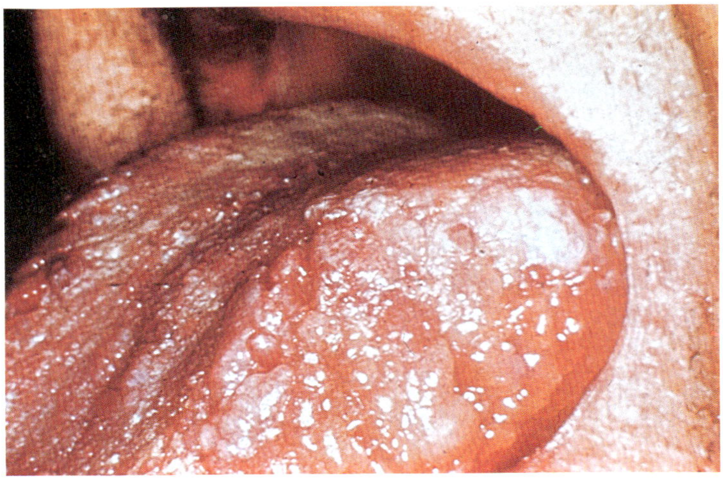

C

AMYLOIDOSIS continued

LOCALIZED AMYLOIDOSIS

Lesions are limited to the skin. The legs are the usual site of lichenoid and nodular types. In the lichenoid type, lesions are densely aggregated, often translucent, reddish-brown papules (Fig. A) which may fuse to form plaques (Fig. B). Pruritus is common. In the macular type, lesions have a pigmented, reticulated surface. Lesions usually occur on the trunk and extremities. Mixed types occur. The nodular type is rare (Fig. C).

There may be a relationship between macular and lichenoid types.

Microscopic features

1. Microscopic features of various types differ only by the size and position of the amyloid deposits. In lichen amyloidosus (Fig. E) amyloid deposits are limited to the papillary dermis, mainly the dermal papillae. In macular amyloidosis the deposits are smaller and there is no acanthosis and hyperkeratosis of the overlying epidermis, which are often present in lichen amyloidosus. The small deposits resemble colloid bodies.
2. With H&E, the amyloid appears as moderately eosinophilic to moderately basophilic, homogeneous fissured material, separated from the epidermis by a narrow zone of uninvolved collagen (Fig. E).
3. In nodular amyloidosis and primary systemic amyloidosis, deposits of amyloid are also present around sweat glands and within walls of blood vessels. The involved blood vessels may show hemorrhage. Amyloid deposits may be present in the subcutaneous fat around individual fat cells (amyloid rings). Amyloid rings in the fat may be observed in secondary amyloidosis. In macular amyloidosis, amyloid is present in the papillary dermis in foci resembling colloid bodies (see p. 440).
4. Special staining reactions for amyloid are best performed on unfixed, frozen sections.
    a. Congo red: amyloid stains orange-red (Fig. F); when examined with polarized light, amyloid shows greenish (Fig. D) or reddish birefringence (dichroism), depending on the rotation angle of the polarizing discs.
    b. Acid orcein Giemsa stain: amyloid stains a sky-blue color (Fig. G).
    c. Crystal violet or methyl violet: amyloid stains metachromatically.
    d. Thioflavin-T: amyloid appears blue or green when examined with ultraviolet light.

Comment

1. The acid orcein Giemsa stain demonstrates amyloid quite well in routine sections (Fig. G). It is useful for differentiating amyloid (sky blue) from foci of solar elastosis (black).
2. Dichroism is not always easy to demonstrate.
3. *Biphasic amyloidosis* describes coexistence of macular amyloidosis and lichen amyloidosus.

LICHEN AMYLOIDOSUS

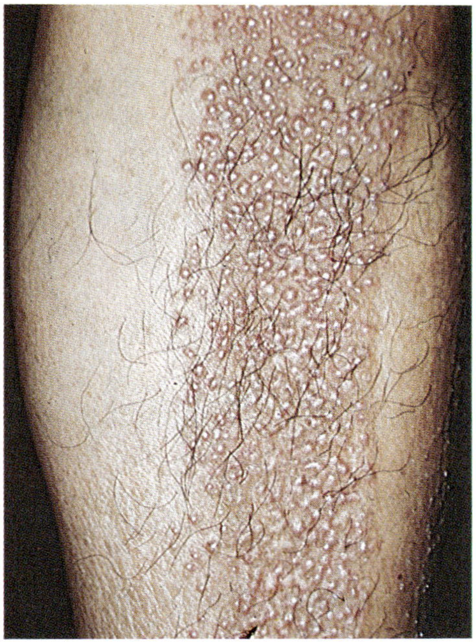

A

Courtesy Dr. Chu-Kwan Wong

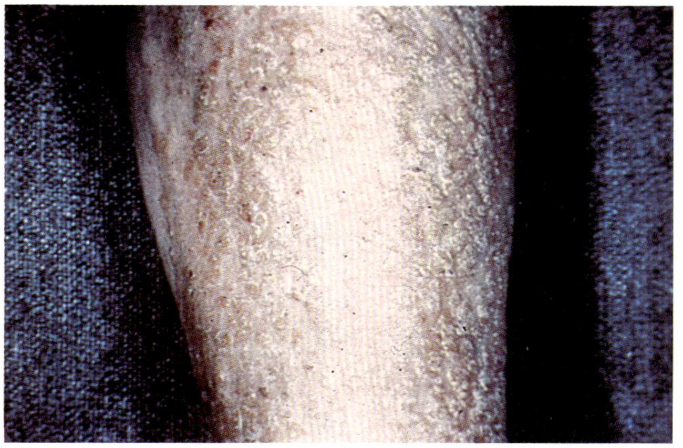

B

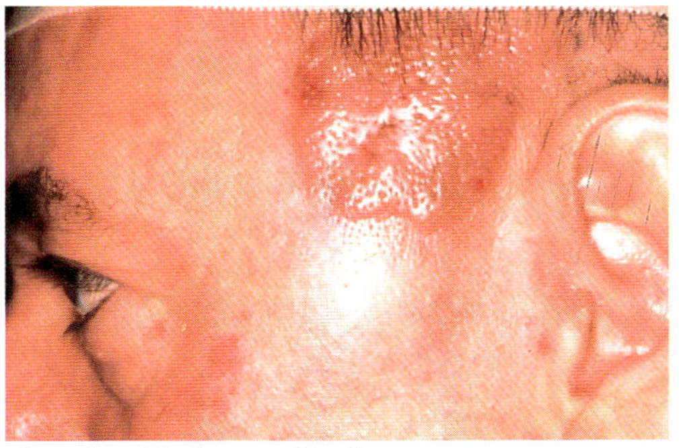

C

Courtesy Dr. Jerome Garden

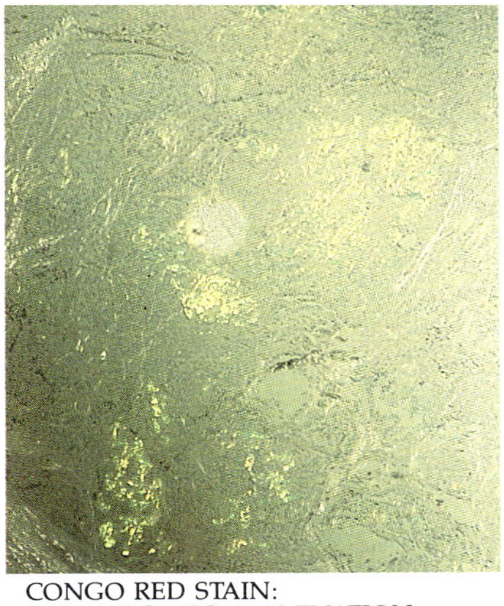

D
X50

CONGO RED STAIN:
POLARISCOPIC EXAMINATION
Courtesy Dr. Simon Hirschl

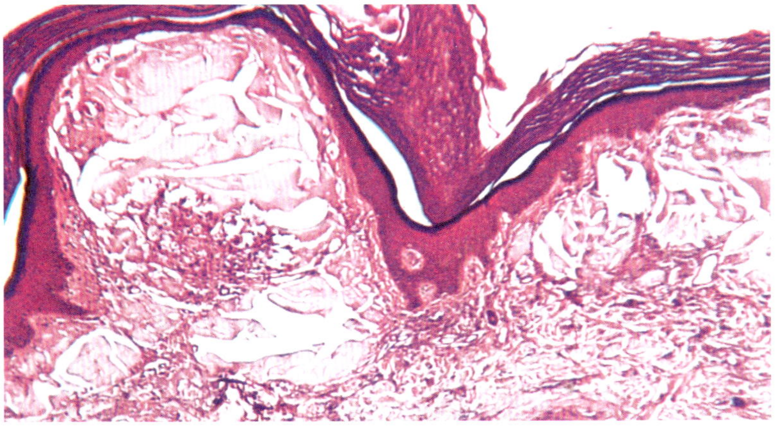

E
X50

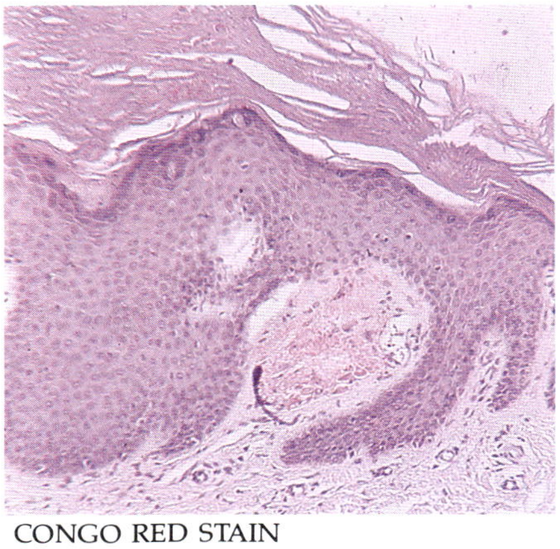

F
X130

CONGO RED STAIN

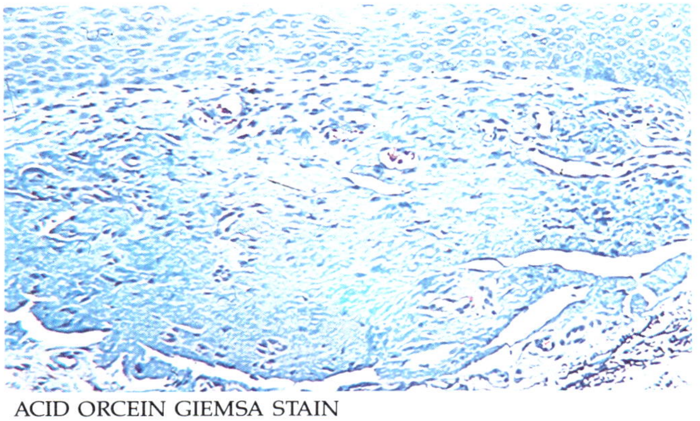

G
X130

ACID ORCEIN GIEMSA STAIN

COLLOID MILIUM

Colloid milia are translucent yellowish papules which tend to occur in clusters on the face (Figs. A,B) and dorsal surfaces of the hands in the adult form. Lesions appearing before puberty (juvenile colloid milium) may be familial. Lesions of this type are numerous and occur mainly on the face. Lesions appearing after puberty are believed to be related to solar damage. Colloid is produced by fibroblasts.

Occasionally, lesions appear as diffuse plaques (colloid degeneration of the skin).

Nodular colloid degeneration of the skin is rare. The nodules can be solitary or multiple and are typically located on the head. There does not seem to be a relationship to sun damage in nodular colloid degeneration of the skin.

Microscopic features

1. Deposits of colloid greatly resemble amyloid with H&E stain. In adult colloid milia, fissured, moderately eosinophilic to moderately basophilic masses are present in the dermal papillae (Figs. C,D). Accumulations of colloid may cause enlargement of papillae. When solar elastosis is present, the elastotic material is beneath the colloid.
2. In juvenile colloid milium, basal cells are transformed into colloid bodies. Colloid is seen in the papillary dermis and sometimes in the epidermis. There are "melanophages" and fibroblasts.
3. In nodular colloid degeneration of the skin, the material is diffusely distributed throughout the dermis.

Microscopic differential diagnosis

Light microscopic differentiation of colloid from amyloid is not possible. It was previously believed that differentiation could be made with special stains. However, recent studies have shown that colloid and amyloid are histochemically identical. Colloid may be a form of amyloid. There are differences that can be seen with electron microscopy.

COLLOID MILIUM

A

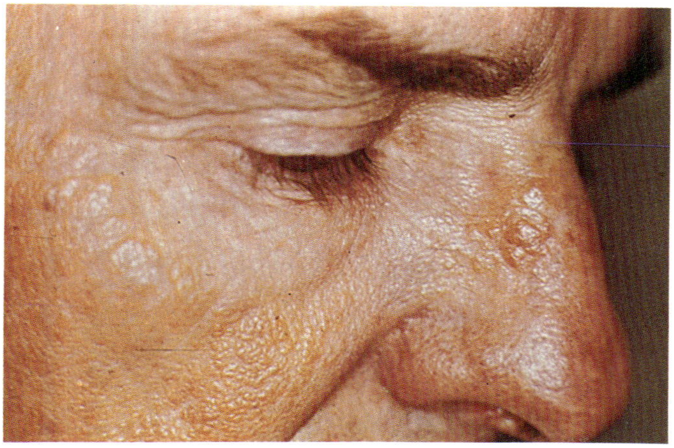

Courtesy Dr. Ken Hashimoto

B

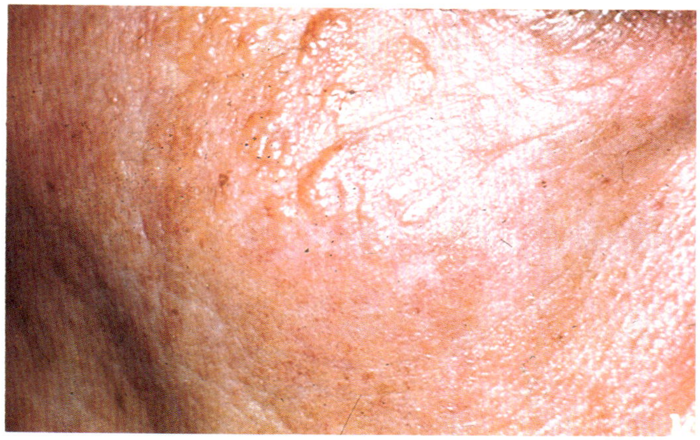

Courtesy Dr. K. Inaba

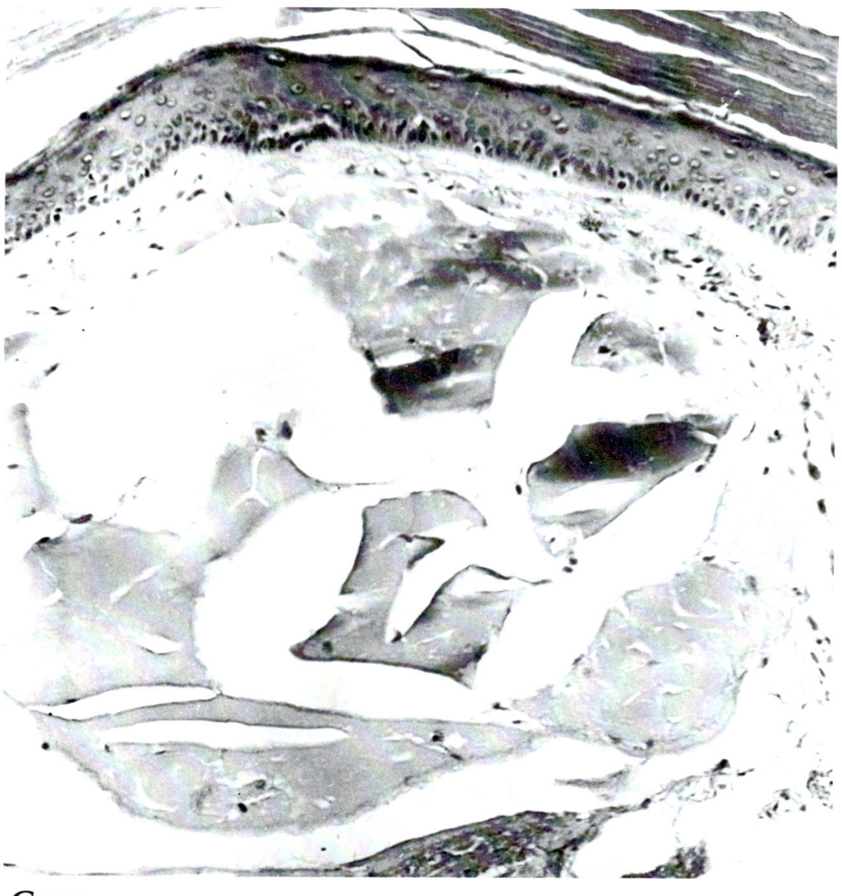

C X180

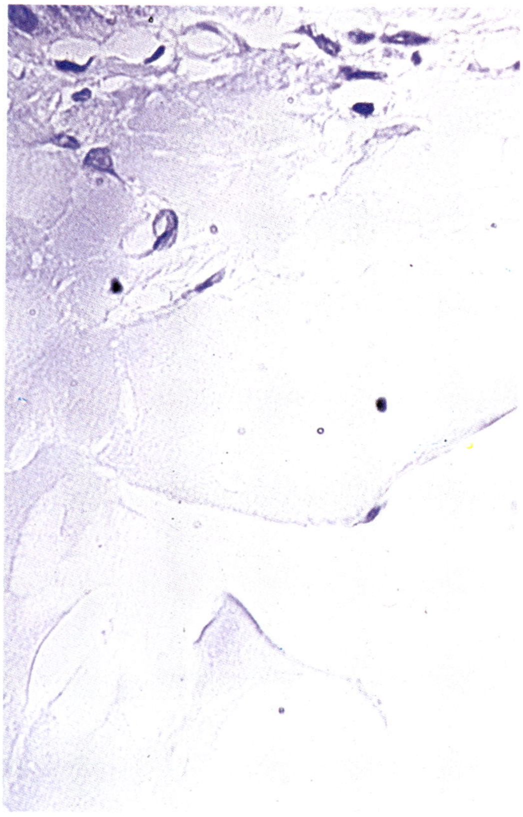

D X720

LIPOID PROTEINOSIS (HYALINOSIS CUTIS ET MUCOSAE)

Lipoid proteinosis is characterized by deposition of amorphous hyaline material in the skin, oral mucosa, and larynx. Other areas, including the gastrointestinal tract, genitourinary tract, and cerebral cortex may be involved.

There is some evidence that the disorder is inherited as an autosomal recessive trait.

Cutaneous lesions are varied. They include translucent papules involving the face (particularly the margins of the eyelids [Fig. A]), neck and hands, morphea-like lesions, ulcerations, and hyperkeratotic, infiltrated areas on the elbows and knees. Diffuse induration of the skin of the face and pitted scars may produce a "pigskin leather" appearance. The eyelid lesions are diagnostic.

Mucous membranes may show diffuse thickening and induration (Fig. B); the tongue may be limited in mobility due to infiltration of the frenulum. Involvement of the larynx may result in hoarseness. Convulsive seizures may occur. The hyaline material is a glycoprotein; lipid deposition and hyaluronic acid deposition are secondary.

The hyalin is mainly type IV collagen containing a glycoprotein.

Microscopic features

1. The dermis is increased in depth. In its upper portion, there is widely distributed eosinophilic, hyaline material, arranged as clustered fibrils. The glycoprotein deposits may also involve the arrectores pilorum.
2. In the papillary dermis, the hyaline fibrils are perpendicular to the epidermis (Fig. C). In the lower dermis, the hyaline deposits are more sparse. They may surround blood vessels and atrophic eccrine glands.
3. The hyaline material is PAS-positive and diastase-resistant; it also may stain slightly for acid mucopolysaccharides. Reaction with fat stains is variable. If lipid is present, it appears as droplets within hyaline material. Elastic fibers are absent within the hyaline material.
4. The epidermis may show hyperkeratosis, acanthosis, and papillomatosis.

LIPOID PROTEINOSIS

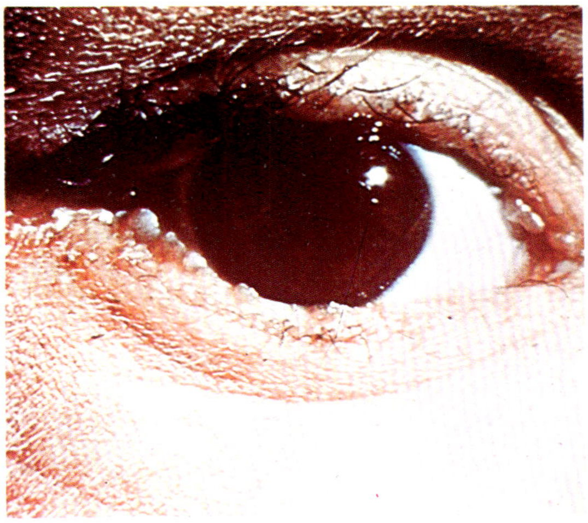

A

Courtesy Dr. John Knox

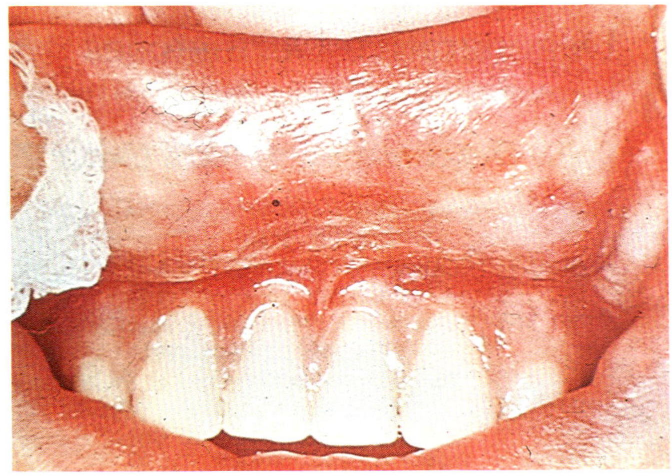

B

Courtesy Dr. Robert Gorlin

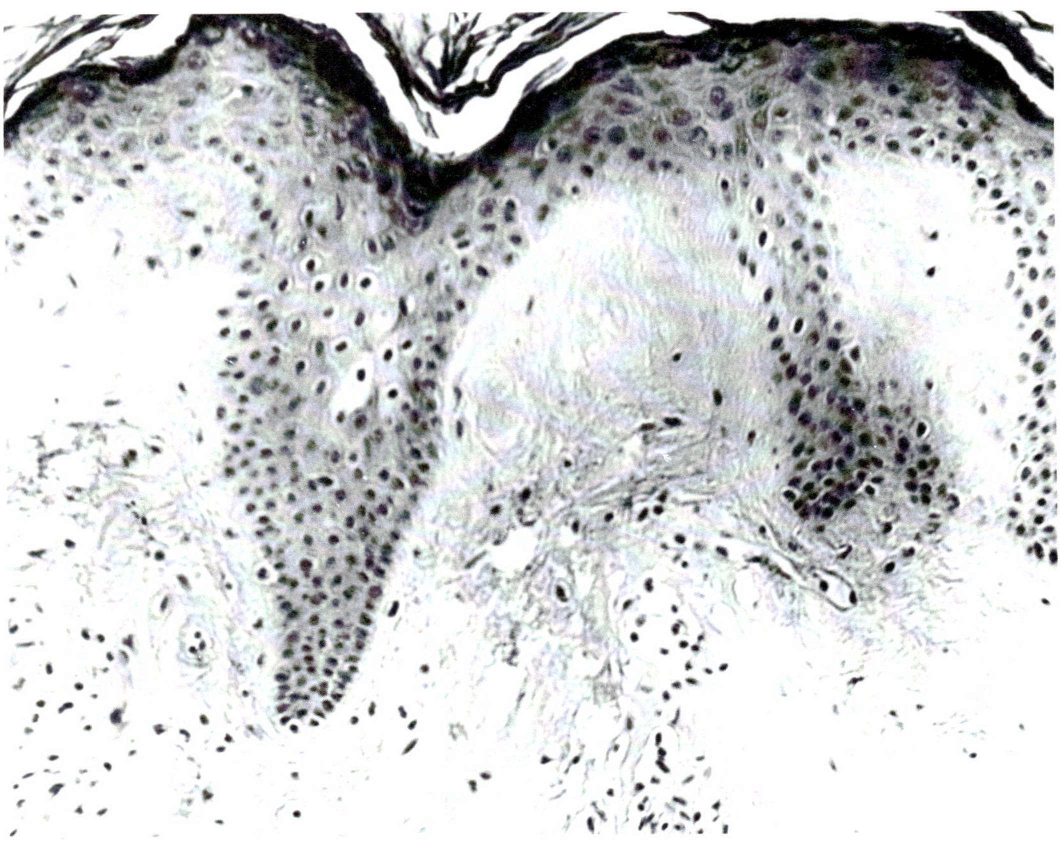

C
X300

689

Suggested Reading

Christianson, H. Elastosis perforans serpiginosa: Association with congenital anomalies: Report of 2 cases. *South. Med. J.*, 59:15, 1966.

Davis, W. Wilson's disease and penicillamine-induced anetoderma. *Arch. Dermatol.*, 113:976, 1977.

Degos, R. et al. Pemphigus chez un malade traité par pénicillamine pour maladie de Wilson. *Bull. Soc. Fr. Dermatol. Syph.*, 76:751, 1969.

Eide, J. Elastosis perforans serpiginosa with widespread arterial lesions: A case report. *Acta Derm. Venereol.* (Stockh.), 57:553, 1977.

From, E. and Fredericksen, P. Pemphigus vulgaris following D-penicillamine. *Dermatologica*, 152:358, 1976.

Goldschmidt, H. and Sherwin, W. Reactions to ionizing radiation. *J. Am. Acad. Dermatol.*, 3:551, 1980.

Greenblatt, M. Elastosis perforans serpiginosa. *Arch. Pathol.*, 75:177, 1963.

Greer, K., Askew, F. and Richardson, D. Skin lesions induced by penicillamine. *Arch. Dermatol.*, 112:1267, 1976.

Guilaine, J., Benhamon, J. and Molas, G. Élastome perforant verruciforme chez un malade traité par pénicillamine pour maladie de Wilson. *Bull. Soc. Fr. Dermatol. Syph.*, 79:450, 1972.

Hashimoto, K., McEvoy, B. and Belcher, R. Ultrastructure of penicillamine-induced skin lesions. *J. Am. Acad. Dermatol.*, 4:300, 1981.

Hitch, J. and Lund, H. Elastosis perforans serpiginosa. *Arch. Dermatol.*, 79:407, 1959.

Katz, R. Penicillamine-induced skin lesions. *Arch. Dermatol.*, 95:196, 1967.

Kirsch, N. and Hukill, P. Elastosis perforans serpiginosa induced by penicillamine: Electron microscopic observations. *Arch. Dermatol.*, 113:630, 1977.

London, I. et al. Elastosis perforans serpiginosa with systemic involvement. *South. Med. J.*, 67:225, 1974.

Marshall, J. and Lurie, H. Keratosis follicularis serpiginosa (Lutz). *Dermatologica*, 113:13, 1956.

Mehregan, A. Elastosis perforans serpiginosa. *Arch. Dermatol.*, 97:381, 1968.

Pedro, S. and Garcia, R. Disseminate elastosis perforans serpiginosa. *Arch. Dermatol.*, 109:84, 1974.

Rasmussen, J. Disseminated elastosis perforans serpiginosa in 4 mongoloids. *Br. J. Dermatol.*, 86:9, 1972.

Reed, W. and Pidgeon, J. Elastosis perforans serpiginosa with osteogenesis imperfecta. *Arch. Dermatol.*, 89:342, 1964.

Reymond, J. et al. Penicillamine induced elastosis perforans serpiginosa: An ultrastructural study of two cases. *J. Cutan. Pathol.*, 9:352, 1982.

Schamroth, J., Kellen, P. and Grieve, T. Elastosis perforans serpiginosa in a patient with renal disease. *Arch. Dermatol.*, 122:82, 1986.

Schneider, W. and Bock, H. Elastosis perforans serpiginosa. *Hautarzt*, 27:117, 1976.

Tsambaos, D. and Berger, H. Elastosis perforans serpiginosa. Licht und elektronenmikroskopische Befunde. *Z. Haut.*, 55:563, 1979.

Ueda, K. et al. A case of elastosis perforans serpiginosa: An ultrastructural study. *J. Cutan. Pathol.*, 10:217, 1983.

Volpin, D. et al. Ultrastructural and biochemical studies on a case of elastosis perforans serpiginosa. *Dermatologica*, 156:209, 1978.

Whyte, H. and Winkelmann, R. Elastosis perforans (perforating elastosis): The association of congenital anomalies, salient facts in the histology, studies of enzyme digestion and a report of necropsy in a case. *J. Invest. Dermatol.*, 35:113, 1960.

Woerdeman, M., Bour, D. and Bijlsma, J. Elastosis perforans serpiginosa: Report of a family with a chromosomal investigation. *Arch. Dermatol.*, 92:559, 1965.

Perforating Calcific Elastosis

Hicks, I., Carpenter, C., Jr. and Reed, P. Periumbilical perforating pseudoxanthoma elasticum. *Arch. Dermatol.*, 115:300, 1979.

Lund, H. and Gilbert, C. Perforating pseudoxanthoma elasticum. *Arch. Pathol.*, 100:544, 1976.

Schwartz, R. and Richfield, D. Pseudoxanthoma elasticum with transepidermal elimination. *Arch. Dermatol.*, 114:279, 1978.

James, W. and Odom, R. Late subcutaneous fibrosis following megavoltage radiotherapy. *J. Am. Acad. Dermatol.*, 3:616, 1980.
Jolles, B. X-ray skin reactions and the protective role of normal tissues. *Br. J. Radiol.*, 14:110, 1941.
Kurban, A. and Farah, F. Effects of x-irradiation on the skin. I. Histochemistry of acute changes in the epithelial structure. *Acta Derm. Venereol.*, 49:64, 1969.
Ledoux-Corbusier, M. and Achten, G. Elastosis in chronic radiodermatitis: An ultrastructural study. *Br. J. Dermatol.*, 91:287, 1974.
Ridley, C., Hope-Stone, H. and Fountain, R. Fibrosis of skin and subcutaneous tissue following megavoltage radiotherapy. *Trans. St. John's Hosp. Dermatol. Soc.*, 57:190, 1971.
Saunders, T. and Montgomery, H. Chronic roentgen and radium dermatitis: An analysis of 259 cases. *JAMA*, 110:23, 1938.
Sweet, R. Acute accidental superficial X-ray burns: An interim report of 11 cases. *Br. J. Dermatol.*, 74:392, 1962.
Teloh, H., Mason, M. and Wheelock, M. A histopathologic study of radiation injuries of the skin. *Surg. Gynecol. Obst.*, 90:335, 1950.
Wolbach, S. The pathological histology of chronic X-ray dermatitis and early X-ray carcinoma. *J. Med. Res.*, 21:415, 1909.
——. A summary of the effects of repeated roentgen-ray exposures upon the human skin, antecedent to the formation of carcinoma. *Am. J. Roentgenol.*, 13:139, 1925.

Poikiloderma

Allison, J. A benign variant of poikiloderma. *Trans. St. John's Hosp. Dermatol. Soc.*, 40:55, 1958.
Dowling, G. and Freudenthal, W. Dermatomyositis and poikiloderma atrophicans vasculare: A clinical and histological comparison. *Br. J. Dermatol.*, 50:519, 1938.
Downing, J., Edelstein, J. and Fitzpatrick, T. Poikiloderma vasculare atrophicans: Report of a case with observations at autopsy. *Arch. Dermatol. Syph.*, 56:740, 1947.
Guy, W., Grauer, R. and Jacob, F. Poikilodermatomyositis. *Arch. Dermatol. Syph.*, 40:867, 1939.
Horn, R., Jr. Poikilodermatomyositis: Report of a case with complete postmortem examination. *Arch. Dermatol. Syph.*, 44:1086, 1941.
Lane, J. Poikiloderma atrophicans vasculare: Conclusion of previously reported case. *Arch. Dermatol. Syph.*, 8:373, 1923.
——. Poikiloderma atrophicans vasculare: With report of a case by Oliver S. Ormsby, M.D., Chicago. *Arch. Dermatol. Syph.*, 4:563, 1921.
Rook, A., Davis, R. and Stevanovic, D. Poikiloderma congenitale: Rothmund-Thomson syndrome. *Acta Derm. Venereol.*, 39:392, 1959.
Rook, A. and Whimster, I. Congenital cutaneous dystrophy (Thomson's type). *Br. J. Dermatol.*, 61:197, 1949.
Thannhauser, S. Werner's syndrome (progeria of the adult) and Rothmund's syndrome: Two types of closely related heredofamilial atrophic dermatosis with juvenile cataracts and endocrine features: A critical study with five new cases. *Ann. Int. Med.*, 23:559, 1945.
Watsky, M. and Lynnfield, Y. Poikiloderma vasculare atrophicans. *Cutis*, 17:938, 1976.
Weary, P., Manley, W., Jr. and Graham, G. Hereditary acrokeratotic poikiloderma. *Arch. Dermatol.*, 103:409, 1971.
Wolf, D. and Selmanowitz, V. Poikiloderma vasculare atrophicans. *Cancer*, 25:682, 1970.

Acrodermatitis Chronica Atrophicans

Biagini, G. et al. Dermal vessels in acrodermatitis chronica atrophicans. *J. Cutan. Pathol.*, 3:199, 1976.
Burgdorf, W., Worret, W. and Schultka, O. Acrodermatitis chronica atrophicans. *Internat. J. Dermatol.*, 18:595, 1979.
Grimer, H. Akrodermatitis chronica atrophicans. *Z. Haut.*, 36:17, 1964.
Hardmeier, T. Zur Histopathologie der fibroiden Knoten bei Akrodermatitis chronica atrophicans. *Arch. Klin. Exp. Dermatol.*, 232:373, 1968.
Kraus, Z., Matéja, F. and Mazàk, J. Myelogram and cryoglobulins in acrodermatitis chronica atrophicans. *Acta Derm. Venereol.*, 43:163, 1963.

Marshall, J. Acrodermatitis chronica atrophicans (Pick-Herxheimer). Report on a South African case and a discussion of the relationship of acrodermatitis chronica atrophicans to erythema chronicum migrans and lymphadenosis benigna cutis. *S. Afr. Med. J.*, 32:753, 1958.

Montgomery, H. and Sullivan, R. Acrodermatitis atrophicans chronica. *Arch. Dermatol. Syph.*, 51:32, 1945.

Nasemann, T. In Südafrika erworbene Acrodermatitis chronica atrophicans Herxheimer. Z. *Haut.*, 55:310, 1980.

Sweitzer, S. and Laymon, C. Acrodermatitis chronica atrophicans. *Arch. Dermatol. Syph.*, 31:196, 1935.

Weber, K. et al. Zur Klinik und Ätiologie der Acrodermatitis chronica atrophicans. *Hautarzt*, 35:571, 1984.

Anetoderma (Macular Atrophy)

Brenner, W. et al. Non-inflammatory dermal elastolysis. *Br. J. Dermatol.*, 99:335, 1978.

Chargin, L. and Silver, H. Macular atrophy of the skin. *Arch. Dermatol. Syph.*, 24:614, 1931.

Cramer, H. Zur Histopathogenese der Dermatitis atrophicans maculosa. *Derm. Wschr.*, 147:230, 1963.

Davis, W. Wilson's disease and penicillamine-induced anetoderma. *Arch. Dermatol.*, 113:976, 1977.

Feldman, S. Macular atrophy (Schweninger and Buzzi type). *Arch. Dermatol. Syph.*, 38:117, 1938.

Kossard, S. et al. Inflammatory macular atrophy: Immunofluorescent and ultrastructural findings. *J. Am. Acad. Dermatol.*, 1:325, 1979.

Marshall, J., Heyl, T. and Weber, H. Postinflammatory elastolysis and cutis laxa: A report on a new variety of this phenomenon and a discussion of some syndromes characterized by elastolysis. *S. Afr. Med. J.*, 40:1016, 1966.

Miller, W., Ruggles, C. and Rist, T. Anetoderma. *Internat. J. Dermatol.*, 18:43, 1979.

Pusey, W. A case of multiple benign tumor-like new growths of Schweninger and Buzzi. *J. Cutan. Dis.*, 35:582, 1917.

Varadi, D. and Saqueton, A. Perifollicular elastolysis. *Br. J. Dermatol.*, 83:143, 1970.

Venencie, P. and Winkelmann, R. Histopathologic findings in anetoderma. *Arch. Dermatol.*, 120:1040, 1984.

Venencie, P., Winkelmann, R. and Moore, B. Anetoderma: Clinical findings, associations, and long term follow-up evaluations. *Arch. Dermatol.*, 120:1032, 1984.

Striae Distensae

Chernosky, M. and Knox, J. Atrophic striae after occlusive corticosteroid therapy. *Arch. Dermatol.*, 90:15, 1964.

Epstein, N., Epstein, W., and Epstein, J. Atrophic striae in patients with inguinal intertrigo. *Arch. Dermatol.*, 87:450, 1963.

Hauser, W. Zur Frage der Entstehung der Striae cutis atrophicae. *Dermatol. Wochenschr.*, 138:1291, 1958.

Klehr, N. Striae cutis atrophicae: Morphokinetic examinations *in vitro*. *Acta Derm. Venereol.* (Stockh.), 59 (85, suppl.):105, 1979.

Pinkus, H., Keech, M. and Mehregan, A. Histopathology of striae distensae with special reference to striae and wound healing in the Marfan syndrome. *J. Invest. Dermatol.*, 46:283, 1966.

Shuster, S. The cause of striae distensae. *Acta Derm. Venereol.* (Stockh.), 59 (85, suppl.):161, 1979.

Simkin, B. and Arce, R. Steroid excretion in obese patients with colored abdominal striae. *N. Eng. J. Med.*, 266:1031, 1962.

Sisson, W. Colored striae in adolescent children. *J. Pediatr.*, 45:520, 1954.

Zheng, P., Lavker, R. and Kligman, A. Anatomy of striae. *Br. J. Dermatol.*, 112:185, 1985.

Steroid Atrophy

Kelly, E., Jr. The effects of triamcinolone on human skin. *J. Natl. Med. Assoc.*, 55:510, 1963.

Polano, M. et al., eds., Advances in topical corticosteroid therapy. *Dermatologica*, 152 (1, suppl.), 1976.

Chondrodermatitis Nodularis Helicis

Bard, J. Chondrodermatitis nodularis chronica helicis. *Dermatologica*, 163:376, 1981.

Barker, L., Young, A. and Sachs, W. Chondrodermatitis of the ears: A differential study of nodules of the helix and anthelix. *Arch. Dermatol.*, 81:15, 1960.

Ebenius, B. Chondrodermatitis nodularis chronica auriculae. *Acta Radiol.*, 22:563, 1941.

Goette, D. Chondrodermatitis nodularis chronica helicis: A perforating necrobiotic granuloma. *J. Am. Acad. Dermatol.*, 2:148, 1980.

Haber, H. Chondrodermatitis nodularis chronica helicis. *Hautarzt*, 11:122, 1960.

McConnell, E. The histological appearances of chondrodermatitis chronica helicis. *J. Clin. Pathol.*, 10:46, 1957.

Newcomer, V. et al. Chondrodermatitis nodularis chronica helicis: Report of ninety-four cases and survey of literature, with emphasis upon pathogenesis and treatment. *Arch. Dermatol. Syph.*, 68:241, 1953.

Santa Cruz, D. Chondrodermatitis nodularis helicis: A transepidermal perforating disorder. *J. Cutan. Pathol.*, 7:70, 1980.

Shuman, R. and Helwig, E. Chondrodermatitis helicis. *Am. J. Clin. Pathol.*, 24:126, 1954.

Silva, L. et al. Bone formation in chondrodermatitis nodularis helicis. *J. Dermatol. Surg. Oncol.*, 6:582, 1980.

Tennstedt, D. and Lachapelle, J. Acanthome fissuré. Revue de la littérature et diagnostic histopathologique différentiel avec le nodule douloureux de l'oreille. *Ann. Derm. Venereol.*, 106:219, 1979.

Relapsing Polychondritis

Barranco, V., Minor, D. and Solomon, H. Treatment of polychondritis with dapsone. *Arch. Dermatol.*, 112:1286, 1976.

Cohen, P. and Rapini, R. Relapsing polychondritis. *Internat. J. Dermatol.*, 25:280, 1986.

Feinerman, L. et al. Relapsing polychondritis. *Dermatologica*, 140:369, 1970.

Foidart, J. and Katz, S. Relapsing polychondritis. *Am. J. Dermatopathol.*, 1:257, 1979.

Foidart, J. et al. Antibodies to type II collagen in relapsing polychondritis. *N. Eng. J. Med.*, 299:1203, 1978.

McAdam, L. et al. Relapsing polychondritis: Prospective study of 23 patients and a review of the literature. *Medicine*, 55:193, 1976.

Thurston, C. and Curtis, A. Relapsing polychondritis. *Arch. Dermatol.*, 93:664, 1966.

Valenzuela, R. et al. Relapsing polychondritis. *Hum. Pathol.*, 11:19, 1980.

Weinberger, A. and Myers, A. Relapsing polychondritis associated with cutaneous vasculitis. *Arch. Dermatol.*, 115:980, 1979.

Elastosis Perforans Serpiginosa

Abel, M. Elastosis perforans serpiginosa associated with penicillamine. *Arch. Dermatol.*, 113:1303, 1977.

Ayala, F. and Donofrio, P. Elastosis perforans serpiginosa: Report of a family. *Dermatologica*, 166:32, 1983.

Bardach, A., Gebhart, W. and Niebauer, G. "Lumpy-bumpy" elastic fibers in the skin and lungs of a patient with penicillamine-induced elastosis perforans serpiginosa. *J. Cutan. Pathol.*, 6:243, 1979.

Bardach, H. and Gebhart, W. Penicillamininduzierte dermolytische Dermatose bei einer Patientin mit Morbus Wilson. *Dermatologica*, 162:473, 1981.

Carey, T. Elastosis perforans serpiginosa. *Arch. Dermatol.*, 113:1444, 1977.

Charles, R. In discussion of Davis W: Wilson's disease and penicillamine-induced anetoderma. *Arch. Dermatol.*, 113:976, 1977.

Christianson, H. Elastosis perforans serpiginosa: Association with congenital anomalies: Report of 2 cases. *South. Med. J.*, 59:15, 1966.

Davis, W. Wilson's disease and penicillamine-induced anetoderma. *Arch. Dermatol.*, 113:976, 1977.

Degos, R. et al. Pemphigus chez un malade traité par pénicillamine pour maladie de Wilson. *Bull. Soc. Fr. Dermatol. Syph.*, 76:751, 1969.

Eide, J. Elastosis perforans serpiginosa with widespread arterial lesions: A case report. *Acta Derm. Venereol.* (Stockh.), 57:553, 1977.

From, E. and Fredericksen, P. Pemphigus vulgaris following D-penicillamine. *Dermatologica*, 152:358, 1976.

Goldschmidt, H. and Sherwin, W. Reactions to ionizing radiation. *J. Am. Acad. Dermatol.*, 3:551, 1980.

Greenblatt, M. Elastosis perforans serpiginosa. *Arch. Pathol.*, 75:177, 1963.

Greer, K., Askew, F. and Richardson, D. Skin lesions induced by penicillamine. *Arch. Dermatol.*, 112:1267, 1976.

Guilaine, J., Benhamon, J. and Molas, G. Élastome perforant verruciforme chez un malade traité par pénicillamine pour maladie de Wilson. *Bull. Soc. Fr. Dermatol. Syph.*, 79:450, 1972.

Hashimoto, K., McEvoy, B. and Belcher, R. Ultrastructure of penicillamine-induced skin lesions. *J. Am. Acad. Dermatol.*, 4:300, 1981.

Hitch, J. and Lund, H. Elastosis perforans serpiginosa. *Arch. Dermatol.*, 79:407, 1959.

Katz, R. Penicillamine-induced skin lesions. *Arch. Dermatol.*, 95:196, 1967.

Kirsch, N. and Hukill, P. Elastosis perforans serpiginosa induced by penicillamine: Electron microscopic observations. *Arch. Dermatol.*, 113:630, 1977.

London, I. et al. Elastosis perforans serpiginosa with systemic involvement. *South. Med. J.*, 67:225, 1974.

Marshall, J. and Lurie, H. Keratosis follicularis serpiginosa (Lutz). *Dermatologica*, 113:13, 1956.

Mehregan, A. Elastosis perforans serpiginosa. *Arch. Dermatol.*, 97:381, 1968.

Pedro, S. and Garcia, R. Disseminate elastosis perforans serpiginosa. *Arch. Dermatol.*, 109:84, 1974.

Rasmussen, J. Disseminated elastosis perforans serpiginosa in 4 mongoloids. *Br. J. Dermatol.*, 86:9, 1972.

Reed, W. and Pidgeon, J. Elastosis perforans serpiginosa with osteogenesis imperfecta. *Arch. Dermatol.*, 89:342, 1964.

Reymond, J. et al. Penicillamine induced elastosis perforans serpiginosa: An ultrastructural study of two cases. *J. Cutan. Pathol.*, 9:352, 1982.

Schamroth, J., Kellen, P. and Grieve, T. Elastosis perforans serpiginosa in a patient with renal disease. *Arch. Dermatol.*, 122:82, 1986.

Schneider, W. and Bock, H. Elastosis perforans serpiginosa. *Hautarzt*, 27:117, 1976.

Tsambaos, D. and Berger, H. Elastosis perforans serpiginosa. Licht und elektronenmikroskopische Befunde. *Z. Haut.*, 55:563, 1979.

Ueda, K. et al. A case of elastosis perforans serpiginosa: An ultrastructural study. *J. Cutan. Pathol.*, 10:217, 1983.

Volpin, D. et al. Ultrastructural and biochemical studies on a case of elastosis perforans serpiginosa. *Dermatologica*, 156:209, 1978.

Whyte, H. and Winkelmann, R. Elastosis perforans (perforating elastosis): The association of congenital anomalies, salient facts in the histology, studies of enzyme digestion and a report of necropsy in a case. *J. Invest. Dermatol.*, 35:113, 1960.

Woerdeman, M., Bour, D. and Bijlsma, J. Elastosis perforans serpiginosa: Report of a family with a chromosomal investigation. *Arch. Dermatol.*, 92:559, 1965.

Perforating Calcific Elastosis

Hicks, I., Carpenter, C., Jr. and Reed, P. Periumbilical perforating pseudoxanthoma elasticum. *Arch. Dermatol.*, 115:300, 1979.

Lund, H. and Gilbert, C. Perforating pseudoxanthoma elasticum. *Arch. Pathol.*, 100:544, 1976.

Schwartz, R. and Richfield, D. Pseudoxanthoma elasticum with transepidermal elimination. *Arch. Dermatol.*, 114:279, 1978.

Kyrle's Disease

Abele, D. and Dobson, R. Hyperkeratosis penetrans (Kyrle's disease). *Arch. Dermatol.*, 83:277, 1961.

Aram, H., Szymanski, F. and Bailey, W. Kyrle's disease. *Arch. Dermatol.*, 100:453, 1969.

Bardach, H. Dermatosen mit transepithelialer Perforation. *Arch. Dermatol. Res.*, 257:213, 1976.

Bovenmyer, D. Reactive perforating collagenosis: Experimental production of the lesion. *Arch. Dermatol.*, 102:313, 1970.

Carter, V. and Constantine, V. Kyrle's disease. I. Clinical findings in 5 cases and review of literature. *Arch. Dermatol.*, 97:624, 1968.

Constantine, V. and Carter, V. Kyrle's disease II. Histopathologic findings in 5 cases and review of the literature. *Arch. Dermatol.*, 97:633, 1968.

Cunningham, S. et al. Kyrle's disease. *J. Am. Acad. Dermatol.*, 16:117, 1987.

Fischer, R., Stamps, P. and Skipworth, G. A proposed variant of hyperkeratosis penetrans. *Arch. Dermatol.*, 98:270, 1968.

Haensch, R., Hettwer, H. and Meisel, U. Morbus Kyrle (Hyperkeratosis follicularis et parafollicularis penetrans). *Z. Haut.*, 54:99, 1978.

Hood, A. et al. Kyrle's disease in patients with chronic renal failure. *Arch. Dermatol.*, 118:85, 1982.

Mehregan, A. and Coskey, R. Perforating folliculitis. *Arch. Dermatol.*, 97:394, 1968.

Mehregan, A., Schwartz, O. and Livingood, C. Reactive perforating collagenosis. *Arch. Dermatol.*, 96:277, 1967.

Nair, B. et al. Reactive perforating collagenosis. *Br. J. Dermatol.*, 91:399, 1974.

Peterson, W., Jr., Goltz, R. and Hult, A. Hyperkeratosis penetrans (Kyrle's disease). *Arch. Dermatol.*, 88:210, 1963.

Prakken, J. Kyrle's disease: Hyperkeratosis follicularis et parafollicularis in cutem penetrans. *Acta Derm. Venereol.*, 34:360, 1954.

Streitmann, B. Ein Beitrag, zu den das Follikelepithel durchbrechenden Prozessen. *Z. Haut.*, 45:195, 1970.

Tappeiner, J., Wolff, K. and Schreiner, E. Morbus Kyrle. *Hautarzt*, 20:296, 1969.

Thyresson, N. Hyperkeratosis follicularis et parafollicularis in cutem penetrans. *Acta Derm. Venereol.*, 31:287, 1951.

Weiner, A. Reactive perforating collagenosis. *Arch. Dermatol.*, 102:540, 1970.

Perforating Folliculitis

Golitz, L. Follicular and perforating disorders. *J. Cutan. Pathol.*, 12:282, 1985.

Hurwitz, R. et al. Perforating folliculitis in association with hemodialysis. *Am. J. Dermatopathol.*, 4:101, 1982.

Mehregan, A. Perforating dermatoses: A clinicopathologic review. *Internat. J. Dermatol.*, 16:19, 1977.

Mehregan, A. and Coskey, R. Perforating folliculitis. *Arch. Dermatol.*, 97:394, 1968.

Streitmann, B. Ein Beitrag zu den das Follikelepithel durchbrechenden Prozessen. *Z. Haut.*, 45:195, 1970.

White, C. et al. Perforating folliculitis of hemodialysis. *Am. J. Dermatopathol.*, 4:109, 1982.

Reactive Perforating Collagenosis

Bovenmyer, D. Reactive perforating collagenosis. *Arch. Dermatol.*, 102:313, 1970.

Delacrétaz, J. and Gattlen, J. Transepidermal elimination of traumatically altered collagen. *Dermatologica*, 152:65, 1976.

Fretzin, D., Beal, D. and Jao, W. Light and ultrastructural study of reactive perforating collagenosis. *Arch. Dermatol.*, 116:1054, 1980.

Kanan, M. Familial reactive perforating collagenosis and intolerance to cold. *Br. J. Dermatol.*, 91:405, 1974.

Mehregan, A. Perforating dermatoses: A clinicopathologic review. *Internat. J. Dermatol.*, 16:19, 1977.

Mehregan, A., Schwartz, O. and Livingood, C. Reactive perforating collagenosis. *Arch. Dermatol.*, 96:277, 1967.

Mohri, S., Sano, T. and Fukuda, S. An adult case of reactive perforating collagenosis. *J. Dermatol.* (Tokyo), 7:363, 1980.
Patterson, J. The perforating disorders. *J. Am. Acad. Dermatol.*, 10:561, 1984.
Poliak, S. et al. Reactive perforating collagenosis associated with diabetes mellitus. *N. Eng. J. Med.*, 306:81, 1982.
Weiner, A. Reactive perforating collagenosis. *Arch. Dermatol.*, 102:540, 1970.
Woo, T. and Rasmussen, J. Disorders of transepidermal elimination. *Internat. J. Dermatol.*, 24:267, 1985.
Woringer, F. and Laugier, P. Collagenoma perforans verruciforme. *Dermatol. Wochenschr.*, 147:64, 1963.

Granuloma Annulare

Aliaga, A. et al. Perforating granuloma annulare and vitamin D. *Dermatologica*, 164:62, 1982.
Bardach, H. Granuloma annulare with transfollicular perforation. *J. Cutan. Pathol.*, 4:99, 1977.
Barr, R. and Stegman, S. Delayed skin test reaction to injectable collagen implant (Zyderm). *J. Am. Acad. Dermatol.*, 10:652, 1984.
Buechner, S. et al. Identification of T-cell subpopulations in granuloma annulare. *Arch. Dermatol.*, 119:125, 1983.
Burket, J. and Zelickson, A. Intracellular elastin in generalized granuloma annulare. *J. Am. Acad. Dermatol.*, 14:975, 1986.
Burton, J. Granuloma annulare, rheumatoid nodules and necrobiosis lipoidica. *Br. J. Dermatol.*, 97 (suppl.):52, 1977.
Calas, E. et al. Granuloma annulaire généalizé perforant: A propos de 2 observations. *Ann. Dermatol. Venereol.*, 107:165, 1980.
Cherney, K. et al. Leukocyte function in granuloma annulare. *Br. J. Dermatol.*, 101:23, 1979.
Cooper, P. Eruptive xanthoma: A microscopic simulant of granuloma annulare. *J. Cutan. Pathol.*, 13:207, 1986.
Dahl, M. et al. Circulating immune complexes in granuloma annulare. (abstr.). *Clin. Res.*, 27:712A, 1979.
Dahl, M. et al. Elevated heparin precipitable fraction of plasma in granuloma annulare. *Arch. Dermatol.*, 115:1059, 1979.
Delaney, T., Gold, S. and Leppard, B. Disseminated perforating granuloma annulare. *Br. J. Dermatol.*, 89:523, 1973.
Dicken, C., Carrington, S. and Winkelmann, R. Generalized granuloma annulare. *Arch. Dermatol.*, 99:556, 1969.
Dos Reis Gadelha, A. and Talhan, S. Granuloma anular perforante. *Med. Cutan. Iber. Lat. Am.*, 9:101, 1981.
Duncan, W., Smith, J. and Knox, J. Generalized perforating granuloma annulare. *Arch. Dermatol.*, 108:570, 1973.
Ellis, F. and Kirby-Smith, H. Necrobiosis lipoidica and granuloma annulare: A comparative study. *Arch. Dermatol. Syph.*, 45:40, 1942.
Grauer, F. Granuloma annulare: Report of an unusual case. *Arch. Dermatol. Syph.*, 30:785, 1934.
Gross, P. and Shelley, W. The association of generalized granuloma annulare with antithyroid antibodies. *Acta Derm. Venereol.*, 51:59, 1971.
Haim, S., Friedman-Birnbaum, R. and Shafrir, A. Generalized granuloma annulare: Relationship to diabetes mellitus as revealed in eight cases. *Br. J. Dermatol.*, 83:302, 1970.
Haustein, U. Zur Ultrastruktur des Granuloma annulare. *Dermatol. Monatsschr.*, 162:289, 1976.
Hazelrigg, D. Generalized perforating granuloma annulare: A case report and review of the literature. *Cutis.*, 23:813, 1979.
Izumi, A. Generalized perforating granuloma annulare. *Arch. Dermatol.*, 108:708, 1973.
Johnson, W. Necrobiotic granulomas. *J. Cutan. Pathol.*, 12:289, 1985.
Laymon, C. and Fisher, I. Necrobiosis lipoidica (diabeticorum?): A histologic study and comparison with granuloma annulare. *Arch. Dermatol. Syph.*, 59:150, 1949.
Majewski, B. et al. Increased factor VIII-related antigen in necrobiosis lipoidica and widespread granuloma annulare without associated diabetes. *Br. J. Dermatol.*, 107:641, 1982.
Marshall, J., Weber, H. and Kok, S. Granuloma multiforme (Leiker). *Dermatologica*, 134:193, 1967.

Meyers, W., Connor, D. and Shannon, R. Histologic characteristics of granuloma multiforme (Mkar disease): Including a comparison with leprosy and granuloma annulare: Report of first case from Congo (Kinshasa). *Inst. J. Lepr.*, 38:241, 1970.
Modlin, R. et al. Immunopathologic demonstration of T lymphocyte subpopulations and interleukin 2 in granuloma annulare. *Pediatr. Dermatol.*, 2:26, 1984.
Monfrecola, G. and Ayala, F. Granuloma annulare perforante. *Ann. Ital. Derm. Clin. Sperim.*, 34:55, 1980.
Moyer, D. Papular granuloma annulare, *Arch. Dermatol.*, 89:41, 1964.
Muhlbauer, J. Granuloma annulare. *J. Am. Acad. Dermatol.*, 3:217, 1980.
Muhlemann, M. and Williams, D. Localized granuloma annulare is associated with insulin-dependent diabetes mellitus. *Br. J. Dermatol.*, 111:325, 1984.
Nieboer, C. and Kalsbeek, G. Direct immunofluorescence studies in granuloma annulare, necrobiosis lipoidica and granulomatosis disciformis Miescher. *Dermatologica*, 158:427, 1979.
Ogino, A. and Tamaki, E. Atypical granuloma annulare. *Dermatologica*, 156:97, 1978.
Owens, D. and Freeman, R. Generalized perforating granuloma annulare. *Arch. Dermatol.*, 103:64, 1971.
Prunty, F. and Montgomery, H. Granuloma annulare. *Arch. Dermatol. Syph.*, 46:394, 1942.
Radcliffe-Crocker, H. Granuloma annulare. *Br. J. Dermatol.*, 14:1, 1902.
Romaine, R., Rudner, E. and Altman, J. Papular granuloma annulare and diabetes mellitus. *Arch. Dermatol.*, 98:152, 1968.
Rubin, M. and Lynch, F. Subcutaneous granuloma annulare: Comment on familial granuloma annulare. *Arch. Dermatol.*, 93:416, 1966.
Schwartz, M. Necrobiosis lipoidica and granuloma annulare: Simultaneous occurrence in a patient. *Arch. Dermatol.*, 118:192, 1982.
Stankler, L. and Leslie, G. Generalized granuloma annulare: A report of a case and review of the literature. *Arch. Dermatol.*, 95:509, 1967.
Thyresson, H., Doyle, J. and Winkelmann, R. Granuloma annulare: Histopathologic and direct immunofluorescence study. *Acta Derm. Venereol.* (Stockh.), 60:261, 1980.
Umbert, P. and Winkelmann, R. Histologic, ultrastructural, and histochemical studies of granuloma annulare. *Arch. Dermatol.*, 113:1681, 1977.
Wells, R. and Smith, M. The natural history of granuloma annulare. *Br. J. Dermatol.*, 75:199, 1963.
Wolff, H. and Maciejewski, W. The ultrastructure of granuloma annulare. *Arch. Dermatol. Res.*, 259:225, 1977.
Wood, M. and Beerman, H. Necrobiosis lipoidica, granuloma annulare, and rheumatoid nodule. *J. Invest. Dermatol.*, 34:139, 1960.

Annular Elastolytic Granuloma (Actinic Granuloma)

Dahl, M. Is actinic granuloma really granuloma annulare? *Arch. Dermatol.*, 122:39, 1986.
Dowling, G. and Wilson-Jones, E. Atypical (annular) necrobiosis lipoidica of the face and scalp. *Dermatologica*, 135:11, 1967.
Hanke, C., Bailin, P. and Roenigk, H., Jr. Annular elastolytic giant cell granuloma. *J. Am. Acad. Dermatol.*, 1:413, 1979.
McGrae, J., Jr. Actinic granuloma: A clinical, histopathologic and immunocytochemical study. *Arch. Dermatol.*, 122:43, 1986.
Mehregan, A. and Altman, J. Miescher's granuloma of the face. *Arch. Dermatol.*, 107:62, 1973.
Moreno, A. et al. Actinic granuloma: An ultrastructural study of two cases. *J. Cutan. Pathol.*, 11:179, 1984.
Moulin, G. et al. Le granulome actinique de O'Brien. *Ann. Dermatol. Venereol.*, 109:135, 1982.
O'Brien, J. Actinic granuloma. *Arch. Dermatol.*, 111:460, 1975.
——. Is actinic granuloma a specific condition? Another view: Perhaps the concept should be extended. *Am. J. Dermatopathol.*, 1:51, 1979.
Ragaz, A. and Ackerman, A. Is actinic granuloma a specific condition? *Am. J. Dermatopathol.*, 1:43, 1979.
Wilson-Jones, E. Necrobiosis lipoidica presenting on the face and scalp. *Trans. St. John's Hosp. Dermatol. Soc.*, 57:203, 1971.

Necrobiosis Lipoidica

Bauer, M. et al. Necrobiosis lipoidica diabeticorum: A cutaneous manifestation of diabetic microangiopathy. *Arch. Dermatol.*, 90:558, 1964.

Bauer, M. et al. Pigmented pretibial patches. *Arch. Dermatol.*, 93:282, 1966.

Dowling, G. and Wilson-Jones, E. Atypical (annular) necrobiosis lipoidica of the face and scalp. *Dermatologica*, 135:11, 1967.

Ellis, F. Necrobiosis lipoidica: A form of granuloma annulare? *Arch. Dermatol. Syph.*, 43:822, 1941.

Ellis, F. and Kirby-Smith, H. Necrobiosis lipoidica and granuloma annulare: A comparative study. *Arch. Dermatol. Syph.*, 45:40, 1942.

Fisher, E. and Danowski, T. Histologic, histochemical and electron microscopic features of the skin spots of diabetes mellitus. *Am. J. Clin. Pathol.*, 50:547, 1968.

Garcia, E. et al. Nécrobiose lipoidique perforante. *Ann. Dermatol. Venereol.*, 108:891, 1981.

Gray, H., Graham, J. and Johnson, W. Necrobiosis lipoidica: A histopathological and histochemical study. *J. Invest. Dermatol.*, 44:369, 1965.

Hildebrand, A., Montgomery, H. and Rynearson, E. Necrobiosis lipoidica diabeticorum. *Arch. Int. Med.*, 66:851, 1940.

Mehregan, A. and Pinkus, H. Necrobiosis lipoidica with sarcoid reaction: A case report. *Arch. Dermatol.*, 83:143, 1961.

Mobacken, H., Gisslen, H. and Johannisson, G. Granuloma annulare. *Acta Derm. Venereol.*, 50:440, 1970.

Muller, S. and Winkelmann, R. Necrobiosis lipoidica diabeticorum: A clinical and pathological investigation of 171 cases. *Arch. Dermatol.*, 93:272, 1966.

——. Necrobiosis lipoidica diabeticorum: Histopathologic study of 98 cases. *Arch. Dermatol.*, 94:1, 1966.

Parra, C. Transepithelial elimination in necrobiosis lipoidica. *Br. J. Dermatol.*, 96:83, 1977.

Smith, J., Jr. Necrobiosis lipoidica: A disease of changing concepts. *Arch. Dermatol.*, 74:280, 1956.

Ullman, S. and Dahl, M. Necrobiosis lipoidica. *Arch. Dermatol.*, 113:1671, 1977.

Wilson-Jones, E. Necrobiosis lipoidica presenting on the face and scalp. *Trans. St. John's Hosp. Dermatol. Soc.*, 57:202, 1971.

Rheumatoid Nodule

Beatty, E., Jr. Rheumatic-like nodules occurring in non-rheumatic children. *Arch. Pathol.*, 68:154, 1959.

Bennett, G., Zeller, J. and Bauer, W. Subcutaneous nodules of rheumatoid arthritis and rheumatic fever: A pathologic study. *Arch. Pathol.*, 30:70, 1940.

Collins, D. The subcutaneous nodule of rheumatoid arthritis. *J. Pathol. Bacteriol.*, 45:97, 1937.

Dabbous, M. et al. Collagenolytic activity in rheumatoid nodules. I. Effect on acid-soluble tropocollagen. *Acta Derm. Venereol.*, 54:265, 1974.

Dubois, E., Friou, G. and Chandor, S. Rheumatoid nodules and rheumatoid granulomas in systemic lupus erythematosus. *JAMA*, 220:515, 1972.

Hahn, B., Yardley, J. and Stevens, M. Rheumatoid "nodules" in systemic lupus erythematosus. *Ann. Int. Med.*, 72:49, 1970.

Harris, E., Jr. A collagenolytic system produced by primary cultures of rheumatoid nodule tissue. *J. Clin. Invest.*, 51:2973, 1972.

Lowney, E. and Simons, H. "Rheumatoid" nodules of the skin: Their significance as an isolated finding. *Arch. Dermatol.*, 88:853, 1963.

Rao, N. and Font, R. Pseudorheumatoid nodules of the ocular adnexa. *Am. J. Ophthalmol.*, 79:471, 1975.

Rush, P. et al. Chronic arthritis following benign rheumatoid nodules of childhood. *Arthrit. and Rheum.*, 28:1175, 1985.

Taranta, A. Occurrence of rheumatic-like subcutaneous nodules without evidence of joint or heart disease: Report of a case. *N. Eng. J. Med.*, 266:13, 1962.

Watt, T. and Baumann, R. Psuedoxanthomatous rheumatoid nodules. *Arch. Dermatol.*, 95:156, 1967.

Lichen Sclerosus et Atrophicus

Barker, L. and Gross, P. Lichen sclerosus et atrophicus of the female genitalia: A clinical study and diagnostic guide. *Arch. Dermatol.*, 85:362, 1962.

Bart, R. and Kopf, A. Squamous cell carcinoma arising in balanitis xerotica obliterans. *J. Dermatol. Surg. Oncol.*, 4:556, 1978.

Bergfeld, W. and Lesowitz, S. Lichen sclerosus et atrophicus. *Arch. Dermatol.*, 101:247, 1970.

Chalmers, R. et al. Lichen sclerosus et atrophicus: A common and distinctive cause of phimosis in boys. *Arch. Dermatol.*, 120:1026, 1984.

Chernosky, M., Derbes, V. and Burks, J., Jr. Lichen sclerosus et atrophicus in children. *Arch. Dermatol.*, 75:647, 1957.

Clark, J. and Muller, S. Lichen sclerosus et atrophicus in children. *Arch. Dermatol.*, 95:476, 1967.

Fairgrieve, J. and Parker, R. Acquired phimosis in the elderly caused by lichen sclerosus et atrophicus. *Br. J. Urol.*, 31:74, 1959.

Gottschalk, H. and Cooper, Z. Lichen sclerosus et atrophicus with bullous lesions and extensive involvement. *Arch. Dermatol. Syph.*, 55:433, 1947.

Harrington, C. and Dunsmore, I. An investigation into the incidence of autoimmune disorders in patients with lichen sclerosus et atrophicus. *Br. J. Dermatol.*, 104:563, 1981.

Janovski, N. and Ames, S. Lichen sclerosus et atrophicus of the vulva: A poorly understood disease entity. *Obstet. Gynecol.*, 22:697, 1963.

Kindler, T. Lichen sclerosus et atrophicus in young subjects. *Br. J. Dermatol.*, 65:269, 1953.

Laymon, C. Lichen sclerosus et atrophicus and related disorders. *Arch. Dermatol.*, 64:620, 1961.

McAdams, A., Jr. and Kistner, R. The relationship of chronic vulvar disease, leukoplakia, and carcinoma *in situ* to carcinoma of the vulva. *Cancer*, 11:740, 1958.

Mann, P. and Cowan, M. Ultrastructural changes in four cases of lichen sclerosus et atrophicus. *Br. J. Dermatol.*, 89:223, 1973.

Miller, R. Lichen sclerosus et atrophicus with oral involvement: Histopathologic study and dermabrasive treatment. *Arch. Dermatol.*, 76:43, 1957.

Montgomery, H. and Hill, W. Lichen sclerosus et atrophicus. *Arch. Dermatol. Syph.*, 42:755, 1940.

Purres, J. and Krull, E. Lichen sclerosus et atrophicus involving the palms. *Arch. Dermatol.*, 104:68, 1971.

Steigleder, G. and Raab, W. Lichen sclerosus et atrophicus. *Arch. Dermatol.*, 84:219, 1961.

Suurmond, D. Lichen sclerosus et atrophicus of the vulva. *Arch. Dermatol.*, 90:143, 1964.

Thomas, R. and Kennedy, C. The development of lichen sclerosus et atrophicus in monozygotic twin girls. *Br. J. Dermatol.*, 114:377, 1986.

Wallace, H. and Whimster, I. Vulval atrophy and leukoplakia. *Br. J. Dermatol.*, 63:241, 1951.

Wallace, J. Lichen sclerosus et atrophicus. *Trans. St. John's Hosp. Dermatol. Soc.*, 57:9, 1971.

The Genetic Mucopolysaccharidoses

Belcher, R. Ultrastructure and cytochemistry of lymphocytes in the genetic mucopolysaccharidoses, *Arch. Pathol.*, 93:1, 1972.

——. Ultrastructure and function of eccrine glands in the mucopolysaccharidoses. *Arch. Pathol.*, 96:339, 1973.

——. Ultrastructure of the skin in the genetic mucopolysaccharidoses. *Arch. Pathol.*, 94:511, 1972.

De Cloux, R. and Friederici, H. Ultrastructural studies of the skin in Hurler's syndrome. *Arch. Pathol.*, 88:350, 1969.

Freeman, R. A pathological basis for the cutaneous papules of mucopolysaccharidosis II (the Hunter syndrome). *J. Cutan. Pathol.*, 4:318, 1977.

Hambrick, G., Jr. and Scheie, H. Studies of the skin in Hurler's syndrome. *Arch. Dermatol.*, 85:455, 1962.

Horiuchi, R. et al. Mucopolysaccharidosis with special reference to Scheie syndrome. *J. Dermatol.* (Tokyo), 3:171, 1976.

Lasser, A., Carter, D. and Mahoney, M. Ultrastructure of the skin in mucopolysaccharidoses. *Arch. Pathol.*, 99:173, 1975.

McKusick, V. The nosology of the mucopolysaccharidoses. *Am. J. Med.*, 47:730, 1969.

McKusick, V. et al. The mucopolysaccharide storage diseases. In: *The Metabolic Basis of Inherited Disease*, 4th Ed. Stanbury, J. et al., eds., New York, McGraw-Hill, 1978, p. 1282.

Pinell, S. and McKusick, V. The genetic mucopolysaccharides. In: *Dermatology in General Practice*, 2nd Ed. Fitzpatrick, T. et al., eds., New York, McGraw-Hill, 1979, p. 1155.

Prystowsky, S. et al. A cutaneous marker in the Hunter syndrome. *Arch. Dermatol.*, 113:602, 1977.

Pretibial Myxedema

Cheung, H. et al. Stimulation of fibroblast biosynthetic activity by serum of patients with pretibial myxedema. *J. Invest. Dermatol.*, 71:12, 1978.

Cohen, B., Benua, R. and Rawson, R. Localized myxedema involving the upper extremities. *Arch. Int. Med.*, 111:641, 1963.

Gimlette, T. Localized myxoedema and thyroid acropachy. In: *The Thyroid Gland*, Vol. 2, Pitt-Rivers, R. and Trotter, W., eds., London, Butterworth, 1964, p. 198.

Kinger, F. Myxedema in hyperthyroidism. *JAMA*, 194:663, 1965.

Konrad, K., Brenner, W. and Pehamberger, H. Ultrastructural and immunological findings in Graves' disease with pretibial myxedema. *J. Cutan. Pathol.*, 7:99, 1980.

Kriss, J., Pleshakov, V. and Chien, J. Isolation and identification of the long-acting thyroid stimulator and its relation to hyperthyroidism and circumscribed pretibial myxedema. *J. Clin. Endocrinol.*, 24:1005, 1964.

Lynch, P., Maize, J. and Lisson, J. Pretibial myxedema and non-thyrotoxic thyroid disease. *Arch. Dermatol.*, 107:107, 1973.

Noppakun, N., Bancheun, K. and Chandraprasert, S. Unusual locations of localized myxedema in Graves' disease. *Arch. Dermatol.*, 122:85, 1986.

Pillsbury, D. and Stokes, J. Circumscribed myxedema of the skin. *Arch. Dermatol. Syph.*, 24:255, 1931.

Pimstone, B., Hoffenberg, R. and Black, E. Parallel assays of thyrotropin, long-acting thyroid stimulator and exophthalmos-producing substance in endocrine exophthalmos and pretibial myxedema. *J. Clin. Endocrinol.*, 24:976, 1964.

Schermer, D. et al. Relationship of long-acting thyroid stimulator to pretibial myxedema. *Arch. Dermatol.*, 103:62, 1970.

Sunseri, J. Elephantiasic papulonodular myxedema. *Arch. Dermatol. Syph.*, 48:70, 1943.

Truhan, A. and Roenigk, H. The cutaneous mucinoses. *J. Am. Acad. Dermatol.*, 14:1, 1986.

Wortsman, J. et al. Preradial myxedema in thyroid states. *Arch. Dermatol.*, 117:635, 1981.

Generalized Myxedema

Cawley, E. et al. Examination of normal and myxedematous skin. *Arch. Dermatol.*, 76:537, 1957.

Gabrilove, J. and Ludwig, A. The histogenesis of myxedema. *J. Clin. Endocrinol.*, 17:925, 1957.

Pitt-Rivers, R. and Trotter, W. *The Thyroid Gland*. Washington, Butterworth, 1964.

Reuter, M. Histopathology of the skin in myxedema. *Arch. Dermatol. Syph.*, 24:55, 1931.

Werner, S. and Ingbar, S. *The Thyroid*, New York, Harper & Row, 1971.

Lichen Myxedematosus (Variant: Scleromyxedema)

Alligood, T. et al. Scleromyxedema associated with eosophageal aperistalsis and dermal eosinophilia. *Cutis*, 28:60, 1981.

Carli-Basset, C. et al. Apparition retardée d'une globuline monoclonale au cours d'une mucinose papuleuse. *Ann. Dermatol. Venereol.*, 106:175, 1979.

Chanda, J. Scleromyxedema. *Cutis*, 24:549, 1979.

Coskey, R. and Mehregan, A. Papular mucinosis. *Internat. J. Dermatol.*, 16:741, 1977.

Dalton, J. and Seidell, M. Studies on lichen myxedematosus (papular mucinosis). *Arch. Dermatol.*, 67:194, 1953.

Dalton, J. et al. A study of a case of lichen myxedematosus (papular mucinosis). *Arch. Dermatol.*, 81:422, 1960.

Feldman, P. et al. Scleromyxedema. *Arch. Dermatol.*, 99:51, 1969.
Hardie, R. et al. Spontaneous resolution of lichen myxedematosus. *Br. J. Dermatol.*, 100:727, 1979.
Harris, R. et al. Treatment of scleromyxedema with melphalan. *Arch. Dermatol.*, 115:295, 1978.
Ishii, M. et al. The use of improved ruthenium red staining for the ultrastructural detection of proteoglycan aggregates in normal skin and lichen myxedematosus. *J. Cutan. Pathol.*, 11:292, 1984.
Kantor, G. et al. Scleromyxedema associated with scleroderma, renal disease and acute psychosis. *J. Am. Acad. Dermatol.*, 14:879, 1986.
Krebs, A. and Müller, A. Lichen myxoedematosus und multiples Myelom vom Typ IgG/kappa. *Hautarzt*, 31:649, 1980.
Kubba, R. and Champion, R. Scleromyxedematosus. *Br. J. Dermatol.*, 93 (11, suppl.):36, 1975.
Kubba, R., McNeil, N. and Rook, A. Lichen myxedematosus, Crohn's disease and mucinous ovarian carcinoma. *Br. J. Dermatol.*, 93 (11, suppl.):34, 1975.
Lai, A. et al. Scleromyxedema (lichen myxedematosus) associated with paraprotein IgG of type kappa. *Br. J. Dermatol.*, 97:107, 1973.
Lang, E., Zabel, M. and Schmidt, H. Scleromyxödem Arndt-Gottron und assoziierte Phänomene. *Dermatologica*, 160:29, 1984.
McCarthy, J. et al. An abnormal serum globulin in lichen myxedematosus. *Arch. Dermatol.*, 89:446, 1964.
McCuistion, C. and Schoch, E., Jr. Autopsy findings in lichen myxedematosus. *Arch. Dermatol.*, 74:259, 1956.
Montgomery, H. and Underwood, L. Lichen myxedematosus (differentiation from cutaneous myxedemas or mucoid states). *J. Invest. Dermatol.*, 20:213, 1953.
Perry, H., Montgomery, H. and Stickney, J. Further observations on lichen myxedematosus. *Ann. Int. Med.*, 53:955, 1960.
Rudner, E., Mehregan, A. and Pinkus, H. Scleromyxedema: A variant of lichen myxedematosus. *Arch. Dermatol.*, 93:3, 1966.
Sawada, Y. and Ohashi, M. Scleromyxedema. *J. Dermatol.* (Tokyo), 7:207, 1980.
Schnyder, U. and Kaufmann, J. Skleromyxoedema Arndt-Gottron, Plasmozytom (Ig-Kappa-Typ). *Dermatologica*, 159:407, 1979.
Tappeiner, J. Zur Pathogenese des Lichen myxoedematosus: Mucinosis papulosa cutis. *Arch. Klin. Exp. Dermatol.*, 201:160, 1955.
Verity, M. et al. Scleromyxedema myopathy: Histochemical and electron microscope observations. *Am. J. Clin. Pathol.*, 69:446, 1978.

Digital Mucous Cyst

Bourns, H. and Sanerkin, N. Mucoid lesions ("mucoid cysts") of the fingers and toes: Clinical features and pathogenesis. *Br. J. Surg.*, 50:860, 1963.
Goldman, J. et al. Digital mucinous pseudocysts. *Arthrit. Rheum.*, 20:997, 1977.
Johnson, W., Graham, J. and Helwig, E. Cutaneous myxoid cyst. *JAMA*, 191:15, 1965.
——. Cutaneous myxoid cyst: A clinicopathological and histochemical study. *JAMA*, 191:15, 1965.
Johnson, W. and Helwig, E. Cutaneous focal mucinosis. *Arch. Dermatol.*, 93:13, 1966.
MacKee, G. and Andrews, G. The pathologic histology of synovial lesions of the skin. *Arch. Dermatol. Syph.*, 5:561, 1922.
Newmeyer, W., Kilgore, E., Jr. and Graham, W., III. Mucous cysts: The dorsal distal interphalangeal joint ganglion. *Plast. Reconstr. Surg.*, 53:313, 1974.

Mucous Cyst of the Oral Mucosa

Bhaskar, S. et al. Pathogenesis of mucoceles. *J. Dent. Res.*, 35:863, 1956.
Braun-Falco, O. Über ein Schleimgranulom der Zunge. *Hautarzt*, 11:131, 1960.
Ehlers, G. Zur Histogenese der Lippenschleimcysten. *Z. Haut.*, 34:77, 1963.
Lattan, A., Johnson, W. and Graham, J. Mucous cyst (mucocele). *Arch. Dermatol.*, 101:673, 1970.
Nikolowski, W. Schleimcysten und sogenanntes Schleimgranulom der Unterlippe. *Arch. Klin. Exp. Dermatol.*, 203:246, 1956.

Shafer, W. et al. *A Textbook of Oral Pathology*, 4th Ed. Philadelphia, WB Saunders, 1983.
Standish, S. and Shafer, W. The mucus retention phenomenon. *J. Oral Surg.*, 17:15, 1959.
Weir, T. and Johnson, W. Cheilitis glandularis. *Arch. Dermatol.*, 103:433, 1971.

Cheilitis Glandularis

Michalowski, R. Cheilitis glandularis, heterotopic salivary glands and squamous cell carcinoma of the lips. *Br. J. Dermatol.*, 74:455, 1962.
Oliver, I. and Pickett, A. Cheilitis glandularis. *Oral Surg.*, 49:526, 1980.
Ruelens-Van Haeverbeek, A. A propos de la cheilite glandulaire de Puente. *Arch. Belg. Dermatol. Syph.*, 25:147, 1969.
Schweich, L. Cheilitis glandularis simplex (Puente and Acevedo). *Arch. Dermatol.*, 89:301, 1964.
Swerlick, R. and Cooper, P. Cheilitis glandularis: A reevaluation. *J. Am. Acad. Dermatol.*, 10:466, 1984.
Weir, T. and Johnson, W. Cheilitis glandularis. *Arch. Dermatol.*, 103:433, 1971.

Alopecia Mucinosa

Binnick, A., Wax, F. and Clendenning, W. Alopecia mucinosa of the face associated with mycosis fungoides. *Arch. Dermatol.*, 114:791, 1978.
Emmerson, R. Follicular mucinosis: A study of 47 patients. *Br. J. Dermatol.*, 81:395, 1969.
Fan, J., Chang, H. and Mac, B. Alopecia mucinosa simulating leprosy. *Arch. Dermatol.*, 95:354, 1967.
Findlay, G. and Loewenthal, L. Alopecia mucinosa with eosinophil granuloma, lichen spinulosus and chancriform lesions. *Dermatologica*, 120:263, 1960.
Haber, H. Follicular mucinosis: Alopecia mucinosa (Pinkus) *Br. J. Dermatol.*, 73:313, 1961.
Ishibashi, A. Histogenesis of mucin in follicular mucinosis: An electron microscopic study. *Acta Derm. Venereol.* (Stockh.), 56:163, 1976.
Johnson, W., Higdon, R. and Helwig, E. Alopecia mucinosa. *Arch. Dermatol.*, 79:395, 1959.
Kim, R. and Winkelmann, R. Follicular mucinosis (alopecia mucinosa). *Arch. Dermatol.*, 85:490, 1962.
Kurban, A., Farah, F. and Chaglassian, H. Alopecia mucinosa: A histochemical study. *Dermatologica*, 124:398, 1962.
Langner, A., Jablonska, S. and Darzynkiewicz, A. Studies on the origin of the mucin in mucinosis follicularis. *Acta Derm. Venereol.*, 49:76, 1969.
Nickoloff, B. Epidermal mucinosis in mycosis fungoides. *J. Am. Acad. Dermatol.*, 14:83, 1986.
Okun, M. and Chorzelski, T. Metachromatic granules in dendritic cells within epithelial structures in alopecia mucinosa. *J. Invest. Dermatol.*, 45:129, 1965.
Okun, M. and Donnellan, B. Ultrastructural relationship of melanocytes to mast cells and "melanophages" in a lesion of alopecia mucinosa. *J. Invest. Dermatol.*, 59:211, 1972.
Okun, M. and Kay, F. Follicular mucinosis (alopecia mucinosa). *Arch. Dermatol.*, 89:809, 1964.
Pinkus, H. Alopecia: Clinicopathologic correlations. *Internat. J. Dermatol.*, 19:245, 1980.
——. Alopecia mucinosa (Commentary). Additional data in 1983. *Arch. Dermatol.*, 119:698, 1983.
——. Alopecia mucinosa: Inflammatory plaques with alopecia characterized by root-sheath mucinosis. *Arch. Dermatol.*, 76:419, 1957.
——. The relationship of alopecia mucinosa to malignant lymphoma. *Dermatologica*, 129:266, 1964.
Plotnik, H. and Abbrecht, M. Alopecia mucinosa and lymphoma: Report of two cases and review of literature. *Arch. Dermatol.*, 92:137, 1965.
Snyder, R., Crain, W. and McNutt, N. Alopecia mucinosa: Report of a case with diffuse alopecia and normal-appearing scalp skin. *Arch. Dermatol.*, 120:496, 1984.
Wolff, H., Kinney, J. and Ackerman, A. Angiolymphoid hyperplasia with follicular mucinosis. *Arch. Dermatol.*, 114:229, 1978.

Reticular Erythematous Mucinosis

Balogh, E., Nagy-Vezekenyi, K. and Forizs, E. REM Syndrome: An immediate therapeutic response to hydroxychloroquine sulphate. *Acta Derm. Venereol.*, 60:173, 1980.

Kocsard, E. and Munro, V. Reticular erythematous mucinosis (REM syndrome) of Steigleder. *Aust. J. Dermatol.*, 19:121, 1978.

Konrad, K., Brenner, W. and Pehamberger, H. Ultrastructural and immunological findings in Graves' disease with pretibial myxedema. *J. Cut. Pathol.*, 7:99, 1980.

Moulin, G. and Lucas, A. Le REM-syndrome. Erythème reticule avec mucinose. *Ann. Dermatol. Venereol.*, 108:783, 1981.

Perry, H., Kierland, R. and Montgomery, H. Plaque-like form of cutaneous mucinosis. *Arch. Dermatol.*, 82:980, 1960.

Steigleder, G. Plaque-artige Form der cutanen Mucinose (PCM) und retikuläre erythematöse Mucinosis (REM-Syndrom). *Z. Haut.*, 50:25, 1975.

Steigleder, G., Gartmann, H. and Linker, U. REM-syndrome: Reticular erythematous mucinosis (round-cell erythematosis), a new entity? *Br. J. Dermatol.*, 91:191, 1974.

Stevanovic, D. Mucinosis in erythematous plaques of Steigleder and Perry. *Dermatol. Monatsschr.*, 166:736, 1980.

Calcification and Ossification

Albright, F., Forbes, A. and Henneman, P. Pseudopseudohypoparathyroidism. *Trans. Assoc. Am. Phys.*, 65:337, 1952.

Barranco, V. Cutaneous ossification in pseudohypoparathyroidism. *Arch. Dermatol.*, 104:643, 1971.

Basler, R., Taylor, W. and Peacor, D. Postacne osteoma cutis. *Arch. Dermatol.*, 110:113, 1974.

Bendl, B. Subungual exostosis. *Cutis*, 26:260, 1980.

Beninson, J. and Morales, A. Subcutaneous calcifications in leg ulcers: Three cases. *Arch. Dermatol.*, 90:314, 1964.

Brook, C. and Valman, H. Osteoma cutis and Albright's hereditary osteodystrophy. *Br. J. Dermatol.*, 85:471, 1971.

Burgdorf, W. and Nasemann, T. Cutaneous osteomas: A clinical and histopathological review. *Arch. Dermatol. Res.*, 260:121, 1977.

Carey, R. et al. Massive extraskeletal calcification during phosphate treatment of hypercalcemia. *Arch. Int. Med.*, 122:150, 1968.

Combes, F. and Vanina, R. Osteosis cutis. *Arch. Dermatol. Syph.*, 69:613, 1954.

Cornelius, C., Tenenhouse, A. and Weber, J. Calcinosis cutis: Metabolic, sweat, histochemical, X-ray diffraction and electron microscopic study. *Arch. Dermatol.*, 98:219, 1968.

Costello, M. Metaplasia of bone. *Arch. Dermatol. Syph.*, 56:536, 1947.

Delacrétaz, J. and Christeler, A. Les phénomènes d'ossification dans les épithéliomas cutanés. *Dermatologica*, 134:305, 1967.

Delacrétaz, J. and Frenk, E. Zur Pathogenese des Osteo-Naevus Nanta. *Hautarzt*, 15:487, 1964.

Delacrétaz, J. and Koenig, R. Osteoma perforant. *Dermatologica*, 156:251, 1978.

Donaldson, E. and Summerly, R. Primary osteoma cutis and physeal aclasis. *Arch. Dermatol.*, 85:261, 1962.

Duperrat, B. Ostéomes cutanés. *Ann. Dermatol. Syph.*, 88:11, 1961.

Duperrat, B. and Vanbremeersch, F. Ostéome perforant verruciforme post-traumatique. *Ann. Dermatol. Syph.*, 90:37, 1963.

Eisenberg, E. and Bartholow, P., Jr. Reversible calcinosis cutis: Calciphylaxis in man. *N. Eng. J. Med.*, 268:1216, 1963.

Eyre, W. and Reed, W. Albright's hereditary osteodystrophy with cutaneous bone formation. *Arch. Dermatol.*, 104:636, 1971.

Fisher, B. and Dvoretzky, I. Idiopathic calcinosis of the scrotum. *Arch. Dermatol.*, 114:957, 1978.

Forbis, R., Jr. and Helwig, E. Pilomatrixoma (calcifying epithelioma). *Arch. Dermatol.*, 83:606, 1961.

Franke, H. Beitrag zum Krankheitsbild der Osteosis cutis circumscripta. *Hautarzt*, 7:270, 1956.

Gayler, B. and Brogdon, B. Soft tissue calcifications in the extremities in systemic disease. *Am. J. Med. Sci.*, 249:590, 1965.

Greenebaum, E. Metastatic calcification in skin: Exclusive involvement of eccrine sweat ducts. A case report. *Hum. Pathol.*, 11:287, 1980.
Haim, S. and Friedman-Birnbaum, R. Two cases of circumscribed calcinosis. *Dermatologica*, 143:111, 1971.
Helm, F., De La Pava, S. and Klein, E. Multiple miliary osteomas of the skin. *Arch. Dermatol.*, 96:681, 1967.
Hogan, V. and Conway, H. Calcification of burn scars. *Plast. Reconstr. Surg.*, 33:559, 1964.
Hopkins, J. Multiple miliary osteomas of the skin. *Arch. Dermatol. Syph.*, 18:706, 1928.
Jewell, E. Osteoma cutis. *Arch. Dermatol.*, 103:533, 1971.
Kabir, D. and Malkinson, F. Lupus erythematosus and calcinosis cutis. *Arch. Dermatol.*, 100:17, 1969.
Kolton, B. and Pedersen, J. Calcinosis cutis and renal failure. *Arch. Dermatol.*, 110:256, 1974.
Lebowitz, S., Miller, O. and Dickey, R. Subungual exostosis. *Cutis*, 13:426, 1974.
Leider, M. Osteoma cutis as a result of severe acne vulgaris of long duration. *Arch. Dermatol. Syph.*, 62:405, 1950.
Lilga, H. and Burns, D. Osteomatosis cutis. *Arch. Dermatol. Syph.*, 46:872, 1942.
Maclean, G. et al. Connective tissue ossification presenting in the skin. *Arch. Dermatol.*, 94:168, 1966.
Marks, J. Studies with ^{47}Ca in patients with calcinosis cutis. *Br. J. Dermatol.*, 82:1, 1970.
Mason, J., Helwig, E. and Graham, J. Pathology of the nevoid basal cell carcinoma syndrome. *Arch. Pathol.*, 79:401, 1965.
Mehregan, A. Calcinosis cutis: A review of the clinical forms and report of 75 cases. *Semin. Dermatol.*, 3:53, 1984.
Mulligan, R. Metastatic calcification. *Arch. Pathol.*, 43:177, 1947.
O'Donnell, T. and Geller, S. Primary osteoma cutis. *Arch. Dermatol.*, 104:325, 1971.
Perez Lopez, M. and De Moragas, J. Osteoma cutis. *Gac. Dermatol.*, 2:147, 1981.
Pursley, T. et al. Cutaneous manifestations of tumoral calcinosis. *Arch. Dermatol.*, 115:1100, 1979.
Roth, S., Stowell, R. and Helwig, E. Cutaneous ossification: Report of 120 cases and review of the literature. *Arch. Pathol.*, 76:44, 1963.
Rothstein, J. and Welt, S. Calcinosis universalis and calcinosis circumscripta in infancy and in childhood: Three cases of calcinosis universalis, with a review of the literature. *Am. J. Dis. Child.*, 52:368, 1936.
Rotteleur, G. et al. Osteomatose cutanée diffuse du nourrisson. *Arch. Fr. Pediatr.*, 37:397, 1980.
Shapiro, L., Plantt, N. and Torres-Rodriquez, V. Idiopathic calcinosis of the scrotum. *Arch. Dermatol.*, 102:199, 1970.
Tezuka, T. Cutaneous calculus: Its pathogenesis. *Dermatologica*, 161:191, 1980.
Wermer, P., Kuschner, M. and Riley, E. Reversible metastatic calcification associated with excessive milk and alkali intake. *Am. J. Med.*, 14:108, 1953.
Wheeland, R. and Roundtree, J. Calcinosis cutis resulting from percutaneous penetration and deposition of calcium. *J. Am. Acad. Dermatol.*, 12:172, 1985.
Wheeler, C. et al. Soft tissue calcification, with special reference to its occurrence in the "collagen diseases". *Ann. Int. Med.*, 36:1050, 1952.
Whiting, D. et al. Unusual cutaneous lesions in tumoral calcinosis. *Arch. Dermatol.*, 102:465, 1970.
Wilson, C., Wingfield, W. and Toone, E., Jr. Vitamin D poisoning with metastatic calcification: Report of a case and review of the mechanism of intoxication. *Am. J. Med.*, 14:146, 1953.

Subepidermal Calcified Nodule

Eng, A. and Mandrea, E. Perforating calcinosis cutis presenting as milia. *J. Cutan. Pathol.*, 8:247, 1981.
Shmunes, E. and Wood, M. Subepidermal calcified nodules. *Arch. Dermatol.*, 105:593, 1972.
Winer, L. Solitary congenital nodular calcification of the skin. *Arch. Dermatol. Syph.*, 66:204, 1952.
Woods, B. and Kellaway, T. Cutaneous calculi: Subepidermal calcified nodules. *Br. J. Dermatol.*, 75:1, 1963.

Vitiligo

Bazex, A., Balas, D. and Bazex, J. Maladie de Vogt-Koyanagi-Harada. *Ann. Dermatol. Venereol.*, 104:849, 1977.

Bhawan, J. and Bhutani, L. Keratinocyte damage in vitiligo. *J. Cutan. Pathol.*, 10:207, 1983.

Birbeck, M., Breathnach, A. and Everall, J. An electron microscope study of basal melanocytes and high-level clear cells (Langerhans cells) in vitiligo. *J. Invest. Dermatol.*, 37:51, 1961.

Brown, J., Winkelmann, R. and Wolff, K. Langerhans cells in vitiligo. *J. Invest. Dermatol.*, 49:386, 1967.

Cowan, C., Jr. et al. Ocular disturbances in vitiligo. *J. Am. Acad. Dermatol.*, 15:17, 1986.

Grimes, P. et al. Autoantibodies and their clinical significance in a black vitiligo population. *Arch. Dermatol.*, 119:300, 1983.

Howsden, S., Herndon, J., Jr. and Freeman, R. Vogt-Koyanagi-Harada syndrome and psoriasis. *Arch. Dermatol.*, 108:395, 1973.

Klaus, S. and Moellmann, G. Vitiligo. In: Proceedings of the First International Workshop on Vitiligo. *J. Invest. Dermatol.*, 71:165, 1978.

Mishima, Y., Kawasaki, H. and Pinkus, H. Dendritic cell dynamics in progressive depigmentations. *Arch. Dermatol. Forsch.*, 247:67, 1972.

Morohashi, M. et al. Ultrastructural studies of vitiligo, Vogt-Koyanagi syndrome, and incontinentia pigmenti achromians. *Arch. Dermatol.*, 113:755, 1977.

Naughton, G. et al. Detection of antibodies to melanocytes in vitiligo by specific immunoprecipitation. *J. Invest. Dermatol.*, 81:540, 1983.

Nordlund, J. et al. Halo nevi and the Vogt-Koyanagi-Harada syndrome. *Arch. Dermatol.*, 116:690, 1980.

Nordlund, J. et al. The prevalence of vitiligo and poliosis in patients with uveitis. *J. Am. Acad. Dermatol.*, 4:528, 1981.

Ortonne, J-P. et al. *Vitiligo and Other Hypomelanoses of Hair and Skin*. New York, Plenum Press, 1983.

Riley, R. A study of the distribution of epidermal dendritic cells in pigmented and unpigmented skin. *J. Invest. Dermatol.*, 48:28, 1967.

Thurmon, T. et al. Deafness and vitiligo. *Birth Defects*, 12:315, 1976.

Zelickson, A. and Mottaz, J. Epidermal dendritic cells. *Arch. Dermatol.*, 98:652, 1968.

Idiopathic Guttate Hypomelanosis

Falabella, R. et al. On the pathogenesis of idiopathic guttate hypomelanosis. *J. Am. Acad. Dermatol.*, 16:35, 1987.

Amyloidosis

Anokoji, K. and Irisawa, K. Five cases of lichen amyloidosus. *Arch. Dermatol.*, 84:759, 1961.

Beacham, B. et al. Bullous amyloidosis. *J. Am. Acad. Dermatol.*, 3:506, 1980.

Bedi, T. and Datta, B. Diffuse biphasic cutaneous amyloidosis. *Dermatologica*, 158:433, 1979.

Benditt, E. et al. Guidelines for nomenclature. In: *Amyloid and Amyloidosis*. Glenner, G. et al., eds., Amsterdam/Oxford/Princeton, Excerpta Medica, 1980.

Berger, P. Amyloidosis: A complication of pustular psoriasis. *Br. Med. J.*, 2:351, 1969.

Binkely, G. Primary systemic amyloidosis. *Arch. Dermatol. Syph.*, 37:330, 1938.

Black, M. and Wilson-Jones, E. Macular amyloidosis. *Br. J. Dermatol.*, 84:199, 1971.

Bluhm, J., III, Johnson, S. and Norback, D. Bullous amyloidosis. *Arch. Dermatol.*, 116:1164, 1980.

Brandt, K., Cathcart, E. and Cohen, A. A clinical analysis of the course and prognosis of 42 patients with amyloidosis. *Am. J. Med.*, 44:955, 1968.

Breathnach, S. The cutaneous amyloidoses: Pathogenesis and therapy. *Arch. Dermatol.*, 121:470, 1985.

Breathnach, S. and Black, M. Systemic amyloidosis and the skin. *Clin. Exp. Dermatol.*, 4:517, 1979.

Breathnach, S. et al. Immunohistochemical deposition of amyloid P component in skin of normal subjects and patients with cutaneous amyloidosis. *Br. J. Dermatol.*, 105:115, 1981.

Brownstein, M. and Hashimoto, K. Macular amyloidosis. *Arch. Dermatol.*, 106:50, 1972.
Brownstein, M. and Helwig, E. The cutaneous amyloidoses. I. Localized forms. *Arch. Dermatol.*, 102:8, 1970.
——. The cutaneous amyloidoses. II. Systemic forms. *Arch. Dermatol.*, 102:20, 1970.
——. Systemic amyloidosis complicating dermatoses. *Arch. Dermatol.*, 102:1, 1970.
Brunsting, L. and MacDonald, I. Primary systematized amyloidosis with macroglossia: A syndrome related to Bence-Jones proteinuria and myeloma. *J. Invest. Dermatol.*, 8:145, 1947.
Buxbaum, J. et al. Amyloidosis of the AL type. *Am. J. Med.*, 67:867, 1979.
Calkins, E. and Wright, J. Amyloidosis. In: *Principles of Immunologic Diagnosis in Medicine.* Milgrom, F. et al., eds., Philadelphia, Lea & Febiger, 1981, p. 341.
Cathcart, E. et al. Immunoglobulins and amyloidosis. *Am. J. Med.*, 52:93, 1972.
Chapel, T., Birmingham, D. and Malinowski, Y. Nodular primary localized cutaneous amyloidosis. *Arch. Dermatol.*, 113:1248, 1977.
Cohen, A. An update of clinical, pathologic and biochemical aspects of amyloidosis. *Internat. J. Dermatol.*, 20:515, 1981.
Cohen, A. and Wegelius, O. Classification of amyloid 1979–80. *Arthrit. Rheum.*, 23:644, 1980.
Danno, K. and Horio, T. Sulphhydryl and disulphide stainings of amyloid: A comparison with hyaline body. *Acta Derm. Venereol.* (Stockh.), 61:285, 1981.
Danno, K. and Imamura, S. Deposition of complement C1q in primary localized cutaneous amyloidosis. *Br. J. Dermatol.*, 107:129, 1982.
De Pietro, W. Primary familial cutaneous amyloidosis: A study of HIA antigens in a Puerto Rican family. *Arch. Dermatol.*, 117:639, 1981.
Dostrovsky, A. and Sagher, F. Localized amyloidosis of the skin: Report of cases: The intracutaneous congo red test as a diagnostic aid. *Arch. Dermatol. Syph.*, 44:891, 1941.
Ebner, H. and Gebhart, W. Light and electron microscopic differentiation of amyloid and colloid or hyaline bodies. *Br. J. Dermatol.*, 92:637, 1975.
Eisen, H. Primary systemic amyloidosis. *Am. J. Med.*, 1:144, 1946.
Eng, A. et al. Familial generalized dyschromic amyloidosis cutis. *J. Cutan. Pathol.*, 3:102, 1976.
Franklin, E. Amyloid and amyloidosis of the skin. *J. Invest. Dermatol.*, 67:451, 1976.
Furie, A. et al. Mechanism of factor X deficiency in systemic amyloidosis. *N. Eng. J. Med.*, 304:827, 1981.
Gabriel, H. and Lindemayr, W. Amyloidosis cutis nodularis atrophicans. *Dermatologica*, 115:508, 1957.
Glenner, G. Amyloid deposits and amyloidosis: The betafibrilloses. *N. Eng. J. Med.*, 302:1283, 1333, 1980.
Glenner, G., Ein, D. and Terry, W. The immunoglobulin origin of amyloid. *Am. J. Med.*, 52:141, 1972.
Glenner, G. and Page, D. Amyloid, amyloidosis and amyloidogenesis. *Internat. Rev. Exp. Pathol.*, 15:2, 1976.
Goerttler, E. Anton-Lamprecht, I. and Kotzur, B. Amyloidosis cutis nodularis. *Hautarzt*, 27:16, 1976.
Goltz, R. Systematized amyloidosis : A review of the skin and mucous membrane lesions and a report of two cases. *Medicine*, 31:381, 1952.
Goodman, T., Jr., Abele, D. and West, C., Jr. Electron microscopy in the diagnosis of amyloidosis. *Arch. Dermatol.*, 106:393, 1972.
Gottschalk, H., Graham, J. and Kohut, R. Macular amyloidosis with localized amyloidosis of the upper air passages. *Arch. Dermatol.*, 111:1017, 1975.
Greipp, P. et al. Factor X deficiency in amyloidosis : A critical review. *Am. J. Hematol.*, 11:443, 1981.
Hashimoto, K. Diseases of amyloid, colloid, and hyalin. *J. Cutan. Pathol.*, 12:322, 1985.
——. Electron microscopy for diagnosis of selected dermatoses. *Semin. Dermatol.*, 3:36, 1984.
Hashimoto, K., Gross, B. and Lever, W. Lichen amyloidosus: Histochemical and electron microscopic studies. *J. Invest. Dermatol.*, 45:204, 1965.
Hashimoto, K. and Kobayashi, H. Histogenesis of amyloid in the skin. *Am. J. Dermatopathol.*, 2:165, 1980.
Hashimoto, K. and Kumakiri, M. Colloid-amyloid bodies in PUVA-treated human psoriatic patients. *J. Invest. Dermatol.*, 72:70, 1979.
Hashimoto, K. and Onn, L. Lichen amyloidosus: Electron microscopic study of a typical case and a review. *Arch. Dermatol.*, 104:648, 1971.
Heyl, T. Amyloid staining with thioflavine T in dermatopathology. *Trans. St. John's Hosp. Dermatol. Soc.*, 52:84, 1966.

Holden, C. et al. Trauma induced bullae: The presenting feature of systemic amyloidosis associated with plasma cell dyscrasia. *Br. J. Dermatol.*, 107:701, 1982.

Ishibashi, A. Histogenesis of hyalinosis cutis et mucosae. *J. Dermatol.*, 5:265, 1978.

Iverson, L. and Morrison, A. Primary systemic amyloidosis. *Arch. Pathol.*, 45:1, 1948.

Jay, C. and Dacosta, J. Lichen amyloidosus: Clinical study of 40 cases. *Br. J. Dermatol.*, 82:129, 1970.

Kesilevsky, R. and Boudreau, L. Kinetics of amyloid deposition. I. The effects of amyloid-enhancing factor and splenectomy. *Lab. Invest.*, 48:53, 1983.

Kobayashi, H. and Hashimoto, K. Colloid and elastic fiber: Ultrastructural study on the histogenesis of colloid milium. *J. Cutan. Pathol.*, 10:111, 1983.

Kobayasi, T. and Asboe-Hansen, G. Ultrastructure of skin in primary systemic amyloidosis. *Acta Derm. Venereol.* (Stockh.), 59:407, 1979.

Kumakiri, M. and Hashimoto, K. Histogenesis of primary localized cutaneous amyloidosis: Sequential change of epidermal keratinocytes to amyloid via filamentous degeneration. *J. Invest. Dermatol.*, 73:150, 1979.

Kurban, A. et al. Primary localized macular cutaneous amyloidosis: Histochemistry and electron microscopy. *Br. J. Dermatol.*, 85:52, 1971.

Kyle, R. Amyloidosis. *Internat. J. Dermatol.*, 19:537, 1980; 20:20, 1981.

Kyle, R. and Bayrd, E. "Primary" systemic amyloidosis and myeloma: Discussion of relationship and review of 81 cases. *Arch. Int. Med.*, 107:344, 1961.

Leach, W., Vassar, P. and Culling, C. Primary systemic amyloidosis presenting as scleroderma. *Can. Med. Assoc. J.*, 83:263, 1960.

MacDonald, D., Black, M. and Ramnarain, N. Immunofluorescence studies in primary localized cutaneous amyloidosis. *Br. J. Dermatol.*, 96:635, 1977.

MacDonald, D. et al. Localized cutaneous amyloidosis; A clinical review of 100 cases including immunofluorescence studies. In: *Amyloid and Amyloidosis*. Glenner, G. et al., eds., Amsterdam/Oxford/Princeton, Excerpta Medica, 1980, p. 239.

Maeda, H. et al. Epidermal origin of the amyloid in localized cutaneous amyloidosis. *Br. J. Dermatol.*, 106:345, 1982.

Masu, S. Hosokawa, M. and Seiji, M. Amyloid in localized cutaneous amyloidosis: Immunofluorescence studies with antikeratin antiserum. *Acta Derm. Venereol.* (Stockh.), 61:381, 1981.

Natelson, E. et al. Amyloidosis palpebrarum. *Arch. Int. Med.*, 125:304, 1979.

Noren, P. et al. Immunofluorescence and histochemical studies of localized cutaneous amyloidosis. *Br. J. Dermatol.*, 108:277, 1983.

Ogino, A. and Tanaka, S. Poikiloderma-like cutaneous amyloidosis: Report of a case and review of the literature. *Dermatologica*, 115:301, 1977.

Palitz, L. and Peck, S. Amyloidosis cutis: A macular variant. *Arch. Dermatol. Syph.*, 65:451, 1952.

Pearson, B., Rice, M. and Dickens, K. Primary systemic amyloidosis: Report of two cases in Negroes, with special reference to certain histologic criteria for diagnosis. *Arch. Pathol.*, 32:1, 1941.

Potter, B. and Johnson, W. Primary localized amyloidosis cutis. *Arch. Dermatol.*, 103:448, 1971.

Powell, C. and Swan, L. Leprosy: Pathologic changes observed in fifty consecutive necropsies. *Am. J. Pathol.*, 31:1131, 1955.

Puchtler, H., Sweat, F. and Kuhns, J. On the binding of direct cotton dyes by amyloid. *J. Histochem. Cytochem.*, 12:900, 1964.

Puchtler, H., Sweat, F. and Levine, M. On the binding of congo red by amyloid. *J. Histochem. Cytochem.*, 10:355, 1962.

Romland, R. Localized (lichen) amyloidosis of the skin: Report of 2 cases, with vital staining of the amyloid nodules by congo red injected intracutaneously or subcutaneously. *Arch. Dermatol. Syph.*, 33:85, 1936.

Rubinow, A. and Cohen, A. Skin involvement in generalized amyloidosis. *Ann. Int. Med.*, 88:781, 1978.

Rukavina, J. et al. Primary systemic amyloidosis: A review and an experimental, genetic and clinical study of 29 cases with particular emphasis on the familial form. *Medicine*, 35:239, 1956.

Runne, U. and Orfanos, C. Amyloid production by dermal fibroblasts. *Br. J. Dermatol.*, 97:155, 1977.

Saltzer, E., Cranmer, L. and Wilson, J. Lichen amyloidosus and the nature of amyloid: Report of cases. *Arch. Dermatol.*, 98:311, 1968.

Shanon, J. and Sagher, F. Interscapular cutaneous amyloidosis. *Arch. Dermatol.*, 102:195, 1970.
Sweet, J., Bear, R. and Lang, A. Amyloidosis and systemic lupus erythematosus. *Hum. Pathol.*, 12:853, 1981.
Symmers, W. Amyloidosis: Five cases of primary generalized amyloidosis and some other unusual cases. *J. Clin. Pathol.*, 9:212, 1956.
Teilum, G. and Lindahl, A. Frequency and significance of amyloid changes in rheumatoid arthritis. *Acta Med. Scand.*, 149:449, 1954.
Toribio, J. et al. Mixed (lichenoid and macular) cutaneous amyloidoses. *Acta Derm. Venereol.*, 55:221, 1975.
Tsuti, T. et al. Secondary localized cutaneous amyloidosis in solar elastosis. *Br. J. Dermatol.*, 106:469, 1982.
Vasily, D., Bhatia, S. and Uhlin, S. Familial primary cutaneous amyloidosis. Clinical, genetic, and immunofluorescent studies. *Arch. Dermatol.*, 114:1173, 1978.
Weedon, D. The composition of amyloid. *Aust. J. Dermatol.*, 20:133, 1979.
Weedon, D. and Shand, E. Amyloid in basal cell carcinomas. *Br. J. Dermatol.*, 101:141, 1979.
Weitzner, S., Keen, P. and Doughty, W. Primary localized amyloidosis of the glans penis. *Arch. Dermatol.*, 102:463, 1970.
Westermark, P. Amyloidosis of the skin: A comparison between localized and systemic amyloidosis. *Acta Derm. Venereol.* (Stockh.), 59:341, 1979.
——. Skin involvement in secondary amyloidosis. *Acta Pathol. Microbiol. Scand.*, 79A:79, 1971.
Westermark, P. and Stenkvist, B. A new method for the diagnosis of systemic amyloidosis. *Arch. Int. Med.*, 132:522, 1973.
Westermark, P. et al. Bullous amyloidosis. *Arch. Dermatol.*, 117:782, 1981.
Wright, J. and Calkins, E. Clinical-pathologic differentiation of common amyloid syndromes. *Medicine* (Baltimore), 60:429, 1981.
Wright, J. et al. Relationship of amyloid to aging: A review of the literature and systematic study of 83 patients derived from a general hospital population. *Medicine*, 48:39, 1969.
Yanagihara, M., Mehregan, A. and Mehregan, D. Staining of amyloid with cotton dyes. *Arch. Dermatol.*, 120:1184, 1984.

Colloid Milium

Dupre, A. et al. Paracolloid of the skin. *J. Cutan. Pathol.*, 6:304, 1979.
Ebner, H. and Gebhart, W. Colloid milium: Light and electron microscopic investigations. *Clin. Exp. Dermatol.*, 2:217, 1977.
——. Vergleichende Untersuchungen bei juvenilem und adultem Colloid Milium. *Arch. Dermatol. Res.*, 261:231, 1978.
Graham, J. and Marques, A. Colloid milium: A histochemical study. *J. Invest. Dermatol.*, 49:497, 1967.
Guin, J. and Seale, E. Colloid degeneration of the skin (colloid milium): A report of seven cases. *Arch. Dermatol.*, 80:533, 1959.
Harris, R. Colloid degeneration of the skin occurring in brother and sister. *Br. J. Dermatol.*, 72:324, 1960.
Hashimoto, K., Miller, F. and Bereston, E. Colloid milium: Histochemical and electron microscopic studies. *Arch. Dermatol.*, 105:684, 1972.
Hashimoto, K. et al. Electron microscopical and biochemical analysis of colloid milium. *Arch. Dermatol.*, 111:49, 1975.
Heyl, T. Amyloid staining with thioflavine T in dermatopathology. *Trans. St. John's Hosp. Dermatol. Soc.*, 52:84, 1966.
Holzberger, P. Concerning adult colloid milium. *Arch. Dermatol.*, 82:711, 1960.
Percivel, G. and Duthie, D. Notes on a case of colloid pseudomilium. *Br. J. Dermatol.*, 60:399, 1948.
Prakken, J. Colloid and senile degeneration of the skin. *Acta Derm. Venereol.*, 31:713, 1951.
Reuter, M. and Becker, S. Colloid degeneration (collagen degeneration) of the skin. *Arch. Dermatol. Syph.*, 46:695, 1942.
Sullivan, M. and Ellis, F. Facial colloid degeneration in plaques. *Arch. Dermatol.*, 84:816, 1961.
Zoon, J., Jansen, L. and Hovenkamp, A. The nature of colloid milium. *Br. J. Dermatol.*, 67:212, 1955.

Lipoid Proteinosis (Hyalinosis Cutis et Mucosae)

Bauer, E. et al. Lipoid proteinosis: *In vivo* and *in vitro* evidence for a lysosomal storage disease. *J. Invest. Dermatol.*, 76:119, 1981.

Bravo-Piris, J., Unamuno Perez, P. and Armijo, M. Hylinose cutanéo-muqueuse chez des jumelles monzygotes. *Ann. Dermatol. Venereol.*, 112:235, 1985.

Burnett, J. and Marcy, S. Lipoid proteinosis. *Am. J. Dis. Child.*, 105:81, 1963.

Caplan, R. Visceral involvement in lipoid proteinosis. *Arch. Dermatol.*, 95:149, 1967.

Cowan, M. et al. Case of lipoid proteinosis. *Br. Med. J.*, 2:577, 1961.

Dupré, A. et al. Étude ultrastructurale d'un cas de hyalinose cutanéo-muqueuse. *Ann. Dermatol. Venereol.*, 108:1003, 1981.

Findlay, G. Studies in morphogenetic dermatology: The brain calcifications of lipoid proteinosis. *Trans. St. John's Hosp. Dermatol. Soc.*, 60:152, 1974.

Findlay, G., Scott, F. and Cripps, D. Porphyria and lipoid proteinosis: A clinical, histological and biochemical comparison of 19 South African cases. *Br. J. Dermatol.*, 78:69, 1966.

Fleischmajer, R., Nedwich, A. and Ramos e Silva, J. Hyalinosis cutis et mucosae. *J. Invest. Dermatol.*, 52:495, 1969.

Fleischmajer, R. et al. Hyalinosis cutis et mucosae: A basal lamina disease (abstr.). *J. Invest. Dermatol.*, 76:314, 1981.

Fleischmajer, R. et al. Ultrastructure and composition of connective tissue in hyalinosis cutis et mucosae skin. *J. Invest. Dermatol.*, 82:252, 1984.

Grosfeld, J. et al. Hyalinosis cutis et mucosae: Lipoid proteinosis (Urbach-Wiethe). *Dermatologica*, 130:239, 1965.

Harper, J. et al. Oropharyngeal and laryngeal lesions in lipoid proteinosis. *J. Laryngol. Otol.*, 97:877, 1983.

Hashimoto, K., Klingmüller, G. and Rodermund, O. Hyalinosis cutis et mucosae. *Acta Derm. Venereol.*, 52:179, 1972.

Ishibashi, A. Histogenesis of hyalinosis cutis et mucosae. *J. Dermatol.*, 5:265, 1978.

——. Hyalinosis cutis et mucosae. *Dermatologica*, 165:7, 1982.

Kint, A. A comparative electron microscopic study of the perivascular hylaine from porphyria cutanea tarda and from lipoid proteinosis. *Arch. Klin. Exp. Dermatol.*, 239:203, 1970.

Laymon, C. and Hill, E. An appraisal of hyalinosis cutis et mucosae. *Arch. Dermatol.*, 75:55, 1957.

Leonard, J. et al. CT scan appearances in a patient with lipoid proteinosis. *Br. J. Radiol.*, 54:1098, 1981.

McCusker, J. and Caplan, R. Lipoid proteinosis (lipoglycoproteinosis): A histochemical study of two cases. *Am. J. Pathol.*, 40:599, 1962.

Meenan, F. et al. Lipoid proteinosis: A clinical, pathological and genetic study. *Q. J. Med.*, 47:549, 1978.

Ramos e Silva, J. Lipoid proteinosis (Urbach-Wiethe). *Arch. Dermatol. Syph.*, 47:301, 1943.

Rasiewicz, W., Rubisz-Brzezinska, J. and Konecki, J. Hyalinosis cutis et mucosae (Urbach-Wiethe): Report of a case and results of histochemical studies. *Dermatologica*, 130:145, 1965.

Ungar, H. and Katzenellenbogen, I. Hyalinosis of skin and mucous membranes (Urbach-Wiethe's lipoid proteinosis): Histochemical study of a case twenty-eight years after its first publication. *Arch. Pathol.*, 63:65, 1957.

Van der Walt, J. and Heyl, T. Lipoid proteinosis and erythropoietic protoporphyria: A histological and histochemical study. *Arch. Dermatol.*, 104:501, 1971.

Wood, M., Urbach, F. and Beerman, H. Histochemical study of a case of lipoid proteinosis. *J. Invest. Dermatol.*, 26:263, 1956.

Chapter 12
Metabolic Dermatoses

GOUT

Gout is a disorder characterized by hyperuricemia. It may be a primary disorder, or it may be secondary to a variety of conditions, including psoriasis. Primary gout usually affects men. Some cases of primary gout are familial. Primary gout can be related to enzymatic overproduction of uric acid or to decreased excretion of uric acid.

The dominant symptoms are recurrent attacks of acute arthritis, and in the late stages, chronic arthritis with destructive changes in the joints. In the late stages of gout, salmon-colored nodules (tophi) develop in the skin and subcutaneous tissue. These frequently involve the ears and areas overlying the elbow joints and the digits (Fig. A). Tophi may discharge a chalky material. Accumulation of uric acid crystals in the kidney may cause damage.

Microscopic features

1. With formalin fixation, sodium urate appears as cleft-like spaces within amorphous material, surrounded by a foreign body granuloma (Figs. B,C). The crystalline structure is better preserved with absolute alcohol fixation than formalin fixation. The crystals are brownish in color; they are birefringent with polarized light.
2. The crystals occasionally show a positive Von Kossa reaction (Fig. D), indicating the presence of calcium urate.

GOUT

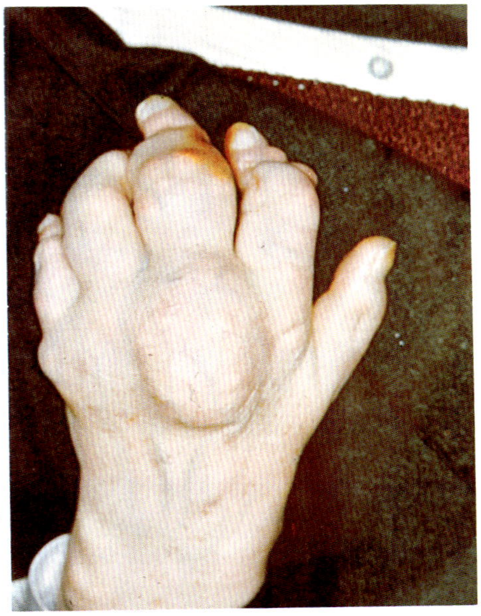

A

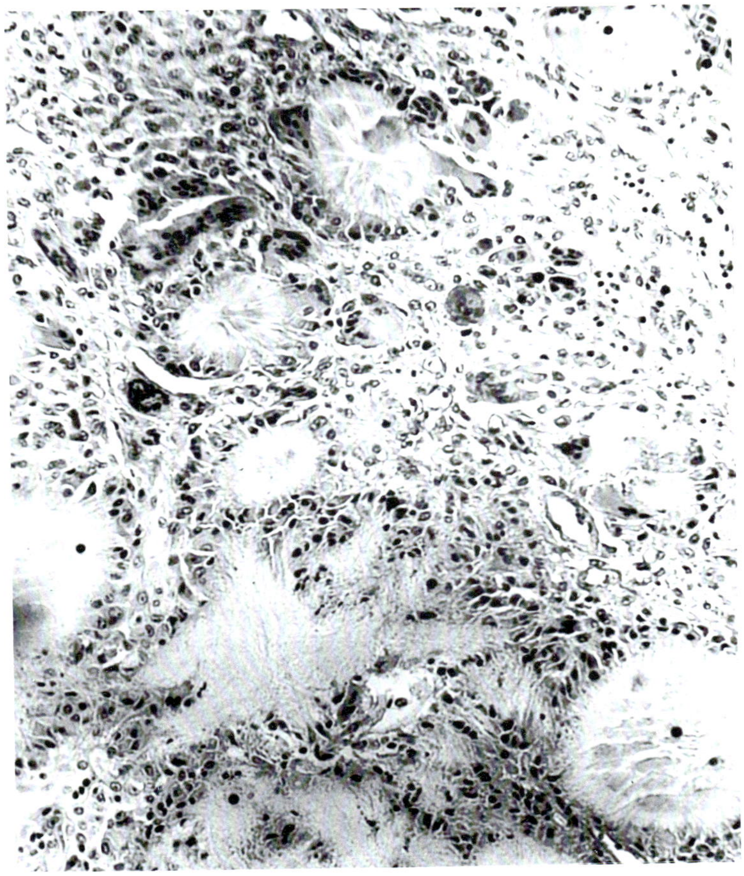

B
X175

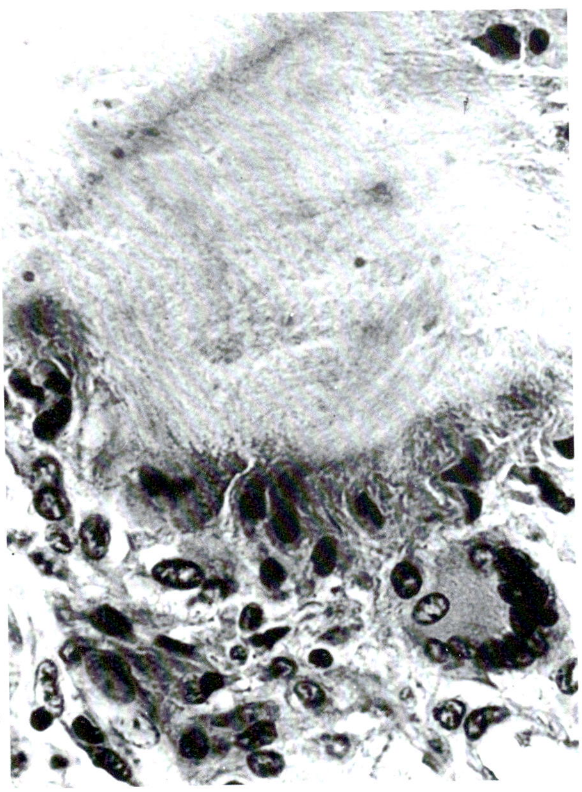

C
X550

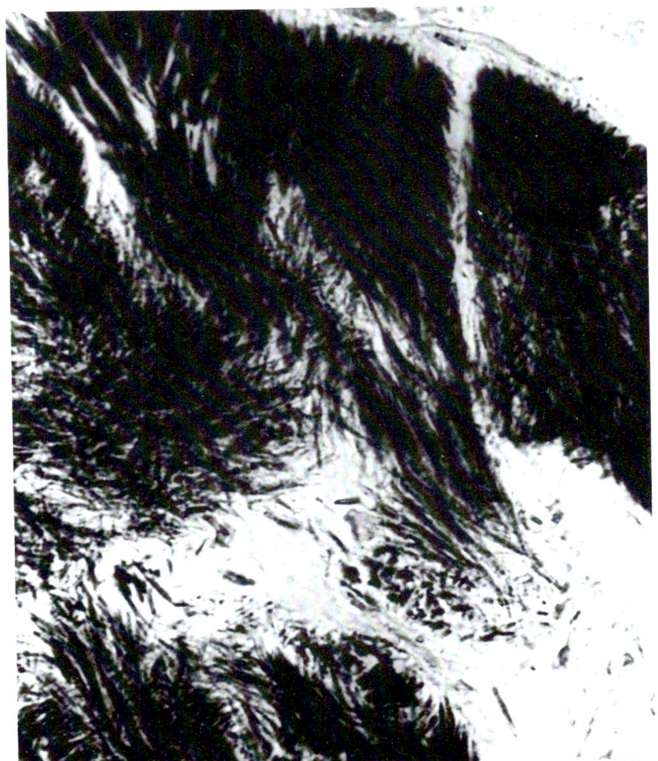

D
X650

VON KOSSA STAIN

IDIOPATHIC HEMOCHROMATOSIS

In idiopathic hemochromatosis there is a deposition of iron in various tissues, leading to fibrosis. The basic cause is believed to be excessive absorption of iron from the gastrointestinal tract.

The liver and pancreas are frequently involved; involvement of the pancreas leads to diabetes (bronze diabetes). Involvement of the myocardium may lead to cardiac failure.

The skin is diffusely brownish (Fig. A) or slate-colored; this hyperpigmentation is most pronounced in the sun-exposed areas. Mucous membranes may also be hyperpigmented. The hyperpigmentation is due principally to an increase in cutaneous melanin, although some authors have attributed the bluish component to hemosiderin deposits.

Microscopic features

1. Refractile, yellowish-brown granules of hemosiderin are present in the basement membrane of eccrine glands (Fig. B) and in the area around blood vessels. Granules may also be scattered through the dermis and are occasionally present in the basal layer of the epidermis. Some of the hemosiderin may be in macrophages.
2. The presence of hemosiderin can be confirmed with Perls reaction (Fig. C). Hemosiderin may also give a positive Fontana-Masson reaction (Fig. D).
3. There is increased melanin, both in the basal layer of the epidermis, and in dermal "melanophages."

Comment

1. A liver biopsy is considered to be more reliable than a skin biopsy as a diagnostic procedure for hemochromatosis. Determination of serum iron, iron-binding capacity, and the degree of saturation of transferrin with iron are of value.

   Skin biopsies should not be taken from the legs, where hemosiderin is commonly present in the absence of hemochromatosis.
2. Associated skin changes that may be seen include atrophy and ichthyosis. There may be nail abnormalities or alopecia.

IDIOPATHIC HEMOCHROMATOSIS

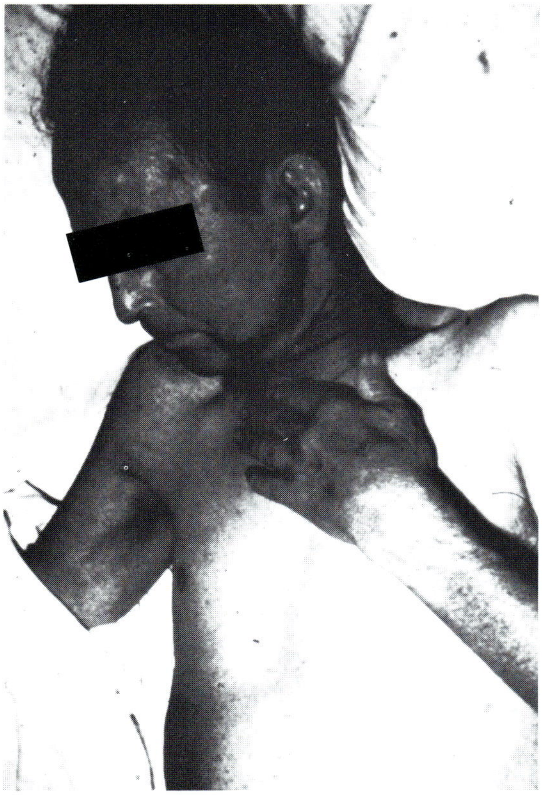

A

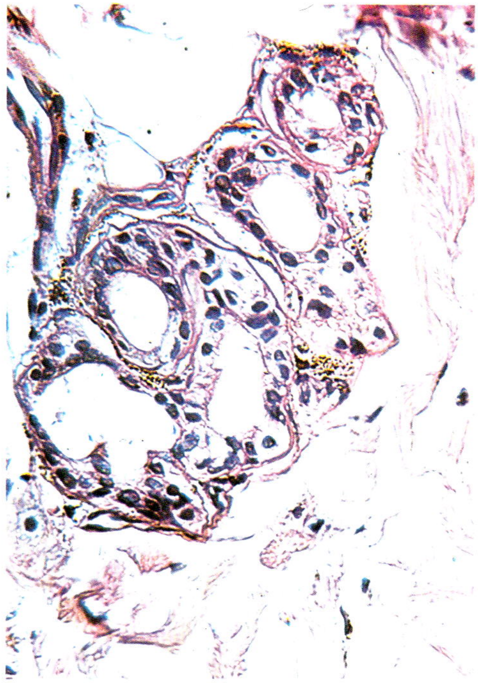

B
X200

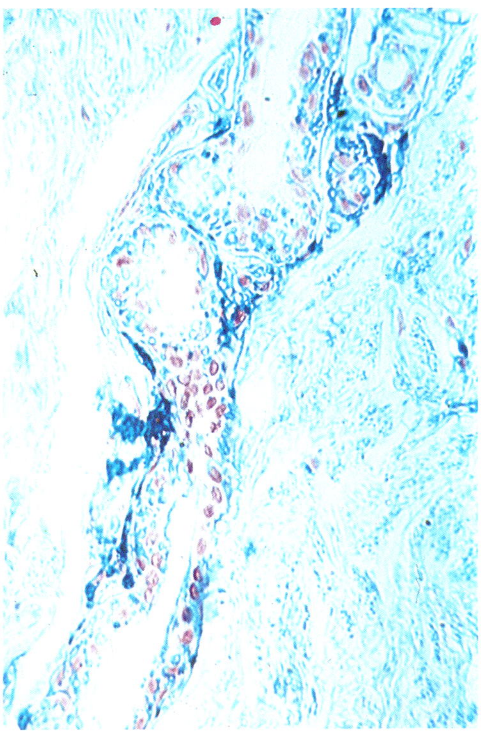

C
X200
PERLS STAIN

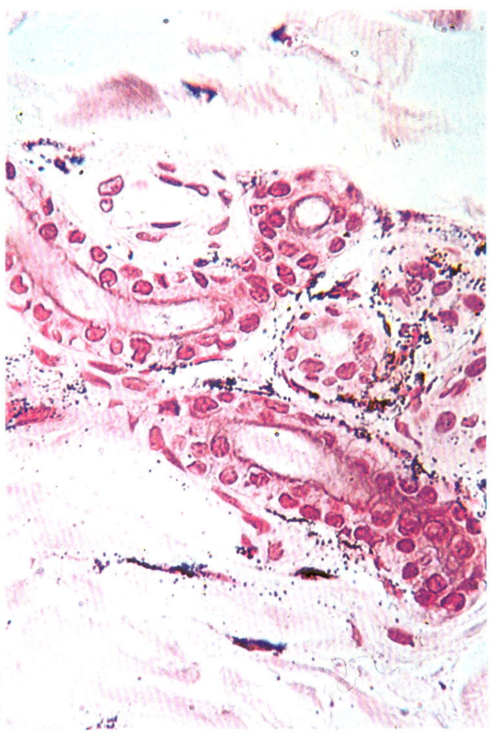

D
X200
FONTANA-MASSON STAIN

Lipidoses

Lipidoses are disorders characterized by deposits of lipid in tissue.
The following is Lever's classification:

1. *Systemic Lipidoses with Altered Serum Lipoprotein Values*
   Hyperlipoproteinemia, types I to V
   Tangier disease
2. *Tissue Storage Lipidoses*
   Niemann-Pick disease
   Gaucher's disease
   Angiokeratoma corporis diffusum (Fabry's disease), fucosidosis
   Lipogranulatomatosis (Farber's disease)
3. *Histiocytosis X*
   Xanthoma disseminatum
4. *Predominantly Cutaneous Lipidoses*
   Diffuse normolipemic plane xanthoma
   Verruciform xanthoma
   Juvenile xanthogranuloma
   Necrobiotic xanthogranuloma with paraproteinemia
   Reticulohistiocytosis
   Congenital self-healing reticulohistiocytosis
   Progressive nodular histiocytoma
   Generalized eruptive histiocytoma

Angiokeratoma corporis diffusum, histiocytosis X, histiocytoma, juvenile xanthogranuloma, and reticulohistiocytosis are discussed elsewhere.

Table from *Histopathology of the Skin*, 6th Edition, by Walter F. Lever and Gundula Schaumburg-Lever, Lippincott, Philadelphia, 1983.

HYPERLIPOPROTEINEMIA

In hyperlipoproteinemia a range of clinical and laboratory manifestations can be observed. The following is Lever's classification:

Biochemical and Clinical Data in Hyperlipoproteinemia

	I	IIA	IIB	III	IV	V
	Hyperchylo-micron	**Hyperbeta**	**Combined**	**Broad-Beta**	**Pre-Beta**	**Mixed Pre-Beta Chylomicron**
Chylomicrons	↑					↑
Pre-Beta (VLD)			↑	↑	↑	↑
Beta (LD)		↑	↑	↑		
Cholesterol	(+)	++	+	++	+	+
Triglycerides	+++		+	++	++	+++
Supernatant **Infranatant**	Creamy Clear	Clear	Slightly turbid	Turbid	Milky	Creamy Turbid
Eruptive Xanthoma	+		(+)	+	++	+
Tuberous Xanthoma		+	(+)	+	(+)	
Tendon Xanthoma		++	(+)	+		
Xanthelasma		++		+		
Plane Xanthoma		(+)		+		
Cardiovascular		++	+	++	+	+
Diabetes			+	+	++	+
Hepatomegaly **Pancreatitis**	+				(+)	

VLD = very low density; LD = low density.

Table from *Histopathology of the Skin*, 6th Edition, by Walter F. Lever and Gundula Schaumburg-Lever, Lippincott, Philadelphia, 1983.

LIPIDOSES continued ⇨

HYPERLIPOPROTEINEMIA

Hereditory Transmission of Hyperlipoproteinemia

I: recessive
II: dominant
III: recessive
IV: dominant
V: uncertain

Skin lesions occur in all types of hyperlipoproteinemia. There are five variants of cutaneous xanthoma observed in hyperlipoproteinemia:

Xanthelasma. Xanthelasmata are soft yellowish plaques of the eyelids (Fig. A). They are commonly seen in type IIA hyperlipoproteinemia, but can be seen in type III. They are very common in persons with normal lipoprotein levels.

Tuberous xanthoma. Tuberous xanthomas are reddish-orange nodules or plaques, often located on the elbows (Figs. B,C), knees, fingers, or buttocks. They are commonly observed in types II and IIIA and infrequently in types IIB and IV. Patients with these types of hyperlipoproteinemia may also develop *tendon xanthomas;* these occur most often in the Achilles tendons and the extensor tendons of the fingers.

Eruptive xanthomas. These are widely distributed reddish-orange to yellow papules (Fig. D) which tend to come and go with fluctuation of plasma concentration of triglycerides. Eruptive xanthomas are typical of triglyceridemia; they occur in all types of hyperlipoproteinemia except type IIA.

Plane xanthomas. These are flat yellowish lesions that tend to develop in skin folds, especially palmar creases. They occur in type III hyperlipoproteinemia and in biliary cirrhosis producing type IIA.

DIFFUSE NORMOLIPEMIC PLANE XANTHOMA

The condition is characterized by diffuse areas of yellowish-orange discoloration of the skin or more circumscribed whitish areas. The principal sites are the face and upper trunk.Lesions may be secondary to pre-existing erythroderma (e.g., atopic dermatitis, leukemia-lymphoma group) or idiopathic. There may be an association with paraproteinemia. The most common association is with multiple myeloma.

VERRUCIFORM XANTHOMA

This is a rare condition, typically occurring on the oral mucosa. Similar lesions can be secondary to benign papillomas, such as epidermal nevus. There are foam cells in the dermal papillae.

LIPIDOSES

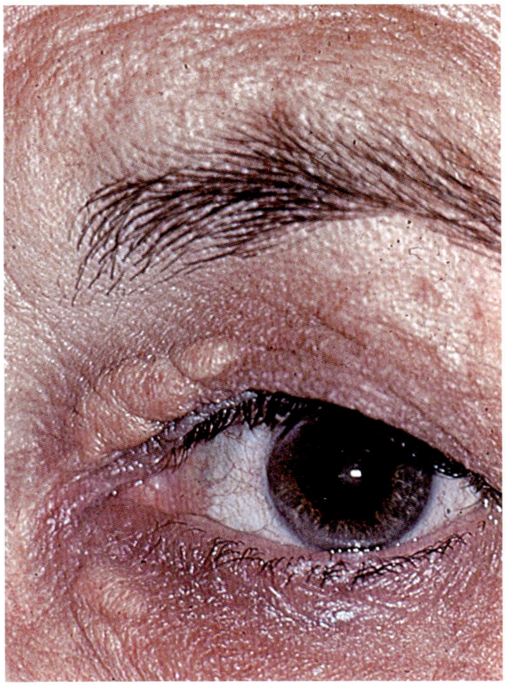

A

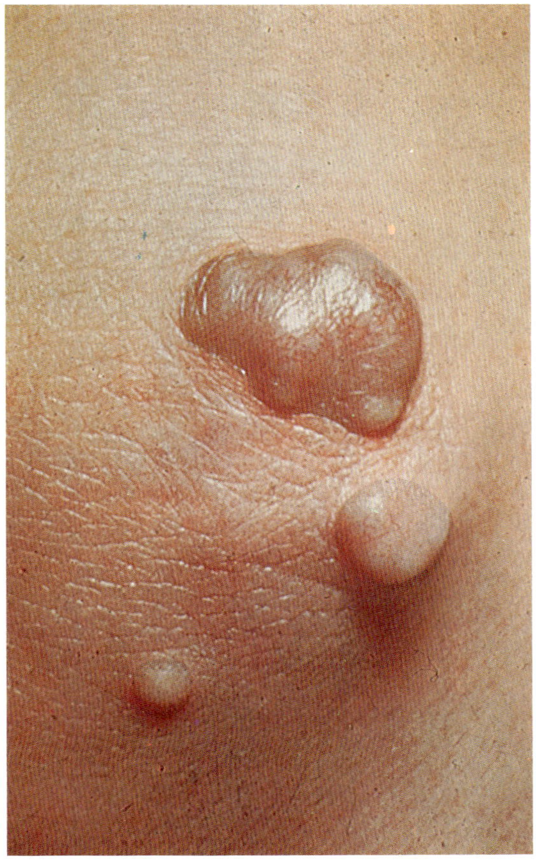

B

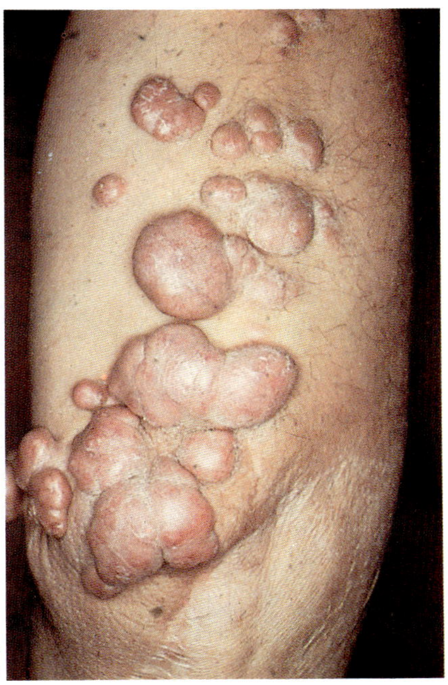

C

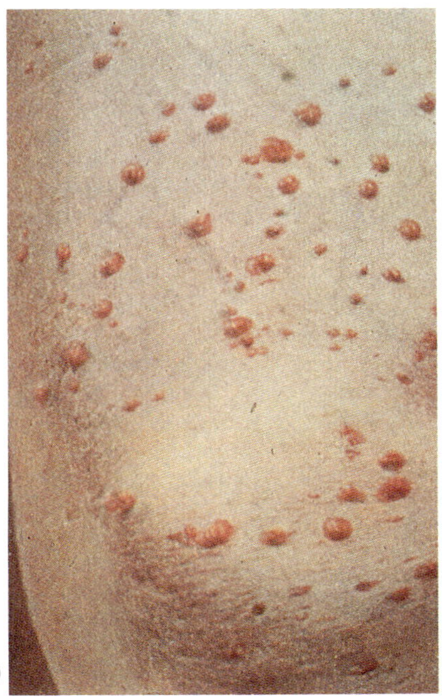

D

LIPIDOSES continued ⇨

Lipidoses

Microscopic features

1. All cutaneous xanthomata are characterized by the accumulation of lipidized histiocytes (foam cells) (Figs. A,B). Foam cells are round or oval cells with a small central nucleus. In paraffin sections, the lipid has been removed, leaving a finely reticular, foamy cytoplasm.
2. In frozen sections the lipid may be directly visualized with fat stains. With scarlet red, the lipid has a reddish-brown color when there is a high percentage of cholesterol. The cholesterol produces birefringence with polarized light. When there is a low level of cholesterol, the lipid stains a reddish-orange color, and there is no birefringence with polarized light (as in eruptive xanthomas).
3. Lipidized giant cells containing a central ring of nuclei (Touton giant cells) (Fig. B, inset) are often present.
4. Early xanthomata (especially eruptive xanthomata) may have an admixture of inflammatory cells, and longstanding lesions may show extensive fibrosis (Figs. C,D).
5. Tuberous and tendonous xanthomata show large sheets and masses of foam cells. Eruptive xanthomata show fewer foam cells and often a larger admixture of inflammatory cells. Plane xanthomata show scattered foam cells rather than large aggregates or masses of foam cells. In xanthelasma palpebrarum the foam cells have a rather superficial location.

Microscopic differential diagnosis

1. Differentiation of xanthomata of hyperlipoproteinemia from highly lipidized dermatofibromas (histiocytomas) may be difficult. Usually differentiation can be made on the basis of the fibroblastic component in histiocytomas, as well as by the hemosiderin that may be present in these tumors.
2. Nevoxanthoendotheliomas (juvenile xanthogranulomas) usually have a higher proportion of nonlipidized histiocytes than xanthomas of hyperlipoproteinemia and have fairly distinctive lipidized giant cells with a perfect ring of nuclei (wreath giant cells). A mixed inflammatory reaction containing eosinophils is often present.
3. With paraffin sections, balloon cell nevi may greatly resemble xanthomas. However, differentiation can be made readily with frozen sections, since balloon cells do not contain lipid.
4. Tumor cells of granular cell Schwannoma resemble foam cells, but with high magnification a granular rather than foamy cytoplasm can be seen. The granules may be PAS-positive.

LIPIDOSES

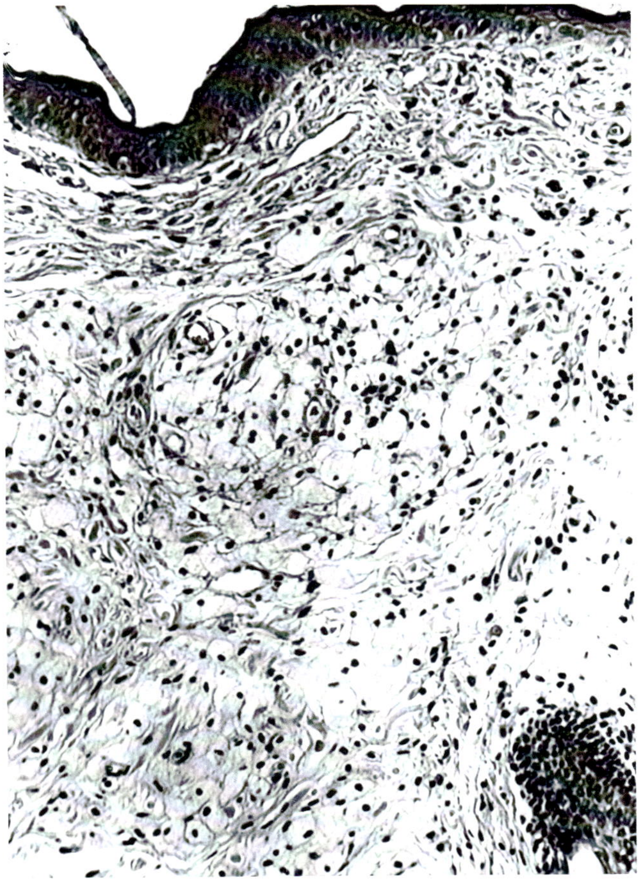

A
X210

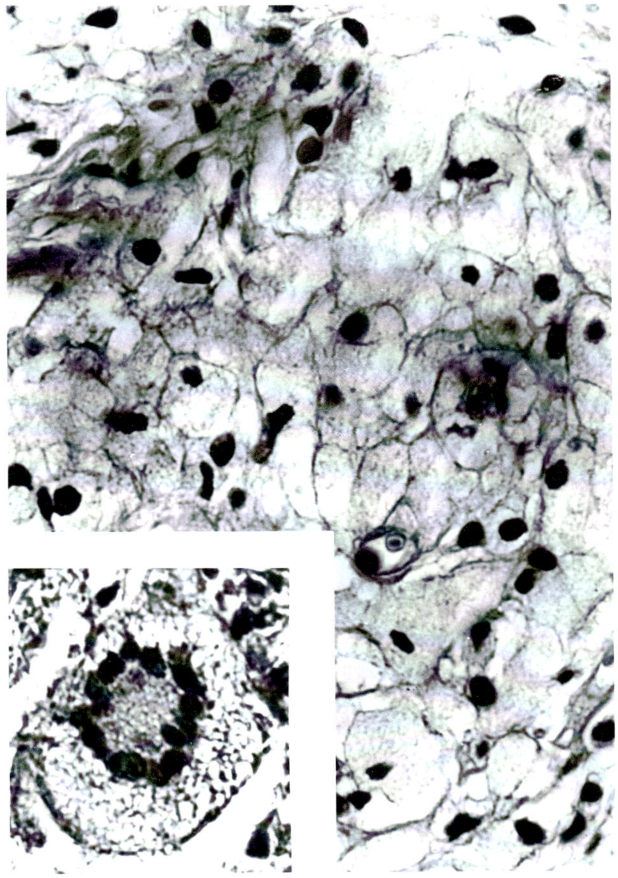

B
X520

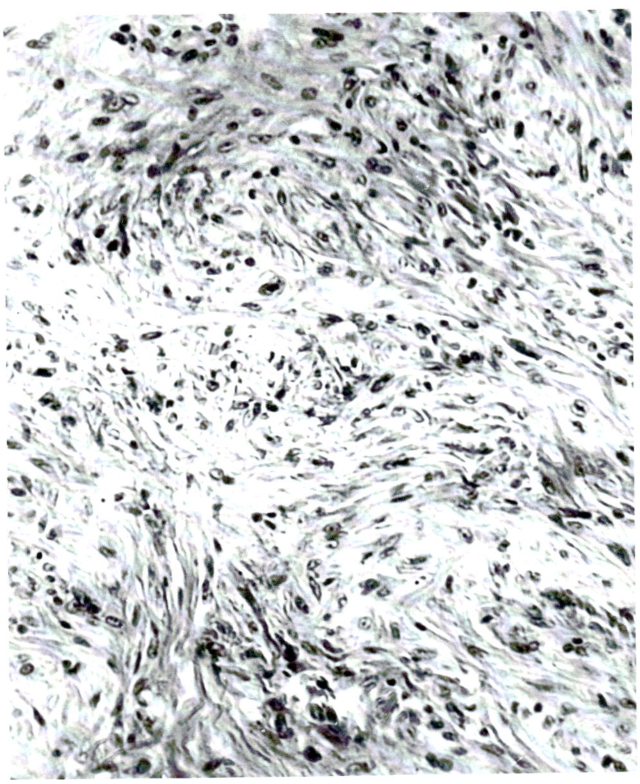

C
X260

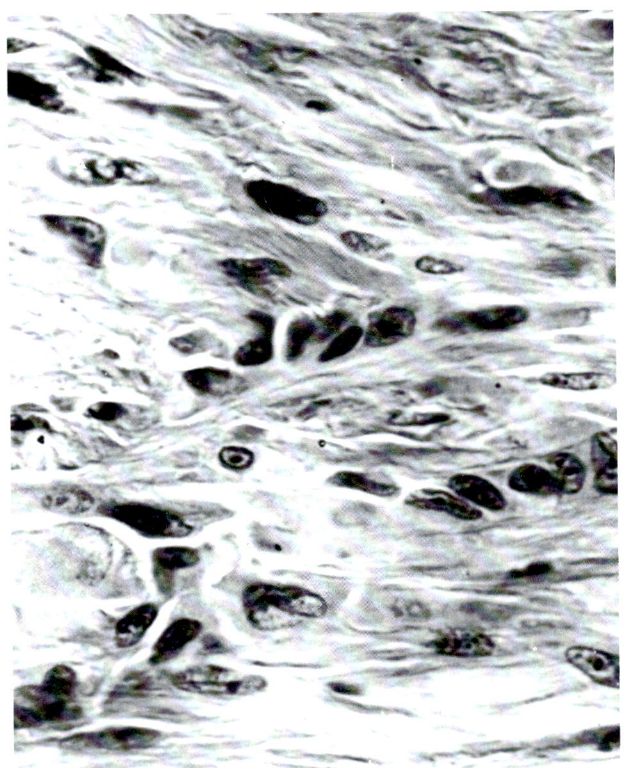

D
X780

Lipidoses

Microscopic differential diagnosis

5. Lipidized histiocytes of lepromatous leprosy (lepra cells) can be distinguished from foam cells of xanthomata by the demonstration of lepra bacilli with acid-fast stains.
6. Surprisingly, the presence of patches of somewhat damaged foam cells in eruptive xanthoma produces a resemblance to granuloma annulare of the diffuse histologic type. The damaged foam cells resemble damaged collagen. Fat stains with frozen sections may not help in the differentiation, since there can be extracellular lipid in granuloma annulare.

Clinical and laboratory data are important in the differential diagnosis of xanthomas.

Suggested Reading

Metabolic Dermatoses

Gout

Chetrick, A. Co-existent sarcoidosis, erythema nodosum, and gout. *JAMA*, 186:950, 1963.

Lichtenstein, L., Scott, H. and Levin, M. Pathologic changes in gout: Survey of eleven necropsied cases. *Am. J. Pathol.*, 32:871, 1956.

Reif, M., Constantiner, A. and Levitt, M. Chronic gouty nephropathy: A vanishing syndrome? *N. Eng. J. Med.*, 304:535, 1981.

Seegmiller, J. Diseases of purine and pyrimidine metabolism. In: *Metabolic Control and Disease*, 8th Ed., Bondy, P. and Rosenberg, L., eds., Philadelphia, WB Saunders, 1980, p. 777.

——. Disorders of purine and pyrimidine metabolism. In: *The Principles and Practice of Medical Genetics*. Emery, A. and Rimoin, D., eds., New York, Churchill Livingstone, 1984, p. 97.

——. Skin manifestations of gout. In: *Dermatology in General Medicine*, 2 Ed., Fitzpatrick, T. et al., eds., New York, McGraw-Hill, 1979, p. 1106.

Simmonds, H. et al. Evidence of a new syndrome involving hereditary uric acid overproduction, neurological complications and deafness. *Adv. Exp. Med. Biol.*, 165 (pt. A):97, 1984.

Sokiloff, L. The pathology of gout. *Metabolism*, 6:230, 1957.

Sorensen, L. The pathogenesis of gout. *Arch. Int. Med.*, 109:379, 1962.

Talbott, J. *Gout*. 2nd Ed., New York, Grune & Stratton, 1964.

Wyngaarden, J. and Kelley, W. Gout. In: *The Metabolic Basis of Inherited Disease*. 3rd Ed., Stanbury, J., Wyngaarden, J. and Fredrickson, D., eds., New York, McGraw-Hill, 1972, p. 889.

Yü, T. et al. Renal function in gout. V. Factors influencing the renal hemodynamics. *Am. J. Med.*, 67:766, 1979.

Zimmer, J. and Demis, D. Associations between gout, psoriasis, and sarcoidosis (with consideration of their pathogenetic significance). *Ann. Int. Med.*, 64:786, 1966.

Hemochromatosis

Cartwright, G. et al. Hereditary hemochromatosis. Phenotypic expression of the disease. *N. Eng. J. Med.*, 301:175, 1979.

Cawley, E. et al. Hemochromatosis and the skin. *Arch. Dermatol.*, 100:1, 1969.

Chevrant-Breton, J. et al. Cutaneous manifestations of idiopathic hemochromatosis. *Arch. Dermatol.*, 113:161, 1977.

Edwards, C. et al. Hereditary hemochromatosis. *N. Eng. J. Med.*, 297:7, 1977.

Feller, E. et al. Familial hemochromatosis. *N. Eng. J. Med.*, 296:1422, 1977.

Heilmeyer, L. Pathogenesis of hemochromatosis. *Medicine*, 46:209, 1967.

Hellier, F. The nature of the skin pigmentation in hemochromatosis. *Br. J. Dermatol.*, 47:1, 1935.

MacDonald, R. *Hemochromatosis and Hemosiderosis*. Springfield, IL, Thomas, 1964.

Milder, M. et al. Idiopathic hemochromatosis: An interim report. *Medicine* (Baltimore), 59:34, 1980.

Perdrup, A. and Poulsen, H. Hemochromatosis and vitiligo. *Arch. Dermatol.*, 90:34, 1964.

Pollycove, M. Hemochromatosis. In: *The Metabolic Basis of Inherited Disease*. 3rd Ed., Stanbury, J., Wyngaarden, J. and Fredrickson, D., eds., New York, McGraw-Hill, 1972, p. 1051.

Scheinberg, I. The genetics of hemochromatosis. *Arch. Int. Med.*, 132:126, 1973.

Sheldon, J. *Haemochromatosis*. London, Oxford Univ. Press, 1935.

Weintraub, L. et al. Iron excretion by the skin: Selective localization of iron^{59} in epithelial cells. *Am. J. Pathol.*, 46:121, 1965.

Lipidoses (Xanthomatoses)

Ahrens, E., Jr. et al. Primary biliary cirrhosis. *Medicine,* 29:299, 1950.

Altman, J. and Winkelmann, R. Diffuse normolipemic plane xanthoma: Generalized xanthelasma. *Arch. Dermatol.,* 85:633, 1962.

Baes, H. et al. Distribution of various forms of xanthomata in 3 types of primary hyperlipoproteinemia. *Dermatologica,* 136:300, 1968.

Barr, R. and Plank, C. Verruciform xanthoma of the skin. *J. Cutan. Pathol.,* 7:422, 1980.

Brewer, H. et al. Type III hyperlipoproteinemia: Diagnosis, molecular defects, pathology, and treatment. *Ann. Int. Med.,* 98:623, 1983.

Brown, M. and Goldstein, J. Familial hypercholesterolemia: A genetic defect in the low-density lipoprotein receptor. *N. Eng. J. Med.,* 294:1386, 1976.

Buchner, A., Hansen, L. and Merrill, P. Verruciform xanthoma of the oral mucosa. *Arch. Dermatol.,* 117:563, 1981.

Curtis, A. and Blaylock, H. Secondary eruptive xanthomatosis due to myxedema: A genetic and metabolic study. *Arch. Dermatol. Syph.,* 66:460, 1952.

Fisher, W. and Truitt, D. The common hyperlipoproteinemias. (Review). *Ann. Int. Med.,* 85:497, 1976.

Fleischmajer, R. Diagnosis and treatment of familial lipoproteinemias. *Internat. J. Dermatol.,* 10:251, 1971.

——. *The Dyslipidoses.* Springfield, IL, Thomas, 1960.

Fleischmajer, R., Hyman, A. and Weidman, A. Normolipemic plane xanthomas. *Arch. Dermatol.,* 89:319, 1964.

Fredrickson, D. and Levy, R. Familial hyperlipoproteinemia. In: *The Metabolic Basis of Inherited Disease.* 3rd Ed., Stanbury, J., Wyngaarden, J. and Fredrickson, D., eds., New York, McGraw-Hill, 1972, p. 545.

Fredrickson, D., Levy, R. and Lees, R. Fat transport in lipoproteins: An integrated approach to mechanisms and disorders. *N. Eng. J. Med.,* 276:34, 1967.

Grosshans, E. and Laplanche, G. Verruciform xanthoma or xanthomatous transformation of inflammatory epidermal nevus. *J. Cutan. Pathol.,* 8:382, 1981.

Havel, R. Typing of hyperlipoproteinemias. *Atherosclerosis,* 11:3, 1970.

Holiman, J. and Wasserman, A. Autopsy findings in type III hyperlipoproteinemia. *Arch. Pathol.,* 92:415, 1971.

Kraemer, B. et al. Verruciform xanthoma of the penis. *Arch. Dermatol.,* 117:516, 1981.

Lever, W. Lipidoses. In: *Histopathology of the Skin.* 5th Ed., Lever, W. and Schaumburg-Lever, G., eds., Philadelphia, Lippincott, 1975, p. 361.

Lloyd, J. Disorders of serum lipoproteins. II. Hyperlipoproteinemic states. *Arch. Dis. Child.,* 43:505, 1968.

Lynch, P. and Winkelmann, R. Generalized plane xanthoma and systemic disease. *Arch. Dermatol.,* 93:639, 1966.

Marten, R. Xanthomatosis and myelomatosis. *Proc. R. Soc. Med.,* 55:318, 1962.

Pedace, F. and Winkelmann, R. Xanthelasma palpebrarum. *JAMA,* 193:893, 1965.

Polano, M. et al. Xanthomata in primary hyperlipoproteinemia: A classification based on the lipoprotein pattern of the blood. *Arch. Dermatol.,* 100:387, 1969.

Roberts, W., Levy, R. and Fredrickson, D. Hyperlipoproteinemia. *Arch. Pathol.,* 90:46, 1970.

Sanbar, S. *Hyperlipidemia and Hyperlipoproteinemia.* Boston, Little, Brown, 1969.

Santa Cruz, D. and Martin, S. Verruciform xanthoma of the vulva. *Am. J. Clin. Pathol.,* 71:224, 1979.

Schatz, I. Classification of primary hyperlipidemia: Observations on 214 patients. *JAMA,* 210:701, 1969.

Schreiber, M. and Shapiro, S. Secondary eruptive xanthoma. Type V hyperlipoproteinemia. *Arch. Dermatol.,* 100:601, 1969.

Shafer, W. Verruciform xanthoma. *Oral Surg.,* 31:784, 1971.

Thannhauser, S. *Lipidoses: Diseases of the Cellular Lipid Metabolism.* 3rd Ed., New York, Grune & Stratton, 1958.

Walker, A. and Sneddon, I. Skin xanthomata following erythroderma. *Br. J. Dermatol.,* 80:580, 1968.

Zemel, H. et al. The ultrastructural features of normolipemic plane xanthoma. *Arch. Pathol.,* 89:111, 1970.

Glossary

Acantholysis — Loss of cohesion between epithelial cells. The term is usually applied to keratinocytes. Primary acantholysis is due to dissolution of the intercellular cement substance, as in pemphigus vulgaris (see p. 530). Secondary acantholysis is the result of cellular damage, as in viral vesicles (see p. 388).

Acantholytic dyskeratosis — A concomitant process of acantholysis and dyskeratosis with corps ronds and grains (see p. 548).

Acanthosis — Increase in thickness of the epidermis due to proliferation of the prickle cell layer (see p. 102).

Alopecia — Loss of hair (see p. 224).

Apocrine secretion — A secretory process characterized by release of apical portions of cells into glandular lumina. The type of secretion is characteristic of apocrine glands. It is also called "decapitation secretion" (see p. 58).

Apoptosis — A peculiar type of individual cell death. The term is usually applied to death of individual keratinocytes resulting in eosinophilic bodies. This can be the result of direct injury, such as sunburn. It is also seen in conditions characterized by destruction of the basal layer (as in lichen planus and lupus erythematosus [see pp. 440, 492]). The eosinophilic bodies in lichen planus and lupus erythematosus are called *colloid bodies* or *Civatte bodies*. The amyloid in macular and lichenoid amyloidosis, as well as the colloid in juvenile colloid milium derive from basal cells transformed by apoptosis.

Argentaffin — Capable of reducing silver salts to metallic silver. Melanin and, to a lesser extent, hemosiderin, have this property, which can be demonstrated by the Fontana-Masson stain (see p. 1246).

Argyrophil — Capable of being stained by silver impregnation techniques. Melanin, nerves, and reticulum fibers have this property (see p. 32).

Asteroid body — This refers either to a collagenous cytoplasmic inclusion found in giant cells of sarcoidosis (and other conditions) or to a type of spore sometimes found in sporotrichosis (see pp. 356, 422).

Ballooning degeneration — A process of swelling of epithelial cells and loss of intercellular bridges, typical of viral vesicles. Balloon cells usually have multiple nuclei (see p. 388).

Basal lamina (basement membrane) — This is a filamentous band visible with electron microscopy. A basement membrane is present along with the undersurface of epidermal basal cells. Basement membranes also border blood vessels and other structures (see p. 20).

Basement membrane zone — Refers to a band beneath the basal layer of the epidermis, which is visible by light microscopy when the PAS stain is used. It is composed of the basal lamina, lamina lucida, anchoring fibrils, and reticulum fibers (see pp. 20, 32).

Birefringence — Doubly refractive. In dermatopathology the term usually applies to material doubly refractive with polarized light examination (see p. 428).

Bulla — A cutaneous cavity, filled with tissue fluid or plasma; it may also contain inflammatory cells. Bullae typically form within the epidermis or beneath it. Bullae smaller than 5 mm are called *vesicles* (see p. 528).

Burrow — A tunnel in the horny layer of the epidermis produced by the female mite in scabies (see p. 410).

Civatte body (colloid body) — see under *apoptosis*.

Colloid — Homogeneous, eosinophilic material of variable composition, found in colloid milium (see p. 686).

Comedo (pl., comedones) (blackhead) — A dilated follicular opening filled with keratotic material and sebum (see p. 160).

Corps rond — A round dyskeratotic cell found in acantholytic dyskeratosis, including Darier's disease and warty dyskeratoma (see pp. 548, 758).

Crust — A surface accumulation of cellular debris, fibrin, and other serum proteins (see p. 98).

Decapitation secretion — see under *apocrine secretion*.

Dermatopathic lymphadenopathy (lipomelanotic reticulosis) — An enlargement of lymph nodes secondary to a widespread inflammatory process of the skin (see p. 112).

Desmosome — A specialized structure concerned with intercellular attachment of keratinocytes. It is best seen with electron microscopy (see p. 20).

Dyskeratosis — Premature keratinization of individual epidermal cells (see p. 810).

Eczema — The term is synonymous with dermatitis, a nonspecific inflammatory response of the skin with concomitant changes in epidermis and dermis (see pp. 85–113).

Epidermotropism — Migration of malignant cells into the epidermis. The term is applied to mycosis fungoides, in which epidermotropism (without spongiosis) of malignant T-lymphocytes may result in the formation of Pautrier microabscesses (see p. 1338).
Erosion — A superficial ulcer not extending beyond the basal layer (see p. 196).
Excoriation — A superficial ulcer, produced by scratching (see p. 556).
Exfoliative — Referring to extensive or widespread scaling (see p. 450).
Exocytosis — Migration of inflammatory cells into the epidermis, accompanied by spongiosis. It is observed in subacute dermatitis, for example (see p. 98). Exocytosis of mononuclear cells and epidermotropism of mycosis fungoides can be difficult to distinguish.
Fibrinoid degeneration — Deposition in tissue of eosinophilic, fibrillar material resembling fibrin (see p. 652).
Foam cell — A lipidized macrophage (see p. 720).
Foreign body giant cell — A giant cell with multiple nuclei in irregular arrangement. It is commonly observed in foreign body granulomas (see p. 42).
Gottron's sign — Infiltrated lesions over the joints of the hand observed in dermatomyositis (see p. 502).
Grain — An ellipsoid dyskeratotic cell with pyknotic nucleus, observed in acantholytic dyskeratosis, including Darier's disease (see p. 548).
Grenz zone — An uninvolved zone of dermis between the epidermis and a dermal lesion (Grenz = *border* in German). Grenz zones may occur in lepromatous leprosy, granuloma faciale, and other conditions (see p. 138).
Holocrine secretion — A type of glandular secretion in which the secretory product forms by cellular disintegration (e.g., in sebaceous glands) (see p. 56).
Horn pearl — A focus of abnormal keratinization characterized by concentrically arranged epidermal cells with increasing keratinization towards the center (see p. 806).
Hyalinization — Formation of a homogeneous, eosinophilic, glassy material. Hyalin is PAS-positive and diastase-resistant. It can form as a result of excessive basement membrane material (from epithelial or blood vessel basement membranes) (see pp. 200, 578).
Ichthyosis — A disorder of keratinization characterized by fish-like scales (see pp. 232–239).
Keloid — A hypertrophic scar with an extended period of uncontrolled fibroblastic proliferation (see p. 210).
Keratinocyte — A squamous epithelial cell whose product of differentiation is a fibrous protein, keratin (see p. 16).
Keratohyalin — This refers to the deeply basophilic granules of cells of the granular layer of the epidermis (see p. 16).
Koebner phenomenon (isomorphic phenomenon) — Development of linear lesions, usually elicited by scratching. The Koebner phenomenon may be seen in lichen planus, psoriasis, and warts (see pp. 438, 450).
Lacuna — An intercellular space formed by suprabasal acantholysis, observed in acantholytic dyskeratosis, including Darier's disease (see p. 548).
Langerhans cell — A dendritic cell of the epidermis, believed to have a role in contact dermatitis and in mycosis fungoides. The Langerhans cells have cytoplasmic granules, visible with electron microscopy, that are shaped like tennis rackets (see pp. 16, 22).
Langhans giant cell — A giant cell with multiple nuclei in "horseshoe" arrangement. It is commonly found in lesions of tuberculosis, but can also be seen in other conditions (see p. 42).
Leukocytoclasis — Fragmentation of neutrophil nuclei seen in a type of vasculitis (see p. 136).
Lichenification — Exaggeration of the surface markings of the skin, usually due to chronic rubbing and scratching (see p. 100).
Macule — A flat lesion, distinguished by color (see p. 1126).
Max Josef spaces — Subepidermal clefts observed in lesions of lichen planus (see p. 440).
Melanophage — A melanin-containing dermal cell widely believed to be a macrophage which has phagocytosed melanin granules synthesized in epidermal melanocytes. Newer evidence has indicated that many of these cells may actually be dermal melanocytes in which melanin complexes form by autophagy (see p. 28).
Merocrine — A type of glandular secretion in which the secretory material does not contain cells or components of cells (e.g., in eccrine glands) (see p. 60).

Metachromasia — Shift in color of certain blue dyes (to violet) after combination with certain polymerized substrates (see pp. 5, 44).
Miliaria — An inflammation of sweat glands (see p. 180).
Milium (whitehead) — A small, superficial epidermal inclusion cyst (see p. 858).
Munro abscess — Foci of degenerated neutrophils observed in the stratum corneum in lesions of psoriasis (see p. 452).
Myoepithelial cell — A modified epithelial cell with contractile function, found at the periphery of eccrine and apocrine glands (see p. 64).
"Naked" tubercle — Epithelioid tubercle without a surrounding zone of lymphoid cells. "Naked" tubercles are observed in sarcoidal granulomas (see p. 420).
Necrobiosis — Physiologic cell death. The term has been applied to normal death of keratinocytes via keratinization. It has also been applied incorrectly to collagen degeneration in disorders such as granuloma annulare and necrobiosis lipoidica (see p. 639).
Nodule — A large raised lesion (see p. 1204).
Orthokeratosis — Normal keratinization, characterized by cornified cells without nuclei (see p. 16).
Papillomatosis — Wavy projections of the epidermal surface (see p. 728).
Papule — A small raised skin lesion (see p. 178).
Parakeratosis — Incomplete keratinization characterized by retention of pyknotic nuclei by cells of the stratum corneum (see p. 98).
Plaque — A raised, flat lesion. In French it signifies a patch without induration (e.g., parapsoriasis en plaques) (see p. 1336).
Poikiloderma — Atrophy of the skin with telangiectasia as well as mottled hypopigmentation and hyperpigmentation (see p. 616).
Pseudoepitheliomatous (pseudocarcinomatous) hyperplasia — An exaggerated benign reactive hyperplasia of the epidermis resembling well-differentiated squamous cell carcinoma (see p. 212).
Pseudohorn cyst — A tortuous invagination of a hyperkeratotic horny layer which, when cut across, has a resemblance to a horn cyst (see p. 738).
Pustule — A focal accumulation of leukocytes and serum usually within or beneath the epidermis (see p. 180).
Reticular degeneration — A degenerative process characterized by severe intracellular edema, resulting in a multilocular bulla with septa formed by residual epidermal cell walls (see p. 390).
Rosette giant cell — A giant cell with multiple nuclei in ring arrangement observed in dermal and compound nevi (see p. 1132).
Scale — A readily shed layer of incompletely cornified skin (see *Parakeratosis* above and p. 450).
Spongiform pustule (Kogoj pustule) — Accumulations of neutrophils between degenerated keratinocytes observed in lesions of psoriasis, candidiasis, and geographic tongue (see pp. 350, 456).
Spongiosis — Intercellular edema involving squamous epithelium (see p. 98).
Squamous eddy — Concentrically arranged epithelial cells observed in irritated seborrheic keratoses. They resemble horn pearls (see p. 742).
Telangiectasia — Dilatation and possible proliferation of superficial capillaries (see p. 612).
Tophus — A cutaneous nodule occurring in gout (see p. 712).
Touton giant cell — A giant cell with a central ring of nuclei and a peripheral lipidized zone (which appears foamy in routine sections) (see p. 720).
Vesicle — A small bulla (see p. 528).
Villus — A projecting dermal papilla lined by a single row of basal cells (see p. 548).
Wickham's striae — Surface striations found in lesions of lichen planus (see p. 438).
Wreath giant cell — A giant cell with multiple nuclei arranged in a perfect ring. It is typically found in nevoxanthoendothelioma (juvenile xanthogranuloma [see p. 1266]).

INDEX